CONTRIBUTIONS TO HEMOSTASIS

ANNALS OF THE NEW YORK ACADEMY OF SCIENCES
Volume 370

CONTRIBUTIONS TO HEMOSTASIS

Edited by Daniel A. Walz and Lowell E. McCoy

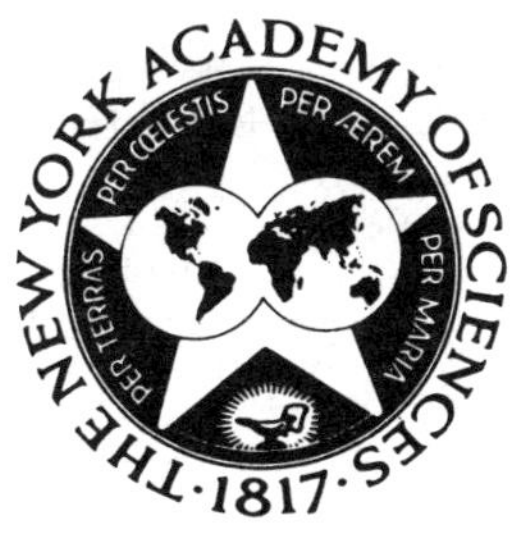

The New York Academy of Sciences
New York, New York
1981

Library of Congress Cataloging in Publication Data

Main entry under title:

Contributions to hemostasis.

(Annals of the New York Academy of Sciences ;
v. 370)
Papers from a conference held by Wayne State
University School of Medicine on May 19-21, 1980, in
Detroit, Mich.
Includes index.
1. Blood--Coagulation--Congresses. 2. Hemostasis
--Congresses. 3. Blood--Coagulation, Disorders of
--Congresses. I. Walz, Daniel A. II. McCoy,
Lowell E. III. Series. [DNLM: 1. Hemostasis--
Congresses. 2. Blood coagulation--Congresses.
Wl AN626YL v. 370 / WH 310 C764 1980]
QP93.5.C68   612'.115   81-11065
ISBN 0-89766-129-X   AACR2
ISBN 0-89766-130-3 (pbk.)

PCP

Printed in the United States of America
ISBN 0-89766-129-x (cloth bound)
ISBN 0-89766-130-3 (paper bound)

ANNALS OF THE NEW YORK ACADEMY OF SCIENCES

VOLUME 370

CONTRIBUTIONS TO HEMOSTASIS *

June 30, 1981

Editors and Conference Chairmen
DANIEL A. WALZ AND LOWELL E. MCCOY

CONTENTS

* This series of papers is the result of a conference entitled Contributions to Hemostasis, held by Wayne State University School of Medicine on May 19–21, 1980 in Detroit, Michigan.

Part III. von Willebrand Factor/Antihemophilic Factor (F VIII)

Part IV. Contact Activation System

Part V. Prothrombin Complex Proteins

Part VI. Prothrombin Activation

Part IX. Diagnostic and Therapeutic Applications

Financial assistance was received from:

- Wayne State University
- Wayne State University School of Medicine

- Abbott Laboratories, Inc.
- Blood Bank, Clinical Center, NIH
- Fogarty International Center, NIH
- General Diagnostics Division, Warner-Lambert Co.
- Heart, Lung, and Blood Institute, NIH
- Hyland Laboratories and Hyland Therapeutics Division of
      Travenol Laboratories, Inc.
- Kabi Group, Inc.
- Eli Lilly and Co.
- Pacific Hemostasis
- Parke-Davis Division, Warner-Lambert Co.
- Pentapharm Ltd.
- Sandoz, Inc.
- The Skillman Foundation
- The Upjohn Company

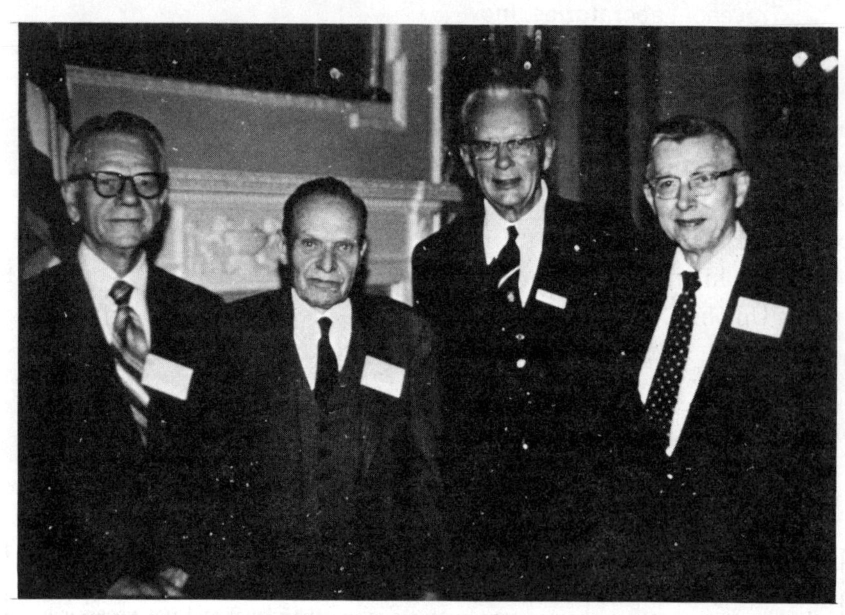

Pictured at this conference, Tuesday May 20, 1980. From the left: Charles A. Owen, Mayo Clinic; Emory Warner, University of Iowa; Walter H. Seegers, Wayne State University; and Kenneth M. Brinkhous, University of North Carolina. (Photo courtesy of Robert Nalbandian).

On May 19–21, 1980 a conference was held in Detroit, Michigan to coincide with the retirement of Professor Walter H. Seegers after 42 years of active research effort on the molecular events of coagulation. It is a fitting tribute to Professor Seegers that over 300 participants from 10 countries attended this conference and witnessed the presentation of 80 oral and poster topics addressing the most recent research problems in the now vast field of blood coagulation. In fact, the title of this volume, *Contributions to Hemostasis,* was selected to acknowledge not only the impact that Professor Seegers' work has had upon hemostasis research but also the magnitude and multiplicity of activity presently being pursued by others.

Professor Seegers began his research efforts on prothrombin and thrombin in the Department of Pathology at the State University of Iowa. He was a member of the research team directed by H. P. Smith, which also included K. M. Brinkhous, E. D. Warner, E. Mertz, and C. A. Owen, Jr. Today, all of these individuals are recognized as prominent scientists in their respective fields. Except for Dr. Mertz, they are pictured together at this conference (see facing page). The initial publications of Seegers *et al.* began with articles on the purification of prothrombin (J. Biol. Chem. **123**: 751–754, 1938) and thrombin (J. Biol. Chem. **126**: 91–95, 1938). Today, some 500 research articles later, Dr. Seegers continues to contribute his insights and interpretations to prothrombin activation, particularly as it relates to a new vitamin K-dependent protein the so-called protein M. In the intervening 42 years Dr. Seegers has developed the technology for the commercial production of Bovine Topical Thrombin, served as the Chairman of the Department of Physiology at Wayne State University and been the pre- and post-doctoral advisor for over 40 students. He has served on both national and international advisory committees for thrombosis and hemostasis study groups.

Throughout his career, Dr. Seegers' research activities have touched upon virtually every aspect of hemostasis. He has frequently been at the forefront with new observations, interpretations, and perspectives. His pursuit of the molecule prothrombin has continued throughout his career. Hence it proved to be a tribute to Dr. Seegers when Dr. Whyte Owen recalled the anecdotal episode of his own assignment to "new" lab space at the University of Iowa. Dr. Owen was surprised to learn that these labs were at one time used by Drs. H. P. Smith and Walter H. Seegers and to his personal pleasure actually discovered a number of samples of prothrombin made and hand-labeled by Dr. Seegers. Dr. Owen took the liberty of using one such ampule for polyacrylamide analysis and, to the pleasure of those in attendance at this meeting showed what was recognized by "prothrombin people" as a typical SDS pattern for prothrombin, prethrombin, and fragments 1 and 2. That in itself sets the tone and underscores the contributions to hemostasis of both Professor Seegers and each of the participants in this conference.

We would like to thank a number of individuals for their assistance in making our task of organizing this conference easier. The greatest appreciation goes to those who directly participated, both for their presentations and also for the excellence of the written contributions. Those people who worked so efficiently behind the scenes include June Snow and Debra McKinley and the unfailing secretarial cooperation of Ruby Beckermeyer and Catherine Smetanka is greatly appreciated. The conference site was professionally managed by the personnel at the Michigan Inn, Southfield, Michigan and the social evening was managed by the personnel at Greenfield Village and the Henry Ford Museum, Dearborn, Michigan. A final word of thanks is extended to Joyce Hitchcock for her patience and cooperation in overseeing the individual manuscripts through the editorial process at the New York Academy of Sciences. None of this would have been possible were it not for the financial assistance of the various sponsors, who are listed separately after the table of contents.

DANIEL A. WALZ
LOWELL E. McCOY

Department of Physiology
Wayne State University
Detroit, Michigan

THE HEMOSTASIS PARADIGM IN 1934 AND IN 1980

L. B. Jaques *

*Department of Physiology
College of Medicine; and the
College of Dentistry
University of Saskatchewan
Saskatoon, Saskatchewan, Canada S7N 0W0*

The best way to contribute to this symposium honoring Dr. Walter Seegers is to compare the concepts current when we began our research careers in the field of hemostasis with those prevalent today. Because Dr. Seegers is best known for his isolation of the trace proteins constituting the enzymes of the prothrombin system,[1] let me point to an instance in that area. In the course in advanced biochemistry that I took at the University of Toronto in 1932–33, our professor assured us that while Sumner had reported isolating jackbean urease and Northrop, pancreatic trypsin as crystalline proteins, whatever enzymes were eventually proved to be, enzymes certainly could not be crystalline proteins (a notion in itself considered irrational by orthodox biochemists at that time). However, the Willstätter school at Munich had established that enzymes were generally trace substances and that adsorption on various alumina gels was an excellent procedure for obtaining them in small amounts.

More specifically in North America, concepts of blood coagulation were dominated by the Howell theory of blood coagulation: prothrombin-antiprothrombin + Ca^{++} + thromboplastin $\rightarrow$ thrombin; fibrinogen $\xrightarrow{\text{thrombin}}$ fibrin.[2] It was not possible to achieve a passing grade in answering a question on blood coagulation in an examination in biochemistry or physiology, without presenting the Howell theory. Quick[3] has reported that his original paper on the prothrombin time was submitted to eight journals before an editor was found who agreed to publish a paper that was thought to be at variance with Howell's theory.

The Howell theory had a serious defect. Different clinicians pointed out to me in the 1930s that it had no meaning (or "relevance," to use the current phrase) for the clinical problems of hemorrhage and thrombosis. Howell's theory suggested that the pathologic conditions of thrombosis and hemorrhage were the result of an imbalance—an excess or deficiency of antiprothrombin. But thrombosis was generally understood, as the result of the work of Aschoff, to be a phenomenon of platelets. Further clinical and experimental observations and practice by Hippocrates, Galen, Paré, Hewson, Virchow, Lister, and, in the 1930s, Tocantins and MacFarlane emphasized that the blood vessel wall played an important and active role in the maintenance of normal hemostasis. Therefore in hemostasis, as in the aspect of thrombosis formulated by Virchow, a triad of physiologic mechanisms exists.

The developments in the 1930s basic to a new understanding of the nature and significance of prothrombin were: (1) the demonstration of its clinical significance as the result of the discovery of vitamin K and dicoumarin, dis-

* Emeritus Professor.

1

0077–8923/81/0370–0001 $01.75/0 © 1981, NYAS

coveries, as emphasized by K. P. Link, based on the development of methods of measurement of prothrombin; and (2) the demonstration of prothrombin as a trace plasma protein and enzyme precursor.

For those in the field of hemostasis research, Walter Seegers' many contributions require little amplification. His work has resulted in a completely new paradigm for prothrombin and its reactions in which it is recognized that the plasma protein enzyme precursor under various influences and conditions undergoes conversion to a number of enzymes that can serve autocatalytic functions.

The antiprothrombin in the Howell theory was a hypothetical concept formulated by Howell in 1911. Howell and Holt[4] in 1918 considered a phospholipid, Baskoff's heparphosphatid prepared from dog liver by MacLean[5] and which Howell and Holt called heparin, to have the action of an antiprothrombin. In 1924, Howell[6] used the same name for an acid polysaccharide previously isolated from dog liver by Doyon.[7] A similar material from beef lung, but much more purified, was produced by Charles and Scott[8] to become the commercial heparin used clinically. Understanding of this material has been slow because of its association with the hypothetical antiprothrombin, although Howell's own experiments showed that the anticoagulant action of heparin was dependent on another plasma protein, referred to today as AT-III. The developmental studies on heparin in Toronto and Stockholm in the 1930s have recently come to a successful conclusion through the formulation of a new paradigm:

> Heparins and related substances are linear anionic polyelectrolytes, with multiple extended chains, constituting a new biochemical species. They are skeleton keys in the key-and-lock analogy, as they show a wide range of biological actions. This is due to their conferring a strong negative charge on proteins, cells and other body constituents. They have a special association with endothelium, macrophages and the RES.[9]

With the identification of the importance of prothrombin and related trace plasma proteins in hemorrhagic conditions and diseases and the control of bleeding with suitable plasma protein fractions, appreciation of the phenomenon of hemostasis has improved, but there still has been resistance to acknowledging its multiple nature. Thus, while the importance of platelets was recognized in the 1920s and 1930s, by 1961 at the meeting in Princeton of the International Committee for Nomenclature of Blood Coagulation Factors (now the International Committee for Hemostasis and Thrombosis), I was a solitary voice in support of Roskam's emphasis upon the significance of platelets and I was appointed a "committee of one" to introduce platelets into the program of the International Committee. Will it take as long before a serious examination of the vascular factor in hemostasis is introduced?

Examination of the vascular factor is possible if one uses the multifactorial approach, an experimental design developed by Fisher and agricultural scientists. While many medical scientists pay lip service to Fisher's statistical formulae, they fail to grasp the significance of the multifactorial approach. This is exemplified in TABLE 1, which summarizes many varied experiments producing spontaneous internal hemorrhage in animals. It can be seen that no single treatment produces hemorrhage. This requires two treatments that act on different hemostatic mechanisms. The principle of multiple causality in these experiments establishes not only that the biological phenomenon of spontaneous hemorrhage is produced by more than one variable, but also that the phenomenon of severe hemorrhage is produced only by the simultaneous operation of two or more variables.[10]

In concluding this brief comparison of the thinking on hemostasis in 1934 with that in 1980 and in the interval between, I would emphasize that while

TABLE 1A

OCCURRENCE OF SPONTANEOUS HEMORRHAGE

Components of Hemostasis	Treatment and Conditions Lowering Hemostatic Efficiency of Components
Group 1: Blood coagulation	(a) Anticoagulants (dicumarol, phenylindanediose, heparin) (b) Deficiencies of coagulation factors as in hemophilia, DIC, and the like
Group 2: Platelets	(a) Thrombocytopenia (b) Drugs affecting platelet function, such as aspirin and reserpine
Group 3: Vascular wall	(a) Stress: frost-bite, hypertonic saline (i.p.), surgery, restraint, physiological saline daily (s.c.), electroshock, insulin convulsions, LSD, anesthetics and depressants (b) Changes in the adrenopituitary axis caused by ACTH, STH, salicylates, histamine, adrenaline, desoxycorticosterone, and adrenalectomy (c) Local pathology: inflammation, bacterial toxins, tumors, and the like.

TABLE 1B

Treatment or Condition:	Treatment of Condition:		
	Group 1	Group 2	Group 3
Group 1	—	+	+
Group 2	+	—	+
Group 3	+	+	—

NOTE: Spontaneous hemorrhage does not result from two treatments that produce a single defect in hemostasis. It results from a combination of treatments, producing multiple defects. Spontaneous hemorrhage (breakdown of hemostasis) has multiple causes.

the changes in knowledge are related to remarkable technical developments in the laboratory, yet even more important are the changes in the intellectual models, the paradigms, that have made use of the information. With prothrombin and the coagulation system, developments have been due to the novel concept of trace proteins with specific properties of interaction; with heparin, empirical advances have resulted from an intuitive appreciation of the properties of linear anionic polyelectrolytes; and with hemostasis, it is the multivariant approach within the whole animal that brings order to the data.

REFERENCES

1. SEEGERS, W. H. 1962. Prothrombin. Harvard University Press. Cambridge, MA.
2. HOWELL, W. H. A Textbook of Physiology for Medical Students and Physicians, 4th ed. W. B. Saunders. Philadelphia, PA.
3. QUICK, A. J. 1974. The Hemorrhagic Disease and the Pathology of Hemostasis. Charles C Thomas. Springfield, IL.
4. HOWELL, W. H. & L. E. HOLT. 1918. Two new factors in blood coagulation—heparin and proantithrombin. Am. J. Physiol. **47:**328–341.
5. McLEAN, J. 1916. The thromboplastic action of cephalin. Am. J. Physiol. **41:** 250–257.
6. HOWELL, W. H. 1922-3. Heparin as an anticoagulant. Am. J. Physiol. **63:** 434–455.
7. DOYON, M., A. MOREL & A. POLICARD. 1911. Estraition directe de l'anti-thrombine du foie. Influence de la congelation. C. R. Soc. Biol. (Paris) **70:** 341.
8. CHARLES, A. F. & D. A. SCOTT. 1936. Studies on heparin. IV. Observation on the chemistry of heparin. Biochem. J. **30:**1927–1933.
9. JAQUES, L. B. 1979. Heparin: An old drug with a new paradigm. Science **206:** 528–533.
10. JAQUES, L. B. 1965. Hemostasis as a total physiological function. Thromb. Diath. Haemorrh. **14:**229–234.

THE REVOLUTION IN CONCEPTS OF COAGULATION *

Charles A. Owen, Jr.

Department of Biochemistry
Mayo Clinic and Mayo Foundation
Rochester, Minnesota 55905

This lecture honors two men, both of whom were pioneers—Dr. Elwood A. Sharp and Dr. Walter Seegers. Doctor Sharp was the physician who developed the first department of clinical investigation in an American pharmaceutical company. For three decades, he was a clinical investigator, applying newly discovered preparations directly to patients: intrinsic factor for pernicious anemia, vitamin K for bleeders, Benadryl® for allergy, Dilantin® for convulsions, and adrenocortical extract for adrenal deficiency, to name only a few. Those acquainted with Doctor Sharp personally knew him to be far more than just a practicing physician; he was an academician and a humanitarian as well.

The other man being honored is retiring after three decades at Wayne State University. But I became acquainted with Dr. Walter Seegers before that, when he was in Iowa City. At that time, the Department of Pathology at the University of Iowa Medical School was headed by Dr. H. P. Smith, a brilliant, hard-driving man who devoted unlimited time to his work. Second in command was Dr. Emory Warner, the "glue" holding the department together. His sense of humor eased many a strain among members of the staff. His surgical technique on animals was superb. A young pathologist by the name of Dr. Kenneth Brinkhous had a driving desire to understand the basic mechanism of hemophilia. He arranged for a hemophiliac to join the department as a glasswasher, not so much to wash glassware as to be able to furnish hemophilic blood at a moment's notice. This was not always possible, because he loved to dance on Saturday evening and not uncommonly had to spend at least Sunday in the hospital with a hemarthrosis. Then Dr. Walter Seegers joined the department. He had just obtained his Ph.D. in biochemistry, and part of Doctor Smith's genius was in recognizing the need for a biochemist.

So Walter Seegers was assigned the task of applying modern biochemical techniques to the study of blood coagulation. The tools of the late 1930s did not include chromatography or electrophoresis or refrigerated centrifuges. The glass electrode pH meter was just being introduced, as was the deep freezer and the walk-in refrigerator. Proteins were isolated and purified by salting out and differential precipitation.

But with these humble tools, Walter Seegers and his associates brought the purification of bovine prothrombin to an amazingly high peak.[1] Soon afterwards, thrombin was purified.[2] With purified preparations of thrombin and fibrinogen, it was quickly found that heparin was not a direct anticoagulant. Some constituent of plasma, but not prothrombin or fibrinogen, had to be present for heparin to interfere with the thrombin-fibrinogen reaction. Heparin cofactor was born.[3] Soon Seegers and colleagues found that heparin cofactor and antithrombin were one and the same.[4]

---

* The Elwood A. Sharp Memorial Lecture.

5

0077-8923/81/0370-0005 $01.75/0 © 1981, NYAS

Doctor Smith's team disintegrated when World War II began. Doctor Warner alone remained at the University of Iowa. Doctor Smith went to Columbia University in New York; Doctor Brinkhous, to the University of North Carolina at Chapel Hill; and Doctor Seegers, to Detroit, first with Parke-Davis and then with the Department of Physiology and Pharmacology at Wayne State University, as it is now called.

One other member of Doctor Smith's department should be mentioned, even though he was in Iowa City only briefly: Dr. Eddie Mertz, a biochemist, who subsequently went to Purdue University. Doctor Mertz is known to the hemostatic world for his early studies on bleeder pigs, now recognized to be suffering from von Willebrand's disease, and for his elegant work on the purification of plasminogen. His acclaim is probably greater, however, for his discovery of high-lysine corn, a complete food, unlike conventional corn. For this he received a nomination for the Nobel prize.

Despite his impressive start, Doctor Seegers did not really bloom until he reached Detroit. He was always surrounded by students, who would ultimately leave to óccupy leading positions in the major coagulation laboratories around the world. He and his students recognized that there is a prothrombin complex in plasma with a number of hemostatic functions, only one of which is to yield thrombin.[5] His group reported [6] that one member of this complex is an anti-coagulant, which was rediscovered many years later as protein C. One could go on and on, but this august audience is already familiar with his work.

Let me now return to the Iowa City days and discuss a problem that arose. In the mid 1930s, two methods for measuring prothrombin were proposed almost simultaneously. Smith's group devised the two-stage test,[7] whereby oxalated plasma was defibrinated and diluted extensively, so that when thrombo-plastin and calcium were added, prothrombin converted slowly into thrombin. The amount of thrombin evolving was measured at intervals by adding a portion of the mixture to a solution of fibrinogen. It was a two-stage test, in that the evolution of thrombin and its measurement were independent.

At about this time, Dr. Armand J. Quick and associates devised a one-stage test,[8] often called "Quick's test" and now universally described as the "pro-thrombin time test." Doctor Quick simply added a potent thromboplastin and then calcium to oxalated plasma and measured the clotting time. Both steps of clotting—the formation of thrombin and the clotting of fibrinogen—were concurrent.

When the two methods were first proposed, no one anticipated disagreement between them. The classic scheme proposed by Morawetz stated that clotting depended solely on prothrombin and fibrinogen when activated by thrombo-plastin in the presence of calcium. Nothing in that theory forewarned of discrepancies that were about to emerge when both prothrombin tests were done on certain samples of plasma.

In 1939, Smith's group [9] reported that the concentration of prothrombin was about the same in the plasmas of rabbit and man. Quick's method indicated that there was five times as much prothrombin in rabbit plasma as in human plasma.[8] The Iowa paper, "Plasma Prothrombin Levels in Various Verte-brates," [9] states that Quick's method "does not differentiate between amount of thrombin and speed of thrombin formation . . . . [and that] the conversion of prothrombin into thrombin is much slower in human plasma than in rabbit plasma." This was the first hint that Morawetz's theory might be incomplete.

However, in 1939, Smith's group [10] suggested that "one is perhaps not justified in concluding that the prothrombin of one species is chemically different from that of another." If the prothrombin molecules varied among species, Morawetz's theory might still be intact.

In 1937, Smith and his associates[11] reported on detection of marked hypoprothrombinemia in newborn infants by means of the two-stage test. The study was repeated with both one- and two-stage tests and was reported on in 1939.[12] Again it was stated that the two-stage plasma prothrombin value was about one-third that in adults and did not reach adult levels for several months. By the one-stage test, however, the newborn's prothrombin was near adult levels. It dropped sharply during the first few days, only to become normal again by about the seventh day. They said that

> [t]he cause of variation in convertibility [of prothrombin] has not been determined. . . . Whether the variable convertibility represents differences in the prothrombin itself, or in the amount of "antiprothrombin" or in other factors must be answered by future research. . . . In newborn infants rapid convertibility of prothrombin compensates for deficient quantity of prothrombin.

In still another paper[13] in 1939, the Iowa team discussed the differences between the two tests of prothrombin: "Since thromboplastin is eliminated as a variable by the test, it follows that some other factor varied, permitting thrombin to be formed with normal speed despite a deficiency in prothrombin."

In supporting the clinical importance of Quick's method, if not its reliability for measuring prothrombin, Smith's group made the following concessions: the Quick test measures "not merely the amount of prothrombin present, but also the ease with which prothrombin can be converted into thrombin. Both the amount of prothrombin and the 'convertibility' vary, but the biological summation of the two is a measure of the tendency to bleed. . . ."[14] "One thus obtains a very practical measure of the tendency to bleed."[15]

In 1941, the Iowa school[16] compared the influence of vitamin K with that of transfusions of whole blood or serum on the hypoprothrombinemia of the newborn. Since serum was believed to be devoid of clotting activity, according to the classic theory, it is surprising that more attention was not paid to the modest but definite shortening of the prothrombin times of babies receiving serum, as much attention, in fact, as that given to their responses to whole blood. This was not the first time that serum was reported to have therapeutic coagulant activity. Roderick[17] had observed that the condition of cattle bleeding from spoiled sweet clover disease improved remarkably after they received transfusions of clotted and defibrinated blood. Even earlier, Sahli[18] and Addis[19] described the shortening of the clotting time of hemophilic plasma when serum was added.

Other discrepancies between the two prothrombin tests were reported in the plasma of patients with pernicious anemia[20] or early liver disease.[21] The same disparity was noted in patients with adrenal failure, but this finding was not published.

How were speculations about altered convertibility of prothrombin accepted outside Iowa City? Quick rejected the two-stage test on technical grounds. It remained for a foreign authority to state that "The [Iowa] authors have strained at the gnat of prothrombin conversion and swallowed a whole camel of physico-chemical objections to their technique."[22]

Part of the real answer to the dilemma was actually at hand. In 1939,

Rhoads and Panzer[23] found that the prothrombin time of banked blood steadily lengthened and attributed this lengthening to a deterioration of prothrombin. But there was no deterioration by the two-stage test.[24] It was several years before Seegers' group discovered Ac globulin[25]; Quick and Stefanini the labile factor[26]; and Owren, factor V.[27] In all likelihood, Fantl and Nance[28] in Australia also discovered it, as did Honorato[29] in Chile; and probably earlier than all the others was Nolf with his "thrombogen."[30]

More was to come. Quick[31] found that the lengthening of the prothrombin time of an animal given dicumarol was different from the lengthening of the prothrombin time due to aging of plasma. He concluded that prothrombin consisted of two components, one susceptible to aging and the other to "dicumarolization."

My own studies in this area were made possible by three things. First, I had the privilege of working with Smith's group while I was a medical student at the University of Iowa; second, I joined Dr. Jesse L. Bollman's Department of Biochemical Research at the Mayo Clinic when interest in dicumarol and vitamin K was at a peak at that institution; and, third, Doctor Seegers very kindly and unselfishly gave me some of his purest preparations of bovine prothrombin.

In studying the plasma of dogs given Dicumarol it became apparent that prothrombin convertibility diminished as the prothrombin time lengthened and accelerated during the recovery phase.[32] A standardized test of convertibility was devised with use of Doctor Seegers' purified prothrombin because this preparation was scarcely convertible to thrombin at all unless plasma was added. Further, it was found that normal serum as well as plasma could correct the hypoconvertible prothrombin in dicumarol-treated dogs.[33] It seemed unlikely that the variability of conversion resided in the prothrombin molecule, since that had been destroyed by clotting during the formation of serum. A convertibility factor, depressed by dicumarol, was proposed and later was called "stable factor."[34] This was subsequently called "serum prothrombin conversion accelerator" (SPCA) by Alexander's group,[35] "proconvertin" by Owren and Bjerkelund,[36] and "factor VII" by Koller and associates.[37] As is now well known, this activity eventually turned out to be two factors, factors VII and X. Factor IX came along and then autoprothrombin IIA, or protein C. With the discovery of the tricarboxyglutamic acid residues in the vitamin K-dependent proteins and this vitamin's role in the carboxylation process, the vitamin K story is brought up to date.

This has been a long and troubled account. At every step, Doctor Seegers' name appears and reappears. At present many biochemists work in all phases of hemostasis, and advances are being made much more rapidly. Perhaps Doctor Seegers was fortunate. In the middle part of this century, he was almost the only biochemist dedicated to the coagulation mechanism. No one can say that he did not make the most of it.

REFERENCES

1. SEEGERS, W. H., H. P. SMITH, E. D. WARNER & K. M. BRINKHOUS. 1938. The purification of prothrombin. J. Biol. Chem. **123:**751–754.
2. SEEGERS, W. H., K. M. BRINKHOUS, H. P. SMITH & E. D. WARNER. 1938. The purification of thrombin. J. Biol. Chem. **126:**91–95.

3. BRINKHOUS, K. M., H. P. SMITH, E. D. WARNER & W. H. SEEGERS. 1939. The inhibition of blood clotting: An unidentified substance which acts in conjunction with heparin to prevent the conversion of prothrombin into thrombin. Am. J. Physiol. 125:683–687.

4. SEEGERS, W. H., E. D. WARNER, K. M. BRINKHOUS & H. P. SMITH. 1942. Heparin and the antithrombic activity of plasma. Science 96:300–301.

5. SEEGERS, W. H., N. ALKJAERSIG & S. A. JOHNSON. 1955. Formation of autoprothrombin in solutions containing purified prothrombin and purified platelet factor 3. Am. J. Physiol. 181:589–594.

6. SEEGERS, W. H. & O. N. ULUTIN. 1961. Antithrombin II anticoagulant (autoprothrombin II-A). Thromb. Diath. Haemorrh. 6:270–281.

7. WARNER, E. D., K. M. BRINKHOUS & H. P. SMITH. 1936. A quantitative study on blood clotting: Prothrombin fluctuations under experimental conditions. Am. J. Physiol. 114:667–675.

8. QUICK, A. J., M. STANLEY-BROWN & F. W. BANCROFT. 1935. A study of the coagulation defect in hemophilia and in jaundice. Am. J. Med. Sci. 190: 501–511.

9. WARNER, E. D., K. M. BRINKHOUS & H. P. SMITH. 1939. Plasma prothrombin levels in various vertebrates. Am. J. Physiol. 125:296–300.

10. WARNER, E. D., K. M. BRINKHOUS & H. P. SMITH. 1939. The prothrombin conversion rate in various species. Proc. Soc. Exp. Biol. Med. 40:197–200.

11. BRINKHOUS, K. M., H. P. SMITH & E. D. WARNER. 1937. Plasma prothrombin level in normal infancy and in hemorrhagic disease of the newborn. Am. J. Med. Sci. 193:475–480.

12. OWEN, C. A., G. R. HOFFMAN, S. E. ZIFFREN & H. P. SMITH. 1939. Blood coagulation during infancy. Proc. Soc. Exp. Biol. Med. 41:181–185.

13. ZIFFREN, S. E., C. A. OWEN, G. R. HOFFMAN & H. P. SMITH. 1939. Control of vitamin K therapy: Compensatory mechanisms at low prothrombin levels. Proc. Soc. Exp. Biol. Med. 40:595–597.

14. ZIFFREN, S. E., C. A. OWEN, G. R. HOFFMAN & H. P. SMITH. 1940. A simple bedside test for control of vitamin K therapy. Am. J. Clin. Pathol. 10 (Techn. Suppl. 4): 13–16.

15. SMITH, H. P., S. E. ZIFFREN, C. A. OWEN & G. R. HOFFMAN. 1939. Clinical and experimental studies on vitamin K. JAMA 113:380–383.

16. WILLUMSEN, H. C., H. E. STADLER & C. A. OWEN. 1941. Comparative effect of vitamin K and whole blood on prothrombin deficiency of newborn infant. Proc. Soc. Exp. Biol. Med. 47:116–121.

17. RODERICK, L. M. 1931. A problem in the coagulation of blood: "sweet clover disease of cattle." Am. J. Physiol. 96:413–425.

18. SAHLI, H. 1910. Weitere Beiträge zur Lehre von der Hämophilie. Deutsch. Arch. Klin. Med. 99:518–556.

19. ADDIS, T. 1911. The pathogenesis of hereditary haemophilia. J. Pathol. Bacteriol. 15:427–452.

20. WARNER, E. D. & C. A. OWEN. 1942. Hypoprothrombinemia in pernicious anemia. Am. J. Med. Sci. 203:187–191.

21. ZIFFREN, S. E., C. A. OWEN, E. D. WARNER & F. R. PETERSON. 1942. Hypoprothrombinemia and liver function. Surg. Gynecol. Obstet. 74:463–467.

22. WITTS, L. J. 1942. Disturbances in the coagulation of the blood. Glasgow Med. J. 137:57–71.

23. RHOADS, J. E. & L. M. PANZER. 1939. The prothrombin time of "bank blood." JAMA 112:309–310.

24. WARNER, E. D., E. L. DeGOWIN & W. H. SEEGERS. 1940. Studies on preserved human blood. V. Decrease in prothrombin titer during storage. Proc. Soc. Exp. Biol. Med. 43:251–254.

25. WARE, A. G., M. M. GUEST & W. H. SEEGERS. 1947. A factor in plasma which accelerates the activation of prothrombin (letter to the editor). J. Biol. Chem. 169:231–232.

26. QUICK, A. J. & M. STEFANINI. 1949. The concentration of component A in blood, its assay and relation to labile factor. J. Lab. Clin. Med. **34:**973–982.
27. OWREN, P. A. 1947. The coagulation of blood: Investigations on a new clotting factor. Acta Med. Scand. (Suppl.) **194:**1–327.
28. FANTL, P. & M. NANCE. 1946. Acceleration of thrombin formation by a plasma component (letter to the editor). Nature **158:**708–709.
29. HONORATO, R. 1947. The plasmatic cofactor of thromboplastin: its adsorption, with prothrombin and fibrinogen, by alumina and tricalcium phosphate gels. Am. J. Physiol. **150:**381–388.
30. NOLF, P. 1938. The coagulation of the blood. Medicine (Baltimore) **17:**381–411.
31. QUICK, A. J. 1943. On the constitution of prothrombin. Am. J. Physiol. **140:**212–220.
32. OWEN, C. A. & J. L. BOLLMAN. 1948. Prothrombin conversion factor of dicumarol plasma. Proc. Soc. Exp. Biol. Med. **67:**231–234.
33. OWEN, C. A. 1947. Experimental alteration of the rate of thrombin formation during blood clotting (abstract). Bull. Am. Coll. Surg. **32:**256.
34. OWEN, C. A., JR., T. B. MAGATH & J. L. BOLLMAN. 1951. Prothrombin conversion factors in blood coagulation. Am. J. Physiol. **166:**1–11.
35. ALEXANDER, B., A. DE VRIES, R. GOLDSTEIN & G. LANDWEHR. 1949. A prothrombin conversion accelerator in serum. Science **109:**545.
36. OWREN, P. A. & C. BJERKELUND. 1949. A new, previously unknown clotting factor (letter to the editor). Scand. J. Clin. Lab. Invest. **1:**162–163.
37. KOLLER, F., A. LOELIGER & F. DUCKERT. 1951. Experiments on a new clotting factor (factor VII). Acta Haematol. (Basel) **6:**1–18.

ELUCIDATION OF THE PLATELET CYTOSKELETON *

Joan C. Mattson and Carol A. Zuiches

Department of Pathology
Michigan State University
East Lansing, Michigan 48824

INTRODUCTION

Morphologic studies of the platelet cytoskeleton at the ultrastructural level have been hampered by the loss of detail that occurs in the process of plastic embedding and thin sectioning. Some of this loss has been ascribed to the action of osmium fixation on filamentous structures, most notably actin.[1] However, the lack of resolution of cytoskeletal elements appears to be an inherent limitation in the approach of using ultrathin sections of material embedded in plastic.[2] The actual structure as well as the interrelationships of a three-dimensional cytoskeleton is difficult to appreciate in ultrathin sections since only perfectly oriented filaments that lie in the plane of the section will appear as filaments. All other orientations will produce oblique or cross-sectional views of filaments, which will appear in micrographs as spherical or ovoid structures. The technique is further hampered by the lack of density differential between the plastic embedding medium and cytoplasmic filaments, which results in almost total obscuration of filaments of finer dimensions. Wolosewick and Porter[2] have demonstrated that if whole cells are processed for electron microscopy without an embedding medium, they can be examined at high voltages (1000 kV) with excellent resolution of minute cytoskeletal details. While these investigators utilized a 1-million volt electron microscope not accessible to the majority of investigators for routine use, other investigators[3,4] have demonstrated that excellent results can be obtained with whole cell preparations utilizing conventional accelerating voltages of 80 to 100 kV. The usefulness of whole cell preparations in studying cytoskeletal architecture has been amplified by the introduction of nonionic detergents to produce partial or complete removal of membranes to yield extracted "cytoskeletons."[5,6]

The study presented here was designed to overcome the inherent difficulties in demonstrating cytoskeletal elements in transmission electron micrographs of sectioned platelets by utilizing whole cell preparations and detergent-extracted cytoskeletons of contact-activated platelets.

MATERIALS AND METHODS

Isolation of Platelets

Whole blood was collected by venipuncture from normal human volunteers who had previously been determined to have normal platelet function. Samples were anticoagulated with 3.8 percent sodium citrate in a ratio of 9 parts whole

* This work was supported by a grant from the Michigan Heart Association.

11

blood to 1 part anticoagulant. Platelet-rich plasma (PRP) was prepared immediately by differential centrifugation at $70 \times g$ for 10 minutes. The resultant PRP was transferred to a clean plastic test tube and allowed to rest for at least 30 minutes, but no more than 1 hour before use in experiments. Whole blood and platelet rich plasma were maintained at room temperature throughout these procedures to avoid cold-induced morphologic alterations. All-plastic labware was used in handling whole blood and platelet-rich plasma to avoid platelet activation by glass or silicone.

Whole Cell Preparations of Contact-Activated Platelets

Whole cell mounts were prepared following a modification of the procedure outlined by Pudney and Singer.[6] Platelets were allowed to settle and spread onto Formvar-coated, carbon-stabilized copper grids that had been briefly pretreated with 0.1 percent polylysine. This was accomplished by placing a drop of PRP onto each prepared grid and allowing the platelets to settle out for 1 hour at room temperature in a moist chamber. Grids were then washed free of nonadherent platelets by briefly rinsing in phosphate-buffered saline (PBS) solution. They were then fixed for 2 hours in 2.5 percent glutaraldehyde in 0.1 M cacodylate buffer pH 7.2, rinsed briefly in distilled water, placed in 30 percent acetone for 10 minutes, stained with 1 percent uranyl acetate in 50 percent acetone for 3 minutes, dehydrated in graded acetones, and dried from CO_2 by the critical point method.

Cytoskeletal Preparations

Cytoskeletal preparations were prepared in an identical fashion, except that a nonionic detergent (Nonedet P40 or Triton X-100) in concentrations from 0.1 to 2 percent was introduced either immediately before fixation for a 2-minute digestion or simultaneously with fixation by placing the appropriate detergent directly into the fixative. In the latter instance, grids containing whole platelets were fixed in the detergent-glutaraldehyde mixture for 15 minutes and then transferred to fresh 2.5 percent glutaraldehyde without detergent for an additional 15 minutes. Grids were then processed as described for whole cell preparations.

Transmission Electron Microscopy (TEM)

The "critical-point-dried" whole platelets were examined on a Philips 201 microscope using a 20-μm objective aperture and operated at an accelerating voltage of 80 kV. Cytoskeletal preparations were examined on the same instrument operated at an accelerating voltage of 60 kV. Selected specimens were photographed as stereoscopic pairs using tilts of $\pm 6°$ from the horizontal to allow study of filament interrelationships. Filaments were measured from photographic prints taken immediately after instrument calibration with a germanium-shadowed carbon replica having 28,800 lines per inch.

Scanning Electron Microscopy (SEM)

Occasional whole-mount preparations were first examined by TEM and then coated with 100 Å of gold and examined by scanning electron microscopy on an ISI Super III scanning electron microscope at an accelerating voltage of 15 kV.

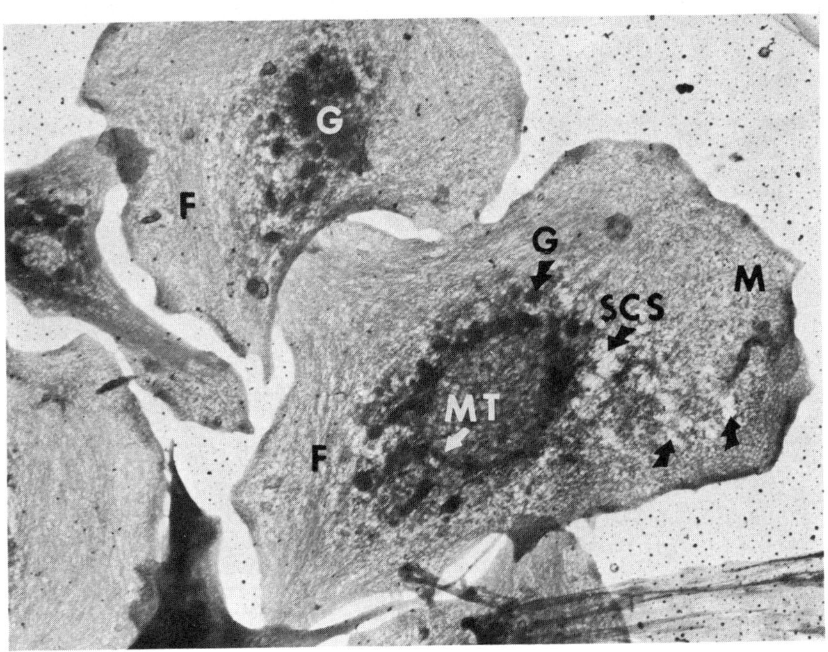

FIGURE 1. Whole cell preparation of platelets allowed to spread for 1 hour prior to fixation. Polygonal cell has centralized granules (G) with closely associated microtubule coil (MT). Fan-shaped cell at upper left also contains aggregated granules (G), but these remain close to the unspread margin of the cell. Clear channels of the surface connecting system (SCS) are visible in close proximity to granules. Occasional channels of SCS extend peripherally into the cytoplasm (*arrows*). The platelet hyalomere contains faintly discernible bundles of filaments (F) interspersed with unstructured areas of cytoplasm having a mat-like appearance (M). (80 kV; original magnification ×11,550; reduced by 15 percent.)

RESULTS

The general features of contact-activated platelets could be appreciated in both whole cell preparations examined at 80 kV and detergent-extracted cytoskeletons examined at 60 kV. Both types of preparations demonstrated that after 1 hour of contact with the substrate, activated platelets spread to produce circular, fan-shaped, polygonal, or angulated configurations (FIGS. 1–6).

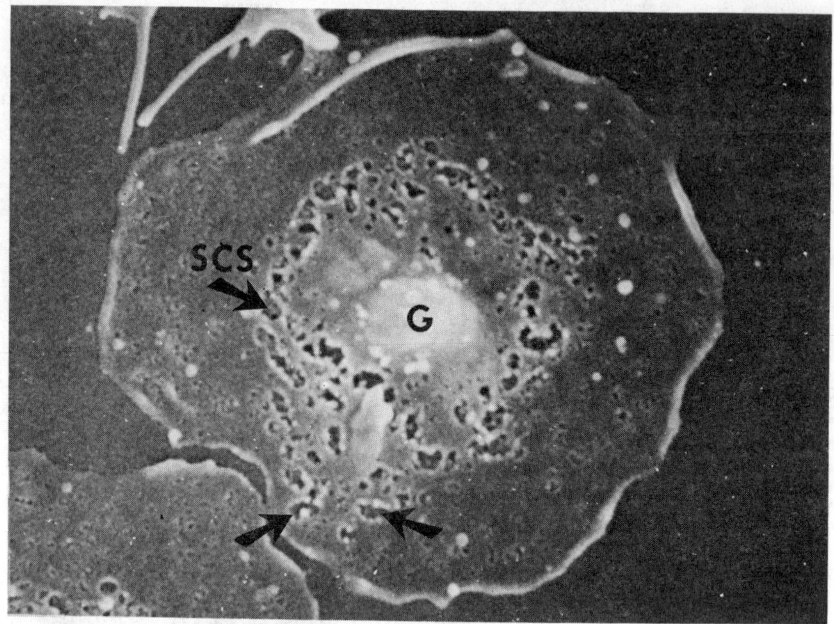

FIGURE 2. Scanning electron micrograph of platelets. The platelet is fully spread with a roughly circular profile. The aggregated granule mass (G) is seen as a hillock in the cell center. Openings of the surface connecting system (SCS) are seen encircling the centralized granules with a few openings extending into the peripheral cytoplasm (*arrows*). Note that fully spread platelets do not contain long pseudopodia or dendritic processes. (15 kV; original magnification ×15,000; reduced by 15 percent.)

Pseudopodia were absent. In 25 randomly selected cells and cytoskeletons, the longest diameters ranged from 5.2 to 10.2 μm. Approximately 25 percent of the platelets were unevenly spread (that is, long and short dimensions differed by 2 μm or more), producing a clearly distinguishable long axis. The mean length along the long axis in this group was 7.8 μm as compared with a mean longest dimension of 6.9 μm in more evenly spread platelets.

In the majority of platelets, granules were found aggregated centrally (FIGURES 1 through 4). However in fan-shaped cells, the aggregated granule mass was found at the unspread, stable margin of the cell (FIG. 5). The morphologic configuration of granules was similar to that seen in thin-sectioned material. They appeared as electron-dense ovoid or spheroid structures that ranged in size from 0.15 to 0.28 μm. However, the density of nonsectioned granules did not allow appreciation of any substructure. In addition, it was not possible to distinguish mitochondria from granules in these preparations.

In both whole cells and in cytoskeleton preparations, channels of the surface connecting system (SCS) were found concentrated near the central granulomere (FIGS. 1, 3, and 5). Surface openings to this system could be seen by scanning electron microscopy to encircle the central granule mass (FIG. 2). In several platelets a few channels of the surface connecting system appeared to extend toward the cell periphery (FIGS. 1 and 3).

Some limited details of the platelet cytoskeleton could be appreciated in whole cell preparations (FIGS. 1–3). Bundles of elongated filaments could be identified interspersed with areas having a more mat-like appearance. At the cell surface, hair-like projections of the glycocalyx were visible in some preparations (FIG. 3, inset). Whole cell preparations examined at an accelerating voltage of 80 kV did not, however, reveal sufficient detail to allow either size of filaments or complex interrelationships to be defined; for this, detergent extraction was required.

In cytoskeletons prepared by partial detergent extraction, the filamentous components were clearly visible (FIGS. 4–8). It was immediately obvious that the cytoskeletons of fully spread platelets have a highly structured organization. All platelets in detergent-treated preparations contained loose bundles of fila-

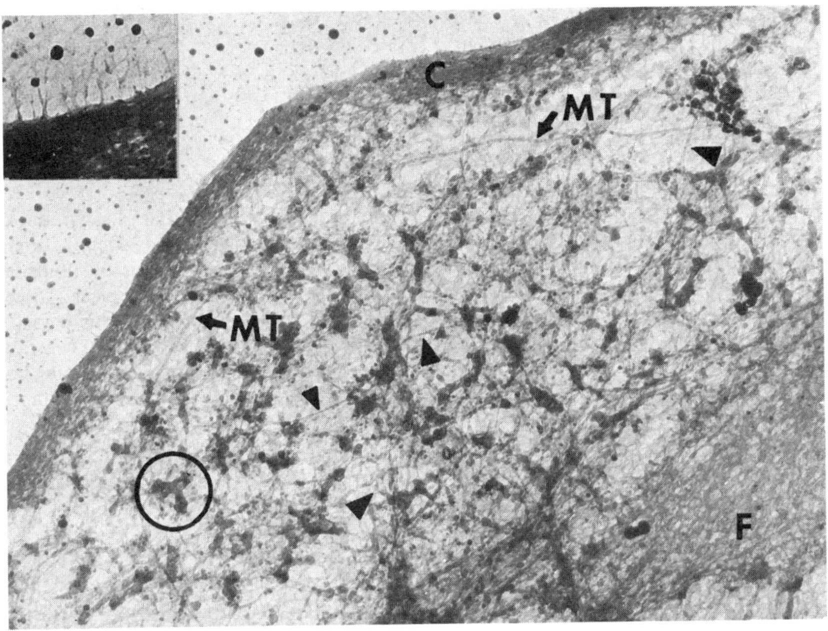

FIGURE 3. Whole cell preparation. Detail from the peripheral hyalomere of a fully spread platelet. A bundle of filaments (F) is seen at the lower right. Resolution of individual filaments in this bundle is insufficient to allow measurements or to judge interrelationships. At the cell periphery, channels of the surface connecting system render the cell more permeable to the electron beam. In this area a network of thin filaments (*arrowheads*) can be distinguished in random array. These become compact at the cell cortex (C). A single microtubule curves through the filamentous network (MT). Irregularly shaped opaque tubular structures (*circle*) are suspended in the interconnecting filaments. On the external surface of the platelet, hair-like projections extend at a 90° angle from the cell surface (*inset*). (80 kV; original magnification ×32,500; reduced by 15 percent.)

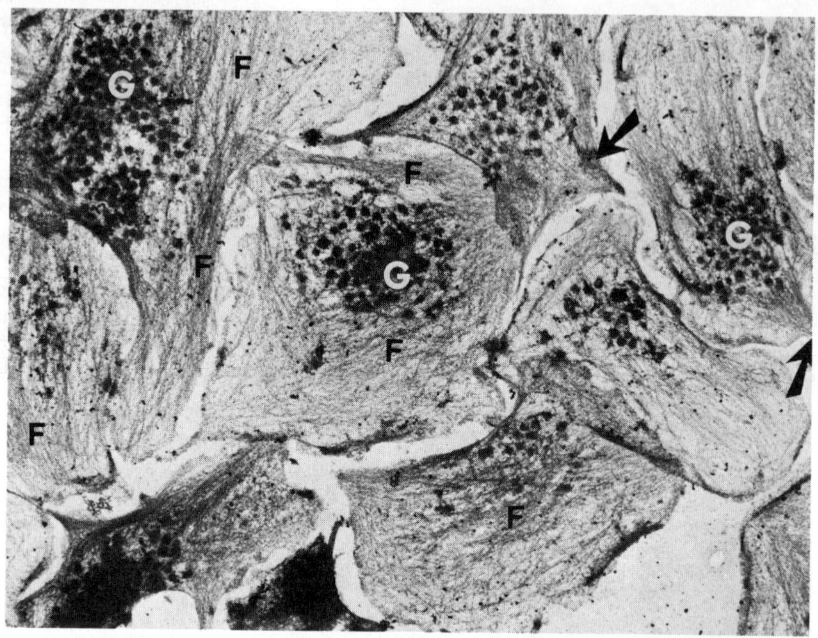

FIGURE 4. Detergent-extracted cytoskeletons produced by partial dissolution of membranes with 2 percent Nonedet P40 in 2.5 percent glutaraldehyde. Details of the cytoskeleton revealed by this technique include prominent loose bundles of elongated filaments (F). In angulated cells, filament bundles coalesce at the apices of cell projections (*arrows*). Note that granules (G) usually remain in place in this partially extracted preparation. As in whole-cell preparations, granules either coalesce centrally or along the unspread margin of incompletely spread platelets. No microtubular coil is identified surrounding granulomeres. (60 kV; original magnification ×4750; reduced by 15 percent.)

ments, which encircled the central granule mass and which were usually oriented in the long axis of the cell (FIGS. 5–7). Individual elongated filaments appeared to come together to form thicker fibrils, then to separate for short distances only to re-form lateral associations with the same or different adjacent filaments (FIG. 7). In this manner an interwoven effect is created within the bundles of long filaments. In angulated cells with short cytoplasmic projections, bundles of filaments often converged and coalesced at the vortex of each projection (FIG. 4). Individual filaments within these bundles ranged in diameter from 60 to 120 Å with occasional larger filaments measuring up to 180 Å. The larger measurements may represent indistinguishable coalescence of two or more thin filaments.

At high magnifications, a filamentous network of thinner, shorter filaments could be seen both interacting with the bundles of long filaments (FIGS. 7 and 8) and extending to the periphery of cells, where it formed the major cytoskeletal framework in areas that contained no filament bundles (FIGS. 5 and 6). This latticework appeared to condense at the cell cortex (FIGS. 3 and 5). Filaments in this network measured from 30 to 85 Å in diameter with occasional thicker segments measuring up to 150 Å. Within this three-dimensional lattice, numerous ovoid or spherical particles measuring 140 to 170 Å could be identified intimately associated with both short and long filaments (FIG. 8). Larger particles measuring up to 280 Å were also found suspended within the filamentous network.

A tight coil of microtubules was rarely found surrounding the central granule mass in any of the whole cells or cytoskeletons examined. Usually, single microtubules were seen coursing in a gently curved fashion through the periphery of the cytoplasm (FIG. 6).

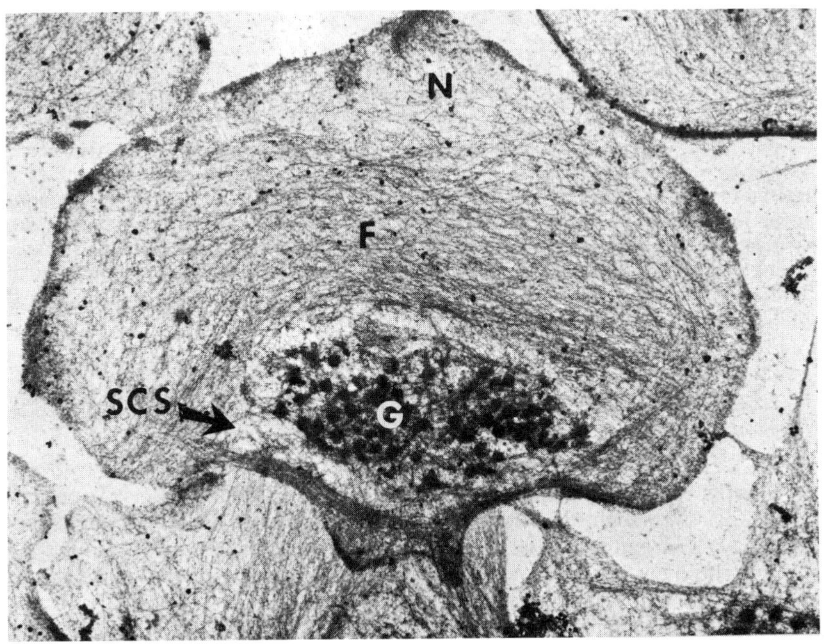

FIGURE 5. Detergent-extracted cytoskeleton. As in whole-cell preparations, channels of the surface connecting system (SCS) appear as clear spaces in close association with the granulomere (G). Filaments are oriented in elongated bundles (F) on the long axis of the cell. Peripheral to the filament bundles is a loosely structured filamentous network (N) which appears to condense at the platelet margin. Note the absence of a microtubular coil surrounding the granulomere. (60 kV; original magnification ×11,375; reduced by 15 percent.

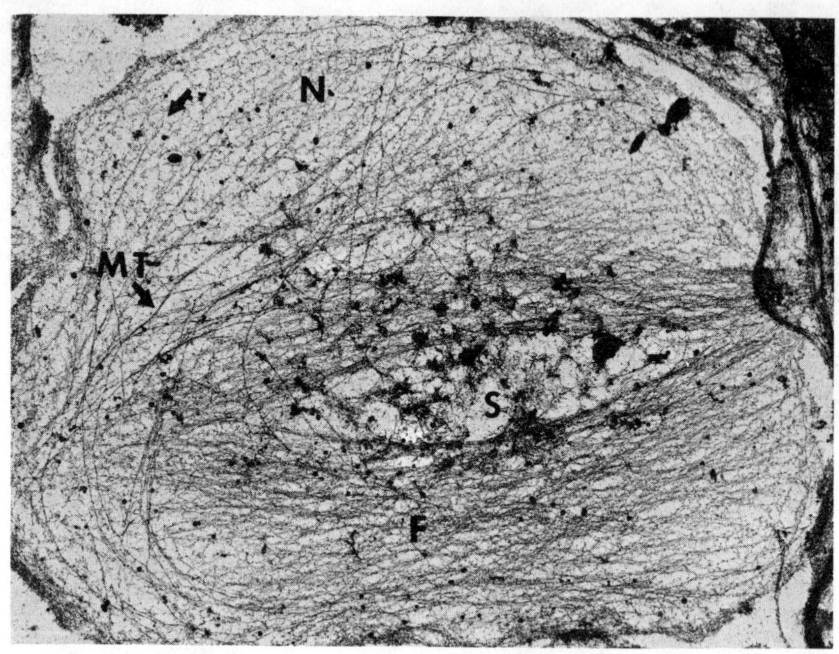

FIGURE 6. Detergent-extracted cytoskeleton. The central granule mass has become dislodged to reveal a set of channels or spaces (S). Loosely structured bundles of elongated filaments (F) surround this central area. Again, filaments (F) are oriented with the long axis of the platelet. At the cell periphery, the cytoskeleton is composed of a more loosely structured filamentous network (N). Single straight and curved microtubules (MT) course through the cell periphery, but these do not appear to be elements of a continuous coil since the ends of some individual microtubules can be identified (*arrow*). 60 kV; original magnification ×12,150; reduced by 15 percent.)

DISCUSSION

By using whole cell preparations and detergent-extracted cytoskeletons, the present work has shown that the spread platelet produced by contact activation contains a well-organized cytoskeleton composed of loose filament bundles and single microtubules intimately associated with a network of short, thin interconnecting filaments. The highly structured organization of the platelet cytoskeleton in these preparations appears to be related to and perhaps responsible for the nonrandom distribution of organelles. Platelet granules were, without exception, found as an aggregate surrounded by filament bundles. The microtubular coil, on the other hand, was generally absent from this location.

Several features of the platelet cytoskeleton as demonstrated in this study are similar to the cytoskeletal components described in other cell systems. Most notably, the fine filamentous latticework, which appears to support organelles and interact with bundles of long filaments and with microtubules, appears to be comparable to the microtrabecular network revealed by high-voltage electron microscopy of cells in culture.[2, 7, 8] Similarly the bundles of elongated filaments have the same dimensions and orientation as the stress fibers of cultured cells.[8] It would be reasonable to suppose that such stress fibers might be a common feature of all cells that are adherent to a substrate. It is also tempting to postulate that the peculiar arrangement of filament bundles around granules in platelets may be critical to the generation of forces that modulate the granule extrusion known to occur during platelet spreading.[9]

It is interesting to note that spread platelets characteristically do not contain a microtubular coil surrounding the granulomere, as is commonly seen in platelets activated in suspension. Instead, individual microtubules were found curving through the peripheral cytoplasm of fully spread platelets. Nachmias [10, 11] has seen microtubular coils in platelet cytoskeletons treated with Triton 45 seconds after contact activation, but has also demonstrated that fully

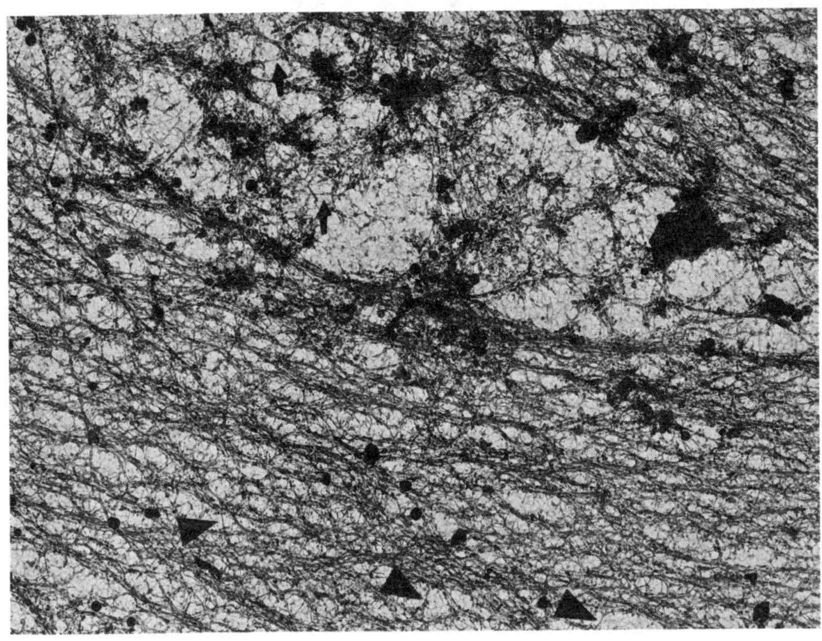

FIGURE 7. Detail of filament bundles from the platelet shown in FIGURE 6. Note that individual thin filaments in these bundles do not run in precise parallel array. Instead, several filaments come together for a short distance, then separate for a distance, and reassociate with the same or different filaments, always maintaining a general orientation along the same axis. This produces an interwoven effect. In the spaces created as bundles separate, thin filaments interconnect long filaments at a roughly 90° angle (*arrowheads*). A similar network of short, thin filaments is also seen within the central space. (60 kV; original magnification ×31,500; reduced by 15 percent.)

spread platelets may not contain this coil. Our interpretation is that microtubule reorientation occurs as platelet spreading progresses.

Further studies are required to identify the precise composition of the platelet cytoskeleton. The platelet cytoskeleton is an extremely complex system that contains multiple components including actin, myosin, tropomyosin, actin-binding protein, α-actinin, and calcium-binding proteins.[12, 13] The adaptation of techniques that allow preservation and visualization of the platelet cytoskeleton is, therefore, an important step toward the ultimate localization of these components and the understanding of their interrelationships. The

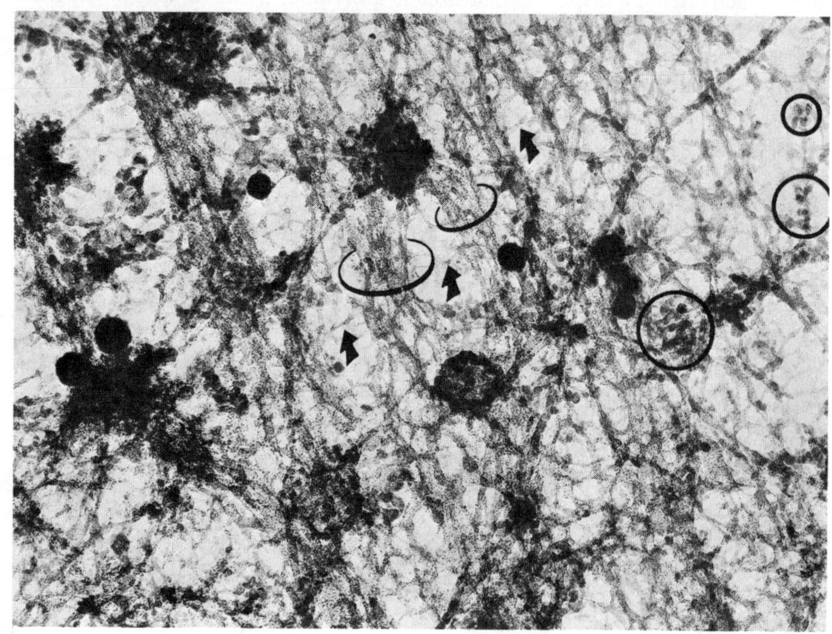

FIGURE 8: High magnification through filament bundles seen in FIGURE 7 shows a detail of the underlying filamentous network. Small groupings of long filaments are encircled. In the spaces between groups of long filaments, short filaments can be seen to cross at right angles (*arrows*). Many long filaments appear to have small spherical or ovoid globules (140 to 180 Å) attached along their surface (*circles*). (60 kV; original magnification ×78,000; reduced by 15 percent.)

excellent preservation of cytoskeletal architecture obtained in this study suggests that this model will provide an appropriate method for biochemical and immunocytochemical studies.

ACKNOWLEDGMENTS

We wish to thank Belinda Oxender for clerical assistance with this manuscript and Dee Jakubiak and Donna Craft for technical assistance in the preparation of the electron micrographs.

[**Note added in proof:** Subsequent to the submission of this manuscript, Lewis *et al.*[14] reported a similar reorientation of platelet microtubules during adhesion and spreading. These authors observed loss of the circumferential band of microtubules during early activation, radially oriented microtubules in the dendritic platelets found in the intermediate stages of spreading, and finally reorientation of microtubules to the cytoplasmic margin in fully spread platelets. These findings support our observations that, in the fully spread platelet, microtubules are seldom found in close association with the central granule mass, but are present in the peripheral cytoplasm where they are oriented parallel to the platelet membrane.]

REFERENCES

1. SZAMIER, P., T. POLLARD & K. FUGIWARA. 1975. Tropomyosin prevents the destruction of actin filaments by osmium. J. Cell Biol. **67:**424a.
2. WOLOSEWICK, J. J. & K. R. PORTER. 1976. Stereo high-voltage electron microscopy of whole cells of the human diploid line, WI-38. Am. J. Anat. **147:** 303–324.
3. KILARSKI, W. & H. KOPROWSKI. 1976. Observation of whole, cultured human brain cells using 100 KV kilovolts electron microscopy. J. Microsc. Biol. Cell. **25:**73–80.
4. BUCKLEY, I. K. & T. R. RAJU. 1976. Form and distribution of actin and myosin in non-muscle cells: A study using cultured chick embryo fibroblasts. J. Micros. (Oxford) **107**(2):129–149.
5. BROWN, S., W. LEVINSON & J. A. SPUDICH. 1976. Cytoskeletal elements of chick embryo fibroblasts revealed by detergent extraction. J. Supramol. Struct. **5:** 119–130.
6. PUDNEY, J. & R. H. SINGER. 1979. Electron microscopic visualization of the filamentous reticulum in whole cultured presumptive chick myoblasts. Am. J. Anat. **156**(3):321–336.
7. BUCKLEY, I. K. 1975. Three dimensional fine structure of cultured cells: Possible implications for subcellular motility. Tissue Cell **7**(1):51–72.
8. BUCKLEY, I. K. & K. R. PORTER. 1967. Cytoplasmic fibrils in living cultured cells. A light and electron microscope study. Protoplasma **64:**349–380.
9. ALLEN R. D., L. R. ZACHARSKI, S. T. WIDIRSTKY, R. ROSENSTEIN, L. M. ZAITLIN & D. R. BURGESS. 1979. Transformation and motility of human platelets. Details of the shape change and release reaction observed by optical and electron microscopy. J. Cell Biol. **83:**126–142.
10. NACHMIAS, V. T., J. SULLENDER, J. FALLON & A. ASCH. 1980. Observations on the "cytoskeleton" of human platelets. Thromb. Haemost. **42**(5):1661–1666.
11. NACHMIAS, V. T. & J. S. SULLENDER. 1978. The cytoskeleton of human platelets at rest and after spreading: Whole mounts viewed at 200 KV correlated with negatively stained specimens examined at 50 KV. Proceedings of the 9th International Congress on Electron Microscopy, Toronto, Canada, Vol. II. :458–459.
12. GOLDMAN, R. D., A. MILSTED, J. A. SCHLOSS, J. STARGER & M.-J. YERNA. 1979. Cytoplasmic fibers in mammalian cells: Cytoskeletal and contractile elements. Ann. Rev. Physiol. **41:**703–722.
13. ADELSTEIN, R. S. & T. D. POLLARD. 1978. Platelet contractile proteins. Prog. Hemostasis Thromb. **4:**37–58.
14. LEWIS, J. C., T. PRATER, R. G. TAYLOR & M. S. WHITE. 1980. The use of correlative SEM and TEM to study thrombocyte and platelet adhesion to artificial surfaces. Scanning Electron Microsc. **III:**189–202.

A COMPARATIVE STUDY OF PLATELET REACTIVITY IN ARTHRITIS *

Jeanne M. Riddle, Gilbert B. Bluhm, Wayne C. Pitchford,
Honora McElroy, Carlina Jimenea, James Leisen, and
Kumar Venkatasubramanian

*Department of Internal Medicine, Division of Rheumatology
Henry Ford Hospital
Detroit, Michigan, 48202*

Thrombosis may represent an important, but relatively unappreciated, event in the pathophysiology of some arthritic disease states. For example, the incidence of myocardial infarction before 50 years of age was found to be significantly increased when 280 patients with primary gout were compared retrospectively with the general population.[1] Hyperuricemia as found in primary gout has been suggested as a potential risk factor for coronary heart disease.[2] Platelet thrombi in association with obliterative microangiopathy and platelet aggregation to altered endothelial surfaces have been demonstrated in histologic studies of active lesions in synovial tissue obtained from patients with early and chronic rheumatoid arthritis.[3, 4] Also, the addition of sera from some patients (29 percent) with seropositive definitive or classical rheumatoid arthritis to platelet-rich plasma isolated from normal subjects induced platelet aggregation.[5]

These studies imply that the reactivity of blood platelets in some types of arthritis is altered. In order to understand more fully the involvement of platelets, we surveyed the level of reactivity shown by platelet populations in five different rheumatic diseases. These findings were compared with values derived from a group of normal subjects.

MATERIAL AND METHODS

The surface response of platelet populations from either normal subjects or patients with a variety of disease states was assessed using our standardized *in vitro* method.[6] In brief, a nonwettable syringe and needle are used to obtain a sample of venous blood that is mixed immediately with 3.8 percent sodium citrate (9 parts blood to 1 part citrate). A microscope slide previously coated with a thin film of Formvar (polyvinyl formal) is covered by the anticoagulated blood sample. The preparation is incubated in a nonwettable vessel placed in a horizontal position for 8 minutes at room temperature. During the period of incubation, platelets adhere to the Formvar film and undergo measurable structural alterations. After 8 minutes, the microscope slide with the attached film and adherent platelets is withdrawn. The film coated with platelets is immediately washed in Tyrode's solution. Next, the specimen is fixed in buffered osmium or buffered glutaraldehyde, rinsed free of contaminating salts in distilled

* This work was supported in part by the Michigan Chapter of the Arthritis Foundation.

22

water, and air-dried. The Formvar film with its attached, stabilized platelets is transferred to 200-mesh stainless steel grids. These specimens are viewed with a transmission electron microscope.

One hundred consecutive, single platelets are classified as either a round, dendritic, or spread type of platelet. The round type is similar to the disc-shaped circulating platelet and has a relatively smooth exterior. The dendritic type shows a minimal amount of surface response as evidenced by the extrusion of cytoplasmic processes (pseudopodia). The spread type exhibits a marked degree of surface activation and shows extensive cytoplasmic spreading between pseudopodia. The total number of aggregates observed during identification of the 100 single platelets is also recorded. The platelet differential count is a combination of the percentages of the different platelet types and the total number of aggregates observed.

RESULTS

We surveyed platelet reactivity in 72 normal subjects who ranged in age from 22 to 70 years. The dendritic type of platelet (FIG. 1) dominated the differential counts of our normal group. In contrast, on the average, only 8 percent of the adherent, individual platelets showed cytoplasmic spreading between adjacent pseudopodia and were therefore classified as the spread type. The mean value for platelet aggregates was 46 per 100 single platelets counted with a range of 0 to 93 (TABLE 1).

Platelet populations from 314 patients with five distinct rheumatic disease states were also surveyed, showing increased surface reactivity in certain patients within each group. The percentage of the spread type of platelet and/or the total number of aggregates was increased more than ± 2 standard deviations from the corresponding mean values for the normal subjects. The number of patients with abnormal differential counts within each group was as follows: normal, 6 of 72 (8 percent); degenerative joint disease, 21 of 52 (40 percent); rheumatoid arthritis, 48 of 84 (57 percent); gout, 89 of 146 (61 percent); scleroderma, 13 of 20 (65 percent); and polymyalgia rheumatica plus temporal arteritis, 9 of 12 (75 percent). The mean values for the spread type of platelet (FIG. 2) and for the total number of platelet aggregates were consistently increased in all of the patient groups when compared with corresponding values in the normal subjects (TABLE 2).

Pair-wise contrasts of the percentage of each platelet type (round, dendritic, and spread) as well as of the total platelet aggregates were performed after an analysis of variance was done (F = 3.66, p = 0.001).

The following differences were found:

1. The mean differential platelet count of the normal subjects was significantly different from that in each of the rheumatic disease states.

2. Platelet populations from patients with polymyalgia rheumatica and temporal arteritis were the most abnormal of the various rheumatic disease states when compared with populations in the normal subjects (FIG. 3).

The following similarities were found:

1. Platelet populations from patients with degenerative joint disease most closely resembled those of the normal subjects (FIG. 4).

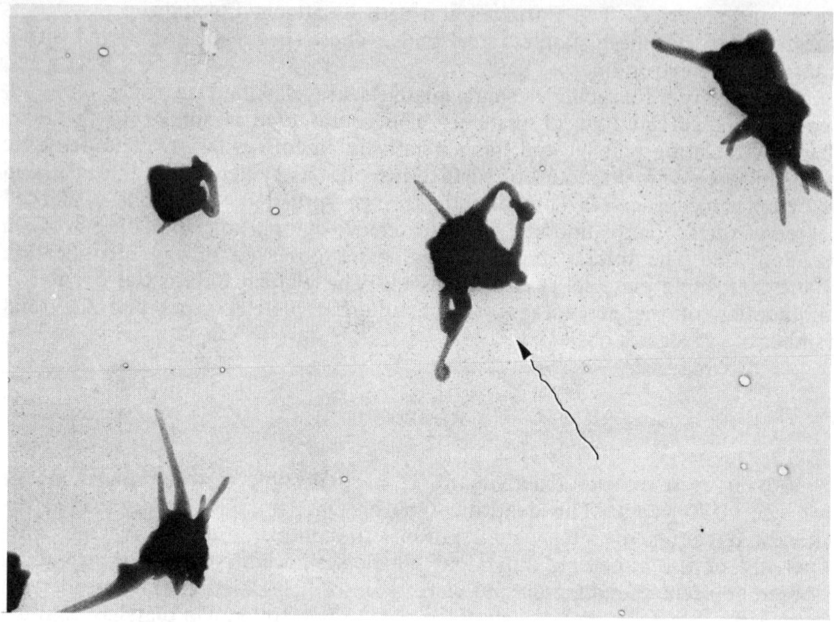

FIGURE 1. Dendritic type platelets (*arrow*) and small aggregate in normal subject. (Original magnification ×7400; reduced by 29 percent.)

2. Platelet populations from patients with scleroderma, rheumatoid arthritis, and gout closely resembled one another (FIG. 5).

DISCUSSION

A variety of platelet alterations has been observed in association with specific types of arthritis. In rheumatoid arthritis, certain patients reportedly have increased numbers of circulating platelets.[6] Platelet populations from some patients with rheumatoid arthritis also have demonstrated reduced adhesiveness,[7] as well as an increased degree of surface activation, or an increased

TABLE 1

MEAN PLATELET DIFFERENTIAL COUNT FOR NORMAL SUBJECTS

Platelet Types	Percent	Range *
Round	7	(0 to 20%)
Dendritic	85	(70 to 100%)
Spread	8	(0 to 20%)
Total aggregates per 100 single platelets counted	46	(0 to 93)

* ±2 standard deviations.

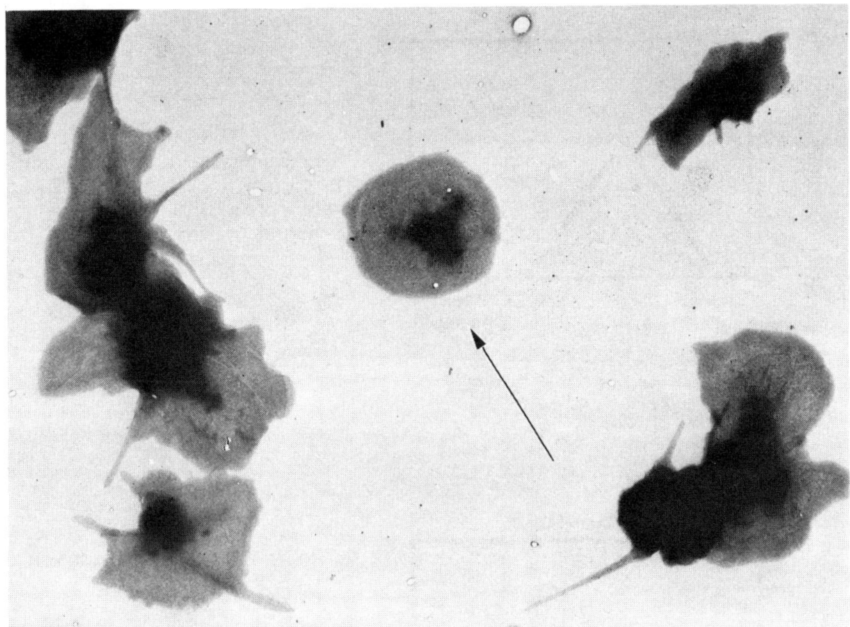

FIGURE 2. Spread type of platelet (*arrow*) and aggregates in a patient with gout. (Original magnification ×7400; reduced by 29 percent.)

TABLE 2

MEAN PLATELET DIFFERENTIAL COUNT FOR
NORMAL SUBJECTS VERSUS THOSE WITH RHEUMATIC DISEASES

Groups Studied	Number of Patients	Type of Platelet (%)			Total Aggregates per 100 Single Platelets
		Round	Dendritic	Spread	
Normal	72	7	85	8	46
Degenerative joint disease	52	9	70	21	82
Polymyalgia rheumatica plus temporal arteritis	12	1	52	47	128
Scleroderma	20	7	72	21	137
Rheumatoid arthritis	84	4	73	23	114
Gout	146	6	64	30	111

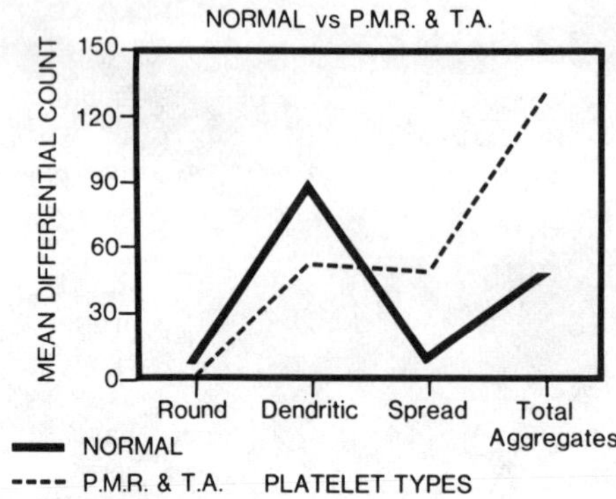

FIGURE 3. Comparison between the mean platelet differential counts in normal subjects and in patients with polymyalgia rheumatica and temporal arteritis.

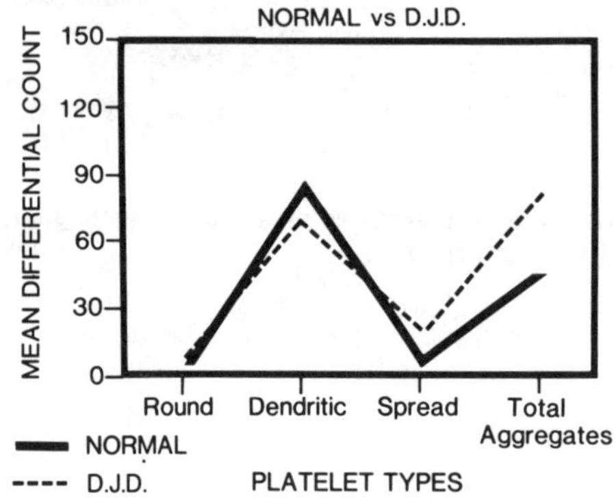

FIGURE 4. Comparison between the mean platelet differential counts in normal subjects and those with degenerative joint disease.

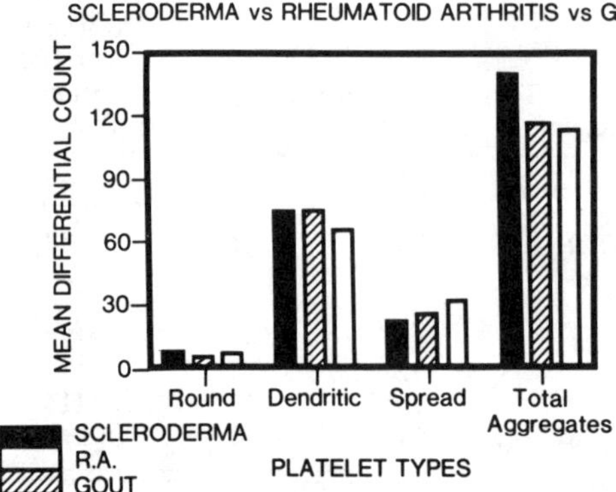

FIGURE 5. Comparison among the mean platelet differential counts in patients with scleroderma, rheumatoid arthritis or gout.

capacity for aggregation, or both.[8] Sera from some patients with adult rheumatoid arthritis also contain immune complexes that are capable of aggregating normal platelet-rich plasma *in vitro*.[5] Biochemical analysis of platelets isolated from patients with rheumatoid arthritis has shown an increased content of acid mucopolysaccharides coupled with low serotonin [9] as well as a diminished protein content, a possible decrease in acid phosphatase activity, and a reduced amount of connective-tissue-activating peptide-III.[10]

In primary gout, platelet survival was found to be decreased.[11] In a previous study, we monitored the surface response of platelets from patients with primary gout and found that the degree of surface activity or amount of aggregation, or both, was increased in more than 50 percent of these patients.[12] The association between hyperactive platelet populations and primary gout may have at least two possible explanations: The first of these is the interaction between platelets and the hyperuricemic state. Normal platelets exposed to increasing concentrations of uric acid *in vitro* showed a progressive amount of surface reactivity which paralleled the plasma urate concentration.[12] Likewise, an infusion of uric acid into the circulation of rats to establish a hyperuricemic state prior to the infusion of adenosine diphosphate (ADP) potentiated platelet aggregation *in vitro* as well as increasing the incidence of pulmonary thrombosis *in vivo*.[13] Finally, the production of hyperuricemia in rats by a dietary modification also resulted in potentiating both ADP- and thrombin-induced platelet aggregation *in vitro*.[14] Crystals of monosodium urate also interact with the blood platelet. Exposure of either washed platelets or platelet-rich plasma to these crystals *in vitro* promoted a two-phase release phenomenon.[15, 16]

A recent view of scleroderma (progressive systemic sclerosis) emphasizes the vascular system as the target organ in this disease state.[17, 18] Histologically, the smaller arteries and arterioles in scleroderma show intimal proliferation and sclerosis with morphologic alterations of endothelial cells. Changing the structural and, probably, the biochemical integrity of endothelial cells predictably leads to alterations in the reactivity of adjacent platelets. Our finding of an increased amount of platelet reactivity in patients with scleroderma may reflect its recognized vascular pathology.

No previous publications in the literature present information about the level of reactivity expressed by platelet populations from patients with polymyalgia rheumatica and temporal arteritis or degenerative joint disease. The functional basis for the high degree of surface activation or increased aggregation, or both, in polymyalgia rheumatica and temporal arteritis may relate to the giant-cell inflammation of the vessel wall, which is the hallmark of this disease state.[19] Those patients with degenerative joint disease whose platelet populations are hyperactive could possibly have a more marked degree of arteriosclerosis, since platelets are now considered to play a role in the development of this vascular alteration.[20]

Our comparative survey of the platelet reactivity in normal subjects and patients with distinct rheumatic diseases has shown that each of the disease states differs from the control. The increased platelet responsiveness within the different forms of the rheumatic diseases may relate to the presence of specific, disease-related components including soluble or insoluble immune complexes, the hyperuricemic state, endothelial deposits of monosodium urate crystals, and atherosclerotic plaques. Our studies suggest that platelets may play an active role and participate in the pathophysiology of some rheumatic diseases by releasing substances *in vivo* that contribute to inflammation, vasculitis, and altered cellular dynamics.

SUMMARY

We utilized a standardized *in vitro* method which employs transmission electron microscopy to monitor the degree of surface activation (cytoplasmic spreading) and amount of aggregation displayed by platelet populations from 314 patients with one of five distinct rheumatic diseases and from 72 normal subjects. The percentage of patients in each group whose platelet populations were hyperactive was as follows: polymyalgia rheumatica, 75 percent; scleroderma, 65 percent; primary gout, 61 percent; rheumatoid arthritis, 57 percent; and degenerative joint disease, 40 percent. Pair-wise contrasts performed after an analysis of variance suggest the following differences and similarities: (1) the mean differential platelet count of the normal subjects differed from that in each disease state; (2) the platelet responsivity in patients with degenerative joint disease most closely resembled that in normal subjects; (3) the platelet response in polymyalgia rheumatica plus temporal arteritis was the most abnormal; and (4) platelet response in scleroderma, rheumatoid arthritis, and gout closely resembled each other. The increased platelet response *in vitro* may reflect the *in vivo* presence of disease-related "risk factors" (hyperuricemia, immune complexes, and atherosclerosis). Those patients with "triggered" platelet populations may be appropriate candidates for antiplatelet therapy.

ACKNOWLEDGMENT

We are indebted to Mr. David W. Smith, Statistical Research Laboratory, University of Michigan, Ann Arbor, who provided assistance for the statistical analysis of the data.

REFERENCES

1. VIOZZI, F. J., G. B. BLUHM & J. M. RIDDLE. 1972. Gout and arterial thrombosis. Henry Ford Hosp. Med. J. **20:**119–124.
2. GERTLER, M. M., S. M. GARN & S. A. LEVINE. 1951. Serum uric acid in relation to age and physique in healthy and coronary heart disease. Ann. Intern. Med. **34:**1421–1431.
3. KULKA, J. P., D. BOCKING, M. W. ROPES & W. BAUER. 1955. Early joint lesions of rheumatoid arthritis. Arch. Pathol. **59:**129–150.
4. SCHUMACHER, H. R. 1975. Synovial membrane and fluid morphologic alterations in early rheumatoid arthritis: Microvascular injury and virus-like particles. Ann. N.Y. Acad. Sci. **256:**39–64.
5. FINK, P. C., V. PIENING, M. FRICKE & H. DEICHER. 1979. Platelet aggregation and aggregation inhibition by different antiglobulins and antiglobulin complexes from sera of patients with rheumatoid arthritis. Arthritis Rheum. **22:**896–903.
6. SELROOS, O. 1973. Thrombocytosis in rheumatoid arthritis. Scand. J. Rheum. **1:**136–140.
7. PAZDUR, J. & M. KOPEC. 1970. Platelets in rheumatoid arthritis. Thromb. Diath. Haemorrh. **23:**276–285.

8. BLUHM, G. B., J. M. RIDDLE, D. G. PICA & G. D. LANGEJANS. 1977. Salicylate effect on platelets and vascular thrombosis in rheumatoid arthritis. Henry Ford Hosp. Med. J. **25:**61–74.
9. KERBY, G. P. & S. M. TAYLOR. 1959. The acid mucopolysaccharide and 5-hydroxytryptamine content of human thrombocytes in rheumatoid arthritis and nonarthritic individuals. J. Clin. Invest. **38:**1059–1064.
10. SMITH, A. F. & W. CASTOR. 1978. Connective tissue activation. XII. Platelet abnormalities in patients with rheumatoid arthritis. J. Rheum. **5:**177–183.
11. MUSTARD, J. F., E. A. MURPHY, M. A. OGRYZLO & H. A. SMYTHE. 1963. Blood coagulation and platelet economy in subjects with primary gout. Can. Med. Assoc. J. **89:**1207–1211.
12. BLUHM, G. B. & J. M. RIDDLE. 1973. Platelets and vascular disease in gout. Semin. Arthritis Rheum. **2:**355–365.
13. NEWLAND, H. 1968. Antagonism of the antithrombotic effect of warfarin by uric acid. Am. J. Med. Sci. **256:**44–52.
14. WINOCOUR, P. D., M. R. TURNER, T. G. TAYLOR & K. A. MUNDAY. 1978. Platelet aggregation in rats in relation to hyperuricaemia induced by dietary single-cell protein and to protein deficiency. Thromb. Haemostas. **39:**346–359.
15. GINSBERG, M. H., F. KOZIN, M. O'MALLEY & D. J. McCARTY. 1977. Release of platelet constituents by monosodium urate crystals. J. Clin. Invest. **60:**999–1007.
16. GINSBERG, M. & F. KOZIN. 1978. Mechanisms of cellular interaction with monosodium urate crystals. Arthritis Rheum. **21:**896–903.
17. NORTON, W. L. & J. M. NARDO. 1970. Vascular disease in progressive systemic sclerosis (scleroderma). Ann. Intern. Med. **73:**317–324.
18. CAMPBELL, P. M. & E. C. LEROY. 1975. Pathogenesis of systemic sclerosis: A vascular hypothesis. Semin. Arthritis Rheum. **4:**351–368.
19. ANDERSON, L. G. & T. B. BAYLES. 1974. Polymyalgia rheumatica and giant cell arteritis. DM. Jan. :3–36.
20. WOOLF, N. 1978. Thrombosis and atherosclerosis. Brit. Med. Bull. **34:**137–142.

ULTRASTRUCTURE OF CIRCULATING AND PLATELET-FORMING MEGAKARYOCYTES: A COMBINED CORRELATIVE SEM-TEM AND SEM HISTOCHEMICAL STUDY

David B. Warheit * and Marion I. Barnhart

*Department of Physiology and
Bargman Foundation Laboratory
for Cell and Molecular Research
Wayne State University School of Medicine
Detroit, Michigan 48201*

INTRODUCTION

For the past two years, we have been investigating the role of the lung as a vascular filter and potential regulator of circulating platelet count. This area of investigation emerged after Aschoff discovered in 1893 that human capillaries contained megakaryocytes (MK).[1] Subsequently, in 1937, Howell and Donahue suggested that the lung might be an important site for the production and release of platelets.[2] Several investigators have since studied the problem, yet virtually all previous studies have presented interpretations regarding the fate of pulmonary megakaryocytes based on counts and light microscopic evaluations of the cells in pulmonary arterial versus venous blood, or anterograde versus retrograde perfusion specimens.[3-5] Thus, the data base has remained largely indirect and circumstantial.

Few reports have dealt with the implications of platelet-shedding pulmonary megakaryocytes, that is, platelet count differences in right and left heart blood. Villalobos *et al.* reported that arterial platelet counts exceeded venous counts when dogs were subjected to conditions of hypothermia.[6] These alterations were attributed to the sequestration of platelets in the portal circulation. Sharnoff and Scardino demonstrated that platelet count differences in the blood of right and left ventricles in rabbits occurred only in animals studied during winter months.[7] Ebbe has suggested that the pulmonary circulation may function as a source of platelets under normal conditions or as a reservoir for platelets in response to stress.[8] We decided to study platelet count differences in normal animals prior to and after a minor thrombin stress. Earlier studies had shown that small doses of thrombin stimulated the egress of megakaryocytes from the bone marrow into the venous circulation, and also reduced the percentage of adult megakaryocytes in bone marrow.[9-11] It was similarly reasoned that thrombin might augment the purported arterial/venous platelet count difference, perhaps as a result of an increased number of megakaryocytes in the circulation.

We have studied the ultrastructure of circulating and pulmonary megakaryocytes, utilizing both scanning electron microscopy (SEM) and transmission electron microscopy (TEM) independently and, more recently, using

* Present address: Laboratory of Pulmonary Function and Toxicology, National Institute of Environmental Health Sciences, Research Triangle Park, North Carolina 27709.

30

correlative SEM-TEM on identical tissues.[10, 11] Attempts to find and identify megakaryocytes through an overview with SEM alone, however, have not been as rewarding as we had hoped. The present study was undertaken to describe the ultrastructural detail and life cycle of megakaryocytes found in circulating blood and lung microvasculature. SEM and TEM correlations are made on identical cells for positive identification of pulmonary megakaryocytes. After confirmation, their surface and internal structural physiology can be examined, and the impact of megakaryocytes on adjacent lung structures can be determined.

One alternative to correlative electron microscopy has surfaced with the advent of scanning electron microscopic cytochemistry and the development of the backscatter detector. Development of this technology by Abraham and DeNee has facilitated the direct correlation in the scanning electron microscope between natural surface topography as viewed in the secondary electron (SE) image, and the underlying histology and cytochemistry as revealed by atomic number contrast in the backscatter electron (BSE) image.[12-14] As a result, certain internal features can be identified and correlated with surface area characteristics of the cell. In our case, it appeared that evaluations based upon SEM-cytochemical preparations of megakaryocytes might be ideal because megakaryocytes have large multilobular nuclei, which presumably would be easily identifiable when stained appropriately and could then be correlated with other megakaryocyte-distinguishing surface features. Hence, we utilized the Becker and Sogard modification[15] of Gomori's methenamine silver stain[16] to permit specific staining of nuclei and other tissue components of cells in both the bone marrow and circulating blood.

This report presents the data gained in studies on 15 dogs with each serving as its own control. As in our earlier work, thrombin was infused to augment the number of megakaryocytes traveling from the bone marrow to the lung.

Materials and Methods

The basic experimental procedure has been described previously.[10] Fifteen normal dogs were anesthetized with 50 mg/kg of Nembutal® (sodium pentobarbital), intubated and ventilated with a Harvard animal respirator. The thorax was opened along the midline and the right apical and cardiac lobes were isolated by placing sutures around the corresponding bronchus, pulmonary artery, and pulmonary vein of each lobe. The control cardiac lobe was ligated and removed prior to the thrombin infusion. Purified bovine thrombin (courtesy of Drs. Seegers, McCoy, and Walz) was then infused at a dose of 100 Iowa U/kg body weight via the femoral vein, over a period of 50 minutes. Arterial and venous blood samples were collected from catheters placed in the aorta and right atrium, respectively, at the following intervals: (1) control; (2) post thoracotomy; (3) immediately after thrombin infusion; (4) 40 to 45 minutes post thrombin; and (5) 2 hours post thrombin. Corresponding arterial and venous platelet counts were made by the methods of Brecher and Cronkite.[17] The second and experimental apical lobe was then ligated 30 to 40 minutes following completion of the thrombin infusion.

Immediately after removal, each isolated lobe of the lung was perfused at physiologic pressures via the pulmonary artery with phosphate-buffered saline solution (PBS, pH = 7.40) followed by 0.06 M cacodylate-buffered 1 percent glutaraldehyde (300 mOsm, pH = 7.2–7.4). The airway and epithelial linings of the pulmonary lobe were similarly exposed to buffered glutaraldehyde (GAH) by instilling the fixative fluid at a constant pressure of 20 cm H_2O above the lobe's hilum. The fixative-filled lobe was kept immersed in fixative for several hours. Then each lobe was cut into 1 cm³ pieces and immersed in buffered 1 percent GAH for 24 hours.

Scanning Electron Microscopy

After completion of fixation by immersion in 1 percent GAH, SEM specimens were cleared in a cacodylate-buffered sucrose solution and then placed through a series of graded dehydration steps in ethanol. Conventional SEM samples were then critical-point-dried using Freon 13. Most specimens were subjected to an ethanol-infiltrated cryofracture technique using liquid nitrogen,[18] and were similarly critical-point-dried. All samples were then placed on stubs, gold-sputtered, silver-plated, and placed in an ETEC-Autoscan® electron microscope for study and photography.

Correlative Transmission Electron Microscopy

Selected cryofractured specimens were mapped by means of SEM micrographs concomitantly with evaluations made from a dissecting microscope. The samples were then infiltrated through a series of graded propylene oxide-Maraglas steps and embedded in Maraglas. The block was trimmed, previously mapped locations were again identified, and ultrathin sections were then cut with a diamond knife. These were doubly stained with uranyl acetate and lead citrate and examined in an RCA-EMU-4 microscope operated at 50 kV.

Light Microscopy

The megakaryocyte count was performed by means of a saponin-hemolysis leukocyte concentration technique. The erythrocytes in the citrated whole blood were hemolyzed according to the method of Kaufman et al.,[3] using a polyvinyl pyrrolidone-formalin-saponin solution. Additional formalin (4 percent) was added following hemolysis. After fixation, the cells were centrifuged at 1100 rpm for 20 minutes and the supernatant decanted. The precipitate was dispersed in PBS and filtered through Millipore® filters (pore diameter 0.45 μm). The retained cells were stained with Harris's hematoxylin and eosin prior to counting.

SEM Histochemistry of Bone Marrow and Blood Megakaryocytes

Whole citrated blood was subjected to a leukocyte concentration technique employing a metrozoate dextran density gradient. The cells retained by the gradient were washed twice with Dulbecco's PBS and fixed in a modified Graham-Karnovsky fixative.[19] The fixative fluid contained 2 percent paraformaldehyde and 0.5 percent glutaraldehyde together in 0.1 M sodium cacodylate buffer (pH = 7.2–7.4) with 0.25 percent $CaCl_2$ added. Blood cell leukoconcentrates and heparinized bone marrow cells were fixed in suspension for 30 minutes, washed several times in Dulbecco's PBS, and placed in a 0.2 M sucrose-cacodylate buffer solution for 24 to 36 hours. Subsequently, the cells were stained for the silver methenamine reaction, according to the methods of Becker and Sogard.[15] The cells were incubated briefly in a methenamine silver solution (GMS [Gomori's methenamine silver]) consisting of 20 ml GMS stock (5 ml of 5 percent nitrate added dropwise to 100 ml of 3 percent hexamethylene tetramin) combined with 20 ml of distilled water and 1.6 ml of 5 percent sodium borate (pH of solution = 8.8–9.0). After initial infiltration, the suspended cells were placed in a water bath (50° C) and stained twice for a period of 45 to 60 minutes each. Following the second staining, the cells were rinsed free with distilled water, cytocentrifuged onto Formvar or plastic coverslips, freeze-dried, glued onto stubs, carbon-coated, and placed in an ETEC-Autoscan electron microscope equipped with an ETEC backscatter detector (3-chip) for study and photography.

RESULTS

Data Obtained from Blood Perfusates

Arterial platelet counts were consistently higher than their venous counterparts. The data on mean corresponding arterial-venous platelet counts can be seen in TABLE 1. Platelet counts were diminished after thrombin administration

TABLE 1

CORRESPONDING MEAN ARTERIAL AND VENOUS PLATELET COUNTS PER μL
WHOLE BLOOD

	Arterial Blood	Venous Blood
n=6		
Control	252,541	219,125
Post thoracotomy	250,541	213,083
Immediately after thrombin infusion	199,375	181,625
40 minutes post thrombin	189,964	172,178
2 hours post thrombin	215,000	180,400

and had not recovered to control values after 2 hours. The ratio of corresponding arterial/venous platelet counts is shown in FIGURE 1a. Control ratio values were augmented following the thrombin infusion, but diminished shortly thereafter. There was little difference between corresponding arterial and venous hematocrit values.

The data on circulating blood megakaryocyte counts from three dogs are shown in FIGURE 16. Circulating megakaryocyte venous counts rose from an average of 7.3 MK/ml to 12.83 MK/ml following thrombin infusion. Mean arterial counts similarly increased from 2.3 MK/ml to 3.8 MK/ml.[11] Therefore, some evidence was gained that increased numbers of megakaryocytes appeared in the venous circulation following the thrombin infusion.

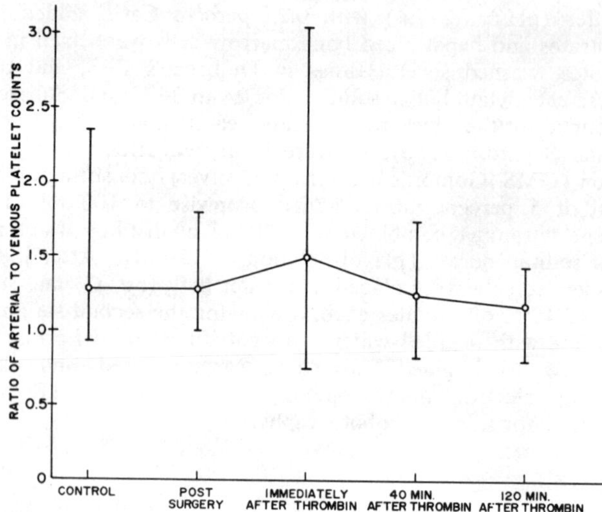

FIGURE 1a. The mean ratio of corresponding arterial to venous platelet counts is plotted as a function of time. Although these ratios are consistently greater than 1.0, there is some variation between counts from dog to dog.

Ultrastructure

Scanning electron microscopy of favorably cryofractured lung tissue revealed mature megakaryocytes, lodged in a vessel and seemingly ready to shed platelets to the circulation (FIGS. 2 and 3). The extensive canalicular system and demarcation membrane system characteristic of mature megakaryocytes is clearly evident. Transmission electron microscopy correlates on the same cell confirmed this description. A large nucleus is discerned, while megakaryocyte cytoplasmic fragmentation appears imminent (FIG. 4).[11]

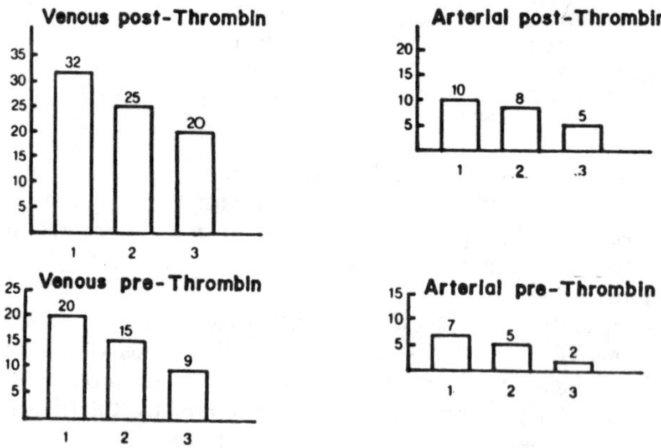

FIGURE 1b. Circulating megakaryocyte counts.

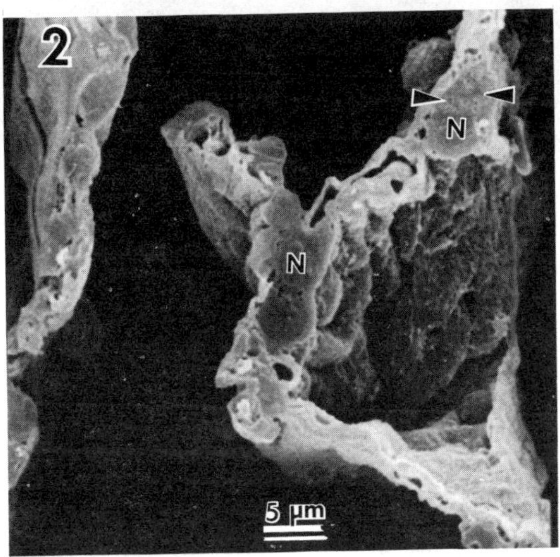

FIGURE 2. Two megakaryocytes are lodged in a cryofractured capillary prior to thrombin infusion. The megakaryocyte nuclei are exposed (N) and a platelet field can be observed (*arrowheads*).

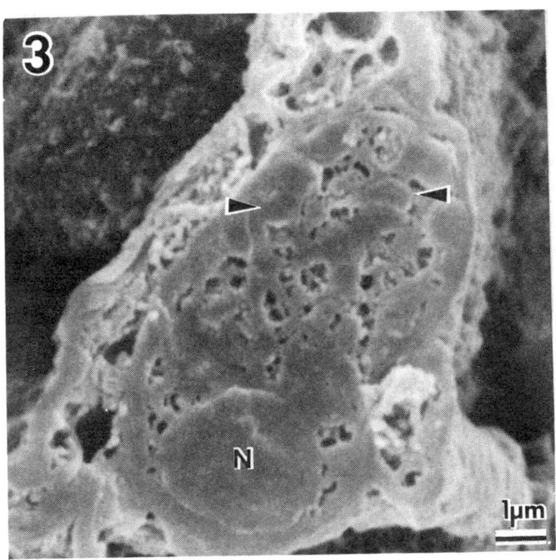

FIGURE 3. Enlargement of a megakaryocyte from FIGURE 2. The exposed nucleus (N) and platelet partitioning (*arrowheads*) are clearly evident.

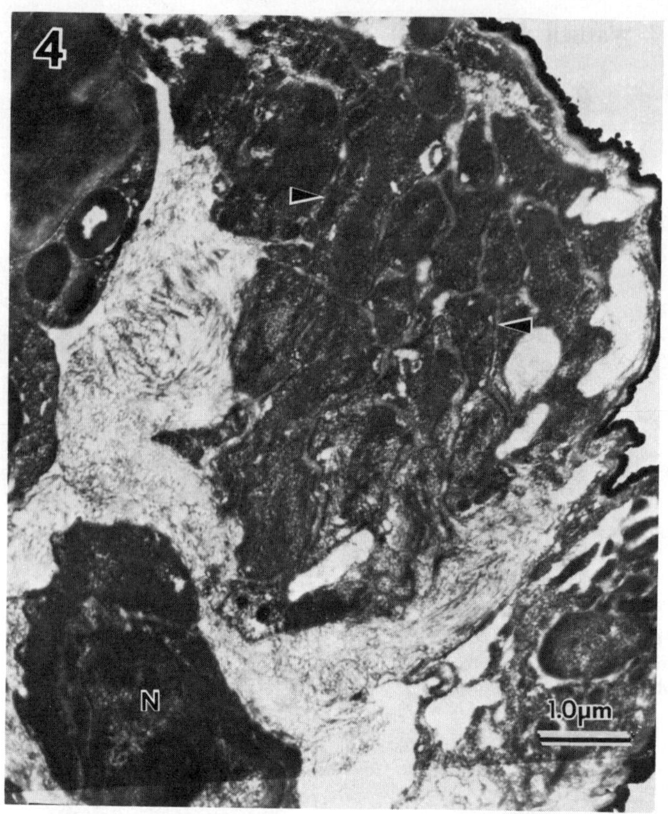

FIGURE 4. A TEM correlation of the megakaryocyte in FIGURE 3. The nucleus (N) and platelet field (*arrowheads*) are confirmed by the ultrathin sections.

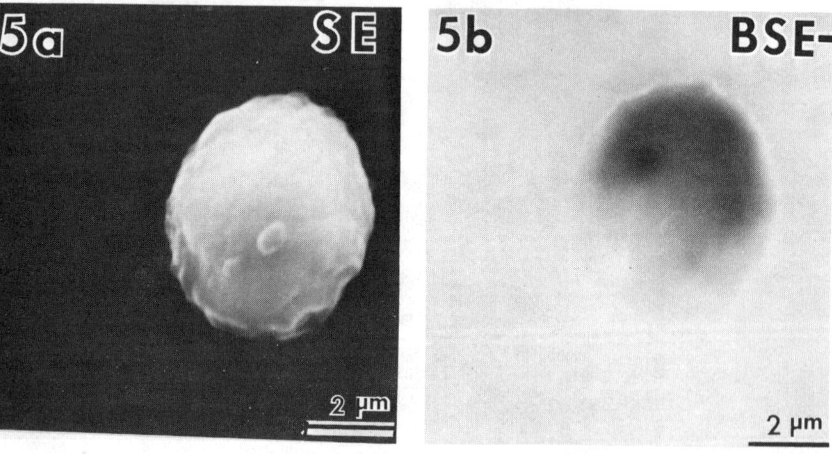

FIGURE 5 a and b. Scanning electron micrographs of a circulating leukocyte prepared for the silver methenamine stain. (a) Surface area in the secondary electron (SE) image. (b) Selective uptake of the silver stain in the backscattered electron reverse polarity image (BSE—).

Light microscopic examination of silver-stained bone marrow and blood cells confirmed the efficacy of the staining procedure. The nuclei of virtually all cells exhibited a dark brown-black staining. Similarly, a leukocyte preparation was utilized to gauge the detectability of the silver stain in the SEM. A secondary electron (SE) image of a blood leukocyte is shown in FIGURE 5a. The corresponding backscattered electron image (FIG. 5b), in which the polarity of the signal was reversed (BSE-), demonstrates the selective uptake of the

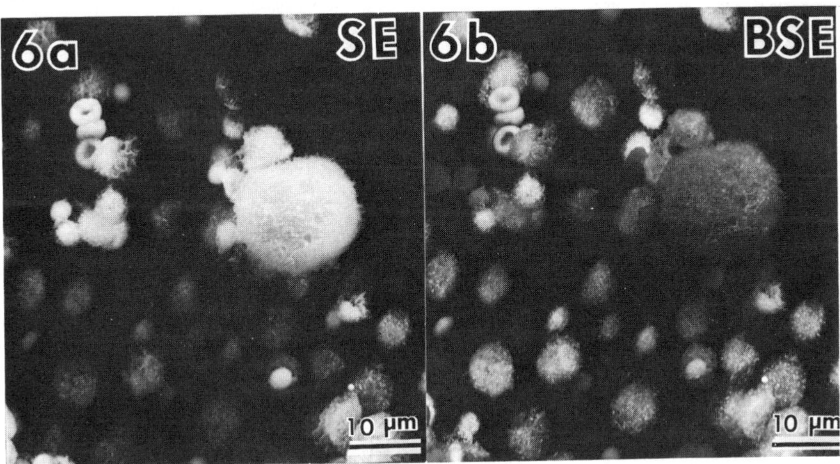

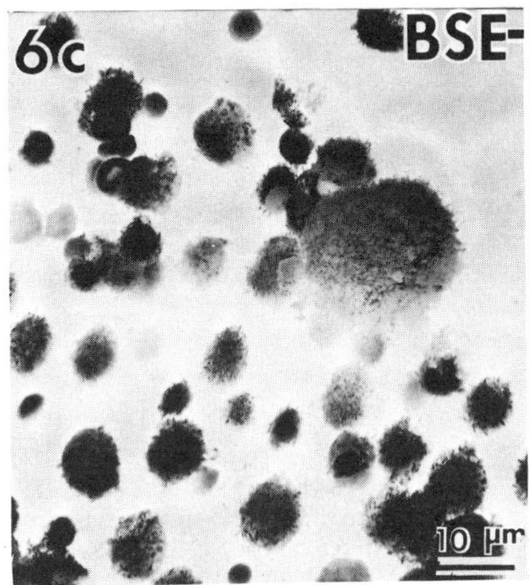

FIGURE 6 a, b, and c. Scanning electron micrograph of a bone marrow megakaryocyte shown in the secondary and backscattered (b and c) electron images. Note the diffuse staining pattern of silver in these cells, in contrast to that of other cells, which display a more discrete uptake of the stain.

silver methenamine stain. The discrete black stain most likely identifies the nucleus, while the diffuse pattern may result from nucleic acids contained within the cytoplasm.

Bone marrow megakaryocytes were easily recognized by virtue of their large size and other distinguishing surface features, including ridges and protrusions and numerous villous formations (FIG. 6a). The brightly stained nuclei of bone marrow cells are evident in the backscattered (BSE) and BSE— images (FIGS. 6b and 6c). The bone marrow megakaryocytes, however, appeared to have

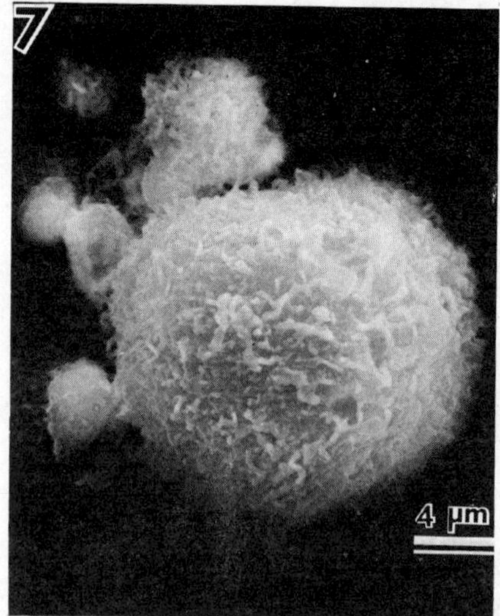

FIGURE 7. An enlargement of mega-karyocyte in FIGURE 6. Note the presence of curly and twisted villous projections extending from the surface of the megakaryocyte.

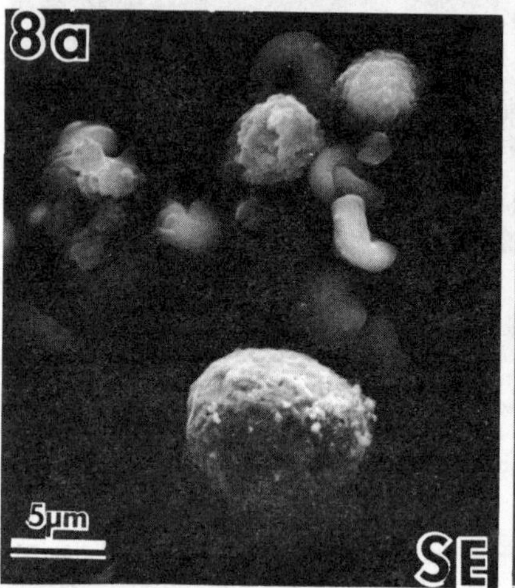

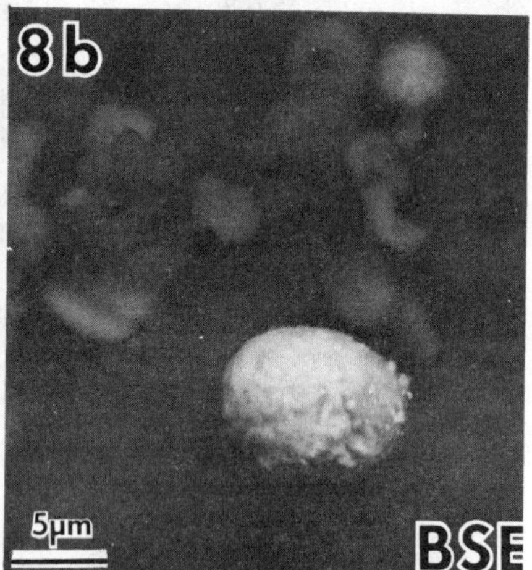

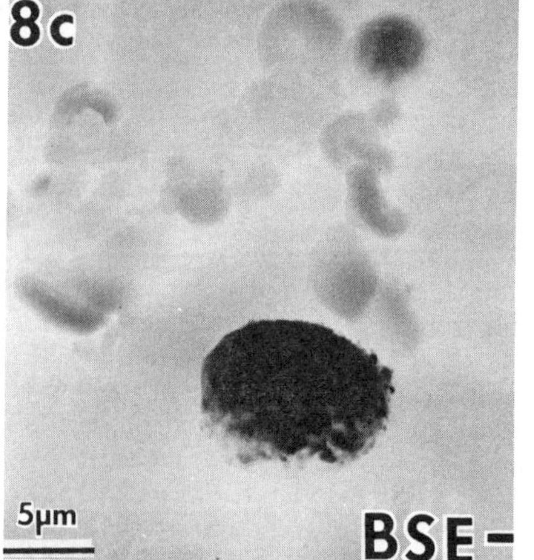

FIGURE 8 a, b, and c. Scanning electron micrograph of a circulating arterial megakaryocyte in the secondary (a) and backscattered (b and c) electron modes. The "naked nucleus" can be identified by its discrete and enlarged staining characteristics. Note that the entire cell appears to be one large nucleus.

little demonstrable uptake of the methenamine stain, when viewed in the backscattered mode, relative to other cells. An enlargement of the preceding figure illustrates the presence of curly and twisted villous projections extending from the surface of the megakaryocytes (FIG. 7); these characteristics correspond well to the surface features of human bone marrow megakaryocytes reported by Djaldetti et al.[20]

Megakaryocytes collected from the aorta were often devoid of cytoplasm and had a barren appearance. Only slight protrusions were noted on the surface of these cells (FIG. 8a). Evaluations made in the backscatter modes facilitated the identification of these cells as "naked nuclei" (FIGS. 8b and c).

DISCUSSION

The results obtained from corresponding arterial/venous platelet counts before and after thrombin administration suggest that platelets are being shed into the circulation from the lung vasculature. Because of the great variation in platelet counts among dogs, these results are not statistically significant, but still give a good indication of platelet count differences in the arterial and venous circulations. The corresponding arterial-venous hematocrits were virtually identical, signifying that little fluid was lost from the circulation after passage through the lungs.

The results obtained on quantitative analysis of circulating megakaryocytes are in close agreement with findings of similar recent studies. Pedersen reported an average of 12 MK/ml of vena caval blood from healthy human donors; arterial counts decreased to 4 MK/ml.[21] These results, together with our own data, convince us that the infusion of thrombin is an effective method for stimulating the movement of megakaryocytes from the bone marrow hematopoietic tissue into the venous circulation, and may provide a good model for the study of megakaryocytes in the lung, although time periods for study may be improved.

In our earlier study,[10] attempts to find and identify megakaryocytes in the lung using SEM were not as rewarding as we had hoped. Absolute identification of in situ megakaryocytes in the lung required SEM-TEM correlations on the same cells. One unfortunate byproduct of this technique centered on the beam damage to the tissue that resulted from the operation of the scanning electron microscope at 20 kV. As a result, TEM thin sections of previously "cooked" SEM samples often appeared dark and somewhat blurred. Although the quality of the transmission micrographs suffered, absolute confirmation of megakaryocytes was made possible.

The evaluations obtained from our SEM-histochemical data confirm the assertion that some megakaryocytes that are devoid of cytoplasm ultimately pass through the lung vasculature into the arterial circulation. Only naked nuclei, as detected by the silver stain, were observed in aortic blood. These results support the view that circulating megakaryocytes shed their platelets after impaction into the alveolar capillaries. It is interesting to note that bone marrow and circulating venous megakaryocytes did not display positive discrete staining characteristics when compared with other nucleated cells. We attribute this phenomenon to our inability to detect the silver stain adequately through the abundant cytoplasm characteristic of platelet-containing megakaryocytes. It is hoped that our capacity to detect backscattered electrons from circulating venous megakaryocytes will be augmented after installation of a more sensitive annular type of backscatter detector.

We have ascertained that platelet-forming megakaryocytes exit from the bone marrow and subsequently become trapped in the pulmonary microvasculature. Our morphologic data strongly suggest that platelets are shed from *in situ* pulmonary megakaryocytes. We believe that this may account, in part, for the higher platelet concentrations that we have shown in central arterial blood relative to central venous blood. We are currently working on TEM enzyme histochemical techniques in an attempt to confirm and extend our work in describing the life cycle of pulmonary megakaryocytes.

ACKNOWLEDGMENTS

The expert technical assistance of Dr. Steve Salley, Rick Kraemer, and Steve Barmatoski was of great value in this project.

REFERENCES

1. ASCHOFF, L. 1893. Veber capillare embolie von riesenkerahaltigen zellen. Arch. Path. Anat. Phys. **134:**11–26.
2. HOWELL, W. H. & D. D. DONAHUE. 1937. The production of blood platelets in the lungs. J. Exp. Med. **65:**177–203.
3. KAUFMAN, R. M., R. AIRO, S. POLLACK & W. H. CROSBY. 1965. Circulating megakaryocytes and platelet release in the lung. Blood **26:**720–731.
4. TINGGAARD PEDERSEN, N. 1974. The pulmonary vessels as a filter for circulating megakaryocytes in rats. Scand. J. Haemat. **13:**225–231.
5. CROSBY, W. H. 1976. Normal platelet numbers—pulmonary-platelet interactions. Ser. Haemat. **8:**89–97.
6. VILLALOBOS, T. J., E. ADELSON, P. A. RILEY, JR. & W. H. CROSBY. 1958. A cause of the thrombocytopenia and leukopenia that occurs in dogs during deep hypothermia. J. Clin. Invest. **37:**1–7.
7. SHARNOFF, J. G. & V. SCARDINO. 1960. Platelet-count differences in blood of the rabbit right and left heart ventricles. Nature **187:**334–335.
8. EBBE, S. 1976. Biology of megakaryocytes. Prog. Hemostasis Thromb. **III:** 211–299.
9. WALSH, R. T. 1968. A study of platelet kinetics in the normal and splenectomized dog. Ph.D. thesis, Wayne State University.
10. WARHEIT, D. B. & M. I. BARNHART. 1979. Megakaryocytes in the lung after thrombin initiated diffuse microthrombosis: A preliminary report on ultrastructure. Scanning Electron Microsc. **III:**801–808.
11. WARHEIT, D. B. & M. I. BARNHART. 1980. Circulating megakaryocytes and the microvasculature of the lung. Scanning Electron Microsc. **III:**255–262.
12. ABRAHAM, J. L. & P. B. DENEE. 1974. Biomedical applications of backscattered electron imaging. One year's experience with SEM histochemistry. Scanning Electron Micros. **I:**251–258.
13. DENEE, P. B., J. L. ABRAHAM & P. A. WILLARD. 1974. Histochemical stains for the SEM: Qualitative and semi-quantitative aspects of specific silver stains. Scanning Electron Micros. **I:**259–266.
14. DENEE, P. B. & J. L. ABRARAM. 1976. Backscattered electron imaging (application of atomic number contrast). *In* Principles and Techniques of Scanning Electron Microscopy: Biological Applications. M. A. Hayat, Ed. Vol. **5:** 144–180.
15. BECKER, R. P. & M. SOGARD. 1979. Visualization of subsurface structures in

cells and tissues by backscattered electron imaging. Scanning Electron Micros. **II**:835–870.

16. GOMORI, G. 1946. A new histochemical test for glycogen and mucin. Am. J. Clin. Pathol. **16**:177–179.

17. BRECHER, G. & E. P. CRONKITE. 1950. Morphology and enumeration of human blood platelets. J. Appl. Physiol. **3**:365–377.

18. HUMPHREYS, W. J., B. O. SPURLOCK & J. S. JOHNSON. 1974. Critical point drying of ethanol-infiltrated cryofractured biological specimens for scanning electron microscopy. Scanning Electron Micros. **I**:275–282.

19. GRAHAM, R. C., JR. & M. J. KARNOVSKY. 1966. The early stages of absorption of injected horseradish peroxidase in the proximal tubules of mouse kidney: Ultrastructural cytochemistry by a new technique. J. Histochem. Cytochem. **14**:291–302.

20. DJALDETTI, M., P. FISHMAN, H. BESSLER & I. NOTTI. 1979. SEM observations on the mechanism of platelet release from megakaryocytes. Thromb. Haemostas. (Stuttgart) **42**:611–620.

21. TINGGAARD PEDERSEN, N. 1978. Occurrence of megakaryocytes in various vessels and their retention in the pulmonary capillaries in man. Scand. J. Haematol. **21**:369–375.

THE INTERACTION OF PLATELETS WITH CULTURED CELLS

Robert I. Handin,* Kathleen D. Curwen, and
Michael A. Gimbrone, Jr.†

*Hemostasis Unit, and Vascular Pathophysiology Laboratory
Brigham and Women's Hospital, and
The Departments of Medicine and Pathology
Harvard Medical School
Boston, Massachusetts 02115*

INTRODUCTION

It is widely recognized that very few platelets adhere to the normal endothelial lining of blood vessels *in vivo*, although the factors that limit adhesion have not been well defined.[1] In contrast, platelets adhere to the subendothelial connective tissue exposed by vascular injury. This reaction is important in the initiation of normal hemostasis as well as in the pathogenesis of thrombosis and vascular disease. The generation of thromboxane A_2 by adherent platelets, coupled with the release of ADP (adenosine diphosphate), recruit additional platelets to form a hemostatic plug on the adherent platelet monolayer.[2] Platelets also release specific proteins and lysosomal enzymes that can modify constituents in the vessel wall. One protein, a platelet-derived growth factor, induces cultured smooth muscle cells to replicate and may enter the wall to modulate both normal vascular repair and early events in atherosclerosis.[3]

Various explanations have been proposed for the nonreactivity of platelets with normal endothelium. First, the luminal surface of endothelial cells does not contain the connective tissue elements that are present in the subendothelium. Secondly, vascular endothelium can degrade substances that may promote aggregation, such as ADP and biogenic amines, and may also secrete substances that directly inhibit platelet-platelet interactions like prostacyclin (PGI_2). This unique cyclic prostaglandin is a potent inhibitor of platelet aggregation and secretion *in vitro* and may also inhibit microthrombus formation *in vivo*.[4] In very high doses, PGI_2 may also block the adhesion of platelets to exposed vascular subendothelium.[5] However, the role of endogenous PGI_2 production in preventing platelet adhesion to normal endothelium remains unclear.

We have developed methods to quantify platelet adhesion to cultured cells and have initiated a study of the biochemical and cell-surface characteristics that modify platelet adhesion to cultured cells.[6] Using this model system, we have observed differences in platelet adhesion to primary cultures of human endothelial cells (HEC), which retain differentiated properties in culture, when compared to virally transformed endothelial cells (SVHEC), which have altered

* Recipient of a National Institute of Health Research Career Development Award.
† Established Investigator of the American Heart Association.

biochemistry and structure. In addition, we have also examined adhesion of platelets to a continuously passaged line of BALB/c 3T3 cells.

MATERIALS AND METHODS

Endothelial Cell Cultures

Human endothelial cells were isolated from umbilical cord veins and cultured as previously described.[7] A line of SVHEC was obtained by transvection of SV 40 DNA.[8] All cells used for the adhesion studies were replicate-plated on 15-mm round Thermonox coverslips in the bottom of 16-mm plastic culture wells (Cluster-24, Costar Plastics, Cambridge, MA). The cells were washed once in a calcium, magnesium-free Hanks balanced salt solution (Microbiological Associates, Bethesda, MD) and the culture media exchanged every two days and then again, approximately one hour prior to the adhesion studies. The HEC reached confluency after 3 to 6 days in culture while the SVHEC and 3T3 cells were confluent after 2 to 4 days. Cultures of SVHEC used in these studies were between the 10th and 20th passage level and the primary cultures were obtained from a pool of two to six umbilical cords. The BALB/c 3T3 (A31 clone) cells were obtained from the American Tissue Culture Collection, Rockville, MD.

Isolation and Labeling of Platelets

Blood was obtained from normal donors, anticoagulated with 0.38% sodium citrate and platelet-rich plasma prepared by centrifugation at $200 \times g$ for 10 min. The platelets were then labeled by incubation with 15 microcuries/ml of [^{3}H]adenine (15–30 Ci/mmol, New England Nuclear, Boston, MA) for 30 min at 37° C. This procedure resulted in incorporation of 70% of the isotope into ATP (adenosine triphosphate) and ADP in the platelet metabolic nucleotide pool. Uptake of unincorporated radioactive adenine by the cultured cells was prevented by including a 100-fold excess of nonradioactive adenine in all incubations, which did not alter platelet adhesion or aggregation.[6]

Platelet Adhesion Assays

Culture wells containing coverslips immersed in either PRP (platelet-rich plasma) or PPP (platelet-poor plasma) were incubated for 30 min at 37° C in a humidified 5% CO_2-air atmosphere. Coverslips that had been pre-incubated with serum-containing tissue culture media were processed in parallel to measure "nonspecific" attachment. The serum and cell-coated coverslips were rinsed free of culture media and platelets and the remaining endothelial cells and adherent platelets were processed for scanning and transmission electron microscopy and liquid scintillation counting as previously described.[6] The radioimmunoassay for released platelet factor four (PF-4) was carried out using previously published techniques.[9]

RESULTS

As shown in FIGURE 1A, when platelet-rich plasma is incubated for 30 min at 37° C with a confluent monolayer of HEC and then rinsed thoroughly, very few platelets remain adherent to the culture monolayer with an average of one adherent platelet noted for each endothelial cell. For comparison, TABLE 1 shows the cell-associated radioactivity and the estimated number of adherent platelets derived from the isotopic adhesion assay. Approximately the same number of adherent platelets are obtained with either method.

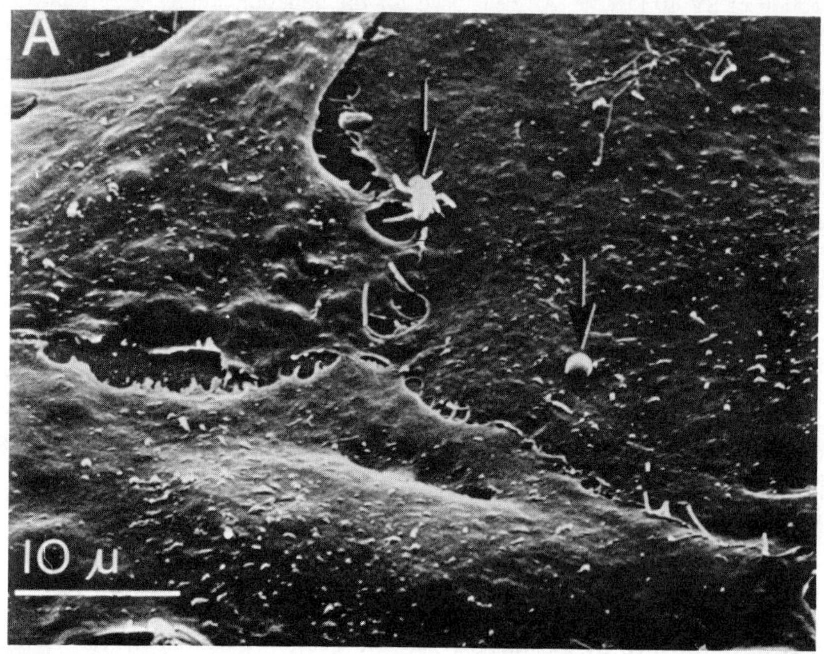

FIGURE 1. Scanning electron micrographs of cultures of primary human endothelial cells, HEC, (A), and virally transformed endothelial cells, SVHEC (B), following incubation with platelet-rich plasma for 30 min and a standardized wash procedure to remove nonadherent platelets.

Platelets (*arrows*) are rarely seen in contact with HEC, while numerous platelets are seen adherent to the surface and overlapping edges of each SVHEC. (Reproduced, by permission, from Curwen *et al.*[6])

FIGURE 1B shows a scanning electron micrograph of an SVHEC monolayer after incubation with platelet-rich plasma. Several differences are readily apparent. First, the surface characteristics of the SVHEC are strikingly different with the ruffled surface and prominent microvilli characteristic of transformed cells. Moreover, there are between 10 and 30 platelets adherent to each SVHEC when measured either by direct examination of the electron micrographs or by quantitation with the isotopic assay (TABLE 1). The adherent platelets are

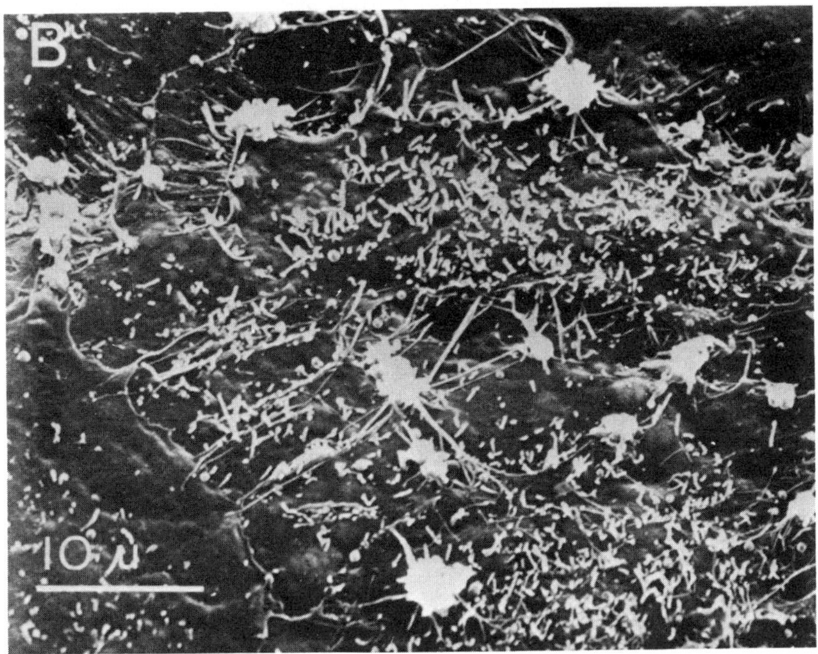

uniformly distributed over the cell surface and are single rather than clustered in microaggregates. Transmission electron micrographs (FIG. 2) demonstrate some platelet pseudopod formation as well as areas where there is distinct inderdigitation between platelet and endothelial cell membranes. However, the platelets do not appear to have degranulated.

There is a marked difference both in the number and the distribution of adherent platelets when BALB/C 3T3 cells are examined (FIG. 3). The platelets attached to the BALB/c 3T3 cells have formed microaggregates on the surface of the cells so that it is impossible to differentiate between adhesion and aggregation. It is not possible to evaluate the degree of secretion or degranulation from the scanning electron micrographs.

In order to define more precisely the events following adhesion, and to

TABLE 1

PLATELET ADHESION TO PRIMARY AND SV 40-TRANSFORMED
HUMAN ENDOTHELIAL CULTURES

Cell Type	cpm [³H] adenine 10⁴ cells *
HEC	228 ± 8
SVHEC	3993 ± 194

* Mean $\pm$ SE for four to six replicate-plated cover slips. Difference between means highly significant ($p < 0.001$). (Modified from Curwen *et al.*[6])

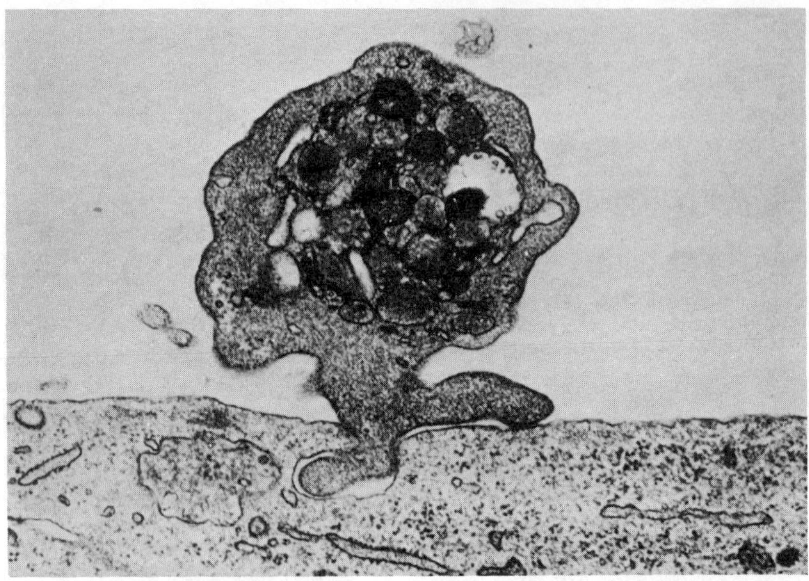

FIGURE 2. Transmission electron micrograph of a platelet adhering to the upper surface of a transformed endothelial cell. Platelet shape change has occurred; note interdigitation of platelet pseudopod with cell membrane.

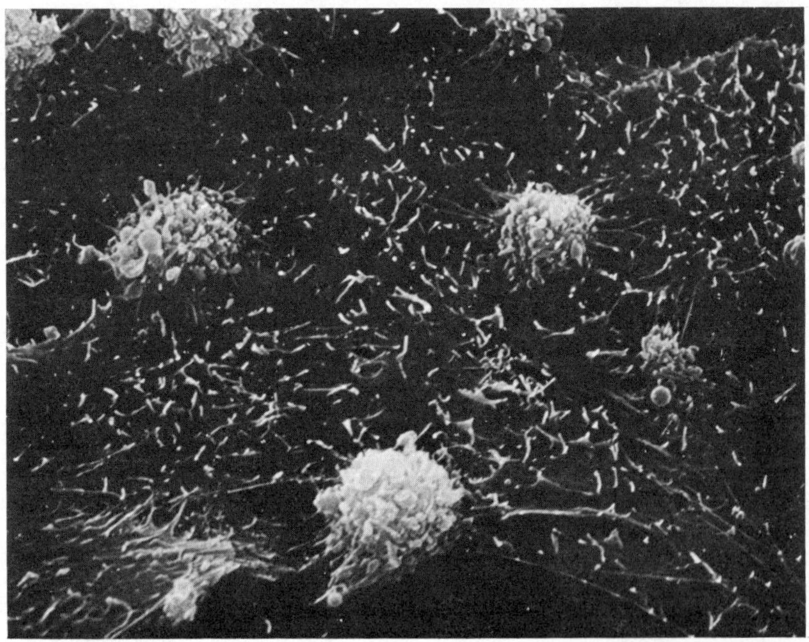

FIGURE 3. Scanning electron micrograph of a BALB/c 3T3 cell culture following a 30-min incubation with platelet-rich plasma. Note attachment of several large platelet aggregates (microthrombi) to the surface of the cultured cells.

quantify secretion induced by the 3T3 cells, a radioimmunoassay for PF-4, a secreted alpha granule protein, was employed in conjunction with the measurement of platelet adhesion to cultured cells. As shown in FIGURE 4, the concentration of PF-4 in platelet-free plasma following exposure of platelets to endothelial cell monolayers was usually quite low. Incubation with HEC (not shown) or SVHEC did not raise the plasma level of PF-4 despite the fact that there was an average 20-fold difference in adhesion between the two cell types. Incubation with smooth muscle cells derived from bovine aorta did raise plasma PF-4 slightly from 10 to 30 ng/ml. Only the 3T3 cells, which had aggregated platelets on their surface, induced release of large quantities of PF-4, with an increase to 100 ng/ml noted.

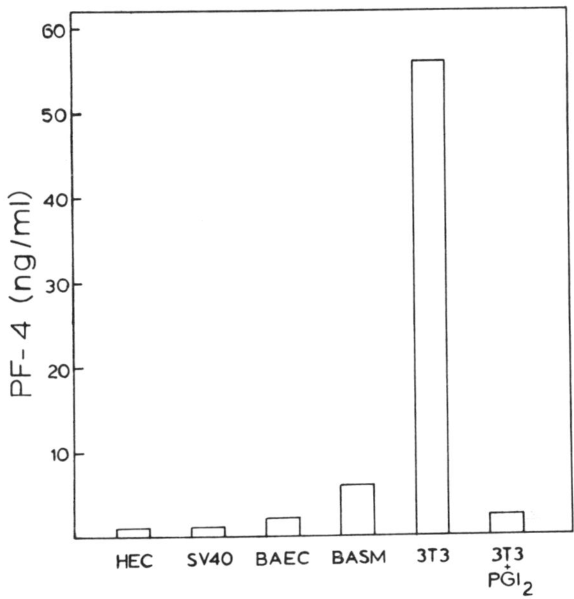

FIGURE 4. Plasma PF-4 levels after incubation of platelet-rich plasma with various cultured cells.
HEC = 1° human endothelial cells; SV40 = SV40 transformed human endothelial cells. BAEC = bovine aortic endothelial cells. BASM = bovine aortic smooth muscle cells. 3T3 = BALB/c 3T3 cells; 1 μM PGI$_2$ was added to PRP prior to incubation with 3T3 cells.

Secretion of PF-4 by platelets interacting with 3T3 cells was then studied in more detail. As shown in FIGURE 5, peak elevation occurred after 5 min of incubation and then progressively declined. PF-4 levels had returned to control levels after 15 min of incubation. This fall in plasma PF-4 is in keeping with other studies demonstrating that PF-4 can bind to cell surface glycosaminoglycans. For comparison, over the same time period, there was no change in plasma PF-4 when platelets were incubated with SVHEC.

The effect of prostacyclin (PGI$_2$) on platelet adhesion and secretion was then examined. As shown in FIGURE 6, the addition of 10^{-8} M PGI$_2$ to PRP

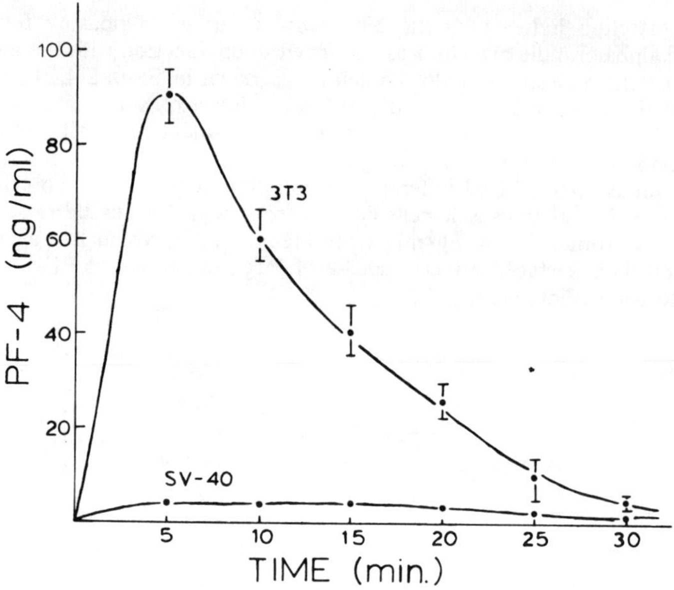

FIGURE 5. Time course of plasma PF-4 elevation after incubation of platelet-rich plasma with SV-40 transformed or BALB/c 3T3 cells. The mean $\pm$ SE for six experiments is depicted.

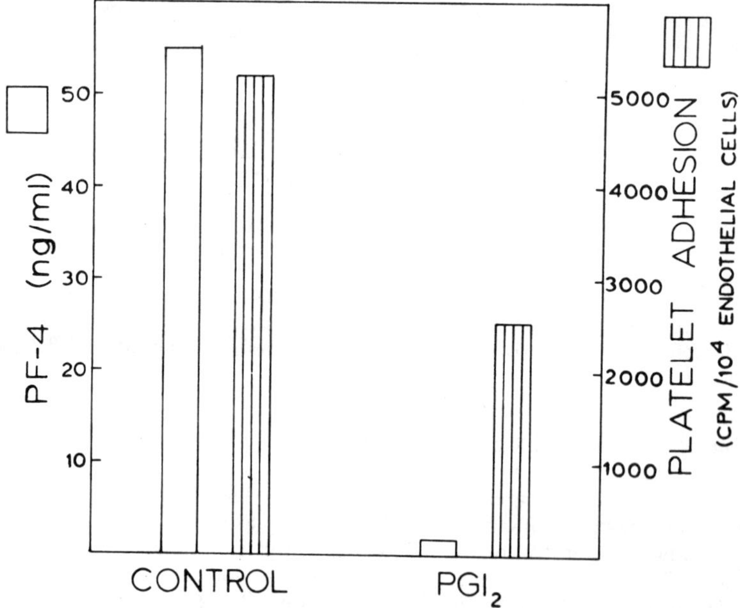

FIGURE 6. Platelet adhesion and release of PF-4 following incubation of platelet-rich plasma with 3T3 cells, 10 nM PGI$_2$ was added to the platelet-rich plasma prior to incubation with the cultured cells.

prior to incubation with 3T3 cells reduced PF-4 secretion at five minutes by 80%. In contrast, this concentration of PGI_2 only reduced adhesion by 45%.

DISCUSSION

The studies outlined here demonstrate that even the small numbers of platelets adhering to primary cultures of vascular endothelium can be quantified with a sensitive isotopic adhesion assay employing [³H]adenine to label the platelet's metabolically active nucleotide pool. The use of this assay, in conjunction with direct morphologic observation by scanning electron microscopy, permits us to analyze both the quantity and distribution of platelets adherent to various cultured cells.

Several important new observations have emerged. First, there is a marked difference in adhesion of platelets to transformed human endothelial cells as compared with primary endothelial cells. However, in either case, platelets adhere as single particles and do not secrete their granule contents following adhesion. Secondly, adhesion to a continuous cell line derived from the BALB/c mouse embryo is associated with microaggregate formation and secretion of large quantities of a platelet alpha granule protein into plasma. Incubation with smooth muscle cells derived from the bovine aorta also induced the secretion of small quantities of PF-4.

The availability of a cultured cell that induces both adhesion and secretion permits us to determine if pharmacologic inhibitors of platelet function can dissociate adhesion from secondary events like secretion of granule contents. The infusion of relatively low doses of a potent inhibitor like PGI_2 markedly reduced secretion but was not able to block the primary event—adhesion to the cell surface. These results are similar to those obtained after *ex vivo* perfusion of balloon de-endothelialized rabbit aorta.[10]

Several laboratories have noted that purified PF-4 adheres to cell surface glycosaminoglycans in a saturable, reversible, concentration-dependent fashion.[11, 12] These studies have been carried out with purified, radiolabeled protein in the absence of plasma. Our studies confirm and extend these studies by demonstrating that the native protein, as secreted from the platelet, rapidly disappears from plasma. On the basis of the previous studies, it seems most likely that released PF-4 is binding to the cultured cells.

The fact that secreted proteins like PF-4 may bind to cultured cells has important implications. For example, this may be the mechanism by which mitogens like the platelet-dependent growth factor enter target cells. Furthermore, other proteins secreted by platelets may regulate cellular metabolism. For example, PF-4 has been shown to inhibit the uptake of low density lipoproteins by cultured fibroblasts.[13] There is also a recent report that another platelet protein, β-thromboglobulin, may inhibit PG12 production by cultured endothelial cells.[14, 15]

We would like to suggest that quantitation of platelet adhesion, aggregation and secretion after incubation with cultured cells of vascular or nonvascular origin provides a useful way to study platelet-cell surface interactions. Future studies can now be carried out to define the cell surface characteristics that promote platelet adhesion. The fact that differences have already been noted between virally transformed and primary cultures of endothelial cells and between 3T3 and endothelial cells provides several useful models for future study.

REFERENCES

1. GIMBRONE, M. A. 1976. Culture of vascular endothelium. Prog. Hemostasis Thromb. **3:** 1–28.
2. MARCUS, A. J. 1978. The role of lipids in platelet function with particular reference to the arachidonic acid pathway. J. Lipid. Res. **19:** 793–812.
3. ROSS, R., J. B. GLUMSET. 1976. The pathogenesis of atherosclerosis. N. Engl. J. Med. **295:** 369–376.
4. MONCADA, S. & J. AMEZCVA. 1979. Prostacyclin, thromboxane A_2 interactions in haemostasis and thrombosis. Haemostasis **8:** 252–265.
5. WEISS, H. J. & V. T. TORITTO. 1979. Prostacyclin inhibits platelet adhesion and thrombus formation on subendothelium. Blood **53:** 244–248.
6. CURWEN, K. D., M. A. GIMBRONE & R. I. HANDIN. 1980. In vitro studies of thromboresistance. The role of prostacyclin (PGI_2) in platelet adhesion to cultured normal and virally transformed human vascular endothelial cells. Lab. Invest. **42:** 366–374.
7. GIMBRONE, M. A., R. S. COTRAN & J. FOLKMAN. 1974. Human vascular endothelial cells in culture. J. Cell. Biol. **60:** 673–680.
8. GIMBRONE, M. A., G. C. FAREED. 1976. Transformation of cultured human vascular endothelium by SV-40 DNA. Cell **9:** 685–691.
9. HANDIN, R. I., M. McDONOUGH & M. LESCH. 1978. Evaluation of platelet Factor 4 in acute myocardial infarction: Measurement by radioimmunoassay. J. Lab. Clin. Med. **91:** 340–344.
10. ADELMAN, B. A., M. STEMERMAN, D. MENNELL & R. I. HANDIN. The interaction of platelets with aortic subendothelium: Inhibition of adhesion and secretion by prostaglandin I_2. Blood. In press.
11. BUSCH, C., J. DAWES, D. S. PEPPER & A. WASTESON. 1980. Binding of platelet Factor 4 to cultured human umbilical vein endothelial cells. Thromb. Res. **19:** 129–134.
12. RYBAK, M. E., R. I. HANDIN & M. A. GIMBRONE. 1980. Platelet Factor 4 binding to vascular endothelial cells. Circulation **62:** III-335.
13. BROWN, M. S., T. F. DEUEL, S. K. BASU, J. L. GOLDSTEIN. 1978. Inhibition of binding of low density lipoprotein to its cell surface receptor in human fibroblasts by positively charged proteins. J. Supramol. Struct. **8:** 223–228.
14. HOPE, W., J. J. MARTIN, C. N. CHESTERMAN, F. J. MORLAN. 1979. Human β-thromboglobulin inhibits PGI_2 production and binds to a specific site in bovine aortic endothelial cells. Nature **282:** 210–212.

ACTIVE-SITE-DEPENDENT, THROMBIN-INDUCED RELEASE OF ADENINE NUCLEOTIDES FROM CULTURED HUMAN ENDOTHELIAL CELLS *

Pete Lollar and Whyte G. Owen

*The Cardiovascular Center and the
Departments of Internal Medicine, Pathology, and Biochemistry
University of Iowa College of Medicine
Iowa City, Iowa 52242*

INTRODUCTION

Thrombin binds to cultured human endothelial cells in a manner similar to that of protein ligand-receptor systems.[1] Binding is rapid, reversible, saturable, and high-affinity. In addition, this binding is active-site-independent, that is, diisopropylphosphoryl-thrombin (DIP-thrombin), which has its active site blocked, binds to endothelium in a manner indistinguishable from that of active thrombin. We have proposed that a function of these binding sites is to protect the circulation from thrombosis by clearing thrombin.[2] Such "receptor"-mediated clearance from circulation has been described for other proteins.[3-5]

Thrombin has a variety of effects on endothelium: mitogenesis,[6-8] inactivation of plasminogen activator,[9] synthesis and release of fibronectin,[10] and release of the prostaglandin prostacyclin, a potent inhibitor of platelet aggregation.[11, 12] Thus it is reasonable to ask whether the effects of thrombin in these phenomena are mediated through the high-affinity binding sites. Recently, Pearson and Gordon [13] showed that thrombin stimulates release of adenine nucleotides from cultured porcine endothelium. Therefore, we asked whether cultured human endothelium responds in a manner analogous to that of porcine endothelium and whether the response involves binding of thrombin to the high-affinity binding sites.

MATERIAL AND METHODS

Materials

Diisopropylfluorophosphate (DFP) (Aldrich Chemical Co., Milwaukee, WI) was diluted to 1 M in dry dimethylformamide before use. Na[^{125}I], 2×10^3 Ci/mmol, and [^{3}H]adenosine, 42 Ci/mmol, were obtained from The Amersham Corp. (Arlington Heights, IL). Unlabeled nucleosides and nucleotides were purchased from Sigma Chemical Co. (St. Louis, MO).

* This work was supported by Grants HL14230–08 and HL22471–02 from the National Heart, Lung and Blood Institute. Pete Lollar is supported by NIH Training Grant P-32-HL-07344–01, and Whyte Owen is a Career Development Awardee from the National Institutes of Health.

51

Endothelial Cell Cultures

Primary cultures of endothelial cells from the human umbilical vein were obtained from the laboratory of Dr. John Hoak and were prepared as described previously [1] as a modification of the method of Jaffe.[11]

Thrombin Preparation

Human thrombin was prepared as described.[14] The product was homogeneous by gel electrophoresis in sodium dodecyl sulfate. In some experiments, thrombin was inactivated at pH 7.5 with 1 mM DFP. Also, in some experiments thrombin was labeled with ^{125}I by the lactoperoxidase method of Thorell and Johansson,[15] as described previously,[1] except that iodination was carried out in chloride-free sodium acetate buffers. This resulted in a product with a clotting activity that was stable at 4° C for at least 1 month.

Assay for Release of Metabolites of [³H]adenosine by Endothelial Cells

Three- or 4-day-old endothelial cell cultures, consisting of confluent monolayers in 16-mm plastic wells, were washed three times with Hanks' balanced salt solution buffered with 15 mM HEPES, pH 7.4 plus 0.1 percent albumin (Buffer A). The cells were incubated with [³H]adenosine in Buffer A (10 μCi/well) and washed three times in Buffer A; then test substances or control solutions were applied in a total volume of 0.5 ml. At intervals, samples (100 μl) were taken and pipetted directly into a toluene-based aqueous scintillation fluid containing Triton X-100 (counting efficiency 33 percent).

Thin-Layer Chromatography

After maximal release of tritium was obtained, the endothelial cell supernatants were removed and samples (25 μl) and standards were analyzed by thin-layer chromatography (TLC) as described previously.[13] Samples were mixed with an unlabeled standard mixture, the strips were developed, and the spots cut out and counted. Also, cell monolayers were analyzed prior to addition of thrombin.

[¹²⁵I]Thrombin Binding to Endothelial Cells

Binding was carried out as described.[1] Binding analysis under these conditions yields a curvilinear Scatchard plot, with $K_D = 3$ nM and $R_0 = 48,000$ sites per cell for the high-affinity sites.

RESULTS

Uptake of [³H]Adenosine by Endothelium

After 1 hour of incubation at room temperature with [³H]adenosine, 50 percent of the radioactivity was cell-associated. When the cells were rinsed with Buffer A, there was less than 100 cpm remaining in the supernatant after the second rinse.

Thrombin-induced Release of Tritium from Endothelium

The addition of thrombin to [³H]adenosine-fed monolayers resulted in a release of tritiated material into the supernatant (FIG. 1). This release began to slow after 10 minutes, but continued for at least 30 minutes. Both the rate and amount of radioactivity released were dependent on the dose of thrombin and were saturable, reaching a maximum at 1 U.S. unit of thrombin per milliliter ($\simeq 10^{-8}$ M). The addition of buffer alone also caused a small release, possibly from mechanical stimulation of the cells by the addition of fluid. Activated factor X (10^{-7} M) did not stimulate release of tritium over control value.

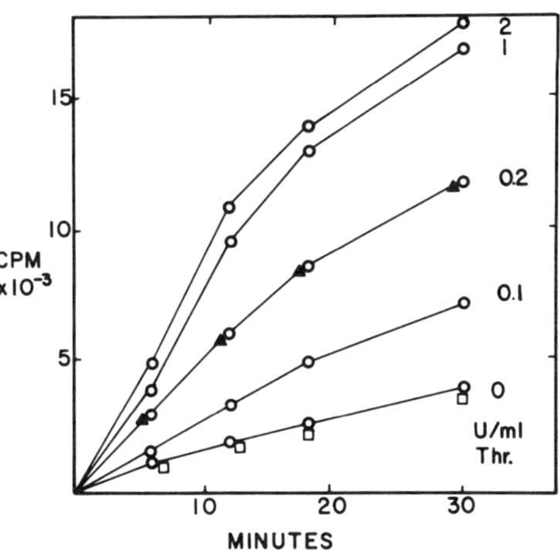

FIGURE 1. Thrombin-stimulated release of tritium by endothelium. Four-day-old endothelial monolayers in 16-mm wells, incubated with [³H]adenosine, were washed three times with Buffer A, and then 0.5-ml samples of varying concentrations of thrombin (Thr.) in Buffer A were added (*open circles*, thrombin concentrations as indicated). In other wells a final concentration of 5 μM DIP-thrombin (equivalent to 50 U/ml) was added along with the control (*open squares*) or with 0.2 U/ml active thrombin (*solid triangles*).

Effect of DIP-Thrombin on Release of [³H]arachidonate and Metabolites

To determine whether the high-affinity thrombin receptor on endothelium is involved in nucleotide metabolism, DIP-thrombin was used. This derivative has a diisopropylphosphoryl group covalently bonded to its active site serine with no other alterations in the structure of thrombin. It neither clots fibrinogen nor cleaves synthetic substrates, but has been shown to bind to endothelium in a manner indistinguishable from that of thrombin.[1] At a concentration of 5×10^{-7} M (equivalent to 50 units/ml), DIP-thrombin caused no release of tritium over control values (FIG. 1, open squares). This concentration is 500 times the amount of active thrombin needed to cause measurable release. However, the presence of 50 units/ml of DIP-thrombin had no effect on the release of tritium by 0.2 unit/ml of thrombin (FIG. 1, solid triangles), even though it caused 98 percent inhibition of the binding of 0.2 unit/ml of [¹²⁵I]thrombin to the high-affinity binding sites (data not shown). Likewise, lower concentrations of DIP-thrombin had no effect.

Analysis of Radiolabeled Products

Supernatants from cells stimulated maximally by thrombin were analyzed by thin-layer chromatography. Greater than 80 percent of the radioactivity had an R_f value corresponding to that of adenosine, when the supernatants were collected 30 minutes after the addition of thrombin. When the monolayers were analyzed before the addition of thrombin, greater than 90 percent of the radioactivity was associated with adenosine diphosphate (ADP) and adenosine triphosphate (ATP). These findings agree with those of Pearson and Gordon, who showed that thrombin induces release of nucleotides followed by extracellular degradation to adenosine.[13]

DISCUSSION

In this paper we have investigated the role of thrombin in nucleotide metabolism in cultured endothelial cells, and have used this system to determine whether the high-affinity thrombin binding sites play a role in adenine nucleotide release. The products released are similar to those described by Pearson and Gordon.[13] Blocking the high-affinity binding sites with DIP-thrombin did not affect thrombin-induced release of adenine nucleotides, which makes it unlikely that this binding is involved. It could be argued that DIP-thrombin blocked less than 100 percent of the binding sites and that occupancy of the remaining small number was responsible for the full effect. This "spare receptors" argument would not be consistent with the dose-response relationship shown in FIGURE 1, where doses of less than 1 U/ml of thrombin result in progressively less release of tritium, while inhibiting binding by 98 percent had no effect on release.

The dose-response to thrombin has a striking similarity to that reported by us for thrombin-stimulated release of arachidonate from endothelium[16] and by Hong and Levine for fibroblasts.[17] Likewise, both the arachidonate[16] and nucleotide systems respond independently of measurable binding of thrombin to high-affinity sites on the cells. On the other hand, tritium release from [³H]adenosine-fed cells continues for at least 30 minutes after stimulation with thrombin, in contrast to arachidonate release, which is complete in 5 minutes.[16] Thus, while it seems likely that the initial stimulus for both processes is the same, the subsequent pathways must diverge.

A high-affinity thrombin receptor has been proposed to be responsible for other effects of thrombin on cells, which include mitogenesis,[6-8] inactivation of plasminogen activator,[9] and release of fibronectin,[10] but cause-effect relationships have neither been demonstrated nor ruled out by experiments similar to those reported in this paper. We have proposed elsewhere that a function of the high-affinity binding of thrombin to endothelium is to clear thrombin from the circulation.[2]

Thus, the initial step on the pathway of thrombin stimulation of prostacyclin production and nucleotide release is not known. Since stimulation is active-site-dependent, proteolytic cleavage of a plasma membrane substrate may be involved. Another possibility is that there is an active-site-dependent receptor for thrombin that is distinct from the receptor that binds both DIP-thrombin and active thrombin. The model for an active-site-dependent receptor would differ from that for the membrane-associated proteolytic substrate in that cellular response would not involve proteolysis of the receptor. If the affinity of thrombin for this receptor were low or the number of receptors smaller than the active-site-independent binding sites, then binding of thrombin to the receptor would be difficult to distinguish from "nonspecific" binding seen in all receptor assay systems.

Regardless of mechanism, the interaction of thrombin with cell membranes is more complex than previously assumed. Caution should be exercised when ascribing cause and effect relationships to the interaction of thrombin with cell surfaces and biological response.

SUMMARY

The effect of thrombin on release of adenine nucleotides is studied in cultured cell monolayers from the human umbilical vein.

Thrombin-induced release of radioactivity from endothelial cells is dose-dependent and saturable with maximal response seen at 1×10^{-8} M thrombin. The products are identified by thin-layer chromatography as adenine nucleotides. Diisopropylphosphoryl thrombin, which is enzymatically inactive, does not cause release of tritium. A 50-fold excess of diisopropylphosphoryl-thrombin, despite causing 98 percent inhibition of binding of ^{125}I-thrombin to its high-affinity binding sites, does not inhibit thrombin-induced release. We conclude that (1) thrombin causes release from endothelial cells of adenine nucleotides and that (2) high-affinity, active-site-independent binding of thrombin is not involved in this process.

ACKNOWLEDGMENTS

We wish to thank Dr. John Hoak for providing the cultured endothelium, Glenna Fry and Connie Schroeder for their technical assistance, and Rhonda Demuth for typing the manuscript.

REFERENCES

1. AWBREY, B. J., J. C. HOAK & W. G. OWEN. 1979. Binding of human thrombin to cultured human endothelial cells. J. Biol. Chem. **254:**4092–4095.
2. LOLLAR, P. & W. G. OWEN. 1980. Clearance of thrombin from circulation in rabbits by high affinity binding sites on endothelium. J. Clin. Invest. **66:** 1222–1230.
3. VANLENTEN, L. & G. ASHWELL. 1971. Studies on the chemical and enzymatic modification of glycoproteins. J. Biol. Chem. **246:**1889–1894.
4. STAHL, P., P. H. SCHLESINGER, J. S. RODMAN & T. DOEBBER. 1976. Recognition of lysosomal glycosidases *in vivo* inhibited by modified glycoproteins. Nature **264:**86–88.
5. STAHL, P. D., J. S. RODMAN, M. J. MILLER & P. H. SCHLESINGER. 1978. Evidence for receptor-mediated binding of glycoproteins, Glycoconjugates, and lysosomal glycosidases by alveolar macrophages. Proc. Nat. Acad. Sci. USA **75:**1399–1403.
6. GOSPODAROWICZ, D., K. D. BROWN, C. R. BIRDWELL & B. R. ZETTER. 1978. Control of proliferation of human vascular endothelial cells. J. Cell. Biol. **77:** 774–788.

7. CARNEY, D. H., & D. D. CUNNINGHAM. 1978. Role of specific cell surface receptors in thrombin-stimulated cell division. Cell **15:**1341–1349.

8. BAKER, J. B., R. L. SIMMER, K. C. GLENN & D. D. CUNNINGHAM. 1979. Thrombin and epidermal growth factor become linked to cell surface receptors during mitogenic stimulation. Nature **278:**743–745.

9. LOSKUTOFF, D. J. 1979. Effect of thrombin on the fibrinolytic activity of cultured bovine endothelial cells. J. Clin. Invest. **64:**329–332.

10. MOSHER, D. F. & A. VAHERI. 1978. Thrombin stimulates the production and release of a major surface-associated glycoprotein (fibronectin) in cultures of human fibroblasts. Exp. Cell Res. **112:**323–334.

11. WEKSLER, B. B., C. W. LEY & E. A. JAFFE. 1978. Stimulation of endothelial cell prostacyclin production by thrombin, trypsin, and the ionophore A23187. J. Clin. Invest. **62:**923–930.

12. CZERVIONKE, R. L., J. B. SMITH, J. C. HOAK, G. L. FRY & D. L. HAYCRAFT. 1979. Use of a radioimmunoassay to study thrombin-induced release of PGI_2 from cultured endothelium. Thromb. Res. **14:**781–786.

13. PEARSON, J. D. & J. L. GORDON. 1979. Vascular endothelial and smooth muscle cells in culture selectively release adenine nucleotides. Nature **281:**384–386.

14. OWEN, W. G., C. T. ESMON & C. M. JACKSON. 1974. The conversion of prothrombin to thrombin. J. Biol. Chem. **249:**594–605.

15. THORELL, J. I. & B. G. JOHANSSON. 1971. Enzymatic iodination of polypeptides with ^{125}I to high specific activity. Biochim. Biophys. Acta **251:**363–369.

16. LOLLAR, P. & W. G. OWEN. 1980. Evidence that the effects of thrombin on arachidonate metabolism in cultured human endothelial cells are not mediated by a high affinity receptor. J. Biol. Chem. **255:** 8031–8034.

17. HONG, S. L. & L. LEVINE. 1976. Stimulation of prostaglandin synthesis by bradykinin and thrombin and their mechanisms of action on MC5–5 fibroblasts. J. Biol. Chem. **251:**5814–5816.

ENDOTHELIAL CELL AND PLATELET BINDING SITES FOR THROMBIN

M. A. Shuman, J. D. Isaacs, T. Maerowitz, N. Savion,
and D. Gospodarowicz

Departments of Medicine and Ophthalmology
University of California Medical Center
San Francisco, California 94143

K. Glenn and D. Cunningham

Department of Microbiology
University of California
College of Medicine
Irvine, California 92717

J. W. Fenton, II
Division of Laboratories and Research
New York State Department of Health
Albany, New York 12201

INTRODUCTION

Traditionally, the endothelium has been considered to be an inert surface which protects against activation of clotting. Until recently, this concept of the endothelium's being unreactive with coagulation factors has predominated. However, it is now clear that there is a dynamic interaction between the endothelium and coagulation and fibrinolytic factors. Much of the information on this subject relates to the effects of thrombin on the endothelium. Thrombin stimulates synthesis and release of prostacyclin by umbilical vein endothelial cells.[1] It also inhibits activation of fibrinolysis by endothelial cells. As shown by ourselves, and others, physiologic concentrations of thrombin markedly inhibit plasminogen activation.[2,3] In these experiments, endothelial cells were grown in tissue culture wells coated with [^{125}I]fibrin, and activation of plasminogen was determined by measuring the amount of [^{125}I]fibrin hydrolyzed. As shown in FIGURE 1, there is a dose-dependent inhibition of fibrinolysis by thrombin. Inhibition occurs at thrombin concentrations as low as 0.033 u/ml (10 ng/ml). When thrombin is added simultaneously with plasminogen to the cells, there is no inhibition. Thus, the cells must be preincubated with thrombin for an inhibitory effect to be achieved. Maximal inhibition occurs when the cells are preincubated with thrombin for 30 to 60 minutes. As indicated later, this is probably the result of the time of incubation necessary for maximal thrombin binding to these cells. At all thrombin concentrations, the inhibitory effect is considerably diminished by 17 hours after the addition of thrombin.

A third effect of thrombin on endothelial cells is that of enhancing the proliferative response of nonconfluent human endothelial cells to fibroblast growth factor (FGF).[4] Thrombin is not, however, mitogenic for endothelial cells. Moreover, it has no effect on FGF-induced mitogenesis of bovine vascular endothelial cells.

The mechanisms involved in these various processes are poorly understood.

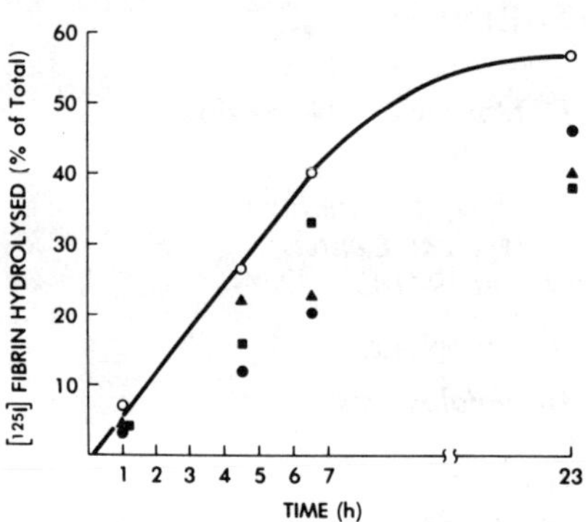

FIGURE 1. Effect of thrombin on bovine corneal endothelial (BCE) cell-mediated fibrinolysis. Cells (1×10^5) were grown for 16 hours on [^{125}I]fibrin-coated tissue culture wells in 2 percent acid-treated calf serum depleted of plasminogen. Human thrombin (●, 2.0 u; ■, 1.0 u; ▲, 0.5 u; ○, control) was added 30 minutes prior to and 45 and 90 minutes after the addition of 5 percent acid-treated calf serum with plasminogen. Aliquots of culture media were removed at the indicated intervals and the percent of hydrolysis of the [^{125}I]fibrin determined. (From Fehrenbacher *et al.*[2] Reproduced by permission.)

Thrombin binds rapidly and reversibly to endothelial cells in a manner similar to that of its binding to platelets and fibroblasts.[5-7] An interesting feature of the binding to both platelets and endothelial cells is that thrombin inhibited at its active serine site binds identically to native thrombin, although the former does not stimulate either cell type.[5, 6, 8, 9] The role of this type of binding in the various thrombin-cell interactions is unknown at this time.

THROMBIN BINDING TO ENDOTHELIAL CELLS

We have studied the interaction between human alpha thrombin and a specific endothelial cell binding site.[10] These experiments have been conducted with pure endothelial cell lines derived from bovine aorta (BAE) and cornea (BCE) in second through fifth passage. Thrombin was radiolabeled by the lactoperoxidase-glucose oxidase technique.[11] There was no significant loss of clotting activity as a result of iodination. The [^{125}I]thrombin was used on the day of preparation. To measure binding, cells were incubated with [^{125}I] thrombin in tissue culture wells, then the reaction stopped by washing the cells several times. The cells were then removed from the wells by solubilization with sodium dodecyl sulfate (SDS) and the amount of [^{125}I]thrombin bound was determined by gamma scintillation spectrometry. Binding could be detected after the shortest incubation, 15 seconds (FIG. 2). Initially, binding was rapid; after 20 to 30 minutes, the amount of thrombin associated with the cells at 37° C continued to increase at a slower rate for at least 3 hours. This slow increase in binding appears to be secondary to internalization of thrombin by the cells. Evidence for this has been obtained by determining the extent to which thrombin that has bound to the cells can be removed by trypsinization; after thrombin has incubated for 30 minutes with the cells, 80 percent of bound thrombin is removed by trypsin; after 1 hour, only 67 percent is trypsinized.

At least 90 percent of binding is specific, as indicated by the marked inhibition by excess unlabeled thrombin. When binding was carried out at 4° C, there was a marked decrease in both thrombin binding and internalization (FIG. 2).

NATURE OF ENDOTHELIAL CELL BINDING SITE

To further characterize the nature of thrombin binding, the solubilized cells were electrophoresed in SDS-10 percent polyacrylamide gel, and autoradiography was performed on the dried gel. As indicated in FIGURE 3, an [125I] thrombin-cell complex of 77,000 daltons was formed (lane 1). The thrombin-cell bond appears to be covalent since it resists disruption by boiling in SDS. Assuming an $M_r = 36,500$ for thrombin, the cellular binding site has a molecular weight of 40,500 daltons. A small amount of thrombin was bound in a smaller complex. This may represent a degradation product of the larger complex or thrombin bound to a second cellular site (FIG. 3).

Thrombin-cell complex formation appears to be specific since a 50-fold excess of unlabeled thrombin completely blocks formation of the radiolabeled complex (lane 2, FIG. 3). Moreover, when the cells were incubated with [125I]thrombin inhibited at its active serine site by diisopropylfluorophosphate ([125I]DIP-thrombin), the 77,000-dalton complex was not formed (lane 3, FIG. 3). There was, however, specific noncovalent binding of [125I]DIP-thrombin since an excess of unlabeled DIP-thrombin reduced the amount of noncovalently bound enzyme (lane 4, FIG. 3).

The thrombin-cell complex (lane 1, FIG. 3) does not appear to be thrombin-bound to antithrombin III (lane 5) in view of the differences in their electrophoretic mobility (77,000 versus 90,000 daltons). Moreover, heparin has no effect on thrombin binding to this cellular site (data not shown).

The amount of [125I]thrombin bound in the 77,000-dalton complex represents approximately 90 percent of the total amount bound to the cells. At

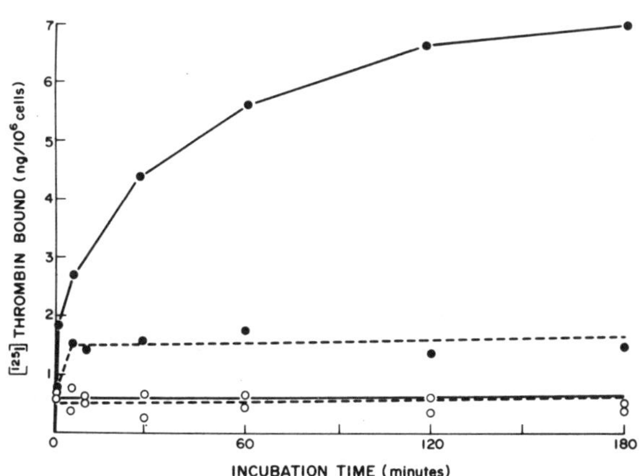

FIGURE 2. Effect of temperature on binding of [125I]thrombin to BCE cells. Confluent BCE cells, 8.5×10^5, were incubated with 0.25 µg/ml [125I]thrombin at 4° (- - - -) and 37° (——). At the indicated intervals, the binding assay was terminated by washing and solubilizing the cells in 2 percent SDS buffer. The amount of [125I]thrombin bound to the cells was determined in a gamma scintillation counter. Each point is a mean of duplicate experiments. ●=binding of [125I]thrombin to BCE cells; ○=binding in the presence of excess unlabeled thrombin (25 µg/ml). (From Isaacs *et al.*[11] Reproduced by permission.)

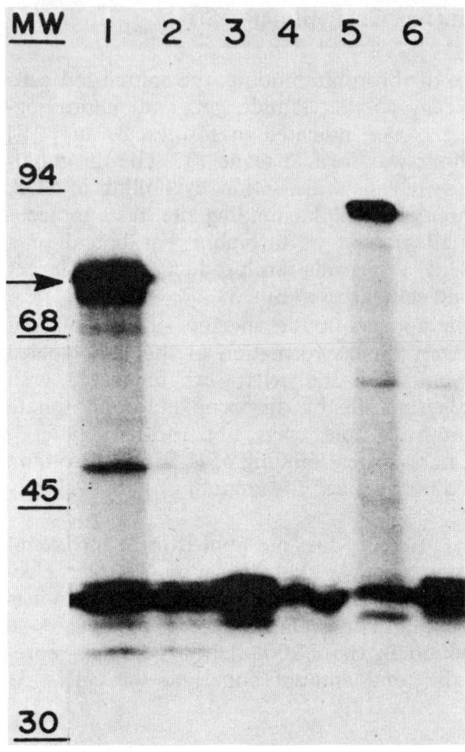

FIGURE 3. Binding of [^{125}I]thrombin to a specific site on confluent BCE cells. [^{125}I]thrombin was incubated with 8.5×10^5 BCE cells for 30 minutes at 37°. After washing and solubilization, the cells were electrophoresed in an SDS-10 percent polyacrylamide gel. An autoradiogram was then made of the gel. Lane 1: [^{125}I]thrombin and BCE cells. Lane 2: [^{125}I]thrombin and BCE cells and 100-fold excess of unlabeled thrombin. Lane 3: [^{125}I]DIP-thrombin and BCE cells. Lane 4: [^{125}I]DIP-thrombin+BCE cells+100-fold excess of unlabeled thrombin. Lane 5: [^{125}I]thrombin and antithrombin III. Lane 6: [^{125}I]thrombin, antithrombin III, and a 100-fold excess of thrombin. The *arrow* indicates the [^{125}I]thrombin-cell complex, $M_r \cong 77,000$. (From Isaacs *et al.*[11] Reproduced by permission.)

saturation, there are between 100,000 and 120,000 molecules of thrombin bound to the surface of BCE cells as part of the 77,000-dalton complex. This does not represent the total amount of thrombin specifically associated with the cells. By 1 hour, approximately one-third of thrombin associated with the cells is intracellular.

The amount of thrombin bound to aortic endothelial cells is markedly influenced by the extent of proliferation of these cells. There is 14-fold more thrombin specifically associated with subconfluent BAE cells than with confluent BAE cells: 67,000 versus 4,700 molecules of thrombin per cell, respectively. This difference is due to a paucity of the cellular binding sites involved in formation of the 77,000-dalton complex in the confluent cells. Thus, it appears that once aortic endothelial cells become confluent in tissue culture, there is a marked reduction in synthesis of these binding sites. In contrast to the binding in vascular endothelial cells, there is no difference in thrombin binding to confluent and subconfluent endothelial cells derived from ocular cornea.

The endothelial cell binding site does not appear to contain intra- or intermolecular disulfide bridges. When the solubilized thrombin-cell complex was treated with dithiothreitol, a reduction in M_r consistent with dissociation of the A from the B chain of thrombin was observed (FIG. 4, lanes 2 and 4).

When the thrombin inhibitor, hirudin, was added to endothelial cells prior to administration of thrombin, there was complete inhibition of thrombin binding (lane 6, FIG. 4). This indicates that thrombin rather than a trace contaminant binds to the cells. In addition, when a 100-fold excess of unlabeled DIP-thrombin was added simultaneously with [^{125}I]thrombin, there was 50 percent inhibition of binding (lane 7, FIG. 4). The inhibition was accounted for by a 0.4 percent contamination of the DIP-thrombin with native thrombin. These results indicate that an intact serine active site is necessary for the apparent covalent binding of thrombin to endothelial cells.

To further characterize the nature of the thrombin-cell bond, the solubilized complex was incubated with hydroxylamine in a final concentration of 1.0 *M* for 6 hours at 37°. As shown in FIGURE 5, there was complete dissociation of both the thrombin-cellular complex and the thrombin-antithrombin III complex. This was not due to the high ionic strength of the hydroxylamine since an equivalent concentration of sodium chloride had no effect on either complex. These results suggest that there is a carboxylic ester bond between thrombin and the cellular binding site similar to that proposed for the thrombin-antithrombin complex.[10]

We have also characterized the [^{125}I]thrombin-cell complex by isoelectric focusing. Thus the isoelectric point of the radiolabeled complex is 8.4 compared with 8.0 for radiolabeled thrombin (FIG. 6).

Once bound to the endothelial cells, thrombin is internalized and hydrolyzed. One hour after [^{125}I]thrombin has bound to the cells, approximately 66 percent appears in the media as small peptides that are not precipitable by trichloracetic acid. Degradation appears to occur in the lysosome since pretreatment of the cells with 50 μM chloroquine completely inhibits degradation of thrombin for at least 2 hours.

Additional evidence that thrombin is bound to the surface of endothelial cells was provided by experiments in which trypsin was added to the cells after the [^{125}I]thrombin had bound and unbound thrombin removed by washing.

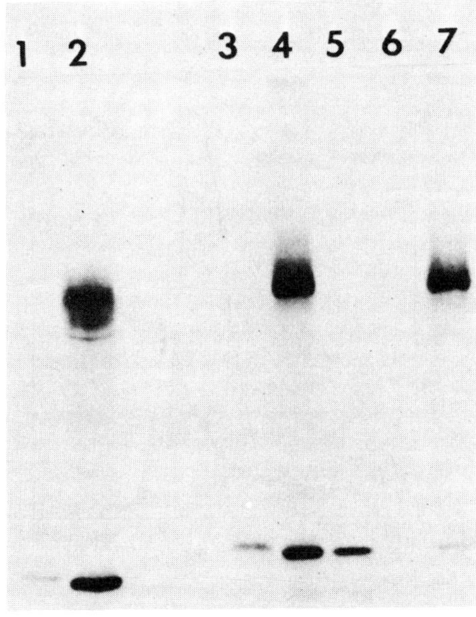

FIGURE 4. Characterization of the [^{125}I]thrombin-cell complex. Autoradiogram of polyacrylamide gel. The [^{125}I]thrombin-BCE cellular complex or [^{125}I]thrombin was treated as follows: Lane 1: [^{125}I]thrombin+0.1 *M* dithiothreitol (DTT). Lane 2: 0.25 μg/ml, [^{125}I]thrombin+cells+0.1 *M* DTT. Lane 3: [^{125}I]thrombin. Lane 4: 0.25 μg/ml [^{125}I]thrombin+cells. Lane 5: 0.25 μg/ml [^{125}I]thrombin +cells+25 μg/ml thrombin. Lane 6: 0.25 μg/ml [^{125}I]thrombin+ cells+hirudin (10 u/ml). Lane 7: 0.25 μg/ml [^{125}I]thrombin+cells+ 25 μg/ml DIP-thrombin. (From Isaacs *et al.*[11] Reproduced by permission.)

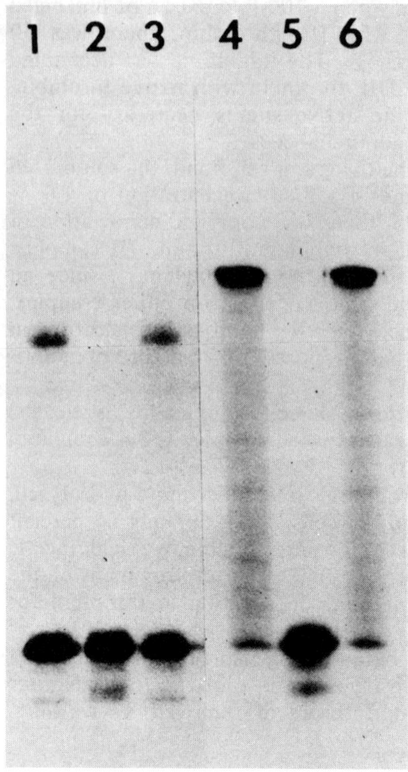

FIGURE 5. Effect of hydroxylamine on [^{125}I]thrombin-antithrombin III and [^{125}I]thrombin-BCE cell complexes. [^{125}I]thrombin was incubated with either antithrombin III or BCE cells as described in FIGURE 3. The samples were solubilized and dialyzed against 0.1 percent SDS, and then hydroxylamine or sodium chloride, final concentration 1.0 M, or isotonic buffer was added for 6 hours at 37°. The samples were again dialyzed against 0.1 percent SDS and then electrophoresed as described in FIGURE 3. Lanes 1–3: [^{125}I]thrombin+BCE cells treated with (1) isotonic buffer, (2) hydroxylamine, or (3) hypertonic sodium chloride. Lanes 4–6: [^{125}I]thrombin+ antithrombin III with (4) isotonic buffer, (5) hydroxylamine, or (6) hypertonic sodium chloride. (From *Isaacs et al.*[11] Reproduced by permission.)

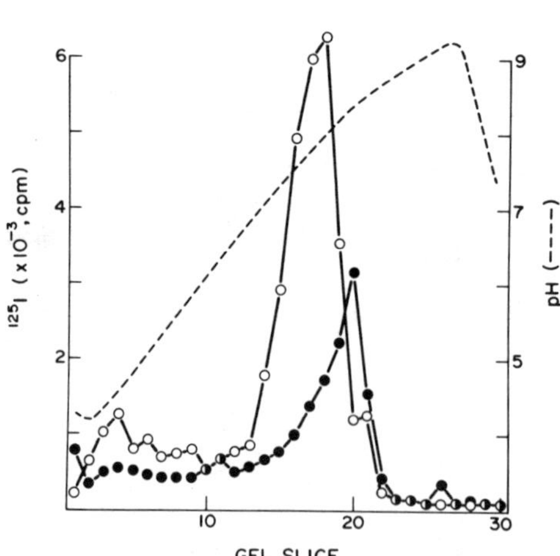

FIGURE 6. Isoelectric focusing of [^{125}I]thrombin and [^{125}I]thrombin-BCE cell complex. BCE cells were incubated with [^{125}I]thrombin as described in FIGURE 3. The cells were washed, solubilized in buffer containing 9.5 M urea, 2 percent (w/v) Nonidet NP40, 2.0 percent Ampholyne (pH range 3.5–10), and 5 percent beta-mercaptoethanol and applied to gels, 60,000 cpm/ gel (●). The samples were electrophoresed at 450 V for 4 hours, and then the gels were cut into 3 mm slices and [^{125}I]-counted by gamma scintillation spectrometry.[13] For comparison, 100,000 cpm/gel of [^{125}I]thrombin was also electrophoresed (○). The pH gradient was measured in individual gel slices (----). (From Isaacs *et al.*[11] Reproduced by permission.)

After a 5-minute incubation with the cells, 90 percent of the bound thrombin was removed by subsequent trypsin treatment. The ability to remove most of the [125I]thrombin with trypsin suggests that the former was bound to the cell surface.

Thrombin Binding to Platelets

We have also studied thrombin binding to human platelets using techniques similar to those used with endothelial cells. [125I]thrombin was incubated with washed human platelets at 37°, then the incubation terminated by centrifugation. The platelets were solubilized and electrophoresed in SDS-8 percent polyacrylamide gels. An autoradiogram from such an experiment is shown in FIGURE 7. There are two radiolabeled [125I]thrombin-platelet complexes, M_r 77,000 and 58,000 (lane 1). Whether the smaller complex represents a degradation product of the larger one or thrombin bound to additional sites is unclear at this time. As noted with endothelial cells, the 77,000-dalton complex and the 58,800-dalton complex did not form between platelets and [125I]DIP-thrombin (lane 2). Addition of unlabeled native thrombin did not result in complex formation between platelets and [125I]DIP-thrombin. This excludes the possibility that these complexes represent dimers of thrombin bound to thrombin by the serine active site.

While a 50-fold excess of unlabeled thrombin completely inhibited binding of [125I]thrombin (lane 3), adding a 50-fold excess of unlabeled DIP-thrombin had no effect on binding (lane 4). This indicates that although DIP-thrombin binds to platelets,[6] it must bind to sites other than those involved in the formation of the 77,000- and 58,800-dalton complexes. These results also indicate that the active site of thrombin is necessary for formation of both platelet complexes.

A further indication of the specificity of this binding reaction is the failure of [125I]thrombin to form similar complexes with red blood cell ghosts (lane 5).

As we observed with endothelial cells, heparin had no effect on formation of the 77,000-dalton complex, nor was there an effect on formation of the 58,800-dalton compex (lane 7).

There are far fewer of these thrombin binding sites associated with intact platelets than with endothelial cells: at saturation there are 600 molecules of thrombin bound per platelet in the 77,000-dalton complex and 400 per platelet in 58,800-dalton complex.

Summary

We have shown that thrombin forms what appears to be a covalent bond with specific sites on both endothelial cells and platelets. The binding characteristics of the platelet and endothelial cell sites involved in the formation of the 77,000-dalton complex appear to be similar. The cellular binding sites do not appear to be antithrombin III in view of the differences in molecular weight, absence of an effect of heparin on thrombin binding, and the failure of an antibody against antithrombin to inhibit thrombin binding to the platelet sites. At this time it is not known whether these complexes represent a physiologic

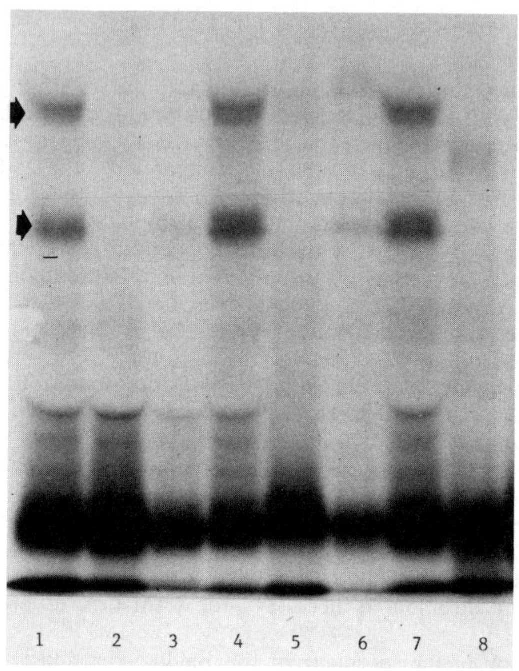

FIGURE 7. Binding of [^{125}I]thrombin to platelets. Washed, human platelets (8×10^8/ml) were incubated with [^{125}I]thrombin (1 u/ml) in 0.15 M NaCl, 30 mM NaH$_2$PO$_4$/Na$_2$HPO$_4$, 5 mM glucose, and 2 mM EDTA for 10 minutes at 37°. The platelets were then isolated by centrifugation at 12,000 $g \times 2$ min, and the pellet solubilized in 2 percent SDS, 15 percent glycerol, 50 mM Tris, pH 7.0, 2 mM EDTA, 2 mM D.F.P., 2 mM N-ethylmaleimide, 2 mM iodoacetic acid, and 0.1 M dithiothreitol. The samples were heated at 65° for 10 minutes, and then electrophoresed in 8 percent polyacrylamide slab gels.[14] After electrophoresis, the gel was dried and an autoradiogram made. Thrombin-platelet complexes are indicated by the *arrows*. Lane 1: Platelets +[^{125}I]thrombin. Lane 2: Platelets+1 u/ml [^{125}I]DIP-thrombin. Lane 3: Platelets +[^{125}I]thrombin+50 u/ml thrombin. Lane 4: Platelets+[^{125}I]thrombin+50 u/ml DIP-thrombin. Lane 5: Red blood cell ghosts (equivalent protein concentration to platelets)+[^{125}I]thrombin. Lane 6: Supernatant from platelet incubation with [^{125}I]thrombin. Lane 7: Platelets+[^{125}I]thrombin+heparin 1 u/ml. Lane 8: [^{125}I]thrombin.

end-product or are the result of SDS-denaturation by disruption of the charge relay system with forcing of the complex to the serine conjugate.

The physiologic significance of these binding sites has yet to be determined. While thrombin binding to these sites may be required for the physiologic effect of the enzyme on these cells, there are features of the reaction that suggest that this is not the case. Thus, although thrombin binds rapidly to endothelial cells, maximal surface binding does not occur for 30 minutes. Maximal prostaglandin synthesis and release is induced by thrombin after only 2 minutes of incubation with endothelial cells.[9] Moreover, only a small amount of 77,000- or 58,000-dalton complex is formed between thrombin and platelets after 1 minute of incubation at 22°, yet platelets have maximally secreted by this time.

The time course of thrombin binding to the endothelium and the concentration at which saturation of surface binding sites occurs correspond closely to the time course and concentration curve for maximal inhibition of plasminogen activation by thrombin. Thus, it may be that thrombin and plasminogen activator compete for binding to the same sites on the endothelial cells. Since activation of plasminogen occurs on the endothelial cell surface, inhibition of binding of plasminogen activator by thrombin would inhibit fibrinolysis.

An alternative physiologic role for these binding sites may be to act as cellular inhibitors of thrombin and possibly other serine proteases. Similar binding of thrombin to fibroblasts has previously been reported.[12] Binding of thrombin by its active serine would result in the inhibition of both its ability to stimulate platelets and endothelial cells and the inhibition of its clotting activity. Thus, binding of thrombin to these cellular sites may serve as an important mechanism for limiting the effects of this enzyme on cell surfaces.

REFERENCES

1. WEKSLER, B. B., C. W. LEY & E. A. JAFFE. 1978. Stimulation of endothelial cell prostacyclin production by thrombin, trypsin, and the ionophore A 23187. J. Clin. Invest. **62:**923–930.
2. FEHRENBACHER, L., D. GOSPODAROWICZ & M. A. SHUMAN. 1979. Synthesis of plasminogen activatior by bovine corneal endothelial cells. Exp. Eye. Res. **29:**219–228.
3. LOSKUTOFF, D. J. 1979. Effect of thrombin on the fibrinolytic activity of cultured bovine endothelial cells. J. Clin. Invest. **64:**329–336.
4. GOSPODAROWICZ, D., K. D. BROWN, C. R. BIRDWELL & B. R. ZETTER. 1978. Control of proliferation of human vascular endothelial cells. Characterization of the response of human umbilical vein endothelial cells to fibroblast growth factor, epidermal growth factor, and thrombin. J. Cell Biol. **77:**774–788.
5. AWBREY, B. J., J. C. HOAK & W. G. OWEN. 1979. Binding of human thrombin to cultured human endothelial cells. J. Biol. Chem. **254:**4092–4095.
6. TOLLEFSEN, D. M., J. R. FEAGLER & P. W. MAJERUS. 1974. The binding of thrombin to the surface of human platelets. J. Biol. Chem. **249:**2646–2651.
7. CARNEY, D. H. & D. D. CUNNINGHAM. 1978. Role of specific cell surface receptors in thrombin-stimulated cell division. Cell **15:**1341–1349.
8. DAVEY, M. G. & E. F. LÜSCHER. 1967. Actions of thrombin and other coagulant and proteolytic enzymes on blood platelets. Nature (London) **216:**857–858.
9. CZERVIONKE, R. L., J. B. SMITH, J. C. HOAK, G. L. FRY & D. L. HAYCRAFT. 1979. Use of a radioimmunoassay to study thrombin-induced release of PGI_2 from cultured endothelium. Thromb. Res. **14:**781–786.
10. ISAACS, J. D., N. SAVION, D. GOSPODAROWICZ, J. W. FENTON, II & M. A.

SHUMAN. 1981. Covalent binding of thrombin to specific sites on corneal endothelial cells. Biochemistry **20:**398–403.

11. HUBBARD, A. L. & Z. A. COHN. 1972. The enzymatic iodination of the red cell membrane. J. Cell Biol. **55:**390–405.

12. BAKER, J. B., R. L. SIMMER, K. C. GLENN & D. D. CUNNINGHAM. 1979. Thrombin and epidermal growth factor become linked to cell surface receptors during mitogenic stimulation. Nature (London) **278:**743–745.

13. O'FARRELL, P. Z., H. M. GOODMAN & P. H. O'FARRELL. 1977. High resolution two-dimensional electrophoresis of basic as well as acidic proteins. Cell **12:** 1133–1141.

14. LAEMMLI, U. K. 1970. Cleavage of structural proteins during the assembly of the head of bacteriophage T4. Nature (London) **227:**680–685.

HYPOTHETICAL MODELS FOR THE THROMBIN-PLATELET INTERACTION

Thomas C. Detwiler

Department of Biochemistry
State University of New York
Downstate Medical Center
Brooklyn, New York 11203

While the exact physiologic role of the thrombin-induced activation of platelets is not clear, the fact that maximal platelet activation is achieved at a thrombin concentration at least ten times lower than that required for detectable coagulation suggests that the thrombin-platelet reaction must be significant. This paper is concerned with the mechanism of the thrombin stimulation of platelets. What is the putative receptor, and what is the mechanism of its reaction with thrombin? While there have been many investigations into this question, there are few definitive answers. In this paper, I will briefly summarize the more important observations, and I will propose several hypothetical models that are intended to better define specific questions and to represent simple statements of complex observations.

A receptor, by definition, exhibits two properties; it forms a complex with an agonist, and it undergoes some change that generates a specific signal. These two properties could, of course, be aspects of a single molecule, or they could involve more than one molecule, either as a complex or as separate molecules, perhaps one on the outer face and one on the inner face of the membrane. Studies of the thrombin-platelet reaction can be considered in three categories: (1) characterization of thrombin stimulation of platelets; (2) analysis of the binding of thrombin to intact platelets; and (3) isolation of membrane components that specifically react with thrombin.

CHARACTERISTICS OF THE THROMBIN STIMULATION OF PLATELETS

Some important characteristics of thrombin-induced platelet activation are listed in TABLE 1. The first three items are consistent with a mechanism that includes an enzyme-catalyzed hydrolysis, the most obvious mechanism for the action of thrombin, a serine protease. Serine proteases have esterase as well as amidase activity, and an esterolytic role in platelet stimulation is as reasonable as a proteolytic role. Seegers *et al.*[4] observed that acetylated thrombin lost its fibrinogen clotting activity but maintained its esterase- and platelet-stimulating activities, while Fenton *et al.*[5] reported that γ-thrombin, a product of partial proteolysis of α-thrombin, retains more activity for ester substrates and platelets than for fibrinogen.

I believe that the most significant observation in TABLE 1 is that in item 4, which suggests that the action of thrombin on platelets may not be catalytic; the rate, but not the extent, of an enzyme-catalyzed reaction should depend on enzyme concentration. This seems to rule out a mechanism that involves thrombin as a catalyst (that is, there is no thrombin "turnover"). There is also

67

0077–8923/81/0370–0067 $01.75/0 © 1981, **NYAS**

TABLE 1

CHARACTERISTICS OF THE THROMBIN STIMULATION OF PLATELETS

1. Catalytically active thrombin is required.[1]
2. The reaction is fast (for example, 4–20 seconds, depending on thrombin concentration.[2,3])
3. Competitive inhibitors, pH, and protease specificity suggest an enzyme-catalyzed reaction.[3]
4. At low concentrations, extent of stimulation depends on thrombin concentration.[2,3]

other, less direct, evidence that the thrombin-platelet interaction might not be an enzyme-catalyzed reaction. Shuman *et al.*[6] reported that exposure of prostacyclin-inhibited platelets to thrombin made the platelets refractory to thrombin after removal of the inhibitor. The degree of refractoriness was time- and temperature-independent, thus not meeting two almost defining characteristics of an enzyme-catalyzed reaction. In their studies of the activation of platelets by immobilized thrombin, Ohning *et al.*[7] observed that platelet activation (but not the responses) was as effective at 4° as at 37° C, whereas little thrombin-catalyzed proteolysis would be expected at 4°. I believe that the absence of a typical enzyme-catalyzed reaction is an almost inescapable conclusion.

BINDING OF THROMBIN TO INTACT PLATELETS

Some of the more important aspects of the binding of thrombin to platelets are listed in TABLE 2. The rates of both association and dissociation are too great to measure by methods that require physical separation of platelet-bound thrombin from free thrombin.[8] The rate of association must, of course, be fast for the binding to be considered significant for platelet stimulation, because the platelet response is so quick. Whether the measured binding represents binding to the receptor is an important question and one without a definite answer. Some of the relevant evidence is listed in TABLE 3 (for a more detailed discussion, see Martin *et al.*[8]). While several correlations are consistent with the high-affinity sites' being the receptors, such correlations cannot constitute proof. In contrast, the failure of inhibited thrombin to inhibit platelet activation while displacing active thrombin seems to be rather solid evidence that the observed binding is not the cause of activation. There must, of course, be binding as an

TABLE 2

CHARACTERISTICS OF THE BINDING OF THROMBIN TO PLATELETS

1. Rapid equilibrium.[8]
2. Site heterogeneity or negative cooperativity.[8,9]
3. Inhibited thrombins binding equally to same sites as active thrombin.[9]
4. More than 80 percent of added thrombin free and active at less than maximal platelet stimulation.[8]

essential first step in platelet stimulation. Whether this constitutes the major portion or an undetectable portion of the observed binding fortunately has no bearing on the most important result of thrombin binding studies (TABLE 2, item 4). Regardless of where on the platelet thrombin binds, most of the added thrombin is *not* bound, even when platelets are only partially activated. This free thrombin retains activity toward platelets and the platelets are responsive to more thrombin.[8] Thus, any explanation of how thrombin activates platelets must account for the fact that an excess of active thrombin only partially activates.

Membrane Components that React with Thrombin

Two isolated membrane components have been shown to react with thrombin. A major surface glycoprotein (glycocalicin) forms a complex with thrombin, thus demonstrating the first aspect of a receptor. No thrombin-

TABLE 3

IS THE OBSERVED BINDING OF THROMBIN TO PLATELETS AT THE RECEPTOR?

Evidence consistent with receptor binding:
1. As the binding affinity is varied by changes in the medium, platelet activation is a function of bound, not total, thrombin.[10]
2. As the rate of binding is slowed, stimulation is slowed.[8]
3. Half-miximal activation corresponds to half saturation of high-affinity sites.[8]

Evidence inconsistent with receptor binding:
1. Active-site-inhibited thrombin is a competitive inhibitor of binding but not activation.[9]

induced change in glycocalicin has been observed, but a receptor function may involve something as difficult to detect as a subtle conformational change. A surface glycoprotein that is hydrolyzed by thrombin has been purified and shown to undergo a cleavage equivalent to the amount of added thrombin.[12] It thus appears to share with intact platelets an interaction with thrombin that involves the enzyme active site but is not catalytic (no turnover of enzyme).

HYPOTHETICAL MODELS OF THE THROMBIN-PLATELET INTERACTION

In an attempt to understand better the implications of some of the observations discussed earlier, we have made simple hypothetical models [2, 3] of the reaction of thrombin (T) with a platelet receptor (R) to form a modified receptor (R*). The simplest mechanism to include the need for active thrombin as well as the lack of turnover is shown by Equation 1,

$$T + R \rightleftharpoons TR \rightarrow TR^* \tag{1}$$

which is analogous to the reaction of thrombin with some esters (forms a stable acyl-enzyme complex) or to the reaction of a protease with a protein inhibitor (for example, thrombin and antithrombin). This model cannot, however, explain how there can be a partial reaction in the presence of free thrombin (Table 2, item 4) since the irreversible step should cause the reaction to proceed until either free thrombin or free receptor has been depleted. We therefore suggested that the modification of the receptor could be reversible[3] (Equation 2),

$$T + R \rightleftharpoons TR \rightleftharpoons TR^*$$ (2)

so that platelet stimulation would have characteristics of both an agonist-receptor equilibrium process (the concentration of TR^* in Equation 2 is a function of the concentration of thrombin) as well as an active site reaction (the modification of the receptor involves a reaction with the active site of thrombin). In this model, it is possible that the reaction continues to the right ($TR^* \rightleftharpoons T + R^*$) as long as it is reversible and the degree of stimulation is a function of $[TR^*]$, not $[R^*]$. This simple model is consistent with essentially all reported observations with intact platelets. While a freely reversible reaction catalyzed by a protease may seem extreme, it should be noted that this is well known for the reactions of proteases with their protein inhibitors.

It is stimulating to consider how a more conventional thrombin-catalyzed hydrolysis of a peptide bond might be reconciled with the observations that there appears to be no thrombin turnover. Two general types of mechanism seem obvious. If the hydrolysis of a substrate were very slow relative to the amount of substrate available (Equation 3),

$$T + R \rightleftharpoons TR \overset{slow}{\longrightarrow} TR^* \rightarrow T + R^*$$ (3)

(stimulation a function of dR^*/dt)

and if the degree of stimulation were a function of the rate of product formation (that is, stimulation proportional to dR^*/dt, not to $[R^*]$), then the degree of stimulation (rate of reaction) would be a function of the concentration of thrombin. This type of mechanism would require a very large excess of receptor and/or a very slow turnover. The glycoprotein described by Berndt and Phillips[12] may meet these criteria, although it should be noted that the slow step must be the first reaction of TR, otherwise the equilibrium would be "pulled" to the right until thrombin was depleted.

A second possible catalytic mechanism, shown in Equation 4,

$$T + R \rightleftharpoons TR \rightarrow TR^* \rightarrow T + R^*$$ (4)

(stimulation a function of $[R^*]_{steady-state}$)

is the same in principle, but involves regeneration of the receptor, either *de novo* or by some type of competing reaction. One could imagine, for example, that thrombin demethylates a receptor and a platelet enzyme remethylates it; the steady-state concentration of the modified receptor would then be a function of thrombin concentration.

The models shown in Equations 2, 3, and 4 have as their major feature, an explanation for (i) how the degree of platelet stimulation is a function of thrombin concentration and (ii) how platelets are only partially stimulated in the presence of free, active thrombin. I favor Equation 2 only because it is the more simple. It suggests a receptor analogous to a protein protease inhibitor; Equations 3 and 4 suggest more traditional enzyme substrate reactions. The model shown by Equation 3 predicts that exposure of platelets to low levels of thrombin should make them less sensitive to subsequent additions of thrombin. There are conflicting reports (from very different types of experiments) on this point,[6, 8] and it is thus a major point to be resolved. None of these models can explain the thrombin-induced refractoriness to thrombin described by Shuman *et al.*[8]

References

1. DAVEY, M. G. & E. F. LUSCHER. 1967. Actions of thrombin and other coagulant and proteolytic enzymes on blood platelets. Nature (London) **216**:857–858.
2. DETWILER, T. C. & R. D. FEINMAN. 1973. Kinetics of the thrombin-induced release of calcium (II) by platelets. Biochemistry **12**:282–289.
3. MARTIN, B. M., R. D. FEINMAN & T. C. DETWILER. 1975. Platelet stimulation by thrombin and other proteases. Biochemistry **14**:1308–1314.
4. SEEGERS, W. H., U. DIEKAMP & L. E. McCOY. 1970. Induction of platelet aggregation with acetylated thrombin. Thromb. Diath. Haemorrh. (Suppl.) **42:** 115–124.
5. FENTON, J. W., II, B. H. LANDIS, D. A. WALZ & J. S. FINLAYSON. 1977. Human thrombins. *In* Chemistry and Biology of Thrombin. R. L. Lundblad, J. W. Fenton, II & K. G. Mann, Eds. :43–70. Ann Arbor Science. Ann Arbor, Mich.
6. SHUMAN, M. A., M. BOTNEY & J. W. FENTON, II. 1979. Thrombin-induced platelet secretion. Further evidence for a specific pathway. J. Clin. Invest. **63**:1211–1218.
7. OHNING, B. L., W. C. WALLACE & H. B. BENSUSAN. 1978. Protein phosphorylation in thrombin-stimulated platelets at 37 and 4 degrees. Fed. Proc. **37**:1143.
8. MARTIN, B. M., W. W. WASIEWSKI, J. W. FENTON, II & T. C. DETWILER. 1976. Equilibrium binding of thrombin to platelets. Biochemistry **15**:4886–4893.
9. TOLLEFSEN, D. M., J. R. FEAGLER & P. W. MAJERUS. 1974. The binding of thrombin to the surface of human platelets. J. Biol. Chem. **249**:2646–2651.
10. SHUMAN, M. A. & P. W. MAJERUS. 1975. The perturbation of thrombin binding to human platelets by anions. J. Clin. Invest. **56**:945–950.
11. OKUMURA, T., M. HASITZ & G. A. JAMIESON. 1978. Platelet glycocalicin. Interaction with thrombin and role as thrombin receptor of the platelet surface. J. Biol. Chem. **253**:3435–3443.
12. BERNDT, M. C. & D. R. PHILLIPS. 1980. Interaction of thrombin with platelets. Purification of the thrombin substrate. This volume.

BIOCHEMISTRY AND IMMUNOLOGY OF PLATELET MEMBRANES WITH REFERENCE TO GLYCOPROTEIN COMPOSITION *

Alan T. Nurden, Dominique Dupuis, Dominique Pidard,
Thomas Kunicki, and Jacques P. Caen

*Unité 150 Inserm
Hôpital Lariboisière
75475 Paris Cedex 10, France*

Increasing evidence points to the platelet membrane's having a specialized structure adapted to meet the functional requirements of the cell. It is the purpose of this report to highlight some of this evidence. During hemostasis the mechanisms of platelet aggregation and adhesion are initiated by the interaction of specific stimuli such as adenosine diphosphate (ADP) or collagen with externally oriented membrane receptors, and concluded through the formation of cohesive forces exposed at the platelet surface. Membrane components must play integral roles in these processes, as they must in binding the different factors that participate in platelet-mediated coagulation and immunologic reactions. Membrane proteins must also carry the platelet alloantigens giving rise to cell specificity, while clot retraction is mediated through the interaction of fibrin with a surface acceptor. Special attention has been given in recent years to the glycoprotein composition of the platelet membrane after the detection of different glycoprotein abnormalities in platelets isolated from patients with hereditary disorders of platelet aggregation or adhesion to subendothelium. In this review of the structure of the platelet membrane we will pay particular attention to the membrane glycoprotein composition and will describe in some detail the glycoprotein deficiencies located in the membranes of abnormal platelets.

MEMBRANE STRUCTURE OF NORMAL HUMAN PLATELETS

Lipid Composition

Studies performed with the use of purified phospholipases added to washed platelet suspensions and to isolated membranes allowed Perret et al.[1] to conclude that 45 percent of plasma membrane phospholipids were located in the outer leaflet of the bilayer and that of the total phospholipids in the membrane, 93 percent of sphingomyelin, 45 percent of phosphatidylcholine, 9 percent of phosphatidylserine, 16 percent of phosphatidylinositol, and 20 percent of phosphatidylethanolamine were exposed at the platelet surface. This asymmetric distribution of phospholipids in the plasma membrane was similar to that observed for other blood cells [2] and is not unique to the platelet. Cholesterol is a significant membrane constituent [3] and there are indications that the cholesterol content may influence platelet plasma membrane fluidity.[4]

* This work was supported by grants from INSERM C.R.L. 78-5-128.1 and from the Thyssen Foundation.

Protein Composition

In an effort to pinpoint the functional proteins of the platelet membrane, the protein composition of isolated platelet membranes is compared in FIGURE 1 with isolated human erythrocyte membranes as analyzed by SDS-polyacrylamide

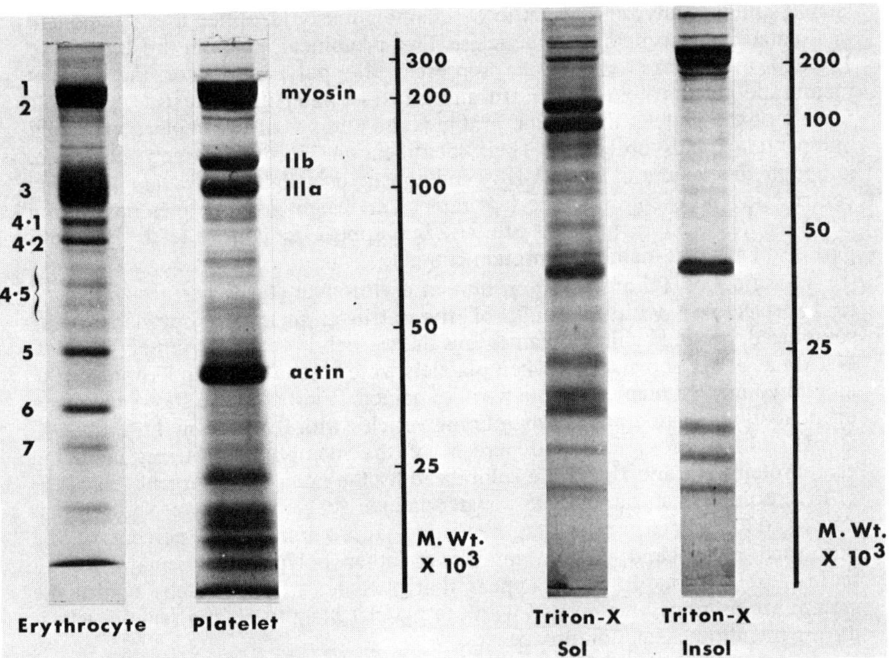

FIGURE 1. Protein patterns of human erythrocyte and platelet membranes as analyzed by SDS-polyacrylamide gel electrophoresis, and of platelet membranes after extraction with Triton X-100. Membranes were isolated from washed red cells according to the procedure of Dodge *et al.*[41] and from washed platelets by the glycerol-lysis method.[3] The washed membranes were solubilized with 2 percent SDS at 100° C for 5 minutes and disulfide bonds reduced with 5 percent 2-mercaptoethanol at 37° C for 1 hour. Samples (100 μg protein) were analylzed on a 1.5-mm thick 7–12 percent exponential gradient acrylamide slab gel using the Laemmli[14] procedure. Protein was located by Coomassie blue staining. Platelet membranes were incubated at 4° C for 30 minutes in the presence of 10 mm Tris, pH 7.0, containing 0.5 percent w/v Triton X-100 and then centrifuged at 100,000 *g* for 1 hour at 4° C, and the Triton X-100 solubilized and insoluble fractions incubated with SDS and 2-mercapto-ethanol as described earlier. Aliquots were analyzed using 7–20 percent exponential gradient acrylamide slab gels to improve the resolution of the low molecular weight polypeptides.

gel electrophoresis. The erythrocyte membrane polypeptides have been numbered according to the nomenclature used by Steck.[5] Prominent are bands 1 and 2 (spectrin), which represent two high molecular weight polypeptides that form a cytoskeletal matrix at the cytoplasmic surface of the red-cell membrane, and band 3, a major transmembrane glycoprotein thought to be involved in anion transport across the membrane. Marchesi[6] should be consulted as a guide to the proposed functional roles of the red cell membrane proteins.

Contractile proteins appear dominant when the protein composition of platelet membranes is assessed. The prominent 45,000 molecular weight band has tentatively been identified as actin associated with the membrane vesicles.[7] The dense 200,000 molecular weight band probably represents myosin heavy chains, although myosin has yet to be unambiguously identified as a component of isolated platelet membrane vesicles. Two prominent bands in the 100,000 to 150,000 molecular weight zone represent the polypeptides of the platelet membrane glycoproteins (GP) IIb and IIIa (see later in the text). A notable feature of the platelet membrane profile is the number of low molecular weight polypeptide bands observed. Their identification is as yet largely uncertain, although the β-subunit of GP IIb[8] and the myosin light chains are probably contributing polypeptides. The low molecular weight polypeptides have often not been resolved in previous studies, but appear to constitute a significant part of the platelet membrane protein content.

The effect of Triton X-100 on human erythrocyte ghosts has been reported to be selective,[5] with the bulk of the intrinsic membrane proteins being solubilized, leaving behind a filamentous matrix rich in the spectrin polypeptides. Nachmias *et al.*[9] showed that when platelets were solubilized with Triton X-100, an interconnected filamentous network remained. FIGURE 1 also shows the effect of incubating isolated platelet membrane vesicles with 0.5 percent Triton X-100 at pH 7.0. Approximately 60 percent of the membrane proteins, including glycoproteins IIb and IIIa, were solubilized by the nonionic detergent. Analysis of the insoluble material by SDS-polyacrylamide gel electrophoresis showed that the 200,000 molecular weight polypeptide, approximately 50 percent of the purported actin band, and a number of other polypeptides remained in a sedimentable form. It would appear that elements of the platelet contractile system are intimately associated with the platelet membrane and remain with it during membrane isolation procedures.

Glycoprotein Composition

Although approximately 30 percent of the membrane carbohydrate groupings are associated with lipids in the form of glycolipids,[10] the bulk of the carbohydrate is associated with the membrane glycoproteins. The glycoprotein composition of the platelet plasma membrane is complex [8, 11–13] with the number of components observed depending largely on the sensitivity of the analytical procedure used. In FIGURE 2 the glycoprotein profiles of isolated membranes are compared with those of intact platelets as analyzed by SDS-polyacrylamide gel electrophoresis. Four major PAS-staining membrane glycoproteins may be observed. When estimated on 6 percent acrylamide gels by means of the Laemmli system of electrophoresis,[14] the apparent molecular weights of these glycoproteins after disulfide bond reduction are 148,000 (Ib), 135,000 (IIb), 116,000 (IIIa) and 93,000 (IIIb). The criteria used for assigning the given nomenclature to the individual bands have been outlined elsewhere.[15] Reference to FIGURE 1 shows that the IIb and IIIa glycoproteins stain strongly with protein-locating reagents while the Ib and IIIb glycoproteins stain weakly, suggesting that the latter have a high carbohydrate content. Comparison of the platelet membrane glycoprotein profiles with those reported for human erythrocyte membranes [5] shows that profound differences exist between the glycoproteins of the membranes of the two cell types. The major glycoprotein (PAS-1 or glycophorin A) of the red cell membrane appears to exist as an 80,000-molecular weight dimer that can be dissociated by heating in the presence of SDS at 100° C (see Marchesi [6]). No changes in the platelet membrane glycoprotein profiles are observed when SDS-polyacrylamide gel electrophoresis is performed using membranes solubilized at 37° C or 100° C. In contrast, a pronounced feature of many of the platelet membrane glycoproteins is that their electrophoretic mobility is changed after reduction as a result of the cleavage of constituent disulfide bonds.[8]

FIGURE 2. Glycoprotein profiles of isolated platelet membranes and whole platelet suspensions. Washed platelets were resuspended at 2×10^9 platelets/ml and solubilized with 2 percent SDS at 100° C for 5 minutes. Isolated platelet membranes were prepared and solubilized as described in FIGURE 1. Disulfide bonds were reduced with 5 percent 2-mercaptoethanol at 37° C for 1 hour and samples (membranes, 100 μg protein; whole platelets, 400 μg protein) analyzed by SDS-polyacrylamide gel electrophoresis using 6 percent acrylamide separating gels and the Laemmli [14] procedure. Glycoprotein was located by periodate-Schiff (PAS) staining and the gels densitometrically scanned at 550 nm. The profile to the left of the vertical arrow represents high molecular weight staining material that was retained in the 3.5 percent acrylamide spacer gel.

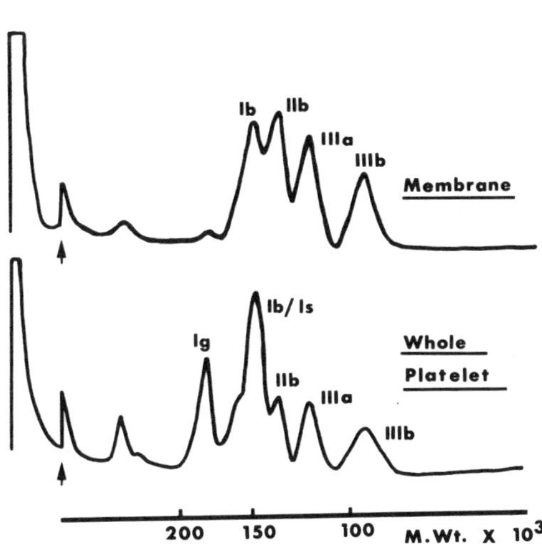

Two pronounced differences may be observed between the glycoprotein profiles obtained after the analysis of isolated membranes or unfractionated platelets (FIGURE 2). A pronounced peak, labeled GP Ig, with an apparent molecular weight of 180,000 after reduction is additionally present on the whole platelet profile. This glycoprotein has been shown to have an intracellular localization, probably in a granule population.[11, 16] In its native form it consists of three polypeptide chains linked by disulfide bonds and has been termed "thrombospondin" by Lawler *et al.*[16] Recent studies [11] suggest that part of GP Ig may become bound to the platelet surface during the thrombin-induced release reaction and that this glycoprotein may be a surface marker after its release. An increased intensity of the GP Ib band relative to the other membrane glycoproteins may also be observed in the whole platelet profile. Okumura and

Jamieson [17, 18] have characterized a glycoprotein that was lost from the platelet surface during platelet homogenization and that accounted for about 10 percent of the total platelet sialic acid. They termed this glycoprotein, glycocalicin; others have called it GP Is.[15] Loss of glycocalicin from the platelet surface was subsequently shown to be inhibited by the addition of EDTA, and a Ca^{2+}-dependent platelet protease has been implicated in the mechanism of its release.[11, 19] Analysis of membranes isolated after platelet lysis performed either in the presence or absence of EDTA [11] suggested that glycocalicin was being derived from an intrinsic membrane glycoprotein precursor, and that this precursor was GP Ib (our nomenclature [15]). This conclusion is supported by recent studies performed using crossed immunoelectrophoresis (see later in the text).

Localization of membrane glycoproteins after SDS-polyacrylamide gel electrophoresis by the periodate-Schiff (PAS) colorimetric reaction is a relatively insensitive procedure, although it is convenient for studying the major glycoproteins. The use of surface-labeling techniques allows an increased sensitivity (see the next section), while McGregor et al.[13] recently detected glycoproteins after electrophoresis by incubating the gels with ^{125}I-labeled lectins. Whole platelet samples were analyzed and the labeled glycoproteins located by autoradiography. ^{125}I-labeled lens culinaris lectin (LCM-B) (specificity : glucose and mannose) bound to 16 bands, the most intensely labeled membrane glycoprotein being GP IIIa. ^{125}I-labeled concanavalin A with a similar sugar specificity predominately bound to GP IIIa. In contrast, ^{125}I-labeled wheat germ agglutinin (specificity: N-acetyl glucosamine and sialic acid), although labeling 10 bands, interacted most intensely with Ib. These studies suggest marked differences in the monosaccharide composition of the major platelet membrane glycoproteins.

PLATELET SURFACE COMPONENTS

Ultrastructural Studies

The external surface of the normal human platelet as studied by freeze-etch electron microscopy shows clusters of spherical particles in a reticular pattern with smooth and regular surface membrane in adjacent areas.[20] Using high-resolution transmission electron microscopy, Skaer et al.[21] have defined the types of contact located within platelet aggregates. Areas of tight contact were apparent, as were 50-nm intercellular spaces spanned by bridges linked to attachment points visualized as blebs extending from the outer surface of the plasma membrane. These images must represent structural components of fundamental importance for the mechanism of platelet aggregation.

Surface-labeling studies prove that the membrane glycoproteins are primary constituents of the platelet surface. Feagler et al.[22] incubated normal human platelets with saturating concentrations of the lectin conjugate, lentil-PHA-ferritin, and studied the distribution of the lectin receptors by freeze-etch electron microscopy. The electron-dense ferritin molecules were seen to be evenly distributed over the platelet surface and arranged in a reticular pattern. The recent studies of McGregor et al.[13] suggest that GP IIIa may have been a major binding site for the lentil-PHA-ferritin conjugate. No obvious relationship was apparent between the arrangement of the lentil-PHA receptor sites on the platelet surface and the intramembranous particles observed within the platelet membrane by freeze-fracture electron microscopy. The latter particles, which probably represent arrangements of intrinsic proteins or glycoproteins traversing or penetrating the membrane, were also observed by Chevalier *et al.*[23] Randomly distributed particles in the 5- to 13-nm size range were observed on the fracture faces of both the outer (EF) and inner (PF) phospholipid leaflets of the bilayer, and particle densities of $925 \pm 52/\mu m^2$ on the E face and $427 \pm 29/\mu m^2$ on the P face were calculated using a computer-linked picture analyzer. Particle size was heterogeneous on both faces.

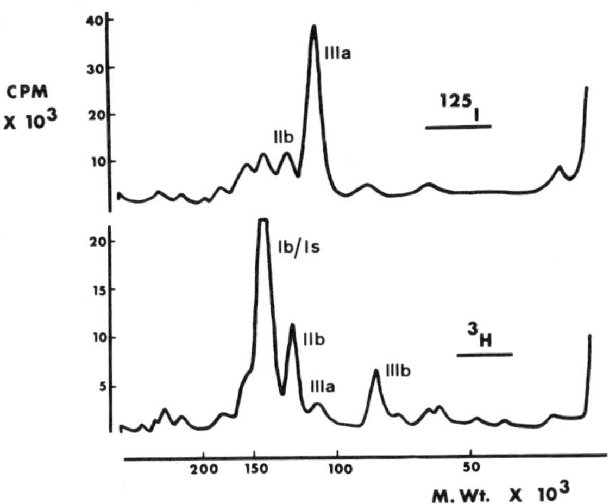

FIGURE 3. Analysis of the polypeptides exposed at the normal human platelet surface. Washed human platelet suspensions were either labeled with ^{125}I using the lactoperoxidase-catalyzed procedure of Phillips and Poh Agin,[8] or treated successively with neuraminidase, galactose oxidase, and sodium [³H] borohydride as described by McGregor *et al.*[12] The labeled platelets were solubilized with SDS, disulfide bonds were reduced with 2-mercaptoethanol, and samples (400 μg protein) were analyzed by SDS-polyacrylamide gel electrophoresis as described in FIGURE 2. After the major glycoprotein bands were located by PAS-staining, the gels were cut into 1-mm slices. The incorporation of ^{125}I into the surface proteins was analyzed by directly counting each slice in a gamma counter. To determine the ³H incorporation, gel slices were solubilized by incubation overnight at 50° C in the presence of 0.1 ml 30 percent v/v hydrogen peroxide, followed by the addition of scintillation fluid and counting in a scintillation spectrometer.

Surface-Labeling Procedures

The method most often used of labeling the platelet surface proteins is the incorporation of ^{125}I by the lactoperoxidase-catalyzed procedure.[8] FIGURE 3 shows that GP IIIa is the major membrane component labeled by this technique, which requires tyrosine or histidine residues accessible to the lactoperoxidase at the platelet surface. The high degree of labeling of IIIa suggests that a large part of the glycoprotein is exposed at the platelet surface. Other authors have used the less specific diazotized diiodosulfanilic acid (DDISA) as a means for incorporating ^{125}I into surface proteins.[11] By this method GP IIb and GP IIIa are labeled equally well, confirming that GP IIb is also a prominent surface glycoprotein. FIGURE 3 also shows those glycoproteins containing carbohydrate groups labeled with ^{3}H after the sequential treatment of platelets with neuraminidase, galactose oxidase, and sodium [^{3}H]borohydride. Galactose and *N*-acetylgalactosamine are the sugars labeled by this method, which was first applied to platelets by Phillips and Poh Agin.[24] A large proportion of the incorporated radioactivity was associated with GP Ib, thus confirming its high carbohydrate content and surface orientation. GP IIb and IIIb are also well labeled, but IIIa was poorly labeled by this procedure. The low amount of ^{3}H incorporated into GP IIIa contrasts with its high affinity for ^{125}I-lens culinaris lectin or for ^{125}I-concanavalin A,[13] suggesting that mannose and/or glucose are important components of the oligosaccharide chains of this glycoprotein.

In addition to labeling the surface-exposed oligosaccharides with ^{3}H, Marchesi and Chassis [25] incubated platelets with [32]Pi and subsequently isolated the major glycoproteins by either lectin-affinity chromatography after SDS-solubilization or by lithium diiodosalicylate extraction followed by gel chromatography. Evidence was presented to show that at least three of the major membrane glycoproteins were phosphorylated. It was concluded that the phosphorylation occurred at the cytoplasmic surface of the membrane and that the glycoproteins have polypeptide chains which traverse the bilayer.

Immunology

The platelet surface proteins contain a whole range of antigenic specificities. The presence of the disaccharide α-D-galactosyl-(1-3)-*N*-acetyl-D-galactosamine, the immunodominant group of the Thomsen-Friedenreich antigen (T-antigen), has been demonstrated within platelet plasma membranes.[10] The receptor was found only after neuraminidase treatment indicating that it is normally a cryptic antigen, that is, is masked by sialic acid in the native membrane. A recent study demonstrating a membrane glycoprotein defect in the platelets of patients with the Tn-syndrome has shown that this antigen is primarily located on membrane GP Ib.[26] Although platelets have been reported to carry the antigens of the ABO blood group system,[27] Glöckner *et al.*[10] were unable to detect the MN blood group antigens on the platelet surface. At least six platelet-specific antigen systems (for example, Pl[A1], Pl[E1], KO[a]) have been detected.[27] Kunicki and Aster [28] isolated the protein carrying the Pl[A1] (Zw[a]) antigen and showed that the antigenic specificity was associated with GP IIIa. Virtually all of the Pl[A1] activity appeared to be located on the external platelet membrane where the activity appeared to involve a polypeptide sequence of GP IIIa. Pl[A1] was the first alloantigen to be assigned to a specific platelet membrane constituent. HLA antigens are also important components of the human platelet surface; deoxycholate-solubilized HLA antigens have been isolated from platelets and shown to be composed of a mixture of 43,000 and 39,000 molecular weight polypeptide chains associated with β_2-microglobulin.[29] As with other surface-oriented proteins, the HLA antigens are glycosylated and are therefore glycoproteins.

ANALYSIS OF ABNORMAL PLATELET MEMBRANES

Glanzmann's thrombasthenia and the Bernard-Soulier syndrome are hereditary platelet disorders associated with defined abnormalities of the platelet membrane. Molecular deficiencies of different platelet membrane glycoproteins are characteristic for each disorder and suggest specific roles for surface oriented glycoproteins in the mechanisms of platelet aggregation and adhesion.

Glanzmann's Thrombasthenia

A disease with an autosomal recessive inheritance, Glanzmann's thrombasthenia (GT) is characterized by the absence of platelet aggregation in response to ADP and all physiologic aggregation-inducing agents.[30] Abnormalities in the membrane glycoprotein composition of GT platelets were first described by Nurden and Caen,[31] who noted a severely reduced carbohydrate staining intensity of the GP II band (1974 nomenclature), and a lower than normal staining intensity of the GP III band after SDS-polyacrylamide gel electrophoresis. These and subsequent early studies performed on the platelets of a large number of patients in several laboratories have been reviewed elsewhere.[15] Current studies suggest that GT platelets are either missing or have severely reduced amounts of membrane glycoproteins IIb and IIIa. (FIGS. 4 and 5). In FIGURE 4 a two-dimensional SDS-polyacrylamide gel electrophoresis procedure has been used to separate the ^{125}I-labeled surface components of normal human and thrombasthenic platelets. In this procedure, first introduced by Phillips and Poh Agin,[8] the first-dimension electrophoresis is performed using nonreduced samples. Subsequent reduction of disulfide bonds results in the cleavage of low molecular weight polypeptides from Ib, IIb, and from an additional membrane glycoprotein, Ic.[8] The released low molecular weight polypeptides have been termed β-subunits.[8] The β-subunits of Ic and IIb are labeled with ^{125}I and may be observed as weak spots on the lower part of the autoradiograph illustrated for ^{125}I-labeled control platelets in FIGURE 4. A slower rate of migration of GP IIIa after reduction has been suggested to be due to its containing intramolecular disulfide bonds and to its having an altered molecular conformation in its reduced state.[8] In summary, the nonreduced/reduced two-dimensional system of SDS-polyacrylamide gel electrophoresis makes use of the different contents of inter- or intramolecular disulfide bonds in the individual membrane glycoproteins to improve the resolution achieved using single-dimension electrophoresis alone (compare with FIG. 3). Additional surface glycoproteins resolved include Ia, Ic, and IIa, according to the nomenclature of Phillips and Poh Agin.[8] Examination of the autoradiograph obtained after the analysis of ^{125}I-labeled GT platelets shows the specific absence of zones of radioactivity in the IIb and IIIa positions. No spot corresponding to the β-subunit of IIb was observed.

FIGURE 5 illustrates the analysis of ^{125}I-labeled GT and normal human platelets by crossed immunoelectrophoresis (CIE) using a polyspecific rabbit antiserum prepared against normal human platelets. Analysis of membrane proteins by CIE was first adapted to platelets by Hagen *et al.*[32] A major ^{125}I-labeled precipitate, previously termed band 16,[32, 33] is severely diminished in intensity in the GT platelet profile. The other major ^{125}I-labeled precipitates were present in their normal positions and were of normal intensity. Platelets from nine patients with Glanzmann's thrombasthenia have now been analyzed by CIE in our laboratory, and the results obtained for three of these patients (as reported by Hagen *et al.*[33]) as well as for those studied subsequently all show either the absence of band 16 or its presence in severely reduced quantities (<15 percent). Analysis by SDS-polyacrylamide gel electrophoresis of band 16 eluted from the agarose gel after its precipitation by either (1) the poly-

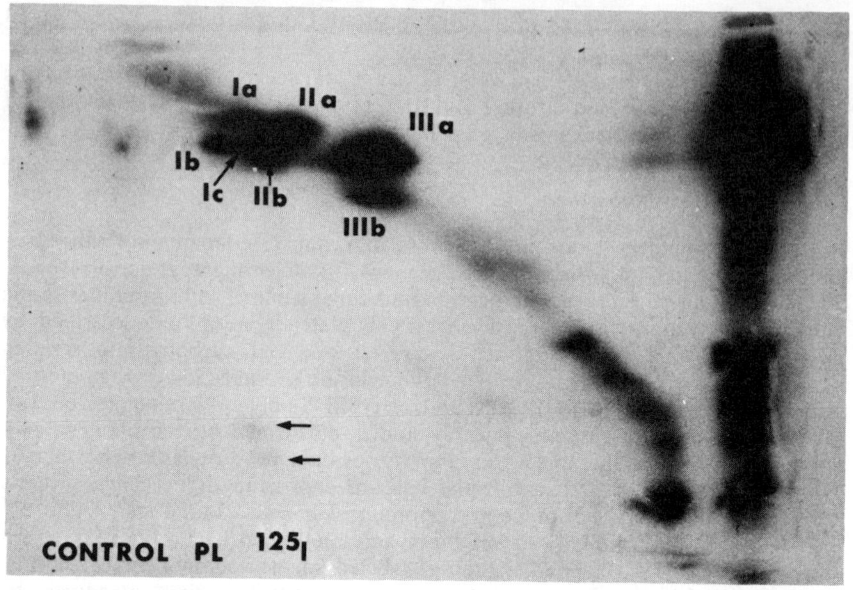

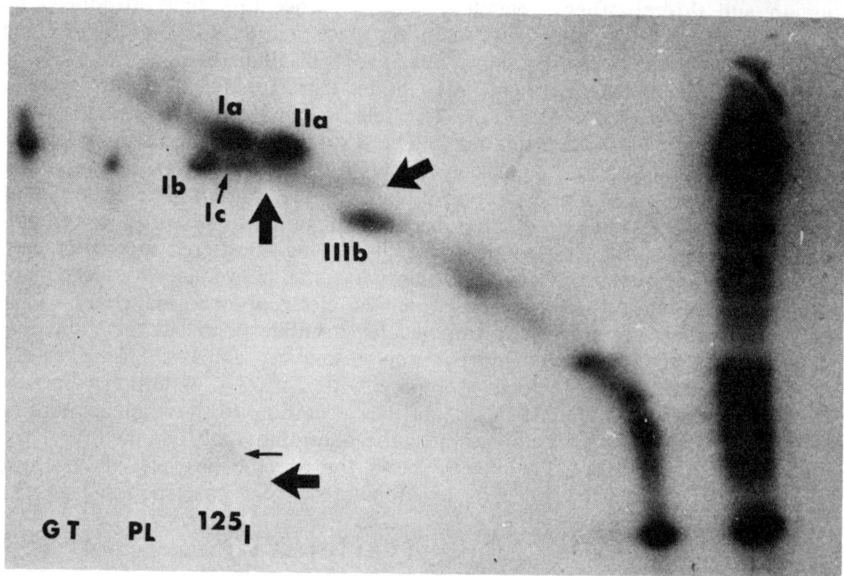

FIGURE 4. Glycoprotein defects in thrombasthenic (GT) platelets. Washed normal human and GT platelets were labeled with ^{125}I by the lactoperoxidase-catalyzed procedure. Two-dimensional SDS-polyacrylamide gel electrophoresis was performed according to the procedure of Phillips and Poh Agin.[8] The first-dimension study was performed using 7 percent acrylamide gels and samples solubilized at 100° C for 5 minutes in the presence of 2 percent SDS and 5 mM N-ethylmaleimide. After electrophoresis the polypeptides were reduced by incubating the gels for 1 hour in the presence of 5 percent 2-mercaptoethanol. Second-dimension electrophoresis[8] was performed by layering the gel containing the now-reduced polypeptides onto a 7–12 percent exponential gradient acrylamide slab gel. The ^{125}I-labeled proteins were detected on dried, protein-stained gels by autoradiography using Kodak® X-Omat MA film. The two horizontal arrows towards the base of the control gel point to the positions of the β-subunits of Ic and IIb, respectively. Typical autoradiographs are illustrated.

specific rabbit antihuman platelet antibody preparation [33] or (2) a monospecific alloantibody, IgG L (unpublished studies), has shown the presence of GP IIb and IIIa as the platelet antigens giving rise to this precipitate. Our current studies suggest that IIb and IIIa exist as a complex after their extraction from the membrane by Triton X-100; whether they also exist as a complex in the native plasma membrane of normal human platelets remains to be learned.

Kunicki and Aster [34] were the first to show that the alloantigen Pl[A1] was deleted in thrombasthenia, and it is now clear that this deletion is due to the absence of the glycoprotein that normally carries the Pl[A1] specificity, namely, GP IIIa.[28] Further support for this conclusion was provided by van Leeuwen *et al.*,[35] who showed that the allelic counterpart of Pl[A1], Pl[A2] (Zw[b]), was also

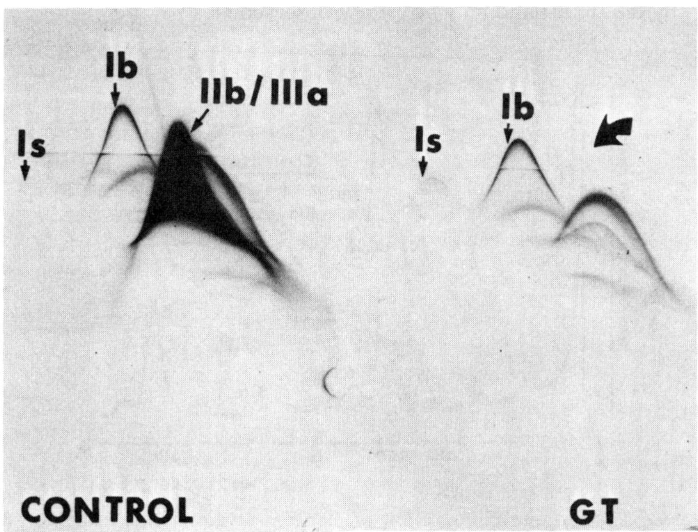

FIGURE 5. Analysis of ^{125}I-labeled normal human and thrombasthenic (GT) platelets by crossed immunoelectrophoresis (CIE). The platelets were solubilized in the presence of 1 percent Triton X-100 and CIE was performed according to the procedures of Hagen *et al.*[32, 33] The immunoglobulin fraction of a multispecific rabbit antiserum prepared against washed, normal human platelets was incorporated into the superior gel for the second dimension. Autoradiography of the dried, protein-stained plates, was performed using Kodak X-Omat MA film. Typical autoradiographs are illustrated.

absent from GT platelets. A different alloantigen (BaK[a], phenotype frequency 90.2 percent) was also absent from the platelets of four patients studied, which strongly suggests that this alloantigen is also located on the IIb/IIIa complex. In contrast, the alloantigens of the Ko-system were normally expressed on GT platelets.

Bernard-Soulier Syndrome

A second platelet disorder with an autosomal recessive inheritance, the Bernard-Soulier (B-S) syndrome is characterized by a moderate to severe thrombocytopenia, the presence of unusually large platelets on blood smears, and a number of proposed platelet function abnormalities.[15, 30] The primary hemostatic defect appears to be a markedly reduced platelet capacity to adhere to subendothelium.[36, 37]

A specific glycoprotein abnormality in B-S platelets was first described by Nurden and Caen,[38] who observed a much decreased carbohydrate staining intensity of the predominant band in the GP I region after the analysis of isolated B-S platelet membranes on SDS-PAGE. Further studies confirmed the abnormality by use of unfractionated platelets.[37] These and other early studies on the glycoproteins and proteins of B-S platelets have been discussed previously.[15] FIGURE 6 shows a typical PAS-profile of platelets isolated from a patient with the B-S syndrome; the absence of PAS-staining in the zone normally occupied by the Ib/Is band may be clearly observed.

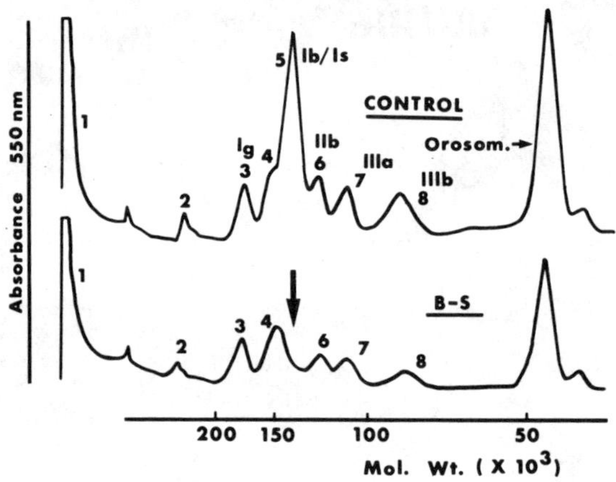

FIGURE 6. Glycoprotein composition of Bernard-Soulier (B-S) platelets. Washed normal human platelets and those isolated from a patient with the B-S syndrome were analyzed by SDS-polyacrylamide gel electrophoresis, as described in FIGURE 2. The glycoproteins were located by PAS-staining and an internal standard (orosomucoid) was added prior to the electrophoresis. To facilitate comparison of the profiles, the major platelet glycoprotein bands are labeled 1 through 8 on the figure.

The amount of radioactivity incorporated into GP Ib during lactoperoxidase-catalyzed ^{125}I-labeling of the platelet surface is small compared with the amounts of radioactivity incorporated into the other major membrane glycoproteins. An electrophoresis procedure giving a high resolution of the membrane glycoproteins is therefore required in order to detect modifications in the ^{125}I-labeling of Ib alone. FIGURE 7 illustrates the analysis of ^{125}I-labeled B-S platelets by means of the nonreduced/reduced two-dimensional system of SDS-polyacrylamide gel electrophoresis. No radioactivity was located in the Ib position on the B-S platelet autoradiograph; note also the apparent normal labeling of the other major membrane glycoproteins. Coomassie blue staining confirmed the absence of Ib from the B-S platelet gel, and in particular the absence of the small molecular weight β-subunit normally cleaved from Ib during disulfide bond reduction (data not shown). In our experience the

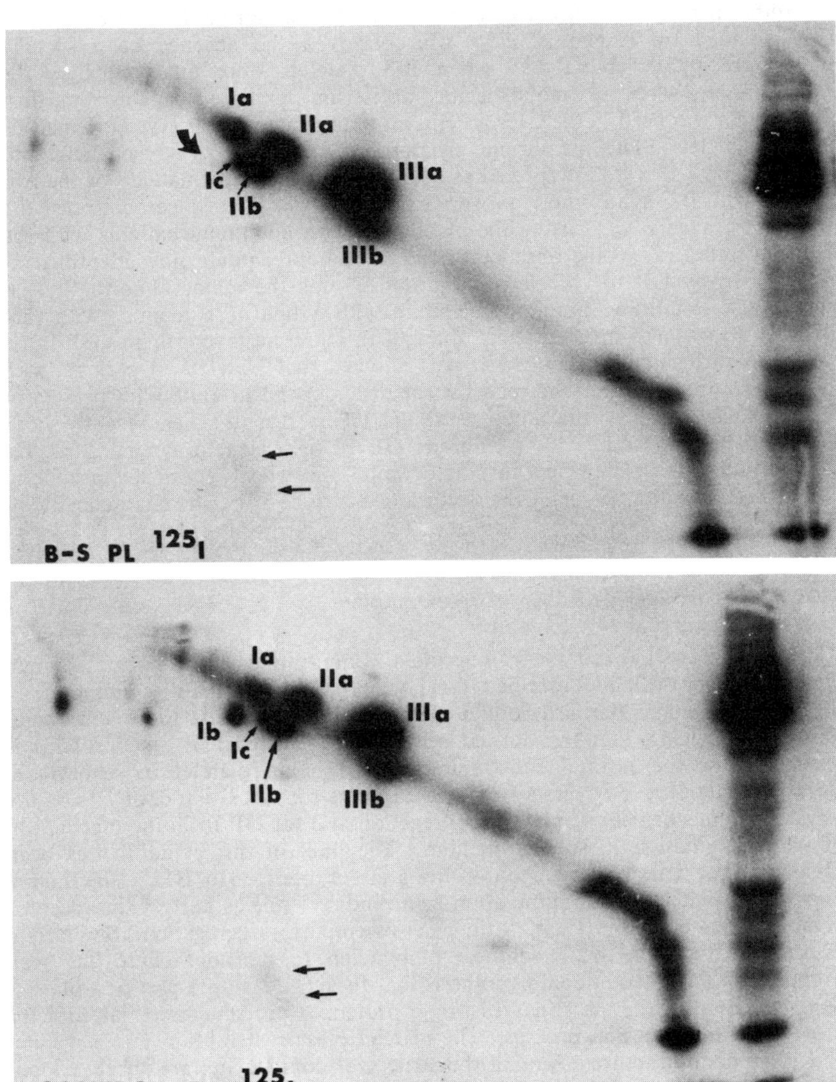

FIGURE 7. Surface defect of Bernard-Soulier (B-S) platelets. Washed normal human and B-S platelets were labeled with 125I and two-dimensional SDS-polyacrylamide gel electrophoresis was performed as described in FIGURE 4. Autoradiography of the dried gels was performed and is illustrated.

β-subunit of Ib is rarely located on autoradiographs, those of Ic and IIb only regularly showing detectable spots.

Additional evidence for a specific glycoprotein abnormality in B-S platelets was provided by Hagen et al.,[33] who observed the absence of a specific immunoprecipitate (band 13) when B-S platelets were analyzed by CIE. Furthermore, when a monospecific antiserum prepared against purified glycocalicin was used in the CIE system, no precipitate was observed on analysis of B-S platelets. The membrane glycoprotein precursor of glycocalicin and glycocalicin itself were interpreted as being missing from the platelets of the two patients with B-S syndrome who were examined. We have since confirmed the results of Hagen et al.[33] using the platelets of two additional patients with the B-S syndrome: a specific absence of the immunoprecipitate now identified as being given by GP Ib (labeled in FIGURE 5) was the major abnormality. A small, faster-migrating immunoprecipitate with a line of coidentity with that given by Ib was also missing and is thought to represent glycocalicin (GP Is).[19]

In an earlier study, Kunicki et al.[39] showed that platelets in patients with the B-S syndrome lacked the receptor for drug-dependent antibodies present in the platelets of all normal subjects tested. This receptor has recently been shown to be associated with membrane GP Ib or a structural analog of this glycoprotein as isolated by chromatography on wheat germ lectin affinity columns.[40] The absence of this receptor appears to be a specific characteristic of the B-S platelet surface.

CONCLUSIONS

We have emphasized the glycoprotein composition of the normal human platelet membrane and described the glycoprotein abnormalities observed in thrombasthenic and Bernard-Soulier platelets. It is clear that these abnormalities show, at least, that the normal presence of the deficient glycoproteins is necessary for the normal functioning of the blood platelet in hemostasis. Certain evidence also suggests fundamental roles for GP IIb and/or IIIa in the physiologic mechanism of platelet aggregation and for GP Ib in the mechanism of platelet adhesion to subendothelium. The bulk of this evidence has been reviewed elsewhere [15] and suggests either a direct role for IIb/IIIa in the linking together of platelets after stimulation or an indirect role as part of the receptor complex for a cofactor (Ca^{2+}, fibrinogen) essential for aggregation. Similarly a direct role for Ib in the attachment of platelets to subendothelium has been proposed, with the additional hypothesis that Ib may constitute part of a platelet receptor complex for the von Willebrand protein, a probable essential cofactor protein for the adhesion process. The platelet plasma membrane has a distinct and individual structure. Among the structural components are those responsible for the functional specificity of this remarkably active cell.

REFERENCES

1. PERRET, B., H. J. CHAP & L. DOUSTE-BLAZY. 1979. Asymmetric distribution of arachidonic acid in the plasma membrane of human platelets. A determination using purified phospholipases and a rapid method for membrane isolation. Biochim. Biophys. Acta 556:434–446.
2. CHAP, H. J., R. F. A. ZWAAL & L. L. M. VAN DEENEN. 1977. Action of highly

purified phospholipases on blood platelets: Evidence for an asymmetric distribution of phospholipids in the surface membrane. Biochim. Biophys. Acta **467**:146–164.

3. BARBER, A. J. & G. A. JAMIESON. 1970. Isolation and characterisation of plasma membranes from human blood platelets. J. Biol. Chem. **245**:6357–6365.

4. INSEL, P. A., P. NIRENBERG, J. TURNBULL & S. J. SHATTIL. 1978. Relationships between membrane cholesterol, α-adrenergic receptors, and platelet function. Biochemistry **17**:5269–5274.

5. STECK, T. L. 1974. The organization of proteins in the human red blood cell membrane. J. Cell Biol. **62**:1–19.

6. MARCHESI, V. T. 1979. Functional proteins of the human red blood cell membrane. Semin. Hematol. **16**:3–20.

7. TAYLOR, D. G., V. M. WILLIAMS & N. CRAWFORD. 1976. Platelet membrane actin. Solubility and binding studies with ^{125}I-labelled actin. Biochem. Soc. Trans. **4**:156–160.

8. PHILLIPS, D. R. & P. POH AGIN. 1977. Platelet plasma membrane glycoproteins. Evidence for the presence of nonequivalent disulfide bonds using nonreduced-reduced two-dimensional gel electrophoresis. J. Biol. Chem. **252**:2121–2126.

9. NACHMIAS, V., J. SULLENDER & A. ASCH. 1977. Shape and cytoplasmic filaments in control and lidocaine-treated platelets. Blood **50**:39–53.

10. GLOCKNER, W. M., H. D. KAULEN & G. UHLENBRUCK. 1978. Immunochemical detection of the Thomsen-Friedenreich antigen (T-antigen) on platelet plasma membranes. Thrombs. Haemostas. **39**:186–192.

11. GEORGE, J. N., R. K. MORGAN & P. C. LEWIS. 1978. Studies on platelet plasma membranes. IV. Quantitative analysis of platelet membrane glycoproteins by (^{125}I)-diazotized diiodosulfanilic acid labeling and SDS-polyacrylamide gel electrophoresis. J. Lab. Clin. Med. **92**:430–446.

12. McGREGOR, J. L., K. J. CLEMETSON, E. JAMES & M. DECHAVANNE. 1979. A comparison of techniques used to study externally orientated proteins and glycoproteins of human blood platelets. Thromb. Res. **16**:437–452.

13. McGREGOR, J. L., K. J. CLEMETSON, E. JAMES, T. GREENLAND & M. DECHAVANNE. 1979. Identification of human platelet glycoproteins in SDS-polyacrylamide gels using ^{125}I-labelled lectins. Thromb. Res. **16**:825–831.

14. LAEMMLI, U. K. 1970. Cleavage of structural proteins during the assembly of the head of bacteriophage T4. Nature **227**:680–685.

15. NURDEN, A. T. & J. P. CAEN. 1979. The different glycoprotein abnormalities in thrombasthenic and Bernard-Soulier platelets. Semin. Hematol. **16**:234–250.

16. LAWLER, J. W., H. S. SLAYTER & J. E. COLIGAN. 1978. Isolation and characterisation of a high molecular weight glycoprotein from human blood platelets. J. Biol. Chem. **253**:8609–8616.

17. OKUMURA, T. & G. A. JAMIESON. 1976. Platelet glycocalicin. I. Orientation of glycoproteins of the human platelet surface. J. Biol. Chem. **251**:5944–5949.

18. OKUMURA, T., C. LOMBART & G. A. JAMIESON. 1976. Platelet glycocalicin. II. Purification and characterisation. J. Biol. Chem. **251**:5950–5955.

19. SOLUM, N. O., I. HAGEN, C. FILION-MYKLEBUST & T. STABAEK. 1980. Platelet glycocalicin: Its membrane association and solubilisation in aqueous media. Biochim. Biophys. Acta. **597**: 235–246.

20. TAN, M. K., M. HARRISON & L. CORASH. 1978. Demonstration of the outer surface of freeze-etched normal human platelets: Correlation with buoyant density. Brit. J. Haematol. **40**:289–298.

21. SKAER, R. J., J. P. EMMINES & H. LE B. SKAER. 1979. The fine structure of cell contacts in platelet aggregation. J. Ultrastruct. Res. **69**:28–42.

22. FEAGLER, J. R., T. W. TILLACK, D. D. CHAPLIN & P. W. MAJERUS. 1974. The effects of thrombin on phytohemagglutinin receptor sites in human platelets. J. Cell Biol. **60**:541–553.

23. CHEVALIER, J., A. T. NURDEN, J. M. THIERY, E. SAVARIAU & J. P. CAEN. 1979.

Freeze-fracture studies on the plasma membranes of normal human, thrombasthenic and Bernard-Soulier platelets. J. Lab. Clin. Med. **94:**232–246.

24. PHILLIPS, D. R. & P. POH AGIN. 1977. Platelet plasma membrane glycoproteins. Identification of a proteolytic substrate for thrombin. Biochem. Biophys. Res. Commun. **75:**940–948.

25. MARCHESI, S. L. & J. A. CHASIS. 1979. Isolation of human platelet glycoproteins. Biochim. Biophys. Acta **555:**442–459.

26. CARTRON, J. P. & A. T. NURDEN. 1979. Galactosyltransferase and membrane glycoprotein abnormality in human platelets from Tn-syndrome donors. Nature **282:**621–623.

27. MUELLES-ECKHARDT, C. 1975. Immune reactions of platelets and their clinical significance. Klin. Wochenschr. **53:**889–897.

28. KUNICKI, T. J. & R. H. ASTER. 1979. Isolation and immunologic characterisation of the human platelet alloantigen, Pl^{A1}. Mol. Immunol. **16:**353–360.

29. TRAGARDH, L., L. KLARESKOG, B. CURMAN, L. RASK & P. A. PETERSON. 1979. Isolation and properties of detergent-solubilised HLA antigens obtained from platelets. Scand. J. Immunol. **9:**303–314.

30. HARDISTY, R. H. 1977. Disorders of platelet function. Brit. Med. Bull. **33:**207–212.

31. NURDEN, A. T. & J. P. CAEN. 1974. An abnormal platelet glycoprotein pattern in three cases of Glanzmann's thrombasthenia. Brit. J. Haematol. **28:**253–260.

32. HAGEN, I., O. J. BJERRUM & N. O. SOLUM. 1979. Characterisation of human platelet proteins solubilised with triton X-100 and examined by crossed immunoelectrophoresis. Reference patterns of extracts from whole platelets and isolated membranes. Eur. J. Biochem. **99:**9–22.

33. HAGEN, I., A. T. NURDEN, O. J. BJERRUM, N. O. SOLUM & J. P. CAEN. 1980. Immunochemical evidence for protein abnormalities in platelets from patients with Glanzmann's thrombasthenia and the Bernard-Soulier syndrome. J. Clin. Invest. **65:**722–731.

34. KUNICKI, T. J. & R. H. ASTER. 1978. Deletion of the platelet-specific alloantigen Pl^{A1} from platelets in Glanzmann's thrombasthenia. J. Clin. Invest. **61:**1225–1231.

35. VAN LEEUWEN, E. F., G. T. E. ZONNEVELS, L. E. RIESZ, C. S. P. JENKINS, J. A. VAN MOURIK & A. E. G. KR. VON DEM BORNE. 1979. Absence of the complete platelet-specific alloantigens $Zw(Pl^{A1})$ on platelets in Glanzmann's thrombasthenia and the effect of anti-Zw^a antibody on platelet-function. Thromb. Haemostas. **42:** 422(abstr.).

36. WEISS, H. J., T. B. TSCHOPP, H. R. BAUMGARTNER, I. I. SUSSMAN, M. M. JOHNSON & J. J. EGAN. 1974. Decreased adhesion of giant (Bernard-Soulier) platelets to subendothelium—further implications on the role of the von Willebrand factor in hemostasis. Am. J. Med. **57:**920–925.

37. CAEN, J. P., A. T. NURDEN, C. JEANNEAU, H. MICHEL, G. TOBELEM, S. LEVY-TOLEDANO, Y. SULTAN, F. VALENSI & J. BERNARD. 1976. Bernard-Soulier syndrome: A new platelet glycoprotein abnormality. Its relationship with platelet adhesion to subendothelium and with the factor VIII von Willebrand protein. J. Lab. Clin. Med. **87:**586–596.

38. NURDEN, A. T. & J. P. CAEN. 1975. Specific roles for platelet surface glycoproteins in platelet function. Nature **255:**720–722.

39. KUNICKI, T. J., M. M. JOHNSON & R. H. ASTER. 1978. Absence of the platelet receptor for drug-dependent antibodies in the Bernard-Soulier syndrome. J. Clin. Invest. **62:**716–719.

40. KUNICKI, T. J., N. RUSSELL, A. T. NURDEN, R. H. ASTER & J. P. CAEN. Further studies of the human platelet receptor for quinine- and quinidine-dependent antibodies. J. Immunol. In press.

41. DODGE, J. T., C. MITCHELL & D. J. HANAHAN. 1963. The preparation and chemical characterisation of hemoglobin-free ghosts of erythrocytes. Arch. Biochem. Biophys. **100:**119–130.

INTERACTION OF THROMBIN WITH PLATELETS: PURIFICATION OF THE THROMBIN SUBSTRATE *

Michael C. Berndt and David R. Phillips †

Department of Biochemistry
St. Jude Children's Research Hospital
Memphis, Tennessee 38101

The molecular mechanism by which α-thrombin activates platelets remains an essentially unsolved problem in hemostasis. Interaction of thrombin with the platelet plasma membrane is sufficient to trigger this event since α-thrombin covalently coupled to agarose beads will activate platelets.[1] The active site of thrombin plays a critical role since active-site-inhibited thrombin (by diisopropyl fluorophosphate [DFP], phenylmethanesulfonyl fluoride [PMSF], and 1-chloro-3-tosylamido-7-amino-L-2-heptanone [TLCK]) will not activate platelets.[2-5] Further, a number of proteases, such as trypsin,[2, 6] papain,[6] and thrombocytin,[7, 8] whose cleavage specificity overlaps that of α-thrombin, will activate platelets. Our working hypothesis for identification of the thrombin receptor on platelets is that interaction of thrombin with its receptor involves a hydrolytic event.

Despite the evidence for a simple hydrolytic mechanism, other aspects of thrombin-platelet interaction suggest a classical agonist-receptor equilibrium[6, 9] in that the amount of dense body secretion is proportional to thrombin concentration.[9, 10] Binding analyses employing ^{125}I-labeled α-thrombin indicate ~500 high-affinity binding sites with a K_d of ~1 nM and ~50,000 low-affinity binding sites with a K_d of ~100 nM.[3, 4, 11-13] Although the precise relationship between the two types of binding sites remains unclear,[4, 14] binding to both classes of sites is freely reversible with $k_{off} \geq 10^{-2}$ sec^{-1}.[4, 15] In contrast, if thrombin is reacted with an excess of platelets, the rate of appearance of catalytically active thrombin may be calculated from the data of Detwiler and Feinman to occur with a first-order rate constant of ~10^{-3} sec^{-1}.[9] Binding analyses using ^{125}I-labeled, active-site-inhibited α-thrombin (by DFP, PMSF and TLCK) yield the same number of binding sites and binding affinities as observed with native α-thrombin.[3, 4, 16] This competition for binding is not reflected in the functional response of platelets, since inhibited thrombin, even in a 1000-fold excess, is without effect on, or enhances, the subsequent response of platelets to catalytically active thrombin.[3, 5, 6]

The simplest explanation for these apparently conflicting results (that is, evidence with both an agonist-receptor equilibrium and hydrolysis) is that the measured thrombin binding does not reflect the functional thrombin receptor on human platelets since this receptor is proteolyzed by active thrombin and poorly recognized by inhibited thrombin. To be fully consistent with the known data, this interpretation further requires the formation of a relatively stable intermediate along the hydrolytic pathway (for example, an acyl enzyme) and that

* This work was suported in part by Grants HL 15616 and HL 21487 from the National Institutes of Health, United States Public Health Service.

† Recipient of Research Career Development Award HL 00080 from the National Heart, Lung and Blood Institute.

87

this intermediate decays or dissociates from the platelet plasma membrane before or as a consequence of the binding measurements.

As a preliminary test of our hypothesis that interaction of thrombin with its receptor involves a hydrolytic event, we have attempted to identify the thrombin substrate(s) on the platelet plasma membrane by utilizing a variety of protein and glycoprotein labeling procedures (FIG. 1). Washed human platelets[17] were labeled by treatment with either neuraminidase-galactose oxidase or periodate, followed by reduction with [³H]sodium borohydride.[18,19] These techniques only permit labeling of glycoproteins exposed on the platelet plasma membrane surface and provide minimal disruption to protein or carbohydrate structures. Thus, it is possible to discriminate between a hydrolytic event(s) on the platelet surface and those proteins lost from the platelet on thrombin treatment as a result of α-granule secretion (compare Refs. 20 and 21). The labeled platelets were incubated at 37° C in the absence and presence of α-thrombin (or other stimulus) for a designated time period. The platelet samples were centrifuged at 800 g for 10 minutes and the supernatant was removed from the platelet pellet and further centrifuged for 5 minutes at 8,730 g in a Beckman microfuge (Beckman Instruments, Inc., Spinco Division, Palo Alto, California). Platelet pellets and supernatants were prepared for electrophoresis by solubilization in 2 percent w/v sodium dodecyl sulfate (SDS) in the presence of 2 percent v/v β-mercaptoethanol and by heating at 100° C for 10 minutes. For one-dimensional analysis, protein was electrophoresed through slab gels according to the method of Laemmli[22] using either a 7.5 percent linear or a 5 to 15 percent exponential gradient of acrylamide in the resolving gel and 3 percent acrylamide in the stacking gel. Two-dimensional electrophoresis was performed according to the method of O'Farrell[23] (isoelec-

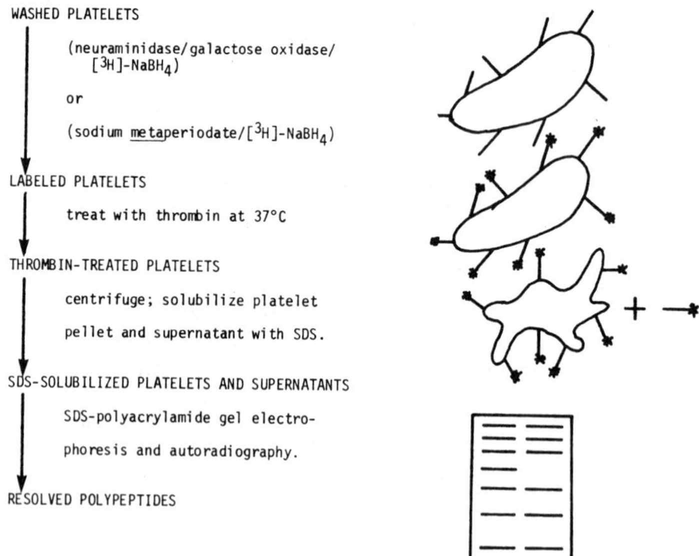

FIGURE 1. Experimental protocol for identification of the thrombin substrate(s) on human platelets.

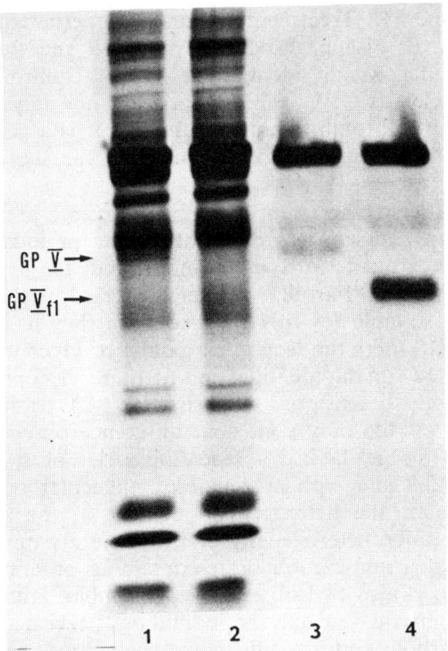

FIGURE 2. Platelet membrane glycoprotein profile upon treatment with α-thrombin. Washed platelets were labeled using sodium periodate and [³H]sodium borohydride. The labeled platelets (10^9/ml) in 0.01 M HEPES, pH 7.6 (0.15 M in sodium chloride, 1 mM in EDTA) were incubated at 37° C for 15 minutes in the absence and presence of 2.0 U/ml of α-thrombin. The platelets were then centrifuged at 800 g for 10 minutes and the supernatant was removed from the platelet pellet and centrifuged at 8,730 g for 5 minutes. Platelet pellets and supernatants were solubilized in 2 percent w/v SDS and electrophoresed according to the method of Laemmli on a 5 to 15 percent exponential gel of acrylamide; the gel was stained for protein and subjected to fluorography. Lane 1, control platelet pellet; lane 2, platelet pellet after thrombin treatment; lane 3, control platelet supernatant; lane 4, platelet supernatant after thrombin treatment.

tric focusing in the first dimension and SDS-polyacrylamide gel electrophoresis in the second dimension using a 5 to 15 percent exponential gradient of acrylamide [22]). Protein was stained with Coomassie brilliant blue, as previously described.[24] The tritium distribution in the dried gels was obtained by fluorography according to the method of Bonner and Laskey.[25]

Treatment of neuraminidase-galactose oxidase-labeled platelets [18, 26] or periodate-labeled platelets [26] (FIG. 2) with α-thrombin (>0.5 U/ml) for 15 min at 37° C caused the loss of only one platelet membrane glycoprotein, glycoprotein V (GPV), since GPV was no longer evident on the membrane (lane 1 versus lane 2) or in the supernatant (lane 4). A hydrolytic fragment, GPV_fl, appeared in the supernatant of the thrombin-treated platelets (lane 4). This is apparently a new molecular species since no band of corresponding mobility occurred in the pellet from control platelets (lane 1 versus lane 4). Trace amounts of GPV were observed in the supernatant of control periodate-labeled platelets (lane 3). Treatment of control supernatants with α-thrombin led to the reduction or disappearance of this band and the appearance of a band with a molecular weight identical to GPV_{f1} confirming that the band from untreated platelets is GPV. This experiment not only suggests that GPV is directly cleaved by α-thrombin, but also that GPV is a peripheral membrane glycoprotein, an observation used to advantage in the subsequent purification of this glycoprotein.

That GPV was the sole apparent thrombin substrate present on the plasma membrane of human platelets was confirmed using periodate-labeled platelets before and after treatment with α-thrombin and the two-dimensional gel electrophoretic system of O'Farrell.[23] Platelets labeled by the galactose oxidase procedure were not suitable for this purpose since they had been treated with neuraminidase, which alters the isoelectric points of glycoproteins.[27] Although this procedure allowed for the identification of more glycoproteins (>30) than were observed by one-dimensional analysis (FIG. 2) or nonreduced-reduced two-dimensional gels,[17] the only consistent difference observed upon thrombin treatment was that this gel lacked a repeating series of spots with isoelectric points from 5.8 to 6.8 and with an apparent molecular weight of GPV. As will be discussed later, the heterogeneity evident in the isoelectric focusing dimension is due to microheterogeneity of the same glycoprotein. Although it remains possible that a non-carbohydrate-containing protein or a glycoprotein in low concentration is also hydrolyzed by α-thrombin, labeling of the platelet membrane by lactoperoxidase-catalyzed iodination [17] revealed no protein moiety not labeled by the carbohydrate-specific methods employed here.

To determine whether glycoprotein V was directly cleaved by α-thrombin and to permit further characterization of this glycoprotein as the potential, functional thrombin receptor, glycoprotein V was purified to >98 percent homogeneity. The purification procedure is summarized in TABLE 1. Washed platelets [17] were prepared from platelet concentrates within 18 hours of venipuncture since clinically expired platelets (>72 hours from venipuncture) were shown to contain little or no detectable GPV. GPV was eluted from the platelet plasma membrane by equilibrating the washed platelets (4×10^9/ml) at 37° C for 24 hours in 0.01 M HEPES, pH 7.6 (0.3 M in sodium chloride, 1 mM in EDTA). After an initial ammonium sulfate fractionation, purification was achieved by successive chromatography on Sephacryl S-200, hydroxylapatite, DEAE- and CM-cellulose, and yielded 0.5–1.0 mg of purified glycoprotein per 100 units of platelet concentrate ($\sim 6 \times 10^{12}$ platelets). Protein eluted from the final CM-cellulose chromatography column as two partially resolved peaks. The first peak consisted of glycoprotein V, the latter fractions of which contained trace amounts of several polypeptides which formed the leading edge of the second partially resolved peak. On the basis of the observed elution profile and densitometric scans of the pooled material from several preparations, we estimate that the impurities constitute by mass no more than 1 to 2 percent of the purified glycoprotein.

The purified glycoprotein was >98 percent homogeneous and appeared identical to GPV from periodate-labeled platelets as judged by SDS-polyacrylamide gel electrophoresis and electrophoresis on O'Farrell gels. Purified GPV was a thrombin substrate and on hydrolysis yielded a major fragment, GPV_{f1}, identical in molecular weight to that previously observed in the supernatant of thrombin-treated periodate-labeled platelets (FIG. 3). GPV existed as at least eight distinct isoelectric forms with pI's ranging from 5.85 ± 0.05 to $6.55 \pm$

0.05. The four principal isoelectric forms had pI's of 6.04 ± 0.04, 6.12 ± 0.05, 6.20 ± 0.05 and 6.28 ± 0.06. At least six other human platelet glycoproteins show a similar pattern of equally spaced spots, suggesting that many of the platelet membrane glycoproteins display microheterogeneity, most likely due to variations in carbohydrate structure, as has been observed with other glycoproteins.[27] GPV and GPV_{fI} had apparent molecular weights of 82,000 and 69,500, respectively, as determined by SDS-polyacrylamide gel electrophoresis on 10 percent acrylamide gels. The purified glycoprotein contained ~48

TABLE 1

PURIFICATION OF HUMAN PLATELET GLYCOPROTEIN V

Step	Total Protein (A_{280})	A_{280}/A_{260}
Washed platelets	12,000	. . .
Extract *	960	1.46
40–50 percent ammonium sulfate fractionation †	91.5	1.69
Sephacryl S-200 ‡	10.5 §	1.45
Hydroxylapatite ‖	4.45 §	1.38
DEAE-cellulose #	1.84 §	1.28
CM-cellulose ¶	0.45–1.00 **	1.29

* Washed platelets, 100 units, 6×10^{12} platelets, 4×10^9/ml, equilibrated for 24 hours at 37° C in 0.01 M HEPES, pH 7.6 (1 mM in EDTA, 0.3 M in NaCl), were centrifuged at 750 g for 30 minutes and the supernatant extract was centrifuged at 35,000 g for 1 hour and dialyzed versus 0.05 M sodium phosphate, pH 6.8 (1 mM in EDTA).

† 40 to 50 percent ammonium sulfate fraction dialyzed versus 0.05 M sodium phosphate, pH 6.8 (1 mM in EDTA).

‡ Column dimensions, 5×75 cm; column buffer, 0.05 M sodium phosphate, pH 6.8 (1 mM in EDTA).

§ All glycoprotein-V-positive fractions pooled.

‖ Column dimensions, 1×20 cm; column buffer, 0.005 M potassium phosphate, pH 6.8 (0.2 mM in EDTA); glycoprotein was eluted with a 300-ml linear gradient, 0.005–0.2 M potassium phosphate (0.2 mM in EDTA).

Column dimensions, 0.7×14 cm; column buffer, 0.02 M sodium phosphate, pH 7.5 (0.2 mM in EDTA); the glycoprotein was coeluted with the flow through.

¶ Column dimensions, 0.7×7 cm; column buffer, 0.01 M sodium acetate, pH 4.5 (0.2 mM in EDTA); glycoprotein was eluted with a 100-ml linear gradient, 0–0.5 M NaCl.

** Corresponding to 0.5–1.0 mg of pure glycoprotein (average of four preparations).

percent carbohydrate by weight, consisting of neutral hexose, hexosamine, and sialic acid in a mole ratio of ~8:2:1. Rabbit antiglycoprotein V antibody gave a single precipitin line against purified GPV, which showed a reaction of complete identity with Triton-solubilized washed platelets.

Several lines of evidence suggest that hydrolysis of GPV may be of physiological significance with respect to thrombin activation of platelets. First, activation of platelets by nonproteolytic stimuli such as collagen, ADP/ fibrinogen and the calcium ionophore, A 23187, did not cause either the loss of GPV from the platelet membrane or the appearance of GPV_{fI} in the supernatant. Similar observations have been recently reported by Mosher and coworkers.[26] Further, hydrolysis of GPV did not occur on treatment of platelets with catalytically inactive, PMSF-inhibited α-thrombin. These results are in accord with hydrolysis of GPV being directly catalyzed by α-thrombin and not a consequence of platelet activation, that is, catalysis by a protease activated upon platelet stimulation. Since reagents that label GPV on intact platelets (sodium periodate, neuraminidase, and galactose oxidase) indicate that GPV is accessible to extracellular proteases and since apparently identical hydrolytic fragments are obtained from thrombin hydrolysis on platelets and with the

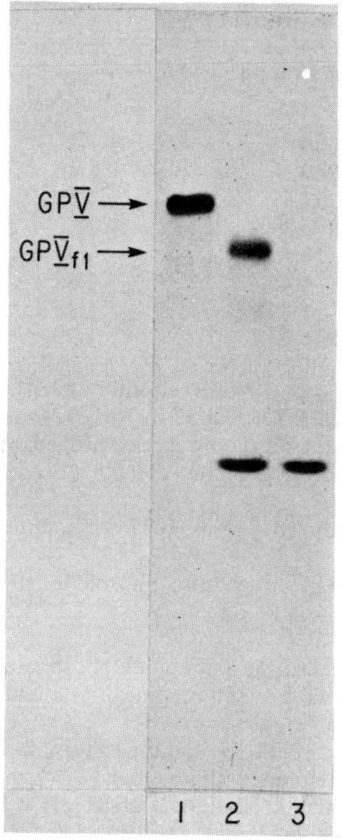

FIGURE 3. SDS-polyacrylamide gel electrophoresis of purified glycoprotein V and the thrombin hydrolytic product. Electrophoresis was performed according to the procedure of Laemmli on a 10 percent linear gel of acrylamide. GPV in 0.1 M sodium phosphate, pH 7.4, was treated with buffer or an equal concentration of α-thrombin for 1 minute at 22° C and solubilized ([glycoprotein V] = 40 μg/ml; [α-thrombin] = 50 U/ml). Lane 1, 2 μg of GPV; lane 2, thrombin digest of 2 μg of GPV; lane 3, α-thrombin.

purified glycoprotein, the available evidence indicates that glycoprotein V-thrombin interaction occurs on the platelet membrane surface.

A second line of evidence came from experiments performed to determine the rate of GPV hydrolysis relative to platelet response, as measured by platelet aggregation. Neuraminidase-galactose oxidase-labeled platelets were equilibrated for 2 min at 37° C with stirring. Thrombin (0.27 U/ml) was then added and aggregation followed, as seen by the change in light transmission in the Chrono-Log Model No. 300 aggregometer (Chrono-Log Corp., Havertown, Pennsylvania). At various time points during aggregation, the reaction was directly quenched by the addition of SDS (2 percent w/v final concentration) and the degree of hydrolysis of GPV quantitated by counting the radioactivity associated with the nonhydrolyzed GPV after SDS-polyacrylamide gel electrophoresis. Within 15 seconds, 70 percent of the maximally observed hydrolysis of GPV was complete and preceded platelet aggregation by 10 to 15 seconds. Quantitation of the other glycoprotein bands observed on SDS-polyacrylamide gel electrophoresis confirmed that the observed loss of GPV was the only significant change in the membrane glycoprotein profile.

To determine whether hydrolysis of GPV occurred over the range of α-thrombin concentrations known to elicit the platelet response, neuraminidase-galactose oxidase-labeled platelets were challenged with α-thrombin (0.005–10 U/ml) and the extent of aggregation followed for 3 minutes. The platelet samples were immediately subjected to rapid centrifugation (30 seconds) and the platelet pellets and supernatants were solubilized in 2 percent w/v SDS and analyzed by SDS-polyacrylamide gel electrophoresis. For one donor, the hydrolytic fragment of GPV, GPV_{fl}, appeared in the supernatant at α-thrombin concentrations of ≥ 0.01 U/ml; for the other donor at α-thrombin concentrations ≥ 0.02 U/ml. However, with both platelet samples, the concentration of thrombin required to observe measurable hydrolysis of glycoprotein V coincided with the concentration of thrombin required to induce an aggregation response.

It has long been recognized that proteases such as trypsin [2] and papain,[6] whose specificity for cleavage overlaps that of α-thrombin, will activate platelets in a manner similar to that of α-thrombin. We therefore examined the changes with time in the membrane glycoprotein profile on treatment of neuraminidase-galactose oxidase-labeled platelets with TPCK-trypsin (trypsin treated with L-1-p-tosylamino-2-phenylethyl chloromethyl ketone to inhibit residual chymotryptic activity). Although GPV was hydrolyzed rapidly under these conditions, it was not possible to correlate a molecular event with platelet activation since all the membrane glycoproteins were hydrolyzed to some extent over the time course of platelet activation. This inability to define a primary hydrolytic event during aggregation was further compounded in corresponding studies with relatively nonspecific proteases such as papain, bromelain, and thermolysin.

The failure of these studies with proteases of broad specificity led us to examine a series of proteases, γ-thrombin, thrombocytin, and α-clostripain, whose specificity of action more closely resembled that of α-thrombin. γ-Thrombin, a product of limited tryptic digestion of α-thrombin,[28] has full esterase activity, virtually no activity towards fibrinogen (clotting activity), and about 1 percent of the platelet-stimulating activity of α-thrombin.[29] Thrombocytin, a serine protease isolated from *Bothrops atrox* venom,[7] is very similar to α-thrombin in many of its activities.[8] It has been shown to activate platelets, causing release of storage granules and aggregation at concentrations of about 10^{-7} M. In contrast to α-thrombin, it has virtually no activity towards fibrinogen or factor VIII, and is not inhibited by hirudin and α_1-antitrypsin.[8] α-Clostripain is a sulfhydryl protease isolated from the culture filtrate of *Clostridium histolyticum*. The enzyme has an absolute requirement for calcium ions and almost total specificity for the carboxyl peptide linkage of arginine, although lysyl bonds are also cleaved, but at a much slower rate.[30, 31] We have found this protease to be a potent activator of platelets, with maximal platelet aggregation occurring at concentrations of enzyme greater than or equal to 1.5×10^{-8} M. Treatment of periodate-labeled platelets in Tyrode's solution at 37° C with α-thrombin (1 U/ml), γ-thrombin (4.7×10^{-7} M), thrombocytin (5.6×10^{-8} M) or α-clostripain (1.5×10^{-8} M) for 15 minutes caused in each case the partial or total cleavage of GPV and the appearance in the supernatant of a fragment with an identical molecular weight to GPV_{f1} as the sole or, in the case of α-clostripain, the major hydrolytic event on the plasma membrane.

The combined results suggest that hydrolysis of GPV may be of physiologic significance with respect to thrombin activation of platelets. GPV was the only detectible membrane surface protein hydrolyzed by thrombin. The purified glycoprotein was a thrombin substrate. Hydrolysis of glycoprotein V occurred only with proteolytic stimuli. Hydrolysis occurred at all physiologically active thrombin concentrations and preceded platelet aggregation by 10 to 15 seconds. Proteases of widely divergent evolutionary origin whose cleavage specificity is similar to that of α-thrombin will aggregate platelets, and all catalyzed the hydrolysis of GPV to GPV_{f1} as the sole or major hydrolytic event. Glycoprotein V thus fulfills several of the requirements expected of the functional thrombin receptor on human platelets.

ACKNOWLEDGMENT

It is a pleasure to acknowledge the generous gifts of α-thrombin and γ-thrombin given by Dr. J. W. Fenton, II, of the New York State Department of Health, Albany, New York.

REFERENCES

1. WORKMAN, E. F., JR., G. C. WHITE, II & R. L. LUNDBLAD. 1976. Platelet-thrombin interactions as assessed by affinity chromatography. Thromb. Res. **9:**491–503.
2. DAVEY, M. G. & E. F. LÜSCHER. 1967. Actions of thrombin and other coagulant and proteolytic enzymes on blood platelets. Nature (Lond.) **216:**857–858.
3. TOLLEFSEN, D. M., J. R. FEAGER & P. W. MAJERUS. 1974. The binding of thrombin to the surface of human platelets. J. Biol. Chem. **249:**2646–2651.
4. WORKMAN, E. F., JR., G. C. WHITE, II & R. L. LUNDBLAD. 1977. Structure-function relationships in the interaction of α-thrombin with blood platelets. J. Biol. Chem. **252:**7118–7123.
5. PHILLIPS, D. R. 1974. Thrombin interaction with human platelets. Potentiation of thrombin-induced aggregation and release by inactivated thrombin. Thromb. Diath. Haemorrh. **32:**207–215.
6. MARTIN, B. M., R. D. FEINMAN & T. C. DETWILER. 1975. Platelet stimulation by thrombin and other proteases. Biochemistry **14:**1308–1314.
7. KIRBY, E. P., S. NIEWIAROWSKI, K. STOCKER, C. KETTNER, E. SHAW & T. M. BRUDZYNSKI. 1979. Thrombocytin, a serine protease from *Bothrops atrox* venom. 1. Purification and characterization of the enzyme. Biochemistry **18:**3564–3570.
8. NIEWIAROWSKI, S., E. P. KIRBY, T. M. BRUDZYNSKI & K. STOCKER. 1979. Thrombocytin, a serine protease from *Bothrops atrox* venom. 2. Interaction with platelets and plasma-clotting factors. Biochemistry **18:**3570–3577.
9. DETWILER, T. C. & R. D. FEINMAN. 1973. Kinetics of the thrombin-induced release of calcium(II) by platelets. Biochemistry **12:**282–289.
10. DETWILER, T. C. & R. D. FEINMAN. 1973. Kinetics of the thrombin-induced release of adenosine triphosphate by platelets. Comparison with release of calcium. Biochemistry **12:**2462–2468.
11. SHUMAN, M. A., D. M. TOLLEFSEN & P. W. MAJERUS. 1976. The binding of human and bovine thrombin to human platelets. Blood **47:**43–54.

12. MARTIN, B. M., W. W. WASIEWSKI, J. W. FENTON, II, & T. C. DETWILER. 1976. Equilibrium binding of thrombin to platelets. Biochemistry **15**:4886–4893.

13. TAM, S. W. & T. C. DETWILER. 1978. Binding of thrombin to human platelet plasma membranes. Biochim. Biophys. Acta **543**:194–201.

14. TOLLEFSEN, D. M. & P. W. MAJERUS. 1976. Evidence for a single class of thrombin-binding sites on human platelets. Biochemistry **15**:2144–2149.

15. TAM, S. W., J. W. FENTON, II, & T. C. DETWILER. 1979. Dissociation of thrombin from platelets by hirudin. Evidence for receptor processing. J. Biol. Chem. **254**:8723–8725.

16. GANGULY, P. 1974. Binding of thrombin to human platelets. Nature (Lond.) **247**:306–307.

17. PHILLIPS, D. R. & P. P. AGIN. 1977. Platelet plasma membrane glycoproteins. Evidence for the presence of nonequivalent disulfide bonds using nonreduced-reduced two-dimensional gel electrophoresis. J. Biol. Chem. **252**:2121–2126.

18. PHILLIPS, D. R. & P. P. AGIN. 1977. Platelet plasma membrane glycoproteins. Identification of a proteolytic substrate for thrombin. Biochem. Biophys. Res. Commun. **75**:940–947.

19. GAHMBERG, C. G. & L. C. ANDERSSON. 1977. Selective radioactive labeling of cell surface sialoglycoproteins by periodate-tritiated borohydride. J. Biol. Chem. **252**:5888–5894.

20. BAENZIGER, N. L., G. N. BRODIE & P. W. MAJERUS. 1972. Isolation and properties of a thrombin-sensitive protein of human platelets. J. Biol. Chem. **247**:2723–2731.

21. LAWLER, J. W., H. S. SLAYTER & J. E. COLIGAN. 1978. Isolation and characterization of a high molecular weight glycoprotein from human blood platelets. J. Biol. Chem. **253**:8609–8616.

22. LAEMMLI, U. K. 1970. Cleavage of structural proteins during the assembly of the head of bacteriophage T_4. Nature (Lond.) **227**:680–685.

23. O'FARRELL, P. H. 1975. High resolution two-dimensional electrophoresis of proteins. J. Biol. Chem. **250**:4007–4021.

24. PHILLIPS, D. R. 1972. Effects of trypsin on the exposed polypeptides and glycoproteins in the human platelet membrane. Biochemistry **11**:4582–4588.

25. BONNER, W. A. & R. A. LASKEY. 1974. A film detection method for tritium-labelled proteins and nucleic acids in polyacrylamide gels. Eur. J. Biochem. **46**:83–88.

26. MOSHER, D. F., A. VAHERI, J. J. CHOATE & C. G. GAHMBERG. 1979. Action of thrombin on surface glycoproteins of human platelets. Blood **53**:437–445.

27. BAUMANN, H. & D. DOYLE. 1979. Localization of membrane glycoproteins by *in situ* neuraminidase treatment of rat hepatoma tissue culture cells and two-dimensional gel electrophoretic analysis of the modified proteins. J. Biol. Chem. **254**:2542–2550.

28. FENTON, J. W., II, B. H. LANDIS, D. A. WALZ & J. S. FINLAYSON. 1977. Human thrombins. *In* Chemistry and Biology of Thrombin. R. L. Lundblad, J. W. Fenton & K. G. Mann, Eds.: 43–70. Ann Arbor Science. Ann Arbor, Mich.

29. CHARO, I. F., R. D. FEINMAN & T. C. DETWILER. 1977. Interrelations of platelet aggregation and secretion. J. Clin. Invest. **60**:866–873.

30. MITCHELL, W. M. & W. F. HARRINGTON. 1968. Purification and properties of clostripeptidase B (clostripain). J. Biol. Chem. **243**:4683–4692.

31. PORTER, W. H., L. W. CUNNINGHAM & W. M. MITCHELL. 1971. Studies on the active site of clostripain. The specific inactivation by the chloromethyl ketone derived from α-N-tosyl-L-lysine. J. Biol. Chem. **246**:7675–7682.

FACTORS AFFECTING THE HIGH-AFFINITY BINDING OF THROMBIN TO PLATELETS *

G. A. Jamieson, S. M. Jung, and A. Ordinas

*American Red Cross Blood Services
Bethesda, Maryland 20014*

Introduction

The binding of thrombin to platelets exhibits complex kinetics [1-3] indicative of either negative cooperativity among a single class of binding sites [4] or the existence of two classes of surface receptor.[5] These studies have shown that platelets appear to have on their surface about 50,000 sites of low affinity for thrombin ($K_d \sim 30$ nM) and about 500 sites of high affinity ($K_d \sim 3$ nM), although there is an apparent 10-fold increase in the number of high-affinity sites when the assay is carried out in cacodylate buffer.[6]

Relationship of Glycoprotein I and Thrombin-Binding

The surface of platelets is rich in carbohydrate and several studies have suggested that surface glycoproteins may be involved in various aspects of the interaction of platelets with thrombin. Glycocalicin (M_r, 150,000) is a glycoprotein that is present on the surface of intact platelets, but is released in soluble form after platelet homogenization.[7] It appears to be closely related to glycoprotein I, which remains bound to the membrane after homogenization. Glycocalicin has been purified to homogeneity [8,9] and shown to inhibit the aggregation of platelets induced by either ristocetin or by thrombin.[10] The fact that Bernard-Soulier platelets were known not to undergo ristocetin-induced aggregation led us to suggest that these platelets would also show defective aggregation with thrombin. This suggestion was confirmed by studies in two persons with the Bernard-Soulier syndrome, in which it was found that there was a reduction in the rate of thrombin-induced aggregation of washed platelets and that this was particularly marked at suboptimal thrombin concentrations of 60 to 120 milliunits/ml.[11] These patients also showed a decrease from 4000 to 1500 in the number of high-affinity sites for thrombin, although the dissociation constant (~4 nM) was unchanged and there was a proportional decrease in the number of low-affinity sites from 24,000 to 8800, although the dissociation constant was again identical with control values (~37 nM).

Several other studies have suggested a relationship between the amount of the glycoprotein I complex present on platelets and the amount of thrombin that will bind to them. First, examination of glycoprotein distribution in sixteen patients with myeloproliferative disease showed a statistically significant reduction in the relative amount of glycoprotein I present on their platelets.[12]

* This work (contribution No. 492 from the American Red Cross Blood Services) was supported in part by Grants HL 20971 and HL 14697 and Biomedical Research Support Grant 2 SO7 RR05737 from the United States Public Health Service.

96

This has been correlated with a decrease in the amount of thrombin bound, although the affinity was unchanged A$K_d \sim 2$ nM), and in their ability to undergo thrombin-induced aggregation,[13] but there was wide individual variation between patients in all of these cases. Second, two unrelated patients, who had been identified with an ill-defined bleeding diathesis, showed a doublet in the region of glycoprotein I comprising a component with a molecular weight equal to that of glycoprotein I, but present in half the normal amount, and another glycoprotein present in the same amount but with a molecular weight 10,000 to 12,000 daltons less.[14] Only one-half the normal amount of thrombin binding was determined in these patients: 2400 high-affinity sites per platelet were calculated as against 5400 for normal control subjects, but the affinity of binding was identical ($K_d = 3.5$ nM). Third, when intact platelets were treated with chymotrypsin, the loss of both glycoprotein I and glycocalicin paralleled the loss in ability to bind thrombin.[15]

ASSOCIATION OF RECEPTORS

The studies described earlier provide circumstantial evidence for a relationship between the amount of thrombin bound to platelets and the amount of glycoprotein I/glycocalicin present on their surface. When the relationship between high-affinity and low-affinity receptors is considered, one possibility is that the affinity might be affected by factors influencing the ability of receptors to associate and dissociate within the plane of the membrane. Receptor clustering has been proposed as the basis for negative cooperativity on theoretical grounds [16] and in relation to the binding of insulin.[17, 18]

Support for the view that similar considerations might be applicable in the case of platelets arose from the observations that changes in membrane microviscosity could affect platelet responsiveness. Specifically, an increase in the membrane microviscosity of platelets by incubation with cholesterol-rich liposomes results in an increase in their sensitivity to aggregating agents such as epinephrine and adenosine diphosphate (ADP),[19] an increase in basal activity of adenylate cyclase,[20] a decreased responsiveness to prostaglandin E_1 (PGE_1),[21] and an increased production of thomboxanes.[22] It is interesting that there is a parallel increase in responsiveness to aggregating agents in patients with type IIa hyperlipoproteinemia.[23] Only in the case of epinephrine-induced aggregation were binding studies carried out, in this case using dihydroergocryptine, which is a specific α-adrenergic antagonist. No difference could be detected between cholesterol-rich and normal platelets with respect to the time course of binding, the affinity of binding ($K_d \sim 4$ nM), or the number of binding sites per platelet ($\sim$350).[24]

In an extension of this work we have found that the ability of platelets to bind thrombin is affected by the relative proportions of cholesterol and phospholipid. After platelets were incubated with liposomes containing a normal ratio of cholesterol and phospholipid (C:P = 0.62), the number of high-affinity sites (3000) was similar to that of normal control subjects, indicating that the incubation procedure itself did not affect the ability of the platelets to bind thrombin. However, when platelets were incubated with cholesterol-rich liposomes, the cholesterol:phospholipid ratio in the platelets was increased to 1.06. In this situation the K_d was essentially unchanged (0.8 nM), but the number of high-affinity sites was increased to 8700. Conversely, the number of high-affinity sites was decreased to 1700 in platelets that had had their cholesterol: phospholipid ratio decreased to 0.45 by incubation with phospholipid-rich liposomes, although the affinity at these sites was unaffected ($K_d = 1$ nM). These results suggest that increases in membrane microviscosity result in increased binding, whereas decreases in microviscosity result in decreased binding. These effects could be due either to the influence of membrane microviscosity on the clustering of receptors or to passive modulation of the exposure of receptors above the membrane surface.[25, 26]

Chemical Crosslinking

We have previously shown that platelets fixed with formaldehyde retain the ability to bind thrombin and that the number of high-affinity sites (3000) and the affinity at those sites ($K_d \sim 3$ nM) is similar to that in control, washed platelets.[15] More recently, we have found that platelets fixed with glutaraldehyde also retain their ability to bind thrombin with high affinity ($K_d = 2.5$ nM). In this case, the number of high-affinity sites is increased to 34,000, which is equal to the total number of low- and high-affinity sites in control platelets. Moreover, low-affinity binding could not be detected in the glutaraldehyde-fixed platelets.

Table 1
High-Affinity Binding of Thrombin in the Presence of Lectins

Lectin	Specificity	Washed Platelets		Formalinized Platelets	
		n_H	K_d	n_H	K_d
None		3300	4.4	1100	4.0
WGA	GlcNAc	14,100	3.9	5800	6.9
Con A	Glc, Man	14,200	5.0	450	6.8
Ricinus communis	Gal	11,200	2.3	2500	4.3
Bandieria simplicifolia	Gal, GalNAc	5,200	3.6	3000	5.0
Lens culinaris	Glc, Man	5,800	4.3	300	1.8

Lectin Effects

Previous studies have shown that the thrombin-binding site of glycoprotein I/glycocalicin is present in the carbohydrate-poor peptide "tail" portion (M_r 45,000) of the molecule and not in the carbohydrate-rich macroglycopeptide. In a further approach to the study of the effects of the association of receptors, we have used lectins on the assumption that they might link the macroglycopeptide portions of glycoprotein I/glycocalicin without blocking the access of thrombin to the binding site.

In the first series of studies blocked (diisopropyl [DIP]) thrombin was used to avoid complications caused by the release reaction. None of the lectins examined affected the affinity of DIP-thrombin for platelets, but wheat-germ agglutinin (WGA), concanavalin A (Con A), and the lectin of *Ricinus communis* caused a four- to five-fold increase in the amount of thrombin bound, and the lectins of *Bandieria simplicifolia* and *Lens culinaris* caused an increase of about two-fold (Table 1). Even with formalinized platelets there was a five-fold increase with WGA and a two- to three-fold increase with *Ricinus communis* and *Bandieria simplicifolia*. Interestingly, there was an apparent decrease in this system in the number of high-affinity sites in the presence of Con A and the lectin of *Lens culinaris* (TABLE 1). Again, there appeared to be no significant change in the affinity of binding with any of the lectins examined.

DISCUSSION

These results suggest that the high-affinity binding of thrombin to platelets is inversely related to the capability for movement of receptors in the membrane. Thus, increases in membrane microviscosity or the use of lectins might be expected to reduce the rate of dissociation of oligomers of receptor molecules, but not to prevent it, and in these cases there is a significant increase in the amounts of thrombin bound. In the case of chemical crosslinking with glutaraldehyde it would be expected that receptor molecules would be fixed in a particular conformation with each other, and in this case there appeared to be a complete conversion of low-affinity sites to high-affinity sites. Obviously, further work is necessary to clarify the relationship between receptor mobility and thrombin binding and to determine whether these changes affect the responsiveness of platelets to thrombin-induced aggregation.

REFERENCES

1. GANGULY, P. 1974. Binding of thrombin to human platelets. Nature **267:** 306–307.
2. TOLLEFSEN, D. M., J. R. FEAGLER & P. W. MAJERUS. 1974. The binding of thrombin to the surface of human platelets. J. Biol. Chem. **249:** 2646–2651.
3. MARTIN, B. M., W. W. WASIEWSKI, J. W. FENTON, II & T. C. DETWILER. 1970. Equilibrium binding of thrombin to platelets. Biochemistry **15:** 4886–4893.
4. WORKMAN, E. F., G. C. WHITE & R. L. LUNDBLAD. 1977. Structure-function relationships in the interaction of α-thrombin with blood platelets. J. Biol. Chem. **252:** 7118–7123.
5. TOLLEFSEN, D. M. & P. W. MAJERUS. 1976. Evidence for a single class of thrombin-binding sites on human platelets. Biochemistry **15:** 2144–2149.
6. SHUMAN, M. A. & P. W. MAJERUS. 1975. The perturbation of thrombin binding to human platelets by anions. J. Clin. Invest. **56:** 945–950.
7. OKUMURA, T. & G. A. JAMIESON. 1976. Platelet glycocalicin. I. Orientation of glycoproteins of the human platelet surface. J. Biol. Chem. **251:** 5944–5949.
8. LOMBART, C., T. OKUMURA & G. A. JAMIESON. 1974. Isolation of a surface glycoprotein of human platelets. FEBS. Lett. **41:** 30–34.
9. OKUMURA, T. & G. A. JAMIESON. 1976. Platelet glycocalicin. II. Purification and characterization, J. Biol. Chem. **251:** 5950–5955.
10. OKUMURA, T. & G. A. JAMIESON. 1976. Platelet glycocalicin: A single receptor for platelet aggregation induced by thrombin ristocetin. Thromb. Res. **8:** 701–706.
11. JAMIESON, G. A. & T. OKUMURA. 1978. Reduced thrombin binding and aggregation in Bernard-Soulier platelets. J. Clin. Invest. **61:** 861–864.
12. BOLIN, R. B., T. OKUMURA & G. A. JAMIESON. 1977. Changes in distribution of platelet membrane glycoproteins in patients with myeloproliferative disorders. Am. J. Hematol. **3:** 63–71.
13. GANGULY, P., S. B. SUTHERLAND & H. R. BRADFORD. 1978. Defective binding of thrombin to platelets in myeloid leukemia. Brit. J. Haematol. **39:** 599–605.

14. BOLIN, R. B., T. OKUMURA & G. A. JAMIESON. 1977. A new polymorphism of platelet membrane glycoproteins. Nature **269:** 69–70.
15. OKUMURA, T., M. HASITZ & G. A. JAMIESON. 1978. Platelet glycocalicin: Interaction with thrombin and role as thrombin receptor of the platelet surface. J. Biol. Chem. **253:** 3435–3443.
16. LEVITZKI, A. 1974. Negative co-operativity in clustered receptors as a possible basis for membrane action. J. Theo. Biol. **44:** 367–372.
17. DE MEYTS, P. 1976. Cooperative properties of hormone receptors in cell membranes. J. Supramol. Struct. **4:** 241–258.
18. KAHN, C. R., K. L. BAIRD, D. B. JARRET & J. S. FLIER. 1977. Direct demonstration that receptor crosslinking or aggregation is important in insulin action. Proc. Natl. Acad. Sci. USA **75:** 4209–4213.
19. SHATTIL, S. J., R. ANAYA-GALINDO, J. BENNETT, R. W. COLMAN & R. A. COOPER. 1975. Platelet hypersensitivity induced by cholesterol incorporation. J. Clin. Invest. **55:** 636–643.
20. SINHA, A. K., S. J. SHATTIL & R. W. COLMAN. 1978. Cyclic AMP metabolism in cholesterol-rich platelets. J. Biol Chem. **252:** 3310–3314.
21. COLMAN, R. W., S. J. SHATTIL & J. S. BENNETT. 1975. Cholesterol-rich platelets are resistant to inhibition by prostaglandin E_1 (PGE_1). Blood **46:** 1033.
22. STUART, M. J., J. M. GERRARD & J. G. WHITE. 1980. Effect of cholesterol on production of thomboxane B_2 by platelets. New Engl. J. Med. **302:** 6–10.
23. CARVALHO, A. C., R. W. COLMAN & R. S. LEES. 1974. Platelet function in hyperlipoproteinemia. New Engl. J. Med. **290:** 434–438.
24. INSEL, P. A., P. NIRENBERG, J. TURNBULL & S. J. SHATTIL. 1978. Relationship between membrane cholesterol, α-adrenergic receptors and platelet function. Biochemistry **17:** 5269–5274.
25. BOROCHOV, H. & M. SHINITZKY. 1976. Vertical displacement of membrane proteins mediated by changes in microviscosity. Proc. Natl. Acad. Sci. USA **73:** 4526–4530.
26. BOROCHOV, H., R. E. ABBOTT, D. SCHACHTER & M. SHINITZKY. 1979. Modulation of erythrocyte membrane proteins by membrane cholesterol and lipid fluidity. Biochemistry **18:** 251–255.

ROLE OF PLATELETS IN TUMOR CELL METASTASES

Simon Karpatkin,* Edward Pearlstein,†
Peter L. Salk,‡ and Ganesa Yogeeswaran §

*Departments of Medicine *† and Pathology,† and
Irvington House Institute †
New York University Medical School
New York, New York 10016; and
Autoimmune and Neoplastic Disease Laboratory,‡ and
Department of Cancer Biology §
The Salk Institute for Biological Studies
San Diego, California 92138*

INTRODUCTION

It has previously been demonstrated that certain animal tumor cells or media conditioned by these cells will induce platelet aggregation *in vitro*.[1-3] The significance of this result is apparent in light of evidence from several laboratories indicating that tumor cells may also aggregate platelets *in vivo*,[4-10] that blood-borne metastatic tumor cells induce thrombocytopenia in the host,[1] and that thrombocytopenia impairs the development of metastasis.[11] Furthermore, a rough correlation can be made between *in vitro* induction of platelet aggregation by certain tumor cells and their propensity for lung metastasis.[1, 6] These observations imply a direct role for the platelet in the pathogenesis of tumor cell metastasis.

In order to define the mechanism of platelet–tumor-cell interaction, an *in vitro* system was developed employing the normal mouse fibroblast cell line 3T3 as a control and the virally transformed SV3T3 cell line as the tumor cell. A technique has been established for extracting platelet-aggregating material (PAM) from the transformed cell. This PAM has been partially characterized and its mechanism of action studied.

A spontaneously metastatic, polyoma-induced PW20 renal sarcoma in the Wistar-Furth rat was also examined *in vivo* and *in vitro* for degree of metastasis, cell-surface sialylation, and *in vitro* platelet-aggregating ability. Ten cell lines from the PW20 transformed parent cell line were selected by tissue and animal passage for their varying ability to develop metastases after subcutaneous injection.[12]

MATERIAL AND METHODS

Cell Culture

A low-passage Balb C/3T3 fibroblast cell line and its SV40 virally transformed derivative (SV3T3) were obtained from stocks at the Imperial Cancer Research Fund, London, and were maintained in Dulbecco's modified Eagle's medium (E4) supplemented with 10 percent fetal calf serum, 2 mM glutamine,

101

100 U/ml penicillin, and 100 μg/ml streptomycin.[13] Cells were "passaged" twice weekly.

The PW20 family of tumor cell lines (TABLE 1) was derived from a culture of the polyoma virus-induced PW20 renal sarcoma in Wistar-Furth rats (obtained from Dr. H. O. Sjögren, University of Lund, Sweden) by varying conditions of passage in tissue culture and passage through syngeneic animals.[14] The R0(L) and R0(H) cell lines represent low and high tissue culture passages, respectively, of the original cell culture. The R1 cell line was obtained by reestablishing a subcutaneous R0(L) tumor in tissue culture, and maintaining the culture for a large number of passages. The R2 cell line was similarly produced by reculturing a subcutaneous R1 tumor and maintaining the resultant

TABLE 1

DERIVATION OF PW20 TUMOR CELL LINES

Derivative Lines	Number of Passages *	Number of *in Vitro* Subcultures Tested †
RO(L)	0	11–19
RO(H)	0	276–283
RO(L)R1	1	18
RO(H)R1	1	3
R1	1	88–92
R2	2	80–84
R2R1	3	6–16
R2L1	3	5–7
R2N1	3	5–6
R2R2	4	6

* Number of passages in the animal since receipt of the original PW20 cell line from Dr. Sjögren.

† Number of subcultures after establishment of each new derivative line. For RO(L) and RO(H) cell line the number represents the number of subcultures after receipt of the original cell line. The numbers listed represent the number of the subculture used for testing of metastatic properties.

culture for a prolonged period. The R0(L)R1, R0(H)R1, R2R1, and R2R2 cell lines were produced by reculturing subcutaneous R0(L), R0(H), R2, and R2R1 tumors, respectively; the R2L1 and R2N1 cell lines were obtained by culturing explanted lung (L) and lymph node (N) metastases that developed from subcutaneous R2 tumors. These latter lines were all tested at low-passage numbers. *In vitro* assays were performed using cells within several passages of those listed in TABLE 1, obtained either from the same cells used for *in vivo* testing or from an aliquot of identical cells preserved in liquid nitrogen. For the *in vitro* assays, the cell lines were maintained as described earlier for the 3T3 fibroblast cell line.

Evaluation of Metastatic Properties

The spontaneous metastatic behavior of the tumor cell lines was evaluated in syngeneic Wistar-Furth rats of both sexes obtained from Microbiological Associates, Inc. Tumorigenic doses of cultured cells were injected subcutaneously in the loose skin of the animals' midback. Tumors were measured at regular intervals after injection and, upon reaching a weight of 2–6 grams, were excised by means of a closed surgical technique. The animals were then observed for the development of palpable regional lymph node metastases and/or clinical signs suggestive of internal metastases to the lung or other organs. Animals with large external metastases or with signs of visceral metastatic growth were sacrificed and a thorough search was conducted for macroscopic metastases to regional lymph nodes or intrathoracic and intraabdominal sites. Asymptomatic animals were similarly sacrificed after a prolonged period of observation. In some experiments the lungs were injected with india ink and fixed according to the method of Wexler[15] in order to facilitate visualization of the metastatic nodules.

Percent Sialylation of Cell-Surface Glycoconjugates

The percentage of sialylation of exposed cell-surface glycoconjugates was determined by the galactose oxidase-sodium borotritide labeling technique, as previously described.[16] This procedure results in the tritiation of terminal galactosyl (Gal) and *N*-acetyl galactosaminyl (GalNAc) groups on exposed cell-surface carbohydrates. Gal and GalNAc groups that are further substituted with sialic acid are protected from labeling. It is therefore possible to determine the percentage of the exposed terminal Gal and GalNAc groups that are sialylated by labeling cells with and without prior incubation with neuraminidase, which cleaves terminal sialic acid residues from the saccharide chains. Galactose oxidase was obtained from A. B. Kabi (Stockholm, Sweden), *Vibrio cholera* neuraminidase was obtained from Calbiochem/Behring (La Jolla, California), and sodium borotritide (4–6 Ci/mmol) was obtained from Amersham/Searle Corp. (Arlington Heights, Illinois).

PAM

Extraction

Cells were grown to confluency on 10-cm tissue-culture dishes and washed twice with Veronal® buffer (11.75 g of sodium diethyl barbiturate, 14.67 g of sodium chloride, 430 ml of 0.1 N HCl, H_2O to 2 L, final pH 7.4). Three milliliters of 1 M urea, dissolved in Veronal buffer, were then added. Dishes were shaken at 30° C for 1 hour in a 5 percent CO_2 atmosphere, the supernatants were spun at 2000 $\times$ g for 5 minutes to remove any floating cells, and the cell-free supernatant was dialyzed against several changes of Veronal buffer for 2 days at 4° C. (Viability of the adherent cells was greater than 90 percent, as judged by trypan blue exclusion after this treatment). After dialysis, the supernatant was concentrated in an Amicon chamber with the use of an XM100 membrane (Amicon Corp., Lexington, Massachusetts) to 1/100 the volume of 1 M urea used in the original extraction (approximately 100 μg/ml protein). In parallel cultures, cells were extracted with E4 or 0.3 mM KCl, and extracts were processed in an identical fashion.

Total Sialic Acid Content

The sialic acid content of PAM was determined by the thiobarbituric acid method of Warren,[17] using N-acetyl neuraminic acid (Sigma Chemical Corp., St. Louis, Missouri) as a standard.

Protein Content

The protein content of PAM was determined by the method of Lowry et al.,[18] using bovine serum albumin as a standard.

Centrifugation

To determine whether PAM was sedimentable, 0.5 ml of extract was spun at $100,000 \times g$ for 1 hour at 4° C in a Beckman L2-65B ultracentrifuge equipped with an SW40Ti rotor (Beckman Instruments, Inc., Fullerton, California). After centrifugation, the supernatant was removed, and the pellet was resuspended in 0.5 ml of Veronal buffer.

Enzyme Treatment

Ten microliters of an enzyme solution were added to 100 μl of PAM (100 μg/ml protein) to give the final enzyme concentration shown in TABLE 5, and the mixture was incubated for 1 hour at 37° C. Enzymes were shown to be active with their respective substrates prior to use. A 50-μl amount of either treated PAM or enzyme alone diluted 1:11 in Veronal buffer was used in the aggregation assay. No enzyme induced aggregation by itself, nor did enzyme treatment of platelets render them unresponsive to 2×10^{-5} M adenosine diphosphate (ADP) or to untreated PAM added simultaneously. To further ensure that the presence of enzyme was not making the platelets specifically unresponsive to PAM, treated PAM was centrifuged as previously described to pellet activity, and the pellet was resuspended in Veronal buffer prior to reacting with the platelets.

Phospholipase-A$_2$ was boiled for 10 minutes prior to use in order to inactivate possible contaminants. Neuraminidase treatment was performed in the presence of 2 mM phenylmethyl sulfonyl fluoride (PMSF) to inhibit any contaminating protease activity.

Preparation of Platelet-Rich and Platelet-Poor Plasma

Rabbits or human subjects were bled by venipuncture directly into a plastic syringe containing a final concentration of 5 U/ml heparin (preservative-free, Connaught Laboratories, Willowdale, Ontario, Canada). Platelet-rich plasma

(PRP) was obtained by centrifugation at $150 \times g$ for 5 minutes at room temperature. Platelet-poor plasma (PPP) was prepared by centrifuging the remaining blood at $2000 \times g$ for 15 minutes. The PRP was allowed to stand at room temperature for 30 minutes in tightly capped plastic tubes prior to testing.

Preparation of Washed Human Platelets

Eighteen milliliters of human blood were drawn into 2 ml of 3.8 percent trisodium citrate. PRP was prepared as described and incubated with 5 mg of apyrase at 37° C for 30 minutes. The platelets were then sedimented as described earlier and resuspended in Ardlie's buffer [19] containing 0.2 U/ml heparin and 0.5 mg/ml apyrase, except that $MgCl_2$ and $CaCl_2$ were omitted from the buffer and 2 mM EDTA was added. The resuspended platelets were again centrifuged, resuspended in half their original PRP volume of Ardlie's buffer (free of $MgCl_2$, $CaCl_2$, heparin, apyrase, and EDTA), and then incubated at 37° C for 45 minutes. In some experiments washed platelets were prepared by gel filtration.[20] These platelets aggregated with 10^{-5} M ADP or 10^{-5} M epinephrine when 2 mg/ml human fibrinogen was added to the suspension. Collagen-induced aggregation did not require fibrinogen, but was enhanced by its addition.

In Vitro Platelet Aggregation

Platelet aggregation was measured turbidometrically [21] with a Bio-Data aggregometer (Bio-Data Corp., Willow Grove, Pennsylvania). In a typical experiment, 0.4 ml of PRP or washed platelets was warmed to 37° C for 3 minutes in a flat-bottomed cylindrical cuvette. The platelets were then stirred in the aggregometer at 1200 rpm, a baseline was obtained on the recorder, and 0.05 ml of PAM was added. Aggregation was recorded as an increase in light transmission, with PPP representing 100 percent transmission. In experiments in which inhibitors of aggregation were assayed, administration of 0.05 ml of inhibitor or 0.05 ml of Veronal buffer was followed by the addition of 0.05 ml of PAM.

Quantitation of the Release with [^{14}C]Serotonin

Serotonin release was determined essentially as described by Gasic *et al.*[3]

RESULTS

Studies on Nontransformed 3T3 and Transformed SV40 3T3 Mouse Fibroblasts

Whole Cells

Intact SV3T3 transformed cells were capable of inducing platelet aggregation after a lag period of 1 to 2 minutes (FIG. 1). When 50 μl of transformed cells at an initial concentration of 10^7 cells/ml were added to 0.4 ml of PRP, the final maximal level of aggregation (optical density change) reached was 80 percent of that achieved by the addition of 2×10^{-5} M ADP. The normal 3T3 line was also capable of inducing moderate aggregation after a slightly longer lag period than that observed with the transformed cell. However, the final percentage of aggregation induced by the normal cell line was approximately 40 percent of that of the ADP control (FIG. 1).

Urea Extract

A urea extract of SV3T3 cells induced platelet aggregation at a final concentration of 40 µg/ml protein (FIG. 2). In contrast, medium conditioned by the same cell type for an identical length of time required an approximately five-fold

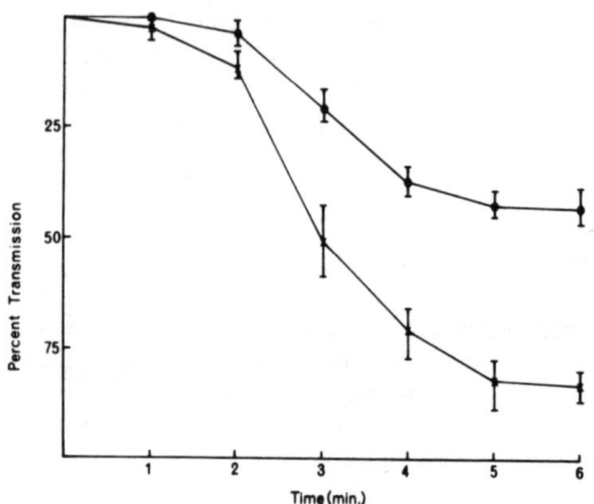

FIGURE 1. Induction of rabbit platelet aggregation in heparinized PRP by 10^7 intact 3T3 (•) or SV3T3 (x) cells. Each point (± SEM) represents the average of four experiments.

to 10-fold higher concentration of protein to induce a similar degree of aggregation (data not shown). Dilution of the extracted SV3T3 cell line PAM by a factor of 20 (from 40 to 2 µg/ml) resulted in a loss of activity (FIG. 2), demonstrating the sensitivity of the system to dilution. Normal 3T3 cell extracts, at 40 µg/ml, were capable of inducing only slight aggregation after a prolonged lag period (FIG. 2).

The transformed cell extract was more effective in heparin-PRP, as were the intact cells, in agreement with the results of others.[3]

Inhibitors of PAM

As shown in TABLE 2, several compounds that inhibit the secondary wave of platelet aggregation[22] also prevented PAM induction of platelet aggregation. Thus 5 mM EDTA, 0.05 mM indomethacin, 0.1 mM adenosine, and 0.1 mM N6,0$^{2'}$-dibutyrl cyclic AMP all inhibited PAM activity.

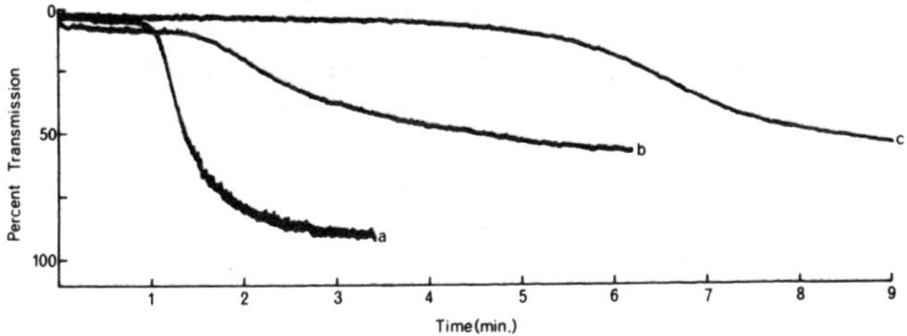

FIGURE 2. Induction of rabbit platelet aggregation in heparinized PRP by 1*M* urea extracts from SV3T3 cells at a final protein concentration of (a) 40 μg/ml or (b) 2 μg/ml and from 3T3 cells (c) at 40 μg/ml. Data are taken from one of 20 experiments with similar results.

Release of [^{14}C]Serotonin

The release reaction was directly measured by quantitating [^{14}C]serotonin release from aggregated platelets. The results, shown in TABLE 3, indicate that PAM accomplishes irreversible aggregation by inducing platelet release.

Noninhibitors of PAM

Certain proteases induce platelet aggregation[23] and tumor cells frequently synthesize higher levels of proteases than do their normal counterparts.[17, 24] Therefore, an attempt was made to inhibit PAM with several specific protease inhibitors known to interfere with transformed cell plasminogen activation.[25] All inhibitors were assayed for activity on appropriate substrates prior to use. For example, 2.5 m*M* disopropyl fluorophosphate (DFP) inhibited thrombin-

TABLE 2

INHIBITION OF PAM-INDUCED AGGREGATION WITH INHIBITORS OF THE
PLATELET-RELEASE REACTION

Inhibitor	Aggregating Agent	Aggregation (%)
Veronal buffer	PAM	100
Veronal buffer	$2 \times 10^{-5}M$ ADP	100
5 m*M* EDTA	PAM	0
0.1 m*M* dBcAMP *	PAM	1–30
0.1 m*M* dBcAMP	$2 \times 10^{-5}M$ ADP	0
0.1 m*M* adenosine	PAM	0
0.1 m*M* adenosine	$2 \times 10^{-5}M$ ADP	0
0.05 m*M* indomethacin	PAM	10

NOTE: All inhibitors were incubated with heparinized rabbit PRP for 6 to 9 minutes at 37° C prior to the addition of PAM, 10 μg/ml. Inhibition concentration is that achieved after dilution of the inhibitor in PRP. Each experiment was performed three or more times.

* dBcAMP = $N^6, O^{2'}$-dibutyrl cyclic AMP.

TABLE 3

RELEASE OF [^{14}C]SEROTONIN AFTER ADDITION OF PAM TO
HEPARINIZED RABBIT PRP

Addition	CPM in Supernatant	Release (%)
Veronal buffer	399	2
$2 \times 10^{-5}M$ ADP	387	2
PAM	10,255	53
Sonication	19,350	100

NOTE: Percentage of release was calculated as radioactivity in PAM-containing supernatant minus background radioactivity (buffer) divided by total radioactivity taken up by the platelet suspension. Results are an average of two determinations.

induced platelet aggregation at a concentration of 0.1 μg/ml. The results given in TABLE 4 clearly indicate that PAM activity is not related to any increase in proteolytic activity associated with transformed cell plasma membranes. Thus epsilon-amino caproic acid (EACA) (0.8 mM), soybean trypsin inhibitor (50–500 μg/ml), Trasylol® (50 units/ml), phenylmethylsulfanylfluoride (PMSF) (2 mM), and diisopropylfluorophosphate (DFP) (2.5 mM) had no significant effect on platelet aggregation.

Centrifugation of PAM

The urea-extracted PAM from SV3T3 cells can be pelleted by centrifugation at 100,000 $\times$ g for 1 hour at 4° C. The results shown in FIGURE 3 clearly demonstrate that all the activity was recoverable in the pellet, with no residual PAM remaining in the supernatant. The ability to pellet the material provided a means of removing enzyme from the enzyme-treated PAM in order to discriminate between the effect of enzyme on PAM and on the platelet surface.

TABLE 4

EFFECT OF PROTEASE INHIBITORS ON PAM-MEDIATED
PLATELET AGGREGATION

Inhibitor	Final Concentration	Aggregation (%)
Veronal buffer	. . .	100
EACA (epsilon-amino-caproic acid)	0.8 mM	95
Soybean trypsin inhibitor	50–500 μg/ml	98
Trasylol	50 U/ml	95
PMSF (Phenylmethylsulfonylfluoride)	2 mM	90
DFP (Diisopropylfluorophosphate)	2.5 mM	82

NOTE: Inhibitors were incubated with PAM for 4–5 min at 20° C prior to addition to PRP. Each experiment was performed 2 or more times.

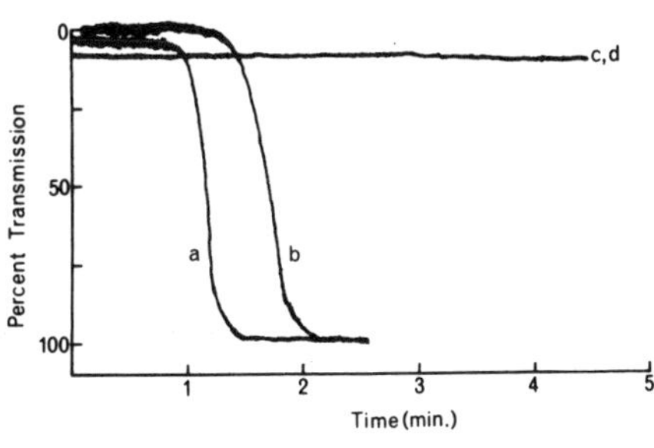

FIGURE 3. Platelet aggregation after sedimentation of PAM by ultracentrifugation. **(a)** original SV3T3 extract; **(b)** resuspended extract pellet in original volume of Veronal buffer after centrifugation at $100,000 \times g$ for 1 hour; **(c)** supernatant after centrifugation; and **(d)** 3T3 extract pellet after centrifugation and resuspension of pellet in Veronal buffer. The difference in lag period between **(a)** and **(b)** is not significant.

Effect of Boiling, Enzymes, Nonionic Detergents, or Sonication on PAM and PRP

The following treatments, listed in TABLE 5, completely destroyed PAM activity: (1) boiling for 15 minutes (partial activity could be restored after boiling by storage for several weeks at 4° C); (2) crystalline trypsin at 1 mg/ml; (3) neuraminidase at 2 mg/ml in the presence of 2 mM PMSF; (4) boiled phospholipase-A$_2$ at 0.1 μg/ml; (5) nonionic detergents, NP-40 (0.1 percent) and Tween-80® (0.1 percent); (6) sonication for 15 seconds at 0° C.

β-Galactosidase at 5 mg/ml had no effect on PAM.

PAM was washed by centrifugation and resuspended in fresh buffer prior to mixing with platelets in order to ensure that these enzymes or compounds did not affect platelets directly, making them unresponsive to PAM. Further-

TABLE 5

EFFECT OF BOILING, ENZYMES, NONIONIC DETERGENTS, AND
SONICATION ON THE ACTIVITY OF PAM

Treatment	Final Concentration or Time	Aggregation (%)	N*
Boiling	15 min	0	3
Boiling and storage at 0° C for 2 weeks	. . .	30–40	2
Trypsin-TPCK	1 mg/ml	0	5
Neuraminidase	2 mg/ml	0	5
Phospholipase-A$_2$	0.1 μg/ml	0	5
NP-40	0.1%	0	3
Tween-80	0.1%	0	3
Sonication	15 sec	0	2
β-Galactosidase	0.5 mg/ml	83	2

NOTE: All enzymes, in 10 μl volumes, were incubated with 100 μl of PAM, 100 μg/ml, for 1 hour at 37° C. PAM was then sedimented at $100,000 \times g$ for 1 hour at 4° C, and the pellet was resuspended in 100 μl of Veronal buffer. Of this material, 50 μl was used for platelet-aggregation studies with heparinized rabbit PRP.

* Number of experiments.

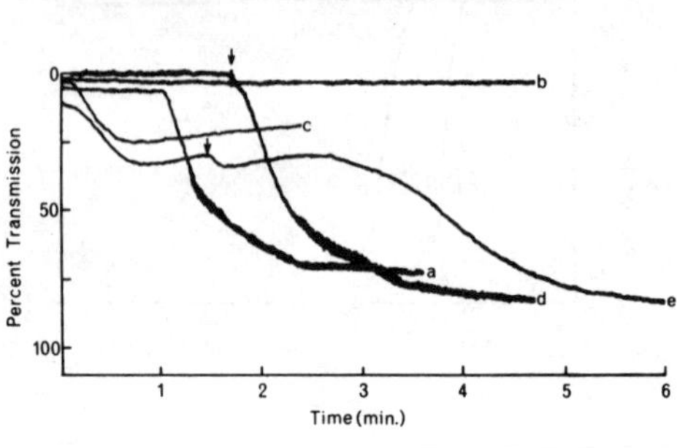

FIGURE 4. Synergistic effect of PAM and epinephrine on platelet aggregation in rabbit PRP. **(a)** 10 μg/ml PAM; **(b)** 1 μg/ml PAM; **(c)** $10^{-5}M$ epinephrine; **(d)** 1 μg/ml PAM followed by $10^{-5}M$ epinephrine; **(e)** $10^{-5}M$ epinephrine followed by 1 μg/ml PAM. Concentrations given are those achieved after dilution of the material in PRP during the assay. Initial additions were done at time zero. Second additions (in **[d]** and **[e]**) are indicated by arrows. Data are taken from one of four experiments with similar results.

more, platelet aggregation could be induced by addition of fresh PAM to PRP containing inactivated PAM. Therefore the effect was directly on PAM, not on platelet receptors for PAM.

PAM Synergism in Rabbit PRP

Dilutions of PAM were prepared that were below the threshold concentration required for platelet aggregation. Epinephrine, ADP, and collagen were also diluted to levels that were incapable of promoting platelet aggregation. By mixing these subthreshold concentrations of aggregating agents with dilute PAM (FIG. 4), we could demonstrate a synergistic effect between PAM and epinephrine at 1 μg/ml and 10^{-5} M, respectively, regardless of the order of addition. Neither ADP nor collagen proved to be synergistic with PAM when assayed in rabbit PRP (data not shown).

Effect of PAM on Washed Platelets

PAM did not aggregate washed platelets in the presence or absence of fibrinogen (FIG. 5, a and b) in most experiments (a small optical density

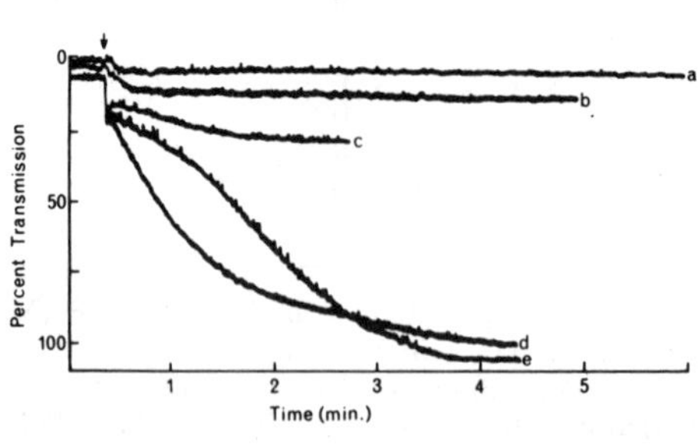

FIGURE 5. Effect of ADP, fibrinogen, and PAM on the aggregation of washed human platelets. Addition of PAM (10 μg/ml) in the **(a)** absence or **(b)** presence of fibrinogen. Addition of ADP $(2 \times 10^{-5}M)$ in the **(c)** absence or **(d)** presence of fibrinogen (2 mg/ml) or **(e)** PAM. Initial incubations were started at time zero, and arrow indicates when additions were made. Data are taken from one of seven experiments with similar results.

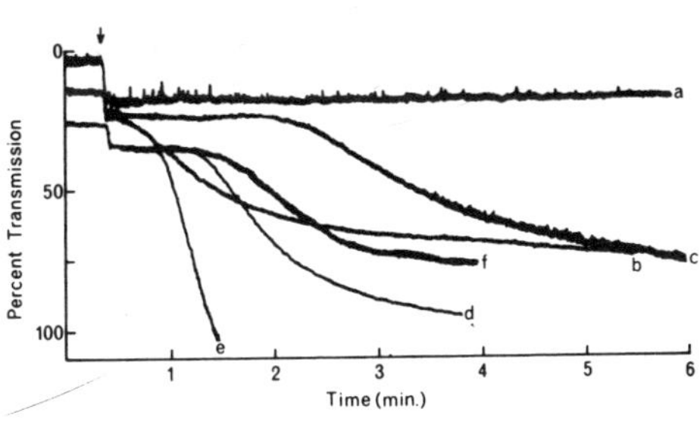

FIGURE 6. Effect of epinephrine, collagen, fibrinogen, and PAM on the aggregation of washed human platelets. Addition of epinephrine $(10^{-5}M)$ in the **(a)** absence or **(b)** presence of fibrinogen or **(c)** PAM. Addition of collagen (1:3200 dilution) in the **(d)** absence or **(e)** presence of fibrinogen or **(f)** PAM. Initial incubations were started at time zero, and arrow indicates when additions were made. Data are taken from one of four experiments with similar results.

change of 10 to 15 percent was occasionally noted in the presence of fibrinogen plus PAM). However, the washed human platelet system developed was responsive to platelet aggregation induced by ADP (FIG. 5, c and d) or epinephrine (FIG. 6, a and b) in the presence of purified human fibrinogen and to collagen (FIG. 6, d and e) in the absence or presence of fibrinogen. Of particular interest was the observation that PAM could replace the fibrinogen requirement for ADP-induced aggregation (FIG. 5, e) or epinephrine-induced aggregation (FIG. 6, c), but not for collagen-induced aggregation (FIG. 6, f).

We have also observed that preincubation of PPP with gel-filtered (washed) platelets, prior to the addition of PAM, restored PAM's ability to induce platelet aggregation (FIG. 7); this effect was concentration-dependent. However, when boiled PPP was employed, no restoration of activity was observed (data not shown).

Further studies on the plasma factor have revealed the following (the details of which will be published elsewhere): (1) incubation of PAM with plasma (1:1) at 37° C for 10 minutes produces an "activated PAM," which abolishes the 1- to 2-minute lag period noted in the absence of prior incubation;

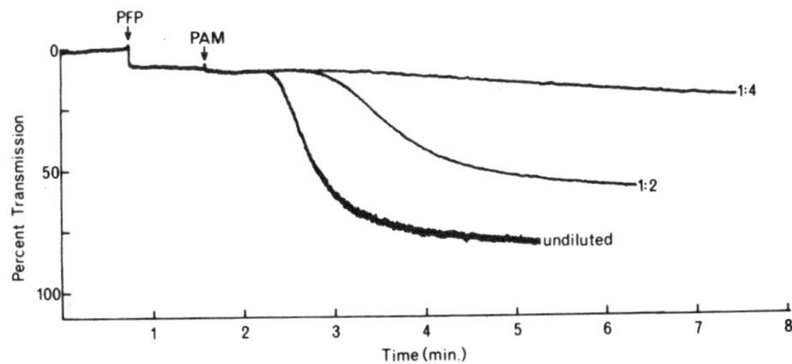

FIGURE 7. Aggregation of gel-filtered platelets in the presence of PPP and PAM. The addition of 50 μl of PPP (*arrow*) to 0.4 ml of gel-filtered platelets prior to the addition of 50 μl of PAM (*arrow*) reconstituted the aggregation-promoting activity of PAM. Dilution of PPP (1:2 and 1:4) with Veronal buffer resulted in a concentration-dependent loss of reconstitution activity. Data are taken from one of three experiments with similar results.

(2) heating of this "activated PAM" at 56° C for 30 minutes does not destroy PAM's activity, whereas heating of plasma at 56° C for 30 minutes does destroy its ability to support PAM-induced aggregation; (3) "activated PAM" loses its ability to aggregate washed platelets if it is separated from plasma by centrifugation at 100,000 g for 1 hour and the plasma supernatant is removed. However, readdition of fresh plasma or of plasma heated to 56° C for 30 minutes restores the activity.

Thus, a heat-labile factor is required to activate PAM and abolish the lag period and a heat-stable factor is required for the "activated PAM" to be operative. Preliminary studies indicate that the heat-labile factor is complement, since treatment of plasma with cobra venom abolishes its ability to activate PAM. Since C4-deficient plasma retains the ability to activate PAM, it appears that the alternative complement pathway is involved. The requirement of complement for tumor cell-induced platelet aggregation has recently been reported by Gasic et al.[26]

Studies on PW20 Renal Cell Sarcoma Variant Cell Lines

Metastatic Properties

The percentage of animals in which one or more spontaneous metastatic lesions developed after primary tumor excision ranged from 0 to 100 percent, with lesions appearing in the lung, mediastinal lymph nodes, abdominal viscera, and external lymph nodes (TABLE 6).

Platelet Aggregation

The maximal average velocity of platelet aggregation induced by PAM ranged from 1.5 to 100 units of light transmission per minute. A significant correlation was observed between the platelet-aggregating activity of PAM and the metastatic potential of the tumor cell lines from which the PAM was derived ($r = 0.68$, $p < 0.03$).

Sialic Acid Content of PAM

The sialic acid content of PAM ranged from 1.5 to 24.7 mg per 100 mg protein. PAM preparations from the three least metastatic cell lines, which were least active with respect to platelet-aggregating ability, contained the lowest levels of sialic acid. A good correlation was observed between the platelet-aggregating activity of PAM and its sialic acid content ($r = 0.60$, $p < 0.06$), and between the metastatic potential of the cell lines and the sialic content of PAM ($r = 0.69$, $p < 0.03$).

Sialylation of Cell-Surface Glycoconjugates

The percentage of sialylation of exposed cell-surface Gal and GalNAc residues ranged from 13 to 77 percent, with the three lowest values observed

TABLE 6

METASTATIC PROPERTIES, PLATELET-AGGREGATING ACTIVITY OF CELL-SURFACE EXTRACTS (PAM), SIALIC ACID CONTENT OF PAM, AND SIALYLATION OF CELL SURFACE GLYCOCONJUGATES OF METASTATIC VARIANT PW20 TUMOR CELL LINES

	Metastases from Primary Subcutaneous Tumors			Platelet-Aggregating Material (PAM)		Cell-Surface Sialylation
Derivative Line	Incidence *	Location †	Percent	Velocity of aggregation (percentage of transmission/min) ‡	Sialic acid content (mg/100 mg protein) §	Percentage sialylation of cell surface Gal and GalNAc ‖
R2N1	13/13	T,A,N	100	73 ± 3	7.1	66 ± 7
R2L1	13/13	T,A,N	100	34 ± 5	16.4	77 ± 7
R1	45/49	T,A,N	92	70 ± 4	15.7	75 ± 3
R2	56/64	T,A,N	88	69 ± 5	24.7	73 ± 5
R2R2	5/7	T,A,–	71	9 ± 2	14.5	36 ± 2
RO(L)R1	4/6	T,–,N	67	63 ± 4	21.4	70 ± 6
RO(L)	6/9	T,A,N	67	100 ± 5	15.8	72 ± 4
R2R1	3/13	T,–,–	23	4 ± 1	5.4	13 ± 2
RO(H)	1/19	–,A,–	5	8 ± 1	5.4	31 ± 7
RO(H)R1	0/5	–,–,–	0	2 ± 1	1.5	10 ± 10

* Number of animals in which one or more metastases developed after primary tumor excision per number of animals surviving surgery.

† T, intrathoracic (lung and/or mediastinal lymph nodes); A, intraabdominal (mesenteric lymph nodes, kidney, adrenal gland, ovary and/or liver); N, superficial lymph nodes (inguinal, axillary, cervical).

‡ Maximal average velocity of platelet aggregation induced by PAM tested at three to five concentrations ranging from 10 to 100 μg/ml. Mean $\pm$ SE of values obtained from two to five independent experiments.

§ Mean obtained from two independent determinations that were very similar.

‖ Mean $\pm$ SE of values obtained from three to seven independent experiments.

in the three least metastatic cell lines. A significant correlation was observed between cell-surface sialylation and metastatic potential ($r = 0.83$, $p < 0.003$) and cell-surface sialylation and the platelet-aggregating activity of PAM ($r = 0.74$, $p < 0.02$).

DISCUSSION

In agreement with the findings of Gasic and coworkers,[1-3, 27] we have demonstrated that viral transformants of established cell lines will cause platelet aggregation, whereas the normal parental line is much less effective (FIG. 1). Indeed, it is conceivable that the low activity of the nontransformed cells could represent initial signs of spontaneous *in vitro* cell transformation. In addition, 1 *M* urea extraction of plasma membrane components from the transformed cells permits this effect to be demonstrated by cell-free extracts (FIG. 3). The extraction of normal cells yields considerably less biologically active PAM. It is of interest that although the intact normal cells contained one-half the platelet-aggregating activity of transformed cells, the urea extract of the normal cells contained 20-fold less PAM.

Both transformed cells and their cell-free extracts cause platelets in PRP to aggregate in a similar fashion: a lag period of 1 to 3 minutes followed by rapid platelet aggregation accompanied by the release reaction. The sensitivity of the tumor cell and the cell-free extract to trypsin was also similar. It is therefore likely that platelet aggregation induced by intact cells and extract is promoted by equivalent factors. PAM operates via the release reaction and requires divalent cation, since inhibitors of the secondary wave of platelet aggregation abolish PAM-induced aggregation of PRP (TABLE 2). PAM operates best in heparin-PRP rather than citrate-PRP and does not operate in the presence of EDTA (TABLE 2).

The mechanism of action of PAM-induced aggregation is unique because PAM aggregates PRP, but does not aggregate washed platelets, which are capable of being aggregated by ADP or epinephrine in the presence of fibrinogen or by collagen in the absence of fibrinogen. However, PAM, like fibrinogen, does support ADP- and epinephrine-induced platelet aggregation and may operate via a mechanism similar to that of fibrinogen in the washed platelet system. It is conceivable that PAM has two activities or sites: one which aggregates platelets in PRP (requiring a plasma factor) and another which supports washed platelet aggregation in the absence of fibrinogen.

The plasma requirement is of interest. A heat-labile factor (probably alternative pathway complement components) is necessary for the activation of PAM and the elimination of the lag period. A heat-stable factor is required for activated PAM to be operative.

Many transformed cells have been shown to have increased levels of proteolytic enzymes,[10, 28] including the transformed lines used in these studies.[29] Because platelets are sensitive to aggregation by specific proteases,[23, 30] we attempted to inhibit PAM-induced aggregation by protease inhibitors known to prevent plasminogen activation by these tumor cells (EACA and soybean trypsin inhibitor) as well as additional protease inhibitors. As shown in TABLE 4, none of these inhibitors prevented platelet aggregation with PAM. This finding is in agreement with a report[3] that showed no correlation between the ability of tumor cells to induce platelet aggregation and their fibrinolytic activity *in vitro*.

We have demonstrated that PAM is a complex mixture of protein, lipid, and carbohydrate assembled in a macromolecular form capable of sedimentation at 100,000 $\times$ g for 1 hour. Destruction of PAM activity by trypsin, neuraminidase, or phospholipase-A_2 indicates that several components interact to produce PAM activity. This interaction may involve maintenance of a vesicular configuration, since sonication will also reduce PAM activity. Attempts to replace lipid by neutral detergents and to maintain activity have been unsuccessful, and it appears that the lipid moiety may play more than a simple structural role in promoting platelet aggregation.

Since fibroblasts synthesize collagen and collagen can induce platelet aggregation *in vitro*,[31] it was necessary to determine whether PAM activity may be related to this protein. Such does not appear to be the case because: (1) treatment of tumor cells with collagenase does not interfere with their aggregation-promoting activity[1]; (2) PAM and collagen are not additive in inducing platelet aggregation; (3) transformation leads to a decrease in collagen biosynthesis[32]; (4) collagen is capable of aggregating washed platelets (FIG. 6, d and e), but PAM is not (FIG. 7, a and b); and (5) treatment of PAM with collagenase does not inhibit PAM-induced platelet aggregation (data not shown).

The involvement of sialic acid is interesting in light of a report demonstrating increased levels of sialic-acid-containing glycolipids in serum samples obtained from mice bearing transplantable mammary carcinomas compared with normal animals.[33] The sialic acid components were shown to be present in the gangliosides. The sensitivity of PAM to neuraminidase but not to β-galactosidase indicates that PAM and the material present in the serum of tumor-bearing animals may be related.

Studies on PW20-Induced Renal Cell Sarcoma Variant Cell Lines

Because the SV40 3T3 fibroblast is not spontaneously metastatic *in vivo*, the pathophysiologic significance of PAM and its relationship to sialic acid was examined in 10 variant cell lines from a spontaneously metastatic PW20 renal cell sarcoma in Wistar-Furth rats. Significant correlations were observed between the metastatic potential of the cell lines, the ability of PAM to aggregate platelets, the sialic acid content of PAM, and the degree of sialylation of the intact tumor cell surface. The correlation between the activity of PAM and its sialic acid content is in accord with our recent report that the activity of PAM obtained from SV3T3 cells is abolished by treatment with neuraminidase[34] and suggests that the sialic acid content of PAM is important in determining its activity. The correlation between the sialic acid content of PAM and the degree of cell surface sialylation is consistent with the evidence suggesting that PAM is composed of membrane vesicles. Interestingly, the total sialic acid content of the cells (data not shown) correlates poorly with the other variables shown in TABLE 6. This finding suggests that the degree of sialylation of the cell surface, which is reflected in the sialic acid content of the extracted PAM, may be a more important determinant of metastatic behavior and platelet-aggregating properties than the overall sialic acid content of the cell.

One cell line (R2R2) appears to be an exception in that it shows relatively low values of PAM activity and cell surface sialylation for its degree of metastasis. Of interest is the observation that this cell line demonstrated a transient incomplete regression of the initially formed tumors *in vivo* followed by delayed progressive growth prior to excision. It is therefore possible that a further immunoselection of highly sialylated cells [35] with enhanced metastatic potential may have taken place from a heterogeneous population of predominantly nonmetastatic poorly sialylated R2R2 cells. In this regard, the reduced *in vitro* adhesiveness and motility of R2R2 cells are also characteristic of the poorly metastatic cell line.[36] If this line were eliminated from the correlation, it would raise the correlation coefficients by an average of 0.06.

The correlation between the spontaneous metastatic behavior of murine tumor cells and their cell-surface sialylation *in vitro* has recently been noted [16, 36] and has now been observed in a total of 32 murine tumor cell lines (data not shown). One mechanism that might be proposed to account for the observed correlation is that elevated levels of sialic acid on the cell surface may reduce the immunogenicity of the tumor cells,[35, 37] thereby increasing their ability to evade immune destruction and establish metastatic foci.[38] Differences in cell-surface sialic acid may also bring about differences in the adhesive properties of the cells,[36, 39] thereby altering their patterns of arrest and implantation at secondary sites.[40] Another mechanism, which is suggested by the results of the present study, is that increased sialylation of the tumor cell surface may enhance the ability of these cells to aggregate platelets, either prior to or after their arrest in the microvasculature.[7, 8, 10] The resulting aggregates may prolong the survival of the tumor cells at the site of arrest.[7, 8, 10] The release of vasoactive substances from the aggregated platelets [41] may facilitate passage of the tumor cells through the vessel wall by promoting endothelial cell damage and enhanced cell adhesion to the subendothelial matrix.

The mechanisms of tumor cell metastasis are inherently complex.[42] The extent to which platelets may be involved in promoting tumor cell metastasis remains to be determined. The variant cell lines employed in this study provide an excellent opportunity to study the role of platelets in tumor cell metastasis. Our data are consistent with the hypothesis that platelets play a role in certain tumor cell metastases and lend support to the therapeutic possibility that certain tumor metastases may be reduced by agents capable of eradicating that property of platelets that promotes metastasis.

SUMMARY

Platelets are required for certain experimental tumor metastases and several lines of tumor cells have been shown to aggregate platelets. We have extracted a sedimentable sialo-lipo-protein, platelet-aggregating material (PAM) from the cell surface of SV40-transformed Balb C3T3 fibroblasts, which aggregates heparinized PRP at 2.5 μg/ml via the release reaction, following a one minute lag period. A similar extract from non-transformed 3T3 cells has barely measurable activity at 40 μg/ml. Gel-filtered platelets (GFP) do not aggregate with PAM. However, PAM aggregation can be restored by addition of 5 percent plasma but not by fibrinogen.

The pathophysiologic significance of PAM has been examined in ten variant cell lines derived from a spontaneously metastatic renal cell sarcoma of rats, initially induced with polyoma virus (PW20 Wistar-Furth parental lines). These lines were selected *in vitro* and *in vivo* from a single line and differed in their capacity to form distant tumors in various organs after subcutaneous injection. These cells were examined for cell surface sialylation, PAM and PAM sialic acid content, since cell surface sialic acid is increased in a variety of tumor tissues and PAM is inhibited by neuraminidase. A good correlation was obtained between *in vivo* metastatic potential and cell surface sialic acid, $r = 0.83$, $p < 0.003$; cell surface sialic acid and PAM, $r = 0.85$, $p < 0.002$; *in vivo* metastatic potential and sialic acid content of PAM, $r = 0.69$, $p < 0.03$; and *in vivo* metastatic potential and PAM, $r = 0.68$, $p < 0.03$. We conclude that platelets may play a role in hematogenous metastasis via the ability of tumor cells to aggregate platelets by cell surface constituents containing sialic acid. The platelet-tumor cell interaction requires activation of the alternate complement pathway and a heat stable plasma factor.

REFERENCES

1. GASIC, G. J., T. B. GASIC, N. GALANTI, T. JOHNSON & S. MURPHY. 1973. Int. J. Cancer **11:**704–718.
2. GASIC, G. J., T. B. GASIC & S. A. JIMENEZ. 1977. Thromb. Res. **10:**33–45.
3. GASIC, G. J., P. A. G. KOCH, B. HSU, T. B. GASIC & S. NIEWIAROWSKI. 1976. Z. Krebsforsch **86:**263–277.
4. GASTPAR, H. 1977. J. Med. **8:**103–114.
5. HILGARD, P. 1973. Br. J. Cancer **28:**429–435.
6. HILGARD, P. & E. C. GORDON-SMITH. 1974. Br. J. Haematol. **26:**651–659.
7. JONES, D. S., A. C. WALLACE & E. F. FRASER. 1971. J. Natl. Cancer Inst. **46:**493–498.
8. SINDELAR, W. F., T. S. TRALKA & A. S. KETCHAM. 1975. J. Surg. Res. **18:**137–161.
9. WARREN, B. A. 1973. J. Med. **4:**150–177.
10. WARREN, B. A. & O. VALES. 1972. Br. J. Exp. Pathol. **53:**301–313.
11. GASIC, G. J., T. B. GASIC & C. C. STEWART. 1968. Proc. Natl. Acad. Sci. USA **61:**46–52.
12. SALK, P. and G. YOGEESWARAN. 1978. Fed. Proc. **37:**1760 (abstract).
13. PEARLSTEIN, E. & J. SEAVER. 1976. Biochim. Biophys. Acta **426:**589–597.
14. HAGMAR, B. & B. BOERYD. 1969. Pathol. Eur. **4:**274.
15. WEXLER, H. 1966. J. Nat. Cancer Inst. **36:**641–645.
16. YOGEESWARAN, G., H. SEBASTIAN & B. S. STEIN. 1979. Int. J. Cancer. **24:**193–202.
17. WARREN, L. 1959. J. Biol. Chem. **234:**1971–1975.
18. LOWRY, O. H., N. J. ROSEBROUGH, A. L. FARR & R. J. RANDALL. 1951. J. Biol. Chem. **193:**265–275.
19. MUSTARD, J. F., D. W. PERRY, N. G. ARDLIE & M. A. PACKHAM. 1972. Br. J. Haematol. **22:**193–204.
20. TANGEN, D. & H. J. BERMAN. 1972. Adv. Exp. Med. Biol. **34:**235–243.
21. KARPATKIN, S. 1978. Blood **51:**307–316.
22. WEISS, H. J. 1975. N. Engl. J. Med. **293:**531–541.
23. DAVEY, M. G. & E. F. LUSCHER. 1966. Thromb. Diath. Haemorrh. Suppl. **20:**283–287.
24. OSSOWSKI, L., J. C. UNKELESS, A. TOBIA, J. P. QUIGLEY, D. B. RIFKIN & E. REICH. 1973. J. Exp. Med. **137:**112–126.
25. HYNES, R. O. & E. PEARLSTEIN. 1976. J. Supramolec. Struct. **4:**1–14.
26. GASIC, G. J., J. L. CATALFAMO, T. B. GASIC & N. AVDALOVIC. *In* Malignancy and Coagulation. M. B. Donati, Ed. Raven Press, New York, N.Y. In press.

27. GASIC, G. J., D. BOETTIGER, J. L. CATALFAMO, T. B. GASIC & G. J. STEWART. 1978. Cancer Res. **38:**2950–2955.
28. GOLDBERG, A. R. 1974. Cell **2:**95–102.
29. PEARLSTEIN, E., R. O. HYNES, L. M. FRANKS & V. J. HEMMINGS. 1976. Cancer Res. **36:**1475–1479.
30. NIEWIAROWSKI, S., A. F. SENYI & P. GILLES. 1973. J. Clin. Invest. **52:**1647–1659.
31. ZUCKER, M. B. & J. BORELLI. 1962. Proc. Soc. Exp. Biol. Med. **109:**779.
32. GREEN, H., B. GOLDBERG & G. J. TODARO. 1966. Nature **212:**631–633.
33. KLOPPEL, T. M., T. W. KEENAN, M. J. FREEMAN & D. J. MORRE. 1977. Proc. Natl. Acad. Sci. USA **74:**3011–3013.
34. PEARLSTEIN, E., L. B. COOPER & S. KARPATKIN. 1979. J. Lab. Clin. Med. **93:**332–344.
35. SALK, P. L. & R. P. LANZA. 1978. J. Supramol. Struct. **9** (Suppl. 3):182 (abstract).
36. RAY, P. K. 1977. Adv. Appl. Microbiol. **21:**227–267.
37. PIMM, M. V. & R. W. BALDWIN. 1978. *In* Secondary Spread of Cancer. R. W. Baldwin, Ed.:163–209. Academic Press. New York, N.Y.
38. WEISS, L. 1963. Exp. Cell Res. **30:**509–520.
39. SINHA, B. K. & G. J. GOLDENBERG. 1974. Cancer **34:**1956–1961.
40. WEISS, L., D. GLAVES & D. A. WAITE. 1974. Int. J. Cancer **13:**850–862.
41. NACHMAN, R., B. WEKSLER & B. FERRIS. 1972. J. Clin. Invest. **51:**549–556.
42. ROOS, E. & K. P. DINGEMANS. 1979. Biochim. Biophys. Acta **560:**135–166.

BACKGROUND AND PRESENT STATUS OF RESEARCH ON PLATELET-ACTIVATING FACTOR (PAF-ACETHER)

B. Boris Vargaftig,* Michel Chignard,* Jacques Benveniste,†
Jean Lefort,* and Françoise Wal *

* *Unité des Venins*
Institut Pasteur
Paris, France
† U 200 INSERM
92240 Clamart, France

HISTORICAL BACKGROUND

A leukocyte-dependent mechanism capable of releasing histamine from platelets was first reported in 1966, and a soluble principal intermediate between rabbit leukocytes and platelets was detected in 1971.[1,2] It was at that time described as "lytic" and was not characterized. One of us described the methodology for obtaining this substance routinely, started its characterization, named it platelet-activating factor (PAF), and showed that it was released from rabbit basophils through an IgE-dependent process.[3] Its presence was subsequently demonstrated in human leukocytes, and aggregation and the release reaction were shown for human platelets.[4] Finally, most of its known physicochemical characteristics, including its phospholipid nature, were described (see refs. in 5). At this stage, we knew that PAF was a glycerophospholipid with a choline polar head group, an ester-linked acyl chain on the carbon 2, and no ester link at the carbon 1 position.[6] A new class of phospholipid mediator was therefore proposed. Finally, the structure of the mediator was elucidated (FIG. 1) as being 1-*O*-alkyl-2-acetyl-glyceryl-3-phosphorylcholine, and its total synthesis was achieved.[7-9] PAF is therefore now termed PAF-acether, since it is an ether-lipid and has an acetate residue. We think it is preferable to keep to the established name, and not to replace it by the initials of the now recognized chemical name, in order to preserve a link with previous accomplishments and reduce literature confusion. For similar reasons prostaglandins or heparin, for instance, were not renamed when structures became available.

Given the numerous substances present in biological fluids and cell supernatants that can activate platelets, it was necessary to define PAF-acether strictly. Even before knowing its structure, we used the following criteria to distinguish it from arachidonic acid, thrombin, ADP or prostaglandins:

(1) aggregation of platelets in the presence of inhibitors of prostaglandin endoperoxide synthetase, such as aspirin or indomethacin, and of ADP scavengers;

(2) elution pattern similar to that of hog leukocyte or synthetic PAF-acether on silicic acid thin-layer or high-pressure chromatography; and

(3) inactivation by phospholipase A2 and resistance to lipase from *Rhizopus arrhizus.*

119

0077–8923/81/0370–0119 $01.75/0 © 1981, NYAS

Cellular Origin of PAF-Acether

Basophils

The release of PAF-acether from rabbit leukocytes by anti-IgE serum suggests its release from basophils. Antigen or anti-IgE, but not anti-IgG serum actively release PAF-acether from human or rabbit buffy coats.[3] Platelets must be carefully eliminated from the leukocyte preparation and bovine serum albumin (BSA) is needed as a carrier in the suspending buffer. Secretion of PAF-acether requires a physiological temperature, the presence of Ca^{2+} and of glucose, and the activation of a membrane serine esterase. "Passive" release of PAF-acether was observed when rabbit, human or hog leukocytes, (as well as

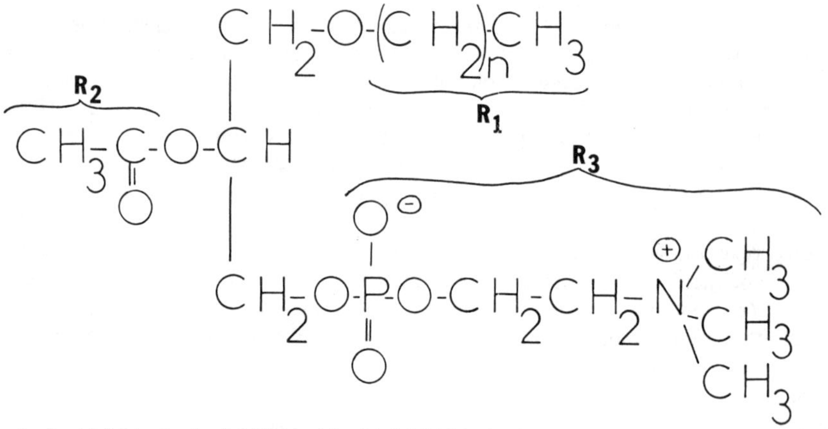

FIGURE 1. Structure of PAF-acether.

all other sources of PAF-acether since described) were placed at room temperature in a BSA-containing Tyrode's solution at pH 9.5. This release was Ca^{2+}-dependent, but was slow, in contrast to the antigen-induced release, which is completed within 5 min.[10] A significant positive correlation between the presence of histamine-releasing leukocytes and the release of histamine was found for the rabbit.[2, 11] Superimposed kinetics for antigen-induced release of PAF-acether and of histamine from sensitized rabbit leukocytes was observed.[11] Direct evidence for basophil-platelet interaction was also provided by electron microscopy studies.[3] Nevertheless, there is controversy concerning the basophil origin of PAF-acether, since a PAF-like material was obtained from 100% pure human basophil preparations from a patient with basophilic leukemia,[12] which has not been confirmed.[13] Moreover, there is evidence both in favor of [14] and opposed to [15, 16] the release of PAF-acether by normal human basophils.

Macrophages

Indirect evidence indicated that PAF-acether might originate from mastocytes.[17, 18] Mastocyte-degranulating agents, such as the compound 48/80, C3a and C5a anaphylatoxins, as well as the neutrophil cationic protein induced the release of PAF-acether from mixed cell populations.[18] Nevertheless, PAF-acether was obtained from macrophages and not from mastocytes from rat and mouse peritoneal cells, upon stimulation with the ionophore A23187, or exposure to phagocytizable particles.[19] Mastocytes release histamine, but not PAF-acether, in the presence of compound 48/80. However, when mixing mastocytes and macrophages to reconstitute the original population, PAF-acether was released by compound 48/80, but in small quantities and at delayed intervals as compared to the release induced by the Ca^{2+} ionophore or that of histamine by compound 48/80.

PAF-acether was obtained from human, rabbit and rat alveolar macrophages.[20] A "PAF-lung" was reported[21] and attributed to mastocytes, but it did not meet the characteristics of PAF-acether. Using the same experimental conditions, we demonstrated release of arachidonate, but not that of PAF-acether. Antigenic challenge induces the release of PAF-acether by peritoneal and alveolar macrophages from immunized rats.[22] Thus the only demonstrated lung source for PAF-acether is the macrophage.

Neutrophils

More recently, PAF-acether was shown to originate from rabbit neutrophils stimulated with opsonized zymosan.[23] PAF-acether, as well as slow-reacting substance of anaphylaxis, can be released from isolated human neutrophils stimulated with the Ca^{2+} ionophore, or with phagocytizable particles.[24] Release of PAF-acether was dissociated from that of lysosomal enzymes, and the well-noted dependence of PAF-acether release on Ca^{2+} was confirmed for the human neutrophil.[25]

The results summarized above show that far from being specific for immediate hypersensitivity, PAF-acether is released by many cells involved with inflammation. It is noteworthy that mechanical or chemical disruption of leukocytes, macrophages or platelets does not result in the release of PAF-acether, indicating that it is not a preformed mediator. Slow reacting substance of anaphylaxis and the eosinophil-chemotactic factor of anaphylaxis were initially considered as mediators of immediate hypersensitivity, and were more recently shown to originate from various unrelated sources, including macrophages and neutrophils. Yet, the release of these mediators by mechanisms implicating mastocytes, but not from the mastocytes themselves, is paradoxical. The release of PAF-acether from reconstituted peritoneal cell populations by compound 48/80 led to the proposal that a mastocyte/macrophage cooperation is operative. On a first step, mastocytes degranulate and then their granules, when ingested by the macrophages, trigger the release, as any phagocytozable particle.[26] It has been recognized since Maximov (1904, cited in 27) that macrophages can phagocytose granules released by nearby mastocytes.

Platelets and PAF-Acether

Platelet activation is mediated by at least three distinct pathways.[28-30] The first one is triggered by ADP, and the second by cyclic endoperoxides and/or thromboxane A2 (TxA2), the potent platelet-aggregating catabolites of arachidonic acid (AA). During platelet aggregation triggered by thrombin or by collagen, ADP is released from the dense bodies, and AA is hydrolyzed from the membrane phospholipids. When ADP is removed with a scavenging system, such as creatine phosphate and creatine phosphokinase (CP/CPK), and formation of the relevant metabolites of AA is prevented by aspirin or indomethacin, aggregation by small amounts of thrombin or of collagen is blocked. Nevertheless, when concentrations of the aggregating agents applied to the platelets are increased, aggregation occurs, despite the presence of the inhibitors of the first two pathways.[28-31] Evidence on the same line was obtained by Charo et al.,[32] who found that collagen and high concentrations of thrombin or of the ionophore A23187 activate platelets by a direct mechanism, which triggers an aggregation-dependent and indomethacin (or aspirin)-insensitive release reaction. This all suggested the existence of other mechanisms and/or mediators to account for ADP- and TxA2-independent platelet activation. The fact that PAF-acether can induce aggregation, even in the presence of the inhibitors of the first and of the second pathways,[33] led us to suggest that PAF-acether might mediate this third pathway.

Formation of PAF-Acether by the Platelets

The hypothesis that PAF-acether may mediate the third pathway of aggregation was substantiated by the finding of a potent aggregating substance in the supernatants of rabbit platelets stimulated with the Ca^{2+} ionophore A23187. This substance was indeed PAF-acether, since it induced aggregation refractory to aspirin and to indomethacin, was destroyed by phospholipase A2 and had an $R_f = 0.35$ on silicic acid TLC developed with chloroform:methanol:water (70:35:7). Formation of PAF-acether was not altered by aspirin or by indomethacin, nor by CP/CPK.[34] Stimulation of rabbit platelets with collagen or thrombin also led to the formation of PAF-acether,[35] which has since been confirmed.[36] The amounts of PAF-acether formed are proportionnal to the concentrations of the aggregating agents added to the platelet suspension.[35] Finally, the kinetics and the amounts of PAF-acether formed are compatible with its hypothesized role as the mediator of the third pathway of platelet aggregation,[35] at least for the rabbit. PAF-acether is in fact also released by human platelets stimulated with A23187[34] or with bovine thrombin.[37]

Mechanisms of PAF-Acether-induced Platelet Aggregation

PAF-acether is the most potent platelet-aggregating agent so far described. Full aggregation of washed rabbit platelets is obtained with a concentration as low as 1 nM,[38] and a threshold activation is obtained with 0.3 nM.[8, 39] Rabbit platelets suspended in plasma are less sensitive, and 60 nM are required to induce aggregation. Moreover, there are large species differences in sensitivity to PAF-acether. Thus guinea-pig platelets are more sensitive than rabbit

platelets, and human platelets are still less sensitive. Rat platelets are refractory
to PAF-acether (TABLE 1 and J. Randon, unpublished). The release reaction,
as measured by the release of serotonin [33, 40] or of ATP [41] to the extra-cellular
medium, accompanies aggregation. Nevertheless the release reaction may not
be necessary for the aggregating effect of PAF-acether, since degranulated
platelets, which lose their dense bodies after stimulation with thrombin, still
aggregate in response to PAF-acether.[33]

Phospholipase A2 activity of rabbit platelets is stimulated by PAF-
acether,[42, 45] and accordingly arachidonate is released, and transformed.[33, 42–45]
This is not the case for guinea-pig or human platelets, which do not release
arachidonate in response to PAF-acether.[41, 45] Human platelets washed under
very mild conditions react poorly to PAF-acether, even in the presence of added
fibrinogen, but the simultaneous addition of subthreshold concentrations of
ADP or of epinephrine results in full aggregation and in a limited release of
arachidonate.[45]

TABLE 1

REACTIVITY TO PAF-ACETHER OF PLATELETS FROM DIFFERENT SPECIES

Species		Guinea-pig	Rabbit	Dog	Human	Rat
Aggregating concentrations	with plasma	2	60	1100	4000	>10,000
in final nM *	without plasma	2	1	—	150	>10,000

* Concentration needed to aggregate by 40–60%.

The physiological significance of the formation of TxA2 by platelets stimulated by PAF-acether is apparently negligible, since aspirin fails to prevent
aggregation.

Analogues of PAF-acether have been tested on platelets.‡ The 1-*O*-octadecyl
and the 1-*O*-hexadecyl compounds are practically equiactive, and 0.6 nM and
0.2 nM, respectively, induce aggregation. Substitution of the ether by an ester
bound in position 1 of the glycerol structure reduces the platelet-aggregating
activity 100-fold, but the substitution of the acetate by a propionate in position 2
increases it 10-fold.[46] Since the lyso derivative is inactive, the pre-incubation
of PAF-acether with phospholipase A2 yields an inactive derivative. This is
used as a tool to discriminate between PAF-acether and other lipo-soluble
platelet-stimulating agents present in a mixture. The optical isomer of PAF-
acether has no intrinsic activity, and any contamination with the active isomer
can be removed by treatment with phospholipase A2 in the presence of
calcium. Phospholipase A2 is very discriminative in its hydrolyzing effect, and
will not hydrolyse the fatty acid of the unnatural phospholipid.

Inhibition of PAF-Acether-induced Aggregation

There is no specific inhibitor of PAF-acether-induced platelet aggregation,
(see below), but PAF-acether itself desensitizes the platelet. This was first

‡ See note on p. 137.

demonstrated for PAF-acether-induced secretion [40] and confirmed for aggregation.[47] Thus platelets pre-incubated with PAF-acether in presence of EGTA do not aggregate when stimulated again with it, in the presence of Ca^{2+}, but are still sensitive to other aggregating agents. Cazenave *et al.*[33] did not observe such a desensitization. Indeed, when the concentration of PAF-acether used for the second stimulation is above that used during the pre-incubation period aggregation can be triggered.[48]

There is evidence for a "specific" site on the platelet membrane, which would bind PAF-acether by a saturable, temperature and concentration-dependent process, independent from Ca^{2+}. A sort of "enzyme-receptor," such as an esterase or a phospholipase A2, was ruled out, since specific inhibitors of these enzymes did not affect the binding of PAF-acether to the membrane.[49] In contrast, an esterase is needed for triggering the biological activity of PAF-acether, and inhibitors of serine-esterases prevent platelet activation by PAF-acether.[50] These are of course nonspecific inhibitors of the latter's effects. Colchicine, which disrupts platelet microtubules, also inhibits the PAF-acether-induced release reaction.[50] A rise in the cyclic AMP content also inhibits platelet activation by PAF-acether, which was shown with prostaglandin E1 and theophylline [50] or prostacyclin.[33, 41, 51] Nonspecific inhibitors of the platelet effects of PAF-acether include the Ca^{2+} chelators EGTA and EDTA, chlorpromazine, reserpine, imipramine, methysergide, lidocaine, methylprednisolone, and mepacrine.[33]

Mode of Formation of PAF-Acether

Formation of PAF-acether by rabbit platelets stimulated with the Ca^{2+} ionophore A23187 is inhibited by bromophenacyl bromide, a phospholipase A2 inhibitor.[30, 52] Other inhibitors of the activation of phospholipase A2, such as dibutyryl cyclic AMP and a compound known under the code number CB874 (Clin Midy) [53] proved to inhibit the synthesis of PAF-acether as well (FIG. 2). EGTA and EDTA were also inhibitory, whereas aspirin was completely inactive (FIG. 2). Similar results were obtained with macrophages.[54]

Stimulated platelets also form a deacetylated derivative, named lyso-PAF-acether. This compound does not aggregate the platelets, and its acetylation yields a compound with biological and chromatographical properties similar to those of PAF-acether.[55] Approximately 100 times more lyso PAF acether is formed than PAF-acether itself in stimulated platelets.[53] The inhibitors mentioned above inhibit as well the formation of lyso-PAF-acether, suggesting that platelet phospholipase A2 is the key enzyme for synthesis of both the lyso- and the acetylated derivative. In the presence of radiolabeled acetate, platelets synthesize PAF-acether with the label on the 2 position.[56] Radiolabeled PAF-acether was also obtained from stimulated murine peritoneal cells incubated with tritiated acetyl CoA or tritiated lyso-PAF-acether.[57, 58] The enzyme responsible is possibly an acetyl CoA:1-alkyl-2-lyso-Sn-glycero-3-phosphocholine acetyl transferase, identical to that described in the spleen, in lungs, lymph nodes, and thymus,[59] and in rat and mouse peritoneal cells.[60] Another enzyme was recently described, namely 1-alkyl-2-acetyl-Sn-glycera-3-phosphocholine: acetylhydrolase, which differs from the phospholipase A2 [61] and transforms PAF-acether into lyso-PAF-acether. The obvious question must be raised: is lyso-PAF-acether the precursor, or is it the inactive catabolite of PAF-acether? (FIG. 3).

PHARMACOLOGY OF PAF-ACETHER

Effects in the Anesthetized Guinea-pig

"Native" or synthetic PAF-acether induce at least two independent acute effects when injected intravenously in the guinea-pig: hypotension, on one

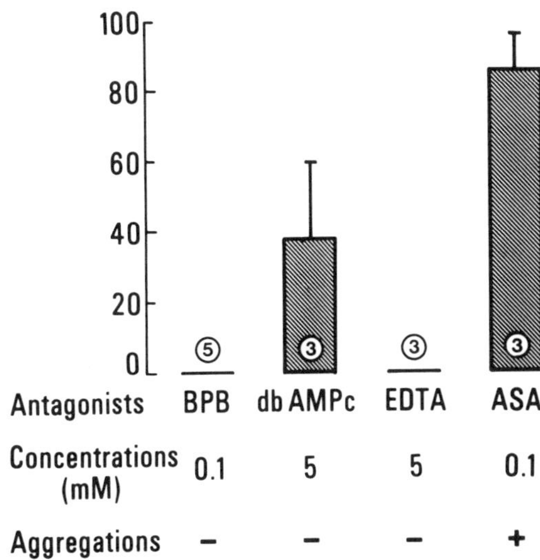

FIGURE 2. Inhibition of the formation of PAF-acether by rabbit platelets stimulated with the Ca^{2+}-ionophore A23187. Rabbit platelets suspended in Tyrode's solution were stimulated with the Ca^{2+} ionophore A23187 (1 μM; for 20 min at 37° C). PAF-acether was then extracted and quantified.[34] In each experiment a control (vehicle) and an experimental tube, containing the potential inhibitors, were run at the same time. The potential inhibitors were bromophenacyl bromide (BPB), dibutyryl cyclic AMP (dbAMPc), EDTA or aspirin (ASA), and were incubated with the platelet suspension at the indicated concentrations for 15 min (BPB) or 5 min (dbAMPc, EDTA and ASA). Each column represents the mean ± S.E.M. for % inhibition of the formation of PAF-acether. Number of experiments is indicated in the circles.

side, and thrombocytopenia with bronchoconstriction, on the other side. Aspirin, up to 50 mg/kg, fails to interfere significantly with these effects, ruling out a direct responsibility of cyclooxygenase derivatives (see below for the combination of aspirin with other antagonists). Bronchoconstriction is suppressed when the guinea-pigs are depleted of circulating platelets with antiplatelet serum, but hypotension persists. Infusions of prostacyclin (PGI_2), just before injecting PAF-acether, prevents thrombocytopenia and bronchoconstriction, and again the hypotensive effect persists. Prostacyclin is not a bronchodilator in the guinea-pig, and in fact it increases the responses to various bronchocon-

ETHER-LINKED PHOSPHOLIPID

(1-alkyl-2-acyl-sn-glycerophosphorylcholine)

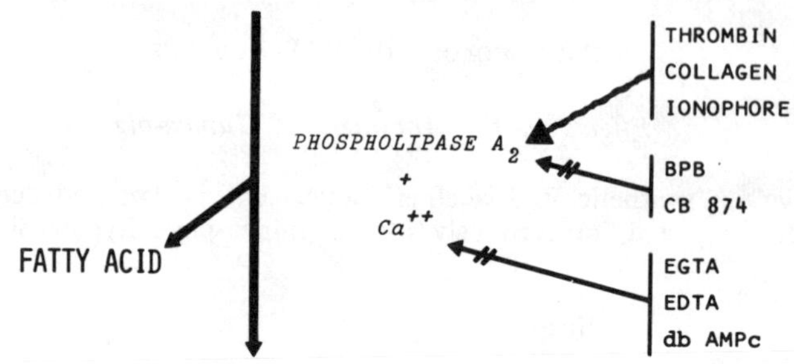

LYSO-PAF-ACETHER

(1-alkyl-2-lyso-sn-glycerophosphorylcholine)

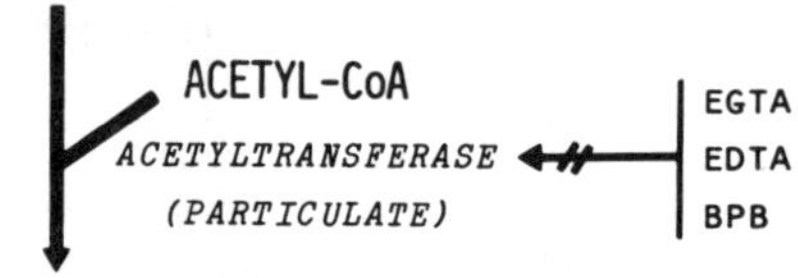

PAF-ACETHER

(1-alkyl-2-acetyl-sn-glycerophosphorylcholine)

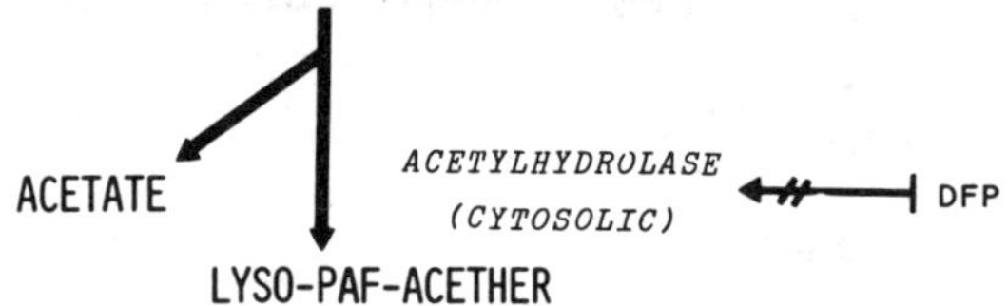

LYSO-PAF-ACETHER

(1-alkyl-2-lyso-sn-glycerophosphorylcholine)

FIGURE 3. Hypothetical pathways for the formation and catabolism of PAF-acether.

strictor agents.[62] The only known site of action of PGI_2, under our experimental conditions, is the platelet. Finally, the correlation between drop in platelet counts and bronchoconstriction in PAF-acether-injected guinea-pigs, illustrated in FIGURE 4, is of r = 0.994. That bronchoconstriction is indirect, and not due to a direct smooth muscle contracting effect of PAF-acether, is further indicated by its failure to contract the parenchyma lung strip, under conditions where $PGF_{2\alpha}$, PGI_2, serotonin, bradykinin or leukotrienes C and D induce reproducible dose-dependent contractions at final concentrations of 1 nM-1 μM. PAF-acether induces a first and small non-dose-dependent contraction, which is not observed again in the same strip. We think that this is due to platelets which remain within the tissue. This marginal effect is not the reflect of the dose-dependent and reproducible effect of PAF-acether in the guinea-pig, obtained already at doses of 50 ng/kg.

The disappearance of free platelets from the blood of PAF-acether-injected guinea-pigs is noted within 10 sec after the injection. Thrombocytopenia is accompanied by the appearance of free ATP in the arterial blood, confirming the intra-vascular platelet release reaction, and demonstrating that PAF-acether is not causing simply platelet sequestration, nor altering the platelet counts by other mechanisms.

We do not know as yet the exact mechanism for the platelet-lung smooth muscle interaction accounting for bronchoconstriction. ATP and ADP are released from the activated platelets, and are effective bronchoconstrictor substances. Nevertheless, bronchoconstriction by ADP and ATP is also platelet-dependent, and that due to the latter is inhibited largely by aspirin. Leukotrienes are very effective bronchoconstrictor substances as well, but their effect in the guinea-pig is inhibited by aspirin, *in vivo* and *in vitro*, ruling out their direct participation for bronchoconstriction by PAF-acether.[63] It might be argued that PAF-acether operates with no need of chemical mediators, simply because of the formation of platelet aggregates within pulmonary vessels, since there is evidence that the mechanical obstruction of lung capillaries with platelet thrombi can evoke bronchoconstriction. This cannot be ruled out at this stage, but we think it unlikely, particularly because of the peculiar interaction between PAF-acether on one side, and sulfinpyrazone or aspirin associated to anti-amine agents, on the other side (see below), which suggests strongly that the platelet release reaction is indeed the cause of bronchoconstriction. The possible involvement of materials extruded by the platelet from its α granules is an open possibility, which was not studied as yet.

Our experiments are performed in propranolol-treated guinea-pigs, in order

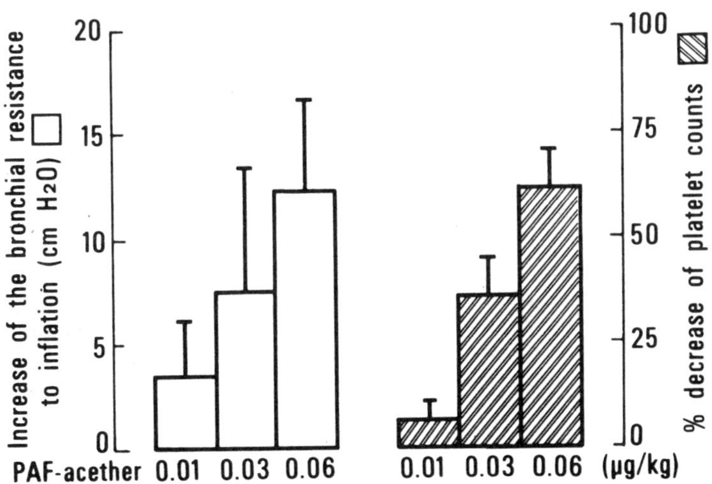

FIGURE 4. Dose-dependent increase in bronchial resistance to inflation and thrombocytopenia induced by PAF-acether in anesthetized guinea-pigs. The maximal increase in bronchial resistance to inflation (*left, open columns*) and the % decrease in platelet counts, measured within one minute after the injection of PAF-acether (*right, double-hatched columns*), were measured in 4–5 guinea-pigs injected intravenously with the indicated doses of PAF-acether.

to counteract the bronchodilator effect of catecholamines released when the animals are under intense bronchoconstriction. The animals are also paralyzed with pancuronium, a neuromuscular blocking agent, used to prevent spontaneous breathing during the experiment. These experimental conditions do not alter the findings, and recent observations made with Drs. F. Berti, G. C. Folco, G. Rossini and C. Omini, from the Department of Pharmacology of the University of Milan, showed that PAF-acether increases the pulmonary resistance and decreases in parallel the lung compliance of spontaneously breathing guinea pigs not treated with propranolol. Again aspirin failed to interfere with the effects of PAF-acether.

Antagonism to PAF-Acether

Mepyramine, an antihistamine agent, methysergide, an antiserotonin agent, or atropine associated with bilateral vagotomy, failed to inhibit the effects of PAF-acether in the propranolol-treated animals. This seemed to rule out the participation of endogenous amines, and of vagal reflexes, to account for these effects. It was therefore surprising to find that the association of aspirin or indomethacin, two nonsteroidal anti-inflammatory drugs which inhibit the synthesis of PGs, or of salicylic acid, an anti-inflammatory agent which does not inhibit this synthesis, with mepyramine and methysergide, blocked bronchoconstriction by PAF-acether (FIG. 5). When this was found, we knew that PAF-acether-induced bronchoconstriction is platelet-dependent, and it was logical to think that the drug association might inhibit at the platelet level. This hypothesis was not supported by the platelet counts performed after the injections of PAF-acether, since thrombocytopenia was present, whereas bronchoconstriction was suppressed by the drug combination. If one equates thrombocytopenia with intravascular aggregation, and the latter with the release reaction, it looked as if the release was not inhibited when bronchoconstriction was suppressed. Nevertheless, since aspirin associated with mepyramine or methysergide had no effect against unrelated bronchoconstrictor substances, such as acetylcholine, which ruled out a direct bronchodilator effect, we decided to investigate more thoroughly the platelet effects of the various drug combinations. Platelet-rich plasma was thus prepared from blood collected from animals treated with the drugs, and aggregation was studied. Results clearly indicated that aggregation was only inhibited to a very limited extent by the drug combinations effective against bronchoconstriction, and for concentrations of PAF-acether near the threshold, but that the release reaction was inhibited by the association of aspirin, indomethacin, or salicylic acid with methysergide and mepyramine (FIG. 6). The doses of methysergide and mepyramine used were very low (0.02–0.2 mg/kg).

The relevance of these drug interactions to physiopathology appears rather obscure. We looked for a drug which would by itself imitate the effects of the drug combinations. Our first choice was sulfinpyrazone, which shows platelet-protective effects unrelated to a feeble anti-cyclooxygenase activity. Sulfinpyrazone is effective against Forssman shock, which involves *in vivo* platelet aggregation.[64]

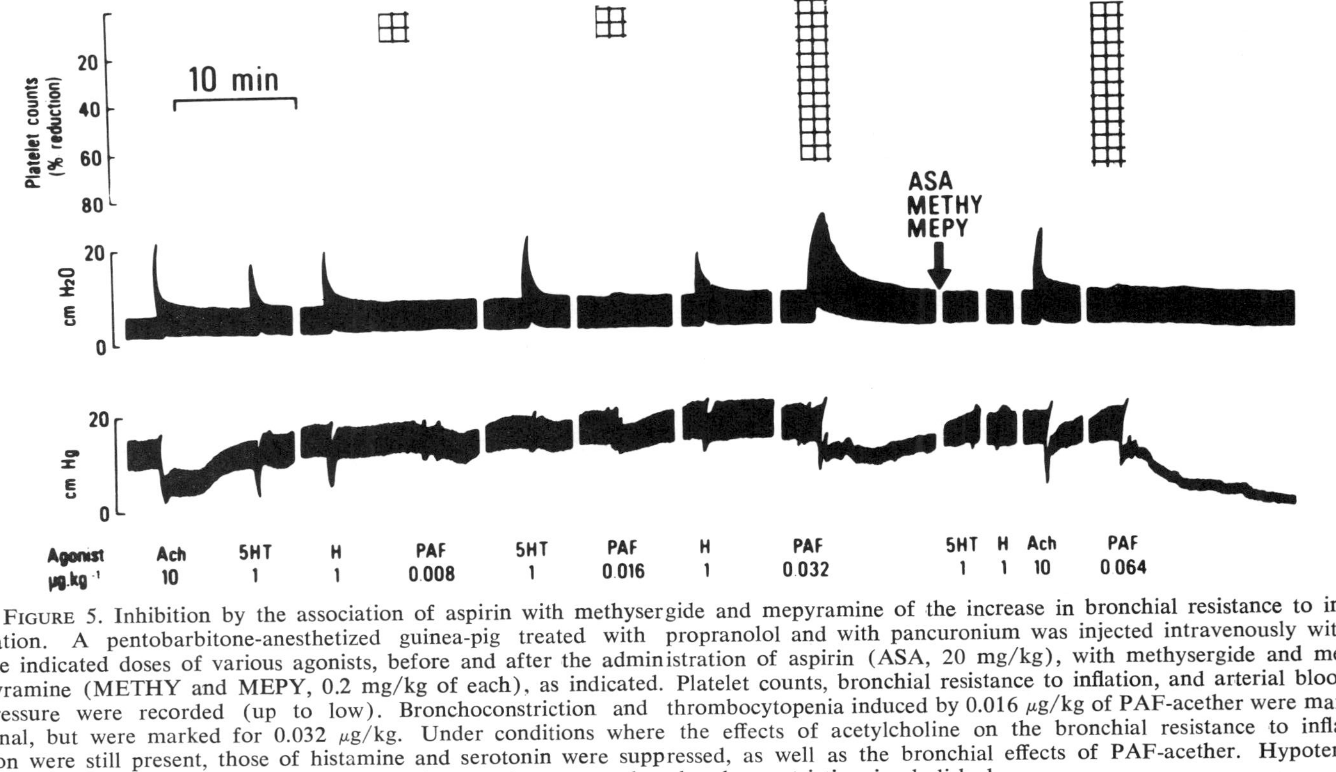

FIGURE 5. Inhibition by the association of aspirin with methysergide and mepyramine of the increase in bronchial resistance to inflation. A pentobarbitone-anesthetized guinea-pig treated with propranolol and with pancuronium was injected intravenously with the indicated doses of various agonists, before and after the administration of aspirin (ASA, 20 mg/kg), with methysergide and mepyramine (METHY and MEPY, 0.2 mg/kg of each), as indicated. Platelet counts, bronchial resistance to inflation, and arterial blood pressure were recorded (up to low). Bronchoconstriction and thrombocytopenia induced by 0.016 µg/kg of PAF-acether were marginal, but were marked for 0.032 µg/kg. Under conditions where the effects of acetylcholine on the bronchial resistance to inflation were still present, those of histamine and serotonin were suppressed, as well as the bronchial effects of PAF-acether. Hypotension and thrombocytopenia due to PAF-acether remain present when brochoconstriction is abolished.

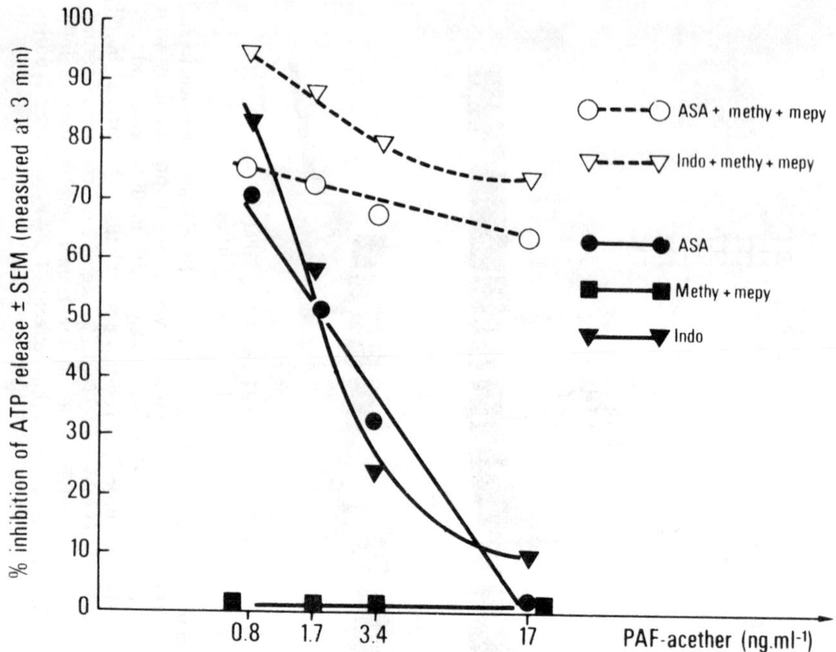

FIGURE 6. Inhibition by the association of aspirin or indomethacin with mepyramine and methysergide of the platelet release reaction due to PAF-acether. Aspirin (ASA, 20 mg/kg) or indomethacin(Indo, 5 mg/kg), methysergide and mepyramine (methy and mepy, 0.2 mg/kg of each), were injected intravenously in guinea-pigs prepared as for the bronchoconstriction experiments. Blood was collected within 3 min, and processed for the preparation of platelet-rich plasma. Aggregation was triggered by the indicated final concentrations of PAF-acether, and the accompanying release of ATP monitored 3 min afterwards. Aspirin and indomethacin inhibit the platelet release reaction due to low amounts of PAF-acether, and inhibition disappears for higher concentrations, whereas inhibition is insurmountable when the anti-inflammatory drugs are associated with mepyramine and methysergide.

Mode of Action of Sulfinpyrazone

When PAF-acether was injected in guinea-pigs 3 min after 30–100 mg/kg of sulfinpyrazone, bronchoconstriction was inhibited (FIG. 7). The higher dose of sulfinpyrazone reduced by around 40% bronchoconstriction by serotonin as well, but this unspecific effect was not seen 13 min later, whereas the effects of PAF-acether were still inhibited. Inhibition persisted less than 1 hour, and disappeared. In contrast, as described by others [65] the anti-cyclooxygenase activity persisted for a much longer time, and was in any case present within 6 hours. Thrombocytopenia due to PAF-acether was not inhibited when the inhibition of bronchoconstriction was at its height. When platelet-rich plasma was prepared from blood collected from animals injected with 100 mg/kg of sulfinpyrazone, aggregation by PAF-acether was reduced, the accompanying release reaction was suppressed for the low concentrations of PAF-acether, and was still inhibited for large increments of it. The effects of arachidonic acid were inhibited as well, but the curve for time and concentration-dependent effects differed from that obtained with PAF-acether. Finally, aggregation by ADP was only marginally reduced (FIGS. 8 & 9).

The *ex vivo* effect detected led us to study whether sulfinpyrazone would stimulate the endogenous formation of prostacyclin. The hypothesis that prostacyclin was released in the presence of sulfinpyrazone was indirectly supported by the fact that when bronchoconstriction by arachidonic acid was inhibited by sulfinpyrazone, the accompanying hypotension, which is attributed to formation of prostacyclin, was unaffected, contrary to what occurs for aspirin, which inhibited thrombocytopenia, bronchoconstriction, and hypotension. In fact, when sulfinpyrazone was incubated with guinea-pig vessels or lung strips, the amounts of anti-aggregating (prostacyclin-like) substances formed were either unchanged, as compared to the controls or reduced; when the concentrations of sulfinpyrazone applied reached 0.5 mM, they inhibited cyclooxygenase directly.

Effects of PAF-Acether on Rats, Rabbits and Dogs

Rat platelets, prepared from citrated or heparinized blood, or suspended in plasma-free buffers, are refractory to PAF-acether, under conditions where ADP is effective. Furthermore, PAF-acether does not potentiate aggregation by ADP or by arachidonic acid (J. Randon, to be published). Finally, the intravenous administration of PAF-acether to anesthetized rats is not followed by thrombocytopenia or by bronchoconstriction, whereas a marked hypotensive response is present for doses of 1–10 μg/kg.[66] The heart frequency of the rat is unaffected by PAF-acether, and hypotension is probably mediated by peripheral direct vasodilatation. Hypotension is not inhibited by aspirin nor by mepyramine, which rules out a role for prostacyclin or for histamine. Nevertheless, the intraplantar administration of PAF-acether to rats induces

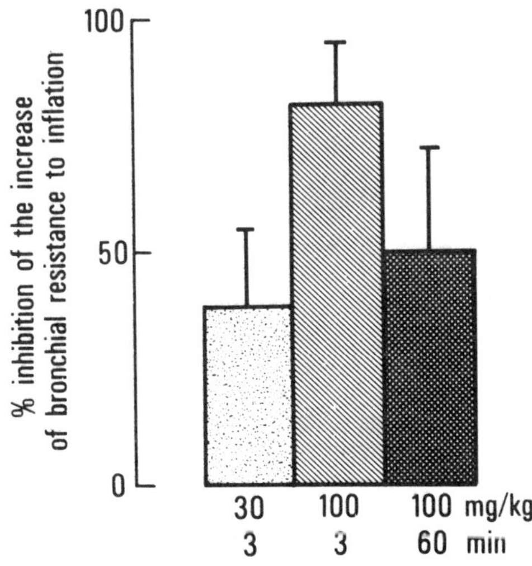

FIGURE 7. Inhibition by sulfinpyrazone of PAF-acether-induced bronchoconstriction in the guinea pig. The bronchoconstrictor effects of 66–132 ng/kg of PAF-acether were measured before and after the intravenous infusion of 30 or 100 mg/kg of sulfinpyrazone. The delay between the end of the infusion and the injection of PAF-acether was 3 or 60 min, as indicated. Results are % inhibition of the brochoconstriction ± S.E.M., for groups of 5–6 guinea-pigs.

edema (FIG. 10) and hyperalgesia,[67, 68] and potentiates the inflammatory effects of carrageenan.[67] Prostaglandins E_1 and I_2 also potentiate the effects of carrageenan,[69] and these effects are not inhibited by aspirin. In contrast, potentiation of edema by PAF-acether is inhibited by aspirin, by indomethacin and by salicylic acid.[67] Since the latter is not an inhibitor of the prostaglandin

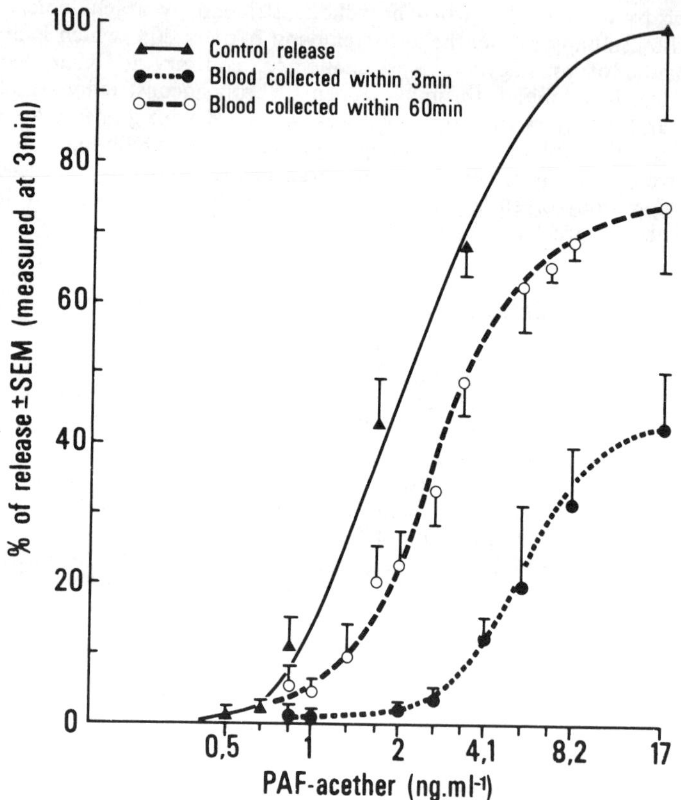

FIGURE 8. Inhibition by sulfinpyrazone of the release of platelet ATP induced by PAF-acether. Sulfinpyrazone was infused intravenously to groups of 5 guinea-pigs, at the dose of 100 mg/kg, and blood was collected for the preparation of platelet-rich plasma, after 3 or 60 min, as indicated. Aggregation was triggered by the indicated concentrations of PAF-acether and the amount of ATP released after 3 min was measured, and compared to that induced by the same concentrations of PAF-acether in a control group of animals, infused with saline. Observe reduction of the platelet release reaction, still present after 60 min and seen for all the concentrations of PAF-acether used.

cyclooxygenase, its effectiveness raises the problem of the correlation between prostaglandins, as causing agents or byproducts, during inflammation.[70] Since PAF-acether may be produced by neutrophils and/or macrophages, during inflammation, (see above) the interaction between both systems—the pharmacologically active phospholipids, and prostaglandins—may be important in the passage from acute to chronic inflammation.

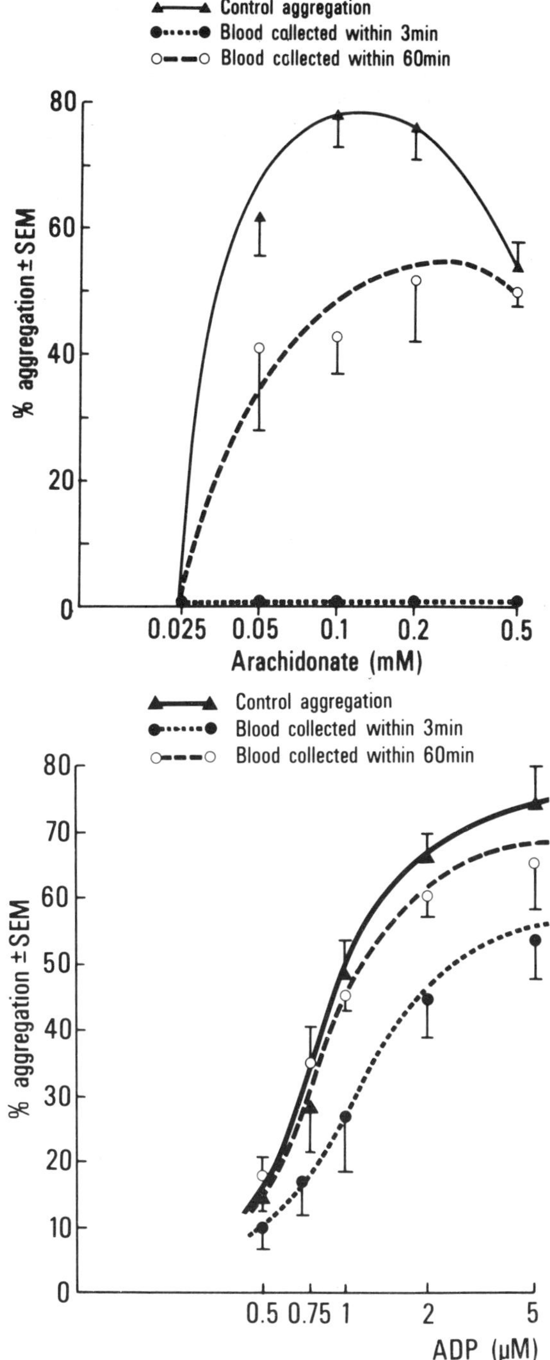

FIGURE 9. Inhibition by sulfinpyrazone of the aggregation of guinea-pig platelets due to arachidonate (A) and to ADP (B). Sulfinpyrazone was injected as indicated in FIGURE 6. Aggregation of the platelets was measured, and compared to that indicated by arachidonate (A) and by ADP (B). Results are % aggregation ± S.E.M.

The intravenous injection of PAF-acether to the anesthetized rabbit is followed by hypotension, accompanied by thrombocytopenia and neutropenia. Both are reversible, when low doses of PAF-acether are used.[38, 71, 72] There is no report on the use of inhibitors against these effects.

Finally, PAF-acether also induces marked cardiovascular effects in the dog,[73] which resemble those of endotoxic shock. Arterial blood pressure decreases, and is accompanied by a long-lasting and platelet-dependent increase in coronary resistance, when PAF-acether is given intravenously at 0.2–20 μg/kg. Metabolic acidosis and a marked elevation of the plasma content in

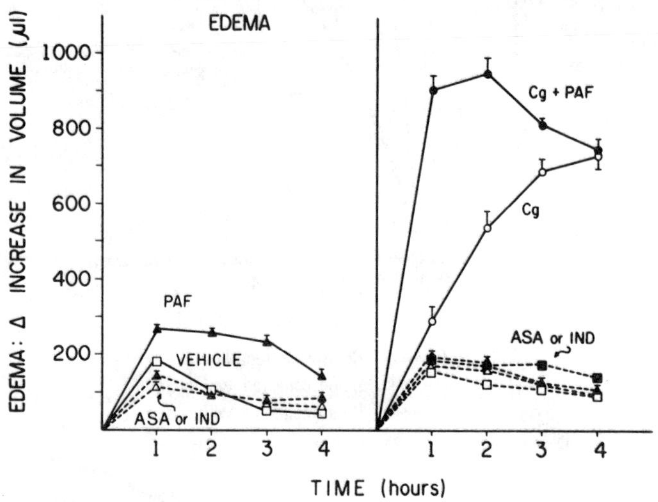

FIGURE 10. Inhibition by aspirin and by indomethacin of PAF-acether induced potentiation of rat paw edema due to carrageenan. The left panel shows the edema induced by 1 μg of PAF-acether injected into the rat paw (*full triangles*). Pretreatment (*dotted lines*) with aspirin (ASA, *open triangles*) or indomethacin (IND, *closed triangles*) reduced the effect to that of the vehicle (*squares*). The right panel shows the effects of carrageenan (Cg, *open circles*) and the potentiation by PAF-acether (Cg + PAG, *full circles*). Pre-treatment (*dotted lines*) with ASA (*triangles*) or with IND (*squares*) inhibits the effects of Cg (*open symbols*) or of the mixture of carrageenan and PAF (*solid symbols*). The points represent the means ± S.E.M. for five paws (From Ferreira & Vargaftig.[67] By permission of the Braz. J. Med. Biol. Res.).

various enzymes indicates tissue injury. Nonsteroidal anti-inflammatory agents fail completely to inhibit these effects.

GENERAL CONCLUSIONS

The initial hypothesis that PAF-acether is involved in anaphylactic shock was extended to a variety of conditions, which include new pathways for platelet aggregation, similarities with endotoxic shock, and hypotensive mechanisms. Presence of PAF-acether under these various conditions, as well as its ability to reproduce the expected effects, is no final proof of its actual involvement as a causative factor. Until inhibitors of the formation and of the effects of PAF-acether become available as specific tools, its role will be only hypothetical and all evidence will be debatable. Nevertheless, PAF-acether has now reached the status of a putative mediator in conditions similar to those of prostaglandins or histamine. Much will be said in the near future and much more will be ruled out, before a final position can be reached concerning the real importance of PAF-acether in physiopathology.

REFERENCES

1. BARBARO, J. F. & N. J. ZVAIFLER. 1966. Proc. Exp. Biol. Med. **122:** 1245.
2. SIRAGANIAN, R. P. & A. G. OSLER. 1971. J. Immunol. **106:** 1252.
3. BENVENISTE, J., P. M. HENSON & C. G. COCHRANE. 1972. J. Exp. Med. **136:** 1356.
4. BENVENISTE, J., J. P. LE COUEDIC & P. KAMOUN. 1975. Lancet **1:** 344.
5. BENVENISTE, J. 1980. *In* Adv. Allergol. Immunol. Oehling, I. Glazer, E. Mathov & C. Arbesman, Eds. Pergamon Press. Oxford and New York.
6. BENVENISTE, J., J. P. LE COUEDIC, J. POLONSKY & M. TENCE. 1977. Nature **269:** 170.
7. BENVENISTE, J., M. TENCE, P. VARENNE, J. BIDAULT, C. BOULLET & J. POLONSKY. 1979. C. R. Acad. Sc. Paris **289:** 1017.
8. DEMOPOULOS, C. A., R. N. PINCKARD & D. J. HANAHAN. 1979. J. Biol. Chem. **254:** 9355.
9. GODFROID, J. J., F. HEYMANS, E. MICHEL, C. REDEUILH, E. STEINER & J. BENVENISTE. 1980. FEBS Lett. **116:** 161.
10. BENVENISTE, J. 1974. Nature **249:** 581.
11. BUSSOLINO, F. & J. BENVENISTE. 1980. Immunology **40:** 367.
12. LEWIS, R. A., E. J. GOETZL, S. I. WASSERMAN, F. H. VALONE, R. H. RUBIN & K. F. AUSTEN. 1975. J. Immunol. **114:** 87.
13. MENCIA-HUERTA, J. M. *et al.* To be published.
14. CAMUSSI, G., M. AGLIETA, R. CODA, F. BUSSOLINO, W. PIACIBELLO & C. TETTA. 1981. Immunology **42:** 191.
15. BETZ, S. J., G. Z. LOTNER & P. M. HENSON. 1980. J. Immunol. **125:** 2749.
16. SANCHEZ-CRESPO, M., F. ALONSO & J. EGIDO. 1980. Immunology **40:** 645.
17. KRAVIS, T. C. & P. M. HENSON. 1977. J. Immunol. **188:** 1569.
18. CAMUSSI, G., J. M. MENCIA-HUERTA & J. BENVENISTE. 1977. Immunology **33:** 523.
19. MENCIA-HUERTA, J. M. & J. BENVENISTE. 1979. Eur. J. Immunol. **9:** 409.
20. ARNOUX, B., D. DUVAL & J. BENVENISTE. 1980. Eur. J. Clin. Invest. **10:** 437.
21. KRAVIS, T. C. & P. M. HENSON. 1975. J. Immunol. **115:** 1677.
22. BENVENISTE, J., J. M. MENCIA-HUERTA & D. DUVAL. 1979. Fed. Proc. **38:** 1168 (Abs.).
23. LYNCH, J. M., G. Z. LOTNER, S. J. BETZ & P. M. HENSON. 1979. J. Immunol. **123:** 1219.
24. JOUVIN, E. & J. BENVENISTE. Submitted.
25. BETZ, S. J. & P. M. HENSON. 1980. J. Immunol. **125:** 2756.
26. MENCIA-HUERTA, J. M. & J. BENVENISTE. Submitted.
27. RILEY, J. F. 1963. Ann. N.Y. Acad. Sci. **103:** 1847.
28. KINLOUGH-RATHBONE, R. L., M. A. PACKHAM, H. J. REIMERS, J. P. CAZENAVE, & J. F. MUSTARD. 1977. J. Lab. Clin. Med. **90:** 707.
29. PACKHAM, M. A., M. A. GUCCIONE, J. P. GREENBERG, R. L. KINLOUGH-RATHBONE & J. F. MUSTARD. 1977. Blood **50:** 915.
30. VARGAFTIG, B. B. 1977. J. Pharm. Pharmacol. **29:** 222.

31. LAPETINA, E. G., K. A. CHANDRABOSE & P. CUATRECASAS. 1978. Proc. Natl. Acad. Sci. USA **75:** 818.
32. CHARO, I. F., R. D. FEINMAN & T. C. DETWILER. 1977. J. Clin. Invest. **60:** 866.
33. CAZENAVE, J. P., J. BENVENISTE & J. F. MUSTARD. 1979. Lab. Invest. **41:** 275.
34. CHIGNARD, M., J. P. LE COUEDIC, M. TENCE, B. B. VARGAFTIG & J. BENVENISTE. 1979. Nature. **279:** 799.
35. CHIGNARD, M., J. P. LE COUEDIC, B. B. VARGAFTIG & J. BENVENISTE. 1979. Br. J. Haematol. **45:** 455.
36. NAMM, D. H. & J. A. HIGH. 1980. Thromb. Res. **20:** 285.
37. CHIGNARD, M. et al. To be published.
38. CHIGNARD, M., B. B. VARGAFTIG, J. BENVENISTE & J. P. LE COUEDIC. 1980. J. Pharmacol. (Paris). **11:** 371.
39. VARGAFTIG, B. B., M. CHIGNARD & J. BENVENISTE. 1981. Biochem. Pharmacol. **30:** 263.
40. HENSON, P. M. 1976. J. Exp. Med. **143:** 937.
41. VARGAFTIG, B. B., J. LEFORT, M. CHIGNARD & J. BENVENISTE. 1980. Eur. J. Pharmacol. **65:** 185.
42. SHAW, J. O., M. P. PRINTZ, K. HIRABAYASHI & P. M. HENSON. 1978. J. Immunol. **121:** 1339.
43. MAC MANUS, L. M., J. O. SHAW & R. N. PINCKARD. 1980. J. Immunol. **125:** 1950.
44. SHAW, J. O., S. J. KLUSICK & D. J. HANAHAN. 1981. Biochem. Biophys. Acta **663:** 222.
45. VARGAFTIG, B. B. et al. To be published.
46. TENCE, M., E. MICHEL, J. POLONSKY & J. BENVENISTE. 1981. Agents and Actions. In press.
47. HENSON, P. M. 1977. J. Clin. Invest. **60:** 481.
48. LALAU-KERALY, C. et al. To be published.
49. SHAW, J. O. & P. M. HENSON. 1980. Am. J. Pathol. **98:** 791.
50. HENSON, P. M. & Z. G. OADES. 1976. J. Exp. Med. **143:** 935.
51. BUSSOLINO, F. & G. CAMUSSI. 1980. Prostaglandins. **20:** 781.
52. CHIGNARD, M., M. TENCE, J. P. LE COUEDIC, B. B. VARGAFTIG & J. BENVENISTE. 1979. Fed. Proc. **38:** 1342 (Abs.).
53. BENVENISTE, J. et al. To be published.
54. MENCIA-HUERTA, J. M., C. AKERMAN & J. BENVENISTE. 1980. Fed. Proc. **39:** 691 (Abs.).
55. POLONSKY, J., M. TENCE, P. VARENNE, B. C. DAS, J. LUNEL & J. BENVENISTE. 1981. Proc. Natl. Acad. Sci. USA **77:** 7019.
56. CHAP, H., G. MAUCO, M. F. SIMON, J. BENVENISTE & L. DOUSTE-BLAZY. 1981. Nature. **289:** 312.
57. MENCIA-HUERTA, J. M., E. NINIO, R. ROUBIN & J. BENVENISTE. 1981. Agents and Action. In press.
58. BENVENISTE, J., J. M. MENCIA-HUERTA & R. ROUBIN. 1981. Monographs in Allergy. In press.
59. WYKLE, R. L., B. MALONE & F. SNYDER. 1980. J. Biol. Chem. **255:** 10256.
60. NINIO, E. et al. To be published.
61. BLANK, M. L., T. C. LEE, V. FITZGERALD & F. SNYDER. 1981. J. Biol. Chem. **256:** 175.
62. VARGAFTIG, B. B. & J. LEFORT. Eur. J. Pharmacol. Submitted.
63. VARGAFTIG, B. B., J. LEFORT & R. C. MURPHY. Agents and Actions. In press.
64. BUTLER, K. D. & A. M. WHITE. In Cardiovascular actions of sulfinpyrazone, Symposia Specialists. 1980. p. 3.
65. BUTLER, K. D., W. DIETERLE, E. D. MAGUIRE, G. F. PAY, R. B. WALLIS & A. M.

WHITE.1980. *In* Cardiovascular actions of sulfinpyrazone, Symposia Specialist. p. 19.
66. BLANK, M. L., F. SNYDER, L. W. BYERS, B. BROOKS & E. E. MUIRHEAD. 1979. Biochem. Biophys. Res. Commun. **90:** 1194.
67. FERREIRA, S. H. AND B. B. VARGAFTIG. Braz. J. Med. Biol. Res. In press.
68. BONNET, J., A. M. LOISEAU, M. ORVOEN & P. BESSIN. Agents and Actions. In press.
69. FERREIRA, S. H. 1981. TIPS. In press.
70. VARGAFTIG, B. B. 1980. TIPS. **1:** 415.
71. PINCKARD, R. N., R. S. FARR & D. J. HANAHAN. 1979. J. Immunol. **123:** 1847.
72. VARGAFTIG, B. B., M. CHIGNARD, J. M. MENCIA-HUERTA, B. ARNOUX & J. BENVENISTE. 1981. *In* Platelets in Biology and Pathology 2. J. L. Gordon, Ed. Elsevier-North Holland. Amsterdam, New York, Oxford. p. 371.
73. BESSIN, P., J. BONNET, D. APFFEL, L. DESGROUX, T. PELAS & J. BENVENISTE. To be published.

[Note added in proof: Hanahan *et al.* (Biochem. Biophys. Res. Commun. **99:** 183, 1981) reported that the enantiomeric forms of PAF-acether show a similar aggregating activity, contrary to our results with guinea-pig and rabbit platelets.]

THROMBOPHLEBITIS IN CANCER PATIENTS

Takeshi Wajima

Departments of Hematology and Medical Oncology
Wilford Hall USAF Medical Center
Lackland AFB, San Antonio, Texas 78236

INTRODUCTION

Migratory thrombophlebitis is a systemic manifestation of a malignant neoplasm. A wide range of clinical abnormalities may develop as a consequence of changes in blood coagulation and platelets.[1-7] No unifying common patho-physiologic mechanism has been found for this disorder. Characteristically in cancer patients thrombophlebitis tends to be migratory or recurrent and it is often resistant to anticoagulant therapy. Stasis due to inactivity and tumor masses may contribute to this thrombophlebitis. A so-called "hypercoagulable state" has been described as a continuing abnormality of hemostasis underlying migratory thrombophlebitis. Heparin is superior to currently available oral anticoagulants for management of this condition.

CASE REPORTS

CASE 1. The patient, a 60-year-old man with undifferentiated carcinoma of the right side and base of the skull, presented with painful swelling of the left leg. The venogram was positive in the deep venous system up to the level of the iliac veins. Prothrombin time (PT) and activated partial thromboplastin time (PTT) were normal. Platelet count was 150,000, fibrinogen 240 mg percent, and thrombin time (TT) 11 seconds. The patient was treated with continuous intravenous infusion of heparin, 36,000 units daily, resulting in PTT greater than 100 seconds for 12 days. Chest X-ray film showed blunting of the left costophrenic angle and subsequent atelectasis of the left lower lobe. A ventilation and perfusion (V/Q) scan showed multiple bilateral perfusion defects without corresponding ventilation defects, con-sistent with multiple pulmonary emboli. Heparin was continued for an additional 12 days and the patient was started on Coumadin® therapy before the heparin was discontinued. Recurrence developed nevertheless. Heparin therapy was resumed and Coumadin continued, maintaining the PT level between 19 and 26 seconds with a control value of 12 to 14 seconds; PTT was maintained greater than 40 seconds throughout the 10 days.

The patient vomited clotted blood, and heparin was discontinued. He became febrile and a left lower lobe infiltrate was noted on X-ray film of the chest. Despite continued anticoagulant and antibiotic therapy, thrombosis of the left leg recurred, and the patient died.

CASE 2. This 66-year-old white woman with undifferentiated large-cell carcinoma of the lung developed pain in the left leg. Platelet count, PT and PTT were normal. Chest X-ray film revealed a left suprahilar mass. A venogram of the left leg revealed deep venous thrombosis in the calf. Heparin therapy was instituted and the dosage gradually increased to 36,000 units per day, but it was difficult to reach adequate anticoagulation as measured by PTT. The antithrombin III (AT-III) level was 65 percent. The patient's symptoms lessened, but her condition became char-

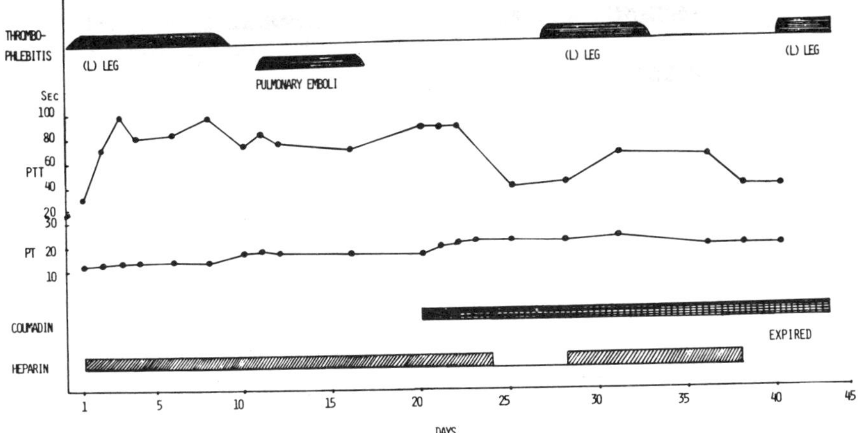

FIGURE 1. *Case 1*. Serial PT, PTT, anticoagulant therapy, and thromboembolic events.

acterized by sepsis. Her right leg became swollen and tender and she died. Findings at autopsy included a large-cell undifferentiated carcinoma, mucin-positive, of the left upper lobe of the lung. Thrombosis of the right iliac vein, extending into the distal inferior vena cava, was also noted.

CASE 3. This 39-year-old man with adenocarcinoma of the lung with metastatic cancer to the right hemisphere of the brain developed superficial thrombophlebitis of the left arm. The left thigh and calf were notably increased in size. Platelet count was 660,000, PT 12 seconds, PTT 25 seconds, thrombin time 11 seconds, and AT-III level 54 percent.

Heparin, 30,000 units per day by intravenous infusion, was given for 18 days, and Coumadin, 10 mg orally per day, was added. Heparin was discontinued five days later, at which time the PT was 20 to 22 seconds and PTT 70 to 80 seconds. Two days later the patient's left leg became swollen, warm, and tender. Subcutaneous

FIGURE 2. *Case 2*. Serial PT, PTT, anticoagulant therapy, and thromboembolic events.

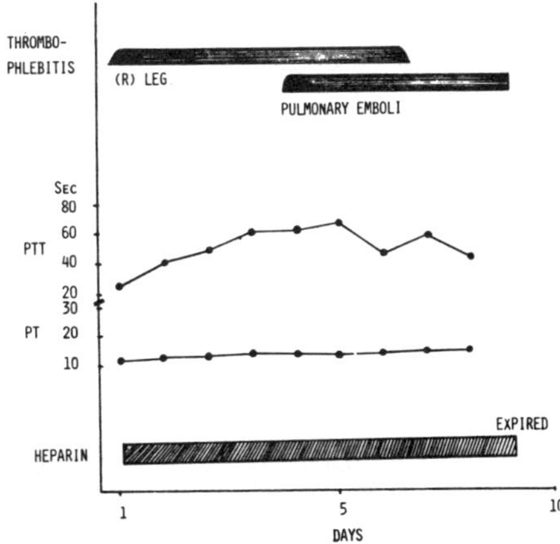

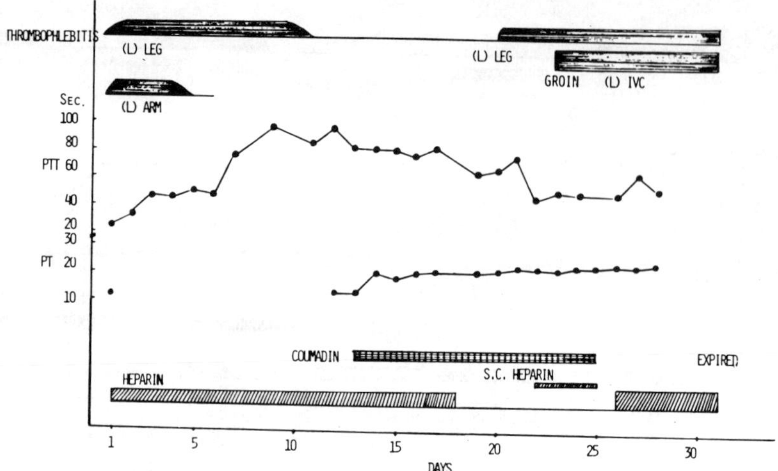

FIGURE 3. *Case 3*. Serial PT, PTT, anticoagulant therapy, and thromboembolic events.

heparin, 5,000 units every 12 hours, was begun, but thrombophlebitis extended to the groin. Coumadin was discontinued, and a full dose of heparin, 36,000 units daily by intravenous infusion, was reinstituted, with partial response. The patient died of central nervous system disease.

CASE 4. A 51-year-old white woman with metastatic breast cancer complained of lethargy and weakness of the right leg. Chest X-ray film revealed infiltration into the left upper lobe of the lung. A V/Q scan showed multiple mismatched defects. Platelet count was 370,000, PT 12 seconds, PTT 28 seconds, fibrinogen 510 mg percent, AT-III level 70 percent, pO_2 60, pCO_2 34, and pH 7.55.

Heparin therapy 30,000 units per day by intravenous infusion, was begun. While the patient was receiving heparin, left iliofemoral thrombophlebitis developed and she died in a state of respiratory failure. Autopsy showed multiple metastases to the lungs, liver, and bone. The main pulmonary artery was occluded by emboli.

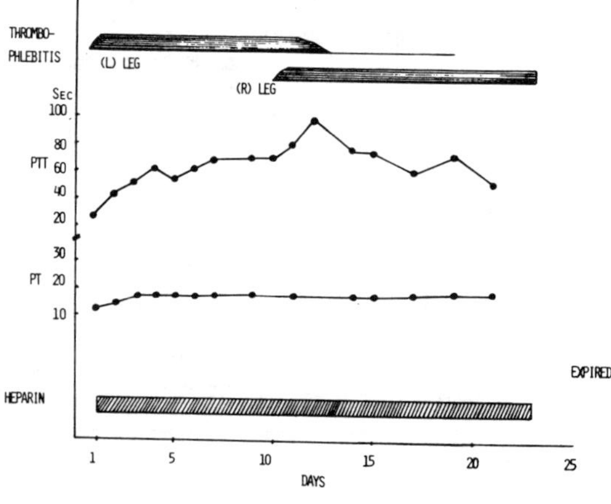

FIGURE 4. *Case 4*. Serial PT, PTT, anticoagulant therapy, and thromboembolic events.

CASE 5. The patient, a 49-year-old white man with metastatic adenocarcinoma of the lung, presented with swelling and pain in the left leg. A venogram demonstrated thrombosis in the deep venous system of this leg. Platelet count was 220,000 and PT, PTT and thrombin time were 12, 28, and 12 seconds, respectively; fibrinogen was 520 mg percent. Heparin, 30,000 units per day, was given by intravenous infusion, and the PTT was 40 to 80 seconds for 18 days. Before heparin was discontinued Coumadin therapy was started. The patient was discharged on a regimen of Coumadin, 5 mg orally per day. Prothrombin time was 20 to 25 seconds (control value, 11 to 13 seconds). Six days later the patient noticed pain in the left ankle with swelling and warmth. Heparin, 30,000 units per day by intravenous infusion, was reinstituted with resolution of symptoms.

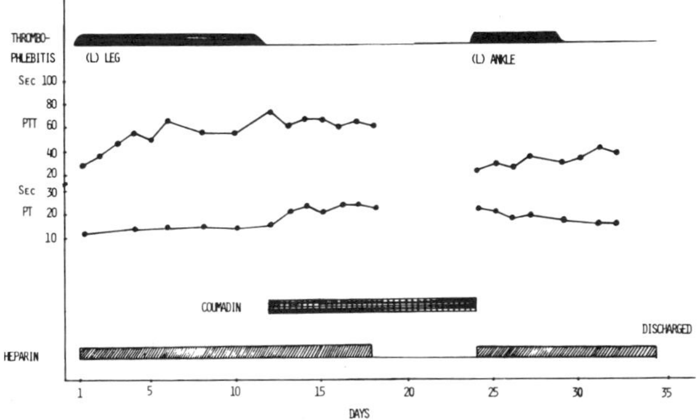

FIGURE 5. *Case 5.* Serial PT, PTT, anticoagulant therapy, and thromboembolic events.

DISCUSSION

The picture of "consumption coagulopathy" was not seen in these patients; platelet counts were consistently normal, and values for PT, PTT, and factor VIII procoagulant activity were in the normal range (TABLE 1). Protamine sulfate test and ethanol gelation test were negative, as was the test for cryofibrinogen. Fragmentation of red blood cells on blood smear was not observed. However, normal to elevated fibrinogen and decreased AT-III levels and slightly increased fibrinogen/fibrin degradation products (FDP) suggest the presence of the "hypercoagulable state" or chronic intravascular coagulation. The syndrome of chronic intravascular coagulation has become well recognized in cases of cancer, particularly in cases of metastatic malignancy.[1, 2, 5, 6] Although levels of clotting factors are commonly depressed in chronic disseminated intravascular coagulation, elevated levels also have been noted in both patients and laboratory animals.[5, 7-9] These patients were perhaps able to compensate for overutilization of the clotting factors and platelets.

Many attempts have been made to identify the factor(s) responsible for initiating this process.[2, 4, 7, 10-13] The "mucus-secreting" nature of several neoplastic tumors resulted in studies of cancer procoagulant activity.[11-13] Some tumors have been shown to alter the fibrinolytic system. These patients had advanced cancer (high tumor mass) and might have had tumor emboli,

TABLE 1

SUMMARY OF RESULTS OF LABORATORY TESTS BEFORE ANTICOAGULATION THERAPY IN FIVE CANCER PATIENTS WITH THROMBOPHLEBITIS

Case No.	Platelet Count ($\times 10^9$/L)	PT (sec)	PTT (sec)	Factor VIII Activity (% of clotting activity)	Fibrinogen (mg %)	TT (sec)	AT-III (%)	(μg/ml) FDP	Protamine Sulfate Test	Ethanol Gel Test	Cryo-fibrinogen
1	150	11	28	100	240	11	70	40–80	—	—	—
2	280	11	26	150	400	11	65	40–80	—	—	—
3	660	12	25	120	600	11	54	40–80	—	—	—
4	370	12	28	100	510	11	70	40–80	—	—	—
5	220	12	28	160	520	12	65	80–160	—	—	—
Normal values	150–400	11–13	25–40	80–150	200–400	11–13	antigenic activity >80	<10	—	—	—

NOTE: PT, Prothrombin time; PTT, activated partial thromboplastin time; factor VIII activity=factor VIII procoagulant activity; TT=thrombin time; AT-III=antithrombin III; FDP=fibrinogen/fibrin degradation products.

thrombosis, or venous obstruction by tumor. Since these patients were hospitalized and bedridden, stasis due to inactivity may also have been a contributing factor.

Heparin acts as a cofactor and accelerates the rate at which AT-III inhibits thrombin and other serine proteases.[15] Changes in the level of AT-III reflect the effect of heparin. If AT-III levels are persistently reduced in cancer patients, the anticoagulant effect of heparin may be diminished, and when heparin is discontinued, thrombosis can occur. In patients in whom thrombosis has already occurred, recurrence is likely when anticoagulation therapy is discontinued.

One patient was treated with subcutaneous heparin and Coumadin, but this therapy failed. Chronic subcutaneous administration of heparin has been used in some patients.[16, 17] No controlled long-term trial of subcutaneous heparin has been carried out, but this therapy may be an effective treatment in this syndrome. Criteria are not well established for discontinuing heparin after control of thrombotic episodes has been achieved.

Oral anticoagulants inhibit only the synthesis of vitamin-K-dependent coagulation factors, and they lead to decreased thrombin generation.[18] Oral anticoagulants were not effective for thrombophlebitis in advanced cancer. Other reviews have consistently emphasized the superiority of heparin in this situation.[6, 19-21]

Summary

Five cancer patients (three with lesions in the lung and one each with breast and head and neck cancer) with multiple metastases developed "migratory thrombophlebitis." These patients were not ambulatory. None of the patients showed a picture of "consumptive coagulopathy," although a "hypercoagulable state" was observed. Fibrinogen levels were normal or increased, FDP were slightly increased, and AT-III was decreased. Prior to heparin therapy, values for PT and PTT were within normal range. Sodium heparin, 30,000 to 36,000 units per day, was administered by continuous intravenous infusion. Despite prolongation of the PTT to twice the baseline levels, signs and symptoms of thrombophlebitis persisted for several days. When thrombophlebitis was controlled with heparin, Coumadin therapy was instituted, but thrombophlebitis recurred at the original site and at new sites, even though the prothrombin time was in the therapeutic range (2 to 2½ times the normal value). The antithrombotic action of heparin depends on a normal quantity of plasma AT-III. Long-term use of heparin is feasible, but the optimal time for discontinuation of heparin treatment has not been established. Heparin is superior to oral anticoagulation therapy to control thrombophlebitis associated with advanced cancer.

References

1. GOODNIGHT, S. H., JR. 1974. Bleeding and intravascular clotting in malignancy: A review. Ann. N.Y. Acad. Sci. **230:** 271–288
2. SACK, G. S., J. LEVEN & W. R. BELL. 1977. Trousseau's syndrome and other manifestations of chronic disseminated coagulopathy in patients with neoplasms: Clinical, pathophysiologic and therapeutic features. Medicine **56:** 1–37.

3. SLICHTER, S. J. & L. A. HARKER. 1974. Hemostasis in malignancy. Ann. N.Y. Acad. Sci. **230:** 252–261.

4. SOONG, B. C. F. & S. P. MILLER. 1970. Coagulation disorders in cancer. III. Fibrinolysis and inhibitors. Cancer **25:** 807–874.

5. SUN, N. C. J., E. J. W. BOWIE, F. J. KAZMIER, L. R. ELVEBACK & C. A. OWEN, JR. 1974. Blood coagulation studies in patients with cancer. Mayo Clin. Proc. **49:** 636–641.

6. MERSKEY, C. 1974. Pathogenesis and treatment of altered blood coagulability in patients with malignant tumors. Ann. N.Y. Acad. Sci. **230:** 289–293.

7. BRUGAROLAS, A., I. B. MINK & E. G. ELIAS. 1973. Correlation of hyper-fibrinogenemia with major thromboembolism in patients with cancer. Surg. Gynecol. Obstet. **136:** 75–77.

8. COOPER, H. A., E. J. W. BOWIE & C. A. OWEN, JR. 1973. Chronic induced intravascular coagulation in dogs. Am. J. Physiol. **225:** 1355–1358.

9. LOSITO, R., P. BEANDRY, J. C., VALDERRAMO, L. COUSINEAU & B. LONGPRÉ. 1978. Antithrombin III and Factor VIII in patients with neoplasms. Am. J. Clin. Pathol. **68:** 258–262.

10. McKAY, D. G. & G. H. WAHLE, JR. 1955. Disseminated thrombosis in colon cancer. Cancer **8:** 970–978.

11. PINEO, G. F., E. REGOECZI, M. W. C. HATTON & M. C. BRAIN. 1973. The activation of coagulation by extracts of mucus. A possible pathway of intravascular coagulation accompanying adenocarcinoma. J. Lab. Clin. Med. **82:** 255–266.

12. PINEO, G. F., M. C. BRAIN, A. S. GALLUS, J. HIRSH, M. W. C. HATTON & E. REGOECZI. 1974. Tumors, mucus production and hypercoagulability. Ann. N.Y. Acad. Sci. **230:** 262–270.

13. GORDON, S. G., J. J. FRANKS & B. LEWIS. 1975. Cancer procoagulant A: A factor X activating procoagulant from malignant tissue. Thromb. Res. **6:** 127–137.

14. BJÖRLIN, G., M. PANDOLFI & B. ÅSTEDT. 1972. Release of fibrinolytic activators from human tumors cultured in vitro. Experientia **28:** 833–834.

15. ROSENBERG, R. D. 1975. Actions and interactions of antithrombin and heparin. N. Engl. J. Med. **292:** 146–151.

16. KAZMIER, F. J., E. J. W. BOWIE, A. B. HAGEDORN & C. A. OWEN, JR. 1974. Treatment of intravascular coagulation and fibrinolysis (ICF) syndrome. Mayo Clinic Proc. **49:** 665–672.

17. STEVENS, W., G. BAELE & G. VERDONK. 1972. Failure of subcutaneous heparin treatment in a case of disseminated intravascular coagulation. Acta Haematol. **48:** 245–250.

18. WESSLER, S. & S. N. GITEL. 1979. Heparin and warfarin therapy. Postgrad. Med. **65:** 103–115.

19. COON, W. W. & P. W. WILLIS, III. 1972. Thromboembolic complications during anticoagulant therapy. Arch. Surg. **105:** 209–212.

20. LIEBERMAN, J. S., J. BORRERO, E. URDANETA & I. S. WRIGHT. 1961. Thrombophlebitis and cancer. JAMA **177:** 542–545.

22. MERSKEY, C. & A. J. JOHNSON. 1966. Diagnosis and treatment of intravascular coagulation. Thromb. Diath. Haemorrh. (Suppl. 21): 556–563.

ESSENTIAL THROMBOCYTHEMIA WITH TRANSITION INTO ACUTE LEUKEMIA

Sundara B. K. Raman, Ahmad Mahmood, Ellis J. Van Slyck,
and Sheikh M. Saeed

Department of Pathology
Division of Hematopathology; and the
Section of Hematology
Division of Hematology/Oncology
Henry Ford Hospital
Detroit, Michigan 48202

Since the syndrome of hemorrhagic thrombocythemia was described by Epstein and Goedel,[1] several subsequent reports have described this disease entity in association with other myeloproliferative disorders, particularly polycythemia vera. Later reviews of the literature by Fanger *et al.*,[2] Gunz,[3] Ozer *et al.*,[4] and Silverstein [5] have established this disease as a distinct clinical entity in the spectrum of myeloproliferative syndromes.

Because of the qualitative and numerical platelet abnormalities found,[6-10] the association of essential thrombocythemia with both hemorrhagic and thrombotic episodes is well recognized. To control these often serious complications, various modalities of treatment have been tried, including ionizing radiation,[11] cytostatic agents,[13, 14] and, recently, thrombocytopheresis.[15, 16]

The few cases of primary thrombocythemia that terminated in acute leukemia [4, 14, 17, 18] were all either treated with ionizing radiation and/or cytostatic agents. The case reported by us is of interest since acute leukemia developed within 16 months after the initial diagnosis of essential thrombocythemia in a patient who did not receive any significant treatment.

CASE REPORT

A 57-year-old black man was first admitted to our hospital in August 1978 with complaints of exertional dyspnea of recent onset and episodes of weakness and abdominal pain of a few weeks' duration. He denied any episodes of gross bleeding. He admitted to heavy ethanol abuse, but not taken no medications.

The physical examination was essentially negative. In particular, there were no palpable lymph nodes or demonstrable enlargement of spleen or liver.

Upon admission laboratory tests showed a hemoglobin of 13.9 gm percent, with slight erythrocytosis (red blood cell count was 6 million/mm^3), hypochromia (mean corpuscular hemoglobin concentration 31.1 percent, mean corpuscular hemoglobin 21.4 pg) and microcytosis (mean corpuscular volume 65 μ^3). The white blood cell count was 8,800/mm^3 with 70 percent polymorphonuclear cells, 1 percent bands, 21 percent lymphocytes, 6 percent monocytes, and 1 percent eosinophils. The platelet count was 1,160,000/mm^3 and the reticulocyte count was 3.7 percent. Examination of Wright-stained peripheral blood smear showed microcytic hypochromic red blood cells and increased platelets. Several platelets were bizarre and hypogranular. A few megakaryocytic fragments were seen. The serum iron was 22 μg/dL and the iron-binding capacity 504 μg/dL, which with the red blood cell indices and red cell morphology supported the diagnosis of iron deficiency. Tests of the stools for

145

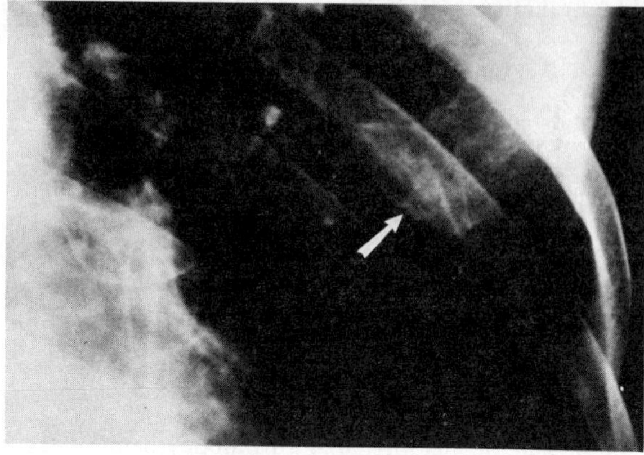

FIGURE 1. Solitary expansile lesion (*arrow*) with sclerotic margins involving the sixth left rib.

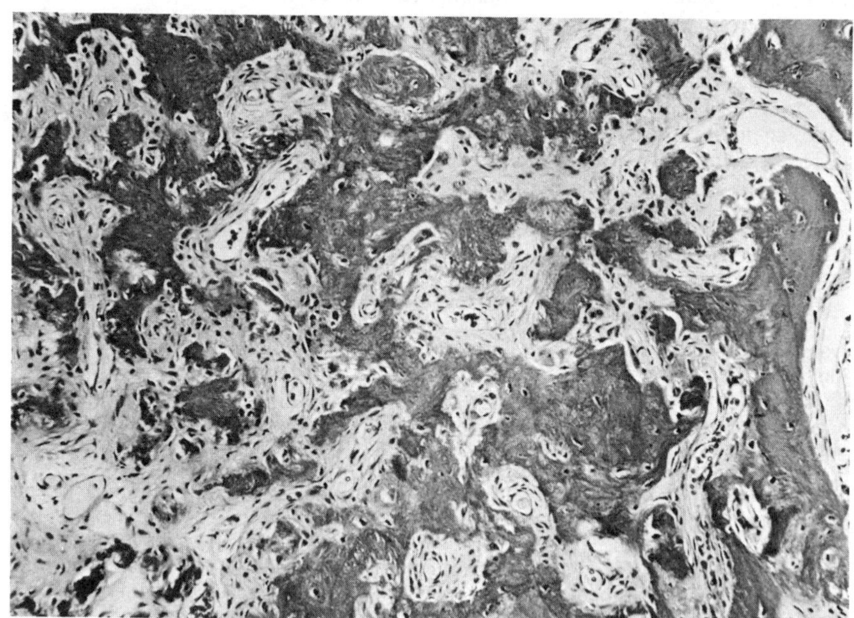

FIGURE 2. Photomicrograph of biopsy specimen of rib lesion showing features of a benign fibrous defect. Note that the bony trabeculae are lined by osteoclasts and osteoblasts, thus differentiating this lesion from the osteomyelosclerotic stage of a myeloproliferative disorder. Hematoxylin and eosin stain; original magnification ×100; reduced by 25 percent.

occult blood gave strongly positive results. Of particular interest were the elevated serum values of potassium (7.3 mEq/L), calcium (11.2 mg/dL), and phosphate (5.3 mg/dL). The plasma values for these substances were normal, indicating that the serum abnormalities were spurious relative to thrombocythemia. Hyperparathyroidism was excluded by reason of normal parathyroid hormone and cyclic AMP values. Leukocyte alkaline phosphatase score was elevated at 188 (normal range 13 to 130).

X-ray studies with barium enema and upper gastrointestinal series were normal. However, the chest X-ray film showed an expansile lesion with sclerotic margins in the left sixth rib (FIG. 1). Biopsy of this lesion indicated a benign fibrous defect (FIG. 2), but the adjacent marrow in the same specimen revealed findings of a myeloproliferative disease, that is, trilineage hyperplasia with mega-

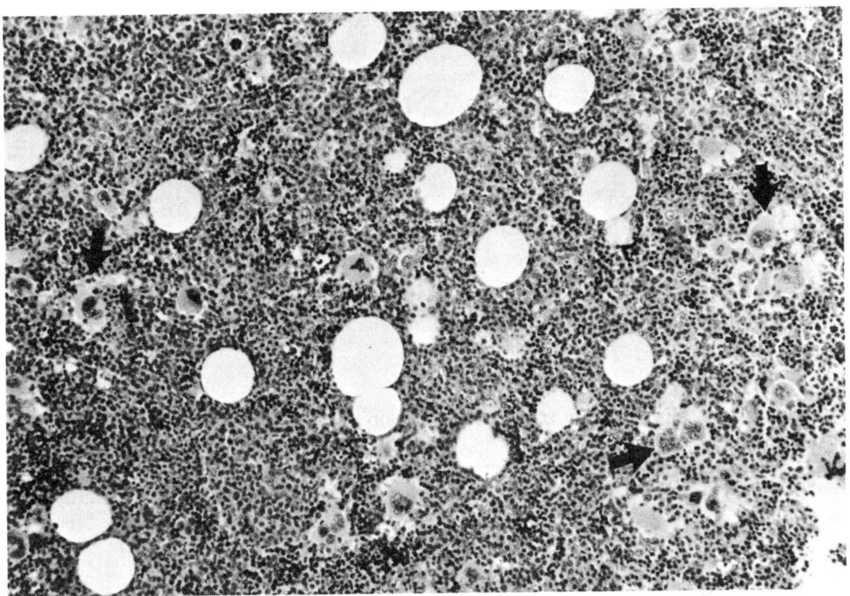

FIGURE 3. Marrow adjacent to the bone defect showing panhyperplasia with megakaryocytic preponderance. Note clusters of megakaryocytes (*arrows*) and atypical forms. Hematoxylin and eosin stain; original magnification ×100; reduced by 25 percent.

karyocytic preponderance and increased reticulin deposition (FIGS. 3 and 4). A bone marrow aspirate and biopsy from the iliac crest confirmed the initial impression of a myeloproliferative disease.

Coagulation studies included bleeding time (Duke), clotting time (Lee-White), activated partial thromboplastin time, prothrombin time, fibrinogen and whole blood clot lysis. All these studies gave results within normal limits. Platelet aggregation studies showed impaired platelet aggregation (FIG. 5) with adenosine diphosphate (ADP) (1 µg/ml, 2 µg/ml and 3 µg/ml) and epinephrine (1 µg/ml, 2 µg/ml and 3 µg/ml). Collagen-induced (0.1 mg/ml) and ristocetin-induced (1.5 mg/ml) aggregation were normal. Other platelet function studies (that is, retention, clot retraction, and prothrombin consumption) revealed no abnormalities.

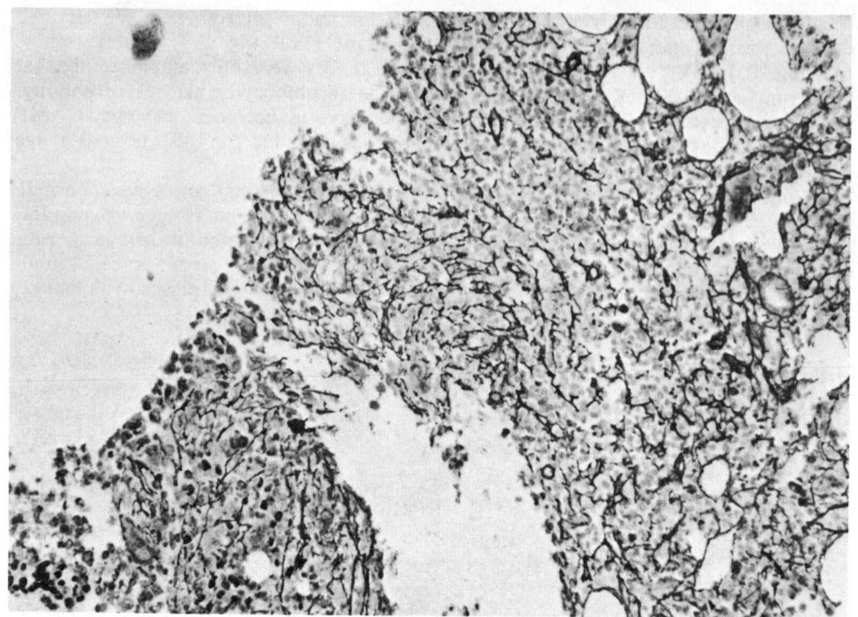

FIGURE 4. Marrow from same site as in FIGURE 3 showing coarse reticulin fibers with condensation. Reticulin stain; original magnification ×100; reduced by 25 percent.

From these clinical laboratory and morphologic data, a diagnosis of essential thrombocythemia was made.

The patient was placed on a regimen of iron therapy and his platelet count increased further to 2,015,000/mm^3. He was started on busulfan, 4 mg daily, on October 26, 1978. A week later his platelet count was 4,000,000/mm^3 and busulfan was increased to 6 mg daily for the next 2 weeks. On November 28, the hemoglobin was 15.9 mg percent, white blood cell count 5,200/mm^3 with a normal differential count, and platelet count 2,340,000/mm^3. At this point, he did not return for further visits or medication and was lost to follow-up study for more than a year.

In January 1980 the patient returned to the clinic with epistaxis and was admitted to the hospital. The laboratory values at this time were as follows: hemoglobin 8.6 gm percent with normal red blood cell indices; white blood cell count 3,400/mm^3, with 7 percent myeloblasts (FIG. 6), 3 percent myelocytes, and 1 percent metamyelocyte; platelet count 9,000/mm^3. Bone marrow biopsy (FIG. 7) and aspirate (FIG. 8) showed a cellularity of 95 percent with 40 percent leukemic stem cells (blast cells 16 percent, promyelocytes 23.5 percent). Megakaryocytes were almost absent. A diagnosis of acute leukemia was made.

Recurrent nose bleeds and upper gastrointestinal hemorrhages necessitated the use of many transfusions with platelets and packed red blood cells over the succeeding 4 months. Chemotherapy for the patient's leukemia is currently under consideration.

DISCUSSION

On the basis of the unitarian concept of the myeloproliferative disorders advocated by Dameshek,[19] essential thrombocythemia is currently accepted within the spectrum of myeloproliferative diseases as a disease entity that contains its own distinct clinical morphologic features. The criteria outlined for diagnosis of this disease by Ozer *et al.*[4] Silverstein,[5] and Gunz[3] include clinical expression of thrombosis, bleeding, or both (more commonly bleeding), frequent splenomegaly, sustained platelet count of more than 1 million/mm³, microcytic hypochromic red cell morphology, usually some neutrophilic leukocytosis, and bone marrow findings of trilineage hyperplasia with megakaryocytic preponderance. Sustained high platelet counts and the bone marrow characteristics were thought to be the most important criteria that we found in our patient (FIG. 1). The slight erythrocytosis seen during his hospitalization could be related to the intermittent bleeding and early iron deficiency anemia.

Abnormal platelet functions have been reported in myeloproliferative disease.[20-24] Studies of platelet aggregation have shown more consistently abnormal findings than have other functional tests in essential thrombocythemia.[6-10, 25] This observation can be used as an aid in differentiating idiopathic thrombocythemia from secondary thrombocytosis.[7-9] Attempts have been made to predict, monitor and even to prevent the hemorrhagic and/or thrombotic complications with the help of platelet aggregation and related tests.[8, 9]

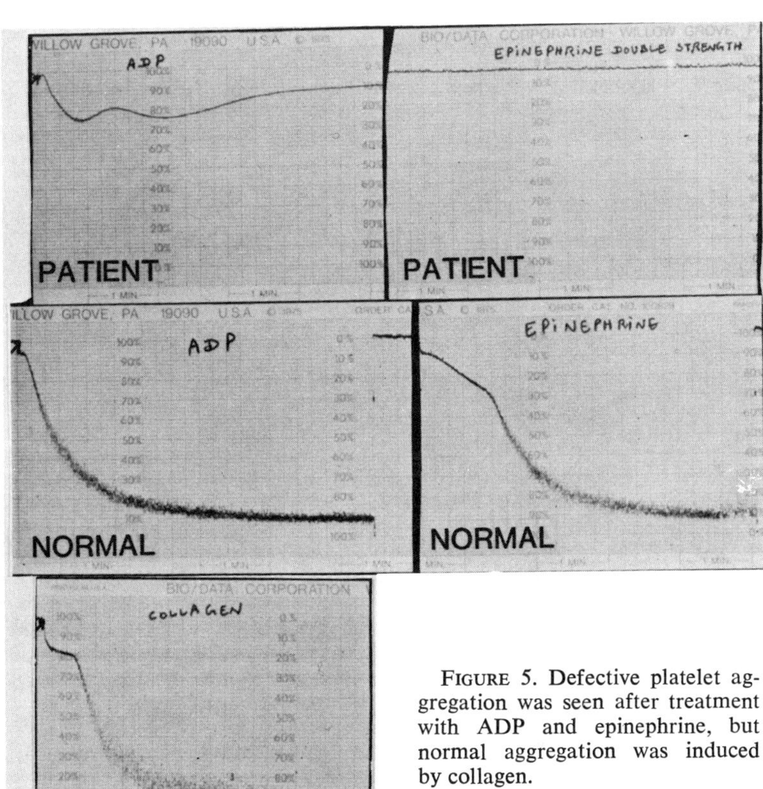

FIGURE 5. Defective platelet aggregation was seen after treatment with ADP and epinephrine, but normal aggregation was induced by collagen.

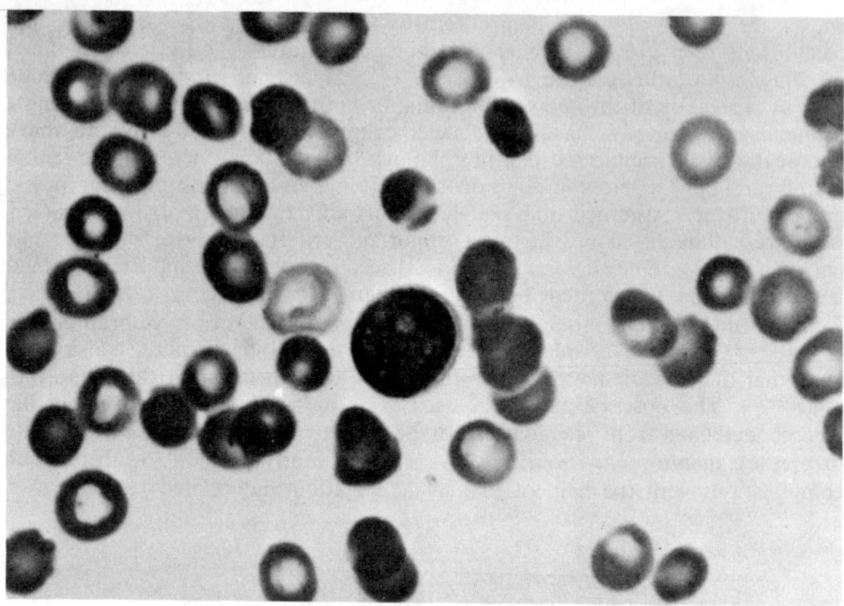

FIGURE 6. Peripheral blood smear showing a myeloblast. Leishman stain; original magnification ×100; reduced by 25 percent.

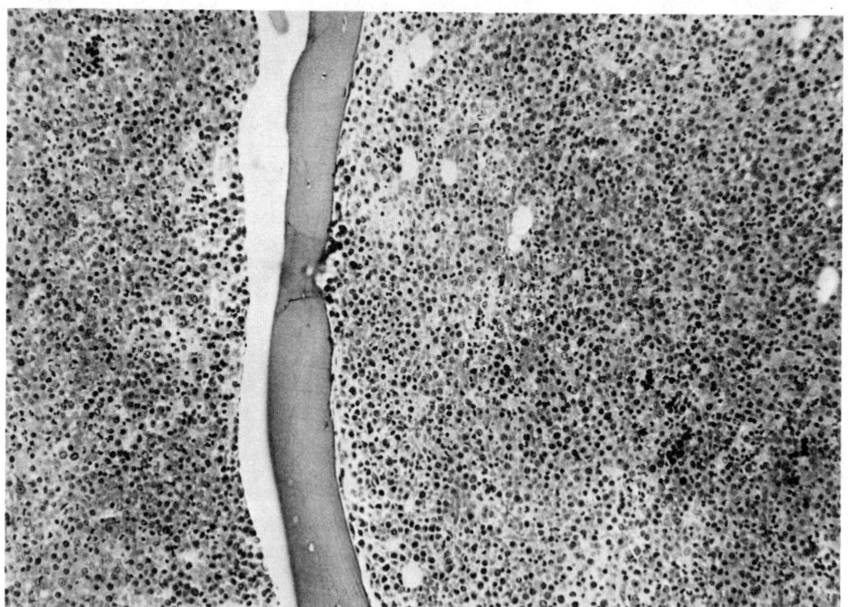

FIGURE 7. Photomicrograph of bone marrow biopsy specimen showing marked hyperplasia with granulocytic bulge and absent megakaryocytes (compare this with FIG. 3). Hematoxylin and eosin stain; original magnification × 100; reduced by 25 percent.

In our patient, platelets showed abnormal aggregation with ADP and epinephrine, but collagen-induced aggregation was normal. Both ADP and epinephrine were used in thrice the threshold concentrations and fresh ADP from a new lot was tried. The abnormalities persisted after all these maneuvers. This aggregation defect pattern was similar to that described by Spaet *et al.*[25] in 1969 in three cases of essential thrombocythemia. These authors suggested that the observed platelet aggregation defect might be specific for essential thrombocythemia. However, subsequently, other patterns of aggregation defects in response to single or multiple aggregating agents have been reported in patients with essential thrombocythemia. Recently, Ts'ao *et al.*[26] described a case with reduced platelet aggregation to four inducers (ADP, collagen,

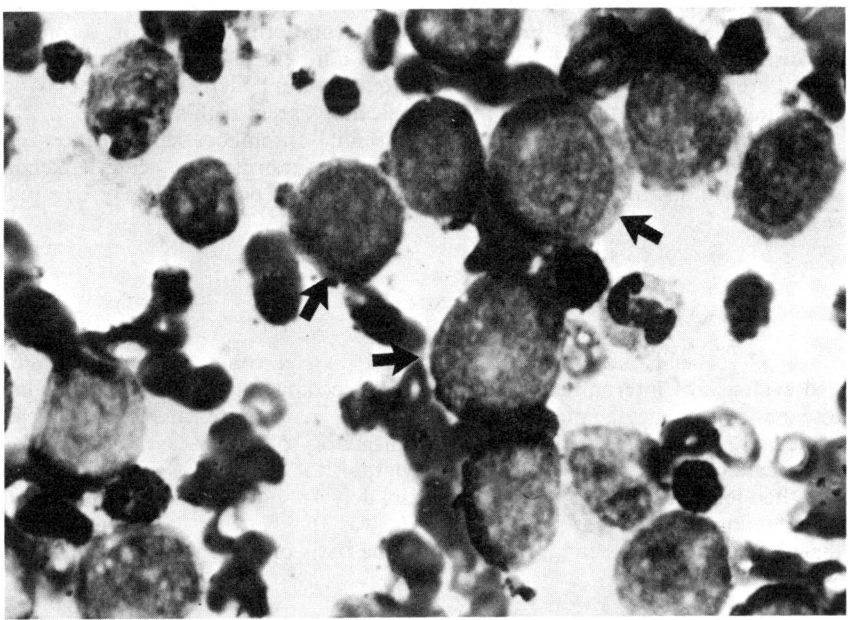

FIGURE 8. Bone marrow aspirate smear showing clusters of myeloblasts (*arrows*) and promyelocytes. Leishman stain; original magnification ×800; reduced by 25 percent.

epinephrine, and ristocetin). They also demonstrated various structural abnormalities of platelets by electron microscope studies. Kaywin *et al.*[27] speculated that the diminished aggregative response to epinephrine that they demonstrated in two patients with essential thrombocythemia might have resulted from the deficiency in α-adrenergic receptors found in the platelets of these patients. Further chemical and ultrastructural studies may unveil the relationship between structural and functional abnormalities in this now well-recognized clinical entity.

Only a few cases diagnosed initially as essential thrombocythemia have terminated in acute granulocytic leukemia.[4, 14, 17, 18] All these cases occurred in patients who had received ionizing radiation and/or cytostatic agents in significant quantities,[18] suggesting a causal role for these agents in the development of leukemia. However, our case was unique in that the patient received a cytostatic agent for only a very short period of time, and, in fact, may actually have received little or no drug because of poor compliance. Onset of leukemia within 16 months after the primary disease was diagnosed reaffirms the fact that the course of the disease is not always indolent and benign.

CONCLUSIONS

1. Essential thrombocythemia is now a well-described, distinct clinical entity with characteristic clinical morphologic features.

2. Platelet functional abnormalities, in particular aggregation defects, have been consistently seen in this disease and have been useful as diagnostic tools to differentiate idiopathic thrombocythemia from other causes of thrombocytosis. Attempts have been made to correlate different functional abnormalities and aggregation patterns with chemical and structural defects. Studies along these lines may help to monitor the complications seen in this disease.

3. Although many of the cases of essential thrombocythemia follow an indolent course, this case emphasizes the fact that transition to acute leukemia with and without therapy with cytostatic agents does occur and may be quite rapid.

SUMMARY

A 57-year-old black man with sustained platelet count of 2 million/mm³ and evidence of intermittent gastrointestinal bleeding was diagnosed as having essential thrombocythemia. Studies of bone marrow morphology, platelet aggregation, and other variables were confirmatory of the disease. The patient was treated briefly with low doses of Myleran® for less than three weeks. He was then lost to follow-up study. Approximately 16 months later he reappeared complaining of recurrent nose bleeds. He was found to be pancytopenic and diagnosis of acute leukemia was made on the basis of bone marrow aspiration.

REFERENCES

1. EPSTEIN, E., & A. GOEDEL. 1934. Hamorrhagische thrombocythamie bei vascularer schrumpfmilz. Virch. Arch. **193:** 233–238.
2. FANGER, H., L. J. CELLA & H. LITCHMAN. 1954. Thrombocythemia: Report of three cases and review of literature. N. Engl. J. Med. **250**(11): 456–461.
3. GUNZ, F. W. 1960. Hemorrhagic thrombocythemia: A critical review. Blood **15:** 706–723.
4. OZER, F. L., W. E. TRUAX, D. C. MIESCH & W. C. LEVIN. 1960. Primary hemorrhagic thrombocythemia. Am. J. Med. **28:** 807–823.
5. SILVERSTEIN, M. N. 1968. Primary or hemorrhagic thrombocythemia. Arch. Intern. Med. **122:** 18–22.
6. HARDISTY, R. M. & H. H. WOLFF. 1955. Hemorrhagic thrombocythaemia: A clinical and laboratory study. Br. J. Hematol. **1:** 390–405.
7. McCLURE, P. D., G. I. C. INGRAM, R. S. STACEY, V. H. GLASS & M. MATCHETT. 1966. Platelet function tests in thrombocythemia and thrombocytosis. Br. J. Hematol. **12:** 478–498.

8. ZUCKER, S. & C. H. MIELKE. 1972. Classification of thrombocytosis based on platelet function tests: Correlation with hemorrhagic and thrombotic complications. J. Lab. Clin. Med. **80:** 385–394.

9. GINSBURG, A. D. 1975. Platelet function with high platelet counts. Ann. Intern. **82:** 506–511.

10. WEINFELD, A., J. BRANEHOG & J. KUTTI. 1975. Platelets in myeloproliferative syndrome. Clin. Haematol. **4**(2): 373–392.

11. FOUNTAIN, J. R. & M. S. LOSOWSKY. 1962. Haemorrhagic thrombocythemia and its treatment with radioactive phosphorus. Quart. J. Med. **31:** 207–220.

12. MODAN, B. & A. M. LILIENFIELD. 1965. Polycythemia and leukemia. The role of radiation treatment. A study of 1222 patients. Medicine **44:** 305–344.

13. BENSINGER, T. A., G. L. LOGUE & R. W. RUNDLES. 1970. Hemorrhagic thrombocythemia: Control of postsplenectomy thrombocytosis with melphalan. Blood **36**(1): 61–69.

14. LEWIS, S. M., L. SZUR & A. V. HOFFBRAND. 1972. Thrombocythemia. Clin. Hematol. **1**(2): 229–357

15. GREENBERG, B. R. & E. J. WATSON-WILLIAMS. 1975. Successful control of life-threatening thrombocytosis with blood processor. Transfusion **15**(6): 620–622.

16. TAFT, E. G., R. B. BABCOCK, W. B. SCHARFMAN & A. P. TARTAGLIA. 1977. Plateletpheresis in the management of thrombocytosis. Blood **50**(5): 927–933.

17. McCABE, W. R., R. M. BIRD & R. A. McLAUGHLIN. 1955. Is primary thrombocythaemia a clinical myth? Ann. Intern. Med. **43:** 182–190.

18. FICKERS, M. & B. SPECK. 1974. Thrombocythaemia: Familial occurrence and transition into blast crisis. Acta Haematol. **51:** 257–265.

19. DAMESHEK, W. 1951. Some speculations on myeloproliferative syndromes. Blood **6:** 372–375.

20. TANGUN, Y. 1971. Platelet aggregation and platelet factors in myeloproliferative disorders. Thromb. Diath. Hemorrh. **25:** 241–251.

21. CARDAMONE, J. M., J. R. EDSON, J. R. McARTHUR & H. S. JACOB. 1972. Abnormalities of platelet function in the myeloproliferative disorders. JAMA **221**(3): 270–273.

22. NEEMAH, J. A. 1972. Quantitation of platelet aggregation in myeloproliferative disorders. Am. J. Clin. Pathol. **57:** 336–347.

23. CAEN, J. P., Y. SULTAN & J. DELOBEL. 1969. Les thrombopathies acquires. Nouv. Rev. F. Hematol. **9:** 553–567.

24. BARBUI, T., R. BATTISTA & E. DINI. 1973. Spontaneous platelet aggregation in myeloproliferative disorders. Acta Haematol. **50:** 25–29.

25. SPAET, T. H., I. LEJNIEKS, E. GAYNOR & M. L. GOLDSTEIN. 1969. Defective platelets in essential thrombocythemia. Arch. Intern. Med. **124:** 135–141.

26. TS'AO, C., E. C. ROSSI & F. C. LESTINA. 1977. Abnormalities in platelet function and morphology in a case of thrombocythemia. Arch. Pathol. Lab. Med. **101:** 526–533.

27. KAYWIN, P., M. McDONOUGH, P. A. INSEL & S. J. SHATTIL. 1978. Platelet function in essential thrombocythemia: Decreased epinephrine responsiveness associated with deficiency of platelet α-adrenergic receptors. N. Engl. J. Med. **299**(10): 505–509.

PLATELET–VESSEL-WALL INTERACTIONS: EXPERIENCES WITH VON WILLEBRAND PLATELETS *

Marion I. Barnhart,† Ross M. Wilkins,†
and Jeanne M. Lusher ‡

*Departments of Physiology † and Pediatrics ‡
Wayne State University School of Medicine
Detroit, Michigan 48201*

INTRODUCTION

In 1926 and 1931, von Willebrand described a congenital bleeding disorder (mucous membrane bleeding) in 23 members of a large family living in the Aland Islands, off the coast of Finland.[1,2] Today, von Willebrand's disease (vWD) is probably the single most common hereditary disorder of hemostasis.[3,4] Still it is not known with certainty exactly how the disorder(s) in vWD account for deficiencies in hemostatic plug formations. The most consistent abnormality in vWD is prolonged bleeding time despite normal platelet count. This bleeding tendency is inherited as an autosomal dominant trait, with variable penetrance accounting for the varying severity of bleeding and the disparity in the laboratory findings for bleeding time and components of the factor (F) VIII plasma protein system. The congenital defect appears to be in the F VIII molecules, which are synthesized by endothelial cells in normal individuals,[5] but not synthesized at all or synthesized in reduced amounts or as abnormal molecules in persons with vWD.[6]

It is only recently recognized that F VIII is a system of three functionally distinct components: F VIII clot-promoting activity, F VIII antigen, and von Willebrand factor activity (which is necessary for a normal bleeding time). Although the nomenclature of the various F VIII activities is still changing, the Working Party on the F VIII Antigens of the International Committee on Hemostasis and Thrombosis designates F VIII clotting activity as VIII:C; the material precipitated by specific rabbit antisera as VIII R:Ag; the activity correcting bleeding time and platelet adhesiveness as VIII:vW; and the ristocetin cofactor activity as VIII:Rcof.[7] Adhesiveness of vWD platelets is known to be abnormal on glass bead columns [8,9] and on exposed subendothelium of rabbit aorta.[10] Our group was the first to demonstrate, using components of human origin only, impaired adhesion of vWD platelets to experimentally injured umbilical vein wall (subendothelium) from cesarean-sectioned normal women.[3,11–13] Recently Sakariassen and associates also reported impaired adhesion using vWD platelets and subendothelium of human renal arteries post mortem.[14] That a plasma factor is essential for normal bleeding time was recognized when Nilsson and colleagues [15] and Cornu *et al.*[16] reported that the prolonged bleeding time of vWD patients could be corrected by transfusion of fresh normal plasma or cryoprecipitate, which we now know contains F VIII: vW.

* This study was partially funded by a grant from the Hemophilia Foundation of Michigan.

154

This communication details our investigation of the hemostatic capabilities (adhesion) of vWD platelets from 15 patients with classic or moderately severe manifestations of von Willebrand's disease using our *ex vivo* umbilical vein perfusion model.[11] Scanning electron microscopy (SEM) was employed to reveal platelet–vessel-wall interactions. Platelets reacted predominantly with subendothelium exposed during a brief hypoxic interval preceding platelet perfusion. Clearly, both qualitative and quantitative differences exist in adhesive ability between platelets from patients with varying degrees of vWD and those of normal adults or fetal specimens. The less-adhesive vWD platelets displayed reduced surface activity and fewer and defective pseudopods as well as limited spreading ability. The deficiencies in adhesion correlated best with the F VIII: Rcof, although F VIII:C and F VIII:Ag were also measured. A monospecific antihuman F VIII:Ag linked to 0.6 μm latex microspheres, upon perfusion through the normal vein model, bound chiefly to exposed subendothelium and partially blocked adhesion of either vWD or normal platelets. In constrasting the abilities of several blood products (cryoprecipitate [American Red Cross, Detroit, MI], antihemophilic factor [Connaught Laboratories, Toronto, Canada] and fresh frozen AB-plasma [American Red Cross, Detroit, MI]) we corroborated the findings of earlier reports that products rich in F VIII:vW were more supportive of adhesion of vWD platelets than were products such as F VIII concentrates (antihemophilic factor), which have little or no F VIII:vW.

MATERIALS AND METHODS

Patients with von Willebrand's Disease

These subjects (10 females and 5 males) were either patients at the Children's Hospital of Michigan (Detroit) or relatives known to have vWD. Informed consent was obtained for use of each vWD subject's platelets. All subjects had documentation of a prolonged bleeding time and deficiencies in one or more of the F VIII components. From a clinical standpoint, most subjects had either classic severe or moderately severe bleeding problems. TABLE 1 summarizes individual F VIII component results from laboratory tests done on the blood specimen drawn immediately prior to perfusion into the umbilical vein model.

Other Platelet Sources

Fetal blood and blood from normal adult volunteers provided sources for the control platelet experiments. The fetal blood was taken immediately from the fresh umbilical vein still attached to the placenta removed during the cesarean section of normal women, who selected this means of delivery for their infants. Such fetal platelets served as the autologous platelet control; vessel-wall interactions were not anticipated because of differences in cell surface antigens. Normal adult volunteers gave blood specimens for other control experiments designed to reveal whether blood type incompatibility played a role in platelet–vessel-wall interactions in the umbilical vein model. Thus far we have no indication that blood type incompatibilities are significant in our model system.[11]

Factor VIII Component Assays

Each assay was performed in triplicate and the average value calculated and reported in units (U) per ml. F VIII:C was determined by the one-stage assay of Simone *et al.*[17] F VIII R:Ag was assayed using quantitative immunoelectrophoresis according to the method of Zimmerman *et al.*[18] F VIII:Rcof was established by means of paraformaldehyde-fixed platelets and aggregometry after addition of ristocetin according to the method of Allain *et al.*[19]

TABLE 1

FACTOR VIII LABORATORY VALUES FOR vWD SUBJECTS AND BLOOD TYPE
INFORMATION FOR EXPERIMENTAL PERFUSIONS

vWD Subjects	F VIII Activities			Blood Types	
	F VIII:C (U/ml)	F VIII R:Ag (U/ml)	F VIII:Rcof (U/ml)	vWD Subjects	Experiment Umbilical Cord
BB	0.48	<0.15	0.54	A+	A+
MB	0.06	<0.15	0.00	O+	A+
VB *	0.95	1.30	1.00	A+	B+
RC	0.35	<0.20	0.00	AB+	O+
AE †	0.70	0.75	0.99	O+	O+
IE †	0.25	0.90	0.90	O+	O+
LF	<0.01	0.00	0.00	A−	O+
SN	0.47	0.27	0.09	A+	A+
DS	0.21	<0.25	0.00	O−	O+
JS	0.35	0.28	<0.01	O+	O+
SS	0.13	<0.25	0.00	O+	O+
AV ‡	0.90	0.45	0.78	O+	B+
CV ‡	0.47	0.68	0.54	O+	O+
JeV ‡	1.00	0.88	0.37	O+	O+
JoV ‡	0.97	0.88	1.00	O+	O+
Normal subjects § (range)	0.60–1.50	>0.50	0.60–1.20		

* Bleeding time, 10 minutes (normal subjects, 3–8 minutes); previous values were 14 minutes, F VIII activities <0.50, and platelet retention test=0. Moderately severe bleeding episodes previously.

† Previous diagnosis in Canada and Florida and history of bleeding problems in six family members.

‡ Family with mild vWD. Platelet aggregation with ristocetin abnormally low.

§ Current laboratory standards.

Rabbit Antibody to F VIII:Ag

Human F VIII concentrate prepared from fresh frozen plasma (Michigan Department of Public Health, East Lansing, MI, lot 256, 2.4 units of F VIII:C/mg protein) was mixed with Freund's complete adjuvant and injected into footpads of adult New Zealand rabbits (2.4 U F VIII:C/kg body weight).

Booster injections were given intramuscularly after 20 days. At 30 days, after development of antibody to F VIII was confirmed by means of micro-ring dilution tests of precipitin formation and quantitative immunoelectrophoresis, the rabbits were exsanguinated by cardiac puncture.[20] The serum containing antibody to F VIII was separated from the clotted whole blood and frozen at —70° C for storage.

Immunoglobulins were later separated by a combination procedure using ethodin followed by ethanol fractionation of the supernatant.[20] A check by immunodiffusion showed that two precipitin bands formed when the antibody was reacted with normal human plasma. Further purification to develop a monovalent anti-F VIII:Ag was accomplished by use of immunoadsorbents coupled by cyanogen bromide (CN-Br) to Sepharose 4B beads.[13] The first immunoadsorbent was von Willebrand plasma from a patient with severe vWD (47 percent F VIII:C, 27 percent F VIII:Ag and 9 percent F VIII:Rcof). Two protein peaks (according to ultraviolet adsorption at 280 nm) existed. The first peak had the strongest precipitin reaction with the original F VIII concentrate, but two precipitin bands were still seen on immunodiffusion. The second immunoadsorbent was purified fibrinogen coupled to CN-Br–activated Sepharose 4B beads. Although effluents from the second immunoadsorbent column still showed two protein peaks, the first peak proved on immunodiffusion and immunoelectrophoresis to have only one precipitin band of identity when reacted with F VIII concentrate and normal plasma. Therefore only this fraction was used as monovalent antibody.

Microsphere-Antifactor VIII:Ag Probe

The monospecific F VIII:Ag just described was covalently linked to 0.6 μm fluorescent carboxylated latex microspheres (Polysciences Co., Warrington, PA) under alkaline conditions by means of carbodiimide.[13] The labeled microspheres were stored at +40° C as a 0.5 percent solid product. Immediately before perfusion into the umbilical vein model, an aliquot of the sonicated stock product was diluted with Dulbecco's phosphate buffered saline (PBS) solution (pH 7.4) to achieve a 0.01 percent solid product. Normal platelets but not vWD platelets were labeled by addition of this latex microsphere-anti-F VIII:Ag probe according to both fluorescent microscopy and SEM. Consequently, we believe that binding of the probe is a reliable indicator of loci for F VIII:Ag and/or F VIII:vW.

Umbilical Vein Perfusions

Human umbilical cords were freshly processed, within minutes after delivery from consenting patients at Hutzel Hospital in Detroit, according to published procedure.[11] Eleven of the cords were from patients with elective cesarean sections and four were from those with normal vaginal deliveries. These 15 cords provided 53 umbilical vein segments for perfusion experiments.

Immediately upon receipt of placenta, the fetal blood was withdrawn from the placenta with a heparinized (2 u/ml) or citrated syringe (1:9, 3.8 percent citrate-to-blood ratio). The cord was then separated from the placenta and the umbilical vein gently flushed with warm, preoxygenated and heparinized (2 u/

ml) Dulbecco's phosphate buffered saline solution containing calcium and magnesium. Each cord was divided into three or four equal-sized pieces, but areas damaged by clamps or manipulation were carefully excluded. These segments were connected to the perfusion pump (explosion-proof, variable-speed drive pump, Cole-Parmer Co., Chicago, Illinois) and the effluent collector. Thereafter, either PBS or platelet-rich plasma (PRP), washed platelets, or whole blood (WB) was continuously pumped through the cord segments until the time selected for fixation. A flow rate of 1 ml per minute at a physiologic pressure of 8 to 10 mm Hg was established and maintained throughout the procedure. The vein was perfusion-fixed by pumping a 300 mOsm solution of 1 percent glutaraldehyde (GAH) in 0.6 M cacodylate buffer, pH 7.3, for at least 15 minutes. Segments were then immersed in fresh buffered GAH, agitated to remove any air bubbles in the vein, and stored at +40° C for 18 to 24 hours.[11] Representative protocols are shown in TABLE 2.

Processing for Scanning Electron Microscopy

Fixed samples were removed from the GAH and transferred to 0.1 M sucrose-cacodylate buffer for SEM preparation or storage. The specimens were dehydrated in increasing concentrations (30 to 100 percent) of ethanol and placed in a 1:1 mixture of 100 percent ethanol and Freon® 113 and finally in two exchanges in Freon 113 alone. Specimens were "critical-point dried" by means of Freon 113 and then mounted on aluminum slugs and sputtered with gold. Edges of the samples were painted with silver paint to reduce charging effects. Slugs were stored in a dessicator for later examination using an ETEC Autoscan R-1 scanning electron microscope, operated at 20 kV with a specimen tilting of 0 to 30 degrees.

TABLE 2

PERFUSION SEQUENCES, TIMING AND PERTINENT PATIENT/SUBJECT DETAILS

PBS-O_2	PBS-O_2	PBS-O_2	PBS-O_2	PBS-O_2
15'	15'	15'	15'	15'
Fetal PRP–O_2	vW PRP-O_2	Fetal WB-O_2	vW WB-O_2	vW WB-O_2
15'	15'	15'	15'	15'
PBS-O_2	PBS-O_2	PBS-O_2	PBS-O_2	PBS-O_2
2'	2'	2'	2'	2'
GAH	GAH	GAH	GAH	Anti-F VIII-MS-O_2
15'	15'	15'	15'	
(#2)	(2#)	(#7)	(7#)	15'
				GAH
	vWD		vWD	vWD
	patient SN		patient AV	patient AV
	blood type		blood type	blood type
	A+		O+	O+

NOTE: *Cord:* #2 fetal blood type A+, elective cesarean section; #7, fetal blood type B+, delivery cord.

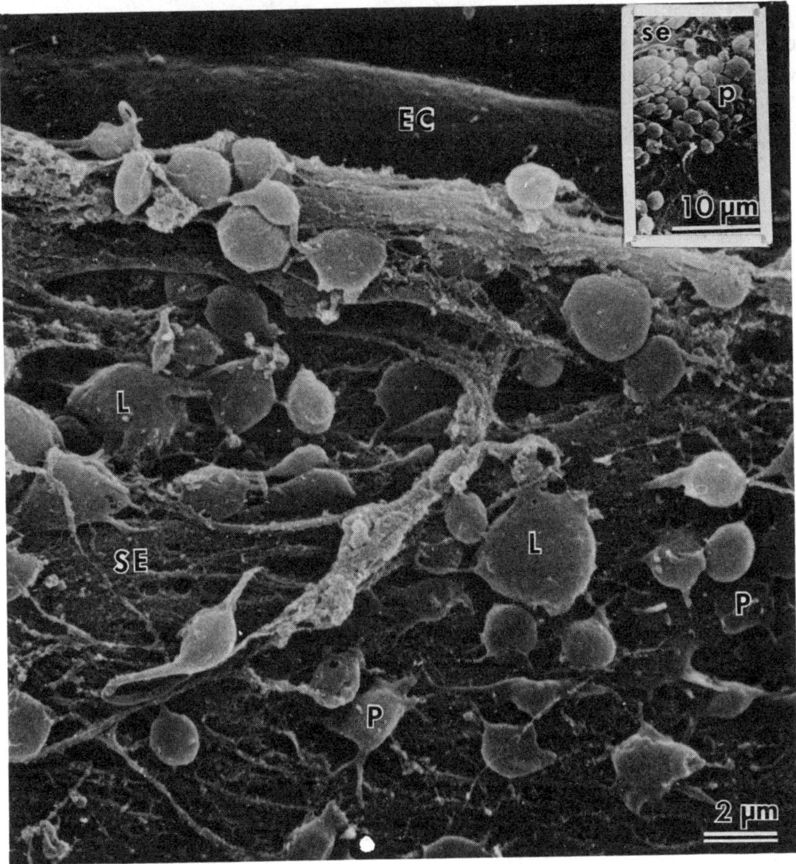

FIGURE 1. Fetal platelets (P and p) adherent to subendothelium (SE and se). Note flattening and spreading platelets as well as extensive pseudopod formation. Inset photograph shows "pavementing." EC = endothelial cell; L = leukocyte.

RESULTS

Adhesiveness of Normal Platelets

Perfusion of four specimens of autologous fetal platelets in PRP through conditioned and essentially normal umbilical vein segments resulted in platelet adhesion to areas of exposed subendothelium, which showed sites of injury that had occurred prior to the platelet perfusion (FIG. 1). Adherent platelets were heterogeneous with respect to size and surface activity. The platelets tended to form a "pavement" over the exposed thrombogenic material by adhering and spreading. Most platelets formed many well-developed dendritic processes (pseudopods) that probably anchor, orient or stabilize the platelet to a surface. Perfusion of three specimens of fetal platelets in whole blood gave morphologically similar results, although some debris and red and white blood cells were adherent to the vessel wall. Perfusion of three specimens of whole blood from normal adult volunteers provided platelet-subendothelial interactions of similar quality and magnitude. Platelet counts per unit area of vessel wall surface averaged 62,803 platelets/cm^2 (TABLE 3).

Adhesiveness of von Willebrand Platelets

Eight subjects previously diagnosed as having classic or moderately severe von Willebrand's disease provided platelets (either as PRP or in whole blood)

TABLE 3

PLATELET ADHESION TO INJURED VESSEL WALL AND
MORPHOLOGY OF ADHERENT PLATELETS

Subjects	VIII:Rcof (U/ml)	Adhesion platelets /cm²	Control (%)	Platelet Morphology
Patients				
JoV	1.00	31,988	51	Multiple pseudopods and spread forms
VB	1.00	28,880	46	Above includes platelet pavement
IE	0.90	29,900	48	As above
CV	0.54	28,812	46	As above
				Discs and spheres Few and stubby pseudopods
SN	0.09	26,964	43	Defective spreading Little or no platelet pavement
JS	<0.01	23,974	38	As above
DS	0	18,722	30	As above
RC	0	12,475	20	As above
MB	0	12,040	20	As above
LF	0	4,404	7	As above
Normal adults (2)	1.00	58,885		Multiple pseudopods
	1.00	68,040		Spreading platelets form pavement
Normal fetal specimens (3)	1.00	72,210		As above
	1.00	57,640		As above
	1.00	62,480		As above
Mean for normals (5) ± SD		62,803 ±5111	100	

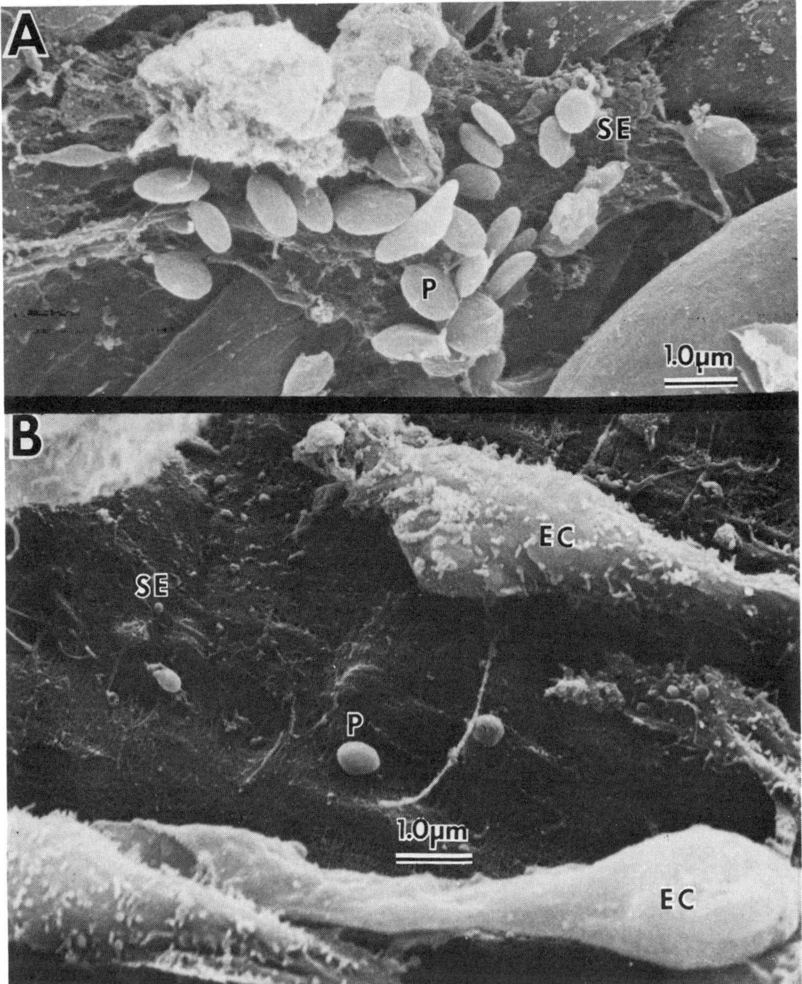

FIGURE 2. **(A)** vW platelets (P) of patient SN appear unactivated and essentially in their native configuration (discoid shape and lacking pseudopods). **(B)** vW platelets (patient MB) which were perfused in citrated whole blood (1:9 ratio, 3.8 percent citrate to blood). The number of adhering platelets (P) was low, but those that did adhere were relatively unactivated. EC = endothelial cell; SE = subendothelium.

for perfusions into umbilical vein segments. The number of vWD platelets adherent to islands of exposed subendothelium was in general reduced (51 percent of control normal platelets). The state of platelet activation was different from that displayed by normal fetal and adult platelets (FIG. 2). For example, adherent vW platelets were seen frequently in their unactivated, native configurations: flat discoid, spherical, and with short abortive-type pseudopods. Moreover, platelets from the patients with the most severe von

Willebrand's disease did not spread to pave the exposed subendothelium. However, vW platelets from two patients in this series behaved like and looked very similar to normal platelets (FIG. 3). Counts of adherent platelets obtained from the eight subjects varied from 4,404 to 31,988/cm² of injured vascular surface (TABLE 3).

Correlation of vW Platelet Morphology with Plasma F VIII:Rcof Levels

It seems evident from this series of patients with von Willebrand's disease that the adhesive ability and especially the morphologic expression of vW platelets correlates best with the level of plasma F VIII:Rcof (TABLES 1 and 3). The most defective platelets with respect to ability to change shape, produce pseudopods, and spread were noted in blood and PRP from patients MB, LF, SN, DS, JS, SS, and JeV. The vWD subjects with plasma levels of F VIII:Rcof > 0.37 U/ml had platelets that upon adhesion to the injured vascular test surface resembled normal platelets in terms of shape and membrane activity. However, defective adhesion capability was notable in platelets from all 15 subjects with vWD since the actual number of vW platelets to adhere was <51 percent of the control normal platelet reference base. Also, with the exception of platelets from patients VB, JoV and CV, the tendency for platelets to pave the exposed subendothelium was poor.

Correction of Adhesion Defects of von Willebrand Platelets

Two experimental approaches were used: substitution for F VIII by admixture of platelets with normal blood products or "bypass" of the F VIII:vW defect by pretreatment of vascular surfaces with thrombin.

Blood Product Experiments

The first blood product substitution experiment utilized lyophilized F VIII concentrate (0.08 mg/ml concentrate produced by the Michigan Department of Public Health) and whole blood from vWD subject JeV. No significant change was noted in platelet adhesion from the baseline value of 12,040 platelets/cm². The adherent platelets remained as smooth-surfaced discs and spheres with rare pseudopods (FIG. 4).

The second substitution experiment employed admixture of whole blood from vWD subject BB (F VIII:C = 0.48, F VIII R:Ag = <0.15, F VIII: Rcof = 0.54) with lyophilized F VIII concentrate (Connaught Laboratories, Toronto, Canada). A partial correction of the platelet adhesion defect was achieved (FIG. 4).

Adhesion of platelets without additives in patient BB was 28,800 platelets/ cm², which represented 46 percent of normal platelet adhesion. Perfusion of an admixture of platelets in patient BB with 15 U of F VIII concentrate resulted in slightly improved adhesion amounting to 58 percent of control normal values.

When cryoprecipitate was added to vW whole blood (patient BB), the vW defect was essentially corrected to achieve a value of normal control platelets

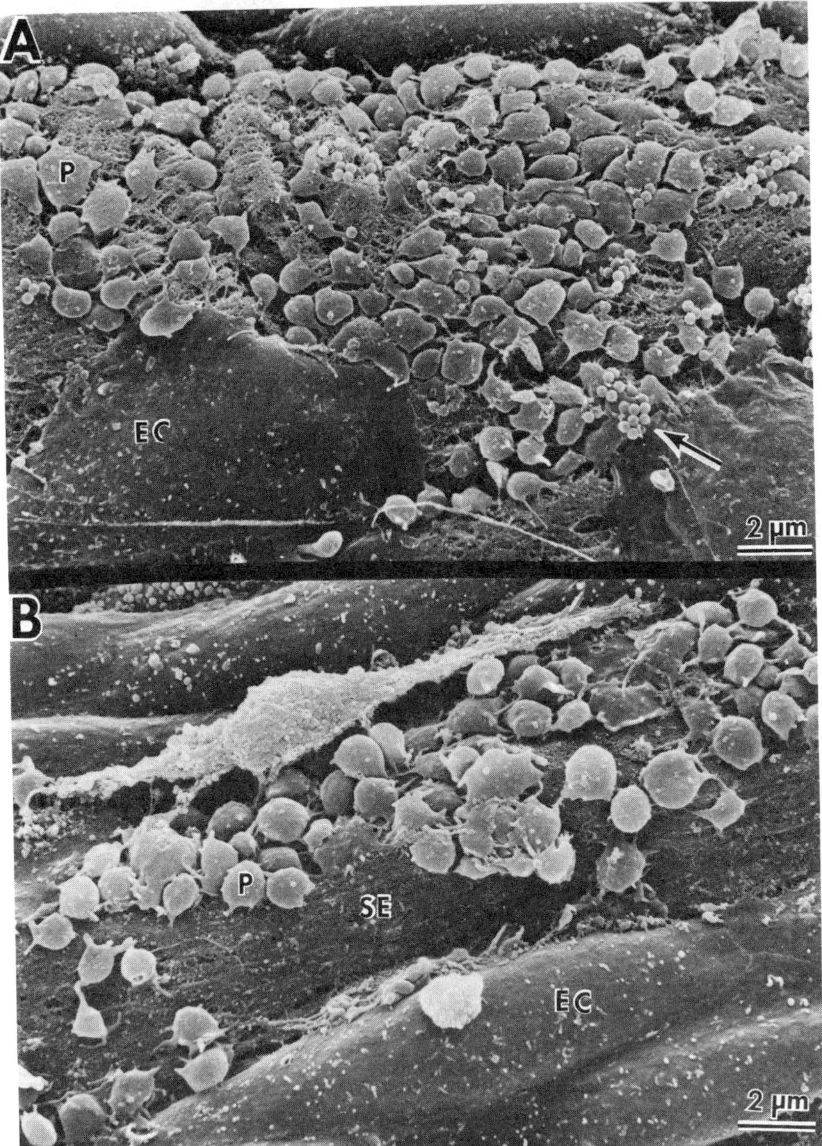

FIGURE 3. **(A)** hypoxic vein after perfusion with vW (patient VB) PRP, followed by addition of anti-F VIII R:Ag microspheres. This patient's F VIII levels were normal at that time. The platelets reacted normally after adhesion, but adhesion was only 46 percent of the normal control. Note microspheres binding to some platelet surfaces (*arrow*). **(B).** vW platelets (P) in whole blood (patient JoV) adhered well to subendothelium (SE) exposed by brief hypoxia. Adhesion was 51 percent of that in normal control platelets. EC = endothelial cell.

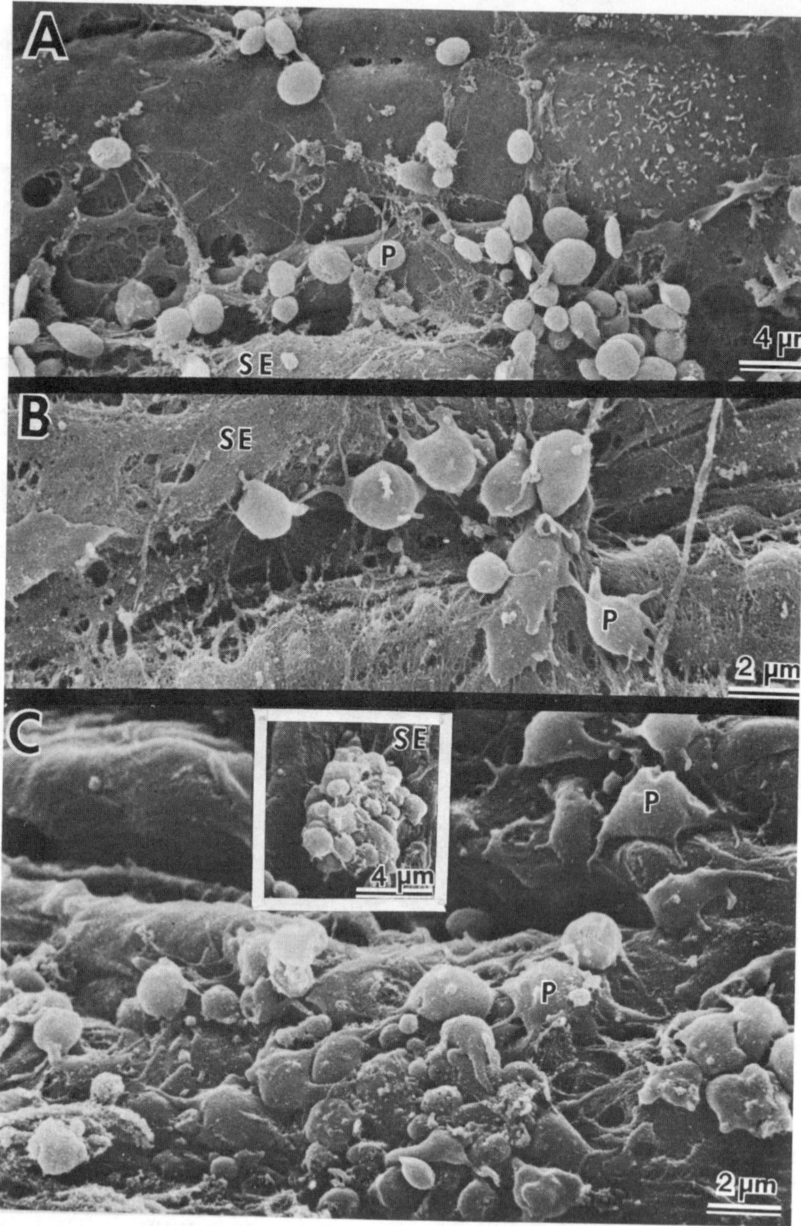

FIGURE 4. Effects of blood products on adhesivity. (A) adhesion defect of patient (JeV) with vWD was not corrected by admixture with F VIII concentrate (produced by the Michigan Department of Public Health). Platelets (P) remain discoid and spherical. (B) partial correction of adhesion defect of platelets from patient BB with severe vWD by F VIII concentrate (Connaught Laboratories). Although pseudopod formation was promoted, it was rare to find platelets (P) on subendothelium (SE). (C) cryoprecipitate added to whole blood of patient BB resulted in a good correction of the platelet (P) adhesion defect with pseudopod formation, spreading, and "pavementing." Some platelet aggregates (*inset*) adhered to subendothelium (SE).

(62,804/cm^2). The number of adherent vW platelets was 66,209 platelets/cm^2. Platelets adhered to the exposed subendothelium, spread, and formed an interlocking "pavement" effect like normal platelets. Also, some aggregative activity seemed to occur, for the platelets appeared to be piling up on each other (Fig. 4).

Finally, fresh frozen plasma (FFP) was tested for possible correction of the adhesion defect: whole blood from a third subject (LF) with severe vWD was admixed with FFP (33 percent). There was a 15 percent decrease in the number of adherent platelets to 3724/cm^2, even though the admixture perfused had been substantially increased in F VIII:Rcof to 0.80 U and F VIII R:Ag to 0.39 U/ml from levels near zero. In the normal control subject (JL), after a similar addition of fresh frozen plasma to the whole blood specimen, platelet adhesion increased by 37 percent.

Thrombin Experiments

Patient RC ($<$0.20 U F VIII R:Ag/ml blood) provided PRP for two sets of experiments that compared the impact of a pretreatment perfusion of 0.1 U purified thrombin/ml oxygenated Dulbecco's phosphate-buffered saline solution followed by perfusion of either vW platelets or autologous fetal PRP (Fig. 5). Decreased numbers of this patient's platelets adhered to injured vascular surface and represented only 20 percent of the autologous fetal platelet adhesive ability. The adherent vW platelets presented a morphologic pattern similar to that of fetal platelets; those in contact with exposed subendothelium had dendrites and often were in spread form. In response to the thrombin-treated vascular surface, this patient's platelets projected more pseudopods and had greater spreading but did not produce a tight pavement. The data were quantified by counting only platelets adherent to exposed subendothelium; only rarely was there adhesion to normal-appearing endothelial cells. Pretreatment of the vessel segments with thrombin made them more attractive or sticky and the number of adherent vW platelets increased by 77 percent over patient RC's baseline values for this set (10,196 platelets/cm^2 exposed subendothelium). However, this value of 18,039 vW platelets/cm^2 was still only 45 percent of that for the control segment pretreated with thrombin and followed by perfusion of fetal PRP.

Factor VIII Activities in Blood and PRP Perfusing the
Test Umbilical Vein Segments

Perfusates of PRP and whole blood were tested for their content of F VIII R:Ag and F VIII:Rcof immediately prior to and post perfusion for 15 minutes through the test umbilical vein segments (TABLE 4). The levels for F VIII:Rcof were elevated in 13 of 15 postperfusion specimens, while those for F VIII R:Ag increased in 10 of 15 specimens. The increases in F VIII:Rcof and F VIII R:Ag were not necessarily parallel. The F VIII R:Ag levels were changed only slightly in contrast to changes in F VIII:Rcof. Averaging the individual data for each group of subjects gave the following results for increased F VIII activities: The increase in F VIII:Rcof was 51.10 percent in vWD specimens versus 26.56 percent in fetal specimens and 7.46 percent in adult postperfusion

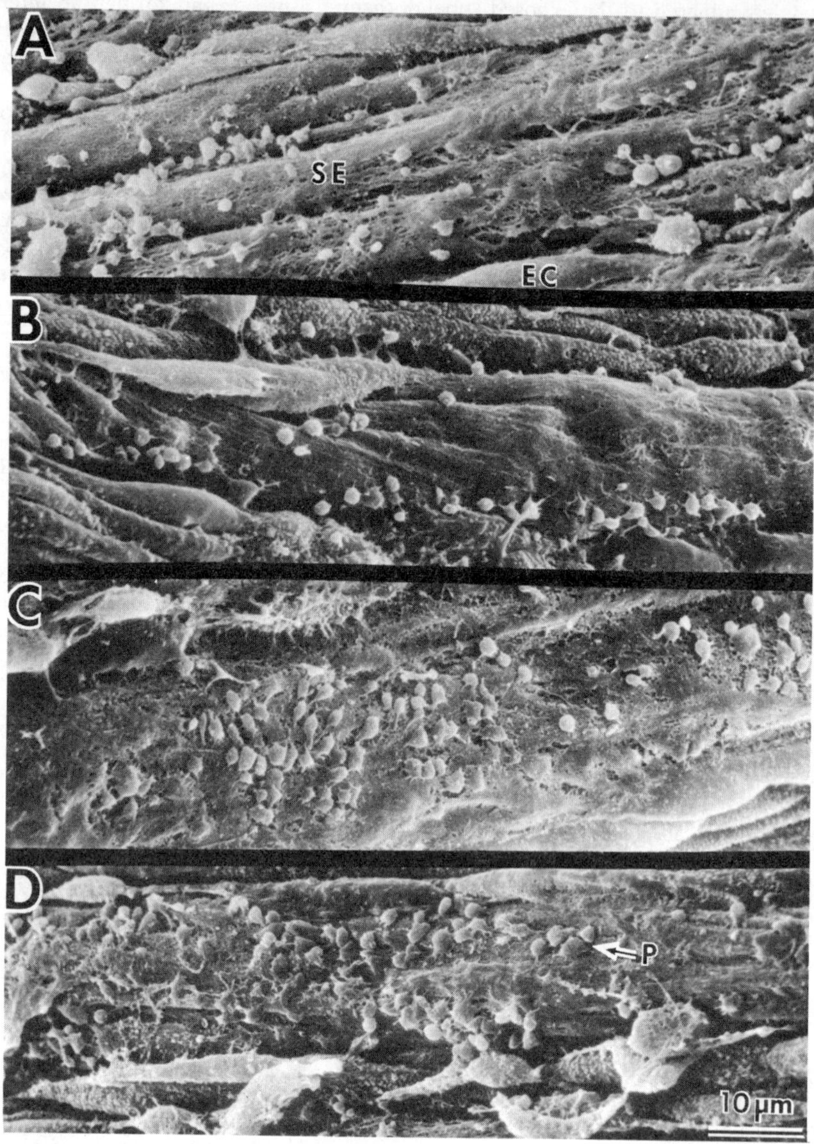

FIGURE 5. Adhesion defect of platelets (P) from patient (RC) with severe vWD was partially corrected by pretreatment of vein with 0.1 U thrombin/ml PBS. **(A)** adhesion of control fetal PRP. **(B)** PRP from patient RC. **(C)** increased adhesion of this patient's platelets, which now show pseudopods and spreading ability. **(D)** adhesion of control PRP after thrombin treatment of vein. EC = endothelial cells; SE = subendothelium.

specimens. On the other hand, F VIII R:Ag levels were insignificantly changed (3.62 percent in those with vWD, 4.62 percent in normal adult subjects, and 7.60 percent in fetal postperfusion specimens). The pre- and postperfusion

TABLE 4

CHANGES IN F VIII ACTIVITIES OF PERFUSATES (BLOOD OR PRP *)
PASSING THROUGH TEST UMBILICAL VEIN SEGMENTS

Experimental Conditions		F VIII R:Ag (U/ml)		F VIII:Rcof (U/ml)	
vWD-VB *	Pre	1.56		1.20	
	Post		1.59		1.80
vWD-IE *	Pre	0.60		0.92	
	Post		0.67		1.40
vWD-SN *	Pre	0.19		0.12	
	Post		0.16		0.17
vWD-AV	Pre	0.70		0.46	
	Post		0.67		1.00
vWD-CV	Pre	0.86		0.78	
	Post		0.62		0.96
vWD-JoV	Pre	1.32		1.00	
	Post		1.71		1.44
Normal-KG	Pre	0.56		1.00	
	Post		0.81		1.00
Normal-JL1	Pre	0.85		0.78	
	Post		0.98		1.00
Normal-JL2	Pre	0.76		1.17	
	Post		0.48		1.17
Fetal-AK1	Pre	0.55		1.50	
	Post		0.67		1.27
Fetal-AK2	Pre	0.48		0.90	
	Post		0.52		1.02
Fetal-RW10 *	Pre	1.53		0.90	
	Post		1.60		1.20
Fetal-RW22	Pre	1.74		1.40	
	Post		1.86		1.00
Fetal-RW32 *	Pre	1.94		1.20	
	Post		2.12		2.04
Fetal-RW43	Pre	0.34		0.84	
	Post		0.31		2.00

NOTE: Pre- and postperfusion specimens were frozen at the same time and within 1 hour of final preparation of the specimen for actual perfusion. Therefore, the F VIII activities do not necessarily correspond with values cited in TABLE 1 for freshly drawn blood.

specimens were frozen ($-70°$ C) at the same time and within 1 hour of final preparation of the specimen for the actual perfusion. Therefore, the preperfusion value is not the same as that given in TABLE 1 for fresh blood specimens frozen at an earlier time on the test day in patients with vWD.

Revelation of F VIII R:Ag Sites on the Subendothelium by a Highly Specific Latex Microsphere Antibody Probe

When the conditioned umbilical vein was perfused with highly specific latex microsphere antibody probes for F VIII R:Ag loci, obviously damaged endothelial cells attracted the microspheres (Fig. 6). Also, microspheres adhered to components in basement membrane and subendothelium exposed by prior injury or normal gestational aging of the fetal umbilical cord near term.

When normal fetal platelets were perfused into the umbilical vein followed by perfusion with anti-F VIII R:Ag microspheres, some platelets adherent to the subendothelium attracted the anti-F VIII R:Ag microspheres (Fig. 6). Adjacent areas of exposed subendothelium and severely damaged endothelial cells also bound the probe.

Perfusion of vW platelets in PRP followed by perfusion of anti-F VIII R:Ag microspheres resulted in very little platelet-microsphere interaction (Fig. 6). Again, primarily damaged endothelial cells attracted the anti-F VIII-labeled microspheres and seemed to do so preferentially. Endothelial cells adjacent to the damaged areas appeared normal and did not attract appreciable numbers of the 0.6 μm microsphere antibody probes.

Attempts to Deplete Umbilical Vein of F VIII R:Ag by Treatment with Epinephrine

Earlier investigators have demonstrated an elevation in F VIII activity after increases in circulating epinephrine.[21] We wondered whether we could measure F VIII release from epinephrine-treated umbilical vein segments, hoping to simulate a vWD vessel if release was significant. However, even after the effluents were concentrated by factors of 5 and 10, neither F VIII R:Ag nor Rcof was measurable in Dulbecco's PBS pre- and postperfusion specimens. Anti-F VIII R:Ag-labeled microspheres were used to localize the cellular sites of release or exposure of F VIII R:Ag on the vascular surface. Four different concentrations of epinephrine (20, 10, 0.5, and 0.05 μg/ml) were employed. Umbilical veins treated with 20 μg epinephrine/ml exhibited extensive endothelial damage and denudation (Fig. 7). The anti-F VIII-labeled microspheres were bound specifically to the injured endothelial cells and to various areas of the exposed subendothelium, but not to uninjured endothelial cells. The vein treated with 10 μg/ml exhibited a lower order of endothelial damage and microsphere binding. In the segments treated with concentrations of 0.5 and 0.05 μg/ml, very few microspheres were attracted to vascular surfaces.

Effect of Controlled Hypoxia on F VIII R:Ag Release and Adhesion of vW Platelets

The endothelium was rendered hypoxic by oxygen deprivation to study the vW platelet reaction to this environment and to measure F VIII release using F VIII R:Ag and Rcof assays as well as labeled anti-F VIII R:Ag microspheres. The labeled microspheres adhered quite specifically to damaged endothelial cells and areas of subendothelium, but not to undamaged endothelial cells. Later-perfused fetal platelets were seen adhering to the subendothelium, where

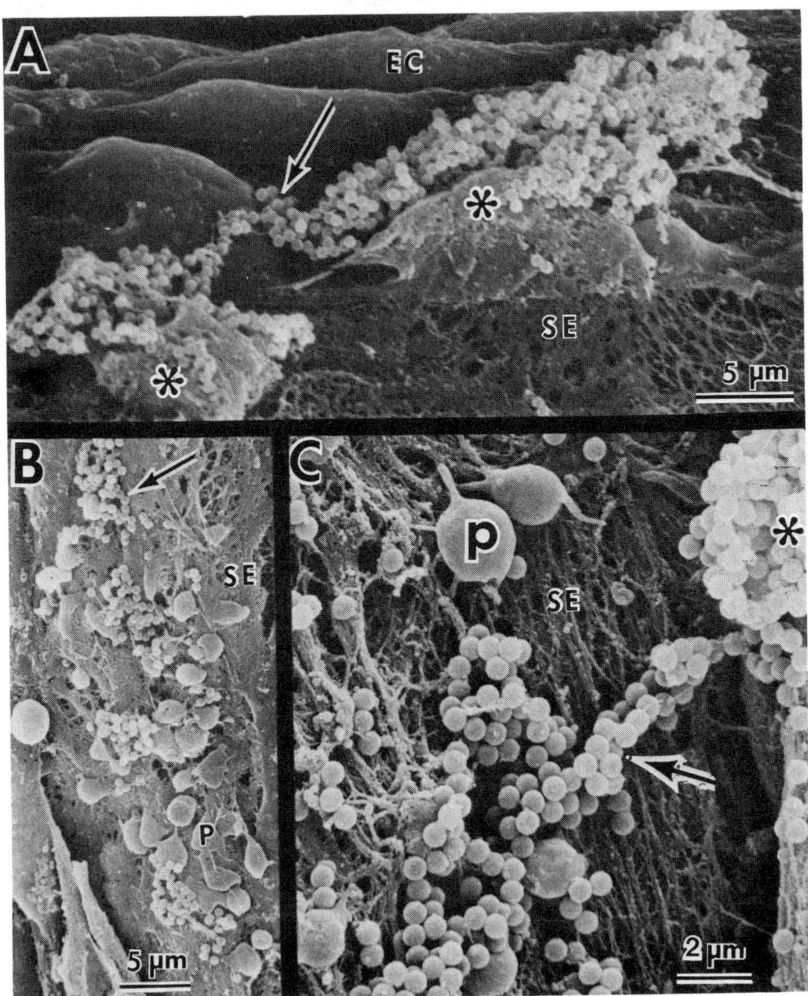

FIGURE 6. Localization of F VIII:Ag-vW sites on damaged endothelial cells (EC) and on subendothelium (SE). **(A)** umbilical vein control segment was perfused with anti-F VIII R:Ag microspheres. Note damaged endothelial cells (*asterisks*) covered by attached microspheres (*arrow*). **(B)** normal fetal platelets were paving the subendothelium. Note microspheres binding to platelets, subendothelium, and damaged endothelial cells. **(C)** Blood from patient AV had some platelets (p) that adhered to the exposed SE. The later-perfused microspheres (*arrow*) deposited on the SE and on damaged EC (*) are seen along the right margin of the micrograph.

they had many pseudopods and spread well. Later-perfused vW platelets of subjects VB and CV also adhered to the exposed subendothelium of hypoxic vein segments. F VIII R:Ag was essentially unchanged in two of three subjects

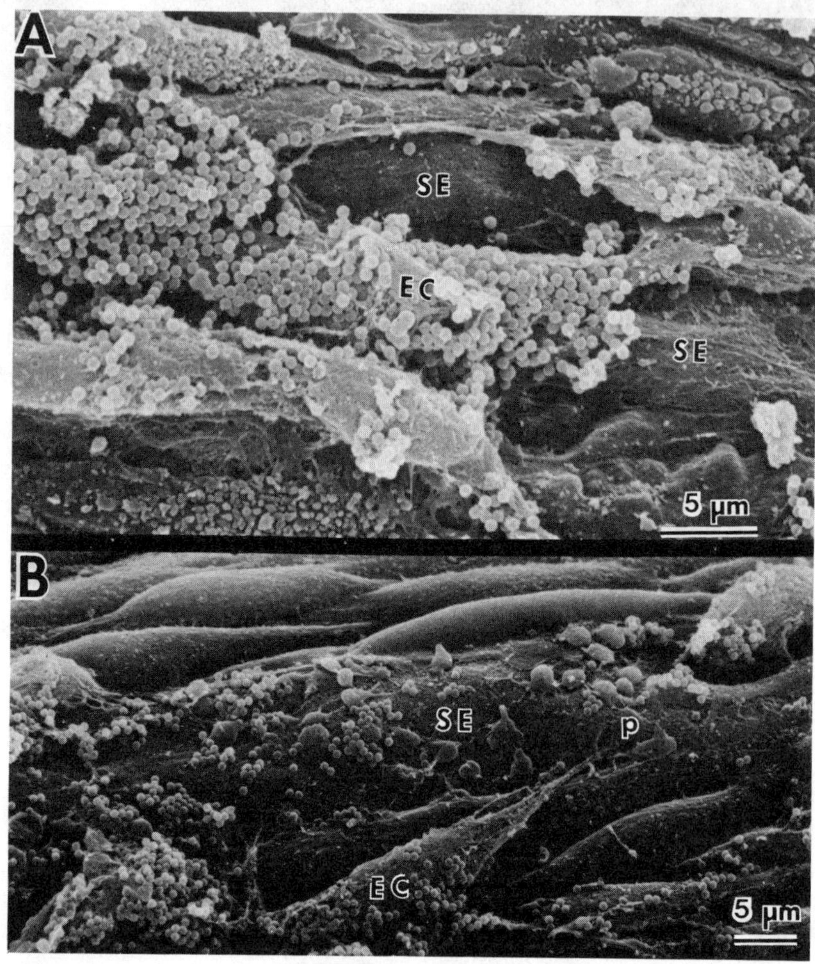

FIGURE 7. Either treatment of the vein with epinephrine (20 μg/ml HEPES buffer) in (A) or a brief period of hypoxia (B) results in a greater labeling of exposed subendothelium (SE) and injured endothelial cells (EC) by microspheres covalently linked to antibody against F VIII R:Ag-vW. Platelets (p) seen in (B) were from fetal PRP perfused before microspheres were added. Note normal pseudopods and spreading.

(VB, CV, and RW10), while F VIII:Rcof increased in all three experiments. Platelets were in either deoxygenated PRP or whole blood for the perfusion and latex microspheres were perfused later.

Influence of Apyrase and Washing of Platelets on Their Vessel Wall Reactivity

Apyrase added to the resuspension medium degrades nucleotides and thus prevents their accumulation. Kinlough-Rathbone *et al.* have shown that F VIII R:Ag-Rcof is removed during apyrase platelet washing.[22] With this procedure we attempted to render normal platelets similar to vW platelets and to study their interaction with the vessel wall.

Fetal platelets washed without apyrase in the final wash were smooth and spherical with obvious areas of membrane damage. Such fetal platelets did not adhere to subendothelial components. Fetal platelets containing apyrase in their final wash reacted normally (that is, with pseudopods and spreading) when exposed to the umbilical vein (FIG. 8).

von Willebrand platelets (patient DS) washed without apyrase exhibited the same morphologic pattern as that of fetal platelets similarly treated. The vW platelets appeared swollen and spherical and showed some membrane damage. There were no vW platelets that adhered to the subendothelium in a normal fashion. vW platelets (patient SS) treated with apyrase throughout the washing procedure (FIG. 8) reacted as vW platelets would normally react, adhering very poorly. When they did adhere, they formed abortive-type pseudopods and failed to spread. There were extensive areas of exposed subendothelium where platelets did not adhere.

The factor assays for the fetal and vW platelets washed with and without apyrase are notable. While there was some measurable F VIII R:Ag and Rcof before perfusion in the apyrase-washed platelets (fetal specimens 116 and 84, respectively, vW 0.14 and 0.16 U/ml), after perfusion there was none present in high enough quantity to measure. It should be noted that the vW platelets used here were from two severely affected patients (TABLE 1).

Blockade of F VIII Sites by Treatment with Antibody Against F VIII R:Ag

In order to block possible F VIII R:vW binding sites for platelets on the subendothelial components, anti-F VIII microspheres or nonparticulate anti-human F VIII R:Ag were perfused through the umbilical veins prior to introducing fetal and vW PRP.

Fetal platelets perfused after the antibody microsphere exposure formed pseudopods well, but overall there was a decrease in the number of platelets adhering when compared with the control (FIG. 9).

The vW platelets (patient JS) exposed to the umbilical vein after the antibody microspheres were perfused exhibited only slight adhesion and only occasional pseudopod formation (FIG. 9). The microspheres were notable, adhering to the subendothelium in sufficient quantity to block platelet access. In the areas of dense microsphere binding, very few platelets adhered (FIG. 9).

The fetal platelets that were exposed to the cord segments pretreated with soluble antihuman F VIII R:Ag were abnormal in several respects. There were very few adherent platelets and they exhibited little spreading or pseudopod formation. Furthermore, the shape of the platelets was atypical: many spherical platelets exhibited abortive-type dendritic processes. There were wide areas of "de-endothelialized" intima without any platelet adhesion.

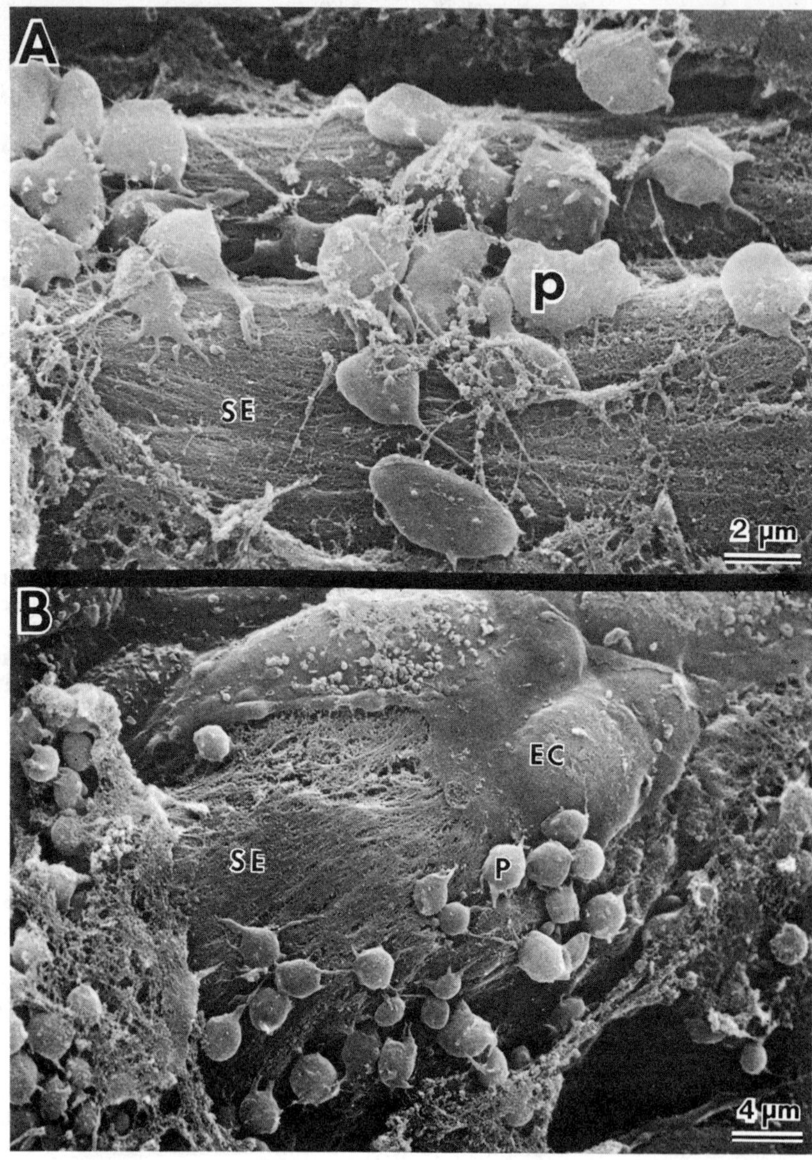

FIGURE 8. Adhesive ability of apyrase-washed platelets (p). **(A)** fetal platelets project pseudopods annd spread to form "pavement" on exposed subendothelium (SE). **(B)** platelets from patient (SS with severe vWD) were defective in ability to pave, but showed more activity upon adhesion than expected from the F VIII component levels. EC = endothelial cell.

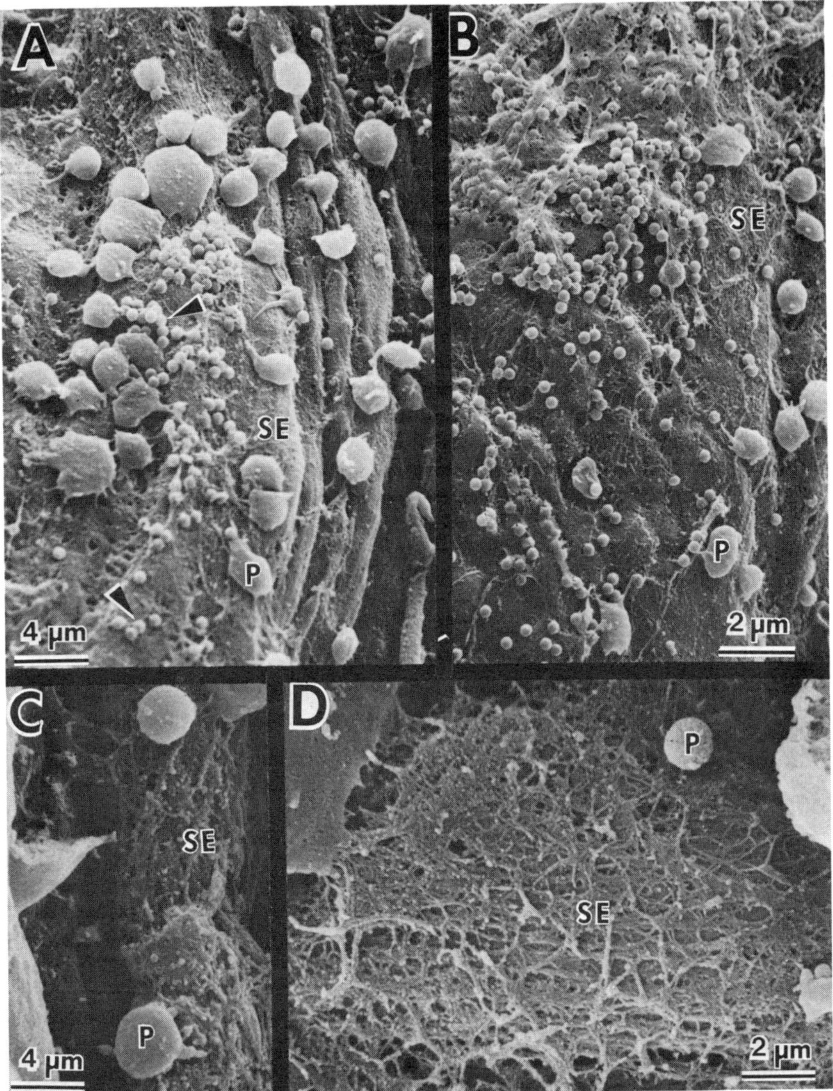

FIGURE 9. Partial blockade of platelet adhesion by pretreatment with microspheres bearing antibody to F VIII R:Ag (*arrows*) and soluble anti-F VIII R:Ag. (A) umbilical vein subendothelium (SE) perfused first with anti-F VIII R:Ag microspheres followed by normal fetal PRP. Although the number of adherent platelets (P) was reduced, those adherent platelets spread and projected pseudopods. Microspheres bind to subendothelium (SE). (B) anti-F VIII R:Ag preceded perfusion of platelets (P) from patient (JS) with vWD. Platelet adhesion was decreased and those adhering were poorly activated. Microspheres bind to subendothelium. (C) vein pretreated with soluble anti-F VIII R:Ag followed by fetal PRP. Note that spherical and relatively unactivated platelets constitute the reduced number adhering. (D) soluble anti-F VIII R:Ag perfusion preceded perfusion of vW platelets of patient MB. Adherent platelets were rare on SE and were unactive spheres or discs.

The vW platelets (patient ME) were perfused into the umbilical vein after treatment with the soluble antihuman F VIII R:Ag. These platelets were difficult to locate because of their scarcity on the subendothelial areas. When encountered, they were sphered and relatively unactivated in appearance, not unlike the fetal platelets in the same environment (FIG. 9). Very many areas of subendothelium existed without a single platelet adhering.

DISCUSSION

The Hemostatic Capabilities of the vW Platelet

From clinical experience and laboratory findings (aggregometry, glass bead retention, electron microscopy of surface adhesiveness), one expects vW platelets to be very defective in their ability to seal damaged vessels. In 1974 Tschopp *et al.* reported that the adhesion of vW platelets to exposed subendothelium in the rabbit aorta model was impaired.[10] Our study, using an all-human materials system and controlled perfusion at physiologic hemodynamic conditions, while corroborating earlier data gained with the rabbit model, considerably extends that information. Most significant is the display by SEM of qualitative as well as quantitive differences in platelet–vessel-wall interactions that correlate best with the plasma level of F VIII:Rcof and to some extent with F VIII R:Ag, but not at all with F VIII:C. This observation is in agreement with the data of Howard and Firkin, who suggested that the F VIII:Rcof level is the most accurate measure of the vW defect.[23]

Few of the platelets from the 15 subjects with vWD were as competent as those from normal subjects (newborn or adult) to participate in platelet-subendothelial interaction. The most competent were platelets from vWD subjects (VB, IE, CV, JoV) who had F VIII:Rcof > 0.53 and F VIII R: Ag > 0.68 U/ml. However, their platelet adhesive ability at best was only 51 percent of that of the normal control platelets to adhere to recently injured vessel wall. At least those adherent vW platelets displayed shape changes (pseudopods, spread forms) resembling those seen by SEM when normal platelets adhere and activate upon subendothelium. The capability of these vW platelets to provide relatively tight coverage, a pavement or temporary vascular lining for the subendothelium, was notable.

In marked contrast, the vW platelets from other patients with lower F VIII: Rcof and F VIII R:Ag levels, although providing nearly the same quantitative information with regard to number of adherent platelets (38 and 43 percent of that of controls), were very ineffective with respect to their ability to change shape and provide an effective pavement on the subendothelium. In support of the experience of others,[10, 24, 25] we found that cryoprecipitate or fresh frozen plasma (both of which contain a high content of F VIII:vW) is corrective of the hemostatic defect exhibited by vW platelets in their own plasma. Not only did cryoprecipitate increase the number of adherent platelets of patient BB toward normal, but also the vW platelets were able to display normal abilities to project pseudopods and to spread to more completely pave the exposed subendothelium.

The question of whether or not the defects in vWD are due entirely to the plasmatic deficiency of F VIII:vW, to impaired or absent platelet membrane receptors for F VIII:vW, or to a combination of the two has not been entirely resolved.

As just mentioned, the degree of vW platelet aberrancy appeared proportional to the deficit in plasma levels of F VIII:Rcof rather than F VIII R:Ag or F VIII:C. These observations tend to support a plasmatic defect. No one will dispute the fact that addition of F VIII:vW and F VIII R:Ag corrects the vW defect in several measurable ways. However, we effectively prevented normal platelet adhesion with specific antibody to F VIII R:Ag perfused before the platelet perfusion. That is, the umbilical vein was treated with the anti-F VIII R:Ag, then flushed with PBS, and finally perfused with fetal or vW platelets. This observation supports the view that F VIII R:Ag-vW, which is bound to the exposed subendothelium, is more crucial than either the F VIII:RAg or F VIII:Rcof level in the perfusate itself. It may be that the plasma factor levels are a poor reflection of the F VIII R:Ag and F VIII:vW content of the subendothelium and platelets. Additional support for this view is provided by the elegant experiments of Sakariassen *et al.* (also in an all-human material model), which demonstrated that normal platelet adhesion to renal arterial subendothelium is mediated by F VIII:vW bound to the subendothelium.[14]

Whether or not vW platelets are intrinsically abnormal remains an intriguing question. Some vW platelets are thought to have abnormal or deficient amounts of membrane glycoprotein Ib, which is known to contain the receptor site for interaction and binding of F VIII:vW.[26] Although the present consensus is that platelet morphology, evident in transmission electron micrographs, is normal in vWD, there are reports that adhesion and spreading on foreign surfaces such as glass, collodion, and Formvar® are abnormal.[3] A plasmatic deficiency of the "bridging" protein F VIII:vW could account for the difficulty that vW platelets show in attaching to the sites on the foreign substrates. Our experiments in which vW platelets were washed in the presence and absence of apyrase and were then ultimately resuspended in HEPES-albumin medium prior to perfusion in the umbilical vein model are of considerable interest. In two experiments, the washed vW platelets of patients DS and SS had unexpectedly high adhesive ability (70 percent) compared to that of the companion washed fetal platelet controls, although surface membrane activity and spreading ability remained abnormal. These results suggest that the handling and washing of platelets from patients with severe vWD may uncover additional membrane receptor sites that facilitate binding to exposed subendothelium. The exact identity of such receptors is not presently known.

Identity of Binding Sites in Subendothelium for vW and Normal Platelets

Our finding that a particulate (latex microspheres) antibody probe for F VIII:Ag-vW binds to freshly exposed subendothelium is strong evidence that F VIII:Ag-vW is already present in or on the subendothelium.[13] The subendothelial binding of anti-F VIII R:Ag-vW appeared to be increased by pretreatment with epinephrine or by a hypoxic interval. Moreover, specific but soluble antibody for F VIII:Ag-vW partially blocked platelet adhesion of both vW and normal platelets. It is therefore suggested that at least one important subendothelial binding site is F VIII:vW. Sakariassen and colleagues convincingly correlate the number of ^{51}Cr-labeled platelets with the increased accumulation of ^{125}I-labeled F VIII:vW on postmortem renal arterial subendothelium.[14] They suggest that on vessel injury the F VIII:Ag-vW synthesized by endothelial cells is released to bind to subendothelium. Rand and associates, using both immunofluorescent and immunoelectron microscopy, have demonstrated the presence of F VIII R:Ag on umbilical vein subendothelium prior to removal of endothelial cells.[27]

SUMMARY

Adhesion of platelets from 15 patients with von Willebrand's disease was tested in an *ex vivo* human umbilical vein model. Experiments employed umbilical veins still in their umbilical cords taken from patients undergoing cesarean section and platelets (fetal, adult and vW) either apyrase-washed or used as platelet-rich plasma or whole blood. F VIII R:Ag, F VIII:Rcof, and F VIII:C were measured in initial fresh plasma and in effluents from the umbilical vein segments. F VIII:Rcof increased in most perfusates. Binding of latex-linked specific antihuman F VIII R:Ag demonstrated that F VIII R:Ag existed on subendothelium and on injured endothelial cells. Scanning electron microscopy three-dimensionally displayed vW platelet–vessel-wall interactions. Although vW platelets adhered to injured vein, both qualitative and quantitative differences existed in comparison with adhesion of normal platelets. The differences correlated best with the plasma F VIII:Rcof level. The best adhesion shown by vW platelets was only 51 percent of the adhesion of control fetal or adult platelets. vW platelets had less surface activity, fewer pseudopods, and little ability to spread and pave the exposed subendothelium. Pretreatment of the vein with F VIII R:Ag antibody partly blocked adhesion. Coperfusion of cryoprecipitate with vW platelets improved their adhesivity, state of activation on subendothelium, and ability to form aggregates. ABO differences in blood cell types of fetal material and platelet donors seemed without effect, which further establishes this model's validity for studies of platelet dysfunction and platelet or endothelial reactive agents.

ACKNOWLEDGMENTS

We wish to thank Dr. Shan-te Chen, Judy Penner, and Ralph Kramer for the technical and photographic assistance that was essential for this research.

REFERENCES

1. VON WILLEBRAND, E. A. 1926. Hereditarpseudohamofili Finsk. Lakarsallsk. Handl. **68:** 87–112.
2. VON WILLEBRAND, E. A. 1931. Uber hereditare pseudohamophilie. Acta Med. Scand. **76:** 521–550.
3. LUSHER, J. M. & M. I. BARNHART. 1977. Congenital disorders affecting platelets. Semin. Thromb. Hemostas. **4:** 123–186.
4. NILSSON, I. M. 1977. von Willebrand's disease—fifty years old. Acta Med. Scand. **201:** 497–508.

5. JAFFE, E. A. 1977. Endothelial cells and the biology of factor VIII. N. Engl. J. Med. **296:** 377–383.

6. HOLMBERG, L., P. M. MANNUCCI, I. TURESSON, Z. M. RUGGERI & I. M. NILSSON. 1974. Factor VIII antigen in the vessel walls in von Willebrand's disease and haemophilia A. Scand. J. Haematol. **13:** 33–38.

7. NILSSON, I. M. 1978. Report on the working party on factor VIII—related antigens. Thromb. Haemostas. **39:** 511–520.

8. BORCHGREVINK, C. F. 1960. A method for measuring platelet adhesiveness in vivo. Acta Med. Scand. **168:** 157–164.

9. SALZMAN, E. W. 1963. Measurement of platelet adhesiveness. A simple in vitro method demonstrating an abnormality in von Willebrand's disease. J. Lab. Clin. Med. **62:** 724–735.

10. TSCHOPP, T. B., H. J. WEISS & H. R. BAUMGARTNER. 1974. Decreased adhesion of platelets to subendothelium in von Willebrand's disease. J. Lab. Clin. Med. **83:** 296–300.

11. BARNHART, M. I. & S. CHEN. 1978. Vessel wall models for studying interaction capabilities with blood platelets. Semin. Thromb. Hemostas. **5:** 112–155.

12. BARNHART, M. I. 1978. Platelet responses in health and disease. Mol. Cell Biochem. **22:** 113–137.

13. WILKINS, R. M. 1978. Von Willebrand platelet-vessel wall interaction. MS dissertation: 1–100. Wayne State University, Detroit, MI.

14. SAKARIASSEN, K. S., P. A. BOLHUIS & J. J. SIXMA. 1979. Human blood platelet adhesion to artery subendothelium is mediated by factor VIII-von Willebrand factor bound to the subendothelium. Nature **279:** 636–638.

15. NILSSON, I. M., M. BLOMBACH & B. BLOMBACH. 1959. Von Willebrand's disease in Sweden. Its pathogenesis and treatment. Acta Med. Scand. **164:** 263–278.

16. CORNU, P., M. J. LARRIEU, J. CAEN & J. BERNARD. 1963. Transfusion studies in von Willebrand's disease: Effect on bleeding time and Factor VIII. Br. J. Haematol. **9:** 189–202.

17. SIMONE, J. V., J. VANDERHEIDEN & C. F. ABILDGAARD. 1967. The semiautomatic one-stage factor VIII assay with a commercially prepared standard. J. Lab. Clin. Med. **69:** 706–712.

18. ZIMMERMAN, T. S., L. W. HOYER, L. DICKSON & T. S. EDGINGTON. 1975. Determination of the von Willebrand disease antigen (Factor VIII-agn) in plasma by quantitative immunoelectrophoresis. J. Lab. Clin. Med. **86:** 152–159.

19. ALLAIN, J. P., H. A. COOPER, R. H. WAGNER & K. M. BRINKHOUS. 1975. Platelets fixed with paraformaldehyde: A new reagent for assay of von Willebrand factor and platelet aggregating factors. J. Lab. Clin. Med. **85:** 318–328.

20. BARNHART, M. I. 1971. Immunologic techniques. *In* Techniques in Thrombosis and Bleeding Disorders. N. Bang, F. Beller, E. Deutsch & E. F. Mammen, Eds.: 457–484. Academic Press. New York, N.Y.

21. RICKLES, F. R., L. W. HOYER, M. E. RICK & D. J. AHR. 1976. The effects of epinephrine injection in von Willebrand's disease. J. Clin. Invest. **57:** 1618–1625.

22. KINLOUGH-RATHBONE, R. L., J. F. MUSTARD, M. A. PACKHAM, D. W. PERRY, H. J. REIVERS & J. P. CAZENAVE. 1977. Properties of washed human platelets. Thromb. Haemostas. (Stuttgart) **37:** 291–308.

23. HOWARD, M. A. & B. G. FIRKIN. 1971. Ristocetin—a new tool in the investigation of platelet aggregation. Thromb. Diath. Haemorrh. **26:** 362–369.

24. WEISS, H. J., H. R. BAUMGARTNER, T. B. TSCHOPP, *et al.* 1978. Correction by factor VIII of the impaired platelet adhesion to subendothelium in von Willebrand's disease. Blood **51:** 267 279.

25. KIMURA, A., E. W. BOWIE, R. J. CAMPBELL & D. N. FASS. 1979. Willebrand factor in hemostasis and in the in vitro bleeding time. Blood **54:** 1347–1357.
26. COOPER, H. A., K. J. CLEMETSON & E. F. LUSCHER. 1979. Human platelet membrane receptor for bovine von Willebrand factor (platelet aggregating factor). An integral membrane glycoprotein. Proc. Natl. Acad. Sci. USA **76:** 1069–1073.
27. RAND, J. H., I. I. SUSSMAN, R. E. GORDON, S. V. CHU & V. SOLOMON. 1980. Localization of F VIII-related antigen in human vascular subendothelium. Blood **55:** 752–756.

PROTEOLYSIS OF HUMAN FIXED, WASHED PLATELETS BY GRAM-NEGATIVE BACTERIAL METALLOPROTEASES: EFFECT ON von WILLEBRAND FACTOR-HUMAN PLATELET INTERACTIONS *

Herbert A. Cooper,†‡ William P. Bennett,‡ Arnold Kreger,§
David Lyerly,§ and Robert H. Wagner ‡

*Department of Pathology and
Center for Thrombosis and Hemostasis ‡
University of North Carolina
Chapel Hill, North Carolina 27514; and the
Departments of Microbiology and Immunology §
Bowman Gray School of Medicine
Wake Forest University
Winston-Salem, North Carolina 27103*

INTRODUCTION

Human platelets fixed with formaldehyde (FWP) retain, during prolonged periods of storage, their ability to aggregate with the von Willebrand factor (vWF) of human and certain animal plasmas. However, they do not aggregate with conventional platelet-aggregating agents such as adenosine diphosphate (ADP), epinephine, collagen, and thrombin.[1] The sudden deterioration of a single batch of FWP, after less than 1 week of storage, led to the studies that form the basis of this report. This preparation of FWP, stored in 0.02 percent sodium azide, lost its ability to aggregate with bovine vWF (platelet-aggregating factor, PAF) or human vWF plus ristocetin. Addition of supernatant fluid from these FWP resulted in a similar loss of aggregability of normal FWP. Further investigation showed that the initial platelet preparation was supporting the growth of a motile gram-negative organism that was identified as *Serratia marcescens*.

Several concentrations of a sterile, culture filtrate of *S. marcescens* were incubated with human FWP and, at intervals, the mixture was tested for its aggregability with bovine vWF or human vWF plus ristocetin. The loss of FWP aggregability was found to be directly related to the concentration of the filtrate and the time of incubation. Within 15 minutes of incubation with undiluted culture filtrate, the FWP completely lost their ability to aggregate with the von Willebrand factor of both species. Incubation of FWP with a 1:100 dilution of the culture filtrate still caused some loss of FWP aggregability. The inhibitory activity of the filtrate was retained after prolonged dialysis in standard Visking tubing, but could be abolished by heating at 60° C for 30 minutes.

These observations and the knowledge that most strains of *S. marcescens*

* This work was supported by Research Grants HL-06350 and HL-16769 from the National Heart, Lung, and Blood Institute, and Research Grant EY-01104 from the National Eye Institute, National Institutes of Health, Bethesda, Maryland.

† Supported by Research Career Development Award HL-00081.

179

produce extracellular proteases suggested that the active material in the culture filtrate was a protease produced by *S. marcescens*. When the culture media of several other gram-negative bacteria were then screened, two other organisms were found to produce similar enzymatic activity. A metalloprotease of *S. marcescens* strain BG was purified and initial testing confirmed that purified *Serratia* protease (SP) abolished the ability of human FWP to aggregate with bovine PAF and human vWF plus ristocetin. Subsequently, highly purified extracellular proteases from two different strains of *Pseudomonas aeruginosa* were also prepared. Studies of the effects of all three proteases on FWP aggregability are reported. For comparison, similar studies were also carried out using more conventional proteolytic agents, such as chymotrypsin and trypsin. In the majority of the experiments, only bovine vWF was used because it allowed a more direct study of the vWF/platelet interaction by obviating the need for any cofactor, such as the antibiotic ristocetin.

MATERIALS AND METHODS

Fixed, Washed Platelets

Platelets from a multidonor pool of recently outdated human platelet concentrates were washed and then fixed with formaldehyde using a modification [2] of the original method.[1] The FWP were adjusted to $8 \times 10^5/\mu l$ and kept at 4° C in storage buffer (0.05 M Tris-HCl, 0.1 M NaCl, 0.001 M EDTA, 0.02 percent sodium azide, pH 6.4). For most of the experiments, platelets were placed in either NH_4HCO_3, Tris, or phosphate-buffered saline without EDTA.

Platelet Aggregability

Platelet aggregability was assayed as previously described.[3] FWP (0.2 ml) and 0.2 ml of buffer (0.05 M Tris-HCl, 0.15 M NaCl, pH 7.4) or test sample were stirred at 1100 rpm, 37° C, in a glass cuvette using a dual-channel aggregometer (Payton Associates, Buffalo, NY) and an Omniscribe recorder (Houston, Inst., Bellaire, TX). After a stable baseline was established ($<$60 sec), 0.2 ml of a standard bovine plasma, diluted 1:8 with 0.05 M Tris-HCl, 0.15 M NaCl, pH 7.0, was added. Unless otherwise stated, bovine plasma was thus used at a final dilution of 1:24 (approximately 0.04 units/ml of vWF). A slope for the test sample was calculated from the steepest part of the aggregation curve and compared with the control slope obtained with FWP and buffer. In experiments concerning human vWF we used dilutions of normal human plasma and initiation of aggregation with ristocetin at a final concentration of 0.8 mg/ml.

Purification of the Bacterial Extracellular Proteases

S. marcescens strain BG and *P. aeruginosa* strains 5–31 and IFO 3455 were cultivated and a protease was purified from each of the three extracellular filtrates as previously described.[4, 5] The purified *S. marcescens* protease (SP) had approximately 50 azocasein units/mg dry weight, whereas those from the two strains of *P. aeruginosa* were eight to nine times more potent (400–450 azocasein U/mg protein). The three proteases did not display any detectable activity of the following enzymes: hexapeptidase, collagenase, lecithinase C, desoxyribonuclease, lipase, and esterase.

Heat Inactivation

Samples of the culture filtrates and the purified protease preparations were brought rapidly to 60° C and maintained for 30 min. Samples were cooled quickly to 23° C and tested for residual protease activity.

PAF Purification

Bovine PAF was purified from blood obtained from adult cows at the time of slaughter, as previously described.[6]

Effect of Protease Digestion on FWP

Ten milliliters of FWP ($8 \times 10^5/\mu l$) in 0.15 M NH_4HCO_3, pH 7.3, were mixed with 10 ml of protease (SP 10 $\mu g/ml$, trypsin 2.5 $\mu g/ml$, or chymotrypsin 100 $\mu g/ml$) in the same buffer. Control FWP (10 ml) were mixed with 10 ml of 0.15 M NH_4HCO_3 buffer, pH 7.3. The mixtures were incubated for 1 hr at 23° C. At the end of the incubation, an aliquot of each platelet mixture was tested for aggregability as previously described and the rate of aggregation (slope) was compared with that of the control platelets, which remained essentially unchanged from preincubation values.

Control and treated platelets were each divided into two 9-ml aliquots and centrifuged at 100,000 g for 1 hr at 4° C. The supernatants were carefully removed and analyzed for protein. The samples from 9 ml of supernatant were then lyophilized with no further treatment. The lyophilized samples were redissolved in 0.25 ml of reducing or nonreducing buffer for polyacrylamide gel electrophoresis. In certain experiments the supernatant was also treated with EDTA to inactivate the metalloenzyme. The inactivated supernatant was then studied for the presence of proteolytic products capable of competing with intact FWP for bovine vWF.

Polyacrylamide Gel Electrophoresis

The platelet pellets were solubilized by heating in a boiling water bath for 30 to 60 min in 2 percent SDS, 0.06 M PO_4, 8 M urea, pH 7.0, with or without 2 percent DTT. The electrophoretic separation of the soluble platelet components was carried out in 0.1 percent SDS, 0.1 M phosphate buffer, pH 7.0, on either 5 percent or 3.5 percent polyacrylamide gels.[7] For reduction, samples from lyophilized supernatants were heated under denaturing conditions in 0.06 M DDT for 2 min at 90° C. All the samples were mixed with bromphenol blue and glycerol prior to application on the gel. For localization of the bands, gels were stained in Coomassie brilliant blue dye for protein and in

PAS (periodic acid Schiff reagent) for carbohydrate. Stained gels were scanned at 540 nm using a Gel Scanner and a U-A5 monitor (Isco, Lincoln, NE). Marker proteins and their assigned molecular weights were as follows: thyroglobulin, 330,000; ferritin; 220,000, albumin, 67,000; catalase, 60,000; and lactic dehydrogenase (LDH) 36,000.

Reagents

Water was deionized and glass-distilled. All chemicals were reagent grade unless otherwise specified. Trypsin was crystalline, lyophilized, and salt-free (Worthington, Freehold, NJ); α-chymotrypsin was prepared from bovine pancreas, thrice crystallized, (Schwartz-Mann, Orangeburg, NY); and ristocetin was obtained as a gift (Abbott Laboratories, Chicago, IL).

RESULTS

Increasing concentrations of highly purified SP were incubated for 15 min at 23° C with a constant concentration of platelets ($4 \times 10^5/\mu$l). After incu-

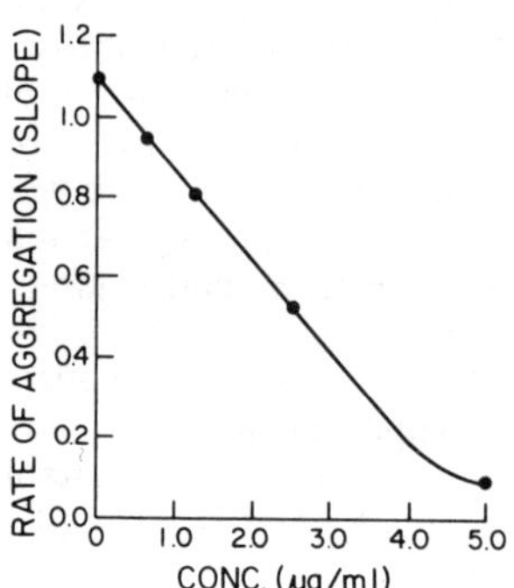

FIGURE 1. SP-induced loss of FWP aggregation as a function of enzyme concentration. Equal volumes of FWP ($8 \times 10^5/\mu$l) and SP were mixed and incubated for 15 min at 23° C. The mixture was then transferred to an aggregation cuvette and the rate of aggregation (slope) determined using 0.04 U/ml of bovine vWF for each SP concentration.

bation, the platelets were compared with untreated platelets for their ability to aggregate with a standard concentration of bovine plasma vWF, approximately 0.04 U/ml. This concentration was selected to give a rate of aggregation (slope) of approximately 1 for the control platelets. When SP (0.625 μg/ml) was mixed in equal volumes with FWP, there was a 13 percent loss of aggregability. Virtually complete loss of aggregability occurred with 5 μg/ml of SP (FIG. 1). The rate of loss of aggregability with SP was reproducible for any given batch of FWP and standard bovine plasma. However, some variation was noted whenever different lots of fixed platelets or bovine plasma were used. Thus, only approximate comparisons between different experiments are possible.

The degree of reduction in the slope of aggregation was related to the length of incubation of SP with the platelets prior to the addition of bovine vWF (FIG. 2). For example, after 30 minutes' incubation, the rate of aggregation of SP-treated FWP was reduced by about 90 percent. At any one time

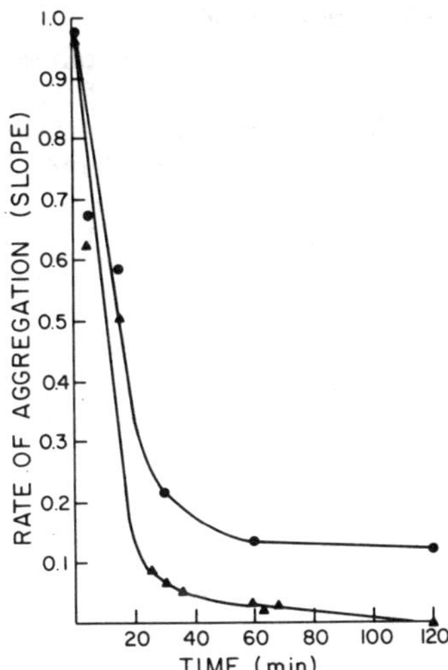

FIGURE 2. Effect of incubation time on the proteolysis of FWP by SP. FWP $(8 \times 10^5/\mu l)$ were mixed in equal volumes with SP giving a final SP concentration of 0.625 μg/ml ($\bullet$—$\bullet$) and 1.25 μg/ml ($\blacktriangle$—$\blacktriangle$). At specified time intervals the mixture was transferred to an aggregometer cuvette and the rate of aggregation (slope) of the treated platelets determined using 0.04 U/ml of bovine vWF.

during the incubation, however, the rate of aggregation could be increased by increasing the concentration of bovine vWF (FIG. 3).

The rate of loss of aggregability of FWP incubated with purified SP was temperature-dependent. It increased with increasing temperatures when tested over a range of 4° C to 40° C. In separate experiments concerning the thermal stability of SP, there was no detectable inactivation of the SP incubated for 20 min at 50° C, but complete inactivation occurred after 30 min at 60° C.

Preliminary experiments with the *S. marcescens* culture filtrate had demonstrated that after incubation with EDTA, the filtrate lost its effect on FWP. In more definitive studies, purified SP, after incubation for 4 hr at 4° C in 10 m*M* EDTA, lost most of its activity (FIG. 4). The slope of aggregation of

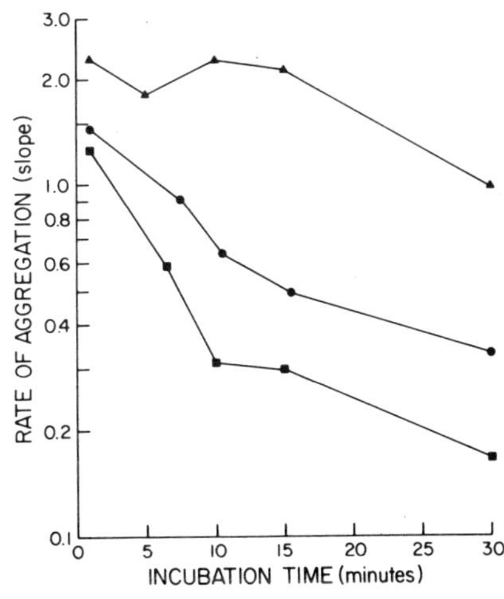

FIGURE 3. SP-induced loss of FWP aggregation as a function of incubation time. Equal volumes of FWP and SP (1 U/ml) preparations were mixed in individual cuvettes and kept at 37° C. After the indicated incubation times, residual aggregability of FWP was tested with three dilutions of standard bovine plasma: undiluted ($\blacktriangle$—$\blacktriangle$); 1:4 ($\bullet$—$\bullet$); 1:8 ($\blacksquare$—$\blacksquare$).

FWP treated with a 1:10 dilution of "inactivated" SP was similar to that obtained with a 1:100 dilution of the untreated SP, that is, the SP had lost more than 90 percent of its activity. Moreover, the addition of Zn^{2+} (2 mM) to the 1:10 dilution of EDTA-treated SP preparation restored activity. Zn^{2+}. at a concentration of 2 mM had a slight effect on the rate of aggregation of the control system. The latter finding was probably reflected in the apparently increased inhibition of FWP aggregation noted with the reactivated SP.

Stock cultures of additional gram-negative organisms were grown in trypticase soy broth. Cell-free filtrates were compared with control sterile trypticase soy broth for their effects on FWP aggregability. Protease activity was found not only in *S. marcescens*, but also in the cell-free filtrates of two strains of *Pseudomonas aeruginosa* and minimal activity was seen in a strain

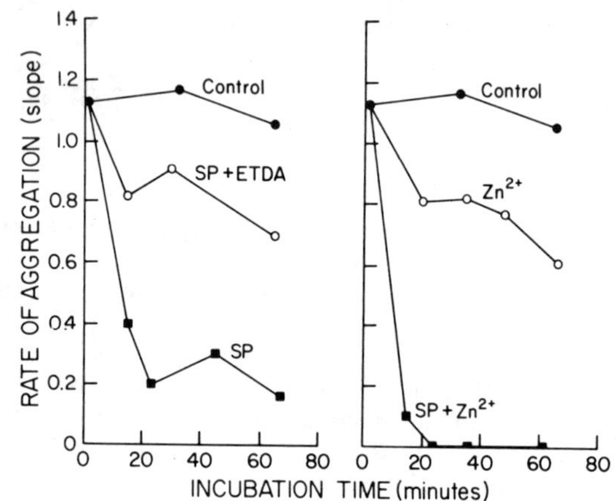

FIGURE 4. Inactivation and restoration of SP-induced loss of FWP aggregation. Test samples were added in equal volumes to FWP and the mixtures tested at intervals in the aggregometer with standard bovine plasma (1:8). (*Left*) SP (100 μg/ml) incubated in 10 mM EDTA for 4 hr, 4° C, pH 6.4, diluted 1:10 (○—○); untreated SP diluted 1:10 (■—■); buffer (0.05 M Tris, 0.15 M NaCl, pH 7.0) (●—●). (*Right*) 2 mM Zn acetate (○—○); EDTA-treated SP in 2 mM Zn^{2+} (■—■); buffer (●—●).

of *Escherichia coli*. Culture filtrates of *Proteus mirabilis*, *Klebsiella pneumoniae*, and *Enterobacter aerogenes* were negative under these conditions.

Purified proteases from *P. aeruginosa*, strains 5–31 and IFO 3455, were incubated with FWP as described earlier for SP, with similar results. When the concentrations of the two *Pseudomonas* proteases were adjusted to the same azocasein units/ml, strain 5–31 caused a greater reduction in the slope of aggregation than IFO 3455. On a weight basis the two *Pseudomonas* proteases caused about the same loss of aggregability as SP, but when compared on the basis of azocasein units/ml, SP was about eight times more potent against FWP as a substrate (TABLE 1).

FWP were incubated for 70 min at 23° C with SP; no aggregation could be detected with bovine plasma. However, these SP-treated platelets, when tested

TABLE 1

EFFECT OF INCUBATION OF FWP WITH EXTRACELLULAR
PROTEASES ON THE SLOPE OF AGGREGATION *

| | Incubation Time (min) | | | |
Protease	0	15	30	60
S. marcescens (0.25 U/ml, 5 μg/ml)	–	0.05	0.04	0.03
P. aeruginosa (2.0 U/ml, 5 μg/ml)				
Strain IFO 3455	–	0.28	0.15	0.07
Strain 5–31	–	0.08	0.07	0.03
Buffer control	1.82	1.62	1.82	1.60

* Average of four experiments.

with polylysine (final concentration 10 μg/ml), gave a slope of aggregation indistinguishable from that obtained with polylysine and control untreated FWP.

The specificity of proteolysis of FWP by SP was studied by comparing its effects with two common serine proteases, trypsin and chymotrypsin. Initially, studies were performed with various concentrations of the three enzymes to establish conditions that would give comparable losses of platelet aggregability (TABLE 2). Trypsin at a final concentration of 1.25 μg/ml and chymotrypsin at 50 μg/ml had a lesser effect on FWP aggregability than SP at 2.5 μg/ml. In order to maximize sensitivity in detecting differences in enzyme specificity, the concentration of SP was doubled. Under these conditions, over a 1-hr period SP cleaved 25 μg/ml of protein, while trypsin cleaved 36 μg/ml and

TABLE 2

EFFECT OF INCREASING CONCENTRATIONS OF ENZYME ON AGGREGATION OF FWP

| | *Percent of Control Slope* | | |
| | Incubation Time (min) | | |
Final Enzyme Concentration (μg/ml)	15	30	60
Chymotrypsin			
150	34	8	7
50	79	52	21
15	100	102	76
Trypsin			
5	21	1	0
2.5	33	18	0
1.25	58	29	19
S. marcescens protease			
5	–	0	0
2.5	8	0	0
1.25 *	52	6	2
0.625 *	53	24	18

* Incubation at 37° C. All other incubations were at 28° C.

TABLE 3

EFFECTS OF PROTEASES ON HUMAN FWP *

Enzyme	Concentration (μg/ml)	Supernatant Protein (μg/ml)	Aggregation (% of Control Slope)
Buffer control	–	16	100
Trypsin	1.25	36 †	18
Chymotrypsin	50.0	132 †	8
S. marcescens protease	5.0	25 †	0

* $4 \times 10^5/\mu$l; 23° C.

† Corrected for enzyme protein and buffer control.

chymotrypsin 132 μg/ml (TABLE 3). The digested platelets were pelleted and the three supernatants lyophilized. They were subsequently reconstituted in 2 percent SDS, 8 M urea, 0.06 M phosphate, pH 7.0, and run both reduced and nonreduced on 5 percent polyacrylamide gels. Densitometric scans of the Coomassie-stained unreduced gels clearly demonstrate the greater specificity of the *Serratia* protease for the FWP membrane (FIG. 5). SP cleaves less protein than either trypsin or chymotrypsin, even at four times the concentration necessary to give a comparable loss of FWP aggregability. The peak of protein at 54,000 in the densitometric scan of the SP supernatant represents added enzyme (FIG. 5c). In addition, SP cleaves more of the 210,000 protein and only minor amounts of other detectable proteins. The gels of all three supernatants had only one protein band that stained positively with PAS. The approximate molecular weight of the carbohydrate-containing band was 210,000. The purified SP appeared to be highly selective for this glycoprotein, cleaving only minor amounts of two or three other, non-carbohydrate-containing surface-oriented proteins.

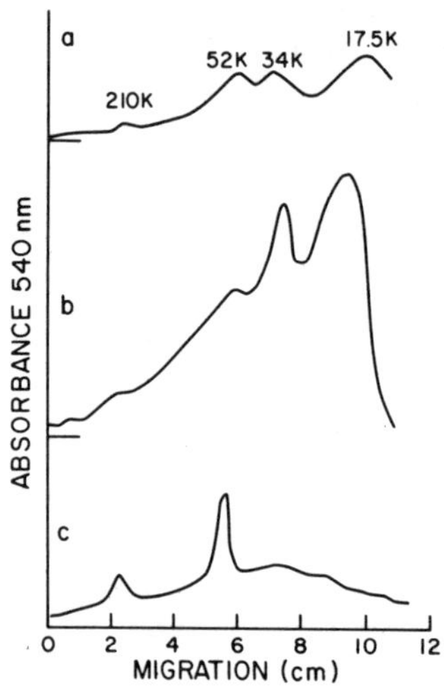

FIGURE 5. The supernatant from 9 ml of FWP ($8 \times 10^5/\mu$l) and SP (5 μg/ml), trypsin (1.25 μg/ml) or chymotrypsin (50 μg/ml) incubated for 1 hr at 37° C were lyophilized and reconstituted in a final volume of 0.25 ml. The samples in denaturing conditions without reduction were run on 5 percent polyacrylamide gels, stained with Coomassie blue dye, and scanned at 540 nm.

Several attempts to demonstrate competitive interference with the aggregation of untreated FWP by the proteolytic fragments in the supernatant have been unsuccessful to date.

Preliminary results of similar studies on fresh, washed platelets and platelet-rich plasma have been obtained. Incubation of bovine plasma for up to 2 hr with purified SP (10 and 20 μg/ml) resulted in essentially no loss of PAF activity, whereas purified bovine PAF at the same concentration was inactivated in less than 1 hr at only 5 μg/ml of SP. Neither human platelet-rich plasma (PRP) nor fresh, washed platelets showed aggregation when tested in the aggregometer with purified SP. At the concentrations of protease reported here, however, fresh, washed platelets also lose their ability to aggregate with both bovine vWF and human vWF plus ristocetin.

DISCUSSION

Our studies demonstrate that extracellular proteases of several species of gram-negative enteric bacteria can digest both fixed and fresh, washed human platelets. Proteolysis, presumably of a specific component(s) of the membrane, renders the platelet unresponsive to human vWF plus ristocetin or to bovine vWF (PAF).

Our initial observations with the sterile filtrate of a pure culture of *S. marcescens* led to a search for a similar effect with culture filtrates from several other gram-negative organisms. These studies resulted in the detection of another strong proteolytic activity in the culture filtrate of *Pseudomonas aeruginosa* and a very weak activity from one strain of *E. coli.* All of the other gram-negative organisms tested showed no effect in our test system.

Three proteases were purified: one from *S. marcescens* and two from different strains of *P. aeruginosa.* They were used to further investigate the proteolytic digestion of human platelets. The majority of the studies reported here were carried out with FWP and the neutral metalloprotease purified from the culture filtrate of *Serratia marcescens* (SP).

Incubation of human FWP with increasing concentrations of purified SP demonstrated that the aggregation response to 0.04 U/ml of bovine vWF decreased as expected over the concentration range of SP used (FIG. 1). If the concentration of SP was held constant (1.25 μg/ml) and the aggregability of the treated FWP to bovine vWF was studied over time, there was greater than 90 percent loss of aggregability within 25 min and the platelets became essentially unaggregable after 2 hours (FIG. 2). However, like untreated platelets, these enzyme-treated platelets would respond with increased rates of aggregation (slopes) when challenged with higher concentrations of bovine vWF (FIG. 3).

SP was compared with the purified proteases of *P. aeruginosa* for the ability to abolish vWF aggregability of FWP (TABLE 1). Results demonstrated a similar ability when comparison was made on the basis of weights. When azocasein was used as a substrate, however, SP was eight times more potent. This discrepancy with different substrates suggests that the enzymes have different specificity. Early reports of partially purified *Serratia* protease enzyme showed no hydrolysis of more than 20 di- and tripeptides except for benzoylglycylleucinamide, which was split at a limited rate into hippuric acid and leucinamide.[8] Against larger substrates, SP cleaved the Gly-Phe bond in bradykinin and the oxidized β chain of insulin at 12 different sites.[8]

The proteolytic effect of SP on the aggregability of FWP was temperature-dependent. The rate of loss of FWP aggregability was reduced at $4°$ C and became optimal around $40°$ C. SP itself was unaffected by temperatures below $50°$ C, but could be completely inactivated by heating at $60°$ C for 30 min.

A number of bacterial proteases are insensitive to inhibitors that react with sulfhydryl groups or serine, but are inactivated by certain metal chelating agents, suggesting that these "neutral proteases" are metalloenzymes.[9] SP in purified form was shown to be inactivated by a variety of such chelating agents, including EDTA and orthophenanthroline at a slightly acidic pH when tested with a casein substrate.[4] The results of the experiment shown in FIGURE 4, in which the FWP membrane was used as the substrate, confirm the inactivation of the enzyme by EDTA. Also, the ability of EDTA-inactivated SP to affect FWP could be restored with Zn^{2+}. The slight inhibitory effect of Zn^{2+} on the mixture of control FWP and bovine vWF is interesting, but no definitive explanation for the effect was found.

The exciting possibility that these proteases could be used as new, more sensitive probes for studying the structure-function relationships at the platelet surface prompted us to begin some comparison studies with serine proteases used in the past for such purposes. Early attempts to study the platelet membrane by enzymatic digestion involved trypsin.[10, 11] These studies, in general, revealed that trypsin routinely cleaved three major glycopeptides from the platelet surface. Trypsin, as well as other commonly used enzymes such as pronase and papain, also destroys platelet vWF aggregability.[12, 13] These enzymes have some distinct disadvantages in platelet studies, however, because they induce platelet aggregation and cause the release of intracellular granules and their contents. The end result is the contamination of the cleaved surface glycopeptides with water-soluble glycoproteins contributed by the release reaction. Chymotrypsin, on the other hand, does not initiate the release reaction,[14] but certain negative aspects of its utility as an enzyme probe make the search for another, more efficient enzyme worthwhile. Our results with chymotrypsin point to a couple of its less attractive aspects. First, it must be used in high concentration compared with that of other enzymes in order to exhibit an effect on FWP aggregability (TABLE 2). This observation is similar to previous experience with fresh, washed platelets.[13, 15] Second, even at these high concentrations, it is difficult to reduce aggregability to extremely low levels, and the selectivity for other substrates on the platelet surface is broad (TABLE 3 and FIG. 5). The initial data presented here would suggest that the metalloenzyme from *S. marcescens* avoids many of these problems. It has a much narrower selectivity than chymotrypsin; it seems to cleave preferentially from FWP a single glycoprotein of about 210,000 mol. wt.; it can be used at low concentrations; and it does not appear to initiate platelet aggregation.

Our data suggest that at least one of the substrates on the human platelet membrane for SP is the vWF receptor. Initial studies with the supernatant of the SP digest failed to demonstrate any ability of the cleaved receptor to competitively inhibit the aggregation of control FWP. The selectivity of SP and its inability to induce platelet aggregation make it a useful new tool in platelet studies, especially of von Willebrand factor-platelet interaction. It may be possible to use these unique proteases to design a procedure for the selective isolation of the vWF receptor or receptor fragments from intact platelets or platelet membranes. Because the partially treated FWP still have some receptor activity, they should prove useful in increasing the sensitivity of vWF membrane receptor assays.[3]

One of the reasons for the widespread use of FWP as a standard reagent for the assay of human and animal vWF is their stability during long-term storage. Therefore, one must be alert for bacterial contamination during this time, particularly by members of the family Enterobacteriaceae. Use of lyophilized uncontaminated platelets would solve this problem.[16] In addition, investigators who prepare FWP from platelet concentrates should keep in mind the possible contamination with *S. marcescens* reported during collection or processing of blood components.[17] The problem is actually the production of extracellular proteases that are inactivated by EDTA. Thus, it would seem reasonable in some situations, to incorporate a chelating agent in the storage buffer.

The application of these findings to a possible *in vivo* role for such extracellular proteases in eliciting some of the hematologic changes observed during gram-negative sepsis is now open to study. Of particular interest would be the relationship of such bacterial proteases to the thrombocytopenia so often seen in such patients. Studies of bleeding times, plasma vWF, vWF-related antigen, vWF platelet aggregability, and platelet survival should be carried out, especially in patients with *S. marcescens* and *P. aeruginosa* septicemia who demonstrate a possible hemostatic defect.

Summary

Fixed, washed platelets (FWP) are usually stable to aggregation with von Willebrand factor (vWF) from human and certain animal plasmas over several months of storage. When one lot of FWP lost its stability in less than 1 week, studies demonstrated contamination with *Serratia marcescens*. Extracellular proteases produced by *S. marcescens,* as well as by *Pseudomonas aeruginosa* and *Esherichia coli,* were found to cause loss of FWP aggregability. Purified proteases were prepared from cell-free culture filtrates of *S. marcescens* and two different strains of *P. aeruginosa*. They were used to study the effect on the interaction of FWP and vWF. All three purified proteases destroyed FWP aggregability in a time- and concentration-dependent fashion. The protease produced by *S. marcescens* (SP) was found to be at least eight times more potent against FWP as a substrate than either of the two *P. aeruginosa* enzymes. The ability of SP to destroy FWP aggregability was prevented by EDTA and could be restored by the addition of Zn^{2+} in slight molar excess. When compared with trypsin and chymotrypsin, SP was found to be highly selective in digesting the FWP membrane, even at concentrations greater than that established to give a similar loss of FWP aggregability. SP does not induce aggregation of fresh, washed platelets or PRP, but renders them unaggregable with vWF. These proteases may be useful research tools for studying membranes and vWF-platelet interactions.

References

1. ALLAIN, J. P., H. A. COOPER, R. H. WAGNER & K. M. BRINKHOUS. 1975. Platelets fixed with paraformaldehyde: A new reagent for assay of von Willebrand factor and platelet aggregating factor. J. Lab. Clin. Med. **85:** 318–328.

2. COOPER, H. A., F. F. REISNER, M. HALL & R. H. WAGNER. 1975. Effects of thrombin treatment on preparations of Factor VIII and Ca^{2+}-dissociated small active fragment. J. Clin. Invest. **56:** 751–760.

3. COOPER, H. A., K. J. CLEMETSON & E. F. LÜSCHER. 1979. Human platelet membrane receptor for bovine von Willebrand factor (platelet aggregating factor): An integral membrane glycoprotein. Proc. Natl. Acad. Sci. USA **76:** 1069–1073.

4. LYERLY, D. & A. KREGER. 1979. Purification and characterization of a *Serratia marcescens* metalloprotease. Infect. Immun. **24:** 411–421.

5. KREGER, A. & L. D. GRAY. 1978. Purification of *Pseudomonas aeruginosa* proteases and microscopic characterization of pseudomonal protease-induced rabbit corneal damage. Infect. Immun. **19:** 630–648.

6. SANTOS, F., P. R. JOHNSON, JR., M. HALL, H. R. CLARK & R. H. WAGNER. 1978. Preparation of bovine platelet aggregating factor (PAF). Thromb. Res. **13:** 741–750.

7. WEBER, K. & M. OSBORN. 1969. The reliability of molecular weight determinations by dodecyl sulfate polyacrylamide gel electrophoresis. J. Biol. Chem. **244:** 4406–4412.

8. MIYATA, K., K. TOMODA & M. ISONO. 1970. Serratia protease. II. Substrate specificity of the enzyme. Agric. Biol. Chem. **34:** 1457–1462.

9. MATSUBARA, H. & J. FEDER. 1971. Other bacterial, mold, and yeast proteases. *In* The Enzymes, Hydrolysis: Peptide Bonds. P. D. Boyer, Ed. Vol. III:765. Academic Press. New York, NY.

10. PHILLIPS, D. R. 1972. Effect of trypsin on the exposed polypeptides and glycoproteins in the human platelet membrane. Biochemistry **11:** 4582–4588.

11. NACHMAN, R. L. & B. FERRIS. 1972. Studies on the proteins of human platelet membranes. J. Biol. Chem. **247:** 4468–4475.

12. COOPER, H. A., K. W. WILKINS, JR., P. R. JOHNSON, JR. & R. H. WAGNER. 1977. Platelet-aggregating factor and the aggregation of fixed washed platelets. J. Lab. Clin. Med. **90:** 512–521.

13. PFUELLER, S. L., C. S. P. JENKINS & E. F. LÜSCHER. 1977. A comparative study of the effect of modification of the surface of human platelets on the receptors for aggregated immunoglobulins and for ristocetin-von Willebrand factor. Biochim. Biophys. Acta **465:** 614–626.

14. DAVEY, M. G. & E. F. LÜSCHER. 1967. Actions of thrombin and other coagulant and proteolytic enzymes on blood platelets. Nature (London). **216:** 857–585.

15. KAO, K. J., S. V. PIZZO & P. A. McKEE. 1979. Platelet receptors for human Factor VIII/von Willebrand protein: Functional correlation of receptor occupancy and ristocetin-induced platelet aggregation. Proc. Natl. Acad. Sci. USA. **76:** 5317–5320.

16. BRINKHOUS, K. M. & M. S. READ. 1978. Preservation of platelet receptors for platelet aggregating factor/von Willebrand factor by air drying, freezing, or lyophilization: New stable platelet preparations for von Willebrand factor assays. Thromb. Res. **13:** 591–597.

17. BLAJCHMAN, M. A., J. H. THORNLEY, H. RICHARDSON, D. ELDER, C. SPIAK & J. RACHER. 1979. Platelet transfusion-induced *Serratia marcescens* sepsis due to vacuum tube contamination. Transfusion **19:** 39–44.

PATHOPHYSIOLOGY OF PLATELET-AGGREGATING VON WILLEBRAND FACTOR: APPLICATIONS OF THE VENOM COAGGLUTININ vWF ASSAY *

K. M. Brinkhous, M. S. Read, R. L. Reddick,
and T. R. Griggs

*Department of Pathology
School of Medicine
University of North Carolina
Chapel Hill, North Carolina 27514*

The term "von Willebrand factor" (vWF) applies to one or more physiological or functional activities of plasma that are deficient in subjects with severe von Willebrand's disease (vWD), excluding the antihemophilic factor (AHF). All of these activities are contained in the macromolecular factor VIII complex. The functional von Willebrand activities are several and include the bleeding time corrective factor, the AHF-stimulating factor, and the platelet-aggregating effect. The first two are recognized by *in vivo* procedures; the latter by *in vitro* procedures. The bleeding time corrective factor is ordinarily determined by the conversion of a long bleeding time to a normal or shortened bleeding time after transfusion of factor VIII into subjects with severe von Willebrand's disease. This corrective action is presumably mediated by adhesion of platelets to injured vessel wall and tissue. It has been proposed that determination of the extent of trapping of platelets in glass bead columns is a possible *in vitro* method for detecting and assessing the amount of this bleeding time factor, but both adhesion of platelets to glass beads as well as trapping of clumps of platelet aggregates occur. The AHF-stimulating factor, like the bleeding time corrective factor, is identified after transfusion of fractions into subjects with severe von Willebrand's disease. The presence of this factor is indicated by a rise in the plasma antihemophilic factor (coagulant factor VIII or VIII:C) 12 to 48 hours later. This late rise in AHF is in contrast to the immediate rise in plasma AHF seen with replacement therapy in both hemophilia and von Willebrand's disease. The platelet-aggregating factor is assayed by one of several *in vitro* methods, as indicated later. In addition to the physiologically based procedures, several immunologic procedures exist for measuring factor VIII-related antigen, which appears to be related to at least two of the functional activities of the macromolecular factor VIII complex, the platelet-aggregating von Willebrand factor and the antihemophilic factor. This presentation will be mainly limited to a consideration of the functional or nonimmunologic aspects of the vWF activities and will discuss a new procedure for studying the platelet-aggregating vWF, the venom coagglutinin test.

* This work was supported by Grants HL01648, HL24609, and HL06350 from the National Institutes of Health and Grant R-804959 from the Environmental Protection Agency.

Bleeding Time Corrective Factor as a Separate Factor

To what extent the three functional vWF activities are separate and distinct or are but different manifestations of the same part of the macromolecular factor VIII complex is uncertain. The bleeding time correction effect, however, has been clearly separated from the platelet-aggregating vWF and the AHF-stimulating factor. This dissociation of the bleeding time corrective factor was observed in a subject with severe von Willebrand's disease during a life-threatening hemorrhagic crisis. He received transfusions on separate occasions of plasma cryoprecipitate and high-potency antihemophilic plasma fraction rich in platelet-aggregating vWF (Fig. 1).[1] After the cryoprecipitate transfusion, bleeding stopped, bleeding time was shortened, the platelet-aggregating vWF was increased, and a delayed rise in AHF occurred. With the purified plasma fraction, the bleeding continued and bleeding time remained prolonged, but the other abnormalities were corrected. These data, with the demonstrated dissociation of the bleeding time corrective factor from other vWF activities as well as AHF, suggest that the former may indeed be separate and attributable to a separate component of the factor VIII complex.

Platelet-Aggregating vWF and the Venom Coagglutinin Assay

The platelet-aggregating vWF is the functional activity that is readily measurable *in vitro* and that can be used to study the pathophysiology of this aspect of the macromolecular factor VIII complex under a variety of circumstances. To distinguish this activity from other activities deficient in von Willebrand disease, we have designated this factor as the platelet-aggregating vWF (PAF/vWF),[2] and will refer to it simply as vWF. This activity was originally studied qualitatively with the use of ristocetin.[3] Quantitatively, vWF was determined by two separate procedures, beginning in 1973. One procedure utilized the vWF "activator," ristocetin, with human plasma and platelets.[4] The other employed no "activator" and is based on the observation that certain animal plasmas, originally bovine and then porcine, cause the vWF-dependent aggregation response in human platelets.[5, 6] Platelet-aggregating vWF measured by the former procedure is often known as ristocetin cofactor, and by the latter procedure simply as platelet-aggregating factor or PAF. The platelet-aggregating vWF proved to have a high degree of species-specificity, as tested by the ristocetin and PAF procedures. Ristocetin had been used mainly with human plasma; the PAF procedure with cow and pig plasmas. When plasmas of other species were investigated with the two tests, most were poorly reactive or completely inactive.[7] For example, plasmas of two species commonly used in investigative studies, the dog and the rat, were essentially inert in both the ristocetin and the PAF tests. This led us to search for an "activator" of the plasma vWF-platelet reaction that would overcome the species limitations and other disadvantages of the existing vWF assay procedures.

A new and apparently universally applicable test procedure for platelet-aggregating vWF was described in 1978, five years after the ristocetin and PAF quantitative assays were introduced. A new venom principle designated as venom coagglutinin, or VCA, which aggregates or agglutinates platelets and whose action is dependent on the presence of vWF, was identified.[2] Without vWF, as in plasmas from patients with severe von Willebrand's disease, no platelet aggregation with VCA occurs. Under controlled conditions, the rate of platelet aggregation is dependent on the dose of vWF. This new venom reagent, VCA, has been used successfully in the clinical laboratory for measuring levels of vWF in plasma, without the disadvantages of ristocetin as a reagent.[8] False-positive and false-negative results may be obtained by the

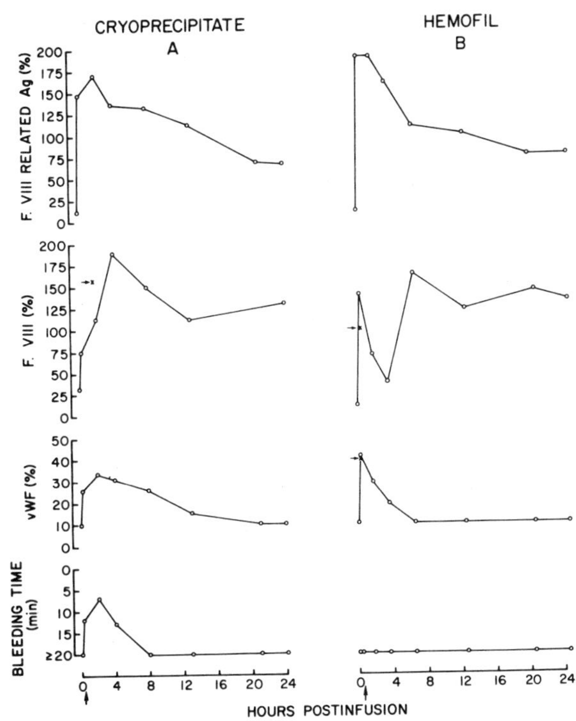

FIGURE 1. Response of a patient with severe von Willebrand's disease to transfusion of cryoprecipitate and high-potency AHF concentrate, Hemofil. **(A)** response to cryoprecipitate, injected at time indicated by arrow. The pretransfusion levels of platelet-aggregating vWF, measured by the ristocetin procedure,[35] factor VIII or AHF measured by the one-stage AHF assay of Langdell *et al.*,[36] and factor VIII-related antigen [37] are indicated at zero time, with the bleeding time being greater than 20 min. All abnormalities were temporarily corrected after transfusion. The AHF-stimulating factor was present in the cryoprecipitate, as indicated by the persistently elevated AHF levels at 24 hours post transfusion. **(B)** response to the high-potency AHF concentrate. The response was similar to that in **(A)**, except that the bleeding time remained prolonged and bleeding continued. (From Blatt *et al.*[1] Reproduced by permission.)

use of ristocetin, because this reagent is a protein precipitant and different plasmas may require different ristocetin concentrations for optimal expression of the aggregation response. In aggregometric assays of vWF with ristocetin and fixed platelets, an initially decreased transmission of light occurs [9]; this artifact is not observed with VCA. The many variables that need to be controlled with vWF assays have been summarized recently.[10]

The VCA reagent effectively overcomes the species barriers that exist with the PAF and ristocetin tests for vWF.[7] It was observed originally that dog plasma, heretofore resistant, could be readily assayed for vWF with the VCA reagent. It was found to contain about three times as much vWF as did human plasma.[2] A large number of different animals, including the cat and rat, were tested, but no species resistance with VCA was encountered.[11] Human platelets in the past had been uniquely fully reactive in both the PAF and ristocetin tests, but platelet preparations of other species were usually poorly or non reactive.[7] With VCA, however, platelets from a variety of species were all rapidly aggregable, regardless of the species of the animal whose plasma was used.[11] Thus, vWF-dependent platelet aggregation was achieved with any homologous or heterologous mixture of plasma or platelets from different species, and this indicates that the VCA reagent had indeed overcome the species barrier that had proved to be such a handicap in past attempts to study the pathophysiology of vWF.

The vWF assays all employ platelets as a reagent. Originally, fresh platelet-rich plasma or isolated and washed fresh platelets were used. The quality control of the platelet preparations was difficult if not impossible to achieve, and new reagents needed to be prepared daily. Three discoveries have corrected this situation and have made available stable and reliable platelet preparations. The first was the finding that fixation of the platelets with formaldehyde preserved the platelet receptor for the plasma von Willebrand factor.[9] (In fact, the fixed platelet was more reactive than the fresh platelet.[12]) The second finding was that the fixed platelets could be lyophilized and retain their ability to react with vWF.[13] The dried platelets appear to be stable for months and possibly years. The third discovery was that animal platelets, either fixed or fixed and lyophilized, could be used successfully in place of human platelets with the VCA assay.[11]

The end-point used in all three assay procedures for vWF is platelet aggregation. The aggregation response is measured either by aggregometry or by determining the macroscopic platelet aggregation time. The use of aggregometry tracing utilizing the VCA test with lyophilized platelets is illustrated in FIGURE 2.[8] Comparison of either the slope of the curve or the maximal aggregation response may be used to judge relative vWF concentration in relation to a normal reference plasma. The macroscopic aggregation time has been determined by different methods, including the microtest flocculation plate [14, 15]

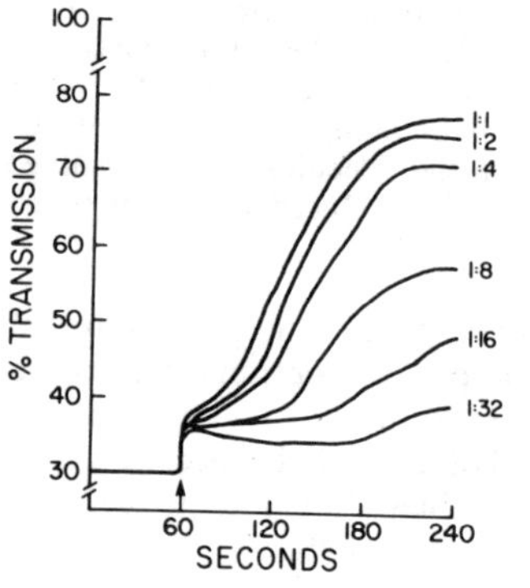

FIGURE 2. Effect of serial dilution of normal human plasma on the rate of aggregation of fixed lyophilized human platelet with VCA as observed with an aggregometry screening test. (From Brinkhous and Read.[8] Reproduced by permission.)

FIGURE 3. Breeding of the male propositus heterozygous for vWD with a normal female. *Squares*=males; *circles*=females; *open symbols*= normal animals; *solid lower half* of symbols=animals heterozygous for vWD. Figures represent plasma vWF level in percent of normal canine reference plasma. Bleeding times of all animals was normal.

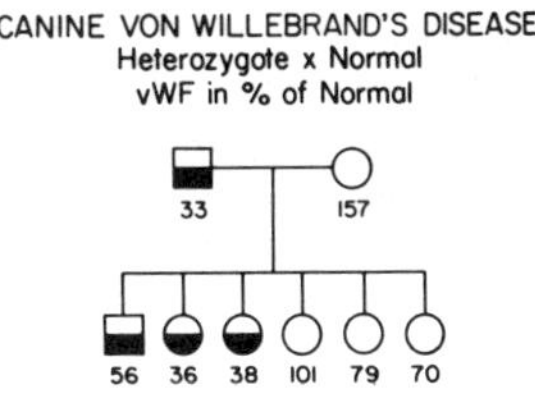

and the "tap tube" test.[8] A comparison has been made between the results of assay of vWF with the two "activators," VCA and ristocetin, using the "tap tube" test. Excellent agreement between the two procedures was obtained.[8]

PATHOPHYSIOLOGIC ASPECTS OF PLATELET-AGGREGATING vWF

Pathophysiologic studies of the von Willebrand factor, made possible in good part by the availability of the new VCA assay procedure, will be summarized in the succeeding sections of this paper. Three main topics will be considered: (1) Genetic studies of plasma vWF in a strain of dogs with von Willebrand's disease and a comparison with pigs with this disease; (2) relationships between endothelial release of vWF and levels of plasma vWF in pigs and rats; and (3) the relative susceptibility of pigs with vWD to induction of accelerated atherosclerosis.

Genetic Studies of vWD in Dogs: Comparison with Swine vWD

The existence of vWD in dogs has been recognized or suspected for many years.[16, 17] In 1973, we examined an adult male Scottish terrier show dog with a history of mild bleeding, especially after trimming of the toenails. History indicated similar mild bleeding in related members of the pedigree, including females. Bleeding time was normal. AHF was determined repeatedly over several months and varied from subnormal values of approximately 50 percent to values in the normal range of 70 to 110 percent. With this single animal a breeding program was started that has now progressed through four generations. Studies of functional plasma vWF were not possible until the VCA test procedure became available. Since 1977, heterozygotes have been reliably identified with plasma vWF determined with VCA and this has permitted an ordered breeding program. The assignment of the canine vWD genotype on the basis of the VCA assay of plasma vWF was reported in 1978.[2] This report provides preliminary data on the establishment of this inbred colony of vWD dogs.

In the first breedings the male propositus was used. His plasma vWF level was 33 percent of normal and he was tentatively classified as a vWD heterozygote. FIGURE 3 depicts the results of one breeding with a normal female with a plasma vWF level of 157 percent of normal. The vWF values of the offspring are indicated in FIGURE 3. From further breeding studies, we found that heterozygotes with few exceptions had vWF levels below 65 percent. On this basis, three of the six puppies were heterozygotes, one male and two females, and three were normal.

The next type of breeding was heterozygote × heterozygote. FIGURE 4 illustrates one such breeding. The parental vWF levels were 56 percent and 43 percent, respectively. The offspring were of two genotypes, heterozygote and homozygote. The homozygotes had no detectable plasma vWF. The bleeding time was indefinitely long, but could be stopped by prolonged application of pressure at the bleeding site. The homozygous animals had a severe bleeding diathesis, which was frequently fatal. The bleeding site was predominantly mucosal, mainly from the nose, mouth, and intestines. AHF levels of bleeder animals ranged between 15 and 30 percent of normal. Inheritance is autosomal. Phenotypically most of the heterozygotes were normal, although a few, like the propositus, were mild bleeders. Whether the inheritance is dominant or recessive is ambiguous.

A colony of swine with von Willebrand's disease, derived from the Missouri strain, has been studied in the laboratory since 1952.[18, 19] The bleeder or homozygous swine are characterized by a severe hemorrhagic diathesis, mainly of mucosal origin. There is a lack of vWF, as indicated by all three platelet-aggregating assay procedures: the PAF test, the ristocetin procedure, and the VCA test. Factor VIII-related antigen and AHF are both low, and the bleeding time is indefinitely prolonged.[6, 20] Except for the lack of species specificity with respect to the several vWF tests in the pig, the heterozygotes have findings similar to those of the canine vWD carriers, and can be identified by reduced levels of plasma vWF. The AHF levels are almost always in the normal range. Carriers rarely have a hemorrhagic diathesis, although we have had one carrier pig with a vWF level of about 15 to 20 percent of normal that died of massive small intestinal hemorrhage.

A comparison of the variables of the disease in the two species of vWD animals, dog and swine, is shown in TABLE 1. The disease is manifest in a similar way in the two species, both symptomatically and with respect to the laboratory values, although the disease appears to be somewhat more severe in the dog. In both species the heterozygotes showed reduced vWF levels, but the values are scattered over a wide range from below 20 percent to low normal values. The AHF values in the carrier vWD swine are within normal limits, a finding previously reported by Owen et al.[21] However, at times the vWD dogs have AHF values below the lower limits of the normal range, but the AHF assay is unreliable for identifying affected animals. Mild bleeding appears somewhat more common in the canine carrier animals than in the swine strain. The homozygotes or bleeder animals of both sexes in the two species are likewise similar. They have an indefinitely prolonged bleeding time, which, if not interrupted, can cause exsanguination of the animal. Bleeding episodes are frequent; vWF is undetectable; AHF levels are reduced; and there is a late posttransfusional elevation in plasma vWF.

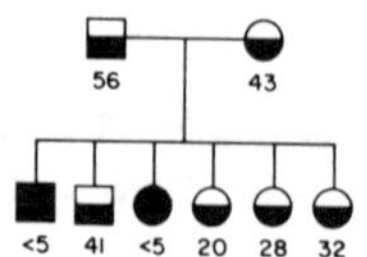

FIGURE 4. Breeding of two animals heterozygous for vWD. *Solid symbols* = animals homozygous for von Willebrand's disease. Bleeding times of these animals was greater than 20 minutes. Other symbols and values as in FIGURE 3.

TABLE 1

COMPARISON OF VON WILLEBRAND'S DISEASE IN PIGS AND DOGS

| Animal | vWD Status | Plasma Values | | | | Bleeding Time (min) | Bleeder State (% of animals) |
		vWF * (%)	AHF † (%)	F VIII-Related Ag (%)	Post-transfusional AHF (%)		
Pig	Heterozygous	42	70–120	Reduced	—	4–6	2
	Homozygous	<5	20–30	Low	75+	>20	100
Dog	Heterozygous	40	50–120	—	—	4–6	4
	Homozygous	<5	20–30	Low	75+	>20	100

NOTE: Data are based on 50 animals of each group, except for homozygous vWD dogs, in which there were 5 animals. Post-transfusion AHF values are from selected animals.

* Mean value.

† Range.

Vascular Endothelium and Plasma vWF

It has been known for many years, from the studies of Jaffe and associates [22,23] and others, that cultured endothelial cells contain factor VIII-related antigen. With functional assays platelet-aggregating vWF is released from the endothelial cells. However, AHF is not released, suggesting that it is not an endothelial cell component. Endothelial cells of many organs and tissues likewise react positively and selectively for factor VIII-related antigen. For example, immunofluorescent microscopy of the liver shows that the sinusoidal lining cells, but not the hepatocytes, are reactive.[24,25] We have studied the relation of the vascular endothelium, with its vWF-positive but AHF-negative reactivities, to the levels of plasma vWF and AHF under two sets of experimental conditions. One is the effect of orthotopic transplantation of normal livers into vWD swine. The other is the effect of hypotonic injury of the endothelium of the pulmonary microvascular bed on the circulating levels of these two factors.

The effect of orthotopic transplantation of the liver in bleeder swine [26] is shown in FIGURE 5. Immediately after the transplanted liver was connected to the circulation, there was an immediate stoppage of diffuse hemorrhagic oozing in the operative bed and with this the long bleeding time immediately converted to the normal range. The platelet-aggregating vWF, measured by the PAF procedure, was likewise converted to normality, or nearly so, throughout the course of the study. Without vWF, the macroscopic aggregation times in the test used were greater than 120 sec, while the normal value was in the range of 20 to 24 secs. The plasma AHF was also elevated. The endothelium of the liver presumably released vWF into the blood on an immediate and then a sustained basis to maintain the plasma vWF. The same would apply to the release of bleeding time corrective factor. The rise in AHF could have

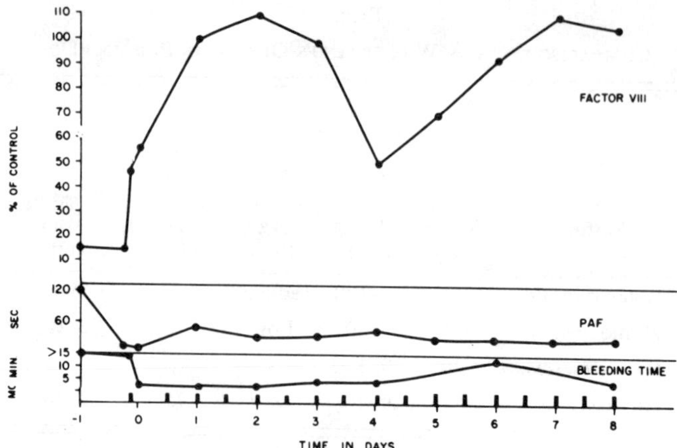

FIGURE 5. Orthotopic transplantation of normal liver to a swine with vWD. Transplanted liver was placed in circulation at 0 time. F VIII (AHF) was determined by the one-stage procedure of Langdell *et al.*[36] Platelet-aggregating vWF was determined by the PAF procedure.[6] Bleeding time was determined by the method of Mertz.[38] (From Webster *et al.*[26] Reproduced by permission.)

been mediated by the release of AHF-stimulating activity, or AHF itself, or both. The pattern of sustained physiological release of the various functional vWF activities from the hepatic sinusoidal endothelium into the circulation may be the same as that which occurs in the normal subject to maintain homeostasis.

Another approach to study the relation of functional plasma vWF to endothelium is to examine induced pathological situations in which there is presumed or demonstrated endothelial damage. A number of clinical studies have demonstrated that in groups of patients with vascular disease there may be elevated factor VIII-related antigen or ristocetin-determined vWF in the circulating plasma.

A direct demonstration of the dynamics of elevation of functional vWF with structurally demonstrated endothelial injury was undertaken in rats.[27] Assay of plasma vWF was carried out with the VCA procedure. An animal model for acute, immediate, and progressive hypotonic injury of the endothelium of the pulmonary microcirculation over a period of a few minutes was utilized.[28] Injury to endothelial cells was determined by transmission electron microscopy. First there was continued cell swelling, which progressed to "blister formation" as the cell was lifted from the basement membrane and finally to actual rupture of the cell membrane. These morphologic events occurred over a time span of 5 minutes. The plasma vWF increased progressively, *pari passu* with the increasing structural damage to the endothelium. The factor VIII coagulant activity or AHF levels did not change over the 5-min period of observation. Illustrative data from one set of experiments are shown in TABLE 2.

In would appear that injury results in release of vWF from pulmonary endothelium in sufficient amounts to elevate the level of plasma vWF to several times the normal level. The finding of no concomitant increase in plasma AHF would appear to confirm the lack of intrinsic AHF activity in endothelial cells.[22] If the capillary endothelium of the lung could be harvested and the total vWF determined, one could arrive at an estimate of what proportion of the endothelial cell vWF was released to give the elevated vWF values found. To what extent the pulmonary capillary endothelium, compared with the liver endothelium, may contribute to the physiological circulating vWF levels in the steady state is a matter for future study. It is evident from these studies in the rat that the extent of increase of plasma vWF over baseline levels (or, what is probably a better indicator, the increase in the vWF:AHF ratio) is a sensitive marker for endothelial pathologic damage.

vWF and Atherosclerosis

In 1978 Fuster and associates [29] reported on the low incidence and extent of atherosclerosis in swine with vWD as compared with normal swine. The difference in incidence between normal animals and those with vWD was observed with two separate dietary regimens—a normal diet and a high-cholesterol diet. It had been postulated for many years that subjects with bleeding disorders should be less susceptible to atherosclerosis than are normal individuals, since it is well known that thrombi complicating atherosclerosis can become incorporated in the atheromatous plaque and may be responsible for much of its mass. However, severe atherosclerosis has been observed in patients with severe hemophilia A with high titer inhibitors.[30] With the recognition of a platelet-derived growth factor that stimulates replication of smooth muscle cells and fibroblasts,[31] another hypothesis appeared more attractive. Von Willebrand factor functionally participates in several reactions of the platelet, either directly or indirectly, including adhesion, aggregation, and release. With vessel injury, vWF-mediated adhesion would be followed by release of the platelet-derived growth factor. Smooth muscle cell proliferation of the intima would follow, initiating and causing enlargement of the atheromatous plaque. In the absence of vWF in the plasma, these platelet responses and the subsequent release of the growth-stimulating factor would be minimized or absent as an atherogenic stimulus. Hence an atheroma should not result.

We have tested this hypothesis in swine with the von Willebrand factor [32, 33]

TABLE 2

ELEVATION IN PLASMA VON WILLEBRAND FACTOR LEVELS AND IN
vWF:AHF RATIO AS AN INDEX OF ENDOTHELIAL DAMAGE

Rat (no.)	Duration of Hypotonic Injury (min)	Endothelial Morphology	VCA-Determined Plasma vWF (%)	AHF (%)	Ratio of vWF:AHF
1	0 (control)	Normal	100	100	1.0
2	1.5	Slight swelling	187	82	2.3
3	3.5	Severe swelling	266	84	3.2
4	5.0	"Blisters" and cell disruption	483	90	5.4

in studies of the aorta and the coronary arteries. Our experiments will be briefly described. Normal, carrier, and bleeder pigs of the Chapel Hill colony from the inbred Missouri strain of von Willebrand's disease were used. The animals were selected so that approximately equal numbers of normal, hetero-zygous, and homozygous vWD pigs were subjected to the atherogenic dietary regimen. An atherogenic diet was started at the age of 4 months and continued for 4 months. The animals were sacrificed at the end of the experimental period.

The entire aorta was stained with Sudan IV dye and the extent of the involvement of the intima by fatty and fibrous lesions was determined on the basis of the relative area involved by lesions. Grossly, the aortic lesions were of three types: (1) those with flat, fatty streaks; (2) raised fatty lesions; and (3) raised lesions with a gray fibrous cap or atheromata. The first two lesions stained uniformly with Sudan IV, giving an orange-red color, while the raised fibrous cap atheromata stained predominantly only at the margins of the raised lesions. Histologically the flat, fatty-streak lesions showed only a few layers of cells in the intima, many of which were lipid-laden "foam" cells. The raised fatty lesion showed great intimal thickening, predominantly due to massive collections of lipid-laden cells. In these lesions no fibrous cap was present, although a few scattered proliferating smooth muscle cells were observed. The third type of lesion showed an intimal smooth muscle cap covering an underlying area of lipid deposition, located both intra- and extra-cellularly. Most sections of these atheromatous lesions showed fragmentation and reduplication of the internal elastic lamina. Some lesions had small areas of calcification in the deeper portions of the lesions.

The animals of each phenotype—normal, carrier, and bleeder—showed each type of aortic lesion. Qualitatively, the lesions were similar in all three groups. However, quantitatively, there appeared to be more lesions of all types in normal animals than in the carriers and bleeders with reduced plasma vWF. For example, in one early experiment, the extent of involvement of the aortic surface by fatty streaks and by raised lesions (type 2 and 3 lesions combined), according to phenotype, was as follows: in normal animals, 62 percent of the aortic area was involved by fatty streaks and 4.7 percent of the area by raised lesions; in carrier pigs, 37 percent fatty streaks, 2.3 per-cent raised lesions; and in bleeder pigs, 33 percent fatty streaks and 2.8 percent raised lesions.[32]

Experimental coronary atherosclerosis was also produced in the normal, carrier, and bleeder vWD pigs. Balloon denudation of the intima of a seg-ment of one or more coronary arteries was carried out [34] followed by the feeding of the atherogenic diet. The bleeder animals received no factor VIII replacement therapy before, during, or after the procedure. The animals with von Willebrand's disease tolerated the procedure well. The balloon pro-cedure has been carried out on more than 50 animals of the three phenotypes. Four months later, the coronary arteries were cut into cross sections throughout their length. Narrowing of the arterial lumen was observed grossly in those segments of the vessels that had been subjected to balloon denudation. All animals of each phenotype showed partially occlusive atherosclerotic lesions. In a few animals the narrowing was marked, with the lumen barely visible grossly.

Histologically, mainly flat, fatty lesions were noted in coronary vessels not subjected to the balloon denudation procedure. In vessels that had been denuded by balloon, the lesions partially occluded the lumen of the vessel. These lesions were characterized by lipid deposition, mainly intracellular, disruption as well as reduplication of the internal elastic lamina, and smooth muscle proliferation, with cap formation. In some instances focal calcification was noted. In this series of animals we have detected no difference qualitatively in the various histologic components of the coronary atheromatous lesions in normal animals, vWD carrier pigs, or in bleeder vWD pigs. Also, the bleeder animals had approximately the same degree of atherosclerosis as the other two groups.

From these data there is evidence for limited protection against the development of atherosclerosis in the aorta of vWD swine, but no protection in the coronary arteries. Our findings suggest that the vWF does indeed play some role in the pathogenetic mechanisms leading to atherosclerosis, but that the vWF pathway is probably but one of several that can lead to platelet activation, adhesion, aggregation, and release. Thus, any protective effect of the lack of vWF on development of atherosclerosis may be masked through alternative pathways of platelet activation.

SUMMARY

Several studies are reported that deal with the pathophysiology of platelet-aggregating von Willebrand factor (vWF), as well as with two other functional activities missing in severe von Willebrand's disease (vWD)—the bleeding time corrective factor and the post-transfusional "stimulating" factor of coagulant factor VIII or antihemophilic factor (AHF). The bleeding time corrective factor was found to be functionally distinct and separable from the other two factors on the basis of transfusion studies of a patient with severe von Willebrand's disease. The platelet-aggregating vWF has been measured in the past by two tests: the ristocetin and the platelet-aggregating factor (PAF) tests. These two tests are highly species-specific so that they cannot be used to measure vWF in most laboratory animals. A new "activator" of the platelet-aggregating vWF has recently been discovered: venom coagglutinin (VCA). This activator provides a means of studying vWF in all animal species tested. This VCA test has many advantages over ristocetin for the assay of vWF in the clinical laboratory and it is used as a simple screening test for vWF deficiencies. The preservation of the vWF receptor in lyophilized platelets, both human and animal, provides for a stable platelet reagent for vWF testing.

Results of three different experimental studies bearing on the pathophysiology of vWF are reported. The first study dealt with the genetic determinants of plasma vWF in a strain of dogs with von Willebrand's disease, and a comparison of the disease in dogs and swine. There is a constant or stereotyped manifestation of severe disease in the canine homozygote which is characterized by a long bleeding time, no detectable vWF, and reduced levels of AHF. In the canine heterozygotes, vWF levels are highly variable from animal to animal. Unlike the case in swine with vWD, the canine vWF is measurable only with the venom coagglutinin procedure. Except for this difference, the homozygous and heterozygous states in the two species with vWD are remarkably similar. The canine heterozygotes may have somewhat lower AHF levels, and phenotypically a mild bleeding syndrome appears to be more common in them.

A second group of studies addressed the question of the relationship between plasma vWF and endothelial cell vWF. Orthotopic transplants of normal liver into swine with vWD immediately corrected the bleeding tendency and caused both immediate and sustained elevation in plasma vWF. There appears to be a regulated physiological release mechanism by which vWF from the hepatic sinusoidal endothelium becomes plasma vWF. Pathologic release of endothelial cell vWF into the plasma was studied in a hypotonic endothelial injury model in the rat. Hypotonic damage of the endothelium of the pulmonary microcirculation was rapid and progressive, and parallel to the cellular damage there was progressive elevation in plasma vWF. Plasma AHF was not increased. Either the elevated plasma vWF levels or the increased vWF/AHF ratios provide a sensitive marker of endothelial damage.

A third group of experiments dealt with the relative susceptibility of normal and vWD pigs to accelerated atherosclerosis. Regardless of genotype, well-developed atherosclerotic lesions developed in the aorta (diet-induced lesions) and in the coronary arteries (caused by balloon injury plus diet) in all animals. However, the aortic lesions in the vWD pigs were less extensive than in normal animals. In contrast, no difference was noted in the severity of coronary atherosclerosis between genotypes. Factors other than the vWF-mediated platelet reaction appear to modify the limited protective effect that lack of vWF has on atherogenesis.

The new VCA assay for vWF is a sensitive and reliable procedure useful for determining variations in plasma vWF in health and in disease.

REFERENCES

1. BLATT, P. M., K. M. BRINKHOUS, H. R. CULP, J. S. KRAUSS & H. R. ROBERTS. 1976. Antihemophilic factor concentrate therapy in von Willebrand's disease. Dissociation of bleeding time factor and ristocetin-cofactor activities. J. Am. Med. Assoc. **236:** 2770–2772.

2. READ, M. S., R. W. SHERMER & K. M. BRINKHOUS. 1978. Venom coagglutinin: An activator of platelet aggregation dependent on von Willebrand factor. Proc. Natl. Acad. Sci. USA **75:** 4514–4518.

3. HOWARD, M. A. & B. G. FIRKIN. 1972. Ristocetin, a new tool in the investigation of platelet aggregation. Thromb. Diath. Haemorrh. **26:** 362–369.

4. WEISS, H. J., L. W. HOYER, F. R. RICKLES, A. VARMA & J. ROGERS. 1973. Quantitative assay of a plasma factor deficient in von Willebrand's disease that is necessary for platelet aggregation. J. Clin. Invest. **52:** 2708–2716.

5. GRIGGS, T. R., H. A. COOPER, W. P. WEBSTER, R. H. WAGNER & K. M. BRINKHOUS. 1973. Plasma aggregating factor (bovine) for human platelets: A marker for study of antihemophilic and von Willebrand factors. Proc. Natl. Acad. Sci. USA **70:** 2814–2818.

6. GRIGGS, T. R., W. P. WEBSTER, H. A. COOPER, R. H. WAGNER & K. M. BRINKHOUS. 1974. Von Willebrand factor: Gene dosage relationships and transfusion response in bleeder swine: a new bioassay. Proc. Natl. Acad. Sci. USA **71:** 2087–2090.

7. BRINKHOUS, K. M., B. D. THOMAS, S. A. IBRAHIM & M. S. READ. 1977. Plasma levels of platelet aggregating factor/von Willebrand factor in various species. Thromb. Res. **11:** 345–355.

8. BRINKHOUS, K. M. & M. S. READ. 1980. Use of venom coagglutinin and lyophilized platelets in testing for platelet-aggregating von Willebrand factor. Blood **55:** 517–520.

9. ALLAIN, J. P., H. A. COOPER, R. H. WAGNER & K. M. BRINKHOUS. 1975. Platelets fixed with paraformaldehyde: A new reagent for assay of von Willebrand factor and platelet aggregating factor. J. Lab. Clin. Med. **85:** 318–328.

10. BRINKHOUS, K. M. 1980. Assay of platelet aggregating von Willebrand factor. *In* CRC Handbook Series in Clinical Laboratory Science. Section I: Hematology. R. M. Schmidt, Ed. **3:** 141–147. CRC Press, Boca Raton, FL.

11. BRINKHOUS, K. M., J. Y. POTTER & M. S. READ. 1979. Venom coagglutinin-lyophilized platelet assay of platelet aggregating factor/von Willebrand factor (PAF/vWF): Commonality of species response. Fed. Proc. **38:** 1272.

12. BRINKHOUS, K. M. 1975. Hemophilia and von Willebrand's disease. Some biological determinants. Am. J. Clin. Pathol. **63:** 609–617.

13. BRINKHOUS, K. M. & M. S. READ. 1978. Preservation of platelet receptors for platelet aggregating factor/von Willebrand factor by air drying, freezing, or lyophilization: New stable platelet preparations for von Willebrand factor assays. Thromb. Res. **13:** 591–597.

14. REISNER, H. M., H. J. KATZ, L. R. GOLDIN, E. S. BARROW & J. B. GRAHAM. 1978. Use of a simple visual assay of Willebrand factor for diagnosis and carrier identification. Br. J. Haematol. **40:** 339–350.

15. BRINKHOUS, K. M., M. S. READ & F. A. DOMBROSE. 1979. Venom coagglutinin and lyophilized platelets for assay of plasma von Willebrand factor: Comparison with ristocetin. Thromb. Haemost. **42:** 407.

16. DODDS, W. J., W. P. WEBSTER, K. M. BRINKHOUS, C. A. OWEN & E. J. W. BOWIE. 1975. Porcine and canine von Willebrand's disease. *In* Handbook of Hemophilia. K. M. Brinkhous & H. C. Hemker, Eds.: 141–148. Excerpta Medica. Amsterdam.

17. DODDS, W. J. 1975. Further studies of canine von Willebrand's disease. Blood **45:** 221–230.

18. BRINKHOUS, K. M., F. C. MORRISON & M. E. MUHRER. 1952. Comparative study of clotting defects in human, canine and porcine hemophilia. Fed. Proc. **11:** 409.

19. MUHRER, M. E., E. LECHLER, C. N. CORNELL & J. L. KIRKLAND. 1965. Antihemophilic factor levels in bleeder swine following infusions of plasma and serum. Am. J. Physiol. **208:** 508–510.

20. GRIGGS, T. R., J. POTTER, S. B. McCLANAHAN, W. P. WEBSTER & K. M. BRINKHOUS. 1977. Macromolecular factor VIII complex: Functional and structural heterogeneity observed in von Willebrand swine with transfusions. Proc. Natl. Acad. Sci. USA **74:** 759–763.

21. OWEN, C. A., E. J. W. BOWIE, P. E. ZOLLMAN, D. N. FASS & H. GORDON. 1974. Carrier of porcine von Willebrand's disease. Am. J. Vet. Res. **35:** 245–248.

22. JAFFE, E. A., L. W. HOYER & R. L. NACHMAN. 1973. Synthesis of antihemophilic factor antigen by cultured human endothelial cells. J. Clin. Invest. **52:** 2757–2764.

23. JAFFE, E. A., L. W. HOYER & R. L. NACHMAN. 1974. Synthesis of von Willebrand factor by cultured human endothelial cells. Proc. Natl. Acad. Sci. USA **71:** 1906–1909.

24. HOYER, L. W., R. P. DE LOS SANTOS & J. R. HOYER. 1973. Antihemophilic factor antigen: Localization in endothelial cells by immunofluorescent microscopy. J. Clin. Invest. **52:** 2737–2744.

25. GRUSON, R. & C. R. RIZZA. 1974. Factor VIII-related antigen in tissues detected by the indirect immunofluorescence technique. Blut **29:** 241–249.

26. WEBSTER, W. P., S. R. MANDEL, L. E. STRIKE, G. D. PENICK, T. R. GRIGGS &

K. M. BRINKHOUS. 1976. Factor VIII synthesis: Hepatic and renal allografts in swine with von Willebrand's disease. Am. J. Physiol. **230:** 1342–1348.

27. BRINKHOUS, K. M., D. L. SULTZER, R. L. REDDICK & T. R. GRIGGS. 1980. Elevated plasma von Willebrand factor (vWF) levels as an index of acute endothelial injury: Use of a hypotonic injury model in rats. Fed. Proc. **39:** 630.

28. NOPANITAYA, W., T. G. GAMBILL & K. M. BRINKHOUS. 1974. Fresh water drowning. Pulmonary ultrastructure and systemic fibrinolysis. Arch. Pathol. **98:** 361–366.

29. FUSTER, V., E. J. W. BOWIE, J. C. LEWIS, D. N. FASS, C. A. OWEN & A. L. BROWN. 1978. Resistance to arteriosclerosis in pigs with von Willebrand's disease. J. Clin. Invest. **61:** 722–730.

30. DALLDORF, F. G., R. E. TAYLOR & P. M. BLATT. 1981. Arteriosclerosis in severe hemophilia—a postmortem study. Arch. Pathol. Lab. Med. In press.

31. ROSS, R., J. GLOMSET, B. KARIYA & L. HARKER. 1974. A platelet-dependent serum factor that stimulates the proliferation of arterial smooth muscle cells in vitro. Proc. Natl. Acad. Sci. USA **71:** 1207–1210.

32. GRIGGS, T. R., D. L. SULTZER, R. L. REDDICK & K. M. BRINKHOUS. 1978. Induced coronary atherosclerosis in von Willebrand disease swine. Fed. Proc. **37:** 841.

33. GRIGGS, T. R., D. L. SULTZER, R. L. REDDICK & K. M. BRINKHOUS. 1979. Induced coronary and aortic atherosclerosis in swine with von Willebrand's disease. Thromb. Haemost. **42:** 271.

34. LEE, W. M. & K. T. LEE. 1975. Advanced coronary atherosclerosis in swine produced by combination of balloon-catheter injury and cholesterol feeding. Exp. Mol. Pathol. **23:** 491–499.

35. BRINKHOUS, K. M., J. E. GRAHAM, H. A. COOPER, J. P. ALLAIN & R. H. WAGNER. 1975. Assay of von Willebrand factor in von Willebrand's disease and hemophilia: Use of a macroscopic platelet aggregation test. Thromb. Res. **6:** 267–272.

36. LANGDELL, R. D., R. H. WAGNER & K. M. BRINKHOUS. 1953. Effect of antihemophilic factor on one-stage clotting tests. J. Lab. Clin. Med. **41:** 637–647.

37. ZIMMERMAN, T. S., L. W. HOYER, L. DICKSON & T. S. EDGINGTON. 1975. Determination of the von Willebrand's disease antigen (factor VIII-related antigen) in plasma by quantitative immunoelectrophoresis. J. Lab. Clin. Med. **86:** 152–159.

38. MERTZ, E. T. 1942. The anomaly of a normal Duke's and a very prolonged saline bleeding time in swine suffering from an inherited bleeding disease. Am. J. Physiol. **136:** 360–363.

CLASSIFICATION OF VARIANT von WILLEBRAND'S DISEASE SUBTYPES BY ANALYSIS OF FUNCTIONAL CHARACTERISTICS AND MULTIMERIC COMPOSITION OF FACTOR VIII/von WILLEBRAND FACTOR *

Zaverio M. Ruggeri † and Theodore S. Zimmerman

Department of Molecular Immunology
The Research Institute of Scripps Clinic
La Jolla, California 92037

Interactions between platelets and factor VIII/von Willebrand factor (F VIII/vWF) induced by the antibiotic, ristocetin, have been used to measure the function of the von Willebrand factor ("bleeding time factor") of this molecule. Decreased ristocetin cofactor activity generally correlates with the prolonged bleeding time seen in various forms of von Willebrand's disease (vWD). However, we have recently described a subtype of von Willebrand's disease in which ristocetin-induced platelet-F VIII/vWF interactions are enhanced.[1] The existence of this group of patients suggests that the ristocetin cofactor activity of F VIII/vWF does not directly reflect the *in vivo* function of the von Willebrand factor. In addition, we have analyzed the multimeric composition of F VIII/vWF in plasma and platelets from patients with different subtypes of vWD and have identified characteristic differences.[2]

Two forms of von Willebrand's disease can be distinguished by different modes of inheritance.[3, 4] The rare, recessive form is inherited from both parents and is characterized by a severe bleeding tendency with extremely low levels of F VIII/vWF protein. The "classical" form of von Willebrand's disease, however, is inherited as an autosomal dominant trait and is clinically less severe. This latter form of the disease can be divided into two main categories on the basis of the nature of the F VIII/vWF phenotype. In von Willebrand's disease Type I, a quantitative defect of F VIII/vWF is reflected by low levels of F VIII procoagulant activity (F VIII:C), F VIII-related antigen (F VIIIR:Ag), and ristocetin cofactor.[3, 4] The F VIII/vWF present appears to be normal when analyzed by crossed immunoelectrophoresis.[5] In von Willebrand's disease Type II, a qualitative abnormality of F VIII/vWF is demonstrated by an abnormal pattern on crossed immunoelectrophoresis with a marked reduction of the larger, less anodic (slower moving) forms of F VIII/vWF.[6–8] The quantitative measurement of F VIII:C and F VIIIR:Ag gives normal or variably reduced levels, whereas ristocetin cofactor activity has characteristically been absent or markedly decreased. The observation that in von Willebrand's disease Type II, ristocetin cofactor activity is decreased and ristocetin-induced platelet aggregation is reduced, even in patients with normal

* Publication number 2148 from The Scripps Clinic and Research Foundation. This work was supported by a grant from the Fondazione Floriana, Milan, Italy, by Grants HL-15491 and HL-16411 from the National Institutes of Health, and by NATO Grant RG 225.80.

† On leave of absence from The Hemophilia and Thrombosis Centre "Angelo Bianchi Bonomi" of the University of Milan Policlinico Hospital, Milan, Italy.

205

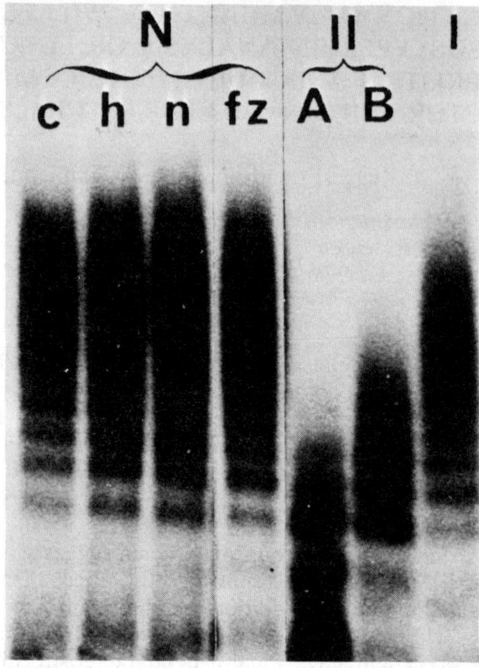

FIGURE 1. SDS agarose gel electrophoresis of factor VIII/von Willebrand factor in plasma. One-μl samples of plasma, containing 1 percent SDS, were applied at the top and electrophoresed in 0.65 percent agarose gels equilibrated with 0.1 percent SDS. After fixing with 10 percent acetic acid and 25 percent isopropanol, the gels were stained with affinity-purified heterologous ^{125}I-anti-factor VIII/von Willebrand factor antibodies and autoradiographs were exposed for 4 to 16 hours. Normal plasma (N) was prepared fresh from blood anticoagulated with citrate (c), heparin (h), and without anticoagulant (n). Citrated plasma stored at $-70°$ C for 6 months was also used (fz). No difference in multimeric composition was seen with different anticoagulants or with storage, suggesting that the observed multimers were not an artefact of preparation of the plasma. Using IgM and its aggregates as markers, the smallest detectable multimer had an apparent M_r of approximately 0.86×10^6. Intervals between adjacent multimers were $0.8–1.1 \times 10^6$. The larger multimers, not resolvable into discrete bands, had an average M_r of 14×10^6. In von Willebrand's disease, three distinct patterns were seen in plasma. In Type I, all the multimers were present in approximately the normal proportion, although all were decreased in quantity. In Type IIA, only the five smallest multimers were present, with relatively increased concentrations of the smallest forms. In Type IIB, intermediate multimers were present in plasma but the largest were missing. (From Ruggeri and Zimmerman.[2] Reproduced by permission.)

levels of F VIIIR:Ag, has supported the contention of a qualitative abnormality of F VIII/vWF in this type of von Willebrand's disease. As a consequence, the measurement of ristocetin cofactor has been considered a reliable index of the *in vivo* function of F VIII/vWF in acting as the "bleeding time factor."

We have now identified a new subtype of von Willebrand's disease Type II (herein called vWD Type IIB) in which F VIII/vWF-platelet interactions show a heightened sensitivity to ristocetin. As in other patients with Type II von Willebrand's disease (herein designated vWD Type IIA), there is a prolonged bleeding time and abnormal crossed immunoelectrophoresis of plasma F VIIIR:Ag with absence of the larger molecular forms.[1]

Twenty patients (nine males and eleven females from five unrelated families) were diagnosed as having vWD type IIB. They had a lifelong hemorrhagic tendency transmitted as an autosomal dominant trait and characterized by spontaneous mucosal and postsurgical bleeding, which could be corrected or prevented by the administration of cryoprecipitates from normal plasma. Ristocetin cofactor activity was normal in four patients and borderline or moderately reduced in most of the remaining patients. Heightened ristocetin-induced F VIII/vWF-platelet interaction was demonstrated by the study of ristocetin-induced platelet aggregation and ristocetin-induced binding of F VIII/vWF to platelets. This heightened interaction was present even in the patients with reduced ristocetin cofactor activity.

All patients with vWD Type IIB demonstrated increased sensitivity to ristocetin when this agent was added to platelet-rich plasma. Thus, the mean ristocetin concentration necessary to induce aggregation with an initial velocity of 30 mm/min was 0.42 mg/ml $\pm$ 0.11 SD in 18 of 20 patients with Type IIB tested as compared with 0.91 mg/ml $\pm$ 0.097 SD in 17 normal subjects. In patients with Type IIA disease, ristocetin usually failed to induce platelet aggregation, even at concentrations as high as 2 mg/ml.

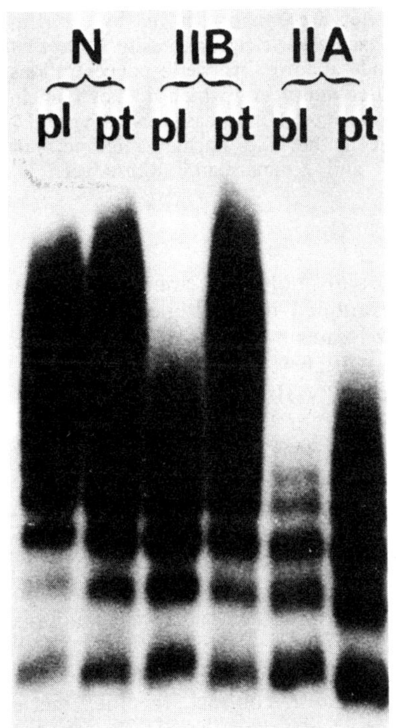

FIGURE 2. Comparison of multimeric composition of plasma and platelet factor VIII/ von Willebrand factor. Note that in Type IIA the larger multimers are missing from plasma and platelets, although some intermediate forms are present in platelets. In Type IIB, all the multimers are present in platelets, although the larger forms are missing from plasma. (From Ruggeri and Zimmerman.[2] Reproduced by permission.)

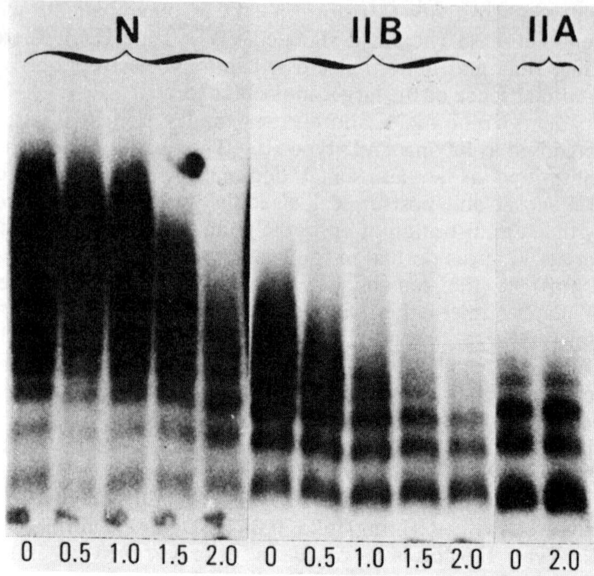

FIGURE 3. Enhanced binding of Type IIB factor VIII/von Willebrand factor to platelets in the presence of ristocetin. Plasma was incubated with platelets and ristocetin at the concentrations shown. The platelets were then removed by centrifugation and the supernatants submitted to SDS-agarose gel electrophoresis. Note that Type IIB factor VIII/von Willebrand factor binds at lower ristocetin concentrations than required for normal binding and that smaller multimers, which do not bind in normal circumstances, bind in the patients with Type IIB disease. No Type IIA factor VIII/von Willebrand factor bound, but neither did normal multimers of similar size ($<4.0 \times 10^6 \ M_r$). (From Ruggeri and Zimmerman.[2] Reproduced by permission.)

In order to better characterize the different molecular abnormalities in Type IIA and Type IIB disease, we have examined the multimeric composition of F VIII/vWF in plasma and in platelet lysates by means of SDS agarose electrophoresis followed by staining with ^{125}I-labeled affinity-purified antibody.[2] In normal plasma and platelet lysates, F VIII/vWF displayed 10 distinct multimers which ranged in apparent M_r from 0.86 to 9.9×10^6. The apparent M_r difference between adjacent bands was $0.8-1.1 \times 10^6$. Larger material, not resolved into discrete bands, was also present with an average M_r of 14.5×10^6 (FIG. 1). No differences were observed between fresh plasma prepared without anticoagulant and fresh or frozen plasma anticoagulated with either citrate or heparin. "Variant" (Type II) von Willebrand's disease could be divided into two subtypes. In subtype IIA, F VIII/vWF in plasma consisted predominantly of the five smaller multimers with trace amounts of the sixth and seventh (M_r up to 4.5×10^6) (FIG. 1). In subtype IIB, all these multimers were easily detected and in addition bands of intermediate size ($M_r = 8.5 \times 10^6$ and smaller) were present. In contrast, the multimeric composition of IIB platelet F VIII/vWF was identical to that of the normal platelet, whereas in subtype IIA the larger multimers were absent from platelets as well as from plasma (FIG. 2). In subtype IIB, binding of factor

VIII/von Willebrand factor to platelets occurred at lower concentrations of ristocetin than normally required and multimers were of smaller size than in normal binding (FIG. 3). On the contrary, in subtype IIA binding corresponded to that of normal F VIII/vWF of equivalent size. Thus, physical as well as functional differences in the two subtypes of "variant" von Willebrand's disease described suggest that different pathogenetic mechanisms underlie the F VIII/vWF abnormalities in these patients.

ACKNOWLEDGMENT

We would like to thank Bobbi Novak for help in the preparation of this manuscript.

REFERENCES

1. RUGGERI, Z. M., F. I. PARETI, P. M. MANNUCCI, N. CIAVARELLA & T. S. ZIMMERMAN. 1979. N. Engl. J. Med. **302:** 1047–1051.
2. RUGGERI, Z. M. & T. S. ZIMMERMAN. 1980. J. Clin. Invest. **65(6):** 1272–1284.
3. ITALIAN WORKING GROUP. 1977. Brit. J. Haematol. **35:** 101–112.
4. SHOA'I, I., J. M. LAVERGNE, N. ARDAILLOU, B. OBERT, F. ALA & D. MEYER. 1977. Br. J. Haematol. **37:** 67–83.
5. ZIMMERMAN, T. S., R. WILSON & T. S. EDGINGTON. 1979. J. Clin. Invest. **64:** 1298–1302.
6. KERNOFF, P. B. A., R. GRUSON & C. R. RIZZA. 1974. Br. J. Haematol. **26:** 435–440.
7. PEAKE, I. R., A. L. BLOOM & J. C. GIDDINGS. 1974. N. Engl. J. Med. **291:** 113–117.
8. GRALNICK, H. R., Y. SULTAN & B. S. COLLER. 1977. N. Engl. J. Med. **296:** 1024–1030.

OBSERVATIONS ON STRUCTURE-FUNCTION RELATIONSHIPS OF HUMAN ANTIHEMOPHILIC/ VON WILLEBRAND FACTOR PROTEIN

Patrick A. McKee

The Howard Hughes Medical Institute Laboratories
Department of Medicine
Duke University Medical Center
Durham, North Carolina 27710

INTRODUCTION

The hemorrhagic diatheses, hemophilia and von Willebrand's disease, have been recognized for years and are the most frequently encountered inherited bleeding disorders. Clinical studies of patients with von Willebrand's disease indicate a close relationship between the plasma antihemophilic factor (factor VIII; FVIII) and the plasma von Willebrand factor (vWF); however, despite an enormous amount of research over the years, we know very little about the structure and function of FVIII and vWF. It seems likely that a definition of the structural features responsible for these two very diverse functions would provide a better understanding of the two corresponding inherited bleeding disorders as well as normal blood clotting. All the other coagulation factors, including newly discovered ones (Protein C and Protein S), have been purified to acceptable criteria and several have now been totally sequenced.[1] Except for relatively minor uncertainties, the complete primary structure of fibrinogen is known,[2] its electron microscopical appearance is established,[3] and now its three-dimensional structure will inevitably be determined by x-ray crystallography. Yet the molecular structure of the complex protein FVIII/vWF is still mysterious. Perhaps unwittingly, many investigators often promote a particular set of biases about the importance of their favorite clotting factor; however, most agree that FVIII/vWF, besides being important to an understanding of its deficiency states, probably occupies a central, pivotal role in the pathogenesis of atherothrombotic disorders.

The intent of this review is to note the major observations made in my laboratory and those made by other investigators regarding certain biochemical features of the FVIII/vWF protein. Some thoughts expressed here will clearly be biased and are not meant to be taken as factual. It is virtually impossible to review all the literature on this subject; except for minor nuances, much of it is repetitious in interpretation. To those whose work I have seemingly ignored, I apologize. I have emphasized my own notions about those areas of FVIII/vWF which I find the most interesting and have arbitrarily selected that work which I believe provides the best information in a rapidly expanding field.

FACTOR VIII(FVIII) PROCOAGULANT ACTIVITY

TABLE 1 lists many of the biochemical properties of the purified human FVIII/vWF protein(s). Virtually all investigators now agree that FVIII pro-

210

0077–8923/81/0370–0210 $01.75/0 © 1981, NYAS

TABLE 1

MAJOR BIOCHEMICAL FEATURES OF HUMAN FVIII/vWF GLYCOPROTEIN

Native molecular weight	10^6–10^7
Subunit molecular weight	2×10^5
Carbohydrate content	15%
Has approximately one ABO(H) blood group per 2×10^5 dalton subunit	
Asialo-FVIII/vWF cleared by hepatocyte	
Amino acid analyses	Good agreement between laboratories; no unusual amino acid ratios
Isoelectric focusing	Probably one type of subunit
Amino terminals	Blocked
Sulfhydryl groups	None when titrated in 6 M guanidine·HCl
Procoagulant function	Very labile
Can be separated from ~99% FVIII/vWF protein by 0.25 M CaCl₂	
Enhanced by trypsin or thrombin	
Spontaneously decays at 25°C	
Destroyed by plasmin or EDTA	
Partially stabilized by bovine serum albumin or 0.25 M CaCl₂	
von Willebrand function	Fairly stable
Ristocetin cofactor activity requires intact carbohydrate side chains on FVIII/vWF	
FVIII/vWF binds to specific platelet receptor	K_d ~0.5–1.0 nM

coagulant activity can be separated from vWF activity by several different techniques, including column chromatography in high salt containing buffers, density gradient ultracentrifugation, or immunoadsorbent chromatography. As recently reviewed by Cooper,[4] most investigators have interpreted such data to indicate that the FVIII/vWF moiety is indeed a complex consisting of either two proteins or two subunits. Except for reports from this laboratory [5,6] and the work of Vehar and Davie,[7] there has been little published on the biochemical characterization of the material associated with isolated or highly concentrated FVIII procoagulant activity. Based on the amount of protein with FVIII procoagulant activity recovered in such experiments, it can be estimated that less than one percent of the mass of the protein initially having both FVIII and vWF activities gives rise to FVIII activity. This clearly presents a problem for the development of an acceptable stoichiometry for the two activities within the range of ratios that usually indicates that a molecule is composed of different subunits.

Vehar and Davie have presented the best evidence to suggest that FVIII/vWF is indeed a complex,[7] in which case the molar relationship between the two different entities may be highly disproportionate. They recovered both a reasonably pure protein of approximately 300,000 daltons by gel filtration in dilute buffer. The protein had a noncovalently linked subunit structure composed of triplet peptides of 85,000, 88,000 and 93,000 daltons. Upon treatment with thrombin, the FVIII procoagulant activity was substantially increased and the triplet bands observed on sodium dodecyl sulfate (SDS) gels were converted to a doublet with molecular weights of 73,000 and 69,000, a faint diffuse-staining band of about 55,000 daltons, and a 38,000 dalton peptide. A rabbit antibody produced against the highly purified protein not only inhibited the FVIII procoagulant activity of the isolated protein, but also the FVIII procoagulant activity of the FVIII/vWF complex. Importantly, the highly purified FVIII protein lacked vWF activity. Vehar and Davie required 125 liters of bovine plasma to recover less than 1 mg of purified FVIII-active protein; this amounted to a yield of 1.4%.[7] Clearly, this latter point is bothersome; it is particularly discouraging when one considers the application of their findings to the isolation of human FVIII. We published SDS-gel analyses of the reduced protein associated with thrombin-activated FVIII procoagulant activity after isolation by gel filtration on 4% agarose in 0.25 M $CaCl_2$.[6] We observed peptides of 79,000, 61,000, 51,000, and 18,000 daltons.[6] Although not purposefully reduced prior to SDS electrophoresis, the bovine FVIII procoagulant protein of Vehar and Davie had been exposed to a reducing agent during purification and it is of interest that they found peptides of 73,000, 69,000, 55,000, and 38,000 daltons following thrombin activation.[7] The differences in molecular weight might be due to species differences if both of our laboratories are working with analogous proteins. At this writing, however, it is evident that this is only speculation and it is clear that much remains to be learned about the structure of FVIII protein.

The major problem that complicates the characterization of FVIII procoagulant protein is its profound susceptibility to proteolysis by a large number of proteases. These affect the expression of FVIII procoagulant activity in different ways. For example, thrombin or trypsin causes a rapid and striking enhancement of FVIII activity that then gradually disappears to levels below preactivation values.[8] In contrast, plasmin quickly destroys FVIII procoagulant activity without any initial enhancement.[8,9] Recent observations in our laboratory indicate that these reactions occur at extraordinarily low concentrations of proteases.[10] Interestingly, if several kinds of protease inhibitor are present in the sodium citrate anticoagulant solution during blood collection and then carried throughout the purification process, a "precursive" form of FVIII procoagulant activity can be isolated.[10] This form of FVIII has very little procoagulant activity until it is exposed to trace thrombin. These observations are in accord with, and more or less resurrect, those of Rapaport *et al.* that FVIII procoagulant activity becomes manifest only in the presence of thrombin or a thrombin-like activity.[11] Obviously, the propensity for FVIII procoagulant activity to be altered so dramatically by trace proteases complicates any isolation method and clouds interpretations of specific activities in relating the latter to intactness of structure.

The interaction of thrombin with the FVIII procoagulant moiety in the isolated FVIII/vWF complex is not simple in the case of usual proteolytic reactions. We find that the proteolytic activation of FVIII by thrombin has features that resemble a stoichiometric interaction more closely than a straight-forward catalytic event.[12] The higher the thrombin to FVIII ratio, the greater the enhancement of FVIII procoagulant activity. A ratio of one thrombin molecule to 20 FVIII/vWF 200,000 dalton subunits caused the greatest enhancement; the lowest discernible activation occurred at about one thrombin molecule per 200,000 FVIII/vWF dalton subunit. Hence, it is apparent that, if very low concentrations of FVIII are exposed to an amount of thrombin that optimizes FVIII activation, more FVIII activity becomes manifest than if the same amount of thrombin is used to activate a larger amount of FVIII. Clearly, this complicates the definition of a "true" level of FVIII activity and essentially precludes comparison of results between laboratories unless one is aware of this problem and precisely defines the ratio of thrombin and FVIII/vWF when the two proteins are incubated together.

The progressive inactivation of FVIII following its activation by thrombin appears to be complicated. Most researchers have assumed that this occurs by continued cleavage by thrombin,[13] although our results strongly suggest that the loss of FVIII activity occurs as a consequence of conformational change instead of further proteolysis.[12] Dansyl-arginine-4-ethylpiperidine amide (DAPA), which is a rapid, potent inhibitor of thrombin, had essentially no effect on the loss of thrombin-enhanced FVIII activity. When thrombin coupled to agarose was used to activate FVIII and then rapidly removed, the enhanced FVIII procoagulant activity deteriorated at the same rate it would have, had thrombin still been present. Hence, we concluded that thrombin-activated FVIII is a highly active, but conformationally unstable, molecule.[12] In keeping with the idea that the manifestation of FVIII activity is highly sensitive to conformational change is the observation that brief exposures of FVIII/vWF proteins to dilute EDTA solutions causes the irreversible loss of FVIII procoagulant activity, but has essentially no effect on vWF activity.[6, 14] We have had no success in restoring the procoagulant activity by the addition of a variety of cations. It therefore seems reasonable to suggest conservative interpretations of data that suggest that FVIII has been "removed" by procedures such as affinity antibody columns and exposure to EDTA solutions. The possibility must be considered that, despite ordinary measures of care with respect to the types of solutions used in laboratory methods, etc., proteolytic degradation or denaturation might result in a conformation that is incompatible with procoagulant function.

We remain attracted to the notion that the FVIII procoagulant function of the FVIII/vWF protein exists *in vivo* in two forms: (1) FVIII procoagulant-*precursive*/vWF and (2) FVIII procoagulant-*inactivated*/vWF. The precursive form of the molecule, besides having the potential to become activated by thrombin or a thrombin-like enzyme, must be extremely sensitive to inactivation by proteolysis (e.g., plasmin) or mild denaturation.[9, 10, 12] Such inactivation, which probably occurs *in vivo* as part of the normal turnover of the complex and *in vitro* due to circumstances already discussed, does not necessarily require prior activation.[12] Based on the results of current methods of FVIII/vWF isolation used by several different investigators, it appears that the plasma concentration of the inactivated-form of the FVIII/vWF protein greatly exceeds the concentration of the precursive form. Most likely, the FVIII procoagulant-activated/vWF species is only generated when the precursive form is exposed to thrombin or a thrombin-like enzyme generated during the earliest stages of blood coagulation. We propose that only the precursive and inactivated forms circulate *in vivo;* it then follows that FVIII procoagulant-activated/vWF protein could result from trace protease activation of the precursive form during the collection and processing of blood. The fact that blood samples, as routinely collected for the measurement of plasma FVIII, are subject to the development of trace protease activity probably explains the wide range of normal FVIII values (50–150%) in the population. The FVIII procoagulant-activated species, whether partially or completely activated, can then be separated from the FVIII procoagulant-inactivated/vWF protein on 4% agarose in 0.25 M $CaCl_2$. In short, our current interpretation is that the FVIII procoagulant-active/vWF species is a derivative of the FVIII procoagulant-precursive/vWF protein. This model then assigns both potential FVIII procoagulant activity and vWF activity to the same parent molecule. If the FVIII procoagulant potential becomes inactivated, then the FVIII procoagulant-inactivated/vWF molecule continues to possess vWF activity, since this latter function is very resistant to protease digestion and mild denaturation.

The application of immunologic techniques cannot be considered to have separated the two "features"—whether they be termed functions or proteins—of the FVIII/vWF complex. Specifically, the extraordinary proclivity of FVIII procoagulant activity to be enhanced or destroyed by minimal proteolytic degradation or by mild denaturation must be considered when interpreting the results from such studies. Studies by Poon and Ratnoff [15] as well as studies from our laboratory suggest that both FVIII procoagulant activity and von Willebrand activity are inhibited by heterologous antisera. Recent unpublished data from our work suggest that the human antibodies to FVIII procoagulant activity have a slight but definite effect on von Willebrand activity as well as on the binding of FVIII/vWF to platelets in the presence of ristocetin. A more direct criticism of immunologic approaches, however, is that no factor VIII procoagulant protein has been isolated and characterized in such studies. Another avenue of investigation that requires consideration as we attempt to understand how FVIII functions is the suggestion by Vehar and Davie that bovine FVIII procoagulant activity may be sensitive to DFP (diisopropyl fluorophosphate).[7] Attempts in our laboratory to reproduce this observation with human FVIII/vWF or FVIII procoagulant activity separated by gel filtration in 0.25 M $CaCl_2$, however, have not been successful.[6] We have concluded that human FVIII procoagulant activity is not DFP sensitive and do not support the notion that FVIII procoagulant protein is a serine protease at this time.

In summary, the human FVIII procoagulant moiety has not been biochemically characterized to anyone's satisfaction. Although several clues have been provided by many different laboratories, there is no clear-cut structural definition of this entity.

THE VON WILLEBRAND ACTIVITY

For some time it has been proposed that as many as five variant forms of von Willebrand's disease exists,[16, 17] but this notion has been recently challenged by Abildgaard *et al.*[18] They performed serial laboratory tests in 50 persons from 25 families with von Willebrand's disease and found that variability in test values over time probably accounted for currently proposed classifications of variant forms of the disease. Only in the homozygous state were test results (bleeding time, FVIII procoagulant activity, vWD Ag level and vWD·Ristocetin cofactor activity) consistently abnormally low. Clearly, the sharpest and most readily accepted laboratory criteria for von Willebrand's disease are the combination of a prolonged bleeding time, a low level of FVIII procoagulant activity, dcreased FVIII/vWF antigen, and impaired platelet aggregation in response to ristocetin. In addition, when transfused with small amounts of either normal or hemophilic plasma, von Willebrand patients respond with an inappropriately prolonged increase of plasma FVIII procoagulant activity.[19, 20] Most agree that a small percentage of patients with symptoms of von Willebrand's disease may have a second form of the disorder characterized by slightly low-to-normal FVIII procoagulant activity, normal levels of FVIII/vWD antigen, a prolonged bleeding time and impaired ristocetin-induced platelet aggregation.

These two forms of von Willebrand's disease are usually separated on the basis of whether the FVIII/vWF protein is decreased or normal ("low" versus "high" antigen forms, respectively). Several years ago, we published a hypothesis that the carbohydrate-side chains on the FVIII/vWF molecule play an important role in defining plasma levels of vWF activity. Essentially, we proposed that this may occur as a consequence of two phenomena: (1) exposure of galactose residues causes the FVIII/vWF molecule to be cleared quickly from the circulation vis-à-vis the Ashwell hepatic lectin receptor;[21] and (2) removal of sialic acid or galactose from the FVIII/vWF glycoprotein results in a decrease in platelet aggregation. We subsequently reported that modification of a carbohydrate on FVIII/vWF did alter its properties.[22] For example, removing sialic acid increased the affinity of FVIII/vWF for the liver asialo-glycoprotein lectin and drastically shortened its plasma survival. Moreover, the removal of sialic acid from human FVIII/vWF diminished its ability to promote platelet aggregating activity by the antibiotic ristocetin to about 40–50% of normal, yet the FVIII procoagulant activity remained unaffected. Later, we observed that removal of the next residue, galactose, nearly restored the affinity of carbohydrate-modified FVIII/vWF for the liver glycoprotein receptor;[23] however, ristocetin-induced platelet aggregating activity was decreased further to about 12% of normal. Again, FVIII procoagulant activity was unaffected. The antigenic properties of the carbohydrate-modified FVIII/vWF species for interacting with rabbit antiserum to native FVIII/vWF continued to be at least normal and, in fact, may have been slightly enhanced. Hence, by modifying the carbohydrate side chains on the FVIII/vWF glycoprotein, we could produce forms of FVIII/vWF that mimicked *in vitro* the results of assays used to define either of the two main forms of von Willebrand's disease. Ultimately, portions of our observations were confirmed in Gralnick's laboratory.[24, 25] Whether or not our results are truly applicable to the human situation remains unanswered: we have not performed carbohydrate studies on FVIII/vWF protein isolated from patients with von Willebrand's disease.

Other laboratories, however, have approached this question about the function of carbohydrate on the FVIII/vWF molecule in patients with von Willebrand's disease. Gralnick *et al.* demonstrated that FVIII/vWF glycoprotein concentrates prepared from each of five von Willebrand patients did not give a positive staining reaction with the periodic acid Schiff (PAS) stain for carbohydrate; they also found that, in two of these five patients, the sialic acid content of the FVIII/vWD glycoprotein was decreased.[26] In contrast, Zimmerman *et al.* found that 15 of 16 von Willebrand patients had FVIII/vWF protein that gave entirely normal PAS staining reactions;[27] it is interesting that the only one of the 16 patients who did have decreased PAS staining was also one of the patients shown by Gralnick *et al.* to have no PAS staining.[26] As far as I know, there has not been any attempt at rigorous quantitation and characterization of the carbohydrate side chains on FVIII/vWF glycoprotein isolated from patients with von Willebrand's disease.

Noting the impaired ability of carbohydrate-modified species of otherwise native FVIII/vWF to support ristocetin-induced platelet aggregation, we decided to determine if this resulted from decreased binding of the carbohydrate-modified FVIII/vWF to platelets. We therefore examined ^{125}I-labeled normal, unmodified FVIII/vWF to determine whether or not it specifically bound to the platelet surface in the presence of ristocetin.[28] The time required for binding to reach equilibrium depended on the number of platelets. When 3 million platelets were used per incubation, approximately 2 hours were required, regardless of the concentration of ristocetin. As the number of platelets was increased, equilibrium could be attained more rapidly, about 100 minutes being required for 5 million platelets. When the incubation time was held constant, the amount of radiolabeled FVIII/vWF that bound to platelets was dependent on the ristocetin concentration, being linear up to ristocetin levels around 1 mg/ml. Above this concentration, binding gradually approached a plateau.

To determine if binding was saturable, two concentrations of ristocetin and a constant number of platelets were used to study the effect of progressively increasing amounts of radiolabeled FVIII/vWF. Results from these experiments clearly showed that the binding of ^{125}I-labeled FVIII/vWF to platelets was saturable and that its specific binding was greater at 1 mg/ml of ristocetin than 0.5 mg/ml. Nonspecific binding, defined by the amount of nondisplaceable bound radiolabeled FVIII/vWF, was determined by adding an excessive amount of cold FVIII/vWF before centrifugation and then determining the number of counts in the platelet pellet. Importantly, nonspecific binding increased linearly with FVIII/vWF concentration and was the same at either ristocetin concentration, suggesting that it was not affected by ristocetin levels up to 1 mg/ml. When these data were subjected to Scatchard analyses, the dissociation constant of binding, K_d, was 0.46 and 0.5 nM for ristocetin levels of 1.0 and 0.5 mg/ml. At the higher ristocetin concentration, the total number of binding sites was estimated to be about 31,000 sites per platelet, assuming only one FVIII/vWF molecule of about 10^6 daltons binds per receptor site. Essentially, the same binding constant and number of binding sites were obtained from competition studies. Although our Scatchard analyses have a slight curvature and several observers have suggested decomposing them to give two classes of binding sites, we have been reluctant to do so, since each of the two dissociation constants generated by this approach would still reflect a high affinity. Were one slope to indicate a low affinity site and the other a high affinity site, then other interpretations would be in order; however, since this is not the case, there seems to be little utility in proposing two high affinity sites.

We examined several other plasma proteins to estimate the specificity of FVIII/vWF binding to platelets in the presence of ristocetin. Only unlabeled human plasma FVIII/vWF competed with the radiolabeled FVIII/vWF for binding. Interestingly, bovine FVIII/vWF did compete with human FVIII/vWF, though it was slightly less potent than the human. Portending a yet unknown significance, the bovine FVIII/vWF did not require ristocetin to compete for the same site to which human FVIII/vWF becomes bound in the presence of ristocetin. Other types of blood cells were also examined; however, it was clear that specific binding was most evident with platelets. There was some binding to red blood cells and polymorphonuclear leukocytes, but the binding could be diminished progressively with additional washes in each case. We thought that this binding most likely represented contamination by platelets; however, in view of our finding that FVIII/vWF has blood group structure attached covalently,[29] there is the possibility that some binding resulted from ABO blood group interactions on the surface of these other cell types, especially since we were using FVIII/vWF isolated from a large pool of donors. We found that the greatest extent of FVIII/vWF binding occurred at physiologic pH; all our binding studies were done at physiologic ionic strengths.

Bound ^{125}I-FVIII/vWF was dissociated extraordinarily slowly from platelets in the presence of a large chase quantity of unlabeled FVIII/vWF. The rate of dissociation could be increased somewhat by decreasing the concentration of ristocetin to 0.1 mg/ml. If formalinized platelets were used, however, it became much more obvious that the binding was dissociable, especially when the ristocetin concentration was diminished from 1 mg to 0.1 mg/ml.

We then determined if the binding of FVIII/vWF to specific sites on platelets correlates with a function, the latter being defined arbitrarily as ristocetin-induced platelet aggregation.[30] We reasoned that ristocetin causes sites on platelets to become accessible for the binding of FVIII/vWF and that the number of these binding sites should depend on the concentration of ristocetin. If binding relates to the rate or extent of platelet aggregation, then the number of available binding sites occupied by FVIII/vWF should have a relationship to platelet aggregation. Therefore, we examined whether or not the extent of FVIII/vWF binding correlates with the initial velocity of platelet aggregation over a range of ristocetin concentrations. Indeed, we found that the initial velocity of platelet aggregation is directly proportional to the amount of FVIII/vWF bound to the platelet receptors. We also showed that both FVIII/vWF binding and platelet aggregation velocity were reduced when platelets were exposed to proteolytic enzymes, having hypothesized that, if the receptor is composed of protein and is on the platelet's exterior, then limited proteolytic digestion should reduce the number of available FVIII/vWF binding sites. Again, we found good correlation between the binding of FVIII/vWF and the initial velocity of platelet aggregation for platelets that had been incubated with different concentrations of trypsin or chymotrypsin and for different lengths of time.

From these same experiments we could conclude with certainty that the receptors are on the platelet's external surface. We then examined a variety of inhibitors of platelet aggregation to determine whether any might affect the binding of FVIII/vWF to its platelet receptor. We proposed that, if the formation of platelet clumps in the presence of FVIII/vWF and ristocetin is dependent on the binding of FVIII/vWF to specific sites on platelets, then inhibitors of ristocetin-induced platelet aggregation should diminish the binding of FVIII/vWF to the platelet. Therefore, known inhibitors of ristocetin-induced platelet aggregation were tested for their effects on the specific binding of FVIII/vWF to platelets in the presence of ristocetin. Platelet aggregation assays and FVIII/vWF binding experiments were done using essentially the same conditions and identical ristocetin concentrations. Results from these experiments clearly demonstrated a highly significant correlation between the extent of FVIII/vWF binding to platelets and the initial velocity of ristocetin-induced platelet aggregation. We concluded that, in the presence of ristocetin, binding of FVIII/vWF to platelets leads to platelet aggregation. From our data we could determine that platelet aggregation occurs only when more than 10% of the total potentially available platelet receptors are occupied in the presence of a ristocetin concentration of 1 mg/ml.

Having defined several major features of the receptor-ligand interaction, we then examined these same binding interactions using carbohydrate-modified species of FVIII/vWF.[31] Our previous studies showed that such forms of FVIII/vWF have substantially less ability to promote ristocetin-induced platelet aggregation; therefore, we proposed that such derivatives may bind to platelets less well than native FVIII/vWF. We tested asialo-FVIII/vWF and galactose-oxidized asialo FVIII/vWF. Clearly, platelet aggregating activity was reduced progressively with removal of sialic acid and even more aggregating activity was lost following galactose modification. However, when the oxidized galactose residues were reduced by potassium borohydride, substantial platelet aggregating activity was restored. The ability of carbohydrate-modified forms of FVIII/vWF to compete for FVIII/vWF receptor sites on platelets was then studied by incubating different amounts of carbohydrate-modified FVIII/vWF with radiolabeled native FVIII/vWF. Binding potency decreased after removal of sialic acid and was decreased substantially more when the terminal galactose residues of asialo-FVIII/vWF were oxidized. Upon reduction of the galactose-oxidized species, however, the ability to compete with native ^{125}I-FVIII/vWF for binding was restored towards that observed for the asialo-FVIII/vWF. To confirm the competitive nature of the binding and to determine the binding affinity of native FVIII/vWF or carbohydrate-modified FVIII/vWF, different concentrations of native FVIII/vWF or carbohydrate-modified FVIII/vWF species were incubated with increasing concentrations of the radiolabeled native FVIII/vWF.

The ability of the unlabeled native or carbohydrate modified species to inhibit the binding of radiolabeled native FVIII/vWF was estimated from Lineweaver-Burke plots. These showed that carbohydrate-modified species of FVIII/vWF compete with native ^{125}I-FVIII/vWF for the same binding site. Binding affinities were then determined by transforming the data into Dixon plots, which showed that the K_i increased from 1.1 nM to 12.3 nM when sialic acid was removed from the molecule. Then, the oxidization of exposed galactose further increased the K_i to 51 nM. Importantly, following potassium borohydride reduction, the marked loss of binding affinity of galactose-oxidized asialo-FVIII/vWF was almost restored to the preoxidization level ($K_i = 18.3$).

Finally, to determine if the function of ristocetin-induced platelet aggregation correlated with binding site occupancy, we tested these two parameters for a potential relationship by expressing them as log functions of each other. Data for native as well as carbohydrate-modified FVIII/vWF species were analyzed by this method. We observed an obvious linear relationship, thereby suggesting strongly that the platelet binding sites for FVIII/vWF are functionally relevant and could therefore be termed platelet FVIII/vWF receptors.

We took advantage of these receptor sites to develop a sensitive and precise radioreceptor assay for plasma levels of human FVIII/vWF.[32] Paraformaldehyde-fixed platelets, which could be prepared and stored, were used as the source of receptors. By this assay, the normal concentration of FVIII/vWF protein ranged from 8.3 to 24.9 μg/ml. Plasma from a patient with classic hemophilia had a significantly higher level and, as expected, plasma samples from patients known to have von Willebrand's disease contained lower amounts.

A recent report has suggested that thrombin might act like ristocetin by causing the platelet receptor for FVIII/vWF to become available.[33] Using final thrombin concentrations of 0.25, 0.5, and 1 unit per ml, we did not observe any enhancement of the rate or extent of aggregation with concentrations of FVIII/vWF up to 4 μg/ml. We also examined the effect of thrombin on the binding of FVIII/vWF to washed platelets and, again, we could show only a marginal effect with high thrombin concentrations, which are unlikely to be present *in vivo* during the initial phases of hemostasis. Still another group of investiagtors has suggested that human asialo-FVIII/vWF induces platelet aggregation without ristocetin having to be present.[34] We could not confirm these results either. We initially added human asialo-FVIII/vWF in concentrations of 0.4, 2, 10, and 20 μg/ml. Then ristocetin was added and, as reported several times previously by our laboratory, we found that the rate of platelet aggregation was proportional to the concentration of asialo-FVIII/vWF. We could not demonstrate that asialo-FVIII/vWF in any concentration caused platelet aggregation; in our experiments, ristocetin had to be present for each of the carbohydrate-modified forms of FVIII/vWF to cause platelet aggregation.

In summary, we have demonstrated the existence of specific, high affinity binding sites for FVIII/vWF on human platelets by a radioligand assay. The binding of FVIII/vWF to platelets is ristocetin dependent; the optimal pH is within a physiologic range. The receptors are membrane located; this is suggested by the loss of binding when platelets are treated with trypsin or chymotrypsin. The binding of FVIII/vWF to its specific sites on human platelets is a prerequisite for ristocetin-induced platelet aggregation; at 1 mg/ml of ristocetin, approximately 10% of the total number of receptors must be occupied before platelet aggregation occurs. The reduced platelet aggregating activity of carbohydrate-modified FVIII/vWF derivatives results from a decreased binding affinity for the platelet receptor. The carbohydrate side-chains of FVIII/vWF must play an important role in platelet aggregating activity and receptor binding since these two properties are closely correlated. We cannot confirm that thrombin is important for FVIII/vWF binding to platelets and do not find that human asialo-FVIII/vWF alone causes platelet aggregation. It is apparent that we have fulfilled the criteria for defining the platelet FVIII/vWF binding site as a receptor. For example, we have shown that the binding site has a high affinity and that its interaction with the FVIII/vWF ligand is rapid and saturable. Under certain circumstances, the binding is dissociable. Using several different approaches, we demonstrated that the biological potency defined by ristocetin-induced platelet aggregation is proportional to the extent of binding. More recently, it has been suggested that, as part of the definition of a receptor, a disease or disorder should occur as a consequence of deranged receptor number or function. It now appears that the Bernard-Soulier syndrome which presents as clinically abnormal bleeding and defective ristocetin-induced platelet aggregation despite normal functional levels of FVIII/vWF, is due to abnormal or absent FVIII/vWF binding sites on platelet membranes.[35]

IMPLICATIONS OF RESEARCH ON FACTOR VIII/VON WILLEBRAND PROTEIN

Rather than make a pretence of being factual, I wish to emphasize that not very many conclusions can be made about the structure-function relationships of FVIII/vWF. It is likely that the two activities circulate as a tightly bound complex or (not yet completely ruled out) as a single molecule with vWF activity and the potential for FVIII procoagulant activity. FVIII procoagulant activity clearly enhances the rate of factor X_a generation [36] and thrombin-activated FVIII causes an earlier and greater acceleration of factor X_a formation than non-thrombin-treated FVIII.[11, 37] Hence, it is likely that the FVIII procoagulant activity of the FVIII/vWF complex requires cleavage by thrombin to maximize the generation of factor X_a and subsequent conversion of prothrombin to thrombin.

Based mostly on the results of Shainoff and Hoyer,[38] the FVIII/vWF complex appears to circulate in plasma as a series of very large multimers with molecular weights in the millions. Zimmerman and colleagues suggest that the highest molecular weight FVIII/vWF multimers have the most vWF activity.[39] Interestingly, the very recent results of Lamb et al. show that the FVIII coagulant antigen, localized by a human radiolabeled FVIII procoagulant antibody, is distributed throughout the population of different sized FVIII/vWF multimers when whole plasma is examined in a crossed immunoelectrophoretic system in 2% agarose under nondenaturing conditions.[40] As stated in an earlier section, isolations of vWF protein or FVIII activity may be due to the separation of derivatives—one having mainly vWF activity and the other mainly FVIII procoagulant activity—from the same parent precursive FVIII/vWF molecule. A specific protease, as yet undefined, may determine the level at which either activity circulates. The exact nature of the FVIII procoagulant moiety remains unknown, with the possible exception of the findings of Vehar and Davie on bovine FVIII/vWF.[7] It is imperative that their observations be confirmed, especially in view of their extraordinarily low yields. Also, as previously speculated upon in this review, they did use a reducing reagent during purification; therefore, it seems reasonable to ask if their results on bovine FVIII procoagulant activity share any similarities with our findings for the reduced protein beneath a separated peak of human FVIII activity.[16]

Hoyer and Trabold have attempted to deduce some of the physicochemical features of the FVIII procoagulant activity before and after exposure to thrombin.[41] They isolated the FVIII procoagulant activity by immunoadsorbent chromatography using a rabbit antibody to FVIII/vWF. Concentrates of FVIII/vWF were then passed through the column and the FVIII procoagulant activity eluted by 0.25 M $CaCl_2$. The FVIII procoagulant activity was then analyzed by Sephadex G-200 gel filtration chromatography before and after exposure to thrombin. Based on peaks of relatively low amounts of FVIII procoagulant activity and FVIII coagulant antigen determinations, they concluded that the molecular weight of the FVIII procoagulant moiety was about 285,000. Following incubation with thrombin, the activated FVIII procoagulant activity was estimated to have a molecular weight of 116,000. Exposure to higher thrombin concentrations caused inactivation of FVIII procoagulant activity and resulted in gel filtration patterns, suggesting that thrombin cleaved FVIII to even lower molecular weight peptides. This interpretation contrasts with our results, which showed that the procoagulant activity of the FVIII/vWF complex could be markedly potentiated by trypsin or thrombin and that DFP or DAPA, the latter an extraordinary rapid and effective thrombin inhibitor, blocked the ability of either enzyme to activate FVIII activity.[12] Yet, once activated by either enzyme, neither DFP nor DAPA prevented the loss of FVIII procoagulant activity. We concluded that proteolysis accounted for activation, but that the subsequent loss of FVIII procoagulant activity occurred by nonproteolytic means. Although of some interest, the molecular weight data of Hoyer and Trabold [41] are incomplete, in that no protein was actually isolated and subjected to even minimal characterization. Their average molecular weight calculations were based on the elution positions of very broad peaks from Sephadex G-200, and therefore must reflect considerable polydispersity of the material giving rise to FVIII procoagulant activity. Moreover, some question must be raised about the sensitivity and specificity of their FVIII procoagulant assays in view of their high calcium concentrations and about whether or not the activity elution profiles could have been affected by the results of these assays. The minimum clotting time in the FVIII assay occurs at a rather narrow calcium ion concentration and, either above or below this level, the clotting time can be prolonged.[42] Hence, if results are to have meaning, the calcium ion concentration, even if not ideal, must be constant in any set of FVIII activity assays, including control assays for setting a standard curve, whether intra- or inter-experimentally determined.

Weinstein has reported that complexes of FVIII procoagulant protein and ^{125}I-labeled antihuman FVIII Fab can be easily detected in whole plasma.[43] Heating at 37°C in the presence of SDS caused the FVIII protein to dissociate from the FVIII/vWF complex, but not from the ^{125}I-labeled Fab fragment. The FVIII protein could then be localized by detecting the mobility of the radioactivity following electrophoresis on SDS gels. Results from his studies suggest that the FVIII procoagulant protein has a molecular weight of about 240,000 and is cleaved by thrombin to a molecular weight of 110,000. These experiments have not been reported in full form and await confirmation. Questions about the completeness of binding of SDS to the protein and whether or not SDS interferes with the antigen-antibody reaction must be considered.

Based on current available information, it seems clear that, at the present stage of research on human FVIII/vWF protein, definitive data have not been provided by any investigator that the FVIII procoagulant protein has indeed been isolated. The effect of thrombin on FVIII procoagulant activity is only partially understood and it must be noted that neither amino-terminal groups nor new peptides have been identified as a consequence of cleavage by thrombin.

Most accept that the endothelial cell does synthesize and release vWF protein,[44-46] but the molecular size and structure of the vWF protein when it is released into circulation have not been determined. The site of synthesis of FVIII procoagulant activity is unknown. Data from tissue culture studies continue to be unsatisfactory because of contaminant proteases and the extraordinary susceptibility of FVIII procoagulant activity to proteolysis.[45] If the FVIII procoagulant activity is not synthesized by the endothelial cell, then how and where the FVIII protein becomes bound to the vWF protein remain to be discovered. Of particular interest, and most likely highly pertinent to *in vitro* studies of FVIII/vWF synthesis, are data that suggest that thrombin binds to a specific receptor on the endothelial cell and then activates protein C, a vitamin K–dependent plasma serine protease, which can very rapidly destroy FVIII procoagulant activity.[47] Exactly what, if any, importance the presence of ABO blood group substances on the FVIII/vWF molecule has in terms of human disease is not clear.[29] It is possible that this has something to do with development of FVIII procoagulant inhibitors in some 10–15% of hemophilic patients following transfusion.

Carbohydrate side chains probably do have relevance to the expression of vWF activity, especially when the latter is measured in the ristocetin-induced platelet aggregation assay. Whether or not the effect of ristocetin mimics *in vivo* phenomena and is therefore truly pertinent to the function of normal vWF glycoprotein is not clear. It may be that impaired ristocetin-induced platelet aggregation is merely an *in vitro* marker of the disorder and has no important *in vivo* implications. It is possible that the vWF protein is only important to the adhesion of platelets to damaged vessel surfaces.[48] Then the aggregation of additional platelets, which is required for adequate primary phase hemostasis, might occur by other mechanisms. Our current opinion is that ristocetin-induced platelet aggregation does have *in vivo* significance, in view of the fact that a decreased response to ristocetin is usually found in the presence of von Willebrand's disease. It appears probable that glycoprotein I of the platelet membrane is the receptor for FVIII/vWF and, as stated earlier about fulfilling criteria for a "receptor," there is a disorder, the Bernard-Soulier syndrome, resulting from its deficiency.[35, 49–51]

It seems sensible to view the binding of FVIII/vWF to platelets as a key link between primary phase hemostasis and the activation of a plasma clotting factor (FVIII) central in the reactions leading to fibrin formation, especially since FVIII/vWF also causes platelet adhesion and aggregation. By collecting on platelet surfaces during platelet plug formation, the FVIII procoagulant moiety is concentrated in a milieu where the slightest trace of thrombin can enhance its activity. The exact structural features of the vWF glycoprotein that account for its binding to platelets, although probably related to its carbohydrate side chains, have not been specifically identified. Assuming that FVIII/vWF is required for *in vivo* platelet aggregation, we still need to define the *in vivo* human counterpart of ristocetin. This need not be a discrete entity, but, instead, could be a phenomenon such as the development of a net electrical charge on certain surfaces to which blood may become exposed. As suggested by some,[52, 53] and based on our own unpublished observations, charge neutralization may be the mechanism by which ristocetin allows specific receptors on human platelets to become accessible to the human FVIII/vWF protein. Certainly not excluded is the possibility that a discrete, definable ristocetin-like substance might circulate in precursive form and become activated or generated during the very earliest stage of hemostasis or be released at the site of tissue injury. The literature is currently virtually devoid of strong leads about the possible existence of such an entity. Of interest are the recent findings of Ruggeri *et al.*, who have observed an unusual situation—the plasmas from a few patients with von Willebrand's disease are hypersensitive to the platelet aggregating effects of ristocetin.[54] They showed that FVIII/vWF protein from those patients had an increased affinity for normal as well as autologous platelets.

In contrast, Takahashi has described patients with clinical findings of von Willebrand's disease, but with an increased sensitivity to ristocetin when their platelets were tested for the ability to bind normal human FVIII/vWF.[55] Each of the patient's FVIII/vWF proteins, however, showed reduced binding to their own platelets as well as to normal human platelets. To date, such subtypes of patients with von Willebrand's disease appear to be rare. But they do give rise to the intriguing possibility of a heightened sensitivity to ristocetin in certain other instances where platelets may become abnormal (e.g., myeloproliferative disorders) and perhaps develop an increase in the amount or affinity of the platelet membrane protein, glycoprotein I, which seems to serve as the receptor for FVIII/vWF.

In summary, I have attempted to touch upon those areas where new information does appear to be developing about structure-function relationships of the human FVIII/vWF glycoprotein. It is likely that answers to the many obvious and important questions about the structural identity and functional features of FVIII/vWF will markedly expand our understanding of normal blood clotting, certain hemorrhagic disorders, thrombo-embolic diseases, and atherogenesis. The steady, albeit slow, progress in the study of this clotting factor promises that these answers will be forthcoming.

REFERENCES

1. SELIGSON, D. & R. M. SCHMIDT, Eds. 1980. Handbook Series in Clinical Laboratory Science, Vol. 3. CRC Press. Boca Raton, Fla.
2. DOOLITTLE, R. F. 1980. Fibrinogen. *In* Handbook Series in Clinical Laboratory Science. D. Seligson & R. M. Schmidt, Eds. Vol. 3: 3–14. CRC Press. Boca Raton, Fla.
3. FOWLER, W. E., L. J. FRETTO, H. P. ERICKSON & P. A. MCKEE. 1980. Electron microscopy of plasmic fragments of human fibrinogen as related to trinodular structure of the intact molecule. J. Clin. Invest. **66:** 50–56.
4. COOPER, H. A. 1980. The factor VIII complex and its associated activities. *In* Handbook Series in Clinical Laboratory Science. D. Seligson & R. M. Schmidt, Eds. Vol. 3: 61–83. CRC Press, Boca Raton, Fla.
5. SWITZER, M. E. & P. A. MCKEE. 1976. Studies on human antihemophilic factor. Evidence for a covalently linked subunit structure. J. Clin. Invest. **57:**925–937.
6. SWITZER, M. E. & P. A. MCKEE. 1977. Some effects of calcium on the activation of human factor VIII/von Willebrand factor protein by thrombin. J. Clin. Invest. **60:** 819–828.
7. VEHAR, G. A. & E. W. DAVIE. 1980. Preparation and properties of bovine factor VIII (Antihemophilic Factor). Biochemistry **19:** 401–410.
8. MCKEE, P. A., J. C. ANDERSEN & M. E. SWITZER. 1975. Molecular structural studies of human factor VIII. Ann. N.Y. Acad. Sci. **240:** 8–33.
9. ANDERSEN, J. C., M. E. P. SWITZER & P. A. MCKEE. 1980. Support of ristocetin-induced platelet aggregation by procoagulant-inactive and plasmin-cleaved forms of human factor VIII/von Willebrand factor. Blood **55:** 101–108.
10. SWITZER, M. E. P., S. V. PIZZO & P. A. MCKEE. 1979. Is there a precursive, relatively procoagulant-inactive form of normal antihemophilic factor (factor VIII)? Blood **54:**916–927.
11. RAPAPORT, S. I., S. SCHIFFMAN, M. J. PATCH & S. B. AMES. 1963. The importance of activation of antihemophilic globulin and proacceleren by traces

of thrombin in the generation of intrinsic prothrombinase activity. Blood **21:** 221–236.

12. SWITZER, M. E. P. & P. A. MCKEE. 1980. Reactions of thrombin with human factor VIII/von Willebrand factor protein. J. Biol. Chem. **255:** 10606–10611.

13. HOYER, L. W. & N. C. TRABOLD. 1981. The effect of thrombin on human factor VIII. Cleavage of the factor VIII procoagulant protein during activation. J. Lab. Clin. Med. **97:** 50–64.

14. WEISS, H. J. 1965. A study of the cation- and pH-dependence of factors V and VIII in plasma. Thromb. Diath. Haemorrh. **14:** 32–51.

15. POON, M. C. & O. D. RATNOFF. 1976. Evidence that functional subunits of antihemophilic factor (factor VIII) are linked by noncovalent bonds. Blood **48:** 87–94.

16. NILSSON, I. M. 1977. Von Willebrand's disease—Fifty years old. Acta Med. Scand. **201:** 497–508.

17. MILLER, C. H., J. B. GRAHAM, L. R. GOLDIN & R. C. ELSTON. 1979. Genetics of classic von Willebrand's disease. I. Phenotypic variation within families. Blood **54:** 117–136.

18. ABILDGAARD, C. F., Z. SUZUKI, J. HARRISON, K. JEFCOAT & T. S. ZIMMERMAN. 1980. Serial studies in von Willebrand's disease: Variability versus "Variants." Blood **56:** 712–716.

19. NILSSON, I. M., M. BLOMBACK & B. BLOMBACK. 1959. von Willebrand's disease in Sweden. Its pathogenesis and treatment. Acta Med. Scand. **164:** 263–278.

20. CORNU, P., M. J. LARRIEU, J. CAEN & J. BERNARD. 1963. Transfusion studies in von Willebrand's disease: effect on bleeding time and factor VIII. Br. J. Haematol. **9:** 189–202.

21. ASHWELL, G. & A. G. MORELL. 1974. The role of surface carbohydrates in the hepatic recognition and transport of circulating glycoproteins. Adv. Enzymol. **41:** 99–128.

22. SODETZ, J. M., S. V. PIZZO & P. A. MCKEE. 1977. Relationship of sialic acid to function and *in vivo* survival of human factor VIII/von Willebrand factor protein. J. Biol. Chem. **252:** 5538–5546.

23. SODETZ, J. M., J. C. PAULSON, S. V. PIZZO & P. A. MCKEE. 1978. Carbohydrate on human factor VIII/von Willebrand factor. Impairment of function by removal of specific galactose residues. J. Biol. Chem. **253:** 7202–7206.

24. GRALNICK, H. R. 1978. Factor VIII/von Willebrand factor protein. Galactose: a cryptic determinant of von Willebrand factor activity. J. Clin. Invest. **62:** 496–499.

25. MORISATO, D. K. & H. R. GRALNICK. 1980. Selective binding of the factor VIII/von Willebrand factor protein to human platelets. Blood **55:** 9–15.

26. GRALNICK, H. R., Y. SULTAN & B. S. COLLER. 1977. Von Willebrand's disease. Combined qualitative and quantitative abnormalities. N. Engl. J. Med. **296:** 1024–1030.

27. ZIMMERMAN, T. S., R. VOSS & T. S. EDGINGTON. 1979. Carbohydrate of the factor VIII/von Willebrand factor in von Willebrand's disease. J. Clin. Invest. **64:** 1298–1302.

28. KAO, K.-J., S. V. PIZZO & P. A. MCKEE. 1979. Demonstration and characterization of specific binding sites for factor VIII/von Willebrand factor on human platelets. J. Clin. Invest. **63:** 656–664.

29. SODETZ, J. M., J. C. PAULSON & P. A. MCKEE. 1979. Carbohydrate composition and identification of blood group A, B, and H oligosaccharide structures on human factor VIII/von Willebrand factor. J. Biol. Chem. **254:** 10754–10760.

30. KAO, K.-J., S. V. PIZZO & P. A. MCKEE. 1979. Platelet receptors for human factor VIII/von Willebrand protein: Functional correlation of receptor oc-

cupancy and ristocetin-induced platelet aggregation. Proc. Nat. Acad. Sci. USA **76:** 5317–5320.

31. Kao, K.-J., S. V. Pizzo & P. A. McKee. 1980. Factor VIII/von Willebrand protein. Modification of its carbohydrate causes reduced binding to platelets. J. Biol. Chem. **255:** 10134–10139.

32. Kao, K.-J., S. V. Pizzo & P. A. McKee. 1981. A radioreceptor assay for quantitating plasma factor VIII/von Willebrand protein. Blood. **57:** 579–585.

33. Ohar, S. & S. J. Hawiger. 1979. Interaction of factor VIII/vWF with human platelets is stimulated by thrombin. Blood **54:** 294a.

34. DeMarco, L., S. S. Shapiro & C. M. Ingerman. 1979. Human asialo-factor VIII: A ristocetin-independent platelet aggregating agent. Blood **54:** 237a.

35. Moake, J. L., J. D. Olson, J. H. Troll, S. S. Tang, T. Funicella & D. M. Peterson. 1980. Binding of radioiodinated human von Willebrand factor to Bernard-Soulier, thrombasthenic and von Willebrand's disease platelets. Thromb. Res. 21–27.

36. Davie, E. W. & K. Fujikawa. 1975. Basic mechanisms in blood coagulation. Annu. Rev. Biochem. **44:** 809–812.

37. Hultin, M. B. & Y. Nemerson. 1978. Activation of factor X by factors IXa and VIII; a specific assay for factor IXa in the presence of thrombin-activated factor VIII. Blood **52:** 928–940.

38. Hoyer, L. W. & J. R. Shainoff. 1980. Factor VIII-related protein circulates in normal human plasma as high molecular weight multimers. Blood **55:** 1056–1059.

39. Ruggeri, Z. M. & T. S. Zimmerman. 1980. Variant von Willebrand's disease. Characterization of two subtypes by analysis of multimeric composition of factor VIII/von Willebrand factor in plasma and platelets. J. Clin. Invest. **65:** 1318–1325.

40. Lamb, M. A., H. M. Reisner, H. A. Cooper & R. H. Wagner. 1980. A sensitive crossed immunoelectrophoresis technique that resolves multimeric forms of factor VIII related antigen. Circulation **62**(II): III–169; personal communication.

41. Hoyer, L. W. & N. C. Trabold. 1981. The effect of thrombin on human factor VIII. Cleavage of the factor VIII procoagulant protein during activation. J. Lab. Clin. Med. In press.

42. Brinkhous, K. M. & F. A. Dombrose. 1980. Partial thromboplastin time. In Handbook Series in Clinical Laboratory Science. D. Seligson & R. M. Schmidt, Eds. Vol. 3: 221–246. CRC Press. Boca Raton, Fla.

43. Weinstein, M. 1980. Factor VIII coagulant antigen—[125]I-labeled antibody complexes analyzed by sodium dodecyl sulfate polyacrylamide gel electrophoresis. Circulation **62**(II): III–107.

44. Jaffe, E. A., L. W. Hoyer & R. L. Nachman. 1974. Synthesis of von Willebrand factor by cultured human endothelial cells. Proc. Nat. Acad. Sci. USA **71:** 1906–1909.

45. Stead, N. W. & P. A. McKee. 1979. The effect of cultured endothelial cells on factor VIII procoagulant activity. Blood **54:** 560–572.

46. Nachman, R. L., E. A. Jaffe & B. Ferris. 1980. Peptide map analysis of normal plasma and platelet factor VIII antigen. Biochem. Biophys. Res. Commun. **92:** 1208–1214.

47. Esmon, C. 1980. Department of Biochemistry, University of Oklahoma Health Sciences Center. Personal communication.

48. Weiss, H. J., H. R. Baumgartner, T. B. Tschopp, V. T. Turitto & D. Cohen. 1978. Correction by factor VIII of the impaired platelet adhesion to subendothelium in von Willebrand's disease. Blood **51:** 267–279.

49. Nurden, A. T. & J. P. Caen. 1979. The different glycoprotein abnormalities in thrombasthenic and Bernard-Soulier platelets. Semin. Hematol. **16:** 234–250.

50. Caen, J. P., A. T. Nurden, C. Jeanneau, H. Michel, G. Tobelem, S. Levy-

Toledana, Y. Sultan, F. Valensi & J. Bernard. 1976. Bernard-Soulier syndrome: a new platelet glycoprotein abnormality. Its relationship with platelet adhesion to subendothelium and with the factor VIII von Willebrand protein. J. Lab. Clin. Med. **87:** 586–596.

51. Sie, P., M. Gillois, B. Boneu, H. Chap, R. Bierme & L. Douste-Blazy. 1980. Reconstitution of liposomes bearing platelet receptors for human von Willebrand factor. Biochem. Biophys. Res. Commun. **97:** 133–138.

52. Coller, B. S. 1978. The effects of ristocetin and von Willebrand factor on platelet electrophoretic mobility. J. Clin. Invest. **61:** 1168–1175.

53. Rosborough, T. K. 1980. Von Willebrand factor, polycations, and platelet agglutination. Thromb. Res. **17:** 481–490.

54. Ruggeri, Z. M., F. I. Pareti, P. M. Mannucci, N. Ciavarella & T. S. Zimmerman. 1980. Heightened interaction between platelets and factor VIII/von Willebrand factor in a new subtype of von Willebrand's disease. N. Engl. J. Med. **302:** 1047–1051.

55. Takahashi, H. 1980. Studies on the pathophysiology and treatment of von Willebrand's disease. IV. Mechanism of increased ristocetin-induced platelet aggregation in von Willebrand's disease. Thromb. Res. **19:** 857–867.

SPECIES SPECIFICITY IN von WILLEBRAND FACTOR–SUPPORTED PLATELET AGGLUTINATION *

Gary S. Johnson † and W. Jean Dodds

Division of Laboratories and Research
New York State Department of Health
Albany, New York 12201

Terry K. Rosborough

Department of Medicine
Veterans Administration Medical Center
Minneapolis, Minnesota 55417

INTRODUCTION

Von Willebrand factor (vWF) causes the agglutination of platelets under a variety of conditions *in vitro*. It has been known for several years that porcine and bovine vWFs agglutinate fresh human platelets [1] and formalin-fixed washed human platelets (FWHP) [2-4] in the absence of ristocetin or other agglutination-inducing agents. A component presumed to be vWF in the plasma of sheep and goats also causes spontaneous agglutination of FWHP.[5] Bovine vWF causes aggregation of guinea pig but not rat platelets.[6] It fails to agglutinate homologous fixed washed platelets and those from the horse, pig, and dog.[5] Porcine vWF weakly agglutinates fixed washed equine platelets but does not agglutinate homologous fixed washed platelets or those from the cow or dog.[5]

The ability of human vWF to support ristocetin-induced agglutination of homologous fresh [7] or fixed washed platelets [2, 8] is the basis for several similar assays used in the diagnosis and study of von Willebrand's disease. However, under some experimental conditions, bovine, porcine, canine, and ursine vWF [9] and rat vWF [6] will not support ristocetin-induced aggregation of homologous fresh platelets; equine and canine vWF fail to support ristocetin-induced agglutination of homologous fixed washed platelets.[5] Other experiments indicate that some of these vWFs (porcine,[10] bovine,[11] and canine [12]) can support ristocetin-induced agglutination of homologous fresh platelets.

Substances that are not structurally related to ristocetin, but induce platelet agglutination dependent upon or augmented by vWF, include hexadimethrine bromide (Polybrene),[13-15] other synthetic polycationic polymers,[16] and coagglutinin, a component in some snake venoms.[17] We recently observed that purified canine vWF supports ristocetin-induced agglutination of both canine and human fresh washed platelets. By contrast, in the presence of ristocetin and purified human vWF, homologous fresh washed platelets do agglutinate, while fresh washed canine platelets are nonreactive.[12] This species-specific pattern for ristocetin-induced vWF-supported platelet agglutination is here compared with that for Polybrene- and coagglutinin-induced agglutination.

* This research was supported by grants HL09902 and HL07173 from the National Heart, Lung, and Blood Institute (PHS/DHHS).

† Present address: Department of Veterinary Pathology, College of Veterinary Medicine, University of Missouri, Columbia, Missouri 65211.

Materials and Methods

Human and canine platelet-rich plasmas (PRP) were prepared from 0.013 M trisodium citrate–anticoagulated fresh blood by 700 g centrifugation for two minutes at room temperature. PRP was equilibrated at room temperature for 30 min before it was tested. Canine von Willebrand's disease (vWD) PRP was obtained from a recently described Chesapeake Bay Retriever whose plasma had no detectable factor VIII–related antigen or ristocetin cofactor.[18] Fresh washed platelets were prepared from human and canine PRP by centrifugation into a single-step Stractan gradient by the method of Corash et al.[19] The FWHP and formalin-fixed washed canine platelets (FWCP) were prepared as previously described.[20]

Human and canine vWF preparations were made from fresh frozen plasma by gel chromatography of cryoethanol precipitates.[20] The protein content of these preparations was determined by the method of Lowry et al.,[21] with bovine serum albumin (BSA) as standard. Coagglutinin was purified from *Bothrops jararaca* venom according to Read et al.,[17] except that the chromatography on DEAE-cellulose was done with a linear gradient of 0.1–0.5 M NaCl in 0.05 M imidazole buffer, pH 7.3. The protein content of the coagglutinin preparation was determined by the method of Schaffner and Weissman,[22] with BSA as standard. The snake venom was obtained from Sigma Chemical Co., St. Louis, Missouri. Ristocetin was purchased from Bio/Data Corp., Horsham, Pennsylvania. Polybrene was purchased from Aldrich Chemical Co., Milwaukee, Wisconsin. Unless otherwise stated, all solutions and dilutions were prepared with 0.125 M NaCl, buffered at pH 7.2 with 0.025 M barbital. This barbital buffered saline (BBS) also contained 0.02% sodium azide.

Platelet agglutination was followed with a Payton aggregometer at 37°C with a stir bar speed of 1200 rpm. Unless otherwise indicated, the final concentrations of the agglutination-inducing agents were: ristocetin 1–2 mg/ml; Polybrene, 0.5 mg/ml; and coagglutinin, 2 μg protein/ml. For experiments with fresh or formalin-fixed washed platelets, the final platelet count was 400,000/μl and the inducers were preincubated with the platelets for three minutes, after which agglutination was initiated by adding vWF.

Results

Platelet-Rich Plasmas

Ristocetin caused the formation of large aggregates in the human PRP, but both normal and vWD canine PRP proved refractory. Polybrene produced large aggregates in normal human and normal canine PRP but much smaller aggregates in vWD canine PRP. Coagglutinin produced large aggregates in the normal PRPs from both species but failed to clump canine vWD PRP (Figure 1).

vWF Preparations

To compare preparations of human and canine vWF, their concentrations were adjusted until they produced approximately equivalent ristocetin-induced agglutination with fixed washed human platelets at all vWF dilutions tested (FIGURE 2). The final concentration of protein from these preparations in all subsequent experiments and in the 1:1 dilution in this experiment was 4 μg/ml for human vWF and 5 μg/ml for canine vWF.

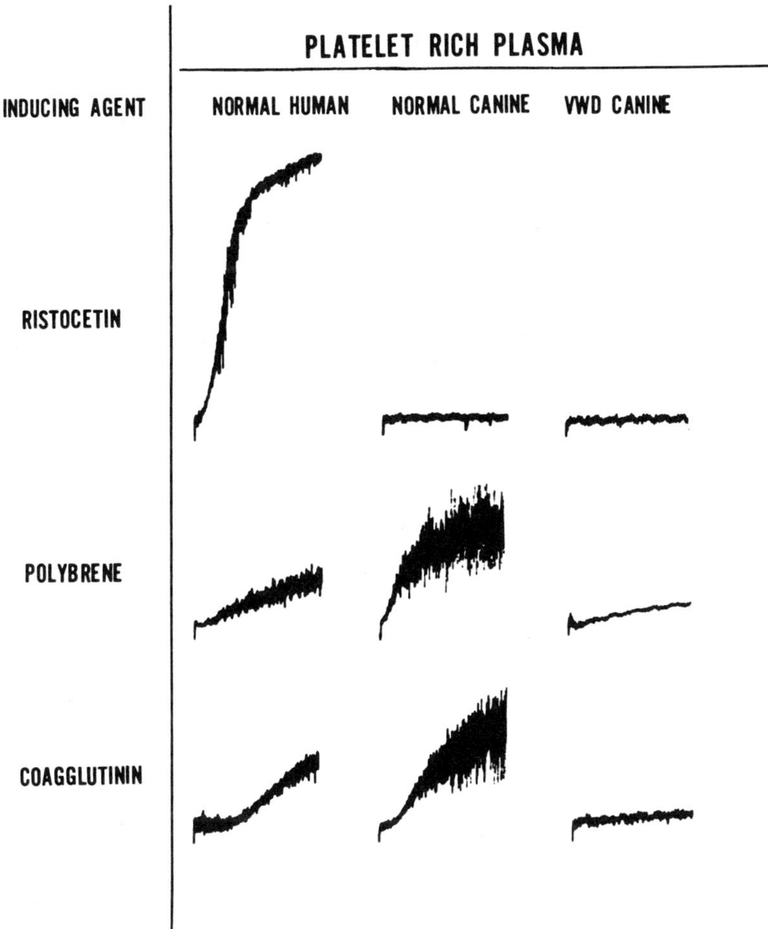

FIGURE 1. Aggregometer tracings produced by the addition of 50 μl ristocetin (15 mg/ml), Polybrene (5 mg/ml) or coagglutinin (20 μg/ml) to a combination of BBS (100 μl) and the appropriate PRP (350 μl).

Fixed Washed Platelets

Ristocetin at 1 mg/ml induced agglutination of FWHP in the presence of both human and canine vWF. Under the same conditions, FWCP did not agglutinate with vWF from either species. A final ristocetin concentration of 2 mg/ml produced more rapid agglutination of FWHP with both human and

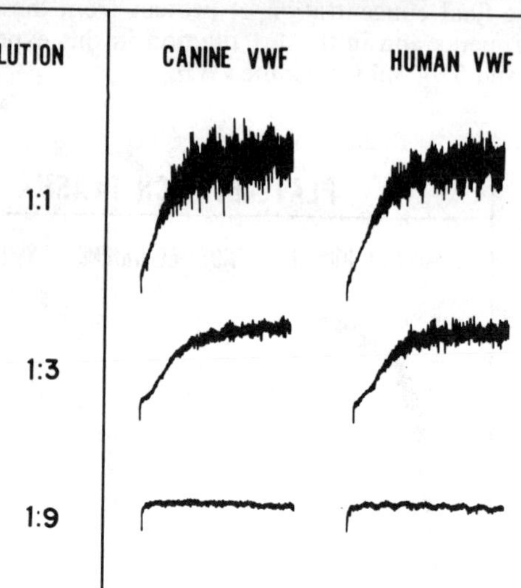

FIGURE 2. Aggregometer tracings produced with human or canine vWF preparations of approximately equal activity. Dilutions of these preparations (100 μl) were added to a preincubated combination of 350 μl FWHP and 50 μl ristocetin (10 mg/ml).

canine vWF. The FWCP failed to agglutinate with human vWF, even at this higher ristocetin concentration, although distinct agglutination was observed with homologous vWF (FIGURE 3).

Polybrene alone caused slight agglutination of FWHP and FWCP. Both canine and human vWF augmented this Polybrene-induced agglutination of FWHP. However, only canine vWF augmented Polybrene-induced agglutination of FWCP. Coagglutinin induced distinct agglutination with all combinations of human or canine vWF and FWHP or FWCP (FIGURE 4).

Fresh Washed Platelets

Human and canine vWF both support ristocetin-induced aggregation of fresh washed human platelets. In contrast, only canine vWF supported ristocetin-induced aggregation of fresh washed canine platelets. Venom coagglutinin induced aggregation of both human and canine fresh washed platelets in the presence of either human or canine vWF (FIGURE 5).

Polybrene alone, at concentrations of 0.62 mg/ml or 0.062 mg/ml, caused the rapid formation of large platelet aggregates in both the fresh washed platelet preparations. Addition of human or canine factor VIII to any of these aggregated suspensions caused the formation of even larger aggregates (not shown).

DISCUSSION

The absence of ristocetin-induced aggregation in canine PRP is consistent with earlier findings that canine plasma does not support ristocetin-induced agglutination of FWHP [5, 20] except when ristocetin concentrations are high relative to the plasma content.[15] This is probably due to plasma protein inhibition, which has been shown to influence ristocetin-induced agglutination with human vWF.[23, 24] Plasma proteins have a much greater inhibitory effect with canine vWF.[12, 20] The failure of some other animal plasmas to support ristocetin-induced agglutination of homologous platelets [5, 9] may be caused by a similar inhibition since, in many of these species, agglutination has been reported when either higher ristocetin-to-plasma ratios or purified vWF were used.[10–12] It is interesting, however, that rat PRP has been shown to be refractory, even

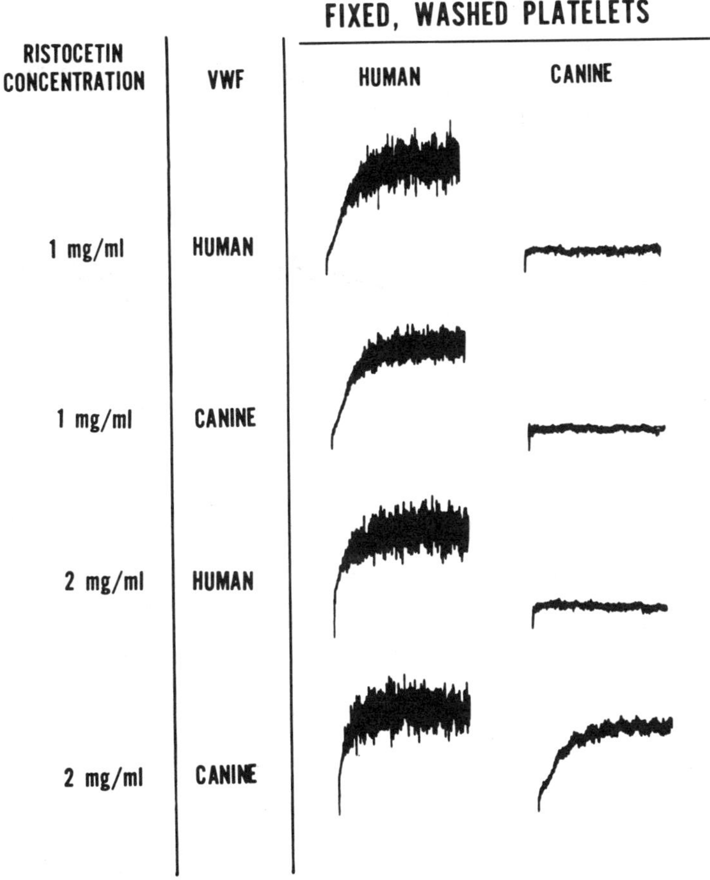

FIGURE 3. Aggregometer tracings produced by the addition of 100 μl human or canine vWF to a preincubated combination of 350 μl FWHP or FWCP and 50 μl ristocetin (10 or 20 mg/ml).

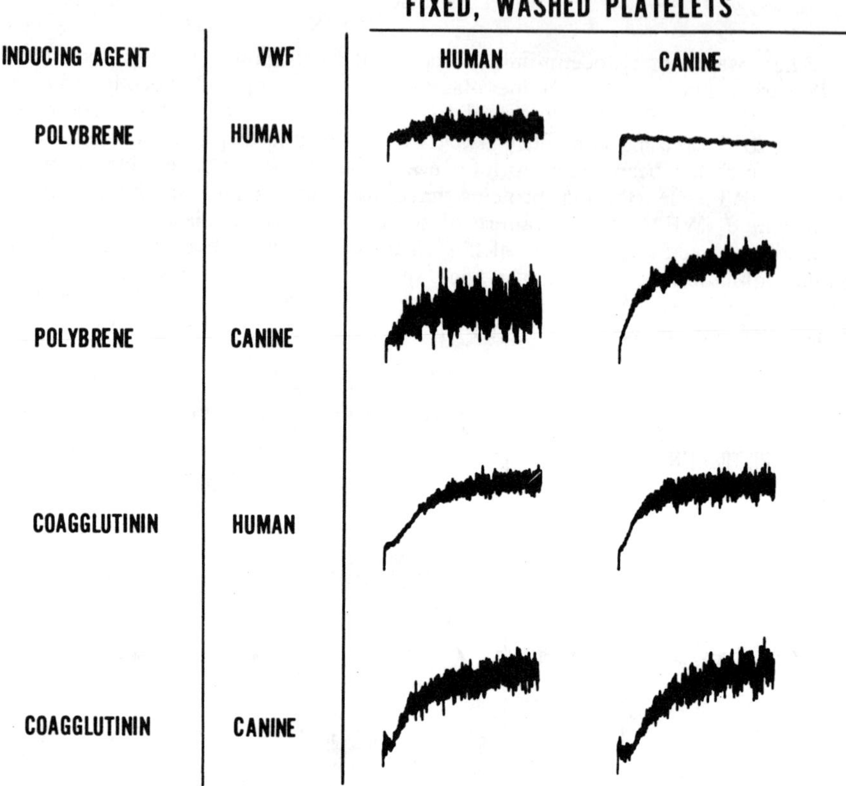

FIGURE 4. Aggregometer tracings produced by the addition of 100 μl human or canine vWF to a preincubated combination of 350 μl FWHP or FWCP and 50 μl Polybrene (5 mg/ml) or coagglutinin (20 μg/ml).

at very high ristocetin concentrations, since rat platelet-poor plasma supported the ristocetin-induced aggregation of fresh washed human platelets.[6]

In contrast to ristocetin, Polybrene and coagglutinin induced distinct agglutination with normal canine PRP. Severe canine vWD PRP was not aggregated with coagglutinin, and only small aggregates formed in this PRP when Polybrene was added. This slight agglutination appears to be vWF-independent, since we have been unable to detect factor VIII–related antigen in plasma from this vWD dog.[18] Consistent with earlier findings, FWHP and FWCP also undergo slight Polybrene-induced agglutination in the absence of added vWF.[13] Both washed human and washed canine platelets form large aggregates in the presence of Polybrene.

Brinkhous et al. found FWCP to be refractory to ristocetin-induced agglutination in the presence of human plasma and the plasma from several animal species, including the dog.[5] Purified human and canine vWF also failed to support ristocetin-induced agglutination at a ristocetin concentration of 1 mg/ml,[12] a finding confirmed in this paper. However, a final ristocetin concentration of 2 mg/ml induced agglutination of FWCP in the presence of canine but not human vWF preparations, although they were equally active when used with FWHP. Even at this high ristocetin concentration, the rate and extent of agglutination were considerably less with canine vWF and FWCP than with canine vWF and FWHP. Thus, it appears that formalin fixation only partially destroys the responsiveness of canine platelets and that the specificity of the residual platelet activity is similar to that found earlier for gel-filtered washed canine platelets.[12]

In this paper, fresh platelets, washed by centrifugation on a Stractan gradient, behaved like gel-filtered washed platelets.[12] Washed human platelets underwent ristocetin-induced aggregation with both purified human and purified canine vWF while washed canine platelets aggregated with canine but not human vWF. In contrast, human and canine vWF both augmented Polybrene-induced agglutination of fresh washed canine platelets. Polybrene-induced agglutination of formalin-fixed platelets had the species specificity seen with ristocetin; both human and canine vWF augmented Polybrene-induced agglu-

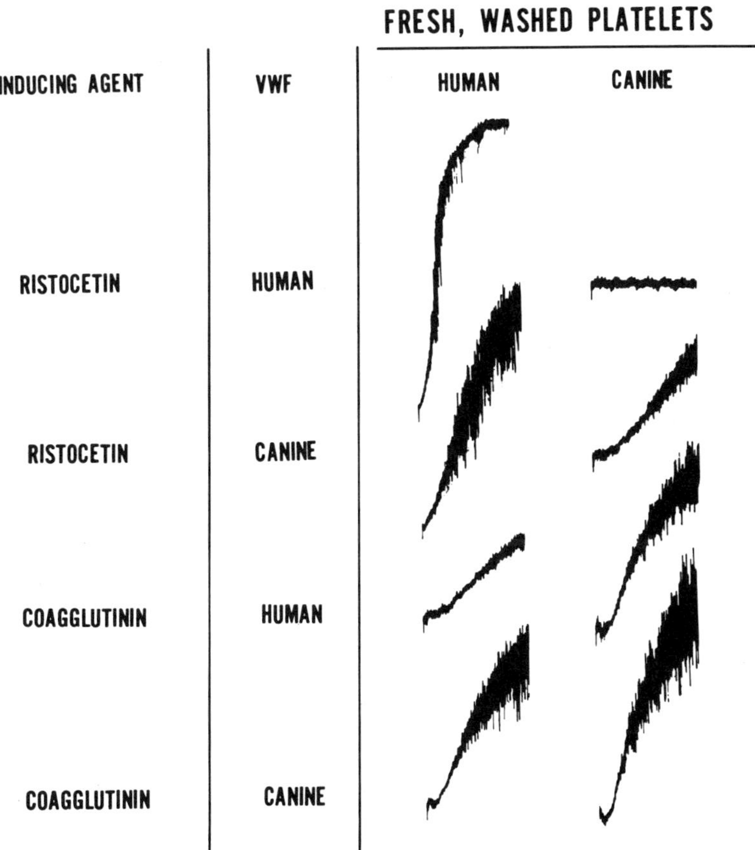

FIGURE 5. Aggregometer tracings produced by the addition of 100 μl human or canine vWF to a preincubated combination of 350 μl fresh washed human or canine platelets and 50 μl ristocetin (10 mg/ml) or coagglutinin (20 μg/ml).

TABLE 1

RESPONSE OF FRESH OR FIXED, WASHED PLATELETS (HUMAN OR CANINE)
TO HUMAN OR CANINE vWF AND AGGLUTINATION-INDUCING AGENTS:
RISTOCETIN, POLYBRENE, OR COAGGLUTININ

		Platelets			
		Fresh Washed		Fixed Washed	
Inducing Agent	vWF	Human	Canine	Human	Canine
Ristocetin	Human	+	−	+	−
Ristocetin	Canine	+	+	+	+/−
Polybrene	Human	+	+	+	−
Polybrene	Canine	+	+	+	+
Coagglutinin	Human	+	+	+	+
Coagglutinin	Canine	+	+	+	+

NOTE: +: Agglutination or aggregation; −: No agglutination or aggregation; +/−: Agglutination at final ristocetin concentration of 2 mg/ml but not 1 mg/ml.

tination of FWHP, but only homologous vWF augmented the agglutination of FWCP. In contrast to ristocetin and Polybrene, coagglutinin agglutinated or aggregated all combinations of fixed or fresh washed human or canine platelets with either human or canine vWF. This is consistent with and extends the earlier findings of Read *et al.*, who showed that FWHP and FWCP undergo coagglutinin-induced agglutination with human, canine, porcine, and bovine plasma.[17]

A summary of the findings for fixed and fresh washed platelets is shown in TABLE 1. It appears that the earlier reported specificity of canine platelets for homologous vWF with ristocetin [12] is only partial with Polybrene and absent with coagglutinin. This variation in specificity suggests that the inducing agents may be acting by different mechanisms. It remains to be determined which, if any, of these three indicators of vWF activity *in vitro* most closely correlates with vWF activity *in vivo*.

REFERENCES

1. FORBES C. D. & C. R. M. PRENTICE. 1973. Aggregation of human platelets by purified porcine and bovine antihemophilic factor. Nature (London) New Biol. **241:** 149–150.
2. ALLAIN, J. P., H. A. COOPER, R. H. WAGNER & K. M. BRINKHOUS. 1975. Platelets fixed with paraformaldehyde: An new reagent for assay of von Willebrand factor and platelet aggregating factor. J. Lab. Clin. Med. **85:** 318–328.
3. KIRBY, E. P. & D. C. B. MILLS. 1975. The interaction of bovine factor VIII with human platelets. J. Clin. Invest. **56:** 491–502.
4. GRIGGS, T. R., J. POTTER, S. B. McCLANAHAN, W. P. WEBSTER & K. M. BRINKHOUS. 1977. Macromolecular factor VIII complex: Functional and structural heterogeneity observed in von Willebrand swine with transfusion. Proc. Nat. Acad. Sci. USA **74:** 759–763.
5. BRINKHOUS, K. M., B. D. THOMAS, S. A. IBRAHIM & M. S. READ. 1977. Plasma levels of platelet aggregating factor/von Willebrand factor in various species. Thromb. Res. **11:** 345–355.

6. DE GAETANO, G., M. B. DONATI, I. R.-D. INNOCENTI & M. C. RONCAGLONI. 1975. Defective ristocetin and bovine factor VIII-induced platelet aggregation in normal rats. Experientia **31:** 500–502.

7. WEISS, H. J., L. W. HOYER, F. R. RICKLES, A. VARMA & J. ROGERS. 1973. Quantitative assay of a plasma factor deficient in von Willebrand's disease that is necessary for platelet aggregation. J. Clin. Invest. **52:** 2708–2716.

8. MACFARLANE, D. E., J. STIBBE, E. P. KIRBY, M. B. ZUCKER, R. A. GRANT & J. MCPHERSON. 1975. A method for assaying von Willebrand factor (ristocetin cofactor). Thromb. Diath. Haemorrh. **34:** 306–307.

9. OLSON, J. D., D. N. FASS, E. J. W. BOWIE & K. G. MANN. 1975. Ristocetin-induced aggregation of gel filtered platelets: A study of von Willebrand's disease and the effect of aspirin. Thromb. Res. **3:** 501–514.

10. BOWIE, E. J. W., D. N. FASS, J. D. OLSON & C. A. OWEN. 1975. Comparison of abnormalities of platelet function in human and porcine von Willebrand's disease. *In* Platelets. N. Ulutin, Ed. :420–423. Excerpta Medica.

11. KALOGJERA, V. & W. G. OWEN. 1978. Identity of bovine platelet aggregating factor and ristocetin-Willebrand factor. Thromb. Res. **13:** 857–864.

12. LEIS, L. A., T. K. ROSBOROUGH, G. S. JOHNSON & G. J. JOHNSON. 1980. Ristocetin-induced aggregation of canine platelets. Thromb. Res. **19:** 309–316.

13. ROSBOROUGH, T. K. & W. R. SWAIM. 1978. Abnormal Polybrene-induced platelet agglutination in von Willebrand's disease. Thromb. Res. **12:** 937–942.

14. COLLER, B. S. 1980. Polybrene-induced platelet agglutination and reduction in electrophoretic mobility: Enhancement by von Willebrand factor and inhibition by vancomycin. Blood **55:** 276–281.

15. ROSBOROUGH, T. K., G. S. JOHNSON, R. E. BENSON, W. R. SWAIM & W. J. DODDS. 1980. Measurement of canine von Willebrand factor using ristocetin and Polybrene: Diagnosis of canine von Willebrand's disease. J. Lab. Clin. Med. **96:** 47–56.

16. ROSBOROUGH, T. K. 1980. Von Willebrand factor, polycations, and platelet agglutination. Thromb. Res. **17:** 481–490.

17. READ, M. S., R. W. SHERMER & K. M. BRINKHOUS. 1978. Venom coagglutinin: An activator of platelet aggregation dependent on von Willebrand factor. Proc. Nat. Acad. Sci. USA **75:** 4514–4518.

18. JOHNSON, G. S., G. E. LEES, R. E. BENSON, T. K. ROSBOROUGH & W. J. DODDS. 1980. A bleeding disorder (von Willebrand's disease) in a Chesapeake Bay retriever. J. Am. Vet. Med. Assoc. **176:** 1261–1263.

19. CORASH, L., H. TAN & H. R. GRALNICK. 1977. Heterogeneity of whole blood platelet subpopulations. I. Relationship between buoyant density, cell volume and ultrastructure. Blood **49:** 71–87.

20. JOHNSON, G. S., R. E. BENSON & W. J. DODDS. 1979. Ristocetin cofactor activity of canine factor VIII: inhibition by plasma proteins. Thromb. Res. **15:** 835–846.

21. LOWRY, O. H., N. J. ROSBOROUGH, A. L. FARR & R. J. RANDALL. 1951. Protein measurement with the folin reagent. J. Biol. Chem. **193:** 265–275.

22. SCHAFFNER, W. & C. WEISSMAN. 1973. A rapid, sensitive method for the determination of protein in dilute solution. Anal. Biochem. **56:** 502–514.

23. BAUGH, R. F., J. E. BROWN & C. HOUGIE. 1975. Plasma components which interfere with ristocetin-induced platelet aggregation. Thromb. Diath. Haemorrh. **33:** 540–546.

24. STIBBE, J. & E. P. KIRBY. 1976. The influence of hemaccel, fibrinogen, and albumin on ristocetin-induced platelet aggregation. Relevance to the quantitative measurement of the ristocetin cofactor. Thromb. Res. **8:** 151–165.

AN AGAROSE GEL METHOD FOR EVALUATING F VIII PROCOAGULANT ELECTROPHORETIC DISTRIBUTION

M. J. Seghatchian

North London Blood Transfusion Centre
Edgware, Middlesex, England

INTRODUCTION

The inherent difficulties with and the lack of specificity of the clotting methods have stimulated considerable interest in developing alternative approaches to the determination of the properties of the F VIII molecular assembly. With the recent progress in uncovering those antibodies which react separately and specifically against different parts of F VIII molecules, immunological assay of F VIII has become the most widely used and productive technique for the evaluation of both F VIII concentration and its molecular heterogeneity.[1] The antigen related to F VIII procoagulant activity (VIII:C) can be identified either by the neutralization activity of an antibody to F VIII or by the radiometric measurement of protein concentrations that have F VIII antigenic determinants, even though they may lack F VIII procoagulant activity.[2]

More recently, an amidolytic method (VIII:Cam), which measures F VIII by its F Xa generation property using a specific F Xa substrate (S2222), has been developed.[3]

In this paper, a newly developed agarose gel method [4] is used to compare the selectivity of the currently used methods for the assay of F VIII-related activity. The binding properties of some antibodies were also investigated, with the aim of characterizing the heterogeneity in the binding of the antibodies to various forms of F VIII in plasma and concentrates.

RESULTS AND DISCUSSION

Comparing Various F VIII–Related Activities

FIGURE 1 shows a representative example of the electrophoretic patterns of F VIII–associated activities determined simultaneously by various methods. Pooled plasma was electrophoresed for 2 hr in barbital buffer, pH 8.6. The gels were sliced in 20 equal sizes, eluted for 2 hr with buffer Tris-saline, pH 7.6, and assayed as previously described.[5]

It is evident that various forms of F VIII are measured disproportionally by these methods. Of particular interest is the second peak of F VIII–like activity measured by both two-stage clotting and amidolytic F VIII:C methods, which are based on the F Xa generation principle. An improvement in sensitivity was detected by performing the amidolytic assay directly on the gel slice without elution with buffer. This method is simple and quantitative and has potential implication in quality control of various preparations.

236

Characterization of F VIII:C Antibodies by the Amidolytic Method

FIGURE 2 shows the VIII:C neutralization properties of two homologous (HO and VL) and one heterologous (RI) IgG obtained by the protein A method (Nilsson *et al.*, to be published).

Normal pooled plasma was incubated for one hour with various IgG. The one-stage method determined that there was enough IgG to neutralize VIII:C in all conditions, while with the amidolytic method, differing specificity is observed in the HO antibody, whether IgG or whole inhibitor plasma was used. A similar experiment was performed using a severe vWD postinfused sample (24 hr after) to identify the binding properties of the newly synthesized F VIII

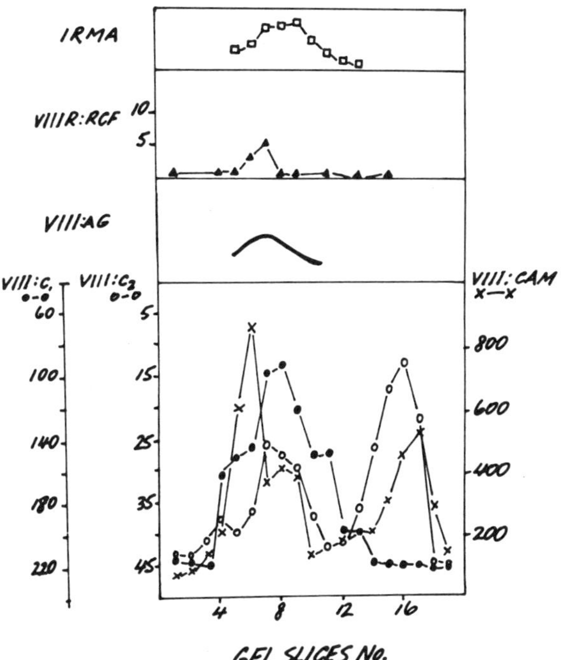

FIGURE 1. The electrophoretic distribution of freshly pooled plasma in 1% agarose (barbital buffer, pH 8.6, containing inhibitors), measured by various techniques.

(not shown). Total neutralization was apparent with VL IgG, while RI consistently led to a nonparallelism and HO led to partial inhibition. The fact that VL seems to inhibit F VIII:Cam completely in all conditions indicates that it has a wider specificity and affinity and/or that its binding is directed to the F VIII:C part by forming a stable complex or leading to the conformational change in the F VIII molecule. Other antibodies bind less specifically and, probably, to a region of the molecule that is less affected than the VIII:Cam.

Distribution of Labeled IgG Incubated with Plasma and Clinical Concentrates

Further information on molecular nature of binding was obtained by use of radiolabeled IgG. FIGURE 3 shows the comparison between the two-stage

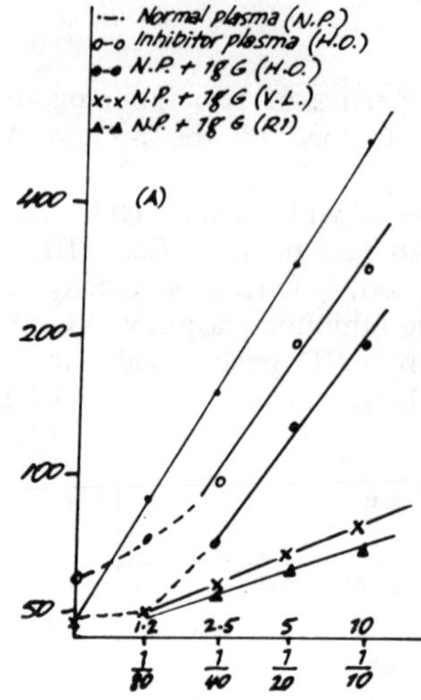

FIGURE 2. VIII:Cam (absorbance at 540 nm). The inhibitory effect of various antibodies, as measured by the chromogenic method (incubation time = 30 min).

VIII:C, VIII:Cam, and radiolabeled IgG distribution patterns. Labeled IgG was usually distributed in the IgG region (fraction 4), but, when it was incubated with plasma or fraction 1–0, which have the same electrophoretic mobility as the native forms of F VIII, there was a shift in the maximum of radiolabeled IgG that coincided with the slow-moving part of the F VIII–related

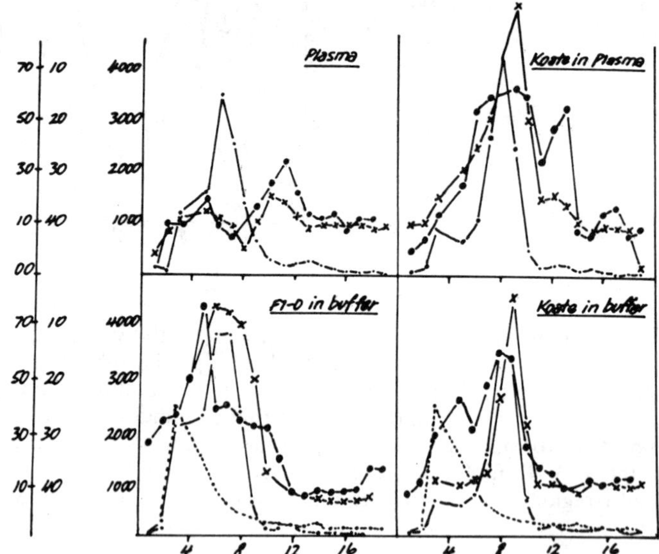

FIGURE 3. A comparison between free labeled IgG (- - -) and F VIII in complex with IgG (——) using fresh plasma, fraction 1–0 (Fl–0), koate in buffer, and koate in plasma. The effluents of the gels were also assayed for VIII:C (·—·) and VIII:Cam (×–×).

activities (fraction 6–7). In koate and koate in plasma, VIIIR:Ag is a fast migrating type and radiolabeled materials also seem to match other F VIII–related activities and migrate faster than fraction 1–0 or plasma alone (fraction 8–9). It is of interest to notice that, in clinical concentrate, both two-stage clotting and chromogenic methods measure activities that are associated with aggregated forms of F VIII, while, under plasma conditions, a second peak of activity is found in a fast moving region. It has been suggested that this peak represents a F VIII subunit.[6]

Distribution of Residual F VIII:Cam Activity

FIGURE 4 shows the patterns obtained in the postinfused severe vWD patient samples treated under conditions strictly identical with those of various antibodies. Three peaks of activity are observed: VL IgG seems to inhibit all forms, while HO is mainly directed to larger forms, leaving the smaller forms

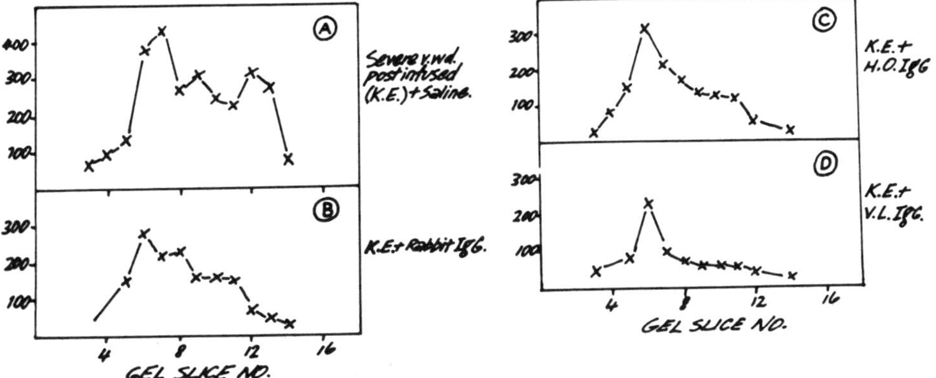

FIGURE 4. VIII:Cam (absorbance at 540 nm). A comparison of the inhibitory effect of three antibodies, incubated for 45 min at 37° C, with a vWD postinfusion sample, measured directly on the gel slice using the chromogenic method.

free, and RI gives a partial inhibition of all three forms, probably because it has a lower affinity for this sample.

CONCLUSION

1. Multiple peaks of F VIII:C and VIII:Cam are identified by quantitative electrophoresis techniques. The intensity of these peaks varies with the method of measurement used.

2. Antibodies for F VIII differ from each other in terms of their mode of action, VIII:Cam neutralization, and electrophoretic distribution of their complex(es). Some antibodies seem to bind tightly to VIII:C and lead to conformational change in the molecular structure while others bind selectively to some forms of F VIII and/or to regions that do not affect the VIII:C part to the same extent.

3. Quantitative electrophoresis in agarose, particularly with the use of labeled IgG, is the method of choice for characterizing the bound and unbound molecules of F VIII. The method has some clinical implications, since, by identifying the type of F VIII required to bind the antibody, it is possible to treat the patient with the right concentrates.

REFERENCES

1. ZIMMERMAN, T. S., J. ROBERTS & T. S. EDGINGTON. 1975. Multiple molecular forms of F VIII in human plasma. Proc. Nat. Acad. Sci. USA **72:** 5121–5125.
2. HOYER, L. W. & M. E. RICK. 1975. Implications of immunological methods for measuring F VIII. Ann. N.Y. Acad. Sci. **240:** 97–109.
3. SEGHATCHIAN, M. J. & M. MILLER ANDERSSON. 1978. A colorimetric evaluation of F VIII potency. Med. Lab. Sci. **35:** 347–352.
4. SEGHATCHIAN, M. J. 1979. Electrophoretic distribution of F VIII:C measured by chromogenic and clotting methods. Thromb. Diath. Haemorrh. **42:** 111.
5. SEGHATCHIAN, M. J., I. M. NILSSON, L. HOLMBERG & M. MILLER ANDERSSON. 1979. Molecular size distribution of native F VIII. Thromb. Res. **14:** 589–598.
6. SEGHATCHIAN, M. J. & K. HIRST. 1979. Evidence for the presence of F VIII subunits in plasma and clinical F VIII concentrates using quantitative electrophoresis. Thromb. Diath. Haemorrh. **42:** 65.

PLATELET-COAGULANT PROTEIN INTERACTIONS IN CONTACT ACTIVATION *

Peter N. Walsh

*Specialized Center on Thrombosis Research
and
Department of Medicine
Temple University School of Medicine
Philadelphia, Pennsylvania 19140*

John H. Griffin

*Department of Immunopathology
Scripps Clinic and Research Foundation
La Jolla, California 92037*

INTRODUCTION

Although a great deal of progress has been made in recent years toward understanding the mechanisms of the interactions of the proteins involved in the contact activation of intrinsic coagulation,[1-12] the mechanisms by which intrinsic coagulation is initiated *in vivo* are largely unknown. At least four plasma proteins are known to be involved in surface-mediated zymogen activations leading to factor IX activation. These proteins include factor XII (Hageman Factor), prekallikrein (Fletcher Factor), high molecular weight (HMW) kininogen (Fitzgerald or Williams Factor), and factor XI.[1-12]

In 1972, we presented the results of investigations on the interactions between platelets isolated by albumin density gradient centrifugation and plasma samples obtained from patients with various coagulation factor deficiencies.[13, 14] These observations suggested that platelets could participate in factor XII activation [13] and also in factor XI activation by mechanisms both dependent upon and independent of factor XII.[14] We suggested that these observations might provide clues to the existence of molecular mechanisms that operate *in vivo* to initiate coagulation in the absence of plasma proteins, such as factor XII, known not to be essential for normal hemostasis.[14, 15] To test these hypotheses directly, we have studied the interactions between isolated platelets and purified proteins of the contact phase of coagulation and here present evidence that platelets can promote the proteolytic activation of factor XII by kallikrein and that of factor XI by mechanisms both dependent upon and independent of factor XII.

METHODS

Preparation of Washed Platelet Suspensions

Blood was collected and platelet-rich plasma obtained as previously described.[16] Platelets were washed by albumin density gradient centrifugation [17, 18]

* This research was supported, in part, by grants from the National Institutes of Health (HL-21544, HL-16411, and HL-14217) and by grant AL-07007 from the Council for Tobacco Research.

241

and then gel filtered according to the method of Tangen *et al.*[19] Platelets were counted by phase contrast microscopy.[20]

Purified Proteins

The following proteins were purified from pooled normal human plasma by procedures previously described and each was more than 95% homogeneous when examined by sodium dodecyl sulfate polyacrylamide gel electrophoresis (SDS-PAGE):[21] Factor XII (specific clotting activity = 82 U/mg protein),[22] kallikrein (30 U/mg),[23] HMW kininogen (12.5 U/mg),[5] and factor XI (250 U/mg).[24] Factor XII and factor XI were radiolabeled with ^{125}I by the insolubilized lactoperoxidase method[25] or by the chloramine T method[26] to 0.5–33 μCi/μg (0.02–1.1 atoms ^{125}I per molecule) and retained 100% of their procoagulant activity after the radiolabeling procedure. The preparations were shown to be in zymogen form and were not contaminated by other coagulation proteins.

Clotting Assays

Incubation mixtures (100–125 μl) containing purified proteins and washed platelet suspensions, as indicated in Results, were assayed for coagulant activity in plasmas deficient in factor XII or factor XI, as previously described.[27]

Polyacrylamide Gel Electrophoresis

Polyacrylamide gel electrophoresis in the presence of sodium dodecylsulfate was carried out on 7.5% gels 8 cm long in 4.5 × 100 mm glass tubes according to the method of Weber and Osborn.[21] Incubation mixtures (100–125 μl) were boiled for 10 min after the addition of 50 μl of a solution containing 10% SDS, 1% β-mercaptoethanol, 8 M urea and 0.01 M ethylenediamine tetraacetic acid (EDTA). Following electrophoresis, the gels were sliced into 1.2 mm sections and counted for radioactivity in a Model 1195 Searle Analytic Gamma Counter. The percentage of factor XII or factor XI cleaved was calculated as the relative amount of radiolabel appearing in the two smaller fragments divided by the amount of radioactivity appearing in all three peaks.

Reagents Used in Experiments

Purified human skin collagen was kindly provided by Dr. George Wilner, Washington University, St. Louis and human α-thrombin by Dr. John W. Fenton, II, New York State Department of Health, Albany, New York. Indomethacin and adenosine diphosphate (ADP) were obtained from Sigma Chemical Company, St. Louis, Missouri; celite (diatomaceous silica), from Johns-Manville; and kaolin, from J. T. Baker Chemical Co., Phillipsburg, New Jersey.

RESULTS

Effect of Platelets on Coagulant Activity and Cleavage of ^{125}I-Factor XII

Washed platelets were incubated with HMW kininogen, ^{125}I-labeled factor XII, collagen or ADP, and kallikrein, after which either the clotting times in factor XII-deficient plasma were determined or the percentage of cleavage of ^{125}I-factor XII was assessed on SDS-PAGE (TABLE 1). When mixtures con-

TABLE 1

CLOTTING TIMES OF FACTOR-XII DEFICIENT PLASMA
AND CLEAVAGE OF ^{125}I-FACTOR XII IN PRESENCE AND ABSENCE
OF PLATELETS, HIGH MOLECULAR WEIGHT KININOGEN, AND KALLIKREIN

Line	Incubation Mixture						Clotting Time (sec) of Factor XII-deficient Plasma	Percentage of Cleavage of ^{125}I-Factor XII
	Platelets	HMWK	FXII	Collagen	ADP	Kallikrein		
1	+	+	+	+	−	+	182	15.5
2	+	+	+	−	+	+	205	12.5
3	+	+	+	−	−	−	258	9.4
4	+	+	+	+	−	−	306	0.2
5	+	+	+	−	+	−	318	0.4
6	+	+	+	−	−	−	332	0.1
7	+	−	+	+	−	+	190	9.6
8	+	−	+	−	+	+	228	6.5
9	+	−	+	−	−	+	241	6.1
10	−	+	+	+	−	+	312	0.8
11	−	+	+	−	−	+	307	0.4
12	−	+	+	celite	−		174	66.5

NOTE: 100 μl washed platelets (5.31×10^8/ml) in calcium-free Tyrode's solution, pH 7.3, with bovine serum albumin (1 mg/ml) or buffer, was incubated in a 10×75 mm siliconized glass tube for 1 min at 37° C with 2 μl (0.54 μg) HMWK (or TBS) and 5 μl (0.2 μg) of a mixture of cold and ^{125}I-labeled factor XII. To this mixture was added 5μl collagen (250 μg/ml), ADP (50 μM), celite (1.35 mg/ml), or TBS pH 7.3 for a further incubation. 5μl kallikrein (1.5 μg) was then added and the mixture was incubated for 20 min at 37° C, after which either clotting times were determined in factor XII–deficient plasma or the percentage of cleavage of ^{125}I-factor XII was determined by SDS-PAGE, as described in METHODS. A background value of 4.5% was subtracted from the total percentage of cleavage to yield a net percentage of cleavage, as described in Methods.

taining platelets and collagen, ADP, or buffer (lines 1, 2, and 3) were compared with similar mixtures not containing platelets (lines 10 and 11), a marked shortening of clotting times (45–113 sec) was observed in association with enhanced cleavage (9.4–15.5%) of ^{125}I-factor XII. When platelets were absent and celite replaced collagen or ADP in the incubation mixture (line 12), the clotting time was shorter and the percentage of the cleavage of factor XII was greater than that of collagen-treated platelets (line 1). In experiments carried out with collagen-treated, ADP-treated, or untreated platelets, both the coagulant activity and the cleavage of factor XII were entirely dependent upon the presence of kallikrein (lines 4, 5 and 6). In contrast, both the coagulant activity and the cleavage of factor XII were only partially dependent upon the presence of HMW kininogen (lines 7, 8 and 9).

The relationship between the coagulant activity and cleavage of factor XII was examined in mixtures containing washed platelets treated with collagen, ADP, or buffer, incubated for 10, 20, or 40 min with HMW kininogen, kallikrein, and ^{125}I-labeled factor XII (FIGURE 1). Both coagulant activity, measured in factor XII-deficient plasma, and factor XII cleavage, measured by SDS-PAGE, are expressed as percentages of those observed in a mixture containing celite without platelets. It is evident that the relative extent of factor XII activation as assessed by clotting assays was greater than the relative extent of cleavage of the molecule on SDS-PAGE. Furthermore, the coagulant activation of factor XII in mixtures containing collagen-treated or ADP-treated platelets occurred within 10 min and increased only slightly thereafter, whereas cleavage of the molecule occurred progressively over a 40 min time course.

Electrophoretic studies were carried out under unreduced and reduced conditions simultaneously in order to ascertain the nature of the factor XII cleavage. When factor XII is cleaved internal to intramolecular disulfide bonds (α Hageman factor), it migrates as a single 80,000 MW protein on unreduced gels and as two polypeptide chains of 52,000 and 28,000 MW on reduced gels. When cleavage occurs outside these disulfide bonds, the protein migrates as two polypeptide chains on both reduced and unreduced gels. It is evident from the results of the experiment shown in TABLE 2 that the percentage of cleaved

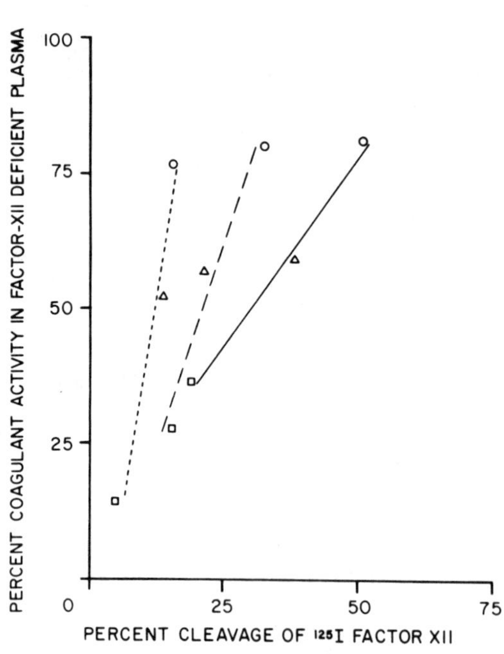

FIGURE 1. The relationship between coagulant activity and cleavage of factor XII. The incubation mixtures, which are identical to those described in TABLE 1 containing washed platelets or buffer; collagen, ADP, celite or TBS; kallikrein, HMW kininogen and ^{125}I-factor XII, were incubated for 10, 20, or 40 min, after which clotting times were determined in factor XII-deficient plasma or the percentage of cleavage of ^{125}I-factor XII was determined by SDS-PAGE. Both coagulant activity and cleavage are expressed as percentages of that observed in the mixture containing celite without platelets. The net percentage of cleavage was calculated as in TABLE 1. Results are shown for platelets incubated with collagen (o), ADP (Δ), or buffer (□) and then with kallikrein, HMW kininogen, and ^{125}I–factor XII for 10 min (– – –), 20 min (— — —) or 40 min (—).

TABLE 2

SDS-PAGE OF ^{125}I-FACTOR XII
IN THE PRESENCE AND ABSENCE OF REDUCING AGENT

Incubation Mixture				Percentage of Cleavage of ^{125}I-Factor XII		Percentage of α Hageman Factor of
Platelets	Collagen	ADP	Celite	Reduced	Unreduced	Total Cleaved
+	+	−	−	36	14	62
+	−	+	−	28	12	58
+	−	−	−	18	8.3	54
−	−	−	+	62	21	66

NOTE: 100 μl washed platelets (5.09 × 10^8/ml) in calcium-free Tyrode's solution, pH 7.3, with bovine serum albumin (1 mg/ml) or buffer, was incubated in a 10 × 75 mm siliconized glass tube for 1 min at 37° C with 2 μl (0.54 μg) HMWK and 5 μl (0.04 μg) of a mixture of cold and ^{125}I-labeled factor XII. To the mixture was added 5 μl of collagen (250 μg/ml), ADP (50 μM), celite (1.35 mg/ml), or TBS, pH 7.3, for a further 5 min incubation. 5 μl kallikrein (1.5 μg) was then added and the mixture was incubated for 30 min at 37° C, after which the percentage of cleavage of ^{125}I-factor XII was determined on SDS-PAGE in the presence or absence of 1% β-mercaptoethanol, as described in METHODS.

factor XII that migrated as a single 80,000 MW protein on reduced gels (*i.e.*, was cleaved internally) ranged between 54% and 62% in the presence of platelets. Similar results were obtained when celite replaced platelets.

Effect of Indomethacin on the Cleavage of ^{125}I-Factor XII

The nonsteroidal anti-inflammatory drug indomethacin is known to inhibit the secretion of stored contents of platelet granules by inhibiting the cyclo-oxygenase enzyme that catalyzes the conversion of arachidonic acid to prostaglandin endoperoxide.[28, 29] It was previously shown that indomethacin at a concentration of 20 μM could inhibit the collagen-dependent secretion of [^{14}C]-5-hydroxytryptamine from platelets washed by albumin density gradient separation.[30] To determine whether inhibition of platelet responses could influence the platelet-dependent cleavage of factor XII by kallikrein, the effect of 20 μM indomethacin on the cleavage of ^{125}I-labeled factor XII was determined (TABLE 3). Indomethacin inhibited the cleavage of factor XII by kallikrein in the presence of collagen-treated or ADP-treated platelets. In a parallel experiment, the release of [^{14}C]-5-hydroxytryptamine from collagen-treated platelets was 80% inhibited by 20 μM indomethacin. In contrast, in control experiments, indomethacin had no effect on the percentage of cleavage of ^{125}I-labeled factor XII in the absence of platelets.

Proteolytic Cleavage of Factor XI.

Effects of Platelets

The conversion of the zymogen, factor XI, to an active serine protease involves the limited proteolytic cleavage of the native molecule (MW = 160,000 without reduction, 80,000 in the presence of reducing agents) to yield two polypeptide chains, of MW = 48,000 and 32,000, which are held together by disulfide bonds.[24] To determine whether the proteolytic activation of factor XII observed in the experiments presented in TABLES 1–3 and FIGURE 1 was accompanied by proteolytic cleavage of factor XI, a series of experiments was carried out in which washed platelet suspensions or Tyrodes' solution were added to collagen, ADP, or buffer and incubated with factor XII, HMW kininogen, kallikrein and ^{125}I-labeled factor XI (TABLE 4). In incubation mixtures containing factor XII, HMW kininogen, kallikrein, and factor XI, only 2.0–4.6% cleavage of ^{125}I-labeled factor XI occurred in collagen-treated, ADP-treated, or buffer-treated samples in the absence of platelets. In contrast, when platelets were present, 26.8% cleavage of ^{125}I-labeled factor XI occurred in the collagen-treated sample, compared with 37.2% cleavage in the celite-treated sample in the absence of platelets. In parallel experiments not reported here, proteolytic cleavage of factor XI was accompanied by evidence of activation, as assessed

TABLE 3

EFFECT OF INDOMETHACIN ON CLEAVAGE OF ^{125}I-FACTOR XII
BY KALLIKREIN IN PRESENCE AND ABSENCE OF PLATELETS

Stimulus	Treatment	Percentage of ^{125}I-Factor XII	
		Platelets Present	Platelets Absent
Collagen	Buffer	41	19
	Indomethacin	27	20
ADP	Buffer	36	19
	Indomethacin	25	20
Buffer	Buffer	28	16
	Indomethacin	26	17
Celite	Buffer	—	66
	Indomethacin	—	65

NOTE: 100 μl washed platelets (6.88 $\times$ 10^8/ml) or buffer was incubated with 5 μl indomethacin (20 μM, final concentration) or with TBS and then with reactants, as indicated in FIGURE 1. 1.5 μg kallikrein was added, after which samples were analyzed by SDS-PAGE, as indicated in METHODS.

by coagulation. These results indicate that collagen-treated, ADP-treated, and buffer-treated platelets promote the proteolytic activation of factor XI in the presence of kallikrein, factor XII and HMW kininogen.

Effects of HMW Kininogen, Kallikrein, Factor XII, and Factor XIIa

A series of experiments was carried out to determine to what extent the proteolytic cleavage of factor XI was dependent upon the presence of HMW kininogen, factor XII, factor XIIa, and kallikrein. In the experiment shown in TABLE 5, either collagen-treated platelets, collagen alone, or celite alone was incubated with various mixtures of HMW kininogen, factor XII or factor XIIa, kallikrein and ^{125}I-labeled factor XI. When collagen was incubated with various mixtures of the purified proteins in the absence of platelets, only

TABLE 4

EFFECTS OF COLLAGEN, ADP, AND CELITE ON CLEAVAGE
OF ^{125}I-FACTOR XI IN PRESENCE AND ABSENCE OF PLATELETS

			Incubation Mixtures				Percentage of Cleavage of ^{125}I-FXI	
							Platelets Present	Platelets Absent
Collagen	ADP	Celite	FXII	HMWK	Kallikrein	^{125}I-FXI		
+	−	−	+	+	+	+	26.8	4.6
−	+	−	−	+	+	+	21.6	3.4
−	−	−	+	+	+	+	14.2	2.0
−	−	+	+	+	+	+	—	37.2

NOTE: A suspension (75 μl) of platelets (6.21 $\times$ 10^8/ml) in calcium-free Tyrode's solution, pH 7.3, containing bovine serum albumin (1 mg/ml) or buffer was placed in a 10 $\times$ 75 mm siliconized glass tube with 5 μl of either collagen (300 μg/ml), ADP (50 μM), celite (1.57 mg/ml), or TBS buffer. To the mixture was added 5 μl of each of the following reactants: factor XII (0.36 μg), HMW kininogen (0.54 μg), kallikrein (1.5 μg), and ^{125}I-Factor XI (0.15 μg). After a 120 min incubation at 37° C, 30 μl of a solution containing 10% SDS, 1% β-mercaptoethanol, 8 M urea, and 0.01 M EDTA was added. The sample was boiled for 10 min, electrophoresed on 7.5% polyacrylamide, and analyzed as described in METHODS.

TABLE 5

EFFECTS OF HIGH MOLECULAR WEIGHT KININOGEN,
KALLIKREIN, FACTOR XII, AND FACTOR XIIa ON THE CLEAVAGE OF ^{125}I-FACTOR XI
IN THE PRESENCE AND ABSENCE OF COLLAGEN-TREATED PLATELETS

	Incubation Mixture					Cleavage (%) of ^{125}I-FXI		
						Platelets + Collagen	Buffer + Collagen	Buffer + Celite
Line	HMWK	FXII	FXII$_a$	Kalli-krein	FXI			
1	+	+	−	+	+	27.3	2.1	45.6
2	−	+	−	+	+	18.2	1.6	24.6
3	+	−	−	+	+	11.2	0.4	2.1
4	+	+	−	−	+	0.2	0.1	0.5
5	+	−	+	−	+	24.1	1.9	34.6

NOTE: 5 μl of each of the reactants indicated or TBS buffer was added to 75 μl of platelet suspension (6.77 $\times$ 10^8/ml) or calcium-free Tyrode's solution, pH 7.3, containing bovine serum albumin (1 mg/ml). The amount of factor XIIa added was 0.36 μg. Otherwise the amount of each reactant added and the experimental conditions are as detailed in the note to TABLE 4.

minimal cleavage of ^{125}I-labeled factor XI (0.1–2.1%) was observed. When collagen-treated platelets were incubated with HMW kininogen, factor XII, kallikrein, and factor XI, the percentage of ^{125}I-labeled factor XI increased 13-fold (27.3%) over the results observed with collagen in the absence of platelets (2.1%), whereas 45.6% cleavage of ^{125}I-labeled factor XI occurred with celite present in the absence of platelets. Generally similar results were obtained when factor XIIa replaced factor XII and kallikrein in the incubation mixture.

When HMW kininogen was excluded from an incubation mixture containing factor XII, kallikrein, and factor XI, the percentage of ^{125}I-labeled factor XI cleaved decreased from 27.3% to 18.2% in the presence of collagen-treated platelets and from 45.6% to 24.6% in the presence of celite alone. When factor XII was excluded from the incubation mixture containing HMW kininogen, kallikrein, and factor XI, only 2.1% of the ^{125}I-labeled factor XI was cleaved in the sample containing celite without platelets. In contrast, 11.2% of the factor XI was cleaved in a similar sample in which collagen-treated platelets were incubated with HMW kininogen, kallikrein, and factor XI in the absence of factor XII. Finally, when kallikrein was excluded from the incubation mixtures, only trace cleavage (0.1–0.5%) of ^{125}I-labeled factor XI occurred in any of the incubation mixtures. It can be concluded from this experiment that the platelet-dependent proteolytic activation of factor XI in mixtures containing factor XII, HMW kininogen, and/or kallikrein required kallikrein and was enhanced 2–3-fold by factor XII, thus demonstrating that significant proteolytic activation of factor XI occurred in the absence of added factor XII.

DISCUSSION

It can be concluded from the experiments presented here that platelets treated with ADP or collagen can promote the proteolytic activation of factor XII in the presence of high molecular weight kininogen and kallikrein; this is shown by three independent criteria: the proteolytic cleavage of factor XII, the development of factor XIIa coagulant activity, and the proteolytic cleavage of added factor XI. Furthermore, platelets treated with collagen participate with high molecular weight kininogen and kallikrein to promote the proteolytic activation of factor XI by mechanisms both dependent upon and independent of factor XII, as shown by the proteolytic cleavage of factor XI and also by the development of factor XIa coagulant activity. It can be further concluded from these experiments that the zymogen activations observed are platelet related, as shown by several lines of evidence: first, the enhanced proteolysis and coagulant activation observed after platelet stimulation; second, the inhibition of proteolytic activation observed when platelet responses were inhibited with indomethethin; third, the absence of proteolytic activation in the absence of platelets or other surfaces; and, finally, the localization of factor XI cleavage products in platelet pellets, as shown in experiments not reported here.

The mechanisms by which platelets contribute to the observed zymogen activations are complex and require further study. Since the platelet-dependent proteolytic activation of factor XII observed here requires the presence of kallikrein, we do not conclude that platelets directly activate factor XII, but rather that they provide a surface similar to that provided by negatively charged substances, such as kaolin or glass, upon which a ternary complex of the proteins kallikrein, HMW kininogen, and factor XII can be assembled, which results in a conformational alteration of factor XII, rendering it more susceptible to proteolytic activation by kallikrein.[1-12] The platelet-dependent proteolytic activation of factor XI in the presence of kallikrein and HMW kininogen occurred by mechanisms both dependent upon and independent of factor XII, from which it can be concluded that platelets provide more than simply a surface. It is possible that platelets provide a factor XII-like protease that can be activated by kallikrein and substitute for added plasma factor XII.

The experiments presented here are consistent with the hypothetical model presented in FIGURE 2. Presently available evidence indicates that prekallikrein circulates in plasma as a complex with high molecular weight kininogen and that it can be activated on a negatively charged surface,[3-5] but whether or not platelets participate in this reaction is unknown.

However, evidence is presented here that platelets can promote the proteolytic activation of factor XII by kallikrein and subsequently give rise to the formation of factor XIa, which remains associated with the platelet surface. Experiments previously reported indicate that factor XIa formed on the platelet surface is protected from inactivation by plasma protease inhibitors.[14, 31] Platelets also possess an intrinsic protein with factor XI activity and antigenic similarities to plasma factor XI.[32] The experiments presented here concern the proteolytic activation of purified plasma factor XI by mechanisms both dependent upon and independent of factor XII. Whether intrinsic platelet factor XI is activated by mechanisms similar to those demonstrated for plasma factor XI remains to be investigated. A final intriguing question relates to the functional significance of platelet factor XI and other platelet-associated contact factors and their possible role in bypassing some of the contact factor activations demonstrated in cell-free systems. Since patients with deficiencies of factor XII, prekallikrein, and high molecular weight kininogen and many patients with deficiencies of plasma factor XI have no problems maintaining normal hemostasis,[33] the ultimate question we will be asking is, How might platelets participate in zymogen activation mechanisms that bypass the plasma system of contact activation?

SUMMARY

Previous studies have suggested that human platelets can promote the activation of factor XI by two different mechanisms, one requiring factor XII and ADP-treated platelets and the other requiring collagen-treated platelets in the apparent absence of factor XII. To investigate these hypotheses, isolated platelets were tested for their capacity to promote the activation and cleavage of purified factors XII and XI in various mixtures of purified factor XII, kallikrein, high molecular weight kininogen, and factor XI. That ADP- or collagen-treated platelets can promote the proteolytic activation of factor XII in mixtures containing kallikrein and HMW kininogen was shown by (1) the proteolytic cleavage of factor XII, (2) the development of factor XIIa coagulant activity, and (3) the proteolytic cleavage of ^{125}I-labeled factor XI. Platelets treated with collagen or thrombin were shown by both coagulant assays and cleavage studies to participate with HMW kininogen and kallikrein in the proteolytic activation of factor XI by mechanisms that are partially dependent

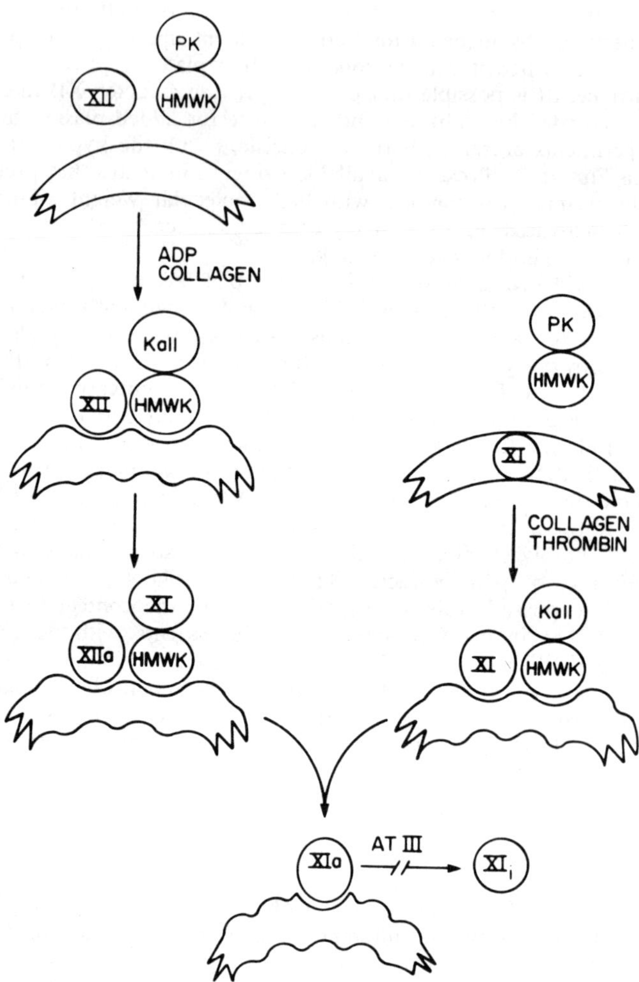

FIGURE 2. A schematic diagram of an hypothesis describing the role of platelets in contact phase activation of intrinsic coagulation. The smooth crescent represents the platelet membrane in the unactivated state, the rough crescent the activated state. Roman numerals refer to coagulation proteins XII and XI, the activated forms of which are indicated by an "a"; XIi is factor XIa complexed to and inactivated by antithrombin III (AT III); and HMWK is HMW kininogen.

upon and partially independent of factor XII. These studies demonstrate that platelets can promote the proteolytic activation of factor XII by kallikrein and of factor XI by both factor XII-dependent and factor XII-independent mechanisms.

ACKNOWLEDGMENTS

We thank Dr. Charles G. Cochrane for helpful advice and support and Eileen Camp, Alice Kleiss, Gregory Beretta, and Kevin Bickford for skillful technical assistance. We are grateful to Connie Moody for typing the manuscript.

REFERENCES

1. COCHRANE, C. G., S. D. REVAK & K. D. WUEPPER. 1973. Activation of Hageman factor in solid and fluid phases. A critical role of kallikrein. J. Exp. Med. **138:** 1564.
2. MCMILLIN, C. R., H. SAITO, O. D. RATNOFF & A. G. WALTON. 1974. The secondary structure of human Hageman factor (factor XII) and its alteration by activating agents. J. Clin. Invest. **54:** 1312.
3. MANDLE, R., JR., R. W. COLMAN & A. P. KAPLAN. 1976. Identification of prekallikrein and HMW kininogen as a circulating complex in human plasma. Proc. Natl. Acad. Sci. USA **73:** 4179.
4. GRIFFIN, J. H. & C. G. COCHRANE. 1976. Mechanisms for the involvement of high molecular weight kininogen in surface-dependent reactions of Hageman factor (coagulation factor XII). Proc. Natl. Acad. Sci. USA **73:** 2554.
5. WIGGINS, R. C., B. N. BOUMA, C. G. COCHRANE & J. H. GRIFFIN. 1977. Role of high molecular weight kininogen in surface-binding and activation of coagulation factor XI and prekallikrein. Proc. Natl. Acad. Sci. USA **74:** 4636.
6. MEIER, H. L., J. V. PIERCE, R. W. COLMAN & A. P. KAPLAN. 1977. Activation and function of human Hageman factor. The role of high molecular weight kininogen and prekallikrein. J. Clin. Invest. **60:** 18.
7. THOMPSON, R. E., R. MANDLE, JR. & A. P. KAPLAN. 1977. Association of factor XI and high molecular weight kininogen in human plasma. J. Clin. Invest. **60:** 1376.
8. FAIR, B. D., H. SAITO, O. D. RATNOFF & W. B. RIPPON: 1977. Detection by fluorescence of structural changes accompanying the activation of Hageman factor (factor XII). Proc. Soc. Exp. Biol. Med. **155:** 199.
9. REVAK, S. D., C. G. COCHRANE & J. H. GRIFFIN. 1977. The binding and cleavage characteristics of human Hageman factor during contact activation. A comparison of normal plasma with plasmas deficient in factor XI, prekallikrein or high molecular weight kininogen. J. Clin. Invest. **59:** 1167.
10. GRIFFIN, J. H. 1978. The role of surface in the surface-dependent activation of Hageman factor (blood coagulation factor XII). Proc. Natl. Acad. Sci. USA **75:** 1998.
11. RATNOFF, O. D. & H. SAITO. 1979. Amidolytic properties of single-chain activated Hageman factor. Proc. Natl. Acad. Sci. USA **76:** 1461.
12. REVAK, S. D., C. G. COCHRANE, B. N. BOUMA & J. H. GRIFFIN. 1978. Surface and fluid phase activities of two forms of activated Hageman factor produced during contact activation of plasma. J. Exp. Med. **147:** 719.
13. WALSH, P. N. 1972. The role of platelets in the contact phase of blood coagulation. Br. J. Haematol. **22:** 237.
14. WALSH, P. N. 1972. The effects of collagen and kaolin on the intrinsic

coagulant activity of platelets. Evidence for an alternative pathway in intrinsic coagulation not requiring factor XII. Br. J. Haematol. **22:** 393.

15. WALSH, P. N. 1974. Platelet coagulant activities and hemostasis: an hypothesis. Blood **43:** 597.

16. WALSH, P. N. 1972. The effect of dilution of plasma on coagulation. The significance of the dilution-activation phenomenon for the study of platelet coagulant activities. Br. J. Haematol. **22:** 219.

17. WALSH, P. N., D. C. B. MILLS & J. G. WHITE. 1977. Metabolism and function of human platelets washed by albumin density gradient separation. Br. J. Haematol. **36:** 281.

18. WALSH, P. N. 1972. Albumin density gradient separation and washing of platelets and the study of platelet coagulant activities. Br. J. Haematol. **22:** 205.

19. TANGEN, O., H. J. BERMAN & P. MARFEY. 1971. Gel filtration. A new technique for separation of blood platelets from plasma. Thromb. Diath. Haemorrh. **25:** 268.

20. BRECHER, G. & E. P. CRONKITE. 1950. Morphology and enumeration of human blood platelets. J. Appl. Physiol. **3:** 365.

21. WEBER, K. & M. OSBORN. 1969. The reliability of molecular weight determination by dodecyl sulfate–polyacrylamide gel electrophoresis. J. Biol. Chem. **244:** 4406.

22. GRIFFIN, J. H. & C. G. COCHRANE. 1976. Human factor XII (Hageman factor). *In* Methods Enzymol. **45:** 56.

23. BOUMA, B. N. & J. H. GRIFFIN. 1977. Human prekallikrein (plasminogen proactivator): Purification, characterization and activation by activated Factor XII. Thrombos. Haemost. **38:** 135.

24. BOUMA, B. N. & J. H. GRIFFIN. 1977. Human blood coagulation Factor XI. Purification, properties, and mechanism of activation by activated Factor XII. J. Biol. Chem. **252:** 6432.

25. DAVID, G. S. & R. A. REISFELD. 1974. Protein iodination with solid state lactoperoxidase. Biochemistry **13:** 1014.

26. McCONAHEY, P. J. & F. J. DIXON. 1966. A method of trace iodination of proteins for immunologic studies. Int. Arch. Allergy. Appl. Immunol. **29:** 185.

27. LIPSCOMB, M. S. & P. N. WALSH. 1979. Human platelets and factor XI. Localization in platelet membranes of factor XI–like activity and its functional distinction from plasma factor XI. J. Clin. Invest. **63:** 1006.

28. SMITH, J. B. & A. L. WILLIS. 1971. Aspirin selectively inhibits prostaglandin production in human platelets. Nature (London) **231:** 235.

29. ROTH, G. J., N. STANFORD & P. W. MAJERUS. 1975. Acetylation of prostaglandin synthase by aspirin. Proc. Natl. Acad. Sci. USA **72:** 3073.

30. WALSH, P. N. 1978. Different requirements of intrinsic factor Xa forming activity and platelet factor 3 activity and their relationship to platelet aggregation and secretion. Br. J. Haematol. **40:** 311.

31. WALSH, P. N. & R. BIGGS. 1972. The role of platelets in intrinsic factor Xa formation. Br. J. Haematol. **22:** 743.

32. TUSZYNSKI, G. P., E. CAMP, S. BEVACQUA & P. N. WALSH. 1979. Factor XI antigen in human platelets. Fed. Proc. Fed. Am. Soc. Exp. Biol. **38:** 1307.

33. RATNOFF, O. D. 1966. The biology and pathology of the initial stages of blood coagulation. Prog. Hematol. **5:** 204.

MECHANISMS FOR HAGEMAN FACTOR ACTIVATION AND ROLE OF HMW KININOGEN AS A COAGULATION COFACTOR

Allen P. Kaplan, Michael Silverberg,
Joseph T. Dunn, and Geraldine Miller *

*Division of Allergy, Rheumatology, and Clinical Immunology
Department of Medicine
State University of New York at Stony Brook
Stony Brook, New York 11794*

INTRODUCTION

Contact activation of plasma sets in motion a series of enzymatic steps leading to blood coagulation, liberation of the vasoactive peptide bradykinin, and conversion of plasminogen to plasmin. Initiation of each of these functional activities is dependent upon a complex interaction between the surface and four plasma proteins, Hageman factor (HF; coagulation factor XII), prekallikrein, factor XI, and high molecular weight (HMW) kininogen. In this review, we will focus our attention upon three important characteristics of these reactions. First, upon binding to surfaces, Hageman factor slowly autoactivates, and our data suggests that this reaction is initiated by traces of activated Hageman factor in our preparations. Second, HMW kininogen is a cofactor required for the activation of both factor XI and prekallikrein by activated Hageman factor. This is accomplished by binding prekallikrein and factor XI to HMW kininogen [1,2] and attaching these complexes to the surface in a conformation that facilitates cleavage by activated Hageman factor. Finally, an optimal rate of initiation of these pathways is achieved by enzymatic activation of Hageman factor by kallikrein; this reaction is indirectly dependent upon HMW kininogen, since it augments the effective concentration of kallikrein/Hageman factor. Recent data pertaining to each of these reaction mechanisms are summarized below.

RESULTS AND DISCUSSION

Activation of Hageman Factor

Human Hageman factor has been shown to exist as an 80,000 dalton single chain molecule,[3] which can be activated enzymatically by plasmin,[4] kallikrein,[5] or trypsin. Griffin has demonstrated that the rate of cleavage of Hageman factor is augmented when it is surface bound regardless which activator is used, indicating that the surface renders Hageman factor a better substrate for enzymatic digestion.[6] Enzymatic activation of Hageman factor has been shown to result in two cleavage products, each of which possesses activity. Cleavage

* Present address: National Cancer Institute, National Institutes of Health, Bethesda, Maryland 20014.

of Hageman factor within a disulfide bridge yields an 80,000 dalton active enzyme consisting of a 52,000 dalton heavy chain disulfide linked to a 28,000 dalton light chain.[7] This molecular species (HFa) represents the coagulant form of activated Hageman factor and remains attached to the surface. Cleavage can also occur external to this critical disulfide bridge so that Hageman factor is cleaved into two pieces. One of these, designated HFf,[8] is a 30,000 dalton fragment that is a potent prekallikrein activator but does not adhere to the surface [3] and has minimal activity as a coagulation enzyme (*i.e.*, activator of factor XI).[8] Since those enzymes which could activate Hageman factor are each products of Hageman factor activation, the mechanism of formation of the initiating active site in Hageman factor is unclear. Ratnoff and Saito have presented evidence that suggests that, upon binding of Hageman factor, a site is exposed to initiating surfaces in the absence of any cleavage.[9] Wiggins and Cochrane, on the other hand, have reported that native rabbit Hageman factor autoactivates and possesses intrinsic proteolytic activity [10] and the ability of native Hageman factor to slowly incorporate ^{3}H-DFP into the serine, which is critical for proteolytic activity,[11] is felt to support such a notion.

Miller *et al.* have reported that binding of highly purified human Hageman factor to kaolin results in autodigestion to form both HFa and HFf. Incorporation of ^{3}H-DFP (^{3}H-diisopropyl fluorophosphate) into each of these products suggested that autoactivation had resulted (FIG. 1) and that the rate of this autoactivation appeared to be dependent upon the concentration of activated Hageman factor present in the starting material.[12] The absence of inhibition by concentrations of trasylol that would rapidly inactivate other enzymes that are known Hageman factor activators lent further support to the hypothesis that this is a result of autoactivation and not of initiation by trace contaminants. However, a definitive demonstration of autoactivation requires a demonstration of an accelerating rate of activated HF formation in which the concentration of activator is continuously increasing. This phenomenon was, therefore, further investigated by Silverberg *et al.*, utilizing the synthetic substrate D-pro-phe-arg-*p*-nitroanilide as a primary assay for activated Hageman factor (either HFa or HFf), and the following results were obtained.[13] First, native Hageman factor that was treated with 10^{-2} *M* DFP for 90 min retained traces of activity upon the synthetic substrate and, upon binding to a glass surface, concave-upward accelerating curves were obtained that were consistent with autoactivation. When placed in a plastic cuvette, a linear progress curve was obtained, the slope of which was proportional to the amount of active enzyme in the preparation.

Further, utilizing the K_m and k_{cat} for the reaction of HFa (or HFf) with the synthetic substrate ($K_m = 200$ μM and $k_{cat} = 18/\text{sec}$) and estimating kinetic constants for the interaction of activated HFf and zymogen HF, we could generate progress curves by computer that had a striking resemblance to our experimental data, if we varied the total protein concentration and/or the ratio of activated HF to total HF. When cleavage of surface-bound HF was examined to determine which molecular species of activated HF was responsible for autoactivation, HFa was found to be effective, but HFf was not.[14] Thus, we view the initial event in our studies to be autoactivation by traces of HFa in Hageman factor preparations. It is our opinion that there are no data available that can unambiguously distinguish whether initiation occurs as a result of intrinsic activity of the zymogen, activity that is seen only upon binding of the zymogen to a surface due to a conformational change, or traces of activated enzyme that might normally circulate. The studies described here are most consistent with this last possibility and we believe that this phenomenon accounts for the results that have been previously reported.[9, 10, 12–14] A diagram illustrating this point is shown as FIGURE 2, in which surface-dependent autoactivation occurs by enzymatic activation of HF by HFa. This reaction appears to be unaffected by the addition of HMW kininogen.

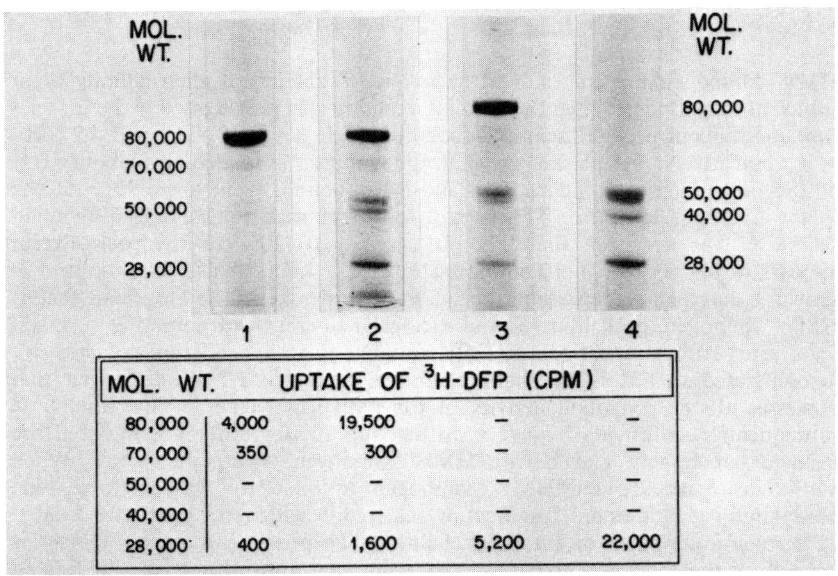

MOL. WT.	UPTAKE OF ^{3}H-DFP (CPM)			
	1	2	3	4
80,000	4,000	19,500	—	—
70,000	350	300	—	—
50,000	—	—	—	—
40,000	—	—	—	—
28,000	400	1,600	5,200	22,000

FIGURE 1. SDS polyacrylamide gel electrophoresis of 10 µg purified HF before and after incubation with kaolin for 10 min at 37° C. Positions 1 and 3 represent HF incubated in buffer and assessed under nonreducing (position 1) and reducing (position 3) conditions. The percentage of activated HF in the preparation (position 3) is 20%. Positions 2 and 4 represent HF bound to kaolin for 2 min, suspended in 3% SDS-8 M urea for 1 min, and assessed under nonreducing (position 2) and reducing (position 4) conditions. Formation of HFf (position 2) and HFa plus (position 4) is rapid, and essentially complete activation is achieved. An identical set of samples was incubated with 50 µCi ^{3}H-DFP (3 Ci/mmole) for 30 min at 37° C prior to electrophoresis. The gels were sliced and counted and the counts corresponding to each band seen are indicated below. The increase from a total of 4750 to 21,400 cpm in gels 1 and 2 indicates that activation had taken place and that, upon reduction, the activity is associated with the light chain (positions 3 and 4).

The Role of HMW Kininogen as a Coagulation Cofactor

Soon after HMW kininogen had been identified as a coagulation factor, it was demonstrated that the substrates of activated Hageman factor, *i.e.*, prekallikrein and factor XI, circulate as bimolecular complexes with HMW kininogen.[1, 2] Thus, HMW kininogen appeared to bind to either prekallikrein or factor XI but not both.[2] Since the concentration of HMW kininogen exceeds the sum of the prekallikrein and factor XI concentrations, there is sufficient

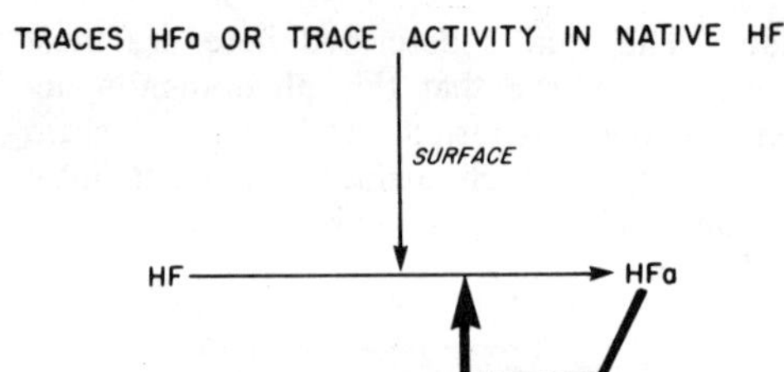

FIGURE 2. A diagram depicting the initiation of the intrinsic coagulation cascade either by traces of activated HF or by intrinsic proteolytic activity present in native HF as it interacts with surface-bound HF. Once HFa forms, autoactivation proceeds as shown by the heavy arrow.

HMW kininogen present to bind each one completely if their affinity is of sufficient magnitude. When this binding reaction was investigated,[15] the association constants of prekallikrein and factor XI were 3.4×10^7 M^{-1} and 4.2×10^8 M^{-1}, respectively. At plasma concentration, it was estimated that about 10% of the prekallikrein would be free and 90% bound, while over 99% of the factor XI would be bound. This is close to the reported values, in that unbound factor XI has not been found in plasma, but 10–20% of the prekallikrein appears to be free and not complexed to HMW kininogen.[16] In FIGURE 3 is shown a diagramatic representation of the manner in which Hageman factor, HMW kininogen, prekallikrein, and factor XI interact with initiating surfaces. Soon after the identification of HMW kininogen as a coagulation cofactor, we demonstrated that it is the light chain of kinin-free HMW kininogen that possesses all the coagulant activity of the native molecule.[17] This result was subsequently confirmed;[18] however, a striking species difference between the behavior of human and bovine HMW kininogen was pointed out. When kallikrein cleaves bovine HMW kininogen to yield the vasoactive peptide bradykinin, an additional fragment is released,[19] which is apparently located at the amino-terminus of the light chain.[20] The presence of this fragment is needed for the coagulant activity of the light chain; thus, the bovine light chain resulting from plasma kallikrein digestion is nonfunctional.[21] The comparable region of human HMW kininogen appears to resist further digestion.[15, 22]

Since prekallikrein and factor XI circulate bound to HMW kininogen, we questioned whether this binding is mediated by the HMW kininogen light chain. When purified heavy and light chains were tested for their ability to bind prekallikrein and factor XI, all the activity was present in the light chain.[15] Wiggins et al. reported that the attachment of prekallikrein and factor XI to surfaces such as kaolin was augmented by HMW kininogen[23] and concluded that the attachment to the surface occurs via HMW kininogen and that the function of HMW kininogen is to facilitate the binding of prekallikrein and factor XI to the surface. This, too, was shown to be a function of the light chain portion of the molecule.[24] Thus, when ^{125}I-prekallikrein was added to HMW kininogen–deficient plasma and the binding to kaolin was assessed, 19% binding was obtained. When the plasma was first reconstituted with HMW kininogen light chain, the binding was augmented to 58%. Reconstitution with

FIGURE 3. Binding of Hageman factor and complexes of HMW kininogen with prekallikrein and factor XI to a surface.

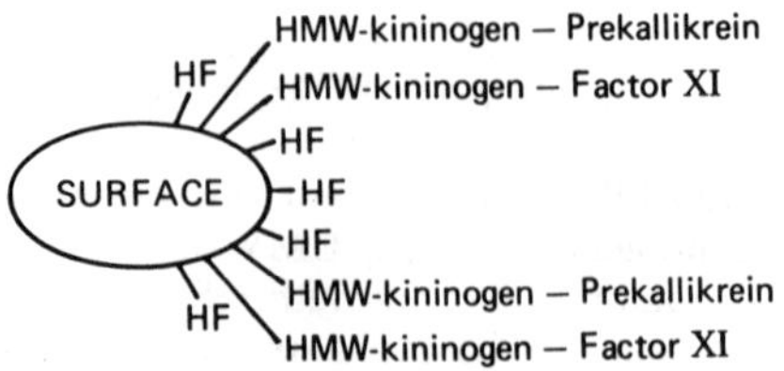

HMW kininogen heavy chain had no effect.[24] This demonstrated that attachment of the Hageman factor substrates to the surface is a property of the HMW kininogen light chain. Thus, this portion of the molecule contains the binding site for the surface as well as for prekallikrein and factor XI. It was of interest, however, that, if this experiment was repeated with a mixture of kaolin, purified ^{125}I-prekallikrein and HMW kininogen, binding of ^{125}I-prekallikrein to the surface was not augmented by HMW kininogen. It appeared that, in a plasma system, the effect of other proteins that might interfere with or compete with prekallikrein for binding is reversed by HMW kininogen. This further suggested that this phenomenon does not represent the critical function of HMW kininogen as a coagulation cofactor, since the activation of the ^{125}I-prekallikrein by Hageman factor in a purified system is augmented by HMW kininogen just as it is in plasma.

We next devised the experiment described in FIGURE 4. An equimolar complex of ^{125}I-prekallikrein and HMW kininogen was first prepared and bound to kaolin. Then a second pellet was prepared by binding the same amount of ^{125}I-prekallikrein to the surface in the absence of HMW kininogen and then adding the HMW kininogen. If complex formation were still to take place, it would be attached to the surface backwards, as shown in the right of FIGURE 4. The mixtures were then added to normal plasma and the cleavage of ^{125}I-prekallikrein was determined. As shown in FIGURE 4, 67% cleavage was obtained when the prekallikrein–HMW kininogen complex was performed and attached to the surface as it normally does, while only 2% cleavage of ^{125}I-prekallikrein was obtained when it was attached directly to the surface, even if HMW kininogen was supplied. Since equal amounts of prekallikrein were bound in each case, any effect of HMW kininogen upon the amount bound is obviated. These data suggest that, for activation of prekallikrein to proceed, it is essential that it be attached to the surface via a HMW kininogen bridge; presumably, it retains a degree of flexibility and/or presents a conformation that is critical for cleavage by activated Hageman factor. When it is bound directly to the surface, activation is actually inhibited. The ability of the kallikrein (or prekallikrein) formed to be eluted from the surface was also examined. When ^{125}I-prekallikrein was bound directly to the surface, it was not activated and none was eluted. When ^{125}I-prekallikrein was bound via HMW kininogen, up to 22% was subsequently found in the fluid phase. This dissociation does not appear to reflect a decreased affinity of kallikrein for HMW kininogen when compared to prekallikrein (although a direct comparison between the two has not been made), but is predicted based upon the known affinity of prekallikrein for HMW kininogen. Cochrane and Revak[25] and Silverberg *et al.*[24] have shown that kallikrein that has dissociated from a surface in this fashion can interact with Hageman factor that is bound to a separate particle and activate it enzymatically. Thus, HMW kininogen presents prekallikrein to surface-bound activated Hageman factor in a fashion optimal for activation, and it allows dissociation of a portion of the kallikrein formed from the surface into the fluid phase; in this way, it indirectly participates in the activation of Hageman factor.

SUMMARY

Our present concept of the initiating reactions of the intrinsic coagulation pathway is outlined in FIGURE 5. Although we remain unsure of the etiology

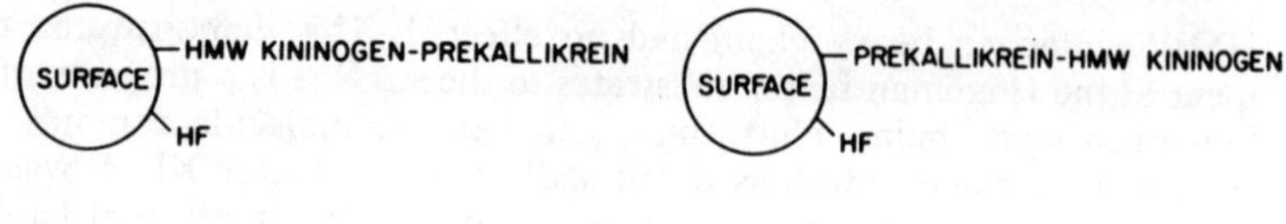

PERCENT
PREKALLIKREIN   67   2
CLEAVAGE

PERCENT
PREKALLIKREIN
ELUTION   22   1
FROM
SURFACE

FIGURE 4. Activation and dissociation of prekallikrein (kallikrein) upon binding to the surface via HMW kininogen compared to direct binding to the surface and subsequent exposure to HMW kininogen. 30 μl ^{125}I-prekallikrein was incubated for 5 min at 37° C with either 10 μl HMW kininogen or 10 μl buffer control. 60 μl kaolin suspension (10 mg/ml) was added and the mixture further incubated for 2 min at 37° C. The mixtures were then centrifuged for 1 min in a microfuge, washed twice in PBS, and the pellets counted. 100 μl normal plasma was added to each pellet and incubated for 3 min at 37° C. The mixture was centrifuged, the pellets were subjected to SDS gel electrophoresis under reducing conditions, the gels were sliced, and the percentage of cleavage was determined. To assess dissociation from the pellets, replicate samples of kaolin-bound ^{125}I-prekallikrein prepared as above were incubated with 60 μl of a 1:4 dilution of normal plasma for varying time intervals. The mixtures were centrifuged for 1 min at 3000 rpm and 50 μl supernatant was then removed and counted.

of the first active site—*i.e.,* traces of activated enzyme, intrinsic activity of the zymogen, or activity created in a small number of molecules upon binding— it appears clear that an accelerating reaction ensues in which native Hageman factor is enzymatically activated by activated Hageman factor. This reaction is independent of HMW kininogen and may be responsible for the gradual autoactivation one observes in prekallikrein-deficient plasma as the time of incubation with surfaces is increased. In normal plasma, HFa converts prekallikrein to kallikrein; this reaction is dependent upon HMW kininogen. As

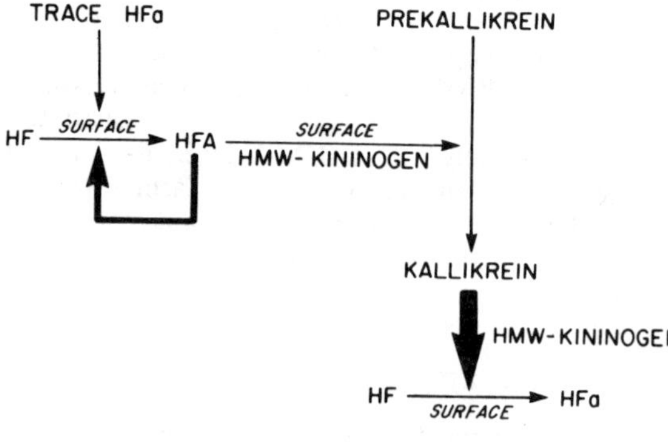

FIGURE 5. A diagrammatic representation of the initiating events of contact activation, including the autoactivation of Hageman factor (reaction 1) and the reciprocal activation of prekallikrein and Hageman factor, in which HMW kininogen functions as a cofactor (reaction 2).

shown in FIGURES 3 and 4, the major function of HMW kininogen is to bind prekallikrein and factor XI in plasma and attach them to surfaces in a conformation that allows activation by HFa. The HMW kininogen–dependent augmentation of the binding of prekallikrein and factor XI to the surface that is seen in plasma (but not buffer systems) would appear to be of lesser importance. Once activated, however, dissociation of kallikrein from the surface allows it to attack adjacent Hageman factor molecules on the same or other particles; this reaction appears to be more rapid than the rate of Hageman factor autoactivation. Thus, the rapid burst of HFa formation seen in normal plasma is kallikrein dependent. It is also dependent upon HMW kininogen, but this appears to be an indirect relationship. The HMW kininogen augments the amount of prekallikrein bound, allows activation to kallikrein, and is needed for kallikrein dissociation from the surface. These three effects all yield a marked increase in the effective ratio of kallikrein/Hageman factor at the surface-fluid interface, and this may be the condition required for rapid HFa formation.

REFERENCES

1. MANDLE, JR., R., R. W. COLMAN & A. P. KAPLAN. 1976. Identification of prekallikrein and HMW-kininogen as a circulating complex in human plasma. Proc. Natl. Acad. Sci. USA **73:** 4179–4183.
2. THOMPSON, R. E., R. MANDLE, JR. & A. P. KAPLAN. 1977. Association of factor XI and high molecular weight kininogen in human plasma. J. Clin. Invest. **60:** 1376–1380.
3. REVAK, S. D., C. G. COCHRANE, A. JOHNSON & J. HUGLI. 1974. Structural changes accompanying enzymatic activation of Hageman factor. J. Clin. Invest. **54:** 619–627.
4. KAPLAN, A. P. & K. F. AUSTEN. 1971. A prealbumin activator of prekallikrein. II. Derivation of activators of prekallikrein from active Hageman factor by digestion with plasmin. J. Exp. Med. **133:** 672–712.
5. COCHRANE, C. G., S. D. REVAK & K. D. WUEPPER. 1973. Activation of Hageman factor in solid and fluid phases. J. Exp. Med. **138:** 1564–1583.
6. GRIFFIN, J. H. 1978. Role of surface in surface-dependent activation of Hageman factor (blood coagulation factor XII). Proc. Natl. Acad. Sci. USA **75:** 1998–2002.
7. REVAK, S. D., C. G. COCHRANE, B. N. BOUMA & J. H. GRIFFIN. 1978. Surface and fluid phase activities of two forms of activated Hageman factor produced during contact activation of plasma. J. Exp. Med. **147:** 719–729.
8. KAPLAN, A. P. & K. F. AUSTEN. 1970. A prealbumin activator of prekallikrein. J. Immunol. **105:** 802–811.
9. RATNOFF, O. D. & H. SAITO. 1979. Amidolytic properties of single-chain activated Hageman factor. Proc. Natl. Acad. Sci. **76:** 1461–1463.
10. Wiggins, R. C. & C. G. Cochrane. 1979. The autoactivation of rabbit Hageman factor. J. Exp. Med. **150:** 1123–1133.
11. GRIFFIN, J. H. & G. BERETTA. 1979. Molecular mechanisms of surface-dependent activation of Hageman factor. *In* Advances in Experimental Medicine and Biology, Vol. 120B-Kinins-II. S. Fuji, H. Moriya, and T. Suzuki, Eds.: 39–51. Plenum Press. New York.
12. MILLER, G., M. SILVERBERG & A. P. KAPLAN. 1980. Autoactivatability of human Hageman factor (Factor XII) Biochem. Biophys. Res. Commun. **92:** 803–810.
13. SILVERBERG, M., J. T. DUNN, L. GAREN & A. P. KAPLAN. 1980. Autoactivation

of human Hageman factor demonstrated by utilizing a synthetic substrate. J. Biol. Chem. **255:** 7281–7286.

14. M. SILVERBERG, J. T. DUNN, G. MILLER & A. P. KAPLAN. 1980. Mechanisms involved in contact activation of plasma. Clin. Res. **28:** 324A.

15. THOMPSON, R. E., R. MANDLE, JR. & A. P. KAPLAN. 1979. Studies of the binding of prekallikrein and factor XI to high molecular weight kininogen and its light chain. Proc. Natl. Acad. Sci. USA **76:** 4862–4866.

16. COLMAN, R. W. & C. F. SCOTT. 1978. Function and immunochemistry of prekallikrein–high molecular weight kininogen complex in plasma. J. Clin. Invest. **65:** 413–421.

17. THOMPSON, R. E., R. MANDLE, JR. & A. P. KAPLAN. 1978. Characterization of human high molecular weight kininogen. J. Exp. Med. **147:** 488–499.

18. KERBIRIOU, D. M. & J. H. GRIFFIN. 1979. Human high molecular weight kininogen. Studies of structure-function relationships and of proteolysis of the molecule occurring during contact activation of plasma. J. Biol. Chem. **254:** 12020–12027.

19. HAN, Y. M., M. KOMIYA, S. IWANAGA & T. SUZUKI. 1975. Studies in the primary structure of bovine high molecular-weight kininogen. J. Biochem. **77:** 55–68.

20. HAN Y. M., H. KATO, S. IWANAGA & T. SUZUKI. 1976. Bovine plasma high molecular weight kininogen: The amino acid sequence of fragment 1 (glycopeptide) released by the action of plasma kallikrein and its location in the precursor protein. FEBS Lett. **63:** 197–200.

21. SCICLI, A. G., N. WALDMAN, J. A. GUIMARAES, G. SCICLI, O. A. CARRETERO, H. KATO, Y. N. HAN & S. IWANAGA. 1979. Relationship between structure and correcting activity of bovine high molecular weight kininogen upon the clotting time of Fitzgerald-Trait plasma. J. Exp. Med. **149:** 847–854.

22. NAKAYASU, T. & S. NAGASAWA. 1979. Studies on human kininogens. I. Isolation and characterization and cleavage by plasma kallikrein of high molecular weight (HMW)–kininogen. J. Biochem. **85:** 249–258.

23. WIGGINS, R. C., B. N. BOUMA, C. G. COCHRANE & J. H. GRIFFIN. 1977. Role of high molecular weight kininogen in surface-binding and activation of coagulation factor XI and prekallikrein. Proc. Natl. Acad. Sci. USA **74:** 4636–4640.

24. SILVERBERG, M., R. THOMPSON, G. MILLER & A. P. KAPLAN. 1980. Initiation of the intrinsic coagulation pathway: Autoactivatability of human Hageman factor and mechanisms by which the light chain derived from HMW-kininogen functions as a cofactor in the activation of prekallikrein, factor XI and Hageman factor. *In* The Regulation of Coagulation. K. Mann & F. Taylor, Jr., Eds.: 531–541. Elsevier North Holland. Amsterdam.

25. COCHRANE, C. G. & S. D. REVAK. 1979. A role of kallikrein in the propagation of contact activation in human plasma. Fed. Proc. Fed. An. Soc. Exp. Biol. **38:** 1271.

REGULATION OF THE FORMATION AND INHIBITION OF HUMAN PLASMA KALLIKREIN *

Robert W. Colman, Marc Schapira, and Cheryl F. Scott

Thrombosis Research Center
Temple University Health Sciences Center
Philadelphia, Pennsylvania 19140

INTRODUCTION AND OVERVIEW

During the past two decades, remarkable strides have been made in defining the mechanisms by which the intrinsic coagulation, fibrinolytic, and kinin-forming pathways are activated. Three proteins, factor XII (Hageman factor), prekallikrein (Fletcher factor), and high molecular weight (HMW) kininogen (Williams, Fitzgerald, Flaujeac factor), have been shown to be the major factors required for the activation of factor XI and prekallikrein. Hereditary deficiencies have been described for each of these contact factors. Methods have been developed for the purification of each of these proteins, and functional and immunochemical assays have been developed for each component. The molecular events occurring during contact activation have been described but are not yet fully understood. Activation has, in each instance, been shown to involve enzymatic digestion; however, the detailed structural features that permit the binding of these reactants to the surface require further study. How the interaction of the enzymes, factor XIIa, factor XIa, and kallikrein with the cofactor-substrate HMW kininogen results in accelerated reaction rates is still unclear.

Each of these three proteins (factor XII, prekallikrein, and HMW kininogen) bears a close functional, and in some cases structural, relationship to the other two. First, factor XII and prekallikrein are each involved in a reciprocal scheme for the activation of the other. Factor XII may be regarded as an essential component of the plasma kinin-forming system, as well as of the intrinsic pathway of coagulation. Thus, addition of kaolin to factor XII–deficient plasma is not followed by the release of either kallikrein or bradykinin,[1, 2] even though this plasma contains adequate quantities of both precursors.[3] The formation of kallikrein is initiated by activation of factor XII (M_r 80,000) (FIG. 1). Two mechanisms have been distinguished. Factor XII may be activated on a surface due to conformational changes[4] and/or cleavage by kallikrein[5] in the presence of HMW kininogen.[6] Initially, in the presence of a surface, a cleavage of factor XII occurs without fragmentation, since the two chains (52,000 and 28,000) are held together by disulfide bridges.

Factor XIIa bound to a surface can then activate either prekallikrein or factor XI bound to the same surface through HMW kininogen. In contrast, cleavage can occur outside the disulfide bridges either after exposure of factor XII to surfaces or during purification. Apparently, the 52,000 chain remains

* This research was supported, in part, by grants from the National Institutes of Health (HL 14217 and HL 24365). M.S. was the recipient of Public Health Service International Research Fellowship FOS TW 02770.

261

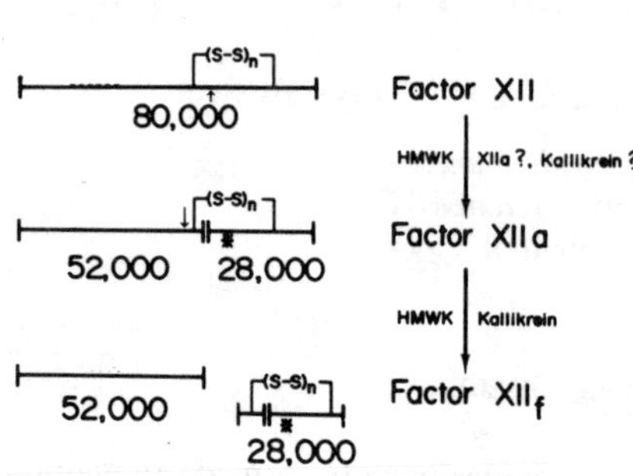

FIGURE 1. Activation scheme of factor XII. *Top:* Zymogen form of factor XII. The dashed area represents a negatively charged surface. The arrow within the disulfide bridges indicates the position of proteolytic cleavage. *Center:* Factor XIIa. The molecule comprises two chains linked by disulfide bridges. The light chain contains the active site serine (asterisk). The heavy chain contains the domain that binds to negatively charged surfaces. The arrow outside the disulfide bridges indicates the cleavage point of factor XIIa by plasma kallikrein. *Bottom:* Factor XII fragments. Factor XIIf (prekallikrein activator), $M_r = 28,000$, is the major activator of prekallikrein in the fluid phase.

attached to a surface, while the prekallikrein activator, or factor XIIf ($M_r = 28,000$),[7, 8] diffuses into the fluid phase. Factor XIIf can also arise from plasmin digestion of factor XII.[5, 9, 10] An activator of intermediate molecular weight has also been isolated.[5, 11] This fragment is resistant to further plasmin digestion and is not an intermediate in the pathway producing the fragments of molecular weight 28,000. These factor XII fragments, although possessing little coagulant activity compared to the parent molecule, have more potent prekallikrein activating ability, on a molar basis, and are responsible for liquid phase activation of prekallikrein.

Prekallikrein ($M_r = 88,000$) cleavage occurs within a disulfide bridge with exposure of an active site serine on the light chain ($M_r = 33,000$) (FIG. 2).[12, 13] The heavy chain ($M_r = 55,000$) remains attached to the surface bridged by HMW kininogen, and, thus, most of the kallikrein remains bound.

Purified HMW kininogen has a molecular weight of 210,000 upon Sephadex G-200 gel filtration, an isoelectric point of 4.3, and a molecular weight of 120,000 when assessed by SDS gel electrophoresis (FIG. 3). The molecular weight is unchanged after reduction, indicating that the HMW kininogen isolated was a single chain. Delineation of the relationship of structure to function has been possible by analysis of the cleavage of HMW kininogen by plasma kallikrein. A loss of peptide material, including bradykinin, of about 15,000 daltons was noted with formation of a heavy chain of 66,000 and a light chain of 37,000 daltons. When human HMW kininogen is cleaved by physiological concentrations of plasma kallikrein, there is no apparent loss in coagulant activity; furthermore, a combination of kallikrein cleavage, reduction and alkylation, and treatment with 6 M guanidine hydrochloride does not inactivate

FIGURE 2. Structure of prekallikrein and kallikrein. *Top:* Prekallikrein. The arrow within the disulfide bridges indicates the position of proteolytic cleavage by factor XIIf (or factor XIIa). *Bottom:* Kallikrein. The molecule comprises two chains linked by disulfide bridges. The light chain contains the active site serine (asterisk).

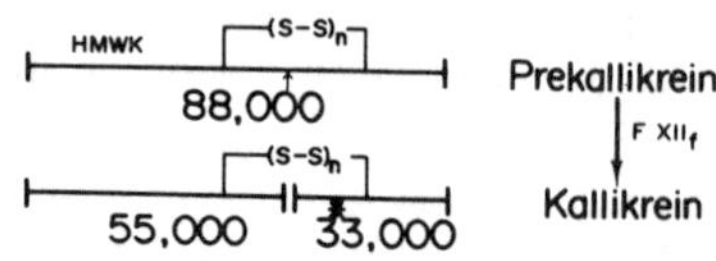

it.[14] All of the coagulant activity is associated with the HMW kininogen light chain. This finding confirms the observations of Colman *et al.*[15] and Schiffman and Lee,[16] who reported that kallikrein cleavage of human HMW kininogen did not diminish its coagulant activity. The light chain also appears to possess the major antigenic determinants that distinguish HMW kininogen from low molecular weight (LMW) kininogen, which is immunologically similar to the heavy chain.

With the discovery of HMW kininogen deficiency, the reciprocal mechanism, in which factor XIIa or XIIf converts prekallikrein to kallikrein, and kallikrein, in turn, activates factor XII, appeared to be an oversimplification. For example, while the addition of factor XIIa to factor XII–deficient plasma causes coagulation in the absence of kaolin by activation of factor XI, the addition of kallikrein to prekallikrein deficient plasma in the absence of a surface does not result in appreciable coagulation. Furthermore, the addition of factor XIIa to HMW kininogen–deficient plasma, even in the presence of a surface, does not significantly shorten its partial thromboplastin time.[17] HMW kininogen therefore appears to be required for the activation of factor XII and/or the expression of factor XIIa activity.

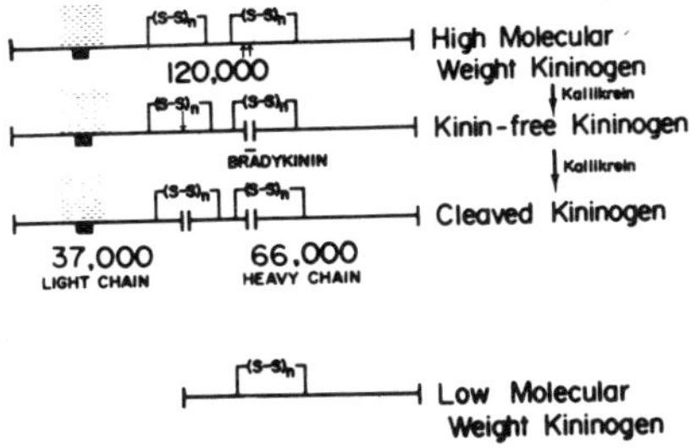

FIGURE 3. Structure of high molecular weight and low molecular weight kininogens. *Top:* High molecular weight kininogen. Limited proteolysis of high molecular weight kininogen by kallikrein leads to the liberation of the nonapeptide bradykinin from a domain located within disulfide bridges. Further digestion of kinin-free kininogen by kallikrein results in the formation of cleaved kininogen containing a 15,000 dalton polypeptide and two major chains. The light chain, $M_r = 37,000$, contains the region responsible for coagulant activity (black rectangle). The heavy chain, $M_r = 66,000$, has no coagulant activity and is immunologically indistinguishable from low molecular weight kininogen. *Bottom:* Low molecular weight kininogen. Low molecular weight kininogen contains the bradykinin region and the heavy chain, but not the light chain of high molecular weight kininogen.

Evidence has been presented that both prekallikrein[18] and factor XI circulate as complexes with HMW kininogen in plasma. The absence of such a prekallikrein–HMW kininogen complex results in an apparent decrease of prekallikrein concentration in the plasma of individuals with no HMW kininogen. Although this association has been suspected to be due to genetic linkage, Scott and Colman have recently demonstrated that the low prekallikrein in those individuals is an artifactual consequence of the functional and immunochemical assays employed.[19] The addition of HMW kininogen to plasma deficient in that protein corrects the apparent prekallikrein deficiency by forming the prekallikrein–HMW kininogen complex, which is more reactive in both functional and immunochemical assays.

However, the events involving kallikrein formation in plasma cannot be fully understood without considering the role of C$\bar{1}$ inhibitor (C$\bar{1}$ INH). This plasma α_2 globulin is the major inhibitor of factor XIIa and factor XIIf, as well as C$\bar{1}$r and C$\bar{1}$s.[20-23] The C$\bar{1}$ INH has been shown to bind and irreversibly inactivate both factor XIIa and XIIf. Moreover, $\overline{C1}$ INH appears to be the major inhibitor of plasma kallikrein.[24] $\overline{C1}$ INH binds to the active site of the enzyme such that all esterolytic and proteolytic activities are inhibited and a 1:1 stoichiometric complex is found.[25, 26]

This paper reports on yet another role of HMW kininogen, the protection of kallikrein from inhibition by C1 INH.

RESULTS AND DISCUSSION

Since the addition of HMW kininogen increased the functional activity of prekallikrein in the plasma of HMW kininogen–deficient individuals, we evaluated the effect of additional HMW kininogen on the kaolin-activated arginine esterase (kallikrein) activity of 13 normal donors' native plasma, as well as plasma in which the inhibitors were inactivated by $CHCl_3$ treatment (FIG. 4).[19] Addition of 0.2 U/ml HMW kininogen to native plasma increased the mean arginine esterase activity (kallikrein) in all plasmas. The difference between the means was significant ($p < 0.001$ by paired Student's t test). The correlation of the activity in the supplemented plasma with activity in the native plasma was excellent ($r = 0.91$). Removal of $\overline{C1}$ INH by $CHCl_3$ treatment yielded an even more striking increase in kallikrein activity. However, no increase in esterase activity occurred after supplementation of the inhibitor-depleted plasma with HMW kininogen, suggesting that the naturally occurring kallikrein inhibitors were limiting the activation or activity.

The effect of the inhibitor is even more evident when factor XIIf is used to activate purified prekallikrein (FIG. 5) in the fluid phase in the absence of kaolin. The rate of prekallikrein activation by XIIf is enhanced by purified HMW kininogen, which prevents surface-induced loss of kallikrein.[27] However, when native prekallikrein-deficient plasma (a source of HMW kininogen and $\overline{C1}$ INH) was added to purified prekallikrein and then activated by XIIf, a maximum of only 30% of its potential activity was reached, as compared to the same amount of purified prekallikrein activated by XIIf in the presence of buffer. A decrease in activity occurred after 1 min; this was a result of the inhibition of kallikrein activity by the $\overline{C1}$ INH in the prekallikrein-deficient plasma. Inactivation of $\overline{C1}$ INH (by acid treatment) in the prekallikrein-deficient plasma before the addition of the purified prekallikrein, and its subsequent activation by XIIf resulted in rapid and complete activation of the prekallikrein. These observations suggested that a deficiency of HMW kininogen

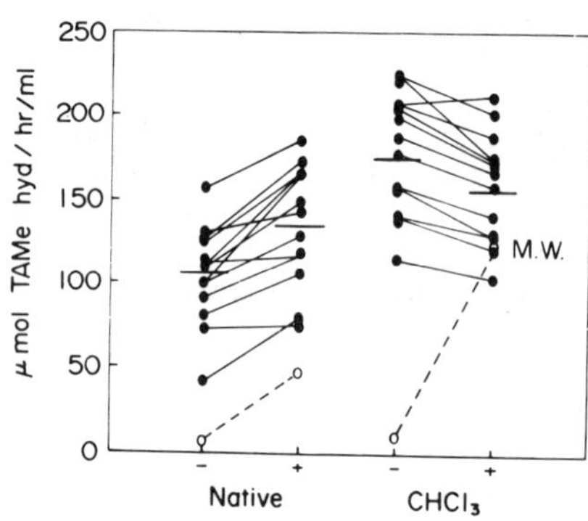

FIGURE 4. Effect of kallikrein inhibitors and HMW kininogen on kallikrein esterase activity in plasma. Native plasma in the absence (−) and presence (+) of additional HMW kininogen (0.2 U/ml) was assayed for TAMe esterase activity.[22] $CHCl_3$-treated plasma was also assayed for TAMe esterase activity in the absence (−) and presence (+) of additional HMW-kininogen (0.2 U/ml). ●: normal donors; ○: kininogen deficient plasma; (M.W.): Mrs. M. Williams.[15]

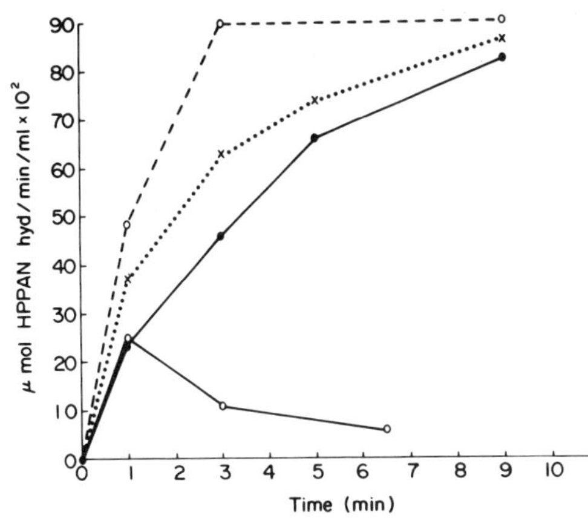

FIGURE 5. Effect of plasma kallikrein inhibitors on kallikrein amidolytic activity. 10 μl (5 μg) of purified prekallikrein was incubated with 100 μl of either buffer (0.1 M sodium phosphate, pH 7.6, containing 0.15 M NaCl and 1 mg/ml bovine serum albumin), native prekallikrein-deficient plasma, or purified HMW kininogen (0.2 U/ml), before addition of 20 μl (1 μg) XIIf. 10 μl aliquots were assayed at various times for the ability to hydrolyze H-D-Pro-Phe-Arg-*p*-nitroanilide-HCl (HPPAN). PK: prekallikrein; ●—●: PK plus buffer; ○—○: PK plus prekallikrein-deficient plasma (native); ○---○: PK plus prekallikrein-deficient plasma (acid-treated); X . . . X: PK plus HMW kininogen. Reproduced from J. Clin. Invest. **65**: 418,[19] with permission.

in plasma can retard the rate of prekallikrein activation long enough to be significantly affected by plasma kallikrein inhibitors.

The functional role of HMW kininogen appears to be in speeding the rate of activation of prekallikrein so as to allow the formation of kallikrein to exceed the rate of its inactivation by plasma inhibitors, in particular $C\bar{1}$ INH. Thus, in inhibitor-depleted normal plasma, activation of prekallikrein by a negative surface proceeds at a similar rate with or without additional HMW kininogen. This finding suggested another role for this cofactor. It is possible that, when HMW kininogen binds to kallikrein, it retards the destruction of the kallikrein activity by competing for binding sites that would otherwise be available to $C\bar{1}$ INH. The importance of $C\bar{1}$ INH is increased when activation proceeds more slowly, as exemplified by experiments using purified XIIf to activate prekallikrein.

Direct evidence for the protection of kallikrein from the action of $C\bar{1}$ INH is shown in FIGURE 6. Purified kallikrein was added to normal plasma or to HMW kininogen–deficient plasma. The rate of inhibition of kallikrein was much greater in the plasma containing no kininogen. This cannot be accounted for by the concentration of $C\bar{1}$ INH, since it was assayed by radial immunodiffusion and adjusted to similar values in normal and kininogen-deficient plasma. Plasma deficient in prekallikrein or factor XII did not show any difference in the inhibition rate of purified kallikrein when compared to normal plasma.

To further delineate this process, we first studied the reaction in a purified system where the only reactants were kallikrein and $C\bar{1}$ INH.[28] The inhibition of kallikrein by $C\bar{1}$ INH was pseudo–first order in the presence of a molar excess of inhibitor. When a double reciprocal plot of the pseudo–first order rate constant versus the concentration of the inhibitor was constructed, the line passed through the origin. This result is consistent with the direct inactivation of kallikrein ($E + I \rightarrow EI^*$) rather than the existence of a prior equilibrium or detectable reversible complex ($E + I \rightleftharpoons EI \rightarrow EI^*$). When similar experiments were performed in the presence of purified HMW kininogen at each concentration of inhibitor, a diminished pseudo–first order rate constant was observed at each concentration of HMW kininogen tested. A decrease in the rate of inhibition was found as the concentration of HMW kininogen was increased, in the physiological range (0.5–2.0 U/ml). The ability of HMW kininogen to compete with C$\overline{1}$ INH for kallikrein suggested that the previous results with kallikrein and C$\overline{1}$ INH obeyed the following kinetic expression:

$$E + I \xrightarrow{k''} EI$$

$$E + C \underset{k_{-1}}{\overset{k_1}{\rightleftharpoons}} EC,$$

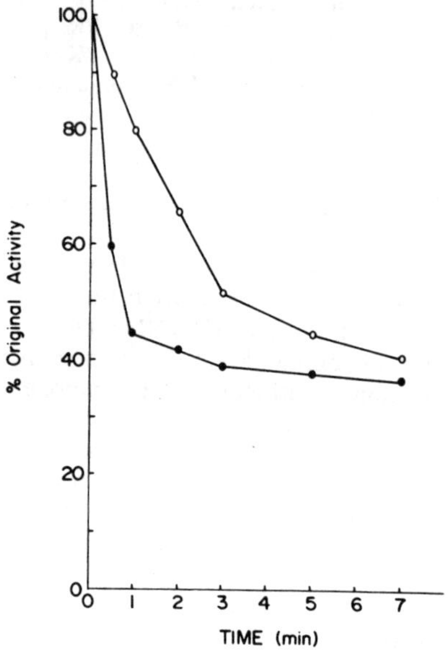

FIGURE 6. Purified kallikrein[15] was incubated at 25° with either normal human plasma (○) or plasma from an individual with HMW kininogen deficiency (●). Aliquots were removed and assayed, at various times, for residual kallikrein activity by an amidolytic assay.

where E = kallikrein, I = C$\overline{1}$ INH, k'' = second order rate constant, C = HMW kininogen, and K_d (dissociation constant for EC complex) = k_1/k_{-1}. Calculation of K_d for the kallikrein–HMW kininogen complex was performed using the following equation:

$$k'_{\text{app}} = \frac{k'}{1 + \dfrac{(C)}{K_d}},$$

where k' = pseudo–first order rate constant (no C) and k'_{app} = pseudo–first order rate constant (with C). The K_d was found to be almost identical to the concentration of HMW kininogen in plasma (80 μg/ml or 0.75 μM). Small changes in HMW kininogen concentration will give potentially large changes in the ratio of bound kallikrein to free kallikrein and thus closely regulate its activity. This value contrasts with the value of 0.029 μM reported by Thompson *et al.*[29] This apparent discrepancy may be due to two experimental differences. The dissociation constant in this report is calculated from kinetic concentrations during the interaction in the fluid phase, while that of Thompson *et al.* measured the binding of prekallikrein to HMW kininogen on a surface where interaction may be strengthened by HMW kininogen surface binding. Also, our constant is determined with kallikrein, the active enzyme, rather than prekallikrein, the zymogen, which may have a different K_d.

To further explore whether the protection of HMW kininogen was due to the formation of a complex between the coenzyme and kallikrein or to a specific effect on C1 INH, we studied the effect of another inhibitor of kallikrein (Fig. 7), soybean trypsin inhibitor (SBTI). Kallikrein (1.5×10^{-8} M) was incubated with various concentrations of SBTI. HMW kininogen decreased the inhibition of kallikrein by this protease inhibitor in a concentration-dependent manner. Since the M_r of SBTI (21,000) is much less than that of C1 INH,

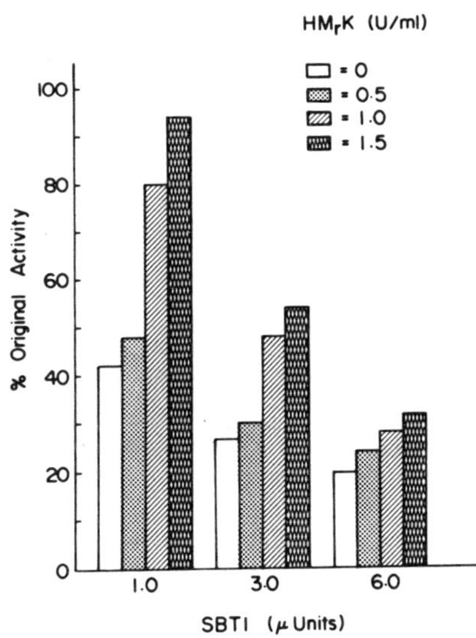

FIGURE 7. Kallikrein inhibition by soybean trypsin inhibitor in the absence and presence of HMW kininogen. Kallikrein was incubated for 1 min with SBTI at a final concentration of 1, 3, and 6 $\mu U/ml$ (1 μU = 0.1 μmol). The residual kallikrein activity was measured with an amidolytic assay in the presence or absence of high molecular weight kininogen (HM_rK).

it appeared that the portion of kallikrein that is involved in HMW kininogen binding might be near the active site of the enzyme.

To further define the mechanism of this reaction, we explored which domains of the components of the reversible complex between kallikrein (enzyme) and HMW kininogen (cofactor-substrate) were responsible for protection against C1̄ INH. Since prekallikrein is transformed to kallikrein when it is cleaved by activated factor XII into a heavy chain (55,000) and a light chain (33,000), which contains the active site serine residue, it would be expected that HMW kininogen would protect against inhibition by diisopropylfluoro phosphate (DFP), which inactivates kallikrein at its active site,[30] if the light chain of kallikrein was involved. A decrease of the rate of inactivation by DFP proportional to the concentration of HMW kininogen was found, indicating either that the binding site is near the active site or that steric hinderance protects the active site.

Since HMW kininogen has two chains after cleavage by kallikrein—the heavy chain, M_r 66,000, which is similar to or identical with LMW kininogen and the light chain, MW 37,000, which contains the portion responsible for coagulant activity and is unique to HMW kininogen—we tested the ability of LMW kininogen to alter the inactivation rate of kallikrein by C$\bar{1}$ INH. No change in the rate of kallikrein inactivation by C$\bar{1}$ INH was found, even at a concentration of LMW kininogen that was 40-fold that concentration of the HMW kininogen which gave protection. These results suggested that the light chain of HMW kininogen might be involved in the binding to kallikrein. Since the bradykinin portion of the molecule is localized in the heavy chain, which is characteristic of both LMW and HMW kininogen, substrate protection of kallikrein against inhibitors seems less likely. In addition, isolated light chain not only decreases the rate of inactivation of kallikrein by C$\bar{1}$ INH but the calculated K_d for the kallikrein-light chain complex is 5-fold lower than for intact HMW kininogen.

To rule out the possibility that an interaction of HMW kininogen with C$\bar{1}$ INH was responsible for the increased activity, we studied plasmin, another serine protease known to be inhibited by this inhibitor. In agreement with the results of Ratnoff [20] and Harpel and Cooper,[22] we found a rapid inhibition of plasmin by C$\bar{1}$ INH, proportional to the concentration of the inhibitor used. However, HMW kininogen (1 U/ml) failed to affect the rate of inhibition, indicating that there is no direct interaction between C$\bar{1}$ INH and HMW kininogen.

CONCLUSIONS

A new role for HMW kininogen appears to be partial protection of the active kallikrein against the action of C$\bar{1}$ INH. This action apparently depends on the formation of a reversible complex of HMW kininogen and kallikrein in the liquid phase with a K_d similar to the concentration of HMW kininogen in plasma. This complex apparently involves the light chain of kallikrein, which contains the active site serine, and the light chain of HMW kininogen, which contains the coagulant activity. No direct interaction between C$\bar{1}$ INH and HMW kininogen was demonstrated, since plasmin, which is inhibited by C$\bar{1}$ INH but does not enter into a complex with HMW kininogen, is not protected. This protective role for HMW kininogen appears not only in purified systems, but also in plasma. This finding constitutes yet another regulatory mechanism for the activation and inhibition of kallikrein, which influences the coagulation, fibrinolytic, and kinin-forming systems.

ACKNOWLEDGMENTS

We thank Ms. Terry Cruice for typing this manuscript. We also thank Ms. Lee D. Silver for preparing purified high molecular weight kininogen.

REFERENCES

1. GIREY, G. J. D., R. C. TALAMO & R. W. COLMAN. 1972. The kinetics of the release of bradykinin by kallikrein in normal human plasma. J. Lab. Clin. Med. **80:** 496–505.

2. MARGOLIS, S. 1960. The mode of action of Hageman factor in the release of plasma kinin. J. Physiol. (London) **15:** 238–245.

3. WEBSTER, M. E. & O. D. RATNOFF. 1961. Role of Hageman factor in the activation of vasodilation activity in human plasma. Nature (London) **192:** 180–181.

4. RATNOFF, O. D. & H. SAITO. 1979. Amidolytic properties of single-chain activated Hageman factor. Proc. Natl. Acad. Sci. USA **76:** 1461–1463.

5. BAGDASARIAN, A., B. LAHIRI & R. W. COLMAN. 1973. Origin of the high molecular weight activator of prekallikrein. J. Biol. Chem. **248:** 7742–7747.

6. COCHRANE, C. G., S. D. REVAK & K. D. WUEPPER. 1973. Activation of Hageman factor in solid and fluid phases. A critical role of kallikrein. J. Exp. Med. **138:** 1564–1583.

7. KAPLAN, A. P. & K. F. AUSTEN. 1970. A prealbumin activator of prekallikrein. J. Immunol. **105:** 802–811.

8. SOLTARY, M. J., H. Z. MOVAT & A. H. OZGE-ANWAR. 1971. The kinin system of human plasma. V. The probable derivation of prekallikrein activator from activated Hageman factor (XIIa). Proc. Soc. Exp. Biol. Med. **138:** 952–958.

9. KAPLAN, A. P. & K. F. AUSTEN. 1971. A prealbumin activator of prekallikrein. II. Derivation of activators of prekallikrein from active Hageman factor by digestion with plasmin. J. Exp. Med. **133:** 696–712.

10. BURROWES, C. E., H. V. MOVAT & M. J. SOLTAY. 1971. The kinin system of human plasma. VI. The action of plasmin. Proc. Soc. Exp. Biol. Med. **138:** 959–966.

11. BAGDASARIAN, A., R. C. TALAMO & R. W. COLMAN. 1973. Isolation of high molecular weight activators of prekallikrein. J. Biol. Chem. **248:** 3456–3463.

12. MANDLE, R. & A. P. KAPLAN. 1977. Hageman factor substrates. Human plasma prekallikrein: Mechanism of activation by Hageman factor and participation in Hageman factor-dependent fibrinolysis. J. Biol. Chem. **252:** 6097–6103.

13. SCOTT, C. F. & R. W. COLMAN. 1979. Human plasma kallikrein: A rapid high yield method for purification. Eur. J. Biochem. **100:** 77–83.

14. THOMPSON, R. E., R. MANDLE, JR. & A. P. KAPLAN. 1978. Characterization of human high molecular weight kininogen. Procoagulant activity associated with the light chain of kinin-free high molecular weight kininogen. J. Exp. Med. **147:** 488–499.

15. COLMAN, R. W., A. BAGDASARIAN, R. C. TALAMO, C. F. SCOTT, M. SEAVEY, J. A. GUIMARAES, J. V. PIERCE & A. P. KAPLAN. 1975. Williams trait. Human kininogen deficiency with diminished levels of plasminogen pro-activator and prekallikrein associated with abnormalities of the Hageman factor-dependent pathways. J. Clin. Invest. **56:** 1650–1662.

16. SCHIFFMAN, S. & P. LEE. 1975. Partial purification and characterization of contact activation cofactor. J. Clin. Invest. **56:** 1082–1092.

17. MEIER, H. K., M. E. WEBSTER, R. MANDLE, R. W. COLMAN & A. P. KAPLAN. 1977. Enhancement of the surface dependent Hageman factor activation by high molecular weight kininogen. J. Clin. Invest. **60:** 18–30.

18. MANDLE, R., R. W. COLMAN & A. P. KAPLAN. 1976. Identification of pre-kallikrein and high molecular weight (HMW) kininogen as a circulating complex in human plasma. Proc. Natl. Acad. Sci. USA **73:** 4179–4183.

19. SCOTT, C. F. & R. W. COLMAN. 1980. Function and immunochemistry of prekallikrein high molecular kininogen complex in plasma. J. Clin. Invest. **65:** 413–421.

20. RATNOFF, O. D., J. PENSKY, D. OGSTON & G. B. NAFF. 1969. The inhibition of plasmin, plasma kallikrein, plasma permeability factor, and the C'1r subcomponent of the first component of complement by serum C'1 esterase inhibitor. J. Exp. Med. **129:** 315–331.

21. FORBES, C. O., J. PENSKY & O. D. RATNOFF. 1970. Inhibition of activated

Hageman factor and activated plasma thrombplastin antecedent by purified C1 inactivator. J. Lab. Clin. Med. **76:** 809–815.

22. HARPEL, P. C. & N. R. COOPER. 1975. Studies on human plasma $C\bar{1}$ inactivator-enzyme interactions I mechanisms of interactions with $C\bar{1}s$ plasmin and trypsin. J. Clin. Invest. **55:** 593–604.

23. SCHREIBER, A. D., A. P. KAPLAN & K. F. AUSTEN. 1973. Inhibition by $C\bar{1}$ INH of Hageman factor fragment activation of coagulation, fibrinolysis and kinin-generation. J. Clin. Invest. **52:** 1402–1409.

24. McCONNELL, D. J. 1972. Inhibitors of kallikrein in human plasma. J. Clin. Invest. **51:** 1611–1623.

25. HARPEL, P. C. 1974. Circulating inhibitors of human plasma kallikrein. *In* Chemistry and Biology of the Kallikrein-Kinin System in Health and Disease, Fogarty International Center Proceedings No. 27. J. J. Pisano & K. F. Austen, Eds. 169–177. U.S. Government Printing Office. Washington, DC.

26. GIGLI, I., J. W. MASON, R. W. COLMAN & K. F. AUSTEN. 1970. Interaction of plasma kallikrein with the C1 inhibitor. J. Immunol. **104:** 574–581.

27. SCOTT, C. F., E. P. KIRBY, P. K. SCHICK & R. W. COLMAN. 1981. Effects of surfaces on fluid-phase prekallikrein activation. Blood **57:** 553–560.

28. SCHAPIRA, M., C. F. SCOTT & R. W. COLMAN. 1981. Protection of human plasma kallikrein from inactivation by $C\bar{1}$-inhibitor and other protease inhibitors. The role of high molecular weight kininogen. Biochemistry. In press.

29. THOMPSON, R. E., R. MANDLE, JR. & A. P. KAPLAN. 1979. Studies of binding of prekallikrein and factor XI to high molecular weight kininogen and its light chain. Proc. Natl. Acad. Sci. USA **76:** 4862–4866.

30. COLMAN, R. W., L. MATTLER & S. SHERRY. 1969. Studies on the prekallikrein (kallikreinogen)-kallikrein enzyme system of human plasma I. Isolation and purification of plasma kallikreins. J. Clin. Invest. **48:** 11–22.

BIOSYNTHESIS OF PROTHROMBIN COMPLEX PROTEINS *

J. W. Suttie, J. McTigue, A. E. Larson, and R. Wallin

Department of Biochemistry
College of Agricultural and Life Sciences
University of Wisconsin–Madison
Madison, Wisconsin 53706

INTRODUCTION

Prothrombin (factor II) and the other vitamin K–dependent plasma clotting factors (VII, IX, and X) are synthesized in the liver in a reaction involving the vitamin K–dependent conversion of specific glutamyl residues of microsomal precursor proteins to γ-carboxyglutamyl (Gla) residues of finished proteins. This conversion is essential for the calcium-dependent clotting factor–phospholipid interaction involved in the physiological action of these proteins. This reaction was first demonstrated in crude microsomal preparations from vitamin K–deficient rats by Esmon et al.[1] and, soon after, was shown to require the reduced form of vitamin K (KH_2) and molecular oxygen. Extensive studies of this activity over the past few years have been recently reviewed;[2, 3] the details of these studies will not be considered here. An indication of the current progress in this area can also be found in the proceedings of a recent symposium on vitamin K–dependent proteins.[4] In addition to the carboxylase, there are other vitamin K–related activities present in microsomes (FIG. 1), and much of the current interest in the field has centered around the possible interrelationship of these activities.

GENERAL PROPERTIES OF THE CARBOXYLASE

Following the initial demonstration of the vitamin K–dependent carboxylase in postmitochondrial supernatants from vitamin K–deficient rat liver, this reaction was studied in washed microsomes and, subsequently, in detergent-solubilized microsomes. Early studies of the carboxylase followed the incorporation of $^{14}CO_3^-$ into precursors of the vitamin K–dependent clotting factors that accumulate in rat liver microsomes when vitamin K action is blocked. Suttie et al. then demonstrated that the pentapeptide, Phe-Leu-Glu-Glu-Val, which is homologous to residues 5–9 of the bovine prothrombin precursor, serves as a substrate for the carboxylase.[5] Low molecular weight peptide substrates are now routinely used to assay carboxylase activity in rat liver microsomes. The properties of this general system are summarized in TABLE 1. The requirement for O_2 is absolute, and other electron acceptors will not substitute. The specificity for the vitamin is limited to 2-methyl-1,4-naphthoquinones with a relatively nonpolar substituent at the 3 position.

* This research was supported, in part, by the College of Agricultural and Life Sciences, University of Wisconsin–Madison and, in part, by grants from the National Institutes of Health, US Public Health Service, nos. AM-14881, DE-07031, and GM-07215.

271

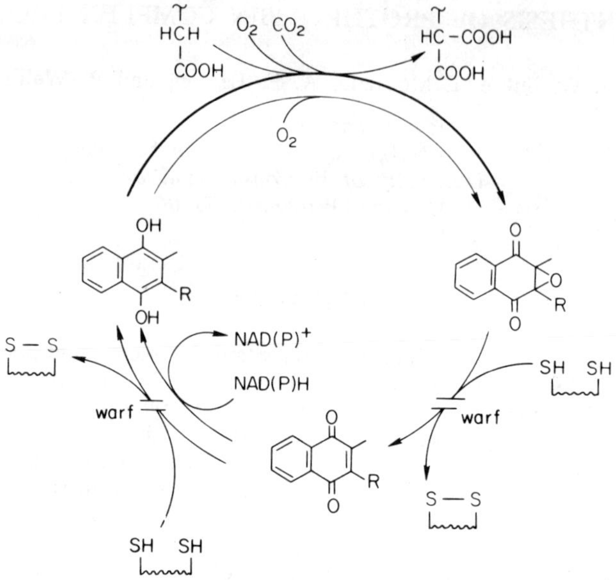

FIGURE 1. Vitamin K–related metabolic activities in rat liver microsomes. The relationship between the carboxylation and epoxidation reactions is discussed in the text. The pathways labeled Warf are those which are most sensitive to the action of the coumarin anticoagulants. The epoxide in *in vitro* studies is reduced by a pathway that uses dithiothreitol (DTT) as a reducing agent. The physiologically active reductant has not been identified. Vitamin K can be reduced to vitamin KH_2 by either a DTT-driven pathway or a NAD(P)H-linked dehydrogenase.

TABLE 1

PROPERTIES OF THE VITAMIN K–DEPENDENT MICROSOMAL CARBOXYLASE

Required	Stimulatory	Inhibitors
Vitamin KH_2	DTT	Chloro K
O_2	High salt	Sulfhydryl poisons
CO_2	Pyridoxal-P	Free radical traps
	Mn^{++} salts	KCN
		Chelating agents
		t-Butyl-OOH
		Glutathione peroxidase

NOTE: Stimulation and inhibition of the carboxylase depends on the system and conditions employed. The general properties indicated here are those observed with detergent-solubilized microsomes, using a low molecular weight peptide as a substrate. Details are available in recent reviews.[2,3]

Phylloquinone or the natural menaquinones have good activity in *in vitro* systems, but shorter isoprenalogs, or even compounds with nonisoprenoid side chains, do have activity. Most preparations studied have considerable vitamin K/NAD(P)H oxidoreductase activity, and the system is active with either vitamin KH_2 or with (vitamin $K + NAD(P)H$). The available data would suggest that CO_2, not HCO_3^-, is the species involved in the carboxylation event.[6] Although the *in vitro* system is strongly stimulated by both pyridoxal-P and Mn^{++} salts, the physiological significance of these compounds is not known. A wide variety of compounds inhibit the action of the carboxylase, and it has not yet been possible to determine the specific site of action of most of them. The system is inhibited only weakly by the coumarin anticoagulants, which is consistent with the data suggesting that the vitamin K epoxide reductase is the important site of action of this class of drugs.[7] The requirements and conditions that are optimal for carboxylation of the endogenous microsomal precursors are similar, but differ somewhat from the peptide substrate system.[8]

Some information on the specificity of the enzyme toward low molecular weight substrates is now available (TABLE 2). Peptides with Glu-Glu sequences are the best substrates, adjacent residues do influence activity, and only free

TABLE 2

SUBSTRATE SPECIFICITY OF THE VITAMIN K–DEPENDENT CARBOXYLASE

Peptide	Activity	Peptide	Activity
Phe-Leu-Glu-Glu-Leu	100	Boc-Glu-Glu-Leu-OMe	107
Phe-Ala-Glu-Glu-Leu	72	Boc-Asp-Asp-Leu-OME	< 1
Phe-Gly-Glu-Glu-Leu	4	Boc-Gln-Gln-Leu-OMe	< 1
Leu-Glu-Glu-Leu	8	Boc-D-Glu-D-Glu-Leu-OMe	< 1
Phe-Glu-Leu-Glu-Leu	< 1	Boc-HGlu-HGlu-Leu-OMe	< 1

NOTE: All peptides were assayed at 1 mM and are compared to the activity of Phe-Leu-Glu-Glu-Leu. HGlu is D,L-homoglutamic acid; all other amino acid residues are L unless indicated. Data taken from Rich *et al.*[9]

Glu residues, and not similar analogs such as glutamine, aspartate, or homoglutamate, are carboxylated. Subsequent studies have shown that only the most amino-terminal of the two Glu residues in these peptide substrates is carboxylated and that a second unidentified modification of the newly formed Gla residue is catalyzed by the same microsomal preparations.[10, 11] Preliminary data suggest that this modification produces a derivatized Gla residue, but the complete characterization of this product is not yet available. The second product is derived by a microsomal enzyme in a non–vitamin K–dependent reaction from the Phe-Leu-Gla-Glu-Leu that was originally formed. Whether the modifications observed in the *in vitro* peptide substrate system are related to the physiologically important modifications involved in prothrombin processing[12] or are some unrelated microsomal activity remains to be demonstrated.

RELATIONSHIP OF CARBOXYLATION AND VITAMIN K EPOXIDATION

The same microsomal preparations that catalyze the vitamin K–dependent carboxylase reaction will also convert the vitamin to its 2,3-epoxide (FIGURE 1).

This enzymatic activity represents that of a typical internal monooxygenase, which utilizes reducing equivalents from the hydroquinone of the vitamin and incorporates molecular oxygen into the epoxide.[13] Willingham and Matschiner first studied this oxygenase and suggested that the vitamin K epoxidase activity of microsomes might be related to the carboxylation reactions.[14] A number of the early observations that supported the hypothesis that these two activities are part of the same activity have been reviewed[15] and confirmed by more recent data. The epoxidase and carboxylase activities have now been shown to be located in the same subcellular fraction, the rough endoplasmic reticulum (FIG. 2), whereas most microsomal hydroxylase/epoxidase activity is a property of the smooth membrane fraction. Carlisle and Suttie have also shown that these activities are associated with tightly-bound membrane proteins that, on the basis of their proteolytic enzyme sensitivity, are apparently located on the luminal surface of the microsomal membrane vesicle.[16]

Another indication of the relationship between these two activities is the demonstration (FIGURE 3) that the oxygen requirement for the two reactions is similar. The apparent K_m for O_2 appears to be about 0.05 atmospheres for both reactions. More direct evidence for the close coupling of these reactions has come from the demonstration that stimulation of carboxylation events through an increase in the concentration of a peptide substrate for the carboxylase also stimulates the epoxidation events in the system (FIGURE 4). The data in FIGURE 4 were obtained using microsomes from vitamin K–deficient rats that were given vitamin K shortly before they were killed. Under these conditions, the concentration of vitamin K–dependent protein precursors in the microsomes is very low. These precursors are carboxylated at a much more rapid rate than the added peptide substrates,[8] and, when the rate of carboxylation and epoxidation in the system is closely followed, it can be seen (FIGURE 5) that there is a burst of epoxide formation that appears to be associated with the rapid carboxylation of endogenous protein, followed by a slower rate of formation, dependent upon the peptide carboxylation.

These data suggest a close relationship between the carboxylation and epoxidation events, but do not indicate any stoichiometric relationship between them. This aspect has been probed by more recent studies. The data in

FIGURE 2. The distribution of vitamin K–dependent activities in rat liver subcellular preparations. The data are expressed as relative specific activities (U/mg protein), with the activity of the rough endoplasmic reticulum (RER) set at 100. The activities shown are: Vitamin K–dependent carboxylation of Phe-Leu-Glu-Glu-Leu (peptide), vitamin K–dependent carboxylation of endogenous microsomal protein (protein), and the vitamin K epoxidase activity. The hatched bars are the activity of the RER fractions, the dark bars the activity of the smooth microsomal fraction, and the shaded bars the activity of the nuclear fraction. The error bars represent SEM for 6–8 rats/group. Data from Carlisle and Suttie.[16]

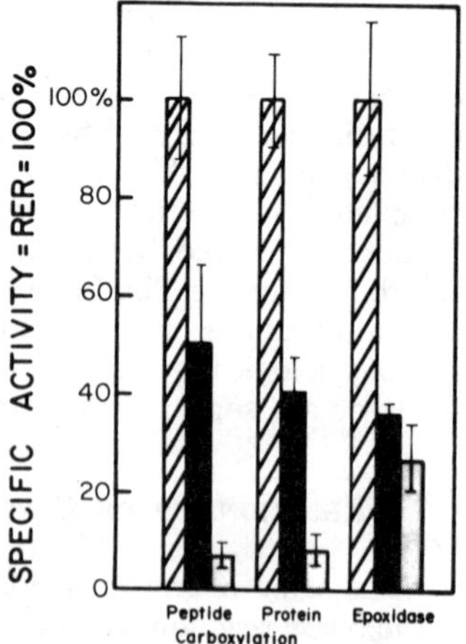

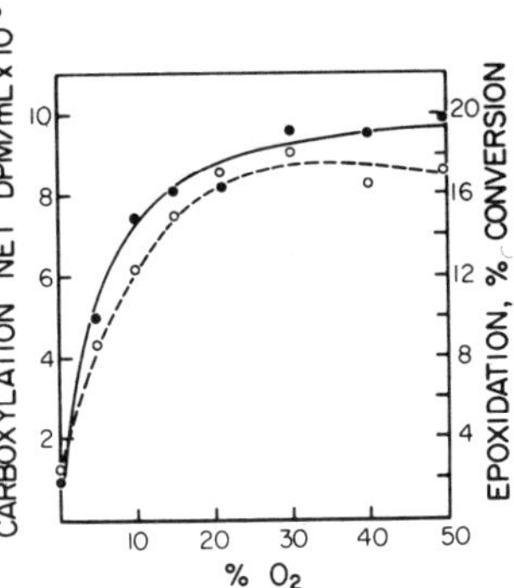

FIGURE 3. Oxygen dependence of the vitamin K–dependent carboxylation and vitamin K epoxidation. Carboxylation was measured as the vitamin KH_2–dependent carboxylation of Phe-Leu-Glu-Glu-Leu and epoxidation as the conversion of ^3H-vitamin KH_2 to the epoxide. The percentage of O_2 in a N_2 atmosphere was varied (McTigue and Suttie, unpublished data).

TABLE 3 demonstrate that the ratio of epoxide formed (KO) to CO_2 fixed is near unity if the extent of carboxylation is varied by increasing the peptide substrate concentration or by the addition of Mn^{++}, a stimulator of the reaction.[18] These reactions can, however, be uncoupled. At low concentrations of CO_2 (data not shown), the ratio can go over 10; when CN^- is added, the amount of CO_2 fixed is altered with little apparent change in epoxidation. Additional data to support the close association between these activities has come from attempts to purify the carboxylase. Although a preparation that is roughly 100-fold purified over intact microsomes in specific activity can be prepared,[19] further purification has been difficult. The results of a number of attempts to purify this activity by column chromatography are shown in TABLE 4. It can be seen that the epoxidase activity closely follows the carboxylase activity during these procedures, even though there has been a significant fractionation of the total protein in the preparation at each step of the purification.

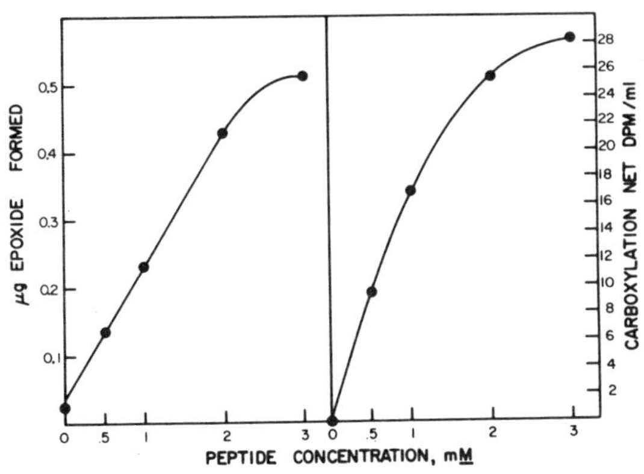

FIGURE 4. The effect of increasing substrate concentration on vitamin K–dependent carboxylation and epoxidation. Microsomes were prepared from vitamin K–deficient rats given vitamin K 30 min before they were killed to reduce endogenous precursor concentrations. The substrate used was Phe-Leu-Glu-Glu-Leu, and epoxidation was measured at the same vitamin K concentration as that used in the carboxylation incubations. For details, see Suttie *et al.*[17]

FIGURE 5. Rates of microsomal vitamin K–dependent carboxylation and vitamin K epoxidation. Vitamin K–dependent carboxylation of the peptide substrate Boc-Leu-Glu-Glu-Leu-OMe (■—■) and of endogenous microsomal protein precursors (●—●) were measured in the same incubation as the epoxidation of vitamin KH_2 (○—○) (McTigue and Suttie, unpublished data).

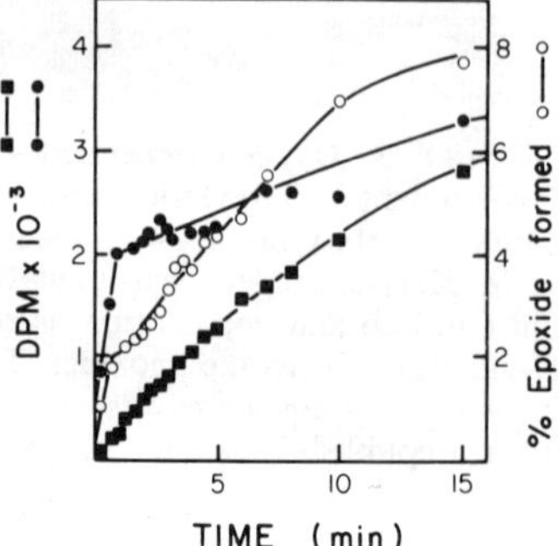

TABLE 3

RELATIONSHIP BETWEEN EPOXIDATION AND CARBOXYLATION

Substrate concentration	Additions	Gla	KO	KO/Gla
		μmol/ml $\times$ 10^{-3}		
1 mM	none	3.8	4.1	1.08
10 mM	none	7.3	6.5	0.89
10 mM	10 mM Mn^{++}	11.7	9.5	0.82
10 mM	10 mM KCN	2.7	6.0	2.22

NOTE: Partially purified microsomal preparation with Phe-Leu-Glu-Glu-Leu as a substrate, 50 μg/ml KH_2, and 5 mM CO_2 (Larson and Suttie, unpublished data).

TABLE 4

FRACTIONATION OF CARBOXYLASE AND EPOXIDASE ACTIVITY

Fraction	% Protein	% Carboxylase	Epoxidase/ carboxylase
Complex A	100	100	23.0
Sepharose-DOC II	60	100	21.3
Sepharose-lipid I	75	97	22.5
Sepharose-heparin I	75	90	20.3
Hydroxylapatite I	66	90	22.1

NOTE: Complex A, a partially purified preparation of the carboxylase [19] was dissolved in 1% Triton X-100 and separated by the four procedures shown into two fractions (I and II). The carboxylase-rich fraction from each column was applied to the next and the recovery of protein and carboxylase activity in each step was calculated as a percentage of that applied to the column. Although both fractions contained a significant amount of protein at each step, the carboxylase activity was present predominately in one fraction. Vitamin K epoxidase activity was also assayed in all the fractions and the ratio of carboxylase activity and epoxidase in each fraction was compared (Wallin and Suttie, unpublished data).

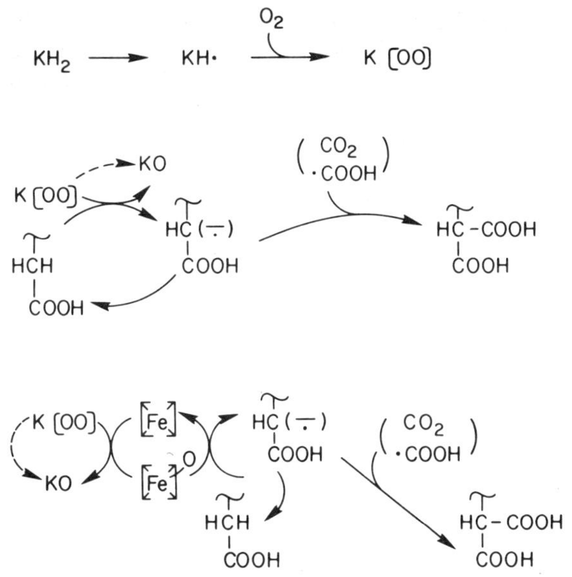

FIGURE 6. A possible molecular role of vitamin K. Current evidence would suggest (I) that some oxygenated intermediate (hydroperoxide or peroxyradical) of the vitamin is formed by attacks of the semiquinone (KH·) on oxygen. An alternate route of formation of this intermediate would be through the generation of superoxide by the vitamin. This intermediate may then be used (IIa) to drive the carboxylation event through hydrogen (proton) abstraction and generate the epoxide. The data available do not distinguish between the formation of a radical or carbanion on the γ-carbon of the glutamyl residue and the electronic nature of the attacking species. It is also possible (IIb) that the vitamin intermediate is used to activate a heme or other reaction center, and that this in turn drives the carboxylation. In either case, it must be possible for the epoxide to form without the carboxylation reaction occurring and for release of the γ-hydrogen to occur without a carboxylation event. Evidence to support any of these reactions is very indirect at this time, and other mechanisms of vitamin action are not ruled out by the available data.

MECHANISM OF THE CARBOXYLATION REACTION

The molecular role of vitamin K in the carboxylation of protein-bound glutamyl residues remains to be determined. The vitamin could function by "activating" or "transferring" CO_2, and considerable unsuccessful effort has been expended by various laboratories in an attempt to prove that it has such a role. The other alternative is that vitamin K functions to remove the hydrogen on the γ-position of the glutamyl residue to allow attack by CO_2 or some CO_2 derivative. Friedman *et al.* have demonstrated that vitamin KH_2 will promote release of a tritium label at the γ-position of the glutamyl residue and that this release is not dependent on the CO_2 concentration of the medium.[20] The data presented above support the hypothesis that epoxide formation is directly associated with the action of the vitamin in driving the carboxylation reaction, presumably this hydrogen abstraction event. Larson and Suttie have considered the possibility that a hydroperoxide of the vitamin would be a logical intermediate of the conversion of the vitamin to its epoxide and have shown that the enzyme glutathione peroxidase, which will reduce many organic hydroperoxides to the corresponding alcohol, will inhibit both the microsomal carboxylation and epoxidation reactions.[21] This indirect evidence for a possible hydroperoxide intermediate suggests that other compounds might substitute for the vitamin in this reaction, and *t*-butyl-OOH has been shown to be a very weak agonist of vitamin K in this reaction. In the presence of vitamin K, *t*-butyl-OOH acts as an apparent competitive inhibitor of the vitamin for both the carboxylation and epoxidation reactions. Although the data represent strong indirect evidence for the involvement of a hydroperoxide intermediate in the reactions, it should be stressed that no such derivative has yet been identified in the reaction mixture.

There are conflicting data [22–24] that support the hypotheses that the initial involvement of oxygen in the reaction is through an attack of the semiquinone of vitamin K on O_2 or that there is a vitamin K–mediated generation of superoxide followed by an attack of $\cdot O_2^-$ on the vitamin. There are no firm data to establish whether the final carboxylation event is ionically or radically mediated; nor is it clear whether the presumed oxygenated intermediate directly functions in the reaction or merely feeds into a heme center in the same way in which the P-450 system can utilize hydroperoxides to carry out its reaction (FIGURE 6). In any event, the role of vitamin K in clotting factor synthesis has been clearly demonstrated to be a cofactor in a postribosomal protein modification and systems are now becoming available that should allow a determination of the mechanism of this reaction at the molecular level.

REFERENCES

1. ESMON, C. T., J. A. SADOWSKI & J. W. SUTTIE. 1975. A new carboxylation reaction. The vitamin K-dependent incorporation of $H^{14}CO_3^-$ into prothrombin. J. Biol. Chem. **250:** 4744–4748.
2. SUTTIE, J. W. 1978. Vitamin K. *In* Handbook of Lipid Research. H. DeLuca, Ed. Vol. **2:** 211–217. Plenum Press. New York.
3. SUTTIE, J. W. 1980. Mechanism of action of vitamin K: Synthesis of γ-carboxyglutamic acid. Crit. Rev. Biochem. **8:** 191–223.
4. SUTTIE, J. W. ED. 1979. Vitamin K Metabolism and Vitamin K–dependent Proteins. University Park Press. Baltimore, Md.
5. SUTTIE, J. W., J. M. HAGEMAN, S. R. LEHRMAN & D. H. RICH. 1976. Vitamin K–dependent carboxylase: Development of a peptide substrate. J. Biol. Chem. **251:** 5827–5830.
6. JONES, J. P., E. J. GARDNER, T. G. COOPER & R. E. OLSON. 1977. Vitamin K–dependent carboxylation of peptide-bound glutamate. The active species of "CO_2" utilized by the membrane-bound preprothrombin carboxylase. J. Biol. Chem. **252:** 7738–7742.

7. WHITLON, D. S., J. A. SADOWSKI & J. W. SUTTIE. 1978. Mechanism of coumarin action: Significance of vitamin K epoxide reductase inhibition. Biochemistry **17:** 1371–1377.

8. SUTTIE, J. W., S. R. LEHRMAN, L. O. GEWEKE, J. M. HAGEMAN & D. H. RICH. 1979. Vitamin K–dependent carboxylase: Requirements for carboxylation of soluble peptide substrates and substrate specificity. Biochem. Biophys. Res. Commun. **86:** 500–507.

9. RICH, D. H., S. R. LEHRMAN, M. KAWAII, H. L. GOODMAN & J. W. SUTTIE. 1979. Rat liver vitamin K–dependent carboxylase: substrate specificity. *In* Vitamin K Metabolism and Vitamin K–dependent Proteins. J. Suttie, Ed.: 471–479. University Park Press. Baltimore, Md.

10. FINNAN, J. L. & J. W. SUTTIE. Carboxylation of low-molecular-weight substrates by the rat liver vitamin K–dependent carboxylase: Characterization of products. 1979. *In* Vitamin K Metabolism and Vitamin K–dependent Proteins. J. Suttie, Ed.: 509–517. University Park Press. Baltimore, Md.

11. RIKONG-ADIE, H., P. DECOTTIGNIES-LE MARECHAL, R. AZERAD & A. MARQUET. 1979. Vitamin K–dependent carboxylation of peptides containing the Glu-Glu sequence: Localization of γ-carboxyglutamic acid. *In* Vitamin K Metabolism and Vitamin K–dependent Proteins. J. Suttie, Ed.: 518–526. University Park Press. Baltimore, Md.

12. GRAVES, C. B., G. G. GRABAU, R. E. OLSON & T. W. MUNNS. 1980. Immunochemical isolation and electrophoretic characterization of precursor prothrombins in H-35 rat hepatoma cells. Biochemistry **19:** 266–272.

13. SADOWSKI, J. A., H. K. SCHNOES & J. W. SUTTIE. 1977. Vitamin K epoxidase: Properties and relationship to prothrombin synthesis. Biochemistry **16:** 3856–3863.

14. WILLINGHAM, A. K. & J. T. MATSCHINER. 1974. Changes in phylloquinone epoxidase activity related to prothrombin synthesis and microsomal clotting activity in the rat. Biochem. J. **140:** 435–441.

15. SUTTIE, J. W., A. E. LARSON, L. M. CANFIELD & T. L. CARLISLE. 1978. Relationship between vitamin K–dependent carboxylation and vitamin K epoxidation. Fed. Proc. Fed. Am. Soc. Exp. Biol. **37:** 2605–2609.

16. CARLISLE, T. L. & J. W. SUTTIE. 1980. Vitamin K–dependent carboxylase: Subcellular location of the carboxylase and enzymes involved in vitamin K metabolism in rat liver. Biochemistry **19:** 1161–1167.

17. SUTTIE, J. W., L. O. GEWEKE, S. L. MARTIN & A. K. WILLINGHAM. 1980. Vitamin K epoxidase: Dependence of epoxidase activity on substrates of the vitamin K–dependent carboxylation reaction. FEBS Lett. **109:** 267–270.

18. LARSON, A. E., D. S. WHITLON & J. W. SUTTIE. 1979. Factors affecting the vitamin K–dependent microsomal carboxylation system. Fed. Proc. Fed. Am. Soc. Exp. Biol. **38:** 876.

19. CANFIELD, L. M., T. A. SINSKY & J. W. SUTTIE. 1980. Vitamin K–dependent carboxylase: Purification of the rat liver microsomal enzyme. Arch. Biochem. Biophys. **202:** 515–524.

20. FRIEDMAN, P. A., M. A. SHIA, P. M. GALLOP & A. E. GRIEP. 1979. Vitamin K–dependent γ-carbon-hydrogen bond cleavage and the non-mandatory concurrent carboxylation of peptide bound glutamic acid residues. Proc. Nat. Acad. Sci. USA **76:** 3126–3129.

21. LARSON, A. E. & J. W. SUTTIE. 1978. Vitamin K–dependent carboxylase: evidence for a hydroperoxide intermediate in the reaction. Proc. Nat. Acad. Sci. USA **75:** 5413–5416.

22. LARSON, A. E., J. J. McTIGUE & J. W. SUTTIE. 1979. Investigation of the role of oxygen in the vitamin K–dependent carboxylase reaction. *In* Vitamin K Metabolism and Vitamin K–dependent Proteins. J. Suttie, Ed.: 413–421. University Park Press. Baltimore, Md.
23. ESNOUF, M. P., A. I. BURGESS, S. J. WALTER, M. R. GREEN, H. A. O. HILL, & M. L. OKOLOW-ZUBROWSKA. 1979. The role of superoxide in the carboxylation of glutamyl residues. *In* Vitamin K Metabolism and Vitamin K–dependent Proteins, J. Suttie, Ed.: 422–432. University Park Press. Baltimore, Md.
24. ESNOUF, M. P., M. R. GREEN, H. A. O. HILL & S. J. WALTER. 1979. The inhibition of the vitamin K–dependent carboxylation of glutamyl residues in prothrombin by some copper complexes. FEBS Lett. **107:** 146–150.

HUMORAL SUBSTANCES REGULATING THE LEVELS OF COAGULATION FACTORS: COAGULOPOIETINS *

Margaret Karpatkin and Simon Karpatkin

Departments of Pediatrics and Medicine
New York University Medical School
New York, New York 10016

Although much is known of the biochemistry of blood coagulation factors, the mechanisms that maintain constant levels of these factors have not been elucidated. We have demonstrated in rabbits that the biological levels of these factors can be modified by humoral substances which we have called coagulopoietins. These coagulopoietins have been demonstrated by lowering one or more clotting factors in a donor animal and then injecting this animal's plasma into a recipient animal. The factor(s) that have been lowered in the donor then rise above base-line in the recipient. Coagulation factors in the donor animals have been depleted by coumadin,[1,2] inducing disseminated intravascular coagulation (DIC),[3] injecting an antiserum against rabbit prothrombin,[4,5] and injecting an antiserum against rabbit factor X.[6,7]

COAGULOPOIETINS IN COUMADIN-TREATED RABBITS

New Zealand white rabbits were given coumadin intramuscularly until factors II, VII, IX, and X were all less than 20% of the pre-injection levels. The animals were then exsanguinated and their plasma separated and stored at $-30°$ C. Plasma from these animals was injected twice daily for 3 to 5 days into recipient rabbits from whom blood samples were drawn daily and the plasma stored at $-30°$ C. At the end of the experiment, factors II, VII, V, IX, and X were measured in the samples and compared to 3 separate base-line samples drawn on 3 separate days before starting the injection schedule. Factors II, VII, V, and X were measured by a biologic assay based upon the one-stage prothrombin time. Factor IX was measured by a method based on the partial thromboplastin time.

Factors II, VII, IX, and X rose significantly in the recipient animals when compared to the base-line values; factor V did not rise. Injection of as little as 0.25 ml of donor plasma twice a day for 3 days resulted in a significant rise of the vitamin K-dependent clotting factors in a recipient. Control recipient animals received plasma from donors who had been injected with saline instead of coumadin. Coagulation factors did not rise above base-line in the controls (FIGURE 1).

COAGULOPOIETINS IN ANIMALS SUBJECTED TO DISSEMINATED INTRAVASCULAR COAGULATION

Rabbits received a large intravenous injection of goat serum. Immediately following the injection, fibrinogen, platelets, and factors II, VII, V, and X all

* Supported by the National Science Foundation grant PCM 7918282 and the National Heart, Lung, and Blood Institute grant 13336-10.

281

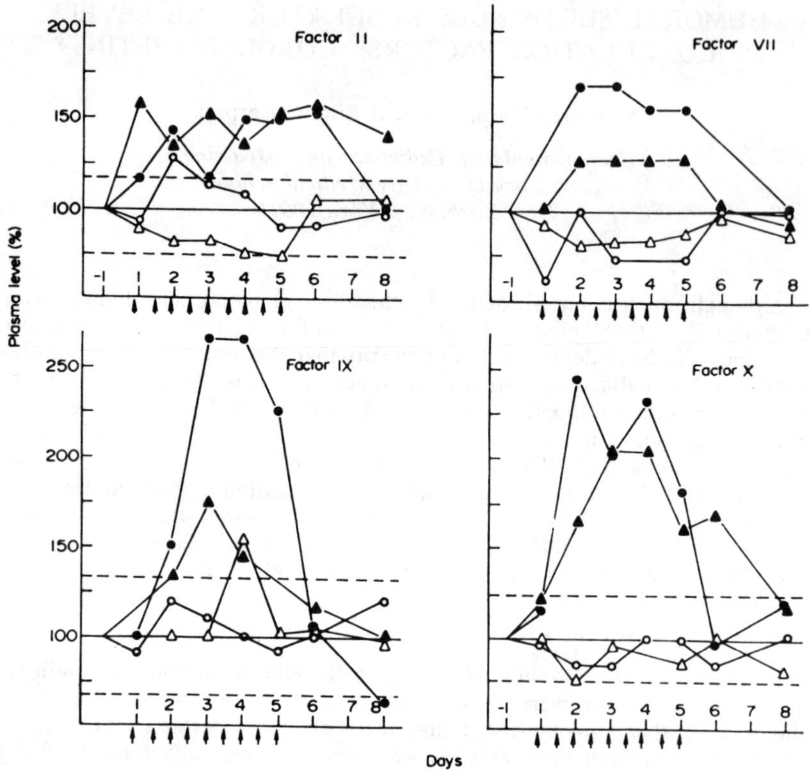

FIGURE 1. Changes in vitamin K-dependent coagulation factors in test and control recipient rabbits following injection of donor test and control plasma. Test animals had received i/m coumadin and control animals i/m saline. Arrows refer to intravenous injections of 4 ml of either test or control donor plasma, twice daily for 4½ days. Horizontal interrupted lines refer to ±2 SD for the assay. The symbols refer to test recipient 1, ●; test recipient 2, ▲; control recipient 1, ○; control recipient 2, △.

fell dramatically and then returned to above base-line values within 12–36 hours. These rabbits were exsanguinated 48 hours after receiving the intravenous serum and their plasma given intravenously twice a day to recipient rabbits for 4 days. Blood samples were drawn and compared to base-line values as described for the coumadin-treated animals. All coagulation factors measured (factors II, V, VII, and X) rose significantly above base-line in the recipients. Control recipient animals were similarly injected with normal rabbit plasma; their coagulation factors remained at base-line (FIGURE 2).

A COAGULOPOIETIN SPECIFIC FOR PROTHROMBIN (FACTOR II)

Rabbit prothrombin was purified as described by Morrison and Esnouf [8] and used to raise an antibody in a goat. The antibody gave one line on immunodiffusion and immunoelectrophoresis and when incubated with normal rabbit plasma, removed prothrombin activity without altering levels of factors V, VII, and X. The antiserum was partially purified by precipitation with 50% ammonium sulphate and was infused slowly (13.5 ml/kg over 1 to 2 hours) into the lateral ear vein of a rabbit. At the end of one hour the rabbit's prothrombin level was 48% of base-line and at 6 hours it was 60%. Levels of factors V, VII, and X, fibrinogen, and platelets did not vary significantly from base-line values. At the end of 6 hours this animal was exsanguinated. The plasma was injected into recipient animals and blood samples were drawn in a similar manner to that described for the coumadin and DIC experiments. Prothrombin rose significantly above base-line in the recipients, while factors V, VII, and X did not change (FIGURE 3). Control recipient animals were given plasma from a donor animal that had received normal goat serum partially purified with ammonium sulphate; prothrombin did not rise in these control recipient animals. Thus a coagulopoietin for one specific coagulation factor, prothrombin was demonstrated.

Prothrombin in 5 test and 5 control recipient animals was measured by an immunological technique.[9] The results in FIGURE 4 show that the increase above baseline levels was significantly less than the increase in biologic activity measured in the same samples of plasma.

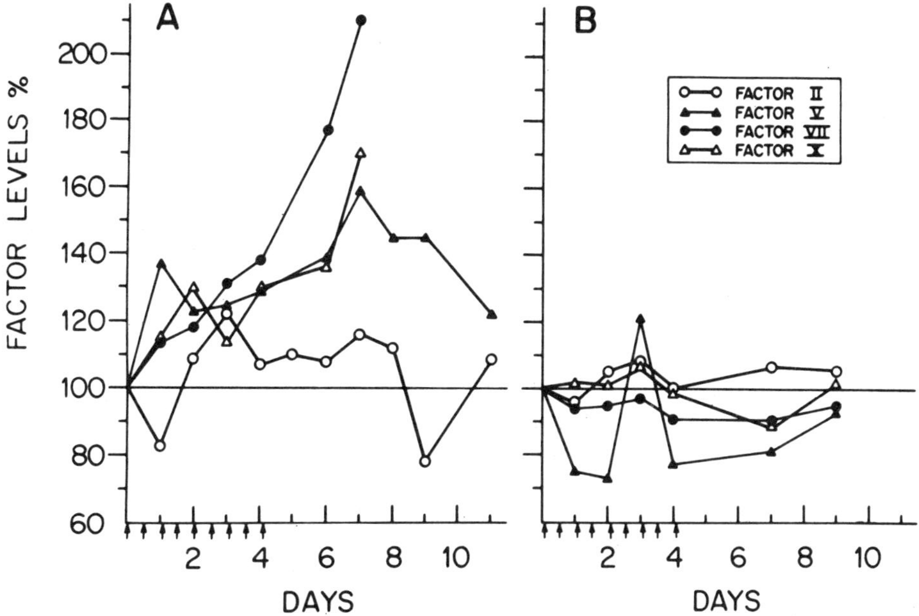

FIGURE 2. A. Response of seven normal recipient rabbits to the intravenous injection of plasma from rabbits given goat serum containing anti-rabbit factor II (five recipients) or normal goat serum (two recipients). The combined mean of seven experiments is given. The arrows refer to the intravenous injection of 1–4 ml plasma; O—O, factor II; ▲—▲, factor V; ●—●, factor VII; △—△, factor X. The 100% value refers to the mean of three samples drawn on each animal on three separate days prior to starting the injection schedule. B. Response of four normal recipient rabbits to the intravenous injection of plasma from normal rabbits. Protocol and symbols are the same as in A.

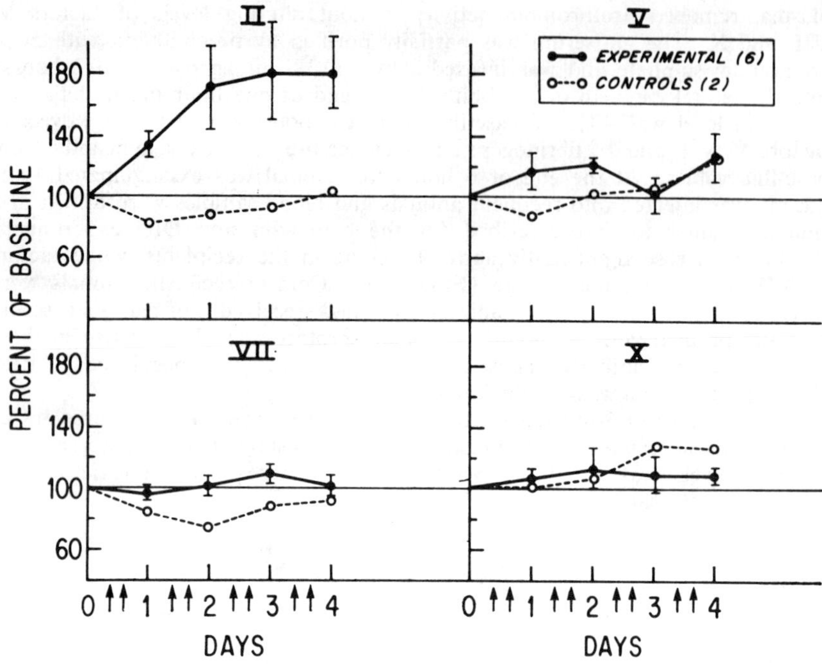

FIGURE 3. Coagulation-factor response of recipient rabbits to injection of experimental donor plasma and control donor plasma. Prothrombin in experimental donors had been lowered by infusion of goat antiserum, control donors had received normal goat serum. Three baseline samples were drawn on 3 different days before starting the injection schedule. Arrows indicate intravenous injection of 3 ml plasma. Samples were drawn on mornings of days 2, 3, 4, and 5. The SEM and number of experiments (*n*) are given.

Donor plasma was boiled for 30 minutes, the precipitate spun down, and the supernatant injected into recipient animals as in the previous experiments. Factor II rose significantly above base-line while V, VII, and X did not, thus demonstrating that the coagulopoietin for factor II is stable to boiling (FIG. 5).

Boiled donor plasma was gel filtered on a G-50 Sephadex column. The void volume and the retained volume were collected and injected into different recipient animals. In the animals who received the retained-volume prothrombin rose significantly. The void volume had no such effect. This suggests that the molecular weight of the coagulopoietin for factor II is <30,000.

Prothrombin production in an *in vitro* liver-mince system was studied. Minced liver from a freshly killed rabbit (35 mg/ml wet weight) was incubated at room temperature in Dulbecco's modification of Eagle's medium and 10% fetal calf serum. At the end of 5 hours the medium was changed and prothrombin was measured in the supernate over a 40 hour period by a two-stage technique.[10] Prothrombin activity in the supernatant rose over the period of study indicating that the liver was secreting prothrombin into the medium. Addition of cycloheximide, 5 mg/ml, to the medium inhibited prothrombin production. When coagulopoietin (boiled donor plasma 20 μg/ml) was added to the medium, more prothrombin appeared in the supernatant compared to a control with normal plasma added. Cycloheximide only partially inhibited the production of prothrombin associated with the coagulopoietin (FIGURE 6).

A COAGULOPOIETIN SPECIFIC FOR FACTOR X

Rabbit factor X was purified and used to raise an antibody in a sheep. Antiserum, partially purified by ammonium sulphate, was used to specifically lower factor X in a donor animal in a similar manner to the lowering of factor II by the goat antiserum. Factors II, V, VII, fibrinogen, and platelets were not affected. Six hours after commencing the infusion the animal was exsanguinated and this plasma was injected into normal recipients. Factor X was measured in the recipients by 3 different biologic assays (one-stage assay using bovine factor VII- and X-deficient plasma and Russell's viper venom; one-stage assay using human factor X-deficient plasma and thromboplastin; and chromogenic substrate and Russell's viper venom) and by immunoassay.[8] All four assays demonstrated an increase in factor X; the differences between the biologic assays were not statistically significant but the immunoassay showed an increase that was significantly lower than that demonstrated by the biological techniques (FIGURE 7). Factors II, V, and VII did not increase in the recipient animals (FIGURE 8).

The coagulopoietin for factor X, like that for prothrombin, was resistant to boiling for 20 minutes (FIGURE 9).

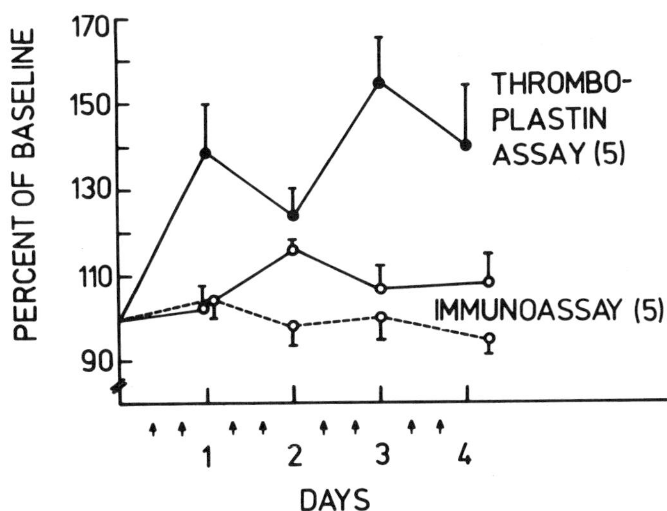

FIGURE 4. Comparison of biologic and immunologic activity±SEM of 5 rabbits injected with coagulopoietin II. Biologic activity of experimental animals (●—●), controls not shown; immunologic activity of experimental samples (○—○); control samples (○- - -○) p < 0.01 on day 2.

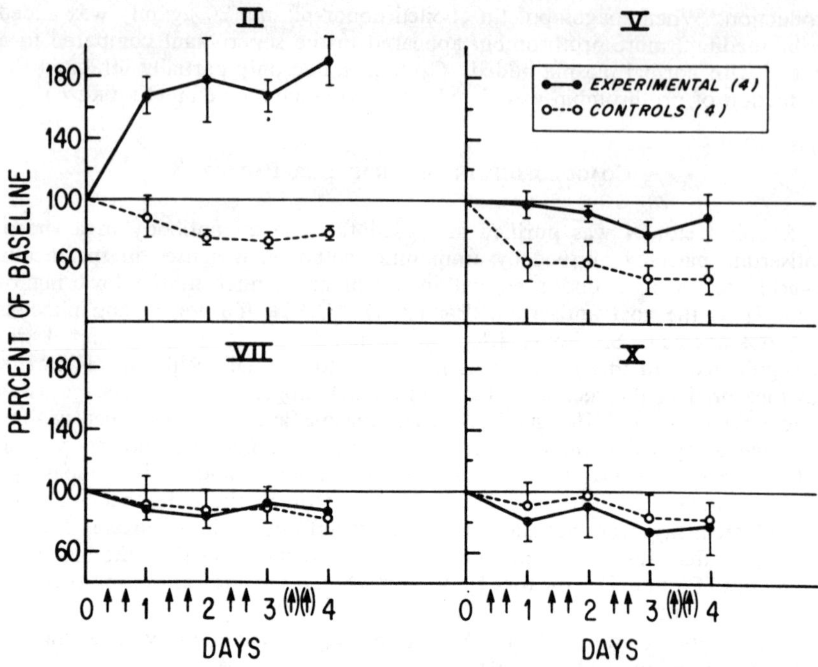

FIGURE 5. Coagulation factor response of recipient rabbits to injection of boiled experimental donor plasma and boiled control donor plasma. Prothrombin in experimental donors had been lowered by infusion of goat antiserum, control donors had received normal goat serum. Three baseline samples were drawn on 3 different days before starting the injection schedule. Arrows indicate intravenous injection of 3 ml plasma. In some experiments, the injections were omitted on day 4. Samples were drawn on mornings of days 2, 3, 4, and 5. The SEM and number of experiments (*n*) are given.

EFFECT OF COAGULOPOIETINS UPON CARBOXYLATION OF GLUTAMIC ACID RESIDUES

Vitamin K-dependent carboxylation was studied using the method of Esmon and co-workers.[11] A rabbit was given on injection of 30 mg of coumadin and sacrificed 18 hours later. The liver was removed and the microsomes prepared and solubilized in triton. The incorporation of $H^{14}CO_3^-$ into a trichloroacetic acid (TCA) precipitate was measured in the presence of vitamin K, NADH, and dithiothreitol. There was a linear increase in incorporation over a 40-minute time period and, as reported by others, incorporation was significantly greater when the experiment was performed at 21° C than at 37° C. If vitamin K was omitted from the reaction system, there was no incorporation of $H^{14}CO_3^-$ into microsomal protein. Plasma from an animal that had received coumadin was added to the system and compared to the addition of plasma from the same rabbit before coumadin. There was no difference in rate or amount of incorporation of $H^{14}CO_3^-$ into TCA-precipitable microsomal protein. Similar results were obtained when a specific antibody for prothrombin was employed to precipitate counts prior to TCA precipitation, indicating no difference in incorporation of $H^{14}CO_3^-$ into prothrombin-precipitable protein.

DISCUSSION

Data have been presented that demonstrate that humoral factors (coagulopoietins) raise the plasma levels of vitamin K-dependent coagulation factors in rabbits. Specific coagulopoietins have been demonstrated for prothrombin (coagulopoietin II) and factor X (coagulopoietin X). Both these coagulopoietins are stable to boiling and coagulopoietin II is retained in a G-50 Sephadex column suggesting a molecular weight of less than 30,000.

The data suggest that coagulopoietins operate by increasing the specific activity of the coagulation proteins. The evidence for this is: (1) When factors II and X were measured immunologically the increases in the recipient animals

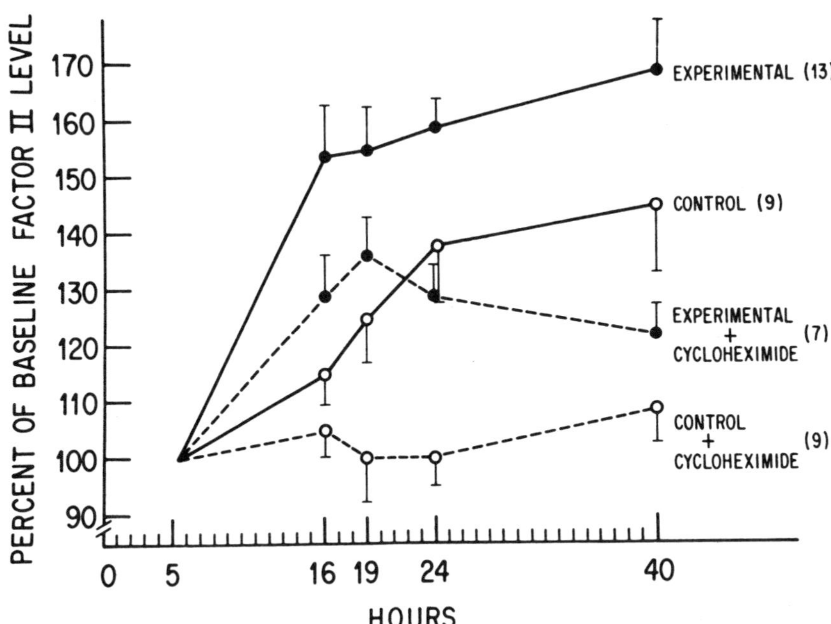

FIGURE 6. Prothrombin (factor II) response of an *in vitro* liver-mince system to incubation with boiled experimental plasma (●—●) or boiled control rabbit plasma (○—○). Boiled experimental and cycloheximide 5 mg/ml (●- - -●) and boiled control plasma and cycloheximide 5 mg/ml (○- - -○). Prothrombin in experimental rabbits had been lowered by infusion of goat antiserum, control rabbits had received normal goat serum. Liver mince (35 mg/ml, wet weight) was incubated in Dulbecco's modification of Eagle's medium, containing 10% fetal calf serum and 1.6 mg gentamicin per ml, in 95% O_2/5% CO_2. The medium was changed after 5 h and base-line samples were taken. Thereafter, 0.1-ml samples were taken at 16, 19, 24, and 40 h and assayed for factor II by the two-stage technique. Boiled control of experimental rabbit plasma containing 20 μg of protein per ml was added to the medium. Data are shown as mean ±SEM.

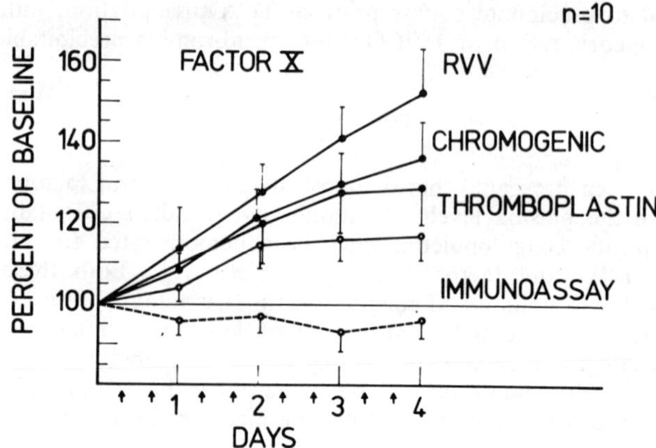

FIGURE 7. Assay of factor X by four different methods in 10 different rabbits. The separated plasma samples were frozen in portions at $-30°$ C. These were assayed with bovine factor VII- and X-deficient plasma and Russell's viper venom (RVV); human factor X-deficient plasma and thromboplastin; chromogenic substrate; and immunoassay (Laurell technique). The differences between the first three assays were not statistically significant. The differences between the immunoassay and these three assays were significant on days 2 ($p < 0.05$), 3 ($p < 0.01$), and 4 ($p < 0.05$). Control samples for the immunoassay were obtained from 10 rabbits injected with normal plasma. Differences between control (○- - -○) and experimental immunoassays were statistically significant on days 2 ($p < 0.05$), 3 ($p < 0.01$), and 4 ($p < 0.05$). SEM is given.

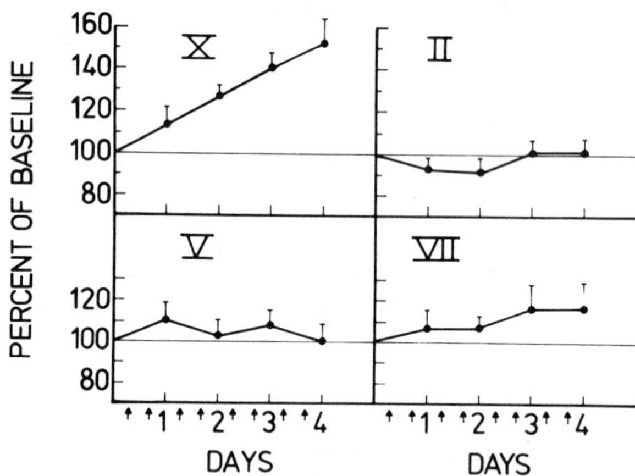

FIGURE 8. Effect of donor plasma from a rabbit partially depleted of factor X on coagulation factor levels in 10 recipient rabbits. Donor rabbits were infused with globulin fractions of goat anti-rabbit factor X (13 ml/kg) over a 1-h period. The donor animal was bled at 6 h and the plasma separated and frozen. 3 ml of donor plasma was injected intravenously, twice daily (arrows) for 4 d, and samples collected at midday on 4 different days. These were assayed for coagulation factor activity and were expressed as percentage fof the average of three base-line samples collected on 3 or more days before infusion of the experimental plasma. SEM is given.

were less than the increases in biological activity in the same plasma samples (FIGURES 4 and 7). (2) When prothrombin in a liver-mince system was studied, prothrombin was secreted into the medium by the liver cells in the presence of cycloheximide when plasma containing coagulopoietin II was present in the medium. When normal plasma was added to the medium in control experiments no prothrombin was secreted in the presence of cycloheximide. In further support, our data have been confirmed by Shah and co-workers using vitamin K-deficient rats as donor animals. They demonstrated a rise in prothrombin in the recipient animals using a two-stage biological assay but no rise by immunoassay.[12]

This relative lack of increase in protein synthesis suggests that coagulopoietins are inducing the secretion into the plasma of clotting factors with

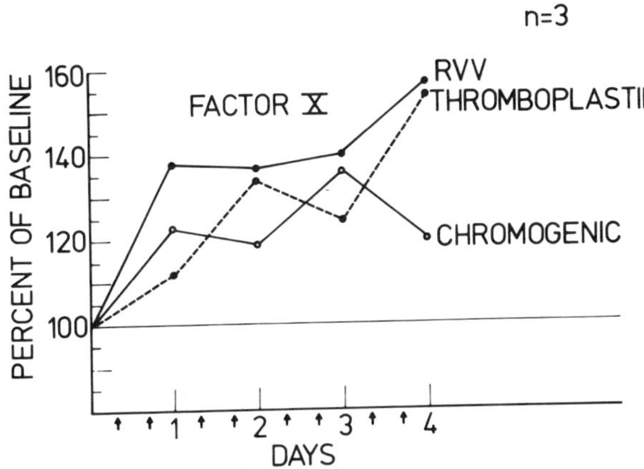

FIGURE 9. Effect of boiled experimental plasma on factor X activity in recipient rabbits. Three different coagulopoietin X plasma samples were placed in a boiling water bath for 20 min. The denatured protein was discarded after centrifugation and the supernate injected, as in FIGURE 8, into three different animals. The average values are given for the measurement of factor X activity by three different methods: bovine factor VII- and X-deficient plasma and Russell's viper venom (RVV); human X-deficient plasma and thromboplastin; and chromogenic substrate.

increased specific activity. This could result from the complete carboxylation of a partially carboxylated molecule. We postulated that normal rabbits secrete into their plasma a population of partially carboxylated molecules as has been described in warfarin-treated humans [13] and that injection of coagulopoietin increased the carboxylation of these proteins. In order to test this hypothesis, we carried out the experiments with $H^{14}CO_3^-$ incorporation into microsomal protein reported here. In this experimental model we were unable to demonstrate increased carboxylation in the presence of coagulopoietins. However, Suttie using a rat *in vivo* system has shown increased γ-carboxylation by the livers of recipient animals.[14] These data would suggest that coagulopoietin enhances the synthesis or activity of microsomal vitamin K-dependent carboxylase.

ACKNOWLEDGMENTS

The expert technical assistance of Karen Moroch and Ray-Jen Chang is gratefully acknowledged.

REFERENCES

1. KARPATKIN, M. H. & S. KARPATKIN. 1971. A new hormone, "coagulopoietin-K." J. Clin. Invest. **50:** 52a. (Abstr.)
2. KARPATKIN, M. H. & S. KARPATKIN. 1973. Evidence for a humoral agent capable of raising vitamin K-dependent coagulation factors in rabbits. Br. J. Haematol. **24:** 553–561.
3. FRIEDMAN, E. W., M. H. KARPATKIN & S. KARPATKIN. 1976. Evidence suggesting the regulation of coagulation factor levels in rabbits by a transferable plasma agent. Blood **48:** 949–954.
4. KARPATKIN, S., M. H. KARPATKIN & H. ALTSZULER. 1978. Identification of a coagulopoietin for prothrombin. Trans Assoc. Am. Physicians **91:** 351–357.
5. KARPATKIN, M. H. & S. KARPATKIN. 1979. Humoral factor that specifically regulates prothrombin (factor II) levels (coagulopoietin-II) Proc. Natl. Acad. Sci. USA **76:** 491–493.
6. KARPATKIN, M. H. & S. KARPATKIN. 1979. Humoral substance regulating the level of coagulation factors: coagulopoietins. Evidence for a specific coagulopoietin for prothrombin. *In* Vitamin K-Eighth Steenbock Symposium. J. W. Suttie, Ed.: 576–587. University Park Press. Baltimore, Md.
7. TRAUBER, D., K. HAWKINS, M. H. KARPATKIN & S. KARPATKIN. 1979. Humoral factor that specifically regulates factor X levels in rabbits (coagulopoietin X). J. Clin. Invest. **64:** 1713–1716.
8. MORRISON, S. A. & M. P. ESNOUF. 1973. The nature of the heterogeneity of prothrombin during dicumarol therapy. Nature New Biology **242:** 92–94.
9. LAURELL, C. B. 1966. Quantitative estimate of proteins by electrophoresis in agarose gel containing antibodies. Anal. Biochem. **15:** 45–52.
10. SHAPIRO, S. S. & D. F. WAUGH. 1966. The purification of human prothrombin. Thromb. Diath. Haemorrh. **16:** 469–473.
11. ESMON, C. T., J. A. SADOWSKI & J. W. SUTTIE. 1975. A new carboxylase reaction. The vitamin-K dependent incorporation of $H^{14}CO_3^-$ into prothrombin. J. Biol. Chem. **250:** 4744–4748.
12. SHAH, D. V., L. J. NYASI, J. C. SWANSON & J. W. SUTTIE. 1979. Studies of a humoral factor influencing prothrombin levels in the rat. *In* Vitamin K-Eighth Steenbock Symposium. J. W. Suttie, Ed.: 584–588. University Park Press. Baltimore, Md.
13. FRIEDMAN, P. A., R. D. ROSENBERG, P. V. HAUSCHKA & A. FITZ-JAMES. 1977. A spectrum of partially carboxylated prothrombins in the plasmas of coumarin-treated patients. Biochim. Biophys. Acta **494:** 271–276.
14. SHAH, D. V., L. J. NYASI, J. C. SWANSON & J. W. SUTTIE. 1980. Effect of a humoral factor on plasma prothrombin and vitamin K dependent liver carboxylase levels in the rat. Thrombos. Res. **19:** 111–118.

PRELIMINARY CHARACTERIZATION OF A
"FACTOR VIII BYPASSING COAGULANT"

D. L. Aronson and J. Bagley

Bureau of Biologics
Bethesda, Maryland 20205

In the last decade there has been growing interest in the use of concentrates of the vitamin K-dependent factors in the treatment of patients who form antibodies against factor VIII.[1-6] This "bypassing activity" not only has clinical importance, it also implies a hitherto undescribed mechanism for the activation of the later stages of coagulation. While increased levels of factors VIIa, IXa, and Xa have been found in the "activated" factor IX concentrates,[7,8] there are strong arguments against any of these activated components being the responsible molecular species. Indeed the only formal trial showing efficacy of factor IX complex used nonactivated preparations.[6]

The *in vitro* operational definition of the "bypassing activity" is that it shortens the activated partial thromboplastin time (APTT) of hemophilic plasma but is presumably neither thrombin nor activated factor X. Its presence in factor IX concentrates implies that it is a vitamin K-dependent coagulant containing γ-carboxyglutamyl residues.

The studies reported here were done in an effort to produce a more characterized standard-reference preparation for the control of commercially produced concentrates recommended for the treatment of patients who acquire an inhibitor to factor VIII. In producing this material, several assumptions were made, including that the "bypassing activity" is adsorbable on barium, activated during clotting, and stable in the presence of plasma protease inhibitors.

MATERIAL AND METHODS

Measurement of the ability to shorten the APTT of hemophilic plasma was done by incubating 0.1 ml of hemophilic plasma, 0.1 ml of the sample, and 0.1 ml of ellagic acid activator (Dade, Miami, FL) at 37° C. After 3 minutes, 0.1 ml of prewarmed 0.025 M $CaCl_2$ was added and the clotting time measured.

Factor X was assayed by the method of Denson[9] using factors VII–X-deficient plasma obtained from Sigma Chemical Co. (St. Louis, MO); factor VII measurements were done as described by Clyne and Nemerson.[10] Prothrombin measurements of the fractionated material were done by a one-stage method using prothrombin-deficient plasma supplied by Dade (Miami, FL) and Ortho thromboplastin. The prothrombin measurements of the samples from the dog experiments were done using the same reagents but the thromboplastin was diluted 1:25 in 0.025 M $CaCl_2$ in order to increase the sensitivity of the assay. Fibrinogen measurements were done by the method of Clauss.[11] The activated partial thromboplastin time (APTT) was measured using a silica activator (Platelin Plus, General Diagnostics, Morris Plains, NJ). All clotting assays were standardized against fresh frozen human plasma stored at −70° C.

Assays that employed chromogenic substrate were done using a Gilford

291

recording spectrophotometer with a thermostatted cuvette holder maintained at 30° C. The substrates were in a final concentration of 0.5 mM in 0.05 M Tris, 0.05 M NaCl, pH 8.0. All synthetic peptide substrates were obtained from Kabi.

A reagent containing both factor X and prothrombin (II–X reagent) was made by a previously described method.[12] Citrated plasma was adsorbed by the addition of $BaCl_2$ (15 g/l) and the protein adsorbed to the resulting barium precipitate was eluted and subsequently precipitated by the addition of ammonium sulfate. After desalting on G-25 Sephadex, the eluted proteins were chromatographed on IR-50 in 0.15 M NaCl, 0.05 M cacodylate buffer, pH 6.0. The eluted protein contained 20 U/ml of prothrombin and 10 U/ml of factor X.

On the basis of the assumptions noted above, the following purification scheme was devised to isolate "bypassing activity" from plasma (FIGURE 1). It is to be noted that because of the presence of varying quantities of thrombin and factor Xa all assays of activity done during the earlier purification are presumed to be inaccurate.

Serum was produced by the addition of celite (10 g/l) and $CaCl_2$ (final concentration 0.025 M) to citrated human plasma prewarmed to ambient temperature (20–23° C). After 1.5 h the clot was removed, 4 g/l of sodium citrate added, followed by $BaCl_2$ (15 g/l). The resulting precipitate was washed successively with 0.1 M $BaCl_2$ and H_2O and the proteins eluted with $(NH_4)SO_4$. The eluted proteins were precipitated by the addition of $(NH_4)_2SO_4$ to a final concentration of 60% saturation. This precipitate was redissolved in a minimal volume of H_2O, applied to a G-25 Sephadex column equilibrated in 0.05 M NaCl, 0.0066 M Tris-HCl, pH 7.4, and subsequently chromatographed on a heparin–agarose column equilibrated in the same buffer containing 2 mM $SrCl_2$. A linear gradient was run starting with the equilibration buffer and finishing with a 1 M NaCl, 0.13 M Tris-HCl pH 7.4 containing 2 mM $SrCl_2$ (250 ml of each buffer).

The elution profile is illustrated in FIGURE 2. While the breakthrough peak could correct the clotting time of hemophilic plasma this was, at least in part, due to its content of thrombin. After the elution of the majority of the protein with low ionic strength buffer material with potent ability to clot, hemophilic plasma was eluted. For example, throughout this region a 1/100 dilution would clot hemophilic plasma in 15 sec or less and a 1/1000 dilution would clot hemophilic plasma in 30 sec.

The fractions with the highest coagulant action from the heparin–agarose column were pooled, soybean trypsin inhibitor (SBTI) added (0.1 mg/ml), dialyzed overnight against 0.10 M NaCl, 0.013 M Tris-HCl, pH 7.4, applied to a 2 cm $\times$ 100 cm column of DEAE-cellulose (DE-52, Whatman), and a linear gradient from 0.10 M NaCl, 0.013 M Tris to 0.5 M NaCl, 0.066 M Tris-HCl, pH 7.4 (250 ml/reservoir) applied. FIGURE 3 demonstrates the profile. The "bypassing activity" elutes as a shoulder following a major protein peak. The residual thrombin activity is eluted in the breakthrough peak.

RESULTS

The purification procedure for the "bypassing activity" was based on available data concerning its presence in concentrates of the vitamin K-dependent

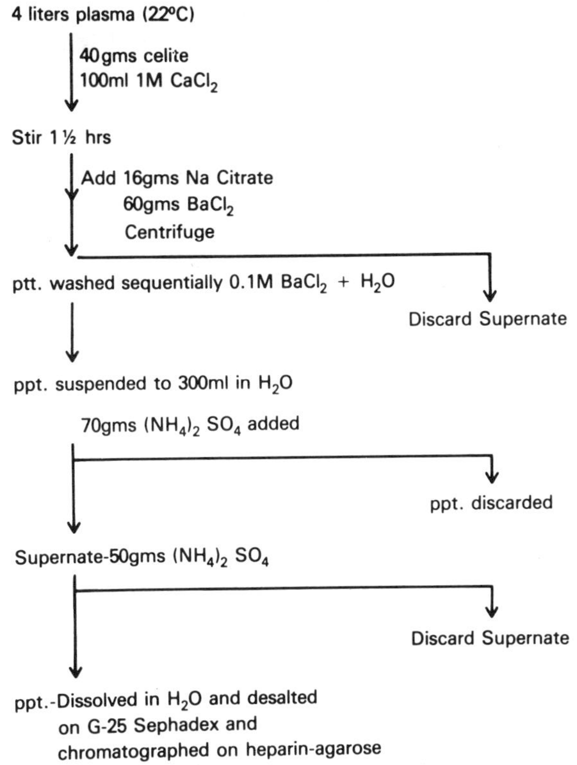

FIGURE 1. Flow diagram for the production of the barium eluate from serum.

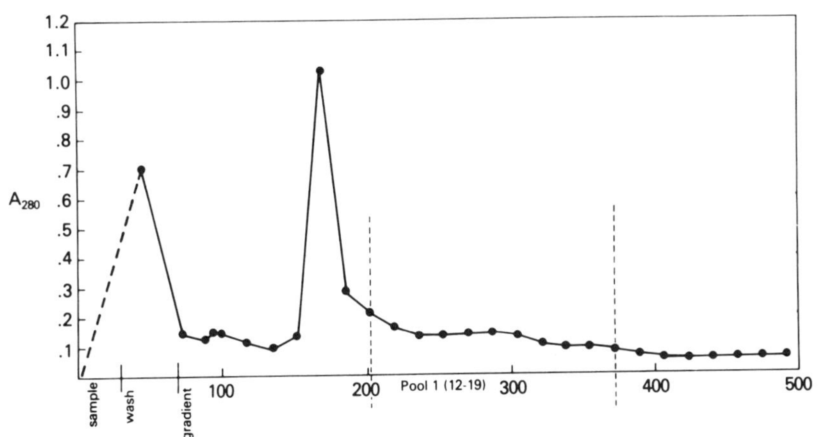

FIGURE 2. Chromatography of serum barium eluate on heparin–agarose. Fractions between the vertical lines were pooled for further purification.

factors [13] and its binding characteristics to heparin–agarose.[14] It was further assumed that it was activated during coagulation and is relatively stable in the presence of plasma protease inhibitors.

FIGURE 4 demonstrates the APTT shortening in hemophilic plasma as a function of dilution of the "bypassing activity." This dose-response curve is somewhat steeper than a comparable experiment for a commercial product (Autoplex, Hyland Laboratories). One possible explanation is that the inclusion of heparin in this commercial preparation leads to a prolongation of clotting time particularly with the more concentrated solutions. The "bypassing activity" in these two preparations is not substantially inhibited by SBTI.

Preincubation of the "bypassing activity" in the hemophilic plasma for

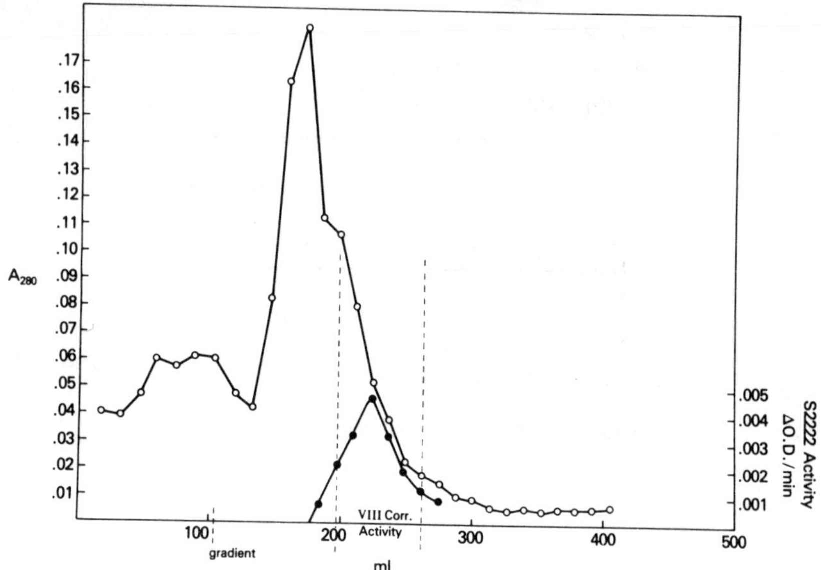

FIGURE 3. Chromatography of heparin–agarose pool on DEAE-cellulose. Fractions between the vertical lines were pooled for further study. The solid circles represent the S-2222 hydrolytic activity generated when these fractions were incubated with the II–X reagent (25 μl/ml sample + 25 μl/ml of the II–X reagent). Twenty-five μl of this mixture was then added to 0.475 ml of 0.5 mM S-2222.

increasing periods of time leads to a progressive decrease in the coagulant activity with loss of half of the activity in 5 min (FIGURE 5).

TABLE 1 gives the apparent content of coagulants in a lot that was prepared as a potential standard. It contains 100 units of "bypassing activitiy" where the unit is defined as the activity that will correct APTT of hemophilic plasma to 30 sec, i.e. 0.1 ml of a 1/100 dilution of this control will shorten the APTT to 30 sec. The content of prothrombin, factor VII, and factor X is very low. The "apparent" content of factor IX is high as is expected for a coagulant that acts later in the sequence than "true" factor IXa. The dose-response slope in IX-deficient plasma is steeper than when normal plasma dilutions are used as a source of factor IX. No factor VIII C ag was found in this product.

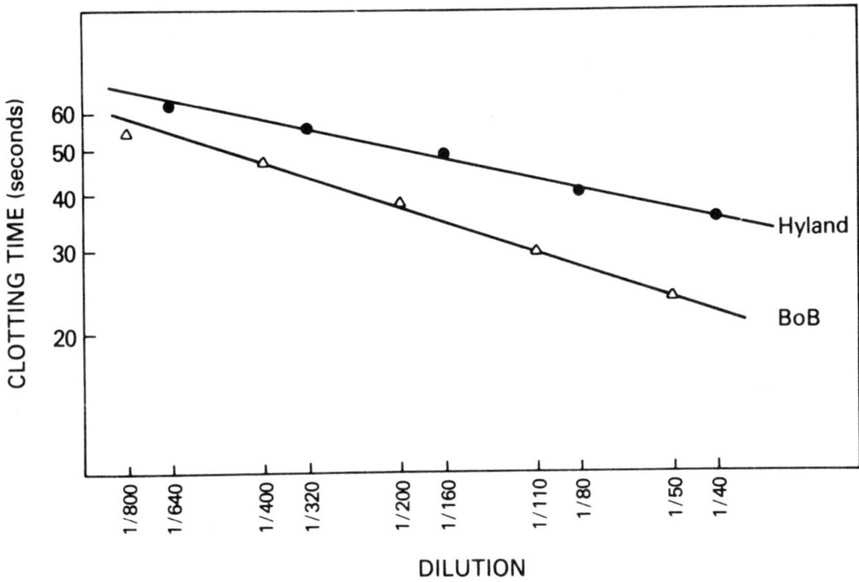

FIGURE 4. The relationship between dilution of sample and the clotting time of hemophilic plasma. The open circles are for the serum derived "bypassing activity," closed circles are for the commercial "bypassing activity."

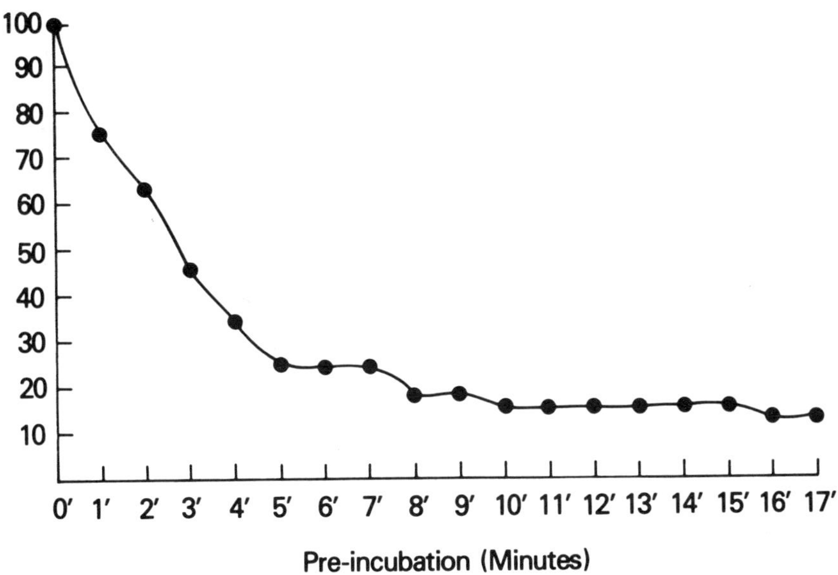

FIGURE 5. Inhibition of serum derived "bypassing activity" by preincubation in hemophilic plasma.

TABLE 1

APPARENT COAGULANT CONTENT IN PURIFIED "BYPASSING ACTIVITY"

Coagulant	U/ml
Prothrombin	0
Factor VII	0.25
Factor X	0.05
Factor IX	50–100
Factor VIII Coagulant Antigen	0

The coagulant fraction derived from serum shows variable amounts of activity against all the synthetic peptide substrates tested (S-2238, S-2222, S-2266, S-2302). However, all of these amidolytic activities, in contrast to the coagulant activity, are essentially completely inhibited by soybean trypsin inhibitor except some S-2266 hydrolase activity. None of these peptidase activities consistently parallels the coagulant activitiy.

A possible mechanism for "bypassing activity" would be a direct activator of prothrombin. When the DEAE fraction is incubated with the II–X reagent there develops the ability to hydrolyze the thrombin substrate S-2238. However this activity can be completely blocked by the addition of SBTI. These results imply that there is no direct prothrombin activation but there might be an activation of factor X.

The "bypassing activity" was tested for its ability to activate factor X by incubating (50 μl/ml) with 50 μl/ml of the II–X reagent. As soon as possible and after a half hour incubation, 25 μl was transferred to a cuvette containing 475 μl of 0.5 mM S-2222. TABLE 2 demonstrates that the combination of "bypassing activity" and a source of factor X generates S-2222 hydrolase activity. The presence of Ca^{2+} is not necessary. More surprising is the fact that after 0.5 h incubation there is no further increase in S-2222 hydrolase activity.

This surprising result is confirmed by the dose-response relation seen in FIGURE 6. There is a linear increase in hydrolysis of S-2222 as a function of the quantity of "bypassing activity" added that does not increase with increasing

TABLE 2

GENERATION OF S-2222 HYDROLYTIC ACTIVITY BY "BYPASSING ACTIVITY"

Interaction of AICC with Factor X Reagent

		Δ O.D./min	
		T_0	T_{30}
1	100μl X, Ca	0.0003	0.0005
2	50μl AICC, Ca	0.0013	0.00092
3	50μl AICC, 100μl X	0.0083	0.0085
4	50μl AICC, 100μl X, Ca	0.0092	0.0103

time. Maintaining the concentration of the "bypassing activity" constant and varying the factor X content shows that at high concentrations of factor X there is a linear reduction in the S-2222 hydrolysis (FIGURE 7). The maximum level of S-2222 hydrolase activity generated by the combination of factor X with "bypassing activity" is very small, being 1/150 the activity generated by Russell's viper venom (RVV) activation of the same factor X.

The activation of factor X cleaves a sialic acid-rich activation peptide of about 11,000 from the heavy chain of factor X. Incubating "bypassing activity" with tritium-labeled human factor X[15] does not however yield TCA-soluble ^{3}H as found with other factor X activators.[16, 17] In contrast, when the "bypassing activity" is incubated with ^{3}H-labeled factor X and submitted

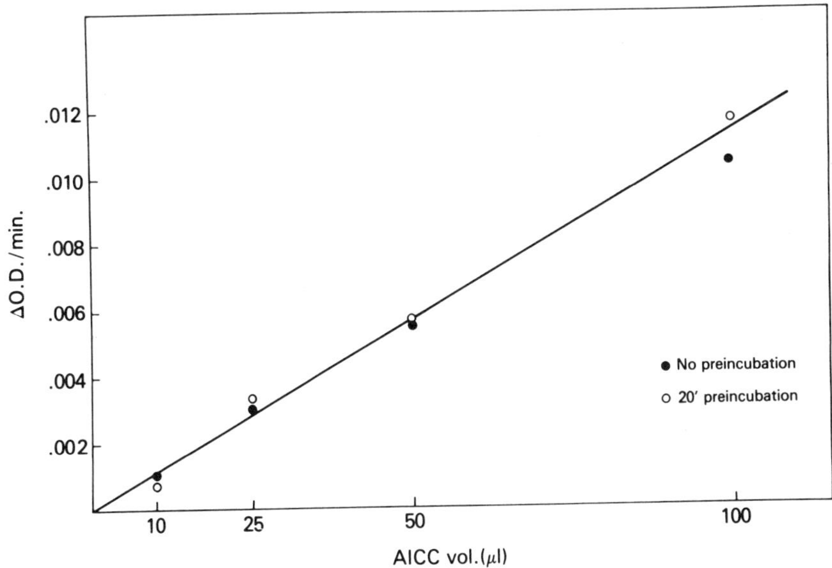

FIGURE 6. Hydrolysis of S-2222 after pretreatment of II–X reagent with serum derived "bypassing activity." Varying quantities of the "bypassing activity" were incubated with 25 μl/ml of the II–X reagent. Immediately after mixing and after 20 min incubation (22° C) 25 μl were introduced into a cuvette containing 475 μl of 0.5 mM S-2222.

to SDS-PAGE, there is a significant shift in the position of the label (FIGURE 8). The migration of the label after treatment with "bypassing activity" is identical to the position of the heavy chain of Xa after RVV activation, both when reduced and nonreduced. In contrast to other mechanisms of factor X activation no evidence of the activation peptide can be found. However, if after treatment with "bypassing activity" RVV is added, the activation peptide promptly appears.

INFUSION EXPERIMENTS

If this fraction is related to the materials used therapeutically, it must not only have potent *in vitro* coagulant activity but also be safe and effective for

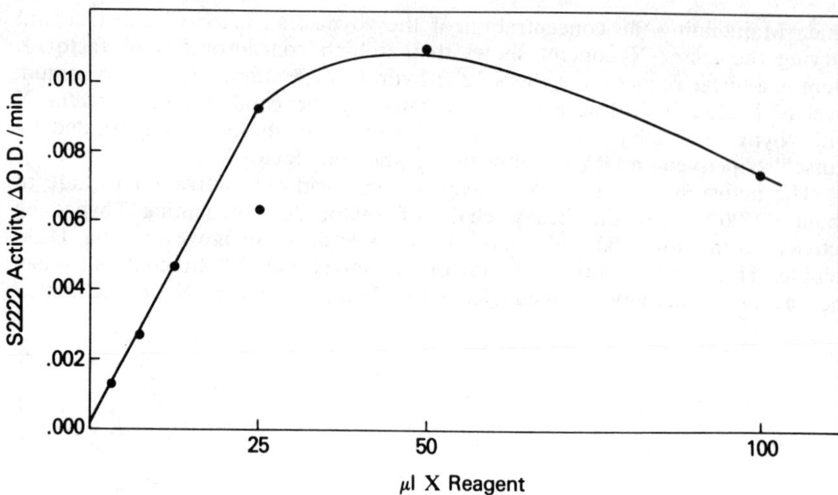

FIGURE 7. Hydrolysis of S-2222 by mixture of II–X reagent with serum derived "bypassing activity." Conditions the same as in FIGURE 5 except the "bypassing activity" was constant and the quantity of II–X reagent was varied.

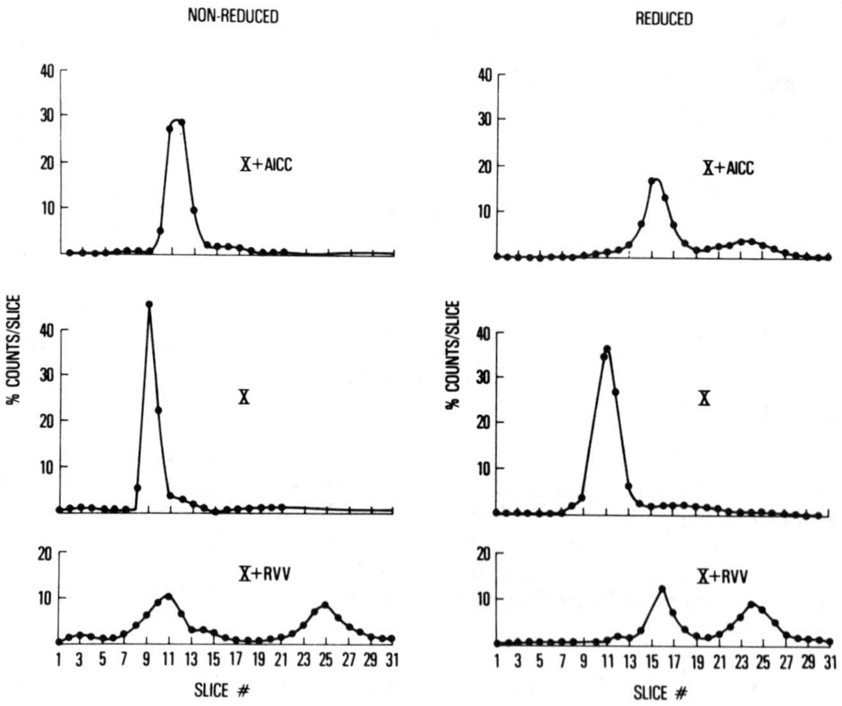

FIGURE 8. Migration of tritium-labeled factor X in SDS-PAGE. Gels were cut into 1.1 mm slices for counting.

in vivo use, i.e. it must not give rise to a state of disseminated intravascular coagulation (DIC) or thrombosis and should arrest hemorrhage in hemophilic recipients.

When 0.3 ml of several preparations containing between 500–1,200 U/ml of "bypassing activity" were injected as a bolus into 20-gm mice, there was no sign of any untoward effect.

A dog model for the study of DIC induced by factor IX concentrates has been well established.[18] This model has been used for safety studies of these fractions. Outbred fox hounds (~15 kg) were anesthetized with sodium pentobarbital and the femoral artery catheterized using a Teflon® catheter. After 0.5 h for stabilization, 200 U/kg of "bypassing activity" in 50 ml of

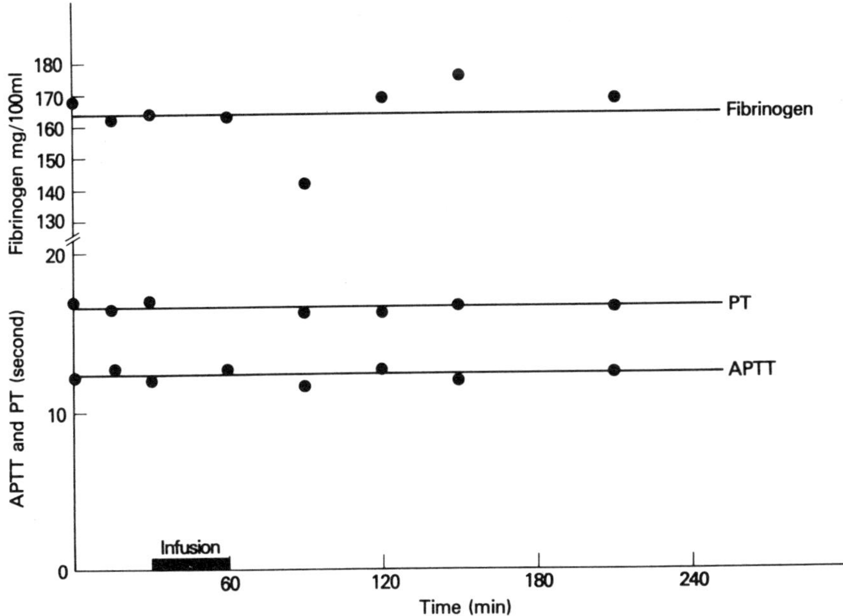

FIGURE 9. The non-effect on the APTT, prothrombin time, and fibrinogen of infusing the 200 units/kg into a dog.

citrate saline was infused via the arterial catheter. Blood samples were removed from the arterial catheter at the indicated times. FIGURE 9 shows the APTT, prothrombin time, and fibrinogen level are stable after infusion of 200 U/kg of this material. No fibrin(ogen)-degradation products were found. No changes of arterial pressure or pulse of any significance were noted nor was there any bleeding from the cutdown for the arterial catheter. Clotted samples of whole blood all had good clot retraction. In contrast after the infusion of either a factor IX complex C (200 U/kg) or "Autoplex" (75 U/kg) changes consistent with disseminated intravascular coagulation were consistently found. Infusion into hemophilic dogs of the purified "bypassing activity" did not stop bleeding from a previously inflicted wound.

DISCUSSION

A material with many *in vitro* attributes of the therapeutic materials used for treating factor VIII inhibitors has been purified from serum. The original assumption that such a material might be slowly inhibited by plasma protease inhibitors seems to be in error since 5 min of incubation in plasma leads to a 50% decrease in the coagulant activity. This finding implies that the activity isolated was generated during the purification process and not during the initial conversion of plasma to serum. An alternate possibility is that we are only isolating a small fraction of the material available. Castaldi and Smith [19] have reported that the inhibition of activated factor IX concentrates is diminished by the presence of platelets.

The "bypassing activity" is either a nonclassic clotting component or a nonclassic pathway of coagulation. Among the possible mechanisms could be an activation of prothrombin, an activation of factor V, or an activation of factor X. Evidence for a direct activation of prothrombin has not yet been explored. However, the "bypassing activity," which is described above, seems to have a direct effect on factor X.

Classically either activated factor VII or factor IX is considered the only plasma enzyme capable of activating factor X. Both of these have almost obligate requirements for cofactors–tissue factor or antihemophilic factor, respectively. While purified factor IXa can partially correct hemophilic plasma, it takes large amounts of purified material. Assuming an extinction coefficient of 10.0 for the partially purified "bypassing activity," 10–50 ng will correct the APTT of hemophilic plasma. A purified human IXa corrects to about 45 sec at a concentration of 300 ng. It has also been proposed that activated factor VII would be a candidate for correcting hemophilic plasma.[7] This suggestion is attractive because of the slow inhibition of activated factor VII in plasma. The material studied above has little apparent factor VII activity and the chromatographic characteristics to the coagulant activity on both DEAE and heparin–agarose are quite different from those reported for factor VII. Finally Nemerson (unpublished data) has found absolutely no shortening of the hemophilic APTT after the addition of 100 ng of 2-chain bovine factor VII.

Several new vitamin K-dependent factors have been described in the last several years—proteins C, S, and M.[20-22] There are no reported data implicating protein C or S as a late-stage coagulant. Walz (unpublished data) has found that purified bovine protein M will shorten the APTT of hemophilic plasma but only at levels of 10 μg and higher.

Two pieces of evidence indicate that this preparation acts directly on factor X. The first is the generation of S-2222 hydrolase activity on mixing with a source of factor X. This activity is similar to Xa in that it is inhibited by SBTI. Further, these experiments imply a stoichiometric activation since there is no increase in S-2222 hydrolase activity with preincubation of the "bypassing activity" and factor X, yet there is a linear relationship between the added "bypassing activity" and the S-2222 hydrolysis. The second piece of evidence indicating a direct activation of factor X is the change in PAGE mobility of factor X after mixing with the "bypassing activity." Two pieces of data however indicate that the proposed factor Xa formed after incubation with "bypassing activity" is a modified form that there is no detectable release of the normal activation peptide, and that the maximum amount of S-2222 hydrolase activity is less than 1% of that measured after RVV activation. This proposed mechanism is somewhat different from that proposed by Vermylen *et al.*[23] These investigators have suggested that "bypassing activity" enhances the activity of a platelet activator of factor X whereas the above experiments, despite the absence of platelets, indicate a direct effect on factor X.

The *in vivo* effect of the "bypassing activity" is amazingly mild compared to its *in vitro* potency. No laboratory evidence of intravascular coagulation has been found. This is in contrast to the experience with regular factor IX concentrates both in animals and in patients.[18, 24] The clinical use of the activated factor IX concentrates does not seem to be associated with substantial thrombo-hemorrhagic problems.[3, 26] The inability of the purified "bypassing activity" to act hemostatically in a bleeding hemophilic dog may simply indicate that the isolated material has no relationship to the hemostatically effective component in the current activated products. It must be noted that 10 times more of the "bypassing" activity was needed to normalize the APTT of dog hemophilic plasma *in vitro* than is needed to normalize human hemophilic plasma.

There may well be no relationship between the material that has been isolated and the therapeutic activity. The only controlled clinical trial unequivocally indicating that factor IX concentrates are effective in treating factor VIII inhibitor patients, utilized non-activated factor IX.[6] Further investigation to establish whether there is a relationship between the *in vitro* activity and a therapeutic effect is urgently needed.

ACKNOWLEDGMENTS

The authors gratefully acknowledge the aid of Dr. John Bacher and his staff for invaluable aid in the dog infusion studies, Mrs. Betsy Poindexter for platelet counts, Dr. Margaret Rick for factor VIII C antigen measurement, and Dr. Henry Kingdon for the infusion studies in hemophilic dogs.

REFERENCES

1. BREEN, F. A. & J. L. TULLIS. 1969. Prothrombin concentrates in treatment of Christmas Disease and allied disorders. J. Am. Med. Assoc. **208:** 1848–1852.
2. FEKETE, L., S. L. HOLST, F. PETOOM & L. L. DEVEBER. 1972. A new approach to treatment of hemophilia A with inhibitor. 14th Cong. Intl. Soc. Haematol. Abstract #295.
3. ELINSGER, F. 1977. Feiba Immuno. A preparation with Factor eight inhibitor activity. Thrombosis and Haemostasis **38:** 346 (abstr.).
4. KURCYNSKI, E. & J. PENNER. 1974. Activated prothrombin concentrate for patients with Factor VIII inhibitors. N. Eng. J. Med. **291:** 164–167.
5. ABILGAARD, C. F., BRITTON & J. HARRISON. 1976. Prothrombin complex concentrate (Konyne) in the treatment of hemophilic patients with Factor VIII inhibitors. J. Pediatr. **88:** 200–205.
6. LUSHER, J. M., S. S. SHAPIRO, J. E. PALASCAK, A. V. RAO, P. H. LEVINE & P. M. BLATT. 1980. Prothrombin complex concentrates in treatment of hemophiliacs with Factor VIII inhibitors-A multicenter therapeutic trial. Clin. Res. **28:** 548A (abstract).
7. SELIGSOHN, U., C. K. KASPER, B. OSTERUD & S. I. RAPAPORT. 1979. Activated Factor VII: Presence in Factor IX concentrates and persistence in the circulation after infusion. Blood **53:** 828–837.

8. HULTIN, M. B. 1979. Activated clotting factors in Factor IX concentrates. Blood **54:** 1028–1038.

9. DENSON, K. W. E. 1961. The specific assay of Prower-Stuart Factor and Factor VII. Acta Haemat. **25:** 105–120.

10. NEMERSON, Y. & L. CLYNE. 1974. An assay for coagulation factor VII using factor VII depleted bovine plasma. J. Lab. Clin. Med. **83:** 301–303.

11. CLAUSS, A. 1957. Gerinnungphysiologische schnell methode zur bestimmung des fibrinogen. Acta Haemat. **17:** 237–246.

12. ARONSON, D. L. & D. MENACHE. 1966. Chromatographic analysis of the activation of human prothrombin with human thrombokinase. Biochemistry **5:** 2635.

13. PEPPER, D. S., D. BANHEGYI, A. HOWIE & J. D. CASH. 1977. *In vitro* thrombo-genicity tests of Factor IX concentrates. Brit. J. Haemat. **36:** 573–583.

14. THOMPSON, A. R. & K. J. SMITH. 1979. Crude, clinical Factor IX concentrates: comparison of Factor IX antigens and demonstration of Factor IX_a. Thrombosis and Haemostastis **42:** 200 (abstract).

15. VAN LENTEN, L. & G. ASHWELL. 1971: Studies on the chemical and enzymatic modification of glycoproteins: a general method for the tritiation of sialic acid-containing glycoproteins. J. Biol. Chem. **246:** 1889–1894.

16. SILVERBERG, S. A., Y. NEMERSON & M. ZUR. 1977. Kinetics of the activation of bovine coagulation factor X by components of the extrinsic pathway. J. Biol. Chem. **252:** 8481–8488.

17. ARONSON, D. & J. BAGLEY. 1978. Regulation of Factor X conversion in plasma. Circulation **58** (Part II): 209 (abstract).

18. CASH, J. D., R. DALTON, S. MIDDLETON & J. SMITH. 1975. Studies on the thrombogenicity of Scottish Factor IX concentrates in dogs. Thromb. Diath. Haemorrh. **33:** 632–639.

19. CASTALDI, P. A. & I. L. SMITH. 1980. The effects of platelets on the in vitro response to prothrombin complex concentrates in F VIII inhibitor plasma. Pathology **12:** 11–18.

20. STENFLO, J. 1976. A new vitamin K-dependent protein. J. Biol. Chem. **251:** 355–363.

21. DISCIPIO, R. G. & E. W. DAVIE. 1979. Characterization of protein S, a γ-carboxyglutamic acid containing protein from bovine and human plasma. Biochemistry **18:** 899–904.

22. SEEGERS, W. H. & A. GHOSH. 1980. Activation of prothrombin and Factor X: Function of previously unrecognized plasma protein. Thrombosis Research **17:** 71–81.

23. VERMYLEN, J., J. SCHETZ, N. SEMERARO, F. MERTENS & M. VERSTRAETE. 1978. Evidence that "Activated" prothrombin concentrates enhance platelet coagulant activity. Brit. J. Haemat. **38:** 235–242.

HUMAN PROTEIN C:
INACTIVATION OF FACTORS V AND VIII IN PLASMA BY THE ACTIVATED MOLECULE *

Richard A. Marlar, Alice J. Kleiss, and John H. Griffin

Department of Molecular Immunology
Scripps Clinic and Research Foundation
La Jolla, California 92037

INTRODUCTION

Human protein C is a vitamin K-dependent serine protease zymogen.[1] The amino acid sequence of bovine protein C is homologous with the procoagulant vitamin K-dependent proteins.[2] Protein C is anticoagulant since it prolongs the clotting time of plasma in an activated partial thromboplastin time (APTT) assay. Until recently, very little was known about human protein C whereas the bovine molecule has been well characterized both physiochemically and functionally.

The anticoagulant nature of the activated form of bovine protein C (termed autoprothrombin II-A) was described over 20 years ago by Seegers and co-workers.[3] They suggested that this potent anticoagulant activity was derived from prothrombin that had been activated by limited proteolysis of thrombin. Indeed, such is not the case. A decade later, Marciniak suggested that human autoprothrombin II-A was not derived from prothrombin but was a separate protein.[4] In 1976, Stenflo [5] isolated an apparently unknown protein, now referred to as protein C, that was then established as the precursor of autoprothrombin II-A.[6] The anticoagulant activity of bovine autoprothrombin II-A was described as a competitive inhibitor of factor Xa.[7,8] Subsequently, it was shown that bovine activated protein C inactivates bovine factors V and VIII:C by limited proteolysis.[9–11] Recently, Kisiel [1] reported the isolation and partial characterization of human protein C and showed that it could be activated by limited proteolysis by thrombin and that this activated form exhibited anticoagulant activity. Current evidence suggests that human protein C is structurally and functionally similar to bovine protein C although the anticoagulant activity of these proteins is highly species-specific since the bovine protein is not active in human plasma and vice versa.

This report summarizes our recent investigations [12,13] that were focused on defining the anticoagulant properties of human protein C in plasma.

* Supported in part by the National Institutes of Health (Grant HL 24891) and the California chapter of the American Heart Association. R. A. M. has been supported by a California Heart Association Fellowship and a National Institutes of Health Fellowship. J. H. G. is a recipient of a National Institutes of Health Research Career Development Award.

303

MATERIAL AND METHODS

Purification of Human Protein C

Human protein C was purified from commercial factor IX concentrate (Proplex®, Hyland Therapeutics) by DEAE–Sephadex and dextran sulfate–Sepharose chromatography and preparative polyacrylamide gel electrophoresis as described elsewhere.[13] Purified protein C was activated using commercial trypsin–agarose beads (Pierce Chemical), soluble α-thrombin, or α-thrombin–Sepharose beads.[13]

Anticoagulant Activity of Protein C

The protein C sample was incubated with normal human plasma plus 58 μg/ml cephalin and 4 mM $CaCl_2$ for 3 min at 37° C. The reaction was stopped by diluting the mixture with EDTA. This mixture was then assayed for the presence of the various clotting factor activities in appropriate deficient human plasmas. In some experiments, buffer replaced protein C, cephalin, or $CaCl_2$ in the preincubation mixture containing normal plasma.

Factor VIII:C Activation and Inactivation

Commercial human factor VIII concentrate (Hemophil®, Hyland Therapeutics) was further purified by gel filtration. Lyophilyzed factor VIII concentrate was reconstituted with buffer, applied at 20° C to a Sepharose 4B column (2.5 × 65 cm), and equilibrated in 0.01 M Imidazole-HCl, 0.15 M NaCl, 0.02% sodium azide, pH 7.4. Factor VIII clotting activity (VIII:C) eluted in the void volume. This partially purified factor VIII:C was activated using α-thrombin–Sepharose beads that were then removed from factor VIII:C by centrifugation. The progress of factor VIII:C activation was monitored by an APTT assay using factor VIII-deficient plasma. Activated protein C was added to either unactivated or activated factor VIII:C, and the remaining factor VIII:C activity was determined using the APTT assay.

RESULTS

Purification of Human Protein C

Human factor IX concentrate (Proplex®) was used as the source for human protein C. The DEAE–Sephadex chromatography not only partially separated protein C from the other vitamin K-dependent coagulation proteins, but also removed the major portion of the proteins. Dextran–sulfate chromatography removed residual factors IX and X, as well as a large bulk of the prothrombin and factor VII. Following preparative polyacrylamide gel electrophoresis, the purified protein C contained no measurable (<0.1%) prothrombin, factor VII, factor IX, or factor X, as measured by clotting assays.

On 10% SDS-polyacrylamide gels in the absence of reducing agent, protein C appeared as a single band (FIGURE 1) with an apparent 62,000 MW, while protein C formed two bands (40,000 MW and 22,000 MW) on SDS-polyacrylamide gels in the presence of a reducing agent (FIGURE 1).

Activation of Protein C

Human protein C was activated with α-thrombin–Sepharose beads. As seen in FIGURE 2, protein C amidolytic activity increased with time and reached a maximum within 60 min. After removing the thrombin–Sepharose by centrifugation, activated protein C remained stable and no thrombin activity was detected. Activated protein C functioned as an anticoagulant in normal plasma. For example, when 3 μg/ml final concentration of this protein was added to an APTT assay of normal plasma, the clotting time was prolonged from less than 50 sec to greater than 240 sec. The unactivated protein C exhibited neither amidolytic nor anticoagulant activity.

Activated protein C was susceptible to the serine protease inhibitor diisopropylfluorophosphate (DFP). An aliquot of the activated protein C was exposed to 5 mM DFP that was then removed by dialysis. Then it was assayed for both amidase and anticoagulant activity. The DFP-treated samples of activated protein C were completely inhibited within 10 min. Moreover, the unactivated protein C was not susceptible to DFP inhibition.

Anticoagulant Activity of Protein C

The effect of activated protein C in plasma on each of the known clotting factors was studied. Factor V and factor VIII:C were the only coagulation

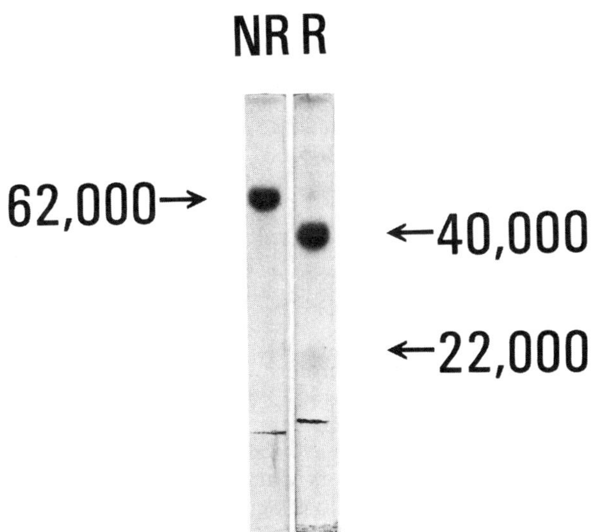

FIGURE 1. Human protein C on 10% polyacrylamide gels in the presence of sodium dodecyl sulfate. NR indicates no reducing agent present; R indicates reducing agent present. Numbers represent apparent molecular weight values. After Marlar *et al.*[13]

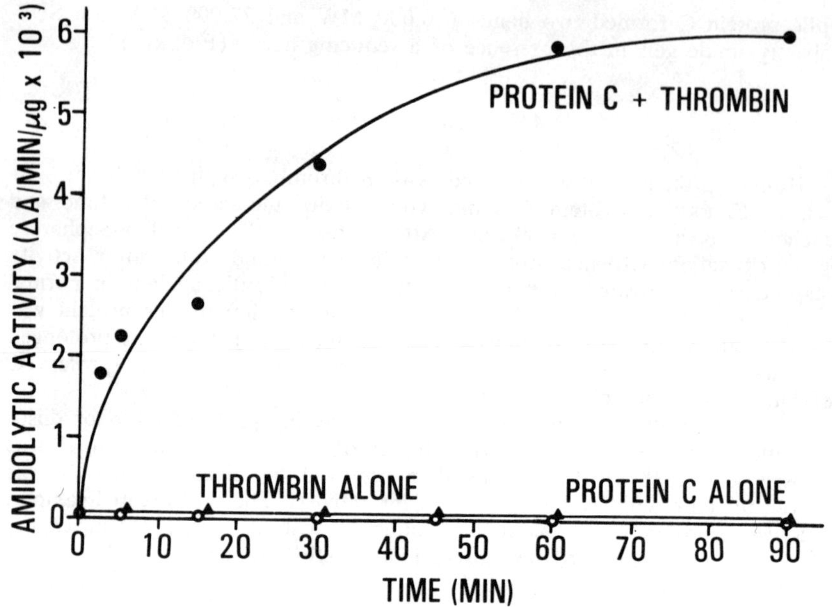

FIGURE 2. Activation of human protein C by insolubilized human α-thrombin. Amidolytic activity of activated protein C was measured spectrophotometrically with the chromogenic substrate, S-2238, Phe-Pip-Arg-*p*-nitroanilide. Protein C was incubated with the thrombin–Sepharose. At various times aliquots were withdrawn from the reaction mixture and, following centrifugation to remove the thrombin-Sepharose, assayed for amidolytic activity (solid circles). Control mixtures contained thrombin–Sepharose alone (triangles) or unactivated protein C (open circles). After Marlar *et al.*[13]

activities reduced by activated protein C (FIGURE 3). Both factors V and VIII:C were reduced to less than 20% of their original values in 3 min and were totally destroyed in 5 min. Neither the vitamin K-dependent coagulation proteins (prothrombin, factors VII, IX, and X) nor the contact activation system proteins (factors XI and XII, prekallikrein and high MW kininogen) were affected (FIGURE 3).

Other forms of protein C were tested for their effect on the clotting activity of factors V and VIII:C (TABLE 1). Unactivated protein C had no anticoagulant activity in plasma and did not reduce the activities of factors V and VIII:C. Likewise, activated protein C, which had been inhibited with DFP (diisopropylphosphoryl-protein C), did not destroy the activity of the two coagulation cofactors tested. Only protein C that had been activated by α-thrombin–Sepharose beads, soluble thrombin, or trypsin–agarose beads decreased the clotting activities of factors V and VIII:C.

Both phospholipid and calcium ions were needed as cofactors for activated protein C to function efficiently as an anticoagulant in an APTT assay. Therefore, these two cofactors were tested to determine their effect on factor V and factor VIII:C inactivation (TABLE 1). For efficient inactivation of each clotting factor, both phospholipid and calcium were needed in con-

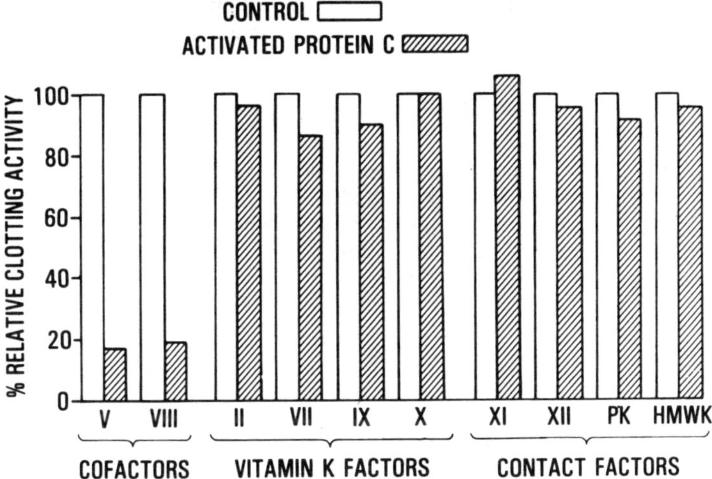

FIGURE 3. Effect of activated human protein C on the various coagulation factors in normal human plasma. Activated protein C (1.5 μg) was combined with citrated normal human plasma (500 μl) in the presence of cephalin (29 μg) and calcium ion (4 mM final concentration). After 3 min at 37° C, EDTA was added and dilutions of the mixture were assayed for individual coagulation factors. The height of each bar represents percent clotting activity compared to the control (open bars). Plasma plus activated protein C is represented by the diagonal lined bars. After Marlar *et al.*[13]

TABLE 1

INFLUENCE OF PROTEIN C, ACTIVATED PROTEIN C, AND DIISOPROPYLPHOSPHORYL-
PROTEIN C ON THE CLOTTING OF FACTOR V AND FACTOR VIII:C IN PLASMA *

	Percent Clotting Activity Remaining	
	Factor V	Factor VIII:C
Control	100 (0.67) †	100 (1.4)
Protein C	100 (0.67)	107 (1.5)
Activated protein C	16 (0.11)	19 (0.27)
Activated protein C Calcium absent	100 (0.67)	100 (1.4)
Activated protein C Cephalin absent	94 (0.63)	100 (1.4)
Diisopropylphosphoryl- Protein C	100 (0.67)	100 (1.4)

* Plasma was incubated with the test sample (3 μg/ml final) for 3 min at 37° C and then assayed for the remaining clotting factor activity using deficient human plasmas. 4 mM CaCl$_2$ and 58 μg/ml cephalin were present unless otherwise indicated. In the control, buffer replaced protein C.

† The values in parentheses are the observed activities in clotting units/ml.

junction with the activated protein since no significant loss of factors V or VIII:C activity was observed in the absence of either cofactor.

Factor VIII:C Activation and Inactivation

Factor VIII:C can be activated to increase greatly its procoagulant activity. Partially purified factor VIII:C was prepared and was free of clottable fibrinogen. In 15 min with thrombin-Sepharose beads, the clotting activity of factor VIII:C increased 20-fold (FIGURE 4). Following removal of the thrombin–Sepharose and upon the addition of activated protein C, phospholipid, and calcium, the clotting activity of thrombin-activated factor VIII:C decreased very rapidly (FIGURE 4). In less than 3 min, greater than 95% of the factor VIII:C activity had disappeared. When the relative rates of inactivation of factor VIII:C and thrombin-activated factor VIII:C were compared,[13] the thrombin-activated factor VIII:C was more rapidly destroyed than was the unactivated factor VIII:C.

DISCUSSION

Human protein C functions as an anticoagulant in human plasma by inactivating coagulation factors V and VIII.[13] The rate of inactivation of these factors in plasma is very rapid with more than 80% of the activity being destroyed within 3 min. Protein C must be activated by another protease to have these anticoagulant properties. Since activated protein C was inhibited with DFP, an active enzyme seems to be required for inactivation of factors V and VIII. The proteolytic activation of protein C [1, 14] and its enzymatic anticoagulant action [9–11, 15] have been demonstrated using purified bovine factors V and VIII:C.

Both factors V and VIII, cofactors that accelerate two enzymatic conversions of the coagulation system, can be activated by thrombin to increase their procoagulant activity from 100- to 1000-fold.[16] Notably, human protein C inactivates thrombin-activated factor VIII:C more rapidly than the untreated form of factor VIII:C. Similarly thrombin-activated factors V and VIII:C in the bovine system are more rapidly inactivated than the native forms by activated bovine protein C.[9–11, 15]

Commercial factor IX concentrate was used as the source for human protein C. This concentrate was also a good source for isolation of other vitamin K-dependent proteins.[16] Factor IX concentrate is used therapeutically in the management of bleeding. It must now be recognized that such commercial products also contain protein C, an anticoagulant serine protease zymogen. The possibility that a commercial concentrate of protein C may possibly be useful for anticoagulant therapy has not escaped our attention.

The human protein C that we prepared from commercial factor IX concentrate [13] seems to be identical to the molecule isolated from plasma by Kisiel.[1] Our work with human protein C substantiates that human protein C is the functional analog of bovine protein.[1, 7, 10, 14] Both molecules contain two disulfide-linked polypeptide chains with similar molecular weights, amino acid and carbohydrate compositions, and sequence homology. Both are anticoagulants in their respective plasmas, and both function by inactivating factors V and VIII. However, the specificity of protein C is such that the human molecule is not anticoagulant in bovine plasma, and bovine protein C is not anticoagulant in human plasma.[1, 4]

Human protein C can be activated by several proteolytic enzymes: the factor X activator of Russell's viper venom, trypsin, or thrombin.[1, 13] Although α-thrombin may be an *in vivo* activator of protein C, this reaction is not particularly efficient. Perhaps some as yet unrecognized cofactor(s) would greatly accelerate the activation of protein C. Or perhaps another enzyme is the physiological activator of protein C. Nothing is yet known about the inhibition of activated protein C.

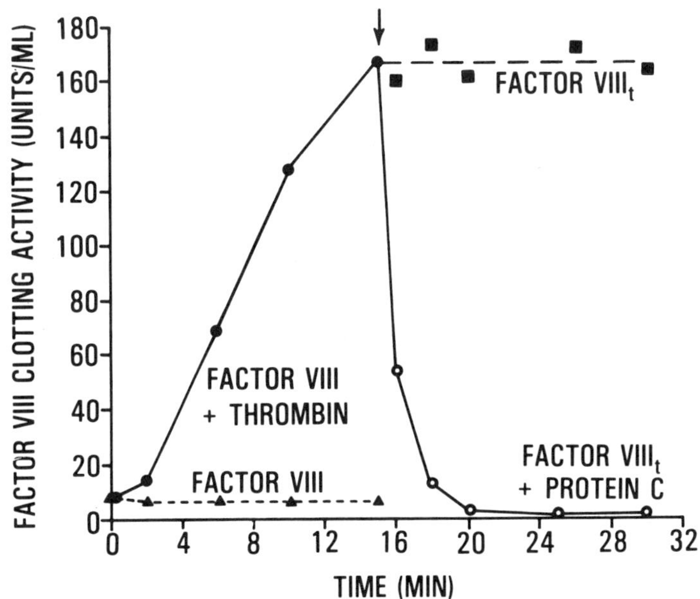

FIGURE 4. Activation and inactivation of human factor VIII:C. Partially purified factor VIII:C was activated with insolubilized human thrombin (solid line, solid circles). At 15 min (arrow), thrombin–Sepharose was removed by centrifugation and activated human protein C, phospholipid, and calcium were added (solid line, open circles). Controls included unactivated factor VIII:C plus buffer (dashed line, solid triangles) and thrombin-activated factor VIII:C (factor VIII$_t$) plus buffer (dashed line, solid squares). After Marlar *et al.*[13]

Human protein C may provide a major control mechanism of blood coagulation. It functions by removing two essential cofactors (factors V and VIII:C) from their respective roles in the enzymatic activation of prothrombin and factor X. If these two cofactors are inactivated by protein C, then the ultimate rate of fibrin formation can be reduced by many orders of magnitude. When factors V and VIII:C are activated by thrombin, their procoagulant activity increases 100- to 1000-fold. Notably, protein C inactivates these activated forms more rapidly than the native forms of factors V and VIII:C, implying a more responsive mechanism for antithrombotic regulation. With protein C functioning in conjunction with protease inhibitors and negative feedback proteolysis, the amount and rate of active coagulation factor formation may be precisely regulated.

ACKNOWLEDGMENTS

The authors thank Jennifer Oldstone for her skillful technical assistance and Dr. T. Yamamoto for assistance in the initial isolation of protein C. We are grateful to Dr. Walter Kisiel, University of Washington, Seattle, Wash. for helpful discussions and for the gift of rabbit anti-human protein C antiserum. We think Hyland Therapeutics, Costa Mesa, Calif., for their generous donation of Proplex and Hemophil.

REFERENCES

1. KISIEL, W. 1979. Human plasma protein C: Isolation, characterization and mechanism of activation by α-thrombin. J. Clin. Invest. **64:** 761–769.
2. FERNLUND, P. & J. STENFLO. 1980. Amino acid sequence of bovine protein C. *In* Vitamin K Metabolism and Vitamin K-dependent Proteins. J. Suttie, Ed.: 84–88. University Park Press. Baltimore, Md.
3. MAMMEN, E., W. THOMAS & W. H. SEEGERS. 1960. Activation of purified prothrombin to autoprothrombin I or autoprothrombin II (platelet cofactor II) or autoprothrombin II-A. Thromb. Diath. Haemorrh. **5:** 218–250.
4. MARCINIAK, E. 1972. Inhibitor of human blood coagulation elicited by thrombin. J. Lab. Clin. Med. **79:** 921–934.
5. STENFLO, J. 1976. A new vitamin K-dependent protein: purification from bovine plasma and preliminary characterization. J. Biol. Chem. **251:** 355–363.
6. SEEGERS, W. H., E. NOVOA, R. HENRY & H. HASSOUNA. 1976. Relationship of "new" vitamin K-dependent protein C and "old" autoprothrombin II-A. Thromb. Res. **8:** 543–553.
7. MURANO, G., W. H. SEEGERS & R. ZOLTON. 1974. Autoprothrombin II-A: A competitive inhibitor of Autoprothrombin C. A review with additions. Thromb. Diath Haemorrh. (Suppl.) **57:** 305–314.
8. SEEGERS, W. H., R. A. MARLAR & D. WALZ. 1978. Anticoagulant effects of autoprothrombin-II-A and prothrombin fragment 1. Thromb. Res. **13:** 233–243.
9. KISIEL, W., W. CANFIELD, L. ERICSSON & E. DAVIE. 1977. Anticoagulant properties of bovine plasma protein C following activation by thrombin. Biochemistry **16:** 5824–5831.
10. ESMON, C., P. COMP & F. WALKER. 1980. Functions for protein C. *In* Vitamin K Metabolism and Vitamin K-Dependent Proteins. J. Suttie, Ed.: 72–83. University Park Press. Baltimore, Md.
11. VEHAR, G. & E. DAVIE. 1980. Preparation and properties of bovine Factor VIII (Antihemophilic Factor). Biochemistry **19:** 401–410.
12. MARLAR, R., A. KLEISS & J. GRIFFIN. 1980. Modes of anticoagulant action of human protein C, a vitamin K-dependent serine protease. Fed. Proc. **39:** 544.
13. MARLAR, R. A., A. J. KLEISS & J. H. GRIFFIN. 1980. Mechanisms of action of human protein C, a thrombin-dependent anticoagulant enzyme. (Submitted for publication.)
14. KISIEL, W., L. ERICSSON & E. DAVIE. 1976. Proteolytic activation of protein C from bovine plasma. Biochemistry **15:** 4893–4900.
15. CANFIELD, W., M. NESHEIM, W. KISIEL & K. MANN. 1978. Proteolytic inactivation of bovine Factor Va by bovine activated protein C. Circulation **58:** 210.
16. DAVIE, E. & K. FUJIKAWA. 1975. Basic mechanisms in blood coagulation. Ann. Rev. Biochem. **44:** 799–879.

TISSUE FACTOR:
A VITAMIN K-DEPENDENT CLOTTING FACTOR?

Leo R. Zacharski,* Robert Rosenstein,† and Philip G. Phillips ‡

*Veterans Administration Medical Center
White River Junction, Vermont 05001; and the
Departments of *Medicine, †Pharmacology/Toxicology, and
‡Biochemistry
Dartmouth Medical School
Hanover, New Hampshire 03755*

INTRODUCTION

Tissues from many organs have long been known to possess a potent initiator of blood coagulation that is not present in plasma.[1] This coagulant, commonly referred to as tissue thromboplastin, is perhaps best known as a laboratory reagent used to perform the one-stage prothrombin time test. The traditional mystique surrounding the supposed nonspecificity of "thromboplastin" has given way to increasingly precise biochemical characterization of this substance [1] and the utility of this term has declined. Reference to the tissue coagulant as "tissue factor" (TF, factor III), rather than thromboplastin, is now more appropriate since it is known to be a specific glycoprotein. TF apoprotein, while lacking coagulant activity itself, becomes a potent coagulant when combined with phospholipid, especially when present in a membrane configuration. TF exerts its coagulant effect upon combining with an activating plasma coagulation factor VII. In so doing, fibrin formation is initiated by way of the so-called extrinsic (or TF-activated) pathway of blood coagulation.[1]

It is not the purpose of this review to present an exhaustive and critical review of the literature on TF. Rather, certain aspects of the cellular biology of TF will be reviewed in order to place in context the recent finding that TF coagulant activity is reduced by warfarin administration. This raises the possibility that TF may be a vitamin K-dependent coagulation factor.

CELL BIOLOGY OF TF

TF is distinct from other coagulants because it is an integral component of cells and does not exist, at least in recognizable form, free in plasma. The resulting difficulties in obtaining TF-containing samples for study have delayed progress in the understanding of its function. In an attempt to overcome these difficulties, various procedures aimed at extraction and purification of TF from tissues have been developed.[1] While these can be used to study TF coagulant activity, they provide little information relative to anatomic localization of TF, its role in the economy of the cell, or its interaction with elements in the environment of the cell. Recently, however, TF protein has been localized in tissues by means of an antibody to TF or by coagulation factor VII to which a histochemical probe has been coupled.[1–4] These substances become fixed to TF

311

in tissues and permit its visualization. Such studies have demonstrated that TF is a component of cell membranes, particularly of vascular endothelial cells. Unfortunately, these techniques afford no information relative to the coagulant activity of TF.

A number of years ago we postulated that cell culture techniques might provide insight into the contribution of cells and tissues to blood coagulation.[5-6] A potent coagulant was, in fact, discovered in a variety of cell types studied in our laboratory and elsewhere.[5-16] While its nature was originally in doubt,[5-6] further study using newer methodologies permitted identification of this coagulant as TF.[10, 11, 16] It was shown to 1) induce rapid coagulation in normal plasma as well as in plasma deficient in either factor VIII, IX, XI or XII; 2) activate factor X in the presence of factor VII but not to induce coagulation in factor VII-deficient plasma; and 3) be inhibited by an antibody to TF protein (provided by Dr. Yale Nemerson).

Identification of this coagulant as TF was followed by work aimed at characterizing this substance in living cells maintained *in vitro*. In general, TF activity is low at the beginning of culture of various cell types but rapidly rises within minutes to hours thereafter.[5-16] This rise in activity is dependent upon intact RNA- and protein-synthesizing mechanisms.[17-18] TF production by fibroblasts is apparently enhanced by the presence of platelets,[19] while TF production by peripheral blood monocytes is enhanced by the presence of lymphocytes [20-22] and certain plasma lipoprotein species.[21] The fifth component of complement may also be involved.[23] A variety of agents stimulate monocyte TF production. These include endotoxin,[15, 23, 24] certain plasma proteins,[25] and antigen-antibody complexes.[22, 25] These inducers may exert their effect on lymphocytes present in mononuclear cell cultures rather than directly on the monocytes.[22] Induction of monocyte TF production is also observed in mixtures of allogeneic leukocytes.[26]

Many pharmacologic agents and metabolic inhibitors modify TF production by cultured cells [27-29] but results apparently vary with the cell type under consideration. However, conditions which increase cyclic AMP are associated with decreased monocyte TF production.[30]

Cell adhesion and spreading appear to be prerequisite for TF synthesis in cells cultured in monolayers.[17, 31] We noticed that the rise in activity in monolayer cultures was independent of cell doubling time but paralleled the period during which the cells were becoming adherent to the floor of the flask. Cells cultured in high concentration (such that a monolayer was formed from the outset and cell spreading on the floor of the flask was restricted) yielded coagulant levels which were about 50% of that of cells cultured in lower concentrations. In addition, the rise in TF observed in stationary cultures was not seen when cell adhesion was prevented by agitation of culture flasks on a mechanical shaker. When flasks of cells were removed from the agitating device after 12 and 24 hours of incubation and placed at rest, TF production commenced as cells became adherent to the floor of the flask. Of various cell types tested, leukocytes cultured in suspension generated lower levels of TF activity than various cell types cultured in monolayer. However, it has been shown that generation of TF by monocytes is also at least partially dependent upon adhesion.[20, 32]

Evidence indicates that TF coagulant activity produced by cultured cells comes to reside on the cell surface.[11, 17, 33] Thus, intact cells, as well as cell homogenates, possessed coagulant activity. Repeated washing of an intact monolayer has been shown to reduce TF activity. Trypsinization (but not neuraminidase treatment) of cultured cells also resulted in reduction of TF activity. The trypsin effect was reversed by soybean trypsin inhibitor. Maynard *et al.*[11] presented evidence that much of the TF activity of the surfaces of cultured cells is present in cryptic form. They showed that activity was increased by freeze-thaw lysis in several cell types. In addition, treatment with very dilute trypsin solutions actually increased (rather than decreased) TF activity. These studies in cultured cells corroborate work by others in which TF was localized to cell membranes using immunohistochemical methods.[2-4]

The relationship of TF to the cell membrane and to adhesion was studied further using the jackbean lectin, concanavalin A (Con A).[33] Con A binds to cell surface alpha-D-glucopyranosyl or alpha-D-mannopyranosyl residues resulting in modification of a variety of surface-related phenomena. However, Con A receptors themselves do not appear to mediate cell adhesion.[34] We demonstrated that Con A inhibits TF activity in a dose-related manner. The inhibitory effect of Con A was observed within five minutes, was maximal within one-half hour, was inhibited by alphamethyl-D-mannopyranoside (AMM), and could not be attributed to an effect of Con A on the assay system. Con A also inhibited the coagulant activity of rabbit brain thromboplastin. Our finding that Con A binds to and inhibits the TF activity of cells in culture was subsequently corroborated by the demonstration of similar binding to and inhibition of partially purified TF.[35]

These results indicate that TF may not, itself, be the cell surface component responsible for cell adhesion but rather that cell adhesion provides the signal for TF production. The possibility exists that this signal is mediated through the microtubular system of the cell. Using peripheral blood monocytes, de Prost *et al.*[36] showed that the cytoskeletal poisons colchicine and vinblastine inhibited TF generation. Muhlfelder and associates [37] found that vinblastine and cytochalasin B (but not colchicine) inhibited TF "release" from cultured leukocytes. Inconsistent results were obtained in studies using these agents in the presence of a variety of cells cultured in monolayer.[28] In the case of peripheral blood monocytes, the microtubular system of the cell may direct the emergence or distribution of TF on the cell surface. Alternatively, the drugs producing this effect may interfere with TF production by a mechanism independent of their effect on microtubules.

IDENTIFICATION OF SALIVARY TF

Although the study of TF by means of cultured cells has yielded useful insights, this approach is cumbersome and artificial, and provides information of uncertain physiologic significance. The desirability of having a readily available source of TF for study is evident. Attention might be directed, in this regard, to body fluids other than blood as potential sources of TF-containing material. While several such fluids (such as amniotic fluid, bile and other intestinal secretions, semen, sweat, tears or various pathologic effusions) may be worth studying, saliva seemed especially suitable because of its ready availability and because it has long been known to possess coagulant activity that had never been fully characterized.

We succeeded in documenting the existence of TF in saliva by four criteria: [38] (1) Saliva induced rapid coagulation in plasmas deficient in either factor VIII, IX, XI or XII. However, less than 1% of the coagulant activity of factors II, VII and X and less than 1% of the factor VIII antigen (determined by Dr. Leon Hoyer) of normal plasma were present in saliva. (2) When incremental volumes of saliva were added to the assay for factor VII, no dose-related reduction of clotting time was observed. Therefore, factor VII was required for the expression of salivary coagulant. (3) Using a two-stage assay system, we showed that the coagulant of saliva activated factor X in the presence of factor VII. (4) The activity of salivary coagulant was eliminated upon addition of an antibody to human TF.

Several experiments led us to conclude that salivary TF resided on cells and cell fragments in saliva. Following hyaluronidase treatment to reduce viscosity, saliva was subjected to graded centrifugation. Reduction in TF activity was in proportion to the force of centrifugation and all activity was eliminated following filtration on filters of 0.2 μ pore size. Greater than 99% of the cells in saliva were buccal epithelial cells and the remainder are neutrophils. No mononuclear leukocytes were observed. Saliva from edentulous individuals (which is devoid of leukocytes) manifested normal levels of TF activity and TF was evident in suspensions of buccal epithelial cells in buffer prepared by scraping the inner surface of the cheek with a spatula. Saliva was rendered cell-free by centrifugation at 1000 $\times$ g for 15 minutes. This procedure resulted in a 78% reduction in TF activity. The remaining particulate material was then pelleted and examined by electron microscopy. Results, presented in FIGURE 1, show that this material consisted of membranous fragments the appearance of which was reminiscent of TF-containing structures observed electronmicroscopically by others.[39, 40]

PATHOPHYSIOLOGIC SIGNIFICANCE OF TF

The development of newer methods for studying TF has permitted certain insights which suggest that its pathophysiologic significance may be profound. For example, Green *et al.*[12] failed to detect TF in fibroblasts cultured from normal synovia. We have confirmed their findings in a synovial fibroblast line studied in our laboratory. It is possible that hemophiliacs whose skin fibroblasts generate normal amounts of TF in culture, are particularly predisposed to hemarthrosis because of absence of synovial TF in addition to absence of circulating factor VIII activity.

Previous reports by us [6] and by Green *et al.*[12] demonstrated no significant difference in TF activity between normal cells and cells cultured from subjects with hemophilia A and B. By contrast, we showed that fibroblasts from the four individuals with von Willebrand's disease yielded activity which was significantly lower than normal.[41] The significance of the TF abnormality and the nature of the defect (whether qualitative or quantitative) in von Willebrand's fibroblasts remain to be determined. The finding of a TF abnormality in von Willebrand's disease together with the well-known abnormality in factor VIII protein which exists in this condition suggests that the formation of these two substances within the cell may, in some way, be linked together.

Goldstein and Niewiarowski [42] recently demonstrated that fibroblasts cultured from the skin of patients with progeria and Werner's syndrome have markedly increased TF activity. These workers postulated that this increased activity is related to the predisposition of these individuals to accelerated atherosclerosis, thrombosis and premature death. Zeldis *et al.*[2] demonstrated TF on the plasma membrane of vascular endothelial cells in various tissues. They speculated that TF on the cell membrane would render it readily available for complexing with plasma coagulation factor VII. TF antigen of plasma membranes of the vascular intima was found to be particularly abundant in the vicinity of atherosclerotic plaques where it virtually encompassed cholesterol crystals. They postulated that TF might initiate coagulation even with minimal endothelial damage or in the event of plaque disruption.

Jensen and associates[43] have recently implicated TF in the hemostatic process which arrests hemorrhage from skin incisions. They demonstrate that factor VIII (and factor V) functional activity greatly increased with time in blood emerging from the incision. They concluded that this rise in activity,

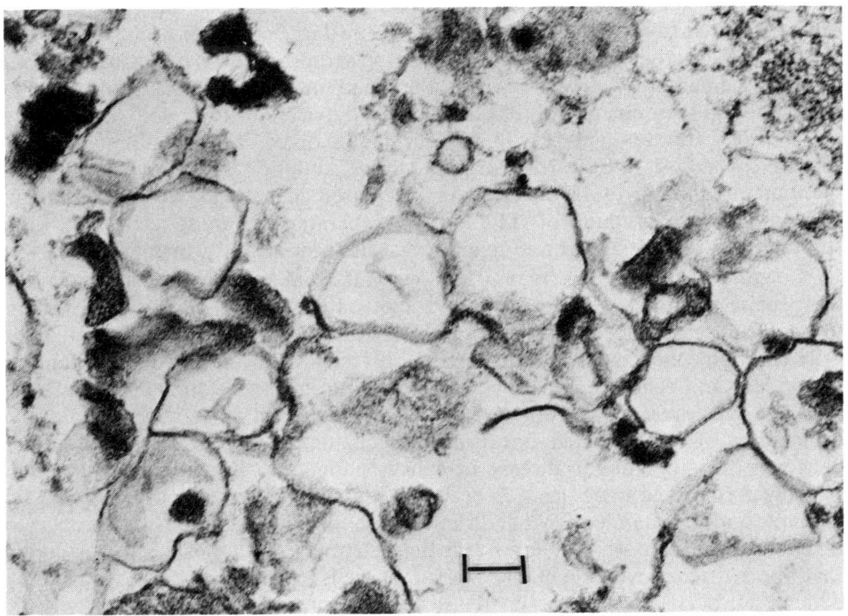

FIGURE 1. Electron microscopic appearance of salivary cell fragments which manifest TF activity. The bar represents 0.1 μm $\times$ 70,000.

which is believed to heighten coagulation, was due to generation of trace amounts of thrombin through the TF pathway. This conclusion was supported by the observation that the rise in VIII activity could be blocked by heparin administration and was not observed in individuals with congenital factor VII deficiency or deficiency of one of the factors in the final common pathway of blood coagulation. In contrast, individuals deficient in factors XII, XI, IX or I, had normal VIII activation. An additional interesting observation was the failure of patients with factor VIII deficiency to generate increased factor V activity. This implies that factor VIII might in some way be involved in the TF pathway.

TF has been implicated in the pathogenesis of several forms of disseminated intravascular coagulation (DIC) such as that observed with malignancy, hemolytic transfusion reactions, amniotic fluid embolism,[1, 44] heat stroke,[45, 46] fat embolism,[47, 48] intravenous infusion of ascitic fluid,[49] and following acute head injury of sufficient severity to cause brain tissue destruction.[50] In these situations, thromboplastin may induce coagulation upon liberation into the circulation. While normal leukocytes contain little or no TF activity, exposure of leukocytes to endotoxin markedly increases their TF content.[15, 23, 24] This increased TF activity might mediate endotoxin-induced DIC. Spontaneously increased leukocyte TF has been discovered in promyelocytic leukemia and incriminated in the development of DIC in this particular disorder.[51–54] TF has also been observed on mononuclear cells infiltrating an organ graft which is undergoing rejection and it has been postulated that such TF is responsible for the deposition of fibrin associated with the rejection reaction.[55] The TF activity generated by peripheral blood mononuclear cells has also been shown to be increased following kidney allografting in dogs.[56] Lerner *et al.*[57] observed increased TF activity in leukocytes recovered from an *in vitro* clot or from an isolated segment of vein into which they had migrated. As a result of the latter finding, they postulated that leukocytes, by virtue of their ability to invade vessel walls and to generate TF, might be involved in the pathogenesis of venous thrombosis. Edwards, Rickles and Cronlund [58] recently found that spontaneous monocyte TF activity was increased in patients with malignancy. In addition, the amount of TF activity generated by these cells following stimulation with antigens or mitogens was also significantly increased.

Coagulant activity has long been recognized in malignant cells.[59] While the precise identity of this coagulant is not entirely clear, it has been shown to be TF at least for certain types of malignancy.[60–63] Migration of malignant cells through vessel walls would expose this cell surface-related coagulant to factor VII and other coagulation proteins in plasma so as to induce clot formation. The presence of this coagulant on malignant cells may explain the occurrence of disseminated intravascular coagulation and the increased incidence of thromboembolic disease in cancer patients.[59] Fibrin-platelet thrombi have been observed in association with local tumor masses in both experimental animals and in man.[59] Since administration of anticoagulants is known to ameliorate the course of many experimental tumors,[59] it has been postulated that the existence of coagulants on tumor cells constitutes a mechanism by which their persistence and ultimate growth and spread is assured.

Giercksky [48] found that human adipose tissue manifested TF activity. A similar coagulant appears in the cerebrospinal fluid which is thought to be a reflection of central nervous system damage.[64] Several workers have studied the TF activity of amniotic fluid in detail.[65–67] This coagulant appears concomitantly with surfactant at about 30 weeks of gestation and gradually increases thereafter.[65] Especially high levels are found with post-mature pregnancies.[67] Both coagulant and surfactant are reduced in the amniotic fluid of patients whose babies subsequently developed the respiratory distress syndrome.[66]

The discovery of TF activity in saliva [38] (with the virtual absence of other coagulant substances) provided a means by which TF could be assessed under a variety of clinical conditions. This "painless biopsy" procedure was applied to a large number of hospitalized patients and individuals with hereditary hemorrhagic disorders in an attempt to discover abnormalities. Despite an extensive search, such abnormalities were not found except in patients on long-term warfarin anticoagulation.[38] Salivary TF activity was significantly reduced in nine patients on long-term warfarin therapy in comparison to that of 34 normal subjects. The mean warfarin dose in these patients was 7.0 mg/d. The depression of TF activity could not be attributed to any other medication being taken or to differences between groups in salivery cell count or protein concentration. Addition of sodium warfarin to saliva in concentrations up to 2 mg/ml failed to alter TF activity.

Salivary TF assays were then performed prior to and during induction of anticoagulation with warfarin in seven patients. Pretreatment activity was indistinguishable from normal. However, in six of the seven patients, a gradual decline in activity (prolongation of clotting times) was observed which paralleled the prolongation of the one-stage prothrombin time. The scatter of data for salivary TF activity was such that linearity versus curvilinearity could not be determined. Therefore, for purposes of illustration, and in order to test the significance of the change in activity, the data were analyzed by linear regression. The regression of TF activity (and the prothrombin time) versus days on warfarin was highly significant ($p \leq 0.01$). At the end of the induction period, the salivary TF activity was similar to that of patients on long-term warfarin therapy, that is about 15 to 20% of pretreatment levels. These results are illustrated in Figure 2. (A change in salivary TF activity was not observed in a patient following initiation of continuous intravenous heparin therapy.) These results suggested that expression of TF coagulant activity might be dependent upon the presence of vitamin K.

DISCUSSION

Fragmentary information about TF collected slowly in recent years is most intriguing but still insufficient to form a clear picture of the *in vivo* significance of this coagulant. One major obstacle to progress is the resistance this substance has shown to efforts at purification.[1] This resistance may be due primarily to the marked hydrophobic properties of TF apoprotein. Another obstacle is the persistent inability to obtain satisfactory samples of tissues suspected of manifesting TF activity and then to determine precisely which cell type within the tissue is responsible for the TF activity. However, the finding that TF activity is reduced with warfarin treatment suggests that it is either directly or indirectly vitamin K-dependent. This observation might allow a new approach to the pursuit of information about TF *in vivo*.

The possibility that TF is a vitamin K-dependent protein deserves critical assessment. A protein may be considered to be vitamin K-dependent if it is modified in the presence of vitamin K deficiency or upon administration of a vitamin K antagonist, or if it can be shown to contain glutamic acid residues which are carboxylated in the γ position (Gla residues).[68, 69] This amino acid imparts to these proteins the ability to bind calcium and to interact with membrane phospholipids.[69] While adipose tissue TF activity has been said to be "slightly reduced" in vitamin K-deficient rats,[48] the vitamin K deficiency state has seldom been studied from the point of view of its effect on TF activity. Bach has shown that purified bovine TF does not contain Gla residues (personal communication) but differences between species may exist in the dependency of various clotting factors on vitamin K.[70] Thus, the only evidence so far available that TF is vitamin K-dependent is that its activity is diminished by the administration of warfarin.[38] This effect has been observed in our laboratory for salivary TF and by Edwards and Rickles [71] in peripheral blood mononuclear cells cultured from subjects on warfarin. We have also observed depression of TF activity upon direct addition of crystalline sodium warfarin in concentrations as low as 10^{-6} M to cultures of mononuclear leukocytes and fibroblasts (unpublished observations).

Several plasma proteins,[72-76] in addition to coagulation factors II, VII, IX and X; and tissue-related proteins [77-79] have recently been shown to be vitamin K-dependent, Gla-containing proteins. In fact, Gla residues are plentiful in many tissues.[80] For example, one of the tissue-related proteins, termed osteocalcin,[77] is apparently present in the intercellular matrix of bone. Still another

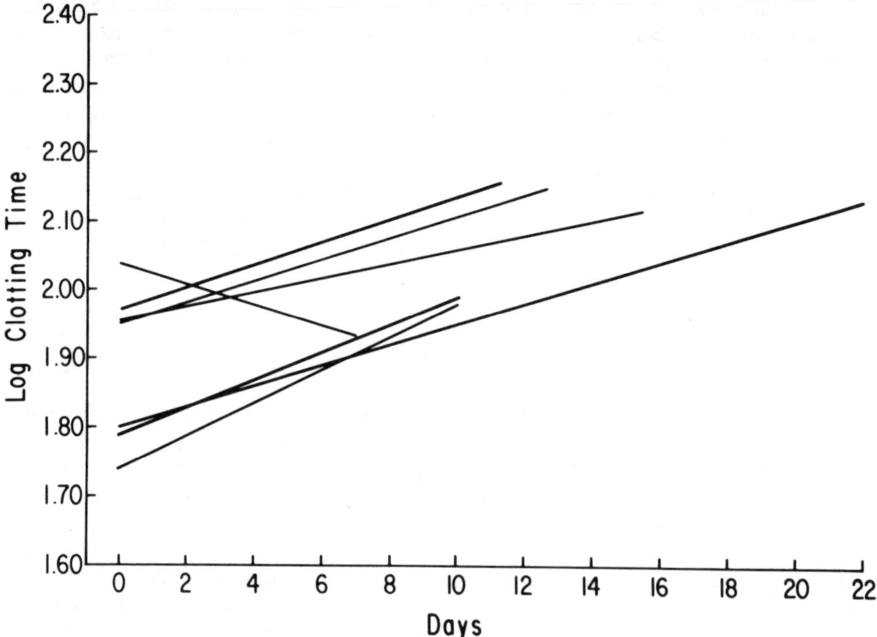

FIGURE 2. Results of one-stage assays for TF in seven patients tested during induction of warfarin anticoagulation. Regression of clotting time (TF assay) versus days on warfarin for the entire group, $p \leq 0.01$.

such protein, the so-called calcium-binding protein (CaBP), is synthesized by the cells of the chick chorioallantoic membrane and comes to reside very superficially on the cell membrane.[78] All of these are different from TF in that they are readily soluble. Should human TF ultimately be found to meet the biochemical criteria for vitamin K-dependency, it would in this respect fall into a class quite different from its relatives. For a vitamin K-dependent protein to be a constituent of cell membranes would be reminiscent of the observation that coumarins inhibit synthesis of certain constituents of plant cell walls.[81]

It must be recognized that depression of TF activity with warfarin does not require that TF be, itself, a vitamin K-dependent protein. In fact, a different protein that serves as an intermediate in TF production may be affected.

Furthermore, warfarin may depress TF activity by a mechanism independent of its ability to antagonize vitamin K-dependent post-translational carboxylation of glutamic acid residues in protein. Stated otherwise, the presence of a coumarin is not necessarily synonymous with a deficiency of vitamin K. For example, evidence exists that both transcription and translation may be influenced (directly or indirectly) by the availability of vitamin K.[82] In addition, Eichbaum *et al.*[83] have recently described the anti-inflammatory properties of warfarin. These properties were unrelated to the anticoagulant properties of this substance and its congeners and, in fact, were also observed for vitamin K_1. These findings suggest that the observed effects of these agents were related more to their fundamental quinone structure than to their involvement in carboxylation reactions. Vitamin K antagonists are known to inhibit mitochondrial oxidative phosphorylation in *in vitro* systems but not *in vivo*.[84–86] They are apparently capable of inducing a variety of ultrastructural changes in hepatic parenchymal cells upon administration to dogs.[87] On the other hand, evidence presented by Edwards and Rickles[71] indicated that, while TF activity was significantly depressed in monocytes from warfarin-treated patients, a variety of other leukocyte functions remained intact. The effect of warfarin on TF was seemingly selective.

Our current understanding of the relationship between vitamin K and TF is obviously limited. Despite existing uncertainties, however, the finding that warfarin anticoagulation is associated with reduced TF activity might provide an important lead to understanding the enigmatic *in vivo* role of TF in humans. Clues to the pathophysiologic significance of TF reviewed above might be reevaluated from this point of view. For example, as suggested by Lerner *et al.*,[57] the beneficial effect of warfarin on venous thrombotic disease might be more related to inhibition of TF generated by leukocytes invading a vessel wall than to inhibition of circulating vitamin K-dependent clotting factors.

Extensive evidence incriminates activation of the clotting mechanism in the growth and spread of malignancy.[59] TF, or a related coagulant present on the tumor cells, may be the initiator of coagulation reactions necessary for persistence of the tumor and metastasis formation. We have recently demonstrated in a controlled, randomized trial that survival in human small cell carcinoma of the lung is significantly prolonged upon administration of warfarin.[88] As predicted, this increased longevity was related to delayed tumor progression rather than to increased tumor regression. One possible mechanism of this beneficial effect is suppression of tumor cell TF activity. Alternatively, a reduction by warfarin of monocyte TF activity may be responsible, as postulated by Edwards *et al.*[58] Conceivably, other types of tumors might be found responsive to warfarin by similar mechanisms.

The role of warfarin in the management of various inflammatory diseases might also warrant further definition. Cellular coagulant activity, which is probably TF, is a feature of mononuclear cells involved in reactions considered to be analogous to delayed hypersensitivity reactions.[89–94] Hedfors[95] described a patient with advanced sarcoidosis who developed thrombophlebitis. Treatment with warfarin was followed by complete resolution of pulmonary infiltrates of sarcoidosis. Fibrin has been observed in sarcoid granulomas[96] and it was postulated that mononuclear cells in these lesions might be responsible for the fibrin deposition by virtue of their TF coagulant activity. The warfarin may have exerted its beneficial effect by inhibition of this TF. Should this be true, a fundamental relationship might exist between induction of local coagulation and the persistence of the granulomas which might be analogous to the proposed relationship between the clotting and certain malignancies.

In conclusion, the discovery of a possible dependency of TF on vitamin K might provide a new strategy for understanding the patho-physiologic significance of TF. Available data provide a basis for the formulation of hypotheses upon which experiments can be designed that promise to expand our understanding of this interesting coagulation factor.

REFERENCES

1. NEMERSON, Y. & F. A. PITLICK. 1972. The tissue factor pathway of blood coagulation. *In* Progress in Hemostasis and Thrombosis. T. H. Spaet, Ed. **1:** 1–37. Grune and Stratton. New York, N.Y.
2. ZELDIS, S. M., Y. NEMERSON, F. A. PITLICK & T. L. LENZ. 1972. Tissue factor (thromboplastin): localization of plasma membranes by peroxidaze-conjugated antibodies. Science **175:** 766.
3. STEMERMAN, M. B., F. A. PITLICK & H. M. DEMBITZER. 1976. Electron microscopic immunohistochemical identification of endothelial cells in the rabbit. Circulation Res. **38:** 146–156.
4. GOLDENFARB, P. B., F. A. PITLICK & Y. NEMERSON. 1973. Factor VII: A biological probe for initiation sites of blood coagulation. J. Clin. Invest. **52:** 34a.
5. ZACHARSKI, L. R., E. J. W. BOWIE, J. L. TITUS & C. A. OWEN, JR. 1968. Synthesis of Antihemophilic factor (factor VIII) by leukocytes: Preliminary report. Proc. Staff Meet. Mayo Clin. **43:** 617.
6. ZACHARSKI, L. R., E. J. W. BOWIE, J. L. TITUS & C. A. OWEN, JR. 1969. Cell-culture synthesis of a factor VIII-like activity. Proc. Staff Meet. Mayo Clin. **44:** 784.
7. ZACHARSKI, L. R. & O. R. McINTYRE. 1971. Characterization of procoagulants produced in cell cultures by tests of coagulation. Thromb. Diath. Haemorrh. **26:** 493.
8. ZACHARSKI, L. R. & O. R. McINTYRE. 1972. Physical stability of cell culture procoagulants detectable in first-stage coagulation factor assays. Proc. Soc. Exp. Biol. Med. **139:** 713.
9. ZACHARSKI, L. R. & O. R. McINTYRE. 1973. Tissue factor (thromboplastin, factor III) synthesis by cultured cells. J. Med. **4:** 118.
10. ZACHARSKI, L. R., L. W. HOYER & O. R. McINTYRE. 1973. Immunologic identification of tissue factor (thromboplastin) synthesized by cultured fibroblasts. Blood **41:** 671.
11. MAYNARD, J. R., C. A. HECKMAN, F. A. PITLICK & Y. NEMERSON. 1975. Association of tissue factor activity with the surface of cultured cells. J. Clin. Invest. **55:** 814–824.
12. GREEN, D., C. RYAN, N. MALANDROCCOLO & H. L. NADLER. 1971. Characterization of the coagulant activity of cultured human fibroblasts. Blood **37:** 47–51.
13. NIEMETZ, J. 1972. Coagulant activity of leukocytes, tissue factor activity. J. Clin. Invest. **51:** 307.
14. RIVERS, R. P. A., W. E. HATHAWAY & W. L. WESTON. 1975. The endotoxin-induced activity of human monocytes. Br. J. Haematol. **30:** 311–316.
15. LERNER, R. G., R. GOLDSTEIN & G. CUMMINGS. 1971. Stimulation of human leukocyte thromboplastic activity by endotoxin. Proc. Soc. Exp. Biol. Med. **138:** 145–148.
16. RICKLES, F. R., J. A. HARDIN, F. A. PITLICK, L. W. HOYER & M. E. CONRAD. 1973. Tissue factor activity in lymphocyte cultures from normal individuals and patients with hemophilia A. J. Clin. Invest. **52:** 1427.

17. ZACHARSKI, L. R. & O. R. McINTYRE. 1973. Membrane mediated synthesis of tissue factor (thromboplastin) in cultured fibroblasts. Blood **41:** 679.

18. NIEMETZ, J. 1971. Role of protein synthesis inhibitors on the procoagulant activity generated by leukocytes. Am. Soc. Hemat. Abst. **13**.

19. SMARIGA, P. E. & J. R. MAYNARD. 1979. Platelets increase human fibroblast thrombogenicity by increasing tissue factor activity and decreasing fibrinolytic activity. Blood **54** (Suppl. 1): 303.

20. EDWARDS, R. L., F. R. RICKLES & A. M. BOBROVE. 1979. Mononuclear cell tissue factor: Cell of origin and requirements for activation. Blood **54:** 359–370.

21. EDGINGTON, T. S., G. A. LEVY, B. S. SCHWARTZ & L. K. CURTIS. 1980. Serum lipoprotein induction of lymphoid procoagulant activity. Fed. Proc. **39:** 544.

22. SCHWARTZ, B. S., G. LEVY & T. S. EDGINGTON. 1980. Induction of monocyte/macrophage procoagulant activity by immune complexes requires lymphocyte collaboration and is restricted by monocyte/macrophage differentiation. Fed. Proc. **39:** 544.

23A. MUHLFELDER, T., J. NIEMETZ, D. KREUTZER, D. BEEBE & P. WARD. 1978. Role of the fifth component of complement related activity (C5ra) on leukocyte generated tissue factor activity (TFa). Fed. Proc. **37:** 545.

23B. NIEMETZ, J. & D. MORRISON. 1976. Role of lipid A on the procoagulant activity of leukocytes. Fed. Proc. **35:** 804.

24. RICKLES, F. R., P. D. RICK & M. VAN WHY. 1977. Structural features of salmonella typhimurium lipopolysaccharide required for activation of tissue factor in human mononuclear cells. J. Clin. Invest. **59:** 1188–1195.

25. ROTHBERGER, H., T. S. ZIMMERMAN, H. L. SPIEGELBERG & J. H. VAUGHN. 1977. Leukocyte procoagulant activity. Enhancement of productivity *in vitro* by IgG and antigen-antibody complexes. J. Clin. Invest. **59:** 549–557.

26. ROTHBERGER, H., T. S. ZIMMERMAN & J. H. VAUGHN. 1978. Increased production and expression of tissue thromboplastin-like procoagulant activity *in vitro* by allogeneically stimulated human leukocytes. J. Clin. Invest. **62:** 649–655.

27. MAYNARD, J. R., D. J. FINTEL, F. A. PITLICK & Y. NEMERSON. 1976. Tissue factor in cultured cells. Metabolic control. Lab. Invest. **35:** 542–549.

28. MAYNARD, J. R., D. J. FINTEL, F. A. PITLICK & Y. NEMERSON. 1976. Tissue factor in cultured cells. Pharmacologic effects. Lab. Invest. **35:** 550–557.

29. MAYNARD, J. R., D. E. BURKHOLDER & D. J. PIZZUTI. 1978. Comparative pharmacologic effects on tissue factor activity in normal cells and an established cell line. Lab. Invest. **38:** 14–20.

30. TONO-OKA, T., M. NAKAYAMA, E. GOTOHDA & T. TAKEDA. 1979. Prevention of tissue factor generation in mononuclear cells by agents known to increase intracellular cyclic amp. Tohoku J. Exp. Med. **127:** 161–167.

31. ZACHARSKI, L. R. & O. R. McINTYRE. 1971. Procoagulant synthesis by cultured fibroblasts triggered by cell adhesion. Nature, Lond. **232:** 338.

32. VAN GINKEL, C. J. W., W. G. VAN AKEN, J. I. H. OH & J. VREEHEN. 1977. Stimulation of monocyte procoagulant activity by adherance to different surfaces. Br. J. Haematol. **37:** 35–45.

33. ZACHARSKI, L. R., R. ROSENSTEIN & P. G. PHILLIPS. 1974. Concanavalin A inhibition of tissue factor (thromboplastin) activity. Blood **44:** 783–787.

34. STEINBERG, M. S. & I. A. GEPNER. 1973. Are Concanavalin A receptor sites mediators of cell-cell adhesion? Nature (New Biol.) **241:** 249.

35. PITLICK, F. A. 1975. Concanavalin A inhibits tissue factor coagulant activity. J. Clin. Invest. **55:** 175–179.

36. DE PROST, D., E. CRAMER & J. HAKIM. 1979. Inhibition by antimicrotubular agents of the procoagulant activity generated by the blood monocytes: a biochemical and morphological study. Am. J. Hematol. **6:** 229–241.

37. MUHLFELDER, T. W., I. KHAN & J. NIEMETZ. 1978. Factors influencing the release of procoagulant-tissue factor activity from leukocytes. J. Lab. Clin. Med. **92:** 65–72.

38. ZACHARSKI, L. R. & R. ROSENSTEIN. 1979. Reduction of salivary tissue factor (TF) by warfarin therapy. Blood **53**: 366–374.
39. HVATUM, M., T. HOVIG & H. PRYDZ. 1969. Studies on tissue thromboplastin-electron micrography. Thromb. Diath. Haemorrh. **21**: 217–233.
40. HASEGAWA, H., H. NAGATA & M. MURAO. 1977. Studies on the tissue thromboplastin during the coagulation-fibrinolytic process-ultrastructural changes. Thromb. Haemostas. **37**: 541–548.
41. ZACHARSKI, L. R., R. ROSENSTEIN, G. G. CORNWELL, III, W. M. DAVIS & O. R. McINTYRE. 1974. Reduced tissue factor (thromboplastin) activity in von Willebrand's disease. Am. J. Med. **57**: 102–107.
42. GOLDSTEIN, S. & S. NIEWIAROWSKI. 1976. Increased procoagulant activity in cultured fibroblasts from progeria and Werner's syndrome of premature aging. Nature **260**: 711–713.
43. JENSEN, A. H. B., S. BEGUIN AND F. JOSSO. 1976. Factor V and VIII activation *"in vivo"* during bleeding. Evidence of thrombin formation at the early stage of hemostasis. Pathol.-Biol. **24** (Suppl): 6–10.
44. OWEN, C. A., JR., E. J. W. BOWIE, P. DIDISHEIM & J. H. THOMPSON, JR. 1969. *In* The Diagnosis of Bleeding Disorders. Little, Brown. Boston, MA.
45. CORNELL, C. J., JR. S. H. FEIN, B. REILLY & G. G. CORNWELL, III. 1974. Heparin therapy for heat stroke. Ann. Int. Med. **81**: 702.
46. PERCHICK, J. S., A. WINKELSTEIN & R. K. SHADDUCK. 1975. Disseminated intravascular coagulation in heat stroke. Response to heparin therapy. JAMA **231**: 480–483.
47. DINES, D. E., R. L. LINSHEID & E. P. DIDIER. 1972. Fat embolism syndrome. Mayo Clin. Proc. **47**: 237–40.
48. GIERCKSKY, K.-E. 1977. The procoagulant activity of adipose tissue. Scand. J. Haematol. **19**: 385–395.
49. LERNER, R. G., J. C. NELSON, P. CORINES & L. R. M. del GUERCIO. 1977. Intravascular coagulation complicating peritoneo-atrial shunts. Blood **50** (Suppl 1): 274.
50. GOODNIGHT, S. H., G. KENOYER, S. I. RAPAPORT, M. J. PATCH, J. A. LEE & T. KURZE. 1974. Defibrination after brain-tissue destruction. A serious complication of head injury. New Engl. J. Med. **290**: 1043–1047.
51. QUIGLEY, H. J. 1967. Peripheral leukocyte thromboplastin in promyelocytic leukemia. Fed. Proc. **26**: 648.
52. POLLICK, A. 1971. Acute promyelocytic leukemia with disseminated intravascular coagulation. Am. J. Clin. Path. **56**: 155.
53. GOUAULT-HEILMANN, M., E. CHARDON, C. SULTAN & F. JOSSO. 1975. The procoagulant factor of leukaemic promyelocytes: Demonstration of immunologic cross-reactivity with human brain tissue factor. Br. J. Haematol. **30**: 151–158.
54. GRALNICK, H. R. & H. K. TAN. 1974. Acute promyelocytic leukemia. A model for understanding the role of the malignant cell in hemostasis. Human Pathol. **5**: 661–673.
55. HATTLER, B. G., R. E. ROCKLIN, P. A. WARD & F. R. RICKLES. 1973. Functional features of lymphocytes recovered from a human renal allograft. Cell Immunol. **9**: 289–296.
56. ROTHBERGER, H., T. P. MUTTON, J. J. BROWN & J. H. MEREDITH. 1979. Increased production of tissue factor by leukocytes due to effects of transplantation surgery and allograft rejection. Blood **54** (Suppl 1): 300.
57. LERNER, R. G., R. GOLDSTEIN & J. C. NELSON. 1977. Production of thromboplastin (tissue factor) and thrombi by polymorphonuclear neutrophilic leukocytes adhering to vein walls. Thromb. Res. **11**: 11–22.
58. EDWARDS, R. L., F. R. RICKLES & M. CRONLUND. 1980. Neoplasia and fibrin deposition: The role of monocyte tissue factor. Clin. Res. **28**: 414.

59. ZACHARSKI, L. R., W. G. HENDERSON, F. R. RICKLES, W. B. FORMAN, C. J. CORNELL, JR., R. J. FORCIER, H. W. HARROWER & R. D. JOHNSON. 1979. Rationale and experimental design for the VA Cooperative Study of anticoagulation (warfarin) in the treatment of cancer. Cancer **44:** 732–741.

60. GOUAULT-HEILMANN, M., E. CHARDON, C. SULTAN & F. JOSSO. 1975. The procoagulant factor of leukaemic promyelocytes: Demonstration of immunologic crossreactivity with human brain tissue factor. Br. J. Haematol. **30:** 151–158.

61. GRALNICK, H. R. & E. ABRELL. 1973. Studies of the procoagulant and fibrinolytic activity of promyelocytes in acute promyelocytic leukemia. Br. J. Haematol. **24:** 89–99.

62. SAKURAGAWA, N., K. TAKAHASHI, M. HOSHIYAMA, C. JIMBO, K. ASHIZAWA, M. MATUSUOKA & O. YASHIKISA. 1976. Pathologic cells as procoagulant substance of disseminated intravascular coagulation syndrome in acute promyelocytic leukemia. Thromb. Res. **8:** 263–273.

63. SAKURAGAWA, N., K. TAKAHASHI, M. HOSHIYAMA, C. JIMBO, K. ASHIZAWA, M. MATUSUOKA & Y. OHNISHI. 1977. The extract from the tissue of gastric cancer as procoagulant in disseminated intravascular coagulation syndrome. Thromb. Res. **10:** 457–463.

64. GRAEBER, J. E. & M. J. STUART. 1978. Spinal-fluid procoagulant activity: A sensitive indicator of central nervous system damage. Lancet **2:** 285–288.

65. SUZUKI, S., N. WAKE & K. YOSHIAKI. 1976. New neonatal problems of blood coagulation and fibrinolysis. J. Perinat. Med. **4:** 221–226.

66. YAFFE, H., H. BAR-ON, A. ELDOR, M. RON & E. SADOVSKY. 1977. Correlation between thromboplastic activity and lecithin/sphingomyelin ratio in amniotic fluid. Br. J. Obstet. Gyn. **84:** 354–356.

67. YAFFE, H., A. ELDOR, E. HORNSHTEIN AND E. SADOVSKY. 1977. Thromboplastic activity in amniotic fluid during pregnancy. Br. J. Obstet. Gyn. **50:** 454–456.

68. STENFLO, J. Vitamin K, prothrombin and γ-carboxyglumatic acid. New Engl. J. Med. **296:** 624–626.

69. NELSESTUEN, G. L. 1978. Interactions of vitamin K-dependent proteins with calcium ions and phospholipid membranes. Fed. Proc. **37:** 2621–2625.

70. OWEN, C. A., JR. & E. J. W. BOWIE. 1978. Rat coagulation factors V, VIII, XI and XII: Vitamin K dependent. Haemostasis **7:** 189–201.

71. EDWARDS, R. L. & F. R. RICKLES. 1978. Delayed hypersensitivity in man: effects of systemic anticoagulation. Science **200:** 541–543.

72. STENFLO, J. 1976. New vitamin-K-dependent protein; Purification from bovine plasma and preliminary characterization. J. Biol. Chem. **251:** 355–363.

73. SEEGERS, W. H., A. GHOSH, & V. Y. WU. 1979. Function of previously unrecognized plasma protein M in thrombin generation. *In* Vitamin K Metabolism and Vitamin K-Dependent Proteins. J. W. Suttie, Ed. 96–101. University Park Press. Baltimore, MD.

74. DI SCIPIO, R. G. & E. W. DAVIE. 1979. Characterization of protein S a γ-carboxyglutamic acid containing protein from bovine and human plasma. Biochemistry **18:** 899–904.

75. PROWSE, C. P. & M. P. ESNOUF. 1977. The isolation of a new warfarin-sensitive protein from bovine plasma. Biochem. Soc. Trans. **5:** 255–256.

76. KISIEL, W. 1979. Human plasma protein C, isolation, characterization and mechanism of activation by α-thrombin. J. Clin. Invest. **64:** 761–769.

77. HAUSCHKA, P. V. & A. H. REDDI. 1980. Correlation of the appearance of γ-carboxyglutamic acid with the onset of mineralization in developing endochondral bone. Biochem. Biophys. Res. Commun. **92:** 1037–1041.

78. TUAN, R. S., W. A. SCOTT & Z. A. COHN. 1978. Purification and characterization of calcium-binding protein from chick chorioallantoic membrane. J. Biol. Chem. **253:** 1011–1016.

79. Levy, R. J., J. B. Lian & P. Gallop. 1979. Atherocalcin, a γ-carboxyglutamic acid containing protein from atherosclerotic plaque. Biochem. Biophys. Res. Commun. **91:** 41–49.

80. Friedman, P. A., P. V. Hauschka, M. A. Shia & J. K. Wallace. 1979. Characteristics of the vitamin K-dependent carboxylating system in human placenta. Biochem. Biophys. Acta **583:** 261–265.

81. Hara, M., N. Umetsu, C. Miyamoto & K. Tamari. 1973. Inhibition of the biosynthesis of plant cell wall materials, especially cellulose biosynthesis, by coumarin. Plant Cell Physiol. **14:** 11–28.

82. Munns, T. W., M. F. M. Johnson, M. K. Liszewski & R. E. Olson. 1976. Vitamin K-dependent synthesis and modification of precursor prothrombin in cultured H-35 hepatoma cells. Proc. Natl. Acad. Sci. USA **73:** 2803–2807.

83. Eichbaum, F. W., O. Stemer & S. B. Zyngier. 1979. Anti-inflammatory effect of warfarin and vitamin K_1. Arch. Pharmacol. **307:** 185–190.

84. Paolucci, A. M., P. B. R. Rao & C. Johnson. 1963. Vitamin K deficiency and oxidative phosphorylation. J. Nutr. **81:** 17–22.

85. Wosilait, W. D. 1966. Effect of vitamin K deficiency on the adenosine nucleotide content of chicken liver. Biochem. Pharm. **15:** 204–206.

86. Bell, R. G. 1978. Vitamin K and chemical carcinogenesis. Lancet **1:** 1161.

87. Barnhart, M. I., S. M. Noonan & G. F. Anderson. 1969. Action of vitamin K at the cellular level. *In* The Fat Soluble Vitamins. H. F. De Luca & J. W. Suttie, Eds.: 399–430. University of Wisconsin Press. Madison, WI.

88. Zacharski, L. R., W. G. Henderson, F. R. Rickles, W. B. Forman, C. J. Cornell, R. J. Forcier, H. W. Harrower and R. O. Johnson. 1979. Effect of warfarin therapy on survival in small cell carcinoma (SCC) of the lung. Blood **54** (Suppl 1): 227.

89. Colvin, R. B. & H. Dvorak. 1975. Fibrinogen/fibrin on the surface of macrophages: detection, distribution, binding requirements, and possible role in macrophage adherence phenomena. J. Exp. Med. **142:** 1377–1390.

90. Beguin, S., A. Goutner & F. Josso. 1977. Tissue factor activity of rabbit peritoneal macrophages: influence of immune stimulation. Ann. Immunol. **128:** 785–798.

91. Makinen, T., T. H. Totterman, A. Gordin & T. H. Weber. 1977. Migration inhibition factor and the blood clotting system: effects of defibrination, heparin and thrombin. Clin. Exp. Immunol. **29:** 181–186.

92. Sipka, S., I. Boldogh & T. Szilagyi. 1977. Macrophage disappearance reaction induced by lymphokines. Acta Allergol. **32:** 3–7.

93. Meade, C. J., P. L. Lachmann & R. M. Binns. 1976. A mechanism of migration inhibition involving components of the coagulation system. Scand. J. Immuol. **5:** 529–539.

94. Colvin, R. B. & H. F. Dvorak. 1975. Role of the clotting system in cell-mediated hypersensitivity. II Kinetics of fibrinogen/fibrin accumulation and vascular permeability changes in the tuberculin and cutaneous basophil hypersensitivity reactions. J. Immunol. **114:** 377–387.

95. Hedfors, E. 1977. Possible role for anticoagulant treatment in sarcoidosis. Mt. Sinai J. Med. **44:** 745–747.

96. Kataria, Y. P., A. Zafranas & H. M. Sharma. 1975. Immunochemistry of human cutaneous sarcoidosis: A study of nine cases. Human Pathol. **9:** 519–522.

ALTERNATIVE PATHWAYS OF THROMBOPLASTIN-DEPENDENT ACTIVATION OF HUMAN FACTOR X IN PLASMA *

Richard A. Marlar and John H. Griffin

Department of Molecular Immunology
Scripps Clinic and Research Foundation
La Jolla, California 92037

INTRODUCTION

The blood coagulation process involves a series of enzymatic conversions of zymogens to active serine proteases. The coagulation pathways have been represented as two independent systems, the extrinsic and intrinsic, which converge in the latter stages.[1] Classically, the extrinsic system consists of factor VII, which interacts with tissue-bound thromboplastin to activate factor X, the common point of the two pathways. The intrinsic system is more complex, involving at least four major steps. Factor XII is activated by kallikrein in the presence of high molecular weight kininogen and a negatively charged surface. Factor XIIa in turn activates factor XI.[2] In the presence of calcium ions, factor XIa converts factor IX to its active form. Factor IXa, in the presence of factor VIII, phospholipids (presumably platelets), and calcium ions, activates factor X by cleaving a small peptide from the same point as thromboplastin–factor VII. In this formulation of the coagulation pathways, factor X is the converging point of both systems, and all subsequent reactions involving factor V, prothrombin, and fibrinogen are common to both pathways.

However, evidence has been accumulated for possibly more complicated interrelationships of the two pathways. Using the thrombin generation test, Biggs and Nossel[3] observed that diluted thromboplastin would not generate normal amounts of thrombin in plasma deficient in factor VIII or factor IX; however, normal amounts of thrombin were generated in plasma deficient in factor XI or factor XII. Josso and Prou-Wartelle[4] confirmed these results and observed that factor VII was essential for the procoagulant activity of diluted thromboplastin. For many years these critical observations seem to have been overlooked. Osterud and Rapaport used a partially purified system to show that a mixture of partially purified factor VII and thromboplastin could activate purified factor IX.[5] Subsequently, Nemerson and his co-workers described similar findings for the purified bovine system.[6]

Using the new nonclotting assay of factor X activation introduced by Nemerson and his colleagues,[9] we studied factor X activation in human plasmas.[7,8] We observed that factor X activation was decreased in plasmas deficient in factors IX or VIII compared to normal human plasma and factor

* This research was supported in part by grants from the National Institutes of Health (HL 21544 and 16411) and the California chapter of the American Heart Association. R.A.M. is a recipient of a National Institutes of Health Postdoctoral Fellowship and an American Heart Postdoctoral Fellowship. J.H.G. is a recipient of a National Institutes of Health Research Career Development Award.

XI deficient plasma when dilute rabbit thromboplastin was used as an initiator. These data support a new concept of the extrinsic pathway. An alternative extrinsic pathway involving the activation of factor IX and subsequently factor VIII may well be the *in vivo* physiological pathway.

In this paper we review our studies of the role of various intrinsic coagulation factors in the thromboplastin-dependent activation of factor X in plasma.[7,8] To accomplish this, we purified human factor X and tritiated its carbohydrate moiety, which permitted the radiolabeled factor X to be used to measure its rate of activation in plasma. Once this radioassay was validated, the rate of factor X activation could be determined when various dilutions of either commercial rabbit thromboplastin or human thromboplastin were added to different types of deficient plasmas. Our data do not fit the classical formulation of the intrinsic and extrinsic coagulation pathways that converge at the activation of factor X. Rather it is implied that both the intrinsic and extrinsic coagulation pathways converge at the activation of factor IX when human plasma is exposed to low levels of thromboplastin.[7,8]

MATERIALS AND METHODS

Purification of Human Factor X

Human factor X and factor IX were purified from commercial human factor IX concentrate (Proplex®, Hyland Therapeutics) by DEAE-Sephadex and heparin-agarose chromatography and preparative polyacrylamide gel electrophoresis as previously described.[7,8]

Tritium Labeling of Factor X

Human factor X was radiolabeled by a modified method[9] of van Lenton and Ashwell,[10] in which minor changes were incorporated.[7,8] ^{3}H-Labeled factor X has also been prepared by Aronson and Bagley[11] using fresh human plasma as a source of factor X.

Validation of Tritium Assay for Factor X Activation

One hundred μg of ^{3}H-factor X was incubated at 37° C with 0.5 μg of purified factor X activator from Russell's viper venom (generously provided by Drs. B. and B. C. Furie) and 5 mM $CaCl_2$ in a total volume of 500 μl. Samples of 50 μl were removed at various times, diluted with 50 μl of 0.1% BSA in 0.01 M Tris, 0.15M NaCl (TBS/BSA) containing 50 mM EDTA (TBS/BSA/EDTA) and kept on ice. These samples were assayed for factor Xa clotting activity and amidolytic activity. 150 μl of 15% cold trichloroacetic acid (TCA) was added to the diluted sample (300 μl), mixed for 2 min and centrifuged for 3 min. Three 100-μl aliquots of the supernatant were assayed for TCA-soluble tritium. Factor Xa clotting activity was assayed by the method of Jobin and Esnouf.[12] Amidolytic activity of factor Xa was measured spectrophotometrically using the chromogenic substrate S-2222 (Kabi) as previously described.[13]

^{3}H-Factor X Activation Assay

^{3}H-Factor X (160,000 cpm/μg, 2.5 clotting units/ml) was used in all experiments described in this paper. In a typical assay, the mixture contained 30 μl plasma, 10 μl ^{3}H-factor X, 5 μl concentrated rabbit brain cephalin (Sigma), and 30 μl of various dilutions of thromboplastin containing 25 mM $CaCl_2$. To stop the reactions at various times, 255 μl of TBS/BSA/EDTA were added and vigorously mixed. Samples were kept on ice and 170 μl 15% cold TCA was added, mixed at 4° C for 2 min, and centrifuged for 3 min in a Beckman Microfuge 152. Triplicate 100-μl aliquots of the supernate were removed and counted in a liquid scintillation counter. The TCA-soluble radio-activity values for the three samples were averaged.

To determine the maximum tritium release that was arbitrarily defined as 100% release in the thromboplastin experiments, 10 μl of Russell's viper venom (1 mg/ml protein) and calcium ions (4 mM final concentration) were added to 10 μl ^{3}H-factor X and TBS/BSA to a final volume of 75 μl and incubated for 90 min at 37° C. To stop the reaction, 255 μl TBS/BSA/EDTA were added, then 170 μl of cold TCA were added, the mixture was centrifuged and triplicate 100-μl aliquots were counted.

Results

Purification of Human Factor X

Commercial human factor IX concentrate was the source for purified factor X. The final purification step employed preparative polyacrylamide gel electrophoresis, which was usually performed after the tritiation of factor X to help reduce the radioactivity background as well as remove any detectable contaminants. This purified factor X did not contain detectable prothrombin, factor VII, or factor IX as measured by SDS gels and clotting assays (<0.1%). The specific clotting activity of human factor X was 130 clotting units/mg. On 10% SDS polyacrylamide gels without reducing agent, human factor X gave a single band of an apparent molecular weight of 59,000, while on SDS gels in the presence of reducing agent, factor X exhibited two bands of apparent molecular weight of 42,000 and 17,000 (FIGURE 1A).

Tritiation of Human Factor X

Three minor modifications [7, 8] of the tritiation procedure used by Nemerson and coworkers [9] were made. First, the molar ratio of sodium periodate to sialic acid was reduced to 8:1, which apparently eliminated oxidation of components necessary for factor X activity. This was necessary since our initial radio-labeling efforts inactivated the coagulant activity of factor X. Second, tritiated sodium borohydride was used for reduction at both 4° C and room tempera-ture,[9] such that factor X was radiolabeled to a specific radioactivity of 160,000 cpm/μg factor X. Finally, when preparative polyacrylamide gel electrophoresis was performed after tritiation of the factor X, the background tritium remain-ing in the supernatant after precipitation of the ^{3}H-factor X with cold 15% TCA was reduced from 4% to 0.45% of the total radioactivity.

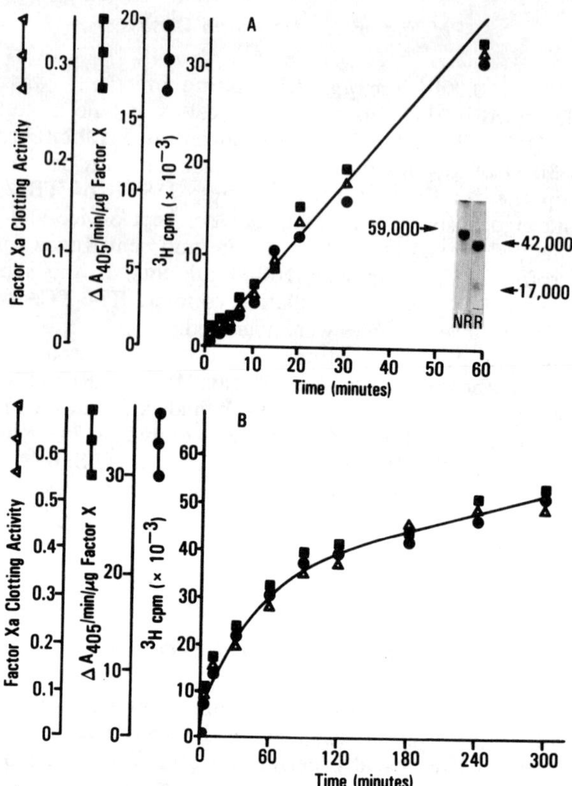

FIGURE 1. Validation of the ³H-labeled factor X activation assay. The release of TCA-soluble tritium is correlated with the appearance of factor Xa amidolytic activity and clotting activity during factor X activation by the factor X activator of Russell's viper venom. Conditions are given in METHODS section. The insert in (A) shows 10% SDS polyacrylamide gels of purified human factor X (10 μg of protein per gel in the absence (NR) or presence (R) of reducing agent). (From Marlar et al.[7, 8] By permission of *Thrombosis and Haemostasis.*)

Validation of Tritium Assay

To determine if the TCA-soluble tritium appeared simultaneously with factor Xa activity, purified factor X activator from Russell's viper venom was used to activate factor X. The results for both short time course incubations (FIGURE 1A) and long time course incubations (FIGURE 1B) showed the appearance of TCA-soluble tritium directly correlated with the appearance of factor Xa clotting and amidolytic activity. The maximum tritium released during factor X activation in buffer or normal plasma varied from 65% to 72% of the total radioactivity in various experiments. These values are in excellent agreement with the predicted value for the amount of sialic acid present on the activation peptide (75%).[14] Thus the release of TCA-soluble tritium from ³H-factor X provides a sensitive and accurate measure of factor X activation.

Rabbit Thromboplastin-dependent Activation of Factor X in Plasma

The kinetics of factor X activation in normal human plasma and plasmas deficient in factor VIII, factor IX, or factor XI were determined at three different dilutions of commercial rabbit brain thromboplastin (Ortho) (FIGURE 2). At 1/5 dilution of the manufacturer's recommended thromboplastin concentration, the initial rate of factor X activation appeared similar in each type of plasma (FIGURE 2, top panel). At the 1/24 dilution of rabbit thromboplastin, plasmas deficient in factor VIII or factor IX exhibited a 50% decrease in the initial kinetics of factor X activation compared to a normal human plasma pool and factor XI deficient plasma (FIGURE 2, middle panel). Also at this dilution, the maximum plateau of factor X activation was reduced by 50% in the hemophilic plasmas. At this dilution of thromboplastin, factor X activa-

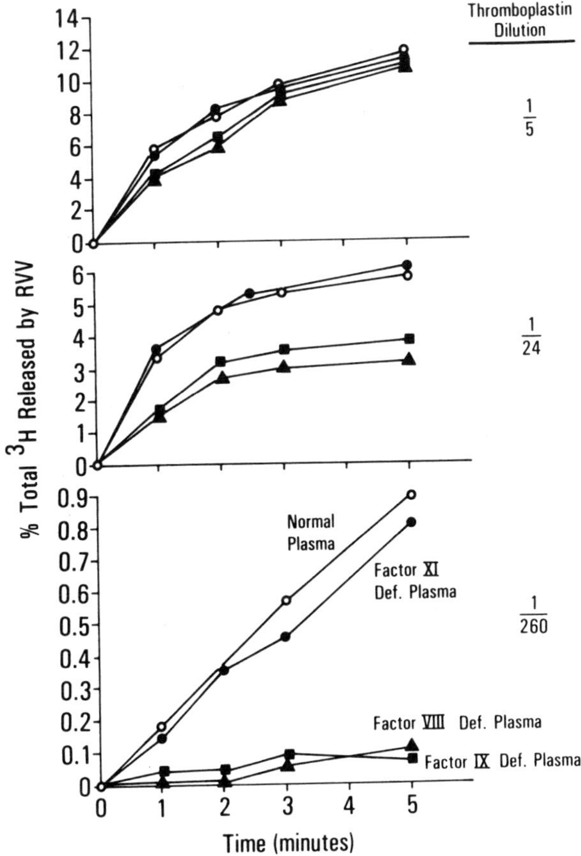

FIGURE 2. Effect of dilution of rabbit thromboplastin on factor X activation in normal human plasma and plasmas deficient in factor VIII, factor IX or factor XI. The 100% value on the ordinate was defined as the maximum TCA-soluble tritium released in 90 min by Russell's viper venom. (From Marlar *et al.*[7, 8] By permission of *Thrombosis and Haemostasis*.)

tion in normal plasma occurred at an initial rate of 3.2% per min. The clotting time of this plasma was 35 sec, at which time only 1.8% of the total factor X in plasma was activated. At the 1/260 dilution of rabbit thromboplastin, the initial rate of factor X activation in plasmas deficient in factor VIII or factor IX was less than 10% of the rate observed for the normal plasma pool and for factor XI deficient plasma (FIGURE 2, bottom panel). Therefore, under these conditions, factors IX and VIII were required for whatever mechanisms determine the activation of factor X.

To determine the generality of these observations, plasmas from five unre-

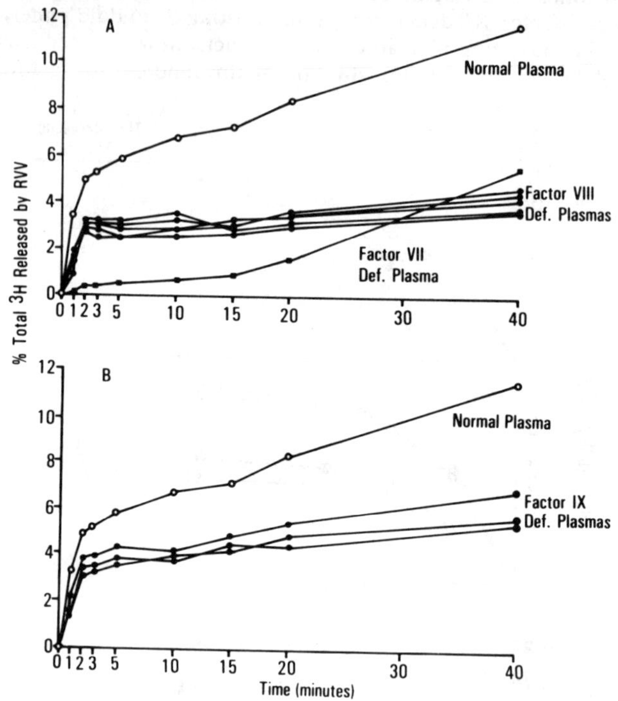

FIGURE 3. ³H-factor X activation by a 1/24 dilution of rabbit thromboplastin in normal plasma, and in plasmas deficient in factor VIII, factor IX, or factor VII. (A) Upper panel, data for plasmas from five unrelated factor VIII deficient patients; (B) lower panel, data for plasmas from three unrelated factor IX deficient patients. (From Marlar *et al.*[7, 8] By permission of *Thrombosis and Haemostasis.*)

lated factor VIII deficient patients were tested for factor X activation at a 1/24 dilution of rabbit thromboplastin. The initial rate of factor X activation was 1.5% per min or 46% of the rate for normal plasma (FIGURE 3A). After 2 min, factor X activation in these factor VIII deficient plasmas reached a plateau that represented less than half the total amount of factor X activation seen in normal plasma. As seen in FIGURE 3A, normal factor X activation required factor VII since this reaction was greatly retarded in factor VII deficient plasma.

In three plasmas from unrelated factor IX deficient patients, the initial kinetics of factor X activation at a 1/24 dilution of thromboplastin was 1.8% per min, or 52% of the rate observed for normal plasma (FIGURE 3B). Factor X activation reached a plateau after an initial 2-minute burst of activation. At this plateau the total amount of factor X activation was half that seen for normal plasma.

In the experiments seen in FIGURES 2 and 3, the normal plasma was a pool of plasma from 25 donors. To determine if a pool of normal plasmas had the same activation characteristics as individual normal plasmas, factor X activation kinetics at a 1/24 dilution of thromboplastin were studied in the normal human pool and in five individual normal human plasmas. All five individual plasmas exhibited similar activation kinetics both in the initial rate and maximal extent of factor X activation. The time course of factor X activation for each of the five normal plasmas was indistinguishable from that for the normal plasma pool.

To determine the contribution of cephalin alone to factor X activation, control experiments containing only rabbit brain cephalin were made using normal plasma and plasmas deficient in factors VIII, IX, or XI. All four plasmas exhibited less than 0.2% factor X activation in 20 min although each had clotted by that time.

When factor VIII deficient plasma was reconstituted with partially purified factor VIII (commercial Hemophil®, Hyland) to 1 clotting unit/ml, the initial rate and maximum plateau of factor X activation paralleled the curve seen for normal plasma (FIGURE 4). However, purified factor IX added to factor VIII deficient plasma did not alter the kinetics of factor X activation.

When purified factor IX equivalent to 1 clotting unit/ml was added to factor IX deficient plasma, the intitial kinetics and maximum extent of factor X activation were similar to those seen for normal plasma (FIGURE 4B). However, the addition of factor VIII to factor IX deficient plasma had no effect on the initial rate or maximum extent of factor X activation. Thus, reconstitution of hemophilic plasmas specifically reconstitutes normal factor X activation.

Human Thromboplastin-dependent Activation of Factor X in Plasma

Using human thromboplastin (British National Standard material kindly provided by Dr. L. Poller) at three different dilutions, factor X activation kinetics were determined for a normal human plasma pool and for plasmas deficient in factors VIII, IX or XI (FIGURE 5).

At a 1/6 dilution of human thromboplastin, the kinetics of factor X activation in all four plasmas appeared similar (FIGURE 5, top panel). At a 1/142 dilution of the human stock thromboplastin, factor VIII deficient and factor IX deficient plasmas exhibited a 40% decrease in the initial rate of factor X activation compared to normal plasma or to factor XI deficient plasma (FIGURE 5, middle panel). In this case, the maximum activation in the hemophilic plasmas was 50% that of normal plasma. At a 1/1420 dilution of human thromboplastin, both hemophilic plasmas appeared very abnormal compared to normal or factor XI deficient plasmas; under these conditions the initial rate of factor X activation in the plasmas deficient in factors IX or VIII was less than 20% of the rate observed for normal or factor XI deficient plasmas. Thus, low levels of human thromboplastin, like rabbit thromboplastin, in the plasma milieu, require factors IX and VIII for optimal activation of factor X.

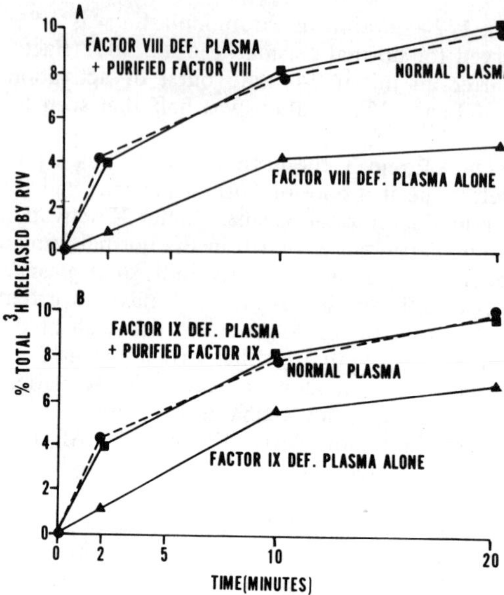

FIGURE 4. ³H-factor X activation in factor IX deficient plasma or factor VIII deficient plasma that had been reconstituted with purified factor IX or with commercial factor VIII concentrate to give 1 clotting unit/ml. A 1/24 dilution of rabbit thromboplastin was used as the initiator of the reaction. Normal human plasma (dashed line) and the deficient plasma alone are also shown. (A) Upper panel, factor VIII deficient plasma; (B) lower panel, factor IX deficient plasma. (From Marlar *et al.*[7, 8] By permission of *Thrombosis and Haemostasis.*)

FIGURE 5. Effect of dilutions of human thromboplastin on factor X activation in normal human plasma and plasmas deficient in factor VIII, factor IX, or factor XI. (From Marlar *et al.*[7, 8] By permission of *Thrombosis and Haemostasis.*)

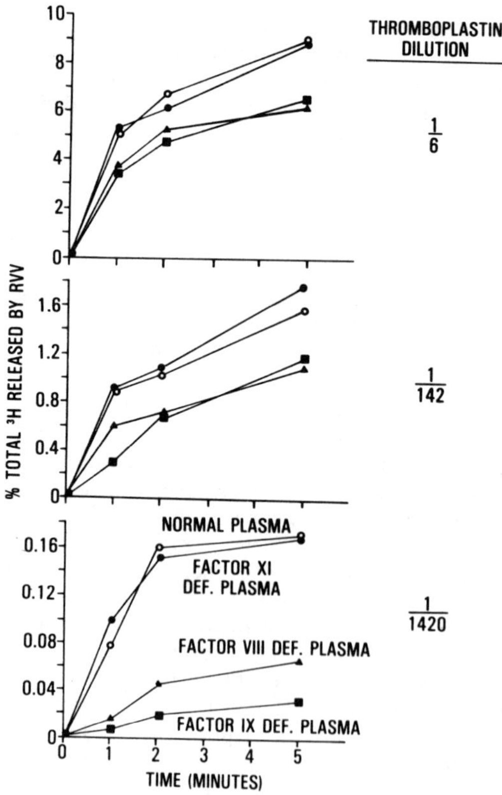

DISCUSSION

Our initial studies were stimulated by the seemingly forgotten observations of Biggs and Nossel[3] and Josso and Prou-Wartelle[4] who found that when diluted thromboplastin was studied, an abnormal and prolonged thrombin generation was observed in plasmas deficient in factors VIII and IX but not in plasmas deficient in factor XI or factor XII. This work suggested an important connection between the extrinsic pathway and factor IX activation. Recently, Osterud and Rapaport[5] demonstrated that purified factor IX was activated by partially purified factor VII and thromboplastin. Hence, we reasoned that low levels of thromboplastin should be studied for their procoagulant activity and ability to activate factor X in normal and various deficient plasmas.

These results summarized here[7, 8] have established that both factor VIII and factor IX are needed for normal factor X activation in human plasma when dilute human or rabbit brain thromboplastin is used as an initiator of coagulation. The more dilute the thromboplastin, the greater the difference in factor X activation between plasmas deficient in factor VIII or factor IX, and normal human plasma. When purified factor IX and factor VIII are added to their respective deficient plasmas, the factor X activation is reconstituted to the kinetic pattern seen for normal human plasma. Both the initial rate and maximum extent of factor X activation is decreased in the hemophiliac plasmas at low levels of thromboplastin.

Nemerson and co-workers[6] using purified bovine proteins and a radioassay for the activation of ^{3}H-factor IX observed that thromboplastin and factor VII can activate factor IX at significant rates. However, further studies by Nemerson et al.[15] and Jesty and Silverberg[16] observed that the rate of activation of factor X by factor VII and thromboplastin was about seven times faster than the activation of factor IX in purified systems[15] or in bovine plasmas.[16] From this they concluded that factor IX activation is not likely to contribute significantly to factor X activation in the bovine system. It will be interesting to see if new studies employing low concentrations of tissue factor in the bovine system confirm what we have observed in the human system or if the bovine coagulation pathways are regulated differently than the human pathways.

From clinical observations, it is apparent that both factor IX and factor VIII are essential for normal hemostasis.[17] Both genetic and acquired deficiencies in coagulation factors VIII or IX result in bleeding disorders. Classical formulations[1] of blood coagulation pathways cannot explain these phenomena because deficiencies in factor XI are often not associated with any bleeding diathesis. Data summarized in this paper[7, 8] as well as work by other investigators[3-5] suggest the existence of an alternative extrinsic pathway that is initiated by low levels of thromboplastin. This alternative extrinsic pathway (depicted in FIGURE 6) requires factors IX and VIII. It cannot be excluded that as yet unknown or unrecognized plasma components also participate in this pathway. This alternative pathway may function physiologically when low levels of thromboplastin are generated in vivo at an injury site. If this new pathway is a major physiologic pathway, it can account for the clinical manifestations of hemophilia since the intrinsic and extrinsic pathways converge at the level of factor IX activation. Hemophiliacs who are deficient in factor IX or factor VIII bleed during traumatic injury because the rate-determining step of coagulation involves factors IX and VIII. In this context it should not be overlooked that recent work has shown that kallikrein[18] or polymorphonuclear leukocytes[19] can also activate factor IX. Hence factor IX may be central to a number of pathways for the generation of coagulant activity. Much further work will be necessary to clarify the regulation of the intermediate stages of blood coagulation.

SUMMARY

To determine the interrelationships of the major coagulation pathways, the activation of ^{3}H-labeled factor X in normal and various deficient human plasmas was evaluated when clotting was triggered by dilute rabbit or human thromboplastin. Various dilutions of thromboplastin and calcium were added to plasma samples containing ^{3}H-factor X, and the time course of factor X activation was determined. At a 1/250 dilution of rabbit brain thromboplastin, the rate of factor X activation in plasmas deficient in factor VIII or factor IX was 10% of the activation rate of normal plasma or of factor XI deficient plasma. Reconstitution of the deficient plasmas with factors VIII or IX, respectively, reconstituted normal factor X activation. Similar results were obtained when various dilutions of human thromboplastin replaced the rabbit

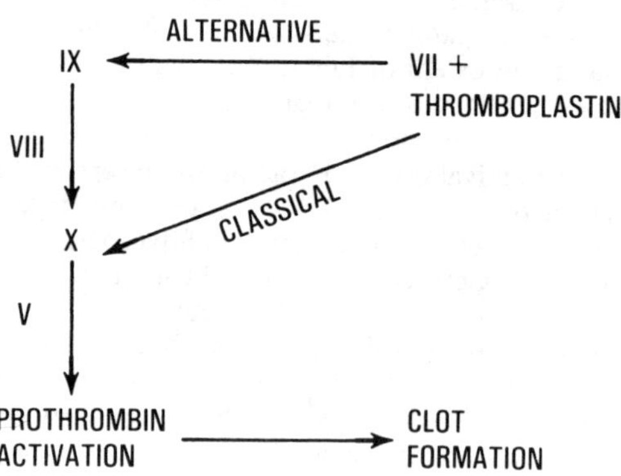

FIGURE 6. Simplified scheme for the extrinsic pathways of blood coagulation. An "alternative" extrinsic pathway that requires factors VII, IX, and VIII for the activation of factor X is suggested by several observations [3-5] and by the data summarized in this paper (FIGURES 2–5).[7, 8] The scheme as depicted is oversimplified since proteolytic activations, feedback proteolysis, and unrecognized plasma components may all contribute significantly to the pathways.

thromboplastin. From these plasma experiments, it is inferred that the dilute thromboplastin-dependent activation of factor X requires factors VII, IX, and VIII. An alternative extrinsic pathway that involves factors IX and VIII may be the physiologic extrinsic pathway and hence help to explain the consistent clinical observations of bleeding diatheses in patients deficient in factors IX or VIII.

ACKNOWLEDGMENTS

The authors thank Jennifer Oldstone and Gregory N. Beretta for their skillful technical assistance, and Alice J. Kleiss for excellent assistance in the isolation of factors X and IX. Helpful discussions with Dr. Yale Nemerson, Dr. David Aronson, and Dr. Theodore Zimmerman are gratefully acknowledged. We acknowledge the gift of purified factor X activator of Russell's viper venom from Drs. Bruce and Barbara Furie, Tufts University, Boston, Mass., and of human thromboplastin from Dr. L. Poller, Manchester, England.

REFERENCES

1. DAVIE, E. W., K. FUJIKAWA, K. KURACHI & W. KISIEL. 1979. The role of serine proteases in the blood coagulation cascade. Adv. Enzymol. **48:** 227–318.
2. GRIFFIN, J. H. & C. COCHRANE. 1979. Recent advances in the understanding of contact activation reactions. Sem. Thromb. Hemost. **5:** 254–273.
3. BIGGS, R. & H. NOSSEL. 1961. Tissue extract and the contact reaction in blood coagulation. Thromb. Diath. Haemorrh. **6:** 1–14.
4. JOSSO, F. & O. PROU-WARTELLE. 1965. Interaction of tissue factor and Factor VII at the earliest phase of coagulation. Thromb. Diath. Haemorrh. (Suppl.) **17:** 35–44.
5. OSTERUD, B. & S. RAPAPORT. 1977. Activation of Factor IX by the reaction product of tissue factor and Factor VII: Additional pathway for initiating blood coagulation. Proc. Natl. Acad. Sci. USA **74:** 5260–5264.
6. ZUR, M., K. SHASTRI & Y. NEMERSON. 1978. Kinetics of the tissue factor pathway of coagulation: Activation of Factor IX. Blood **52:** 198.
7. MARLAR, R., A. KLEISS & J. H. GRIFFIN. 1981. Reevaluation of the extrinsic pathways of blood coagulation. (Submitted.)
8. MARLAR, R., A. KLEISS & J. H. GRIFFIN. 1979. Studies of the activation of human Factor X in plasma. Thromb. Haemost. **42:** 166.
9. SILVERBERG, S., Y. NEMERSON & M. ZUR. 1977. Kinetics of the activation of bovine coagulation Factor X by components of the extrinsic system. J. Biol. Chem. **252:** 8481–8488.
10. VAN LENTEN, L. & G. ASHWELL. 1971. Studies on the chemical and enzymatic modification of glycoprotein. J. Biol. Chem. **246:** 1889–1894.
11. ARONSON, D. L. & J. BAGLEY. 1978. Regulation of Factor X conversion in plasma. Circulation **58:** 209.
12. JOBIN, F. & M. ESNOUF. 1967. Studies on the formation of the prothrombin-converting complex. Biochem. J. **102:** 666–674.
13. AURELL, L., P. FRIBERGER, G. KARLSSON & G. CLAESON. 1977. A new sensitive and highly specific chromogenic peptide substrate for Factor Xa. Thromb. Res. **11:** 595–609.
14. DI SCIPIO, R. G., M. A. HERMODSON, S. G. YATES & E. W. DAVIE. 1977. A comparison of human prothrombin, Factor IX (Christmas Factor), Factor X (Stuart Factor), and Protein S. Biochemistry **16:** 698–706.
15. NEMERSON, Y., M. ZUR, R. BACH & R. GENTRY. 1980. The mechanism of action of tissue factor: A provisional model. *In* The Regulation of Coagulation. K. Mann & F. Taylor, Eds. Vol. **8:** 193–202. Elsevier-North-Holland, New York, N.Y.
16. JESTY, J. & S. SILVERBERG. 1980. The kinetics of Factor VIII action in a bovine plasma system. *In* The Regulation of Coagulation. K. Mann & F. Taylor, Eds. Vol. **8:** 205–212. Elsevier-North Holland, New York, N.Y.
17. HOUGIE, C. 1977. Hemophilia and related conditions-congenital deficiencies of prothrombin (Factor II), Factor V and Factors VII to XII. *In* Hematology. W. Williams, R. Beutler, A. Erslev & R. W. Rundles, Eds. pp. 1404–1422. McGraw-Hill Book Co., New York, N.Y.
18. SELIGSOHN, U., B. OSTERUD, S. F. BROWN, J. H. GRIFFIN & S. I. RAPAPORT. 1979. Activation of human factor VII in plasma and in purified systems. J. Clin. Invest. **64:** 1056–1065.
19. KINGDON, H. S., J. C. HERION & P. G. RAUSCH. 1978. Cellular activation of Factor IX. Thromb. Res. **13:** 501–507.

NONENZYMIC CONTROL OF PROTHROMBIN ACTIVATION *

Kent D. Miller

*Departments of Medicine and Microbiology
University of Miami School of Medicine
Miami, Florida 33101; and
Division of Laboratories and Research
New York State Department of Health
Albany, New York 12201*

Although considerable attention has been given to the enzymic mechanisms of prothrombin activation, Waugh *et al.*[1] suggested that nonenzymic mechanisms should not be ruled out. Landaburu and Seegers had described activation of purified prothrombin in protamine sulfate solutions,[2] a process that, like an extrinsic thromboplastic system,[3] was resistant to (and progressed in) diisopropylfluorophosphate (DFP).[4] Evidence for a nonenzymic control mechanism stemmed from subsequent studies of thrombin generation from purified horse prothrombin mixed with synthetic polylysine (polyLYS) preparations.[5] Activation occurred only within a relatively high, optimum weight ratio of polyLYS to prothrombin. Other characteristics of the polyLYS reaction were a low temperature optimum, high sensitivity to salt, and insensitivity to DFP. Also, the maximum *rate* of thrombin formation at optimum ratios of polyLYS to prothrombin varied with the average molecular weight of each polyLYS preparation and with the concentrations of the two reactants. However, the smallest amount of each polyLYS preparation just sufficient to *initiate* activation was constant despite wide variations in the average molecular weights of the polymers. A number of high-molecular-weight basic compounds substituted for the polyLYS.[4]

The present studies are based on the hypothesis that some basic substances of relatively high molecular weight represent models for a physiologic, nonenzymic substance, the latter substance required for *initiation* of prothrombin activation regardless of the rate of that activation. The studies delineate distinctive parameters of the nonenzymic reaction, unusual solvent effects, and the significance of the purity and species of the prothrombin activated. Activators of known molecular weight are identified that will permit detailed kinetic studies at known molar concentrations of the reactants.

MATERIALS AND METHODS

Reagents and Assay Methods

Horse and cow prothrombins were prepared according to Miller and Phelan.[6] Prothrombin and thrombin were measured by the methods of Ware

* Supported in part by grants from the National Institutes of Health (HE-09902) and the American Red Cross (K-34799).

and Seegers,[7] employing the National Institutes of Health (NIH) thrombin unit as standard. Nitrogen was determined by micro-Kjeldahl methods.[8]

Included among substances examined as potential initiators of prothrombin activation were gifts of the following; Polybrenes of varying average molecular sizes (Abbott Labs.), polyvinylamine (Eastman Research Labs.), viomycin and colistin (Squibb Institute for Medical Research), and circulin (Upjohn Co.). Polymyxin, neomycin, streptomycin, polyLYS, polyornithine (polyORN), polyarginine (polyARG) and other chemicals were from commercial sources.

Identification of Activators and Activation Parameters .

A nonenzymic prothrombin activator is not detectable unless tested within its optimum, sometimes narrow range of activator:prothrombin ratios. Hence, varying amounts of each compound must be mixed with a relatively constant amount of prothrombin. Each potential activator was therefore dissolved in water, the pH adjusted to 7.5, and the nitrogen content determined. Reaction mixtures (1.0 ml) were then prepared, each containing 0.05 Tris buffer, pH 7.5, a varying amount of the substance tested as activator, and 1.5–2.5 mg purified horse prothrombin. The prothrombin was always added last. Reactions were followed by thrombin and prothrombin analyses at 25° C. Controls included mixtures of prothrombin without activator as tests for spontaneous prothrombin activation, and samples of activator with thrombin rather than prothrombin as tests for activator effects on the thrombin titrations. Results were arbitrarily considered negative when no measurable thrombin was formed in 24 hours.

Compounds activating prothrombin in these screening tests were then re-studied at varying activator:prothrombin ratios for determination of the several activation parameters. Those parameters included (a) maximum thrombin yields, (b) rates of activation at optimum activator:prothrombin ratios, and (c) the smallest amount of each activator just required to *induce* thrombin formation. This smallest ratio of activator to prothrombin essential for initia-tion of thrombin formation, termed the A_i/P, is determined by plotting values representative of the rates of activation on an ordinate and the corresponding activator:prothrombin ratios on the abscissa. Since the primary or quaternary amino groups are presumed responsible for the reactivity of each nonenzymic activator, the amount of activator added is usually indicated by the nitrogen it contributes to each reaction. The ascending limbs of the curves are then extrapolated to the abscissa. Thus, each intercept is the A_i/P for that com-pound (or the $A_i(N)/P$ when activator nitrogen content is plotted).[5] Several mixtures of the reactants just below the A_i/P are always examined simultane-ously with the activation solutions to assure localization of the A_i/P.

When screening studies indicated the $A_i(N)/P$ for polybrene was very low, and since polybrene contains quaternary- rather than primary amino groups, a series of studies compared the activation parameters of that substance to those of polyLYS. The $A_i(N)/P$ for polybrenes of average molecular weights 300–600, 600–900, 1600–1800, and 2400–3000 were determined as described above. The activation rates and thrombin yields under optimum conditions were also determined as were the optimum pH and temperature.

Evidence from these polybrene studies confirmed prior experiences with polyLYS samples of varying average molecular weights in that variations in molecular size affected activation rates but not the A_i/P.[5] Further confirmation was sought among partial acid hydrolyzates of a polyLYS preparation of 175,000 average molecular weight, a slow prothrombin activator under its optimum conditions. Fifty mg were hydrolyzed in constant boiling HBr at 25° C for eight days. Samples removed every second day were repeatedly diluted with water and dried *in vacuo*. Each hydrolyzate was then dissolved in water, neutralized, and evaluated as a prothrombin activator. A sample of the 4-day hydrolyzate was streaked on Whatman 3-mm papers. The tri-, tetra-, penta- and hexaLYS peptides were then separated by a butanol-acetic acid-water system, eluted with water, and employed for identification of the smallest lysine peptide capable of supporting prothrombin activation.

Solvent Effects

The effects of methanol, *n*-butanol, ethylene glycol, propanediol glycerol, dimethylsulfoxide (DMSO), dioxane, ethylacetate, dimethylformamide, urea, and guanidine HCl on this so-called nonenzymic phase of prothrombin activation in polyLYS were studied. Final concentrations in separate reaction mixtures ranged from 0.05–2.0 M dependent on the miscibility of each solvent. All reaction mixtures contained 1.7 mg per ml prothrombin, 0.15 mg polyLYS nitrogen per ml, and 0.05 M Tris, pH 8.0. Glycerol and DMSO, solvents enhancing the rate of the polyLYS-prothrombin activation system, were then investigated for possible effects on the A_i/P. Test samples (1.0 ml) contained 1.0 mg prothrombin, 0.05 M Tris (pH 7.8), 1.0 M glycerol or DMSO, and varying amounts of either polyLYS or neomycin.

Prothrombin Concentration, Purity, and Species

The original studies indicated the rates of nonenzymic activation are directly related to the concentrations of polyLYS and prothrombin when held in constant proportions.[5] In the present studies effects of varied prothrombin concentrations on the A_i/P as well as on reaction rates were determined. Three series of tubes, containing, respectively, 0.5, 1.0, and 1.5 mg per ml of horse prothrombin, were reacted with varying amounts of polyARG. Thrombin formation was followed in all tubes, and the A_i/P determined by extrapolation.

Historically, the purity of prothrombin preparations employed in thrombin generation experiments has always been open to question. Therefore several zymogen samples, drawn during the prothrombin purification procedures (purposely impure), were compared to the purified materials as regards activation with polyLYS. In this case the smallest amounts of polyLYS inducing activation of each zymogen were divided by the concentrations of prothrombin in units per ml ($A_i(N)/P$ (units)). Those results would reflect on the specificity and stoichiometry of the reactions as well as on effects of contaminants on the A_i/P. Similar objectives were sought in studies of polyLYS-induced activation of purified horse and cow prothrombins. Prior evidence from these laboratories had indicated twofold differences between molecular weights of the two prothrombins, also reflected in their maximum specific activities.[9] Thus, the activation parameters would again reflect on the stoichiometry of the reactions, either for the weight of each zymogen or for the number of active sites (units) available.

RESULTS

Activation Parameters

FIGURE 1 illustrates the means by which the A_i/P were determined for a group of so-called nonenzymic prothrombin activators. Although the entire optimum range of each series of activator-prothrombin mixtures was studied only the ascending limb of each is plotted on FIGURE 1 for extrapolation to the abscissa, the intercept being the A_i/P. That factor, the smallest amount of substance that initiates prothrombin activation, appears to represent the sensitivity of prothrombin to the specific substance. Thus, based on nitrogen content of each activator, prothrombin is 12 times more sensitive to polybrene

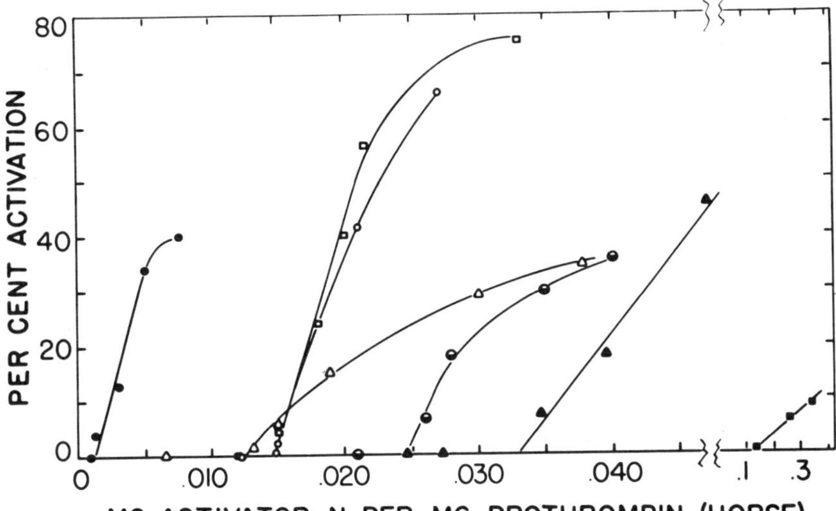

FIGURE 1. Method for determination of A_i (N)/P for several prothrombin-activating substances. Ordinate represents percent activation in 2 hr by all substances except polybrene (4 hr). Horse prothrombin = 1.5–2.5 mg per ml. ● polybrene; □ polyLYS; ○ polyORN; △ neomycin; ◓ polymyxin; ▲ colistin; ■ viomycin.

$(A_i(N)/P = 1.25 \times 10^{-3})$ than to polyLYS and polyORN $(A_i(N)/P = 1.5 \times 10^{-2})$, and 19 times more sensitive to polybrene than to polymyxin $(A_i(N)/P = 2.5 \times 10^{-2})$.

The A_i/P appeared highly reproducible. It was determined more than 20 times for polyLYS using ten different prothrombin preparations (some of reduced purity), four polyLYS preparations, and in solvents such as glycerol and DMSO that enhance activation velocities. In all cases the $A_i(N)/P$ was in the range 0.013–0.016. PolyORN gave the same value as polyLYS (FIG. 1) as expected from its near identical content of primary amino groups.

The two-hour activation values plotted in FIGURE 1 reflected the rates of conversion of prothrombin by many of the more active substances under standard conditions. Notable exceptions were the polybrenes. While prothrombin was most sensitive to the polybrenes the rates of thrombin formation within the optimum polybrene-prothrombin range were substantially lower than those for other substances under identical conditions. Thus, the polybrene-induced activation values plotted in FIGURE 1 represent four-hour reactions. However, those differences in activation rates did not alter the $A_i(N)/P$.

TABLE 1 lists activation parameters for a number of the substances reactive with horse prothrombin under standard conditions. The two-hour and maximum thrombin yields represent the rates and final yields of the reactions at optimum activator-prothrombin ratios. The A_i/P, the so-called sensitivity value, was expressed in a number of ways. To date all substances found to induce prothrombin activation in this system have been basic compounds of relatively high molecular weight (TABLE 1). The activations by polybrenes and polyARG indicate the phenomenon is not restricted to substances with primary amino groups. However it was convenient to have the first A_i/P calculations based on the nitrogen content of each activator ($A_i(N)/P$). One can then take advantage of what is known of the chemistry of the activator and the prothrombin. For example, half the nitrogen atoms of polyLYS and polyORN occur in free amino groups, and 5 of the 16 nitrogens of the cyclic antibiotic, polymyxin, are primary amino groups. Assuming a molecular weight for horse prothrombin of 130,000 [9] the $A_i(\mu\text{mole-NH}_2)/\mu$mole prothrombin for polyLYS, polyORN, and polymyxin were, respectively, 70, 70, and 72.5. On the other hand, colistin, another cyclic peptide antibiotic with 4 of 13 nitrogens in the primary amino group form, gave a value of 94.5.

Polybrene Studies

Special attention was given to the polybrenes because of their very low $A_i(N)/P$. The pH optimum for activation with 2400–3000 MW polybrene was extraordinarily sharp compared to that of polyLYS (FIG. 2). Interestingly, the optimum pH range of this compound, containing quaternary nitrogen groups, is nearer physiologic than that of polyLYS.

TABLE 1

PARAMETERS FOR CHARACTERIZATION OF NONENZYMIC
ACTIVATORS OF HORSE PROTHROMBIN

Activator	$[A_i]\dfrac{\text{mg N/}}{\text{mg Proth.}}$	$[A_i]\dfrac{\text{mg N/}}{\text{unit}}$	$[A_i]\dfrac{\mu\text{mole N/}}{\mu\text{mole Prothrombin}}$	% Activation * 2 Hr	Max
Polybrenes	0.0013	1.18×10^{-6}	12	25 †	66
Polyvinylamine	0.0038	3.45×10^{-6}	35	91	97
PolyARG	0.0052	4.70×10^{-6}	48	75	91
Neomycin	0.013	1.18×10^{-5}	121	65	89
PolyLYS	0.015	1.36×10^{-5}	140	68	76
PolyORN	0.015	1.36×10^{-5}	140	66	71
Polymyxin	0.025	2.27×10^{-5}	233	68	73
Colistin	0.033	3.00×10^{-5}	307	56	64
Viomycin	0.13	1.18×10^{-4}	1210	6	58

* Percent activation at optimum activator:prothrombin ratios.
† Four-hour yield for polybrene.

The range of polybrene-prothrombin mixtures that support activation is broad (Fig. 3) compared to that of polyLYS.[5] Also, as in the case of polyLYS, the *rate* of prothrombin activation at optimum proportions varied with the size of the polybrene polymers (Fig. 3). Indeed, a polybrene preparation of average molecular weight 300–600 was inert in the activation system. However, as with various polyLYS preparations, the $A_i(N)/P$ of each of the three active polybrene polymer sizes tested was the same. This reconfirms the independence of that end-point from some structural variations in the activator.

Activator Size

In a prior study, polyLYS preparations of average molecular-weights 175,000 and 15,000 activated prothrombin more slowly at optimum proportions than did a preparation of 5,000 average molecular weight.[5] In the present case, partial acid (HBr) hydrolysis, for two and four days, increased the rate of activation induced by the 175,000 dalton polyLYS preparation. After the 6th day the hydrolyzed specimen lost potency (Fig. 4). This reconfirmed, as did the polybrene data cited above, the relationship between polymer size and the *rate* of prothrombin activation.

The smallest lysine peptide, purified from the four-day hydrolyzate, that demonstrated significant activating potential was hexaLYS. The molecular weight of that peptide (787) correlates well with other small, basic substances demonstrating the same activity. Those included neomycin (MW 774), polymyxin (MW 1200), colistin (MW 1168), and the smallest effective polybrene preparation (Av. MW 600–900).

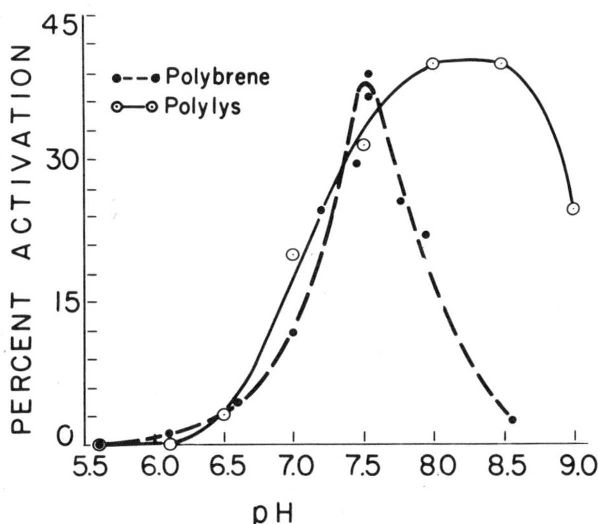

FIGURE 2. pH optima for prothrombin activation by polyLYS and polybrene. ○-Horse prothrombin (1.6 mg per ml) and 0.28 mg polyLYS-N per ml reacted for 45 min. ● Horse prothrombin (3.1 mg per ml) and 0.06 mg polybrene-N per ml reacted for 2 hr.

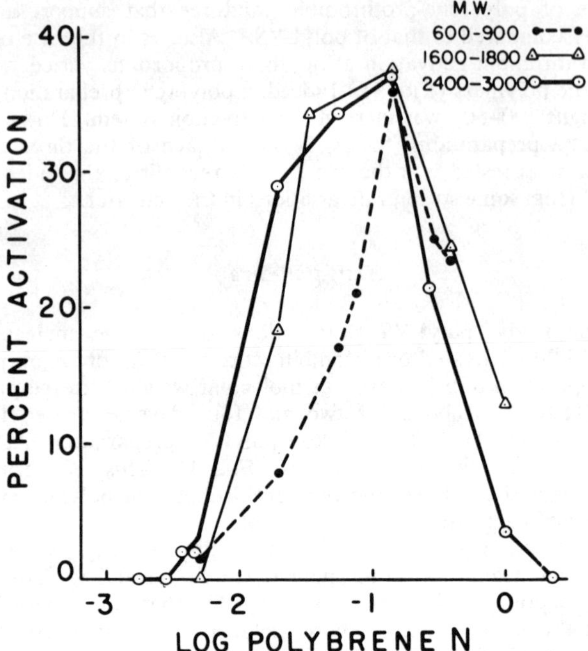

FIGURE 3. $A_1(N)/P$ determination and percent activations of horse prothrombin (2 mg per ml) after 4 hr in varying concentrations of polybrenes of different average molecular weights: ●‒‒● 600–900; △—△ 1600–1800; ○—○ 2400–3000.

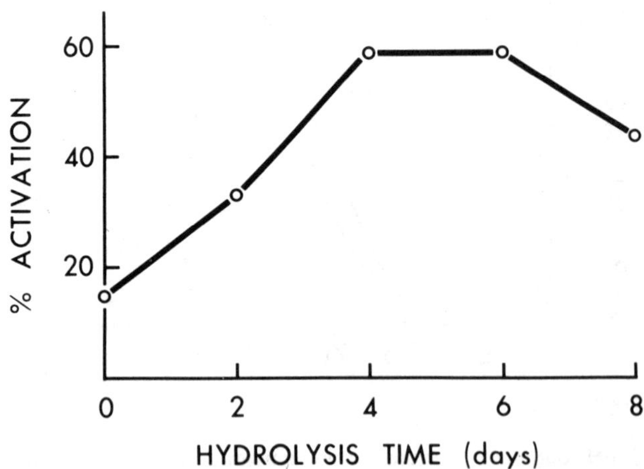

FIGURE 4. Effect of HBr hydrolysis on the rate of prothrombin activation by high-molecular-weight polyLYS. Samples contain 1.9 mg per ml horse prothrombin and 0.15 mg per ml hydrolyzate nitrogen.

Solvent Effects

The rates of polyLYS-induced activation of horse prothrombin were accelerated in 1.0 M solutions of glycerol, propanediol and ethylene glycol, and by DMSO up to 2.0 M (TABLE 2). The phenomenon was particularly important because it led to accomplishment of two major objectives of these studies. The first objective was a so-called nonenzymic activation as rapid as that achieved with an extrinsic tissue thromboplastic system. A mixture of horse prothrombin (1.9 mg per ml) and polyARG (0.1 mg polyARG-N per ml) in 1.0 M glycerol produced a linear, quantitative activation in 60 minutes at pH 8.0 and 25° C. As is the case with the polyLYS-induced reaction the rate of prothrombin consumption in the presence of both the polyARG and 1×10^{-3} M DFP was equal to the rate of thrombin generation in the absence of the DFP.

The second objective was a quantitatively activatable system induced by a substance of known chemical structure, a system which would permit detailed

TABLE 2

CONCENTRATIONS OF SUBSTANCES AFFECTING POLYLYS-
PROTHROMBIN REACTIONS *

Substance	Acceleration	Inhibition
Guanidine HCl	–	0.05 M
Dimethylformamide	–	1.00 M
Urea	–	1.00 M
Ethylene glycol	1.0 M	–
Propanediol	1.0 M	–
Glycerol	0.5–1.0 M	3.00 M
Dimethyl sulfoxide	1.0–2.0 M	3.00 M

* Methanol, dioxane—no effects from 0.05–2.0 M.

kinetic analyses of the activation phenomenon. Such a system was provided by mixtures of horse prothrombin (1.2 mg per ml), neomycin (0.2 mg neomycin-N per ml), and 2.0 M DMSO, at 18–25° C and pH 7.5–8.0. Those activations were complete in 2–3 hr.

Glycerol and DMSO appear to act by enhancement of the activation rates themselves rather than through stabilization of the thrombin formed since the same polyARG and neomycin systems eventually produced quantitative thrombin yields in the absence of the solvents. Neither glycerol nor DMSO altered the A_i/P of the polyLYS, polyARG or neomycin.

Prothrombin Concentration, Purity and Species

The polyARG-prothrombin system behaved the same as did polyLYS-prothrombin mixtures.[5] When the reactants were held in constant proportions the activation rates were linearly related to the concentration of the combined reagents. Also, the $A_i(N)/P$ for the polyARG system, 0.0052, was identical at each prothrombin concentration.

Measurements of the A_i/P using (a) prothrombin specimens of varying purity, and (b) the horse and cow zymogens (believed to have twofold differences in molecular weights and specific activities) provided the opportunities to determine whether the nonenzymic mechanism is directed toward the active sites on the zymogen, toward the total zymogen protein, or toward the zymogen and its impurities. For example, if horse prothrombin is twice the size of cow prothrombin, and has half the specific activity of the latter, one can easily determine whether the horse zymogen requires twice or half as much activator to initiate the reaction. Results employing polyLYS are summarized on TABLE 3. The horse zymogen requires half the polyLYS to initiate activation $(A_i(N)/P = 0.015)$ as does the cow prothrombin $(A_i(N)/P = 0.030)$. Thus, the amount of polyLYS nitrogen required *per unit* of prothrombin is constant

TABLE 3

SPECIES AND SPECIFIC ACTIVITIES OF PROTHROMBIN
AS RELATED TO PolyLYS-INDUCED ACTIVATION

	Units / mg Protein	$[A_i]$ mg N/ mg Prothrombin *	$[A_i]$ mg N/ unit Prothrombin	% Activation 2 Hr	Max
Horse	1100	0.015	1.36×10^{-5}	40	87.5
	1100	0.016	1.45×10^{-5}	74	83
	760	0.014	1.27×10^{-5}	56	75.5
	500	0.015	1.36×10^{-5}	54	87.5
Cow	2200	0.029	1.32×10^{-5}	48	96
	620	0.030	1.36×10^{-5}	73	91.5

* Actual prothrombin content in the sample.

between the species, a relationship that is also true for the purposely contaminated zymogen specimens (TABLE 3). Consequently, it appears the nonenzymic activation reaction, as measured by the A_i/P, is only directed at the components of a prothrombin preparation that are also activatable by the bioassay system.

DISCUSSION

The rates of thrombin formation in the processes reported herein were the most variable of the reaction parameters. Velocities of polyLYS-induced prothrombin activations had previously been found sensitive to ionic strength, activator:prothrombin ratios, concentrations of those reactants when in constant proportions, and size of the activator.[5] The present data corroborate the significance of an optimum size for each activator. The polybrene preparation of 300–600 average molecular weight was inactive in contrast to those of 600–900 and higher average weights. Also, during early stages of partial acid hydrolysis of a high molecular weight polyLYS (Av. MW 175,000) the rate at which that preparation produced thrombin was increased, only to be reduced again on prolonged hydrolysis. Identification of the hexaLYS in those hydrolyzates as the smallest lysine peptide capable of inducing significant prothrombin activation helps delineate the minimum size requirement for a nonenzymic activator. The effectiveness of hexaLYS (MW 787), polybrenes of MW 600–900 and larger, neomycin (MW 774), polymyxin (MW 1200), and colistin (MW 1168), suggests the minimum required size for a basic prothrombin activator is in the range of 700–1000 daltons.

The present studies also identify solvent influences on the rates of prothrombin activation induced by the nonenzymic substances. Seegers had noted stabilization of preformed thrombin in glycerol solutions.[10] However glycerol and DMSO also enhanced the rates of prothrombin activation. In a number of experiments, the thrombin yields in the absence of those solvents eventually reached levels more promptly achieved in their presence. Finally, rates of activation also appear dependent on the monomeric structure of each activator. The most pronounced examples of that phenomenon are the slow prothrombin activations at optimum polybrene concentrations compared to rates of thrombin generation induced by most of the other substances studied.

Slow activations of prothrombin at optimum polybrene concentrations contrasts markedly with the high sensitivity of the zymogen to those synthetic substances, characterized by the lowest A_i/P observed. The contrast illustrates the major distinction between the two parameters of prothrombin activation, rates of activation and the sensitivity characteristic, the A_i/P. The present and prior data[5] indicate the A_i/P is independent of the variety of factors that affect activation rates (i.e., molecular weight of the activator [if greater than 700–1000], temperature, solvent manipulations, purity and concentration of the prothrombin). The A_i/P is highly reproducible and appears characteristic for each activator. To date the only factor found to affect the A_i/P is the presence of a high-molecular-weight polyanion.[4]

Extrinsic thromboplastic systems (calcium ions, tissue factor, and sources of factors V, VII, and Xa) share some common properties with the nonenzymically controlled reactions described herein; namely, low temperature optima, sensitivity to salt concentrations, and resistance to DFP.[3] Also, preliminary studies demonstrate that either polyLYS or a Ca^{++}-brain thromboplastin-accessory factor complex,[11] each carefully equilibrated in an automatic titrator, yield bursts of protons when added to similarly equilibrated prothrombin specimens. In each case the proton burst precedes thrombin formation. This common property implies that a constituent(s) of the complex extrinsic thromboplastic system functions as does the polyLYS in the control of prothrombin activation.

Should one or more constituents of an extrinsic or intrinsic thromboplastic system function by the nonenzymic mechanism, the significance of the various activation parameters will have to be determined. From the standpoint of the etiology of thrombosis, the sensitivity of prothrombin to the activator (i.e., the least amount of activator necessary to form small amounts of thrombin) might be more important than the rate at which that substance supports thrombin formation under optimum conditions. For example, polybrenes might be regarded as poor thromboplastic substances since they induce relatively slow prothrombin activation. However, the polybrenes displayed the lowest A_i/P of any substance tested to date. Likewise, methods for quantitation of coagulation factors are usually based on rates of thrombin formation and attendant clotting times. However, factors required for initiation of prothrombin activation might better be evaluated by a dilution end-point system, one that measures the smallest amount of the substance required to induce a detectable change in that system, an initiating function.

Concerning the mechanism of the nonenzymically controlled prothrombin activations, the activators appear to combine directly with the prothrombin molecules. That is indicated by the constant A_i/P of 1.36×10^{-5} mg poly-LYS-N per unit prothrombin regardless of the purity or species of the prothrombin (TABLE 3), and by the identical A_i/P for polyORN which contributes identical numbers of primary amino groups to the reaction as does polyLYS (TABLE 1). Following this combination of the activator with prothrombin, and the proton burst referred to above, the further role of the substance in thrombin formation needs clarification. It is assumed the prothrombin preparations employed in these studies contained small amounts of factor X or Xa, although three of the crystalline horse preparations were negative in a factor X assay system.[12] All the lyophilized prothrombin preparations were extracted with chloroform:methanol (2:1) for removal of lipids before use,[6] and no calcium salts are added to the nonenzymically induced reactions. Thus, the nonenzymic activators appear to replace the calcium, lipid constituents, and possibly the factor V of the extrinsic system. Hypothetically, the activators may bind to the γ-carboxyglutamyl residues of the fragment $1\cdot2$ portion of the prothrombin [13, 14] in place of a Ca^{++}-lipid-factor V complex, with release of the protons.

At this time one can only speculate on subsequent events. The nonenzymic activators may bring the prothrombin and contaminating factor Xa into close proximity by the coprecipitation that occurs in most, but not all, of the mixtures. Again, activators bound to the prothrombin may, through steric hindrance, restrict factor Xa action to more efficient cleavage of the peptide bond in prethrombin 2 responsible for α-thrombin formation.[15-17] A third mechanism might be the induction of a conformational change in the zymogen beginning at the A_i/P, as suggested by the sharpness and reproducibility of that end point under a variety of conditions. The thrombin formed might participate in other activation mechanisms.[18, 19] Questions concerning the latter mechanism are raised by the DFP-resistance of the polyLYS, polyARG and extrinsic thromboplastic systems. Finally, any discussion of biologic effects of polycations, should include mention of the ability of polyLYS to catalyze decarboxylation reactions.[20]

One goal achieved through these studies was identification of a low-molecular-weight prothrombin activator of known structure, neomycin, which induces quantitative thrombin formation in 2.0 M DMSO, thus permitting detailed kinetic analyses and binding studies. A second goal was identification of a nonenzymic activator that induces the same rapid, complete prothrombin activation as does an extrinsic tissue thromboplastic system. That criterion was met by mixtures of prothrombin with optimum concentrations of polyARG in 1.0 M glycerol. When carried out at 17–20° C in DFP, that system should permit studies of structural changes in the prothrombin during activation complicated by few secondary enzymic alterations in the zymogen.

Finally, the constancy of an A_i/P, and its independence from the variety of factors that affect rates of thrombin formation, offers a unique method for standardization of a prothrombin solution. Following additions of increments of a known activator (i.e., polyLYS) to the zymogen, the smallest amount which induces thrombin formation is determined, and the prothrombin concentration is calculated from the A_i/P (unit).

REFERENCES

1. WAUGH, D. F., D. J. BAUGHMAN & K. D. MILLER. 1960. Thrombin. *In* The Enzymes. P. D. Boyer, H. Lardy & K. Myrback, Eds. **4:** 215–232. Academic Press. New York, N.Y.
2. LANDABURU, R. H. & W. H. SEEGERS. 1958. Activation of prothrombin. Am. J. Physiol. **193:** 169–180.
3. MILLER, K. D. & H. VAN VUNAKIS. 1956. The effect of diisopropyl fluorophosphate on the proteinase and esterase activities of thrombin and on prothrombin and its activators. J. Biol. Chem. **223:** 227–237.
4. MILLER, K. D., W. H. COPELAND & J. F. McGARRAHAN. 1961. Agents providing nonenzymic prothrombin activation. Proc. Soc. Exp. Biol. Med. **108:** 117–119.
5. MILLER, K. D. 1960. The nonenzymic activation of prothrombin by polylysine. J. Biol. Chem. **235:** PC63–64.
6. MILLER, K. D. & A. W. PHELAN. 1967. Purification and crystallization of horse prothrombin. Biochem. Biophys. Res. Commun. **27:** 505–510.
7. WARE, A. G. & W. H. SEEGERS. 1949. Two-stage procedure for the quantitative determination of prothrombin concentration. Am. J. Clin. Pathol. **19:** 471–482.
8. MARKHAM, R. 1942. A steam distillation apparatus suitable for micro-Kjeldahl analysis. Biochem. J. **36:** 790–791.
9. MILLER, K. D. 1971. Horse prothrombin. *In* Biochemical Preparations. J. H. Law, Ed. **13:** 49–55. John Wiley & Sons. New York.
10. SEEGERS, W. H. 1944. Purified prothrombin and thrombin: stabilization of aqueous solutions. Arch. Biochem. **3:** 363–367.
11. MILLER, K. D. 1959. Rivanol, resin and the isolation of thrombins. Nature **184:** 450.
12. BACHMANN, F., F. DUCKERT & F. KOLLER. 1958. The Stuart-Prower Factor assay and its clinical significance. Thromb. Diath. Haemorrh. **2:** 24–38.
13. STENFLO, J., P. FERNLAND, W. EGAN & W. ROEPSTORFF. 1974. Vitamin K dependent modifications of glutamic acid residues in prothrombin. Proc. Natl. Acad. Sci. USA **71:** 2730–2733.
14. MAGNUSSON, S., L. SOTTRUE-JENSEN, T. E. PETERSEN, H. R. MORRIS & A. DOLL. 1974. Primary structure of the vitamin K-dependent part of prothrombin. FEBS Lett. **44:** 189–193.
15. HELDEBRANT, C. M., R. J. BUTKOWSKI, S. P. BAVAN & K. G. MANN. 1973. The activation of prothrombin. J. Biol. Chem. **248:** 7149–7163.
16. ESMAN, C. T., W. G. OWEN & C. M. JACKSON. 1974. The conversion of prothrombin to thrombin. J. Biol. Chem. **249:** 7798–7807.
17. FENTON, J. W., M. J. FASCO, A. B. STACKROW, D. L. ARONSON, A. M. YOUNG & J. S. FINLAYSON. 1977. Production, evaluation and properties of α-thrombin. J. Biol. Chem. **252:** 3587–3598.
18. SEEGERS, W. H. 1971. Theory of blood coagulation: Three basic reactions. Thromb. Diath. Haemorrh. **46:** 63–86.
19. ARONSON, D. L. 1976. Comparison of the actions of thrombin and the thrombin-like venom enzymes Ancrod and Batroxobin. Thromb. Diath. Haemorrh. **36:** 4–13.
20. ROHLFING, D. L. 1967. The catalytic decarboxylation of oxalacetic acid by thermally prepared poly-α-amino acids. Arch. Biochem. **118:** 468–474.

THE PLATELET MEMBRANE AS A CATALYTIC SURFACE IN THROMBIN GENERATION: AVAILABILITY OF PLATELET FACTOR 1 AND PLATELET FACTOR 3 *

Arthur P. Bode,† Frederick A. Dombrose,†¶ Barry R. Lentz,‡
and Harold R. Roberts §

Center for Thrombosis and Hemostasis
University of North Carolina at Chapel Hill
Chapel Hill, North Carolina 27514

INTRODUCTION

The contribution of platelets to blood coagulation can be described in general terms as: the possible site of activation of certain clotting factors; a surface upon which certain clotting factors may selectively bind; and a potential source of coagulant activities.[1] Presumably, the circulating platelet must be activated before it will participate in coagulation. In response to any of several agents (thrombin, ADP, collagen, epinephrine, etc.) platelets undergo morphological and biochemical changes that coincide with the release of several intracellular constituents.[2-4] The appearance (or availability) of platelet coagulant activities seems to follow this release reaction, although some evidence suggests that the appearance of platelet coagulant activities may be associated with the small amount of platelet lysis that accompanies the release reaction.[5]

The contribution of the platelet membrane as a catalytic surface in enhancing thrombin generation can be measured as a clot-promoting activity, which has been defined operationally as platelet factor 3 or PF3. An operational definition has been necessary because PF3 does not appear to result from the contribution of a single molecular component,[6] but is believed to be a generalized chemical property of negatively charged lipids (for reviews see References 7–9). Whether PF3 is an acquired property of the entire platelet plasma membrane or is a distinct membrane component released from activated platelets [10] remains unclear.

The overall catalytic surface activity of activated platelets must include the contribution made by membrane-associated coagulation factors. In this regard, a platelet-associated factor V-like activity (platelet factor 1 or PF1) was first described in detail by Ware, Fahey, and Seegers over 30 years ago.[11] Further

* This work was supported by Grants HL22771–03 and HL06350–18 from the National Heart, Lung, and Blood Institute. This work was done in part during the tenure of an Established Investigator Award to BRL from the American Heart Association and with funds contributed in part by the North Carolina Heart Association. APB received support from a National Institute for General Medical Science Training Grant GM00092.

† Department of Pathology.
‡ Department of Biochemistry.
§ Department of Medicine.
¶ Address all correspondence to FAD.

work by Seegers and his colleagues supported a hypothesis that PF1 was activated factor V intimately associated with the platelet.[12-14] However, several other investigators have reported that PF1 is related to adsorbed factor V.[15, 16] Mann and coworkers [17] have demonstrated that factor V binds to a specific, high-affinity receptor on platelets that appears to be different from a lower affinity binding site provided by negatively charged phospholipid surfaces.[18, 19] It is still unclear as to what extent the availability of a high-affinity factor V receptor may contribute to the PF1 catalytic surface activity of the platelet. The precise contribution of platelet membrane-bound factor V to thrombin generation is not known, although Miletich *et al.*[20-22] have demonstrated a relationship between the high affinity binding of factor Xa and the presence of platelet-bound factor Va.

To investigate the role of the platelet membrane as a catalytic surface in thrombin generation, we have studied the availability of PF1 and PF3 using an adaptation of the partial thromboplastin time test.[23] In this report we demonstrate that PF1 and PF3 in human platelets are available only upon activation and/or lysis. While normal platelets and platelets isolated from a severe factor V-deficient donor have equivalent PF3, only normal platelets have PF1. However, the PF1-deficient platelets will take up factor V from plasma in proportion to the level of platelet activation. These data are interpreted in terms of a model based on the availability of PF1 in normals and of a factor V receptor in PF1-deficient platelets.

MATERIALS

Plasmas. All normal and congenitally factor-deficient human plasmas were obtained through the Clinical Coagulation Laboratory of North Carolina Memorial Hospital from healthy donors after informed consent was obtained. Venipuncture was performed on fasting, healthy donors who reportedly had not ingested aspirin or other drugs for at least 10 days prior to collection. Blood was collected either by the two syringe technique with a 19g needle (1/7 vol. ACD) or by standard double plasmapheresis (1/9 vol. 4% trisodium citrate) after discarding the first 10–15 ml of whole blood. Platelet-rich plasma (PRP) was obtained by immediate centrifugation of the whole blood for 10 minutes at $300 \times g$, 22° C. Platelet-poor plasma (PPP) was obtained by a double centrifugation technique at 4° C (less than 500 platelets/mm^3). PPP was snap frozen and stored at −76° C in capped polypropylene tubes.

Freeze-Thawed Platelets. Aliquots of frozen platelets at 1×10^9 platelets/ ml were thawed quickly in a 37° C water-bath and then snap frozen in a dry ice–alcohol bath. Freeze-thawing was twice repeated and the suspension was centrifuged for 15 minutes at $800 \times g$, 22° C, in conical plastic centrifuge tubes to remove unlysed platelets. The frozen-thawed platelet supernatant (FTPS) was carefully pipetted into plastic tubes and kept in an ice-water bath during the assay procedure.

Platelet Washing Buffer. Platelets were washed by gel-filtration or by centrifugation-resuspension as described in the text using a modification of the buffer described by Baenziger and Majerus [24]: 0.113 M NaCl, 0.0043 M K_2HPO_4, 0.0043 M Na_2HPO_4, 0.0244 M NaH_2PO_4, 0.2 g/liter dextrose, 1 g/liter albumin (bovine, fatty acid-free, or bovine fraction V), 5 mM adenosine, 250 mg/liter theophylline, and 100 ng/ml prostaglandin E_1 (PGE_1).

METHODS

Gel Filtration of Platelet Suspensions. Platelets were harvested from PRP by centrifugation at $700 \times g$ for 15 minutes at 22° C in plastic tubes. The supernatant plasma was decanted and the platelet pellet was gently resuspended in a small volume of platelet washing buffer by slow flushing with a wide bore plastic Pasteur pipet or by swirling of the resuspension tube alone if it proved sufficient. The platelet suspension was then loaded on a 1.5×24 cm bed of Biogel A-150m in a silanized borosilicate glass column and chromatographed in the same buffer. The gel-filtered platelets (GFP) eluted in the void volume fractions without any detectable aggregation.

Centrifugation Washing of Platelets. Platelets were harvested from PRP as above. The platelet pellet was resuspended in the platelet washing buffer to approximately one-half the original plasma volume and centrifuged at $700 \times g$ for 10 minutes at 22° C. The supernatant was decanted and the walls of the centrifuge tube were carefully wiped dry. The resuspension–centrifugation was repeated twice and the platelet count of the final resuspended centrifugation-washed platelets (CWP) determined using an electronic counter. The extent of any platelet aggregation was examined by phase contrast microscopy.

Assay Procedure. Historically, one of the most productive approaches to evolving knowledge of the coagulation cascade has been the use of plasmas from human patients deficient in a specific clotting factor. By taking advantage of this approach, we have devised a whole plasma test system for PF1 and PF3 in which assay conditions are closer to the native state than in other systems constructed from purified components or which employ crude enzyme preparations (Stypven time). Analysis of the assay system and the basis of data interpretation have been described elsewhere;[23] a summary of assay procedure and interpretation is given below:

Reagent A:	Contact-activated PPP	0.1 ml
Reagent B:	Test material (e.g., platelets)	0.1 ml
Reagent C:	Unactivated PPP	0.1 ml

Incubated 60 seconds in a 13×75 mm polystyrene test tube at 37° C.

Reagent D:	0.04 M $CaCl_2$	0.1 ml

Timer started: Additional incubation at 37° for 30 seconds.

High-V: Normal PPP in reagents A and C
Low-V: Factor V-deficient PPP in reagents A and C

Reagent A was a source of activated factor XI. The PPP was activated with 10 mg/ml kaolin for 10 minutes at 37° C after which the kaolin particles were removed by centrifugation at $12,000 \times g$ for 4 minutes at 22° C. The kaolin-free supernatant plasma was quickly transferred to a polypropylene tube and placed in an ice-water bath.

Reagent B was the test material, either whole platelets diluted in the platelet washing buffer or FTPS diluted in Tris-buffered saline.

Reagent C was unactivated platelet-poor plasma which served to balance the level of any desired coagulant activity in the test system.

The level of factor V in the assay was adjusted with reagents A and C using either pooled human normal plasma or plasma from a severe factor V-deficient patient (less than 0.2% of normal activity), which had no detectable cross-reacting antigenic material. To perform the assay, equal parts of reagents A, B, and C were combined in small plastic test tubes and warmed to 37° C before recalcification with reagent D; a timer was started upon the addition of reagent D and the elapsed time to a fibrin clot was recorded.

All data analysis was performed by plotting the logarithm of clotting time versus the logarithm of dilutions employed in each assay. In this analysis, the data showed the following behavior: (1) log(clotting time) increased linearly with log(dilution), where the appropriateness of the straight-line model was accepted if $p > 0.25$; and (2) the "residual" standard deviation of clotting time increased linearly with log(dilution).[25] The first result is expected on the basis of the kinetics of the coagulation cascade, where it has been shown by Savageu[26] that such log–log plots should be an accurate linear description of the clotting process over a narrow range of dilutions and an approximation over a large range (power-law approximation). The linear model provided two parameters: the slope and the intercept. Each parameter was examined under different assay conditions.

RESULTS

Evaluation of PF3 and PF1

FTPS preparations derived from either normal platelets or those obtained from the severe factor V-deficient donor were used as reference curves for measurement of PF3 and PF1. Lines-of-best-fit for normal FTPS (NFTPS) and factor V-deficient FTPS (VdFTPS) are shown in FIGURE 1. Assay data were obtained in a plasma test system with either normal levels of factor V (High-V) or in a factor V-deficient system (Low-V). In the High-V system, both FTPS preparations had the same catalytic surface activity; the clotting times for NFTPS were indistinguishable from those for VdFTPS. The activity measured in the High-V assay system represents the accelerated coagulation of recalcified, contact-activated normal plasma, which by analogy with previous definitions we identify as PF3.

In the Low-V system, a factor V-like activity was observed in NFTPS, which, compared to VdFTPS, was characterized by its marked difference in both activity and log–log slope. While VdFTPS did shorten the clotting time in the Low-V system, the line of best fit for VdFTPS was parallel to bovine brain cephalin.[23] The difference in the log–log slope between these preparations and NFTPS formed the basis for distinguishing PF1 from PF3; the increase in the observed log–log slope for NFTPS was presumably due to the contribution of PF1. This was demonstrated by the fact that the log–log slope obtained for dilutions of plasma factor V (normal plasma diluted in factor V-deficient plasma as reagents A and C, with buffer substituted for reagent B) was the same as the log–log slope obtained for dilutions of NFTPS in the Low-V system. Based on these observations and the fact that no other clotting factor activities were identified in either the NFTPS or cephalin, we concluded that the rate-limiting activity in NFTPS measured in the Low-V system was platelet-associated factor V-like activity, or PF1. Therefore, in this study we used NFTPS for establishing a standard curve for a parallel line assay of either PF1 in the Low-V system, or PF3 in the High-V system. Provided that the sample assay curve was both linear and parallel to this standard,[27] interpolations of

PF1 and PF3 assay data for platelet samples were made directly from the NFTPS reference curve. The activities in 10^9 platelets/ml were reported as a percentage of the standard, where NFTPS prepared from 10^9 platelets/ml had 100% PF1 and 100% PF3.

Washed Platelets

Human platelets were isolated from normal plasma or factor V-deficient plasma by gel filtration or a centrifugation-washing technique. The washed platelets were serially diluted in platelet washing buffer and assayed in the High-V and Low-V systems. Typical assay data obtained for washed platelets from normal donors are shown in FIGURE 2. Since for most preparations of gel-filtered normal platelets (open circles) the clotting times in the High-V assay were not significantly different from the blank time (buffer substituted for

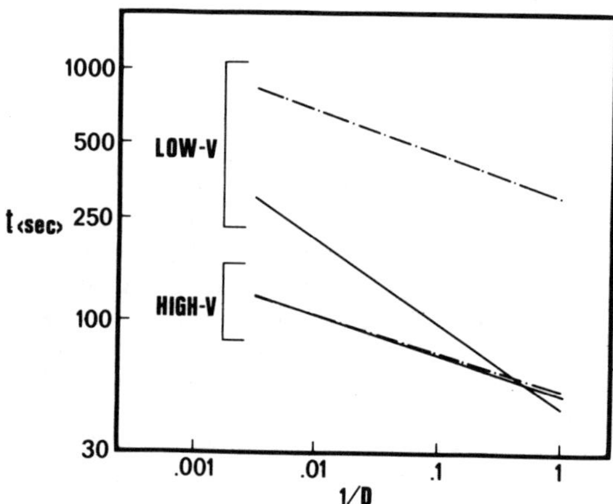

FIGURE 1. Double logarithmic plot of clotting time versus reciprocal of dilution in the High-V and Low-V assay systems, lines of best fit for: solid line, NFTPS; dashed line, VdFT-PS.

platelets) until the platelet concentration reached 10^9/ml, we estimated that normal gel-filtered platelets (NGFP) had less than 1% available PF3 (the lower limit of detection in our assay). In the Low-V system, the log–log slope obtained for these platelets was slightly less than that of the NFTPS reference curve, which probably meant that the assay data was below the limit of sensitivity of the PF1 assay. Since the clotting time for NGFP at 1×10^9 platelets/ml approached the clotting time for 1% NFTPS on the reference curve, we estimated that these platelets had no more than 1% available PF1.

Normal platelets obtained from the centrifugation-washing procedure (filled circles) had considerably more activity than the gel-filtered platelets. The assay data obtained for preparations of normal centrifugation-washed platelets (NCWP) consistently met the parallel-line criteria for assay of PF1 and PF3. Although the values obtained for PF1 and PF3 varied considerably for different preparations of NCWP, they consistently exceeded the activities observed in NGFP prepared from the same donor. We observed as much as 20% available PF1 and 20% available PF3 in NCWP.

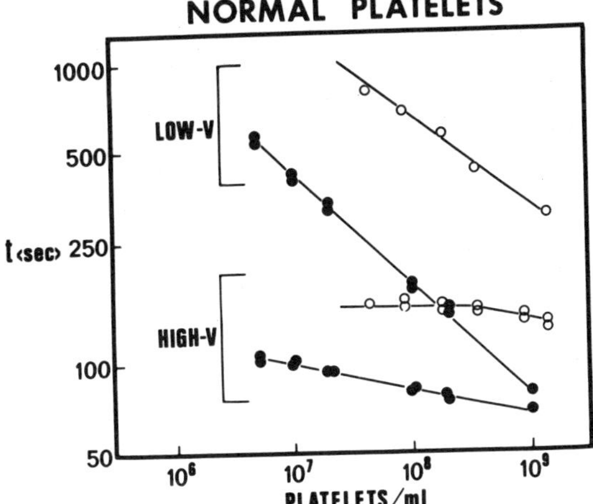

FIGURE 2. Typical High-V and Low-V assay data for washed, human normal platelets: ○, gel filtered platelets (NGFP); ●, centrifugation washed platelets (NCWP).

Typical assay data for platelets prepared from the factor V-deficient donor by gel filtration (VdGFP) or by centrifugation-washing (VdCWP) are shown in FIGURE 3. The VdGFP (open circles) were not different from buffer in either the High-V or Low-V assay system, indicating that no PF1 or PF3 was exposed on the intact Vd platelets. VdCWP (filled circles) produced curves in the High-V and Low-V assay systems that were parallel to those obtained with VdFTPS. Since the log–log slope in the Low-V assay was less than that for NFTPS, there was no evidence for PF1 in these Vd platelet preparations. Compared to the NFTPS reference curve, the VdCWP shown in FIGURE 3 had 10% available PF3 and no detectable PF1.

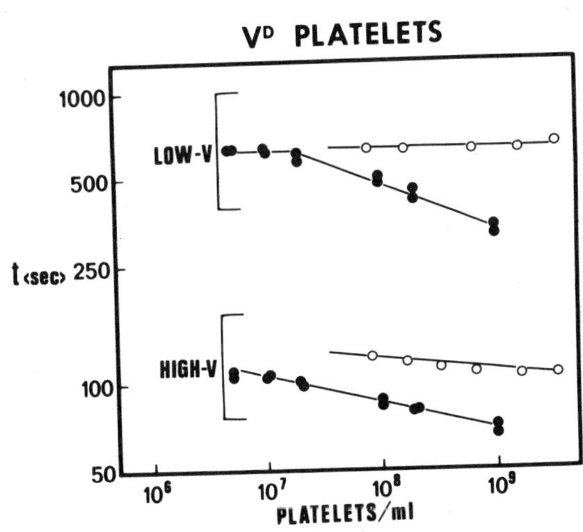

FIGURE 3. Typical High-V and Low-V assay data for washed, human Vd platelets: ○, gel filtered platelets (Vd-GFP); ●, centrifugation washed platelets (VdCWP).

Acquired PF1 in Vd Platelets

To investigate the uptake of factor V by platelets prepared from the factor V-deficient donor, we incubated Vd platelet preparations (approximately 10^9 platelets/ml) in normal human plasma at 37° C and then assayed these platelets for PF1 after suitable washing. The data from these incubation experiments are summarized in TABLE 1. The second line for each table entry shows the activities measured in the FTPS prepared before or after incubation of the whole platelets in normal plasma. Vd platelets were isolated from VdPRP with or without gel-filtration washing and resuspended in normal human plasma for 30 minutes at 37° C. Platelets were then washed by gel filtration and assayed. In both cases, the platelets appeared to have acquired no more than 1% PF1, which was the same as the available PF1 in NGFP. Upon 3× freezing and thawing, these incubated Vd platelets still had less than 1% PF1 (and now 100% PF3) in sharp contrast to the 100% PF1 obtained from 3× freezing

TABLE 1

APPEARANCE OF PF1 IN FACTOR V-DEFICIENT PLATELETS INCUBATED IN
NORMAL PLASMA AT 37° C

Incubated Preparation	Material Assayed	Before Incubation		After Incubation	
		PF1 *	PF3 *	PF1 *	PF3 *
VdGFP	GFP	0%	0–1%	1%	1%
	FTPS	0%	100%	1%	100%
VdCWP	CWP	0%	10%	ND †	ND
	FTPS	0%	100%	20% ‡	100%
VdFTPS	FTPS	0%	100%	100%	100%

* NFTPS was assigned the values 100% PF1 and 100% PF3 and was used as a standard curve for a parallel line assay.

† ND = Assays not done.

‡ Same value was obtained after 2, 5, 10, or 15 minutes incubation of VdCWP.

and thawing of NGFP. These observations suggested that unactivated, PF1-deficient platelets did not take up substantial amounts of factor V-like activity.

This experiment was repeated using a preparation of VdCWP which we estimated had 15% available PF3. These Vd platelets were incubated in normal plasma at 37° C (2, 5, 10, or 15 min) and then washed again by the centrifugation washing technique. The total PF1 in the FTPS derived from any of these incubations was approximately 20% of the limiting 100% PF1 in NFTPS (TABLE 1). The uptake of factor V by VdCWP was the same for each incubation (one-way analysis of variance, $p > 0.50$), suggesting that the uptake of factor V was rapid and apparently saturated.

Compared to the incubation experiment that began with unactivated VdGFP, the results obtained with partially activated VdCWP suggest that the ability of V-deficient platelets to acquire PF1 may be related to the level of platelet activation. To test this working hypothesis, we incubated VdFTPS (which operationally represented membrane material from fully activated platelets) in normal plasma at 37° C for 10 minutes. The entire incubation mixture was then gel-filtered to remove excess plasma factor V. Chromatography conditions were chosen so that the PF1 and PF3 from FTPS eluted in the void volume of a Biogel A-150m column, whereas plasma factor V eluted near the gel total volume. Membrane vesicles were visible only in the void volume fractions both by enhanced phase contrast microscopy and transmission electron microscopy. The void volume fraction obtained after gel filtration of this preparation of originally V-deficient FTPS now had 100% PF1 and 100% PF3. These void volume vesicles were indistinguishable from NFTPS in both the High-V and Low-V systems.

Thrombin-induced PF1 and PF3

In order to demonstrate the availability of PF1 and PF3 in response to physiological stimuli, we have undertaken some preliminary experiments with thrombin activation of washed platelets. NCWP in buffered saline at 10^9 platelets/ml aggregated irreversibly within 20 seconds when incubated with 0.5 NIH units/ml thrombin (Bethesda reagent, lot H1) at room temperature. The platelet aggregates were removed by centrifugation at $800 \times g$ for 15 minutes, and the supernatant was passed over a Biogel A-150m column to separate excess thrombin from released platelet membrane fragments. In all three experiments where aggregation occurred, a small amount of PF1 and PF3 (1–2%) was found in the chromatographed release supernatant. In order to assay thrombin-treated platelets, it was necessary to include platelet aggregation inhibitors. In the presence of adenosine, theophylline, and PGE_1 treatment of normal platelets with 0.1, 0.5, 2.0 units/ml thrombin at 37° C for 10 minutes did not induce aggregation, released no more than 1% of maximum available platelet factor 4 (PF4, measured by RIA, Abbott Laboratories, North Chicago, IL), and did not induce the release of PF1 and PF3 into the supernatant. The small amount of PF4 released into the supernatant increased with increasing levels of thrombin, indicating that the release of alpha granule contents from the platelets was not completely blocked. When these platelets were washed by rapid centrifugation/resuspension (two centrifugations at $12,000 \times g$ for 1 min) and then assayed for PF1 and PF3, the log-log slopes obtained were always greater than the slopes of the standard curves. Also, the clotting times obtained with these platelets were markedly decreased in both test systems; but, because of the altered slopes, PF1 and PF3 could not be quantitated by parallel line assay.

The control NGFP in these experiments had no significant increase in PF1 and PF3 after the washing procedure, suggesting that the decrease in clotting times observed after thrombin treatment was not due to mechanical stimulation of the platelets. Although the decrease in clotting times could have been due to residual thrombin remaining with the platelets after the washing procedure, the washed platelet suspension did not clot a canine fibrinogen solution in 10 mM Ca^{+2} during 9 minutes' incubation at 37° C. However, when hirudin (2000 ATU/mg, Pentapharm Ltd., Basle) was added after the thrombin incubation and prior to the centrifugation/resuspension washing (fourfold excess hirudin over thrombin based on functional activities), the clotting times in the PF1 and PF3 assays were the same as those of the control platelets that were not treated with thrombin. In other words, hirudin completely nullified the decrease in clotting times observed with thrombin treatment of NGFP and VdGFP. Hirudin by itself did not alter already available PF1 and PF3. Therefore, it appears that thrombin treatment of platelet suspensions in the presence of adenosine, theophylline, and PGE_1 did not make PF1 and PF3 available in washed platelet suspensions. The observed decrease in clotting times with thrombin-treated platelet suspensions must have been the result of catalytic quantities of thrombin remaining on the platelet surface. Further evidence for this interpretation was provided by experiments where the thrombin-treated platelets were washed by gel-filtration rather than centrifugation. In these platelets, very little decrease in clotting times was observed over the controls.

We also studied the effect of thrombin treatment in the presence of the inhibitors on the ability of Vd platelets to acquire PF1. When thrombin-treated, unaggregated VdGFP were incubated in normal plasma (under conditions similar to those described in the previous section) and gel-filtered to remove the excess plasma factor V, they acquired less than 1% PF1, which was no more than the amount obtained when untreated VdGFP were incubated in normal plasma. The inhibitors used in this study apparently blocked both the appearance of PF3 and the appearance of the putative receptor for factor V under these conditions.

Conclusions

Normal platelets participate in blood coagulation by providing a catalytic phospholipid surface activity (PF3) and a membrane-associated factor V-like activity (PF1), both of which accelerate the rate of thrombin generation. In this report we have demonstrated that human platelets isolated from normal or a severe factor V-deficient donor by gel filtration had little or no measurable PF3 and PF1. To generate these activities in sufficient amounts to be detectable in our clotting assays, the resting platelet had to be activated (for example, thrombin treatment, centrifugation-washing, or freezing and thawing). Activation of normal platelets induced PF3 and PF1 in proportion to the degree of stimulation; but only PF3 was observed in the PF1-deficient platelets isolated from the severe factor V-deficient donor. However, activated PF1-deficient platelets had the ability to acquire PF1 in proportion to the degree of platelet activation after incubation in normal plasma. Our data support the hypothesis that these platelet-related coagulant activities are expressed only in activated platelet preparations.

Recent reports [28] have further strengthened the argument that intrinsic factor V-like activity in normal human platelets may actually be factor Va,[11] and that normal human platelets contain high-affinity receptors for both factors V and Va.[29] Based on these and our own observations, we believe that the data presented here are consistent with a model wherein PF1-deficient platelets have a receptor(s) induced by activation, which binds plasma factor V (Va), resulting in the appearance of PF1. Our working hypothesis is that this receptor exists in normal platelets and that it is saturated with an intrinsic factor V (Va). We postulate that when normal platelets are activated, the intrinsic factor V(Va)–receptor complex is made available as PF1. In activated, PF1-deficient platelets, only unoccupied receptors are made available which can be saturated with factor V (Va) by incubation in normal plasma.

REFERENCES

1. SIXMA, J. J. 1978. Platelet coagulant activities. Throm. Haemostas. **40:** 163–167.
2. WHITE, J. G. 1979. Current concepts of platelet structure. Am. J. Clin. Pathol. **71:** 363–378.
3. RODMAN, N. F. 1971. The morphological basis of platelet function. *In* The Platelet. K. M. Brinkhous, R. W. Shermer & F. K. Mostofi, Eds. pp. 55–70. Williams & Wilkins Co., Baltimore, Md.
4. HOLMSEN, H., H. J. DAY & H. STORMORKEN. 1969. The blood platelet release reaction. Scand. J. Hematol. Suppl. **8:** 3–26.
5. JOIST, J. H., G. DOLEZEL, J. V. LLOYD, R. L. KINLOUGH-RATHBONE & J. F. MUSTARD. 1974. Platelet factor 3 availability and the platelet release reaction. J. Lab. Clin. Med. **84:** 474–482.
6. MARCUS, A. J. 1972. Recent advances in platelet lipid metabolism research. Ann. N.Y. Acad. Sci. **201:** 102–108.
7. MARCUS, A. J. 1966. The role of lipids in blood coagulation. Adv. Lipid Res. **4:** 1–37.
8. JACKSON, C. M., W. G. OWEN, S. N. GITEL & C. T. ESMON. 1974. The chemical role of lipids in prothrombin conversion. Thromb. Diath. Haemorrh. **17** (Suppl.): 273–293.
9. ZWAAL, R. F. A. 1978. Membrane and lipid involvement in blood coagulation. Biochim. Biophys. Acta **515:** 163–205.
10. SANDBERG, H., L. ANDERSSON & S. HÖGLUND. Particles with platelet factor 3 activity isolated from platelet release supernatant. (Submitted for publication to Biochem. J.)
11. WARE, A. G., J. L. FAHEY & W. H. SEEGERS. 1948. Platelet extracts, fibrin formation and interaction of purified prothrombin and thromboplastin. Am. J. Physiol. **154:** 140–147.
12. McCLAUGHRY, R. I. & W. H. SEEGERS. 1950. Prothrombin, Ac-globulin and platelet accelerator: quantitative interrelationships. Blood **5:** 303–312.
13. DEUTSCH, E., S. A. JOHNSON & W. H. SEEGERS. 1955. Differentiation of certain platelet factors related to blood coagulation. Circulation Res. **3:** 110–115.
14. FELL, C. & W. H. SEEGERS. 1958. Platelet factor 1 related to prothrombin activation. Can. J. Biochem. Physiol. **36:** 645–652.
15. JOHNSON, S. A., W. M. SMATHERS & C. L. SCHNEIDER. 1952. Platelets and their plasma cofactor activity in the activation of purified prothrombin. Am. J. Physiol. **170:** 631–635.
16. HJORT, P., S. I. RAPAPORT & P. A. OWREN. 1955. Evidence that platelet accelerator (platelet factor 1) is adsorbed plasma proaccelerin. Blood **10:** 1139–1150.
17. TRACY, P. B., J. M. PETERSON, M. E. NESHEIM, F. C. McDUFFIE & K. G. MANN. 1979. Interaction of coagulation Factor V and Va with platelets. J. Biol. Chem. **254:** 10354–10361.
18. COLMAN, R. W. 1976. Factor V. *In* Progress in Hemostasis and Thrombosis. T. H. Spaet, Ed. Vol. 3: 109–143. Grune & Stratton, New York, N.Y.
19. BLOOM, J. W., M. E. NESHEIM & K. G. MANN. 1979. Phospholipid-binding properties of bovine Factor V and Factor Va. Biochemistry **18:** 4419–4424.
20. MILETICH, J. P., C. M. JACKSON & P. W. MAJERUS. 1977. Interaction of coagulation Factor Xa with human platelets. Proc. Natl. Acad. Sci. USA **74:** 4033–4036.
21. MILETICH, J. P., D. W. MAJERUS & P. W. MAJERUS. 1978. Patients with congenital Factor V deficiency have decreased Factor Xa binding sites on their platelets. J. Clin. Invest. **62:** 824–831.
22. MILETICH, J. P., C. M. JACKSON & P. W. MAJERUS. 1978. Properties of the Factor Xa binding site on human platelets. J. Biol. Chem. **253:** 6908–6916.

23. DOMBROSE, F. A., A. P. BODE & B. R. LENTZ. 1979. Differentiation of platelet membrane-associated Factor V activity and membrane catalytic surface activity using a new clotting assay. Thromb. Haemostas. (abst.) **42:** 209. (Full manuscript in preparation.)

24. BAENZIGER, N. L. & P. W. MAJERUS. 1974. Isolation of human platelets and platelet surface membranes. Methods Enzymol. **31:** 149–155.

25. KLEINBAUM, D. G. & L. L. KUPPER. 1978. Applied regression analysis and other multivariable methods. Chap. 5–7: 37–94. Duxbury Press, North Scituate, Mass.

26. SAVAGEAU, M. 1976. Biochemical Systems Analysis. Chap. 5: 89–92 and Chap. 13: 217–234. Addison-Wesley Publishing Co., Reading, Mass.

27. COUNTS, R. B. & J. E. HAYS. 1979. A computer program for analysis of clotting factor assays and other parallel-line bioassays. Am. J. Clin. Pathol. **71:** 167–171.

28. ØSTERUD, B., S. I. RAPAPORT & K. K. LAVINE. 1977. Factor V activity of platelets: Evidence for an activated Factor V molecule and for a platelet activator. Blood **49:** 819–834.

29. KANE, W. H., M. J. LINDHOUT, C. M. JACKSON & P. W. MAJERUS. 1980. Factor Va-dependent binding of Factor Xa to human platelets. J. Biol. Chem. **255:** 1170–1174.

MECHANISM OF ACTION OF THE LUPUS ANTICOAGULANT

Sandor S. Shapiro, Perumal Thiagarajan, and Luigi De Marco

The Cardeza Foundation for Hematologic Research
Department of Medicine
Jefferson Medical College of Thomas Jefferson University
Philadelphia, Pennsylvania 19107

The coagulation inhibitor known as the "lupus anticoagulant" was first clearly described in systemic lupus erythematosus (SLE) by Conley and Hartmann in 1952.[1] Since then, numerous inhibitors of this type have been described in SLE and in other conditions.[2] The phenomenon is characterized by prolongation of lipid-dependent coagulation tests, especially the prothrombin time, partial thromboplastin time and Russell's viper venom time, and by variable deficits of one or more coagulation factors, often factors VIII, IX, or XI. In addition, occasional patients with SLE and a lupus anticoagulant have isolated deficits of prothrombin.[3] Although most evidence has pointed to the immunoglobulin nature of these inhibitors, their precise mechanism of action has been difficult to elucidate. Despite the coagulation abnormalities, patients with lupus anticoagulants rarely bleed. This apparent dissociation of laboratory and clinical findings suggested that an understanding of lupus anticoagulants might contribute some insights into the physiology of the hemostatic mechanism.

We have studied a patient with Waldenstrom's macroglobulinemia whose IgMλ paraprotein was a lupus anticoagulant.[4] We were able to demonstrate that this paraprotein had immunologic specificity towards phospholipids with a net negative charge. By virtue of this specificity, the paraprotein interfered with the ability of the vitamin K-dependent, γ-carboxyglutamic acid (gla)-containing, coagulation factors to bind to phospholipid micelles in the presence of calcium ions, accounting for the abnormalities in coagulation tests. We have examined several lupus inhibitors in patients with SLE and have found that these, too, are immunoglobulins possessing specificity towards anionic phospholipids.

The screening studies in our macroglobulinemic patient are shown in TABLE 1. Prothrombin time, partial thromboplastin time, Russell's viper venom time, and Taipan snake venom time, all tests depending upon the presence of phospholipid, are prolonged. In addition, one-stage assays for factors V, VIII, IX, X, and XI, all of which utilize phospholipid, were moderately to severely depressed. In contrast, the *Echis carinatus* time of patient plasma was normal; *Echis carinatus* venom contains an enzyme capable of activating prothrombin directly, without need for phospholipid. Prolongations in these tests were independent of the source of tissue factor or phospholipid. When the patient's IgMλ paraprotein was purified and added to normal plasma, inhibition of all the same tests began to be noted at paraprotein concentrations of 20 mg/dl. This effect is illustrated for the Russell's viper venom time in FIGURE 1. For comparison, concentration of the paraprotein in the patient's own plasma was 2–3 gm/dl. In order to demonstrate the immunologic nature

359

TABLE 1

SCREENING STUDIES

	Patient	Control
Prothrombin time (sec)	18.4	12.4
Partial thromboplastin time (sec)	96.0	61.4
Activated partial thromboplastin time (sec)	76.4	47.8
Russell's viper venom time (sec)	12.8	5.4
Taipan snake venom time (sec)	27.9	15.9
Echis carinatus time (sec)	15.8	16.2

of this inhibition, Fab_μ and $Fc_{5\mu}$ fragments were isolated, after tryptic digestion at $65°\,C$,[5] from patient IgMλ and from a control IgMλ obtained from a macroglobulinemic patient without a lupus inhibitor. Fragments were separated on Sephadex G-200 (FIG. 2) and characterized by SDS gel electrophoresis and by immunologic methods. As can be seen in FIGURE 3, patient Fab_μ prolonged the Russell's viper venom time proportional to the amount added, while patient $Fc_{5\mu}$ and fragments of control IgMλ were without effect.

Binding of radiolabelled prothrombin (FIG. 4) and factor X (FIG. 5) to mixed phospholipid micelles in the presence of calcium was studied by the method of Gitel and coworkers.[6] Patient IgM, but not control IgM, inhibited the binding of these two zymogens to the phospholipid micelles. In another series of experiments, the identical effect was obtained with patient Fab_μ, but not with patient $Fc_{5\mu}$, again indicating the immunologic nature of the inter-action.

Specificity towards phospholipids was studied in several manners, including thin-layer chromatographic identification of specific phospholipids precipitated by patient IgM, and complement fixation after interaction of patient IgM and specific phospholipid liposomes. However, reaction of patient IgM against sonicated preparations of purified phospholipids can be studied directly by

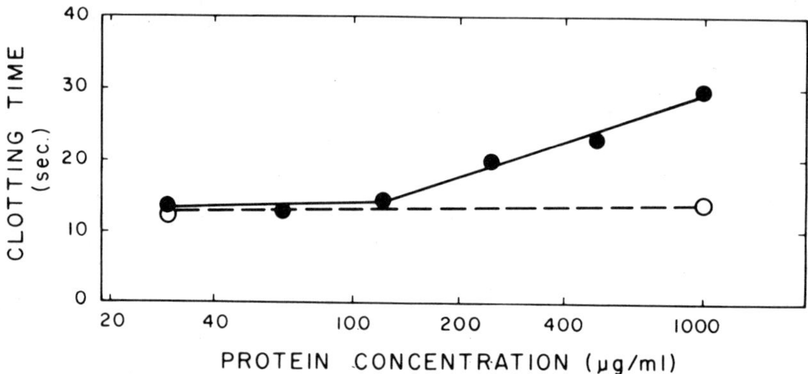

FIGURE 1. The effect of IgM on the RVV time of normal plasma. Normal plasma, RVV and phospholipid were incubated for 30 seconds with varying dilutions of IgM before addition of $CaCl_2$. ●: patient IgM; ○: normal polyclonal IgM.

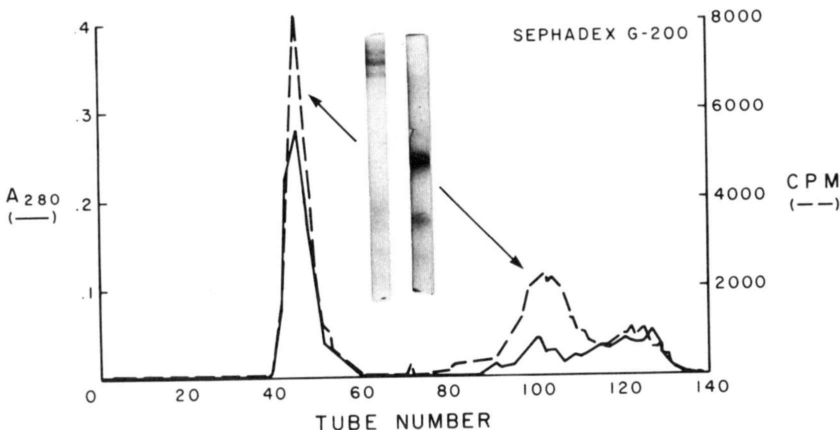

FIGURE 2. Sephadex G-200 gel-filtration of tryptic digest of monoclonal IgM with lupus anticoagulant activity. SDS gels of Fc$_{5\mu}$ (left) and Fab$_\mu$ (right) peaks are shown.

Ouchterlony immunodiffusion. Results obtained with this method were in complete agreement with those obtained by the previously mentioned techniques. Patient IgM reacted with phosphatidylserine (PS), phosphatidylinositol (PI), and phosphatidic acid (PA), but not with phosphatidylethanolamine (PE) or phosphatidylcholine (PC).[4] Furthermore, preincubation of these phospholipids with patient Fab$_\mu$ completely blocked the reaction to patient IgM, again indicating the immunologic nature of the interaction.[4] As shown in FIGURE 6, preincubation of patient IgM with PI inhibited the interaction of patient IgM with PI and partially inhibited the reaction with PS and PA; preincubation of patient IgM with PS, PA, lysophosphatidylserine (LPS), glycerylphosphorylserine (GPS) or with glycerol-3-phosphate (not shown) inhibited the reaction, while preincubation with phosphorylserine (PhS) had no effect. These results

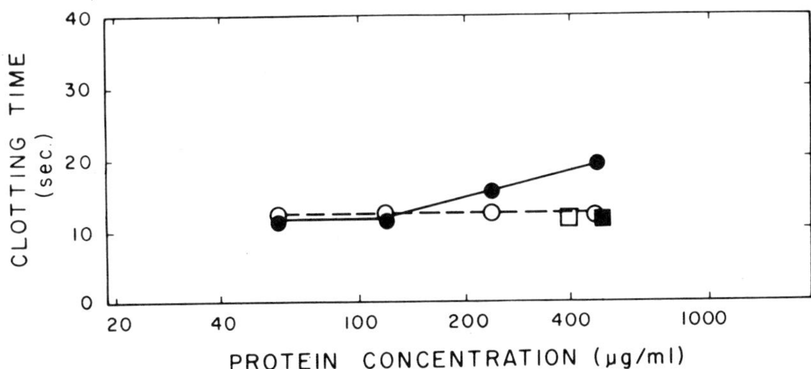

FIGURE 3. The effect of Fab$_\mu$ and Fc$_{5\mu}$ on the RVV time of normal plasma. The conditions were the same as those in FIGURE 1. ●: patient Fab$_\mu$; ○: control monoclonal Fab$_\mu$; ■: patient Fc$_{\mu5}$; □: control monoclonal Fc$_{5\mu}$.

indicate that the antigenic locus on the anionic phospholipid being recognized by the patient IgM involves the net negative charge and perhaps the adjacent C3 of glycerol, but not the C1 or C2 fatty acid chains.

When washed platelets from a normal person or from the patient himself were substituted for phospholipid in clotting assays on the patient's plasma, results of these assays were entirely normal (TABLE 2). Furthermore, when washed platelets were used instead of phospholipid in one-stage assays for specific coagulation factors, the deficits previously seen disappeared. Direct

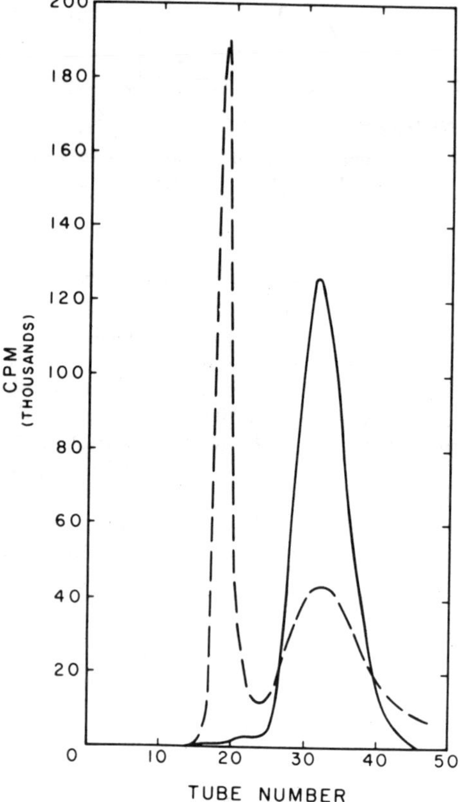

FIGURE 4. Effect of IgM on the Ca++-dependent binding of prothrombin to phospholipid micelles. Cold prothrombin, iodinated prothrombin, IgM and CaCl₂ were incubated with phospholipid at 37° C for 15 minutes in the presence of heparin and antithrombin III. The mixture was gel-filtered on Biogel A 0.5M. ——————— patient monoclonal IgM. －－－－－ control monoclonal IgM.

study of the binding of radiolabelled factor Xa to platelets, as described by Miletich et al.,[7] is consistent with this conclusion. Whereas patient IgM completely blocked binding of factor X to phospholipid micelles, it had no effect on the binding of factor Xa to platelets (TABLE 3). Taken together, these studies indicate the platelets are capable of supporting activation of the coagulation cascade, probably accounting for the lack of bleeding in this patient despite presence of a potent lupus anticoagulant.

Since studying this patient, we have examined several dozen plasmas from normal individuals and from patients with SLE *without* lupus anticoagulants.

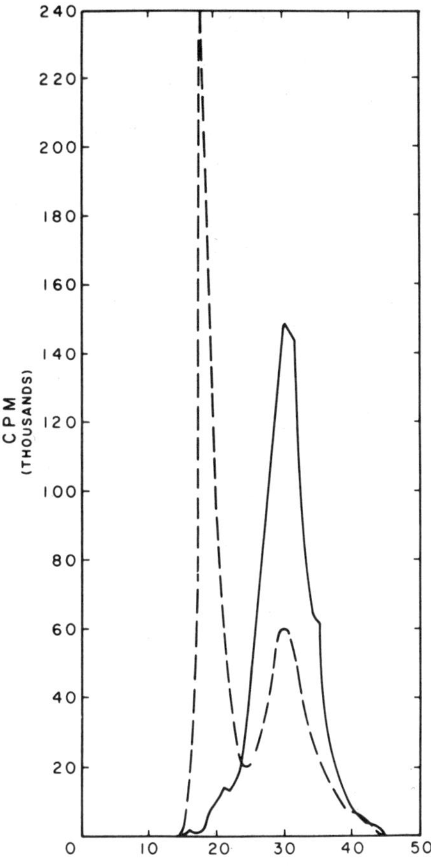

FIGURE 5. Effect of IgM on the Ca⁺⁺-dependent binding of factor X to phospholipid micelles. The conditions were the same as in FIGURE 4, except that factor X was substituted for prothrombin. —— patient monoclonal IgM; – – – control monoclonal IgM.

In no case have we been able to detect antibodies to anionic phospholipids, although several plasmas from SLE patients with false-positive serologies contained antibodies to cardiolipin. In two SLE patients *with* lupus anticoagulants, immunoglobulin fractions of serum reacted in Ouchterlony double diffusion against negatively-charged phospholipids, but not against phosphatidylethanolamine or phosphatidylcholine. Selected coagulation test results in these

TABLE 2

CORRECTION OF PATIENT PLASMA ABNORMALITIES IN THE PRESENCE OF PLATELETS

	Phospholipid	Patient platelets *
Partial thromboplastin time (sec)	85.3	44.2
Russell's viper venom time (sec)	12.8	6.8

* Washed platelets added in volume of 0.1 ml containing 200,000 platelets/μl.

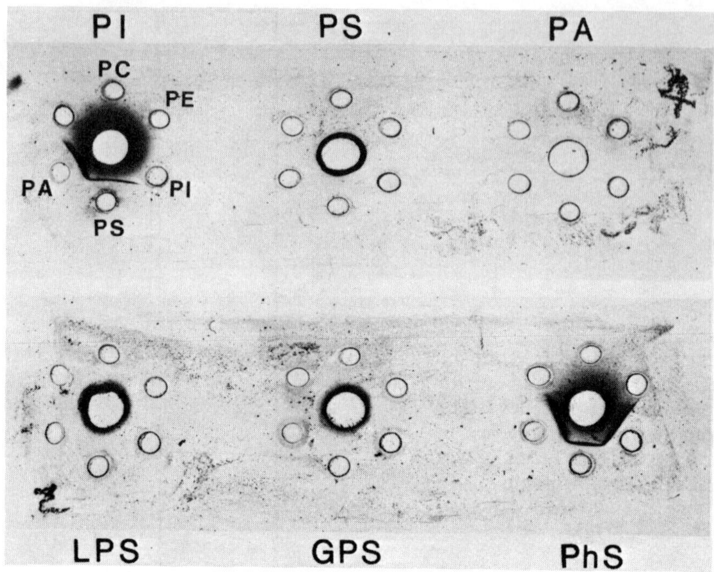

FIGURE 6. Immunodiffusion of patient monoclonal IgM against phospholipids. Peripheral wells were all filled as indicated in pattern at upper left. Center wells contain mixtures of patient IgM and the purified compound indicated.

TABLE 3

BINDING OF ^{125}I-FACTOR XA TO PLATELETS *

Test material	Saturable Binding of Factor Xa (cpm/10^8 platelets)
Buffer	1300
Normal IgM (1 mg/ml)	1150
Patient IgM (1 mg/ml)	1100

* Binding study performed as described by Miletich *et al.*[7]

TABLE 4

PROPERTIES OF LUPUS ANTICOAGULANTS IN TWO PATIENTS WITH SLE

	Phospholipid Specificity	Russell's Viper Venom Time	
		With Phospholipid	With Platelets
SLE No. 1	PI, PS	31.8	24.4
SLE No. 2	PI, PS, PA	30.8	19.9
Normal	—	19.9	20.4

two patients are shown in TABLE 4. Phospholipid-dependent tests were prolonged; these same tests were normalized when performed with washed platelets substituted for phospholipids. Thus it appears likely that the mechanism studied in detail in our macroglobulinemic patient is generally applicable to patients with lupus anticoagulants.

These studies demonstrate that the lupus anticoagulant is in the nature of a laboratory artifact. However, the very nature of this artifact and its disappearance when platelets are substituted for phospholipid, suggests strongly that the major pathway for physiologic activation of the coagulation system is intimately associated with the platelet surface and not with phospholipid micelles. The inability of macroglobulinemic antibody to inhibit factor Xa binding to platelet surfaces is difficult to explain, but suggests that the phospholipid micelle model may not apply exactly to the *in vivo* situation at the platelet surface. Data concerning the presence of anionic phospholipids on the platelet surface, before or after exposure to platelet aggregating agents, are conflicting.[8-11] However, it can be calculated that methods utilized to measure these anionic phospholipids, since they ultimately depend upon detection in thin-layer chromatography, are too insensitive to detect the small numbers of anionic phospholipids that might be associated with each of the 200–300 factor Xa binding sites present on the platelet surface. In addition, large antibody molecules might be sterically hindered from approaching phospholipids closely enough to bind to them. Nevertheless, the use of immunologic probes to study the phospholipid structure of the platelet surface seems promising enough to warrant further investigation, particularly if combined with sensitive chemical probes. Studies along these lines have been initiated in our laboratory.

REFERENCES

1. CONLEY, C. L. & R. C. HARTMANN. 1952. J. Clin. Invest. **31:** 621–622.
2. FEINSTEIN, D. I. & S. I. RAPAPORT. 1972. Prog. Hemostasis Thromb. **1:** 75–95.
3. SCHLEIDER, M. A., R. L. NACHMAN, E. A. JAFFE & M. COLEMAN. 1976. Blood **48:** 499–509.
4. THIAGARAJAN, P., S. S. SHAPIRO & L. DE MARCO. 1980. J. Clin. Invest. **66:** In press.
5. PLAUT, A. G. & T. B. TOMASI, JR. 1970. Proc. Natl. Acad. Sci. USA **65:** 318–322.
6. GITEL, S. N., W. G. OWEN, C. T. ESMON & C. M. JACKSON. 1973. Proc. Natl. Acad. Sci. USA **70:** 1344–1348.
7. MILETICH, J. P., C. M. JACKSON & P. W. MAJERUS. 1978. J. Biol. Chem. **253:** 6908–6916.
8. SCHICK, P. K., K. B. KURICA & G. K. CHACKO. 1976. J. Clin. Invest. **57:** 1221–1226.
9. OTNAESS, A. B. & T. HOLM. 1976. J. Clin. Invest. **57:** 1419–1425.
10. CHAP, H. J., R. F. A. ZWAAL & L. L. M. VAN DEENEN. 1977. Biochem. Biophys. Acta **467:** 146–164.
11. BEVERS, E. M., P. C. COMFURIUS & R. F. A. ZWAAL. 1979. Thromb. Hemost. **42:** 211.

CALCIUM ION–PROTEIN INTERACTIONS IN PROTHROMBIN ACTIVATION

George M. Brenckle, Thomas L. Carlisle, and
Craig M. Jackson

Department of Biological Chemistry
Washington University School of Medicine
St. Louis, Missouri 63110

INTRODUCTION

The activation of prothrombin to thrombin by factor Xa is accelerated in the presence of calcium ions and negatively charged phospholipid. This process involves calcium mediated interaction of prothrombin and factor Xa with the lipid surface and requires the vitamin K dependent carboxylation of 10–14 glutamic acid residues in the 40 amino terminal residues of these proteins. The calcium binding behavior of prothrombin and other vitamin K dependent coagulation proteins is of central importance for understanding the molecular interactions involved in coagulation. An in-depth study of calcium binding to prothrombin and to prothrombin fragment 1 has been undertaken in our laboratory in an attempt to clarify the divergent, although reproducible results reported in the literature,[1-13] and to determine what additional processes might contribute to the apparent cooperative ion binding behavior observed in most laboratories. There is considerable variation in the literature both with regard to the total number of binding sites, (4 to 14), and to the actual shape of the binding curve. Whereas the binding isotherm for the interaction of a negatively charged protein with calcium ions would be expected to exhibit decreased ion affinity upon binding because of decreased electrostatic attraction,[14] pro-thrombin and prothrombin fragment 1 usually exhibit positive cooperativity, indicating that another process must be coupled to the actual binding process.[15, 16]

To explain the cooperative binding behavior, a conformation change which occurs upon the initial binding of divalent ions has been proposed.[5, 13, 17, 18] It is suggested that this conformation change can induce perturbations in the spectral behavior observable by fluorescence,[5, 13, 19, 20] circular dichroism,[21-23] and ultraviolet difference spectroscopy,[24, 25] and is necessary for binding to negatively charged phospholipid vesicles and for accelerating the rate of pro-thrombin activation.[5, 13, 17] While conformation changes undoubtedly occur, it has not been demonstrated that they are responsible either for the observed calcium binding behavior or for the divalent ion induced spectral shifts. In fact, this simple model is difficult to reconcile with the occurrence of both positive and negative cooperativity and with the fact that manganese, which induces the spectral shifts attributed to the divalent ion-induced conformation change, neither induces binding to negatively charged phospholipid nor increases the rate of prothrombin activation.[26] In an attempt to construct a model that is consistent with all reproducible observations, we have tried to determine what process is coupled to calcium ion binding and is responsible for the observed

366

0077-8923/81/0370-0366 $01.75/0 © 1981, NYAS

cooperative behavior, and to elucidate the relationship between the divalent ion induced spectral perturbations and the cooperative ion binding process.

The possible mechanisms that can be responsible for the observed cooperative behavior can be grouped in two classes: intramolecular processes such as a simple conformation change, and intermolecular processes, an example of which is ligand-mediated self association.[15, 27–30] Obviously, the actual cooperative behavior may also result from a combination of both an intra- and an inter-molecular process. Sedimentation and fluorescence polarization studies have established that divalent ion induced dimerization of prothrombin and prothrombin fragment 1 occurs and therefore must influence divalent ion binding behavior.[5, 26] We have investigated the magnitude and direction of the influence of this coupled process by examining the protein concentration dependence of calcium binding to fragment 1 closely.[15, 16] We have also examined the effects of temperature, pH, and ionic strength on calcium binding. A number of different techniques were used including direct mass measurements and various spectral techniques.

Concentration Dependence of Calcium Binding to Fragment 1

The protein concentration dependence of calcium binding was measured using the Hummel-Dreyer column chromatography technique.[31] Columns (0.6 by 60 cm) were packed with Sephadex G-25 and equilibrated with a sodium chloride-Tris buffer containing ⁴⁵Ca-labeled calcium chloride of the desired concentration. Samples of ³H-labeled fragment 1 at various concentrations were injected and 80 fractions were collected in 1/2 dram collection vials. In order to correct for variation in fraction size, the collection vials were weighed before and after sample collection, and placed directly into scintillation vials for counting. A typical elution profile is shown in FIGURE 1. With this technique it was possible to collect data faster and with more precision than with equilibrium dialysis. It was possible to collect binding data at protein concentrations as low as 5 μM ($\simeq 0.1$ mg/ml).

As can be seen in FIGURE 1A, the trough in the calcium elution profile is not symmetrical. This asymmetry has been predicted by Cann and Hinman for ligand-mediated associating systems.[32] As the protein moves down the column, it is removing ligand from the buffer which gives rise to the trough. However, the protein is also being diluted as the band moves down the column. If tight binding is dependent upon high protein concentration, calcium will be released as the protein is diluted leading to an asymmetrical trough.

The binding experiments were conducted in sets using the same calcium-containing elution buffer and injecting fragment 1 samples of varying concentration. The type of concentration dependence observed varied at different calcium concentrations. At low (<200 μM calcium) and very high (>2–3 mM) calcium concentrations, increased protein concentration resulted in decreased binding. At intermediate concentrations ($\simeq 200$ μM to 1 mM) increased protein concentration resulted in increased binding. This variation in behavior indicates that the calcium-mediated dimerization is coupled to the calcium binding in a rather complex manner, both enhancing and inhibiting binding depending upon the variation of other factors. Binding isotherms obtained at different protein concentrations are shown in FIGURE 2. As can be seen, the sigmoidal shape is decreased as the concentration is lowered. These data demonstrate that the

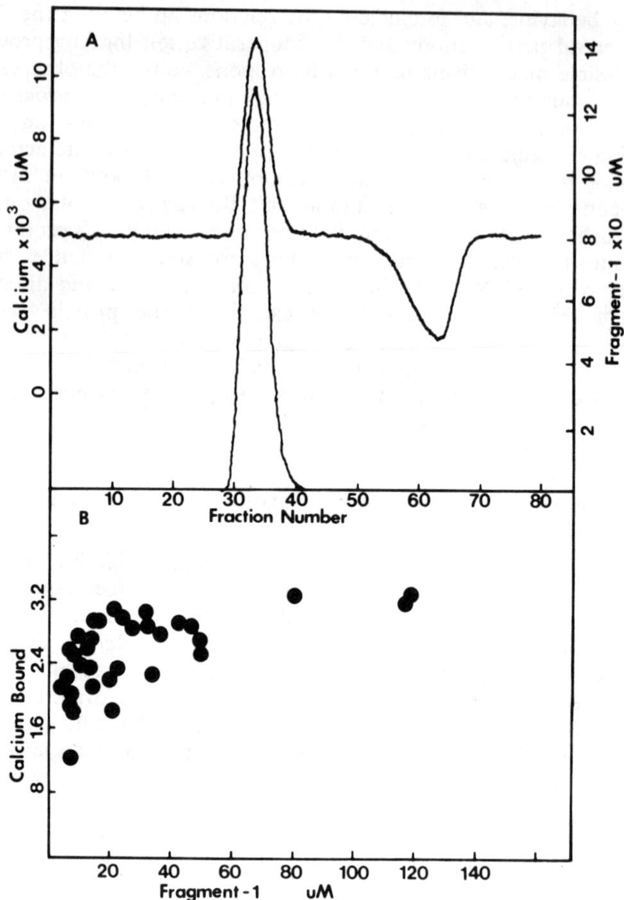

FIGURE 1. (A) Hummel-Dreyer column elution profile for the binding of calcium to bovine prothrombin fragment 1. Sephadex G-25 columns (0.6×60 cm) were equilibrated in buffer, 0.1 M NaCl, 0.01 M Tris-HCl, 0.02% NaN₃, pH=7.5, and calcium chloride of the desired concentration. A sample of Fragment 1 was applied to the column and 80 fractions ($\simeq$0.2 ml) were collected. Binding ratios were calculated for the peak fractions. (B) Calcium binding to Fragment 1 as a function of protein concentration in 0.1 M NaCl, 0.01 M Tris-HCl, 0.02% NaN₃, 225 μM CaCl₂, pH = 7.5. The results of several Hummel-Dreyer column experiments run using the same elution buffer while varying the concentration of fragment 1 injected are shown.

apparent positive cooperativity observed at protein concentrations above 10 μM ($\simeq$0.2 mg/ml) is due to calcium-mediated association of fragment 1.

EFFECT OF TEMPERATURE, pH, AND IONIC STRENGTH

The ionic strength dependence of calcium binding to fragment 1 was found to be extremely large. At low calcium concentrations, less than 300 μM, the binding increased from less than 0.5 gram-atoms of calcium bound per mole of protein at high (0.5–1.0) ionic strength to almost seven gram-atoms per mole as the ionic strength approached zero. At higher calcium concentrations, the change in ionic strength has less effect, since the net negative charge on the protein has decreased considerably because of charge neutralization by bound calcium ions. All the data have been corrected for the Donnan effect, which was found to be negligible. The large ionic strength dependence indicates quite clearly that the binding interaction is mainly electrostatic in nature.

The temperature dependence was found to be extremely small in the range from 4° to 40° C. The direction of change in binding indicates that the enthalpy change is negative as expected for an interaction that is mainly electrostatic. The pH dependence was also found to be small, in contrast to data reported in the literature.[3, 6] However, in previously reported experiments changes in pH were accompanied by rather large shifts in ionic strength. Because of the large effects of ionic strength on the calcium binding behavior, the actual magnitude of pH-induced effects is not clear.

CALCIUM-INDUCED ULTRAVIOLET DIFFERENCE SPECTRAL
TITRATION DATA

Although the binding experiments clearly establish that the calcium-induced dimerization of fragment 1 is responsible for the cooperative binding behavior,

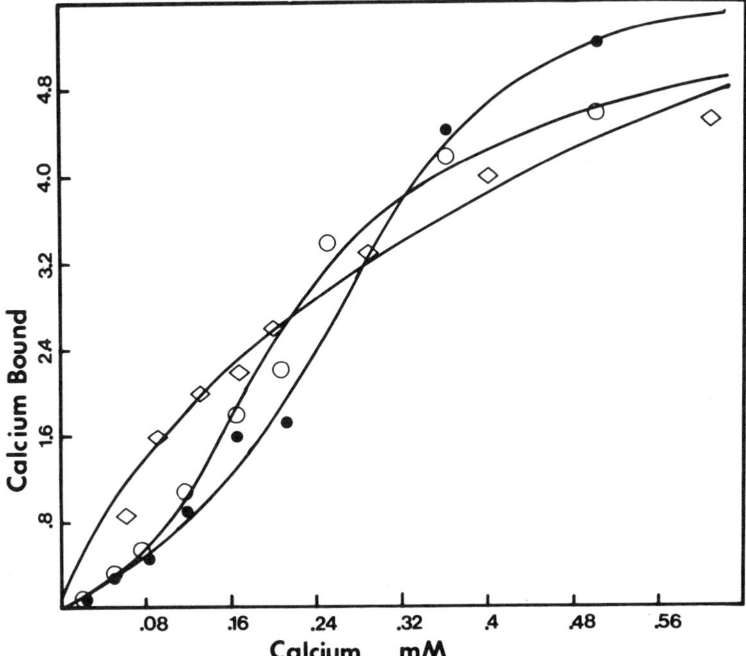

FIGURE 2. Calcium binding isotherms for prothrombin fragment 1 at three different concentrations. The curves were obtained by interpolation of experimental data similar to that in FIGURE 1B. As the protein concentration is lowered, the cooperativity apparent at higher concentrations disappears. ● 100 μM Fragment 1; ○ 10 μM Fragment 1; ◇ 5 μM Fragment 1.

they do not rule out the existence of a required conformation change. Calcium binding has therefore been examined by various spectroscopic techniques in order to investigate the relationship between the calcium-induced spectral changes and the cooperative binding process. Calcium binding induces perturbations in the absorption and emission spectra,[5, 13, 19, 20, 24, 25] which have been attributed to alteration of the environment of tryptophan, with small ($\simeq$6%) contributions from tyrosine.[24] A calcium-induced difference spectrum is shown in FIGURE 3. Using ultraviolet difference spectroscopy or fluorescence, it is possible to follow the perturbations in the tryptophan spectra as a function of calcium concentration.

The use of a spectral technique, such as fluorescence quenching or ultraviolet difference spectroscopy to study protein–ligand interaction has two major limitations. First, the spectral perturbation is measured as a function of total, rather than free, ligand. Although this limitation is not a problem in the limit of low acceptor concentration where the difference between the free and the total ligand concentration is negligible, it is impossible to compare data collected at different protein concentrations. However, since calcium binding data for fragment 1 are available, this limitation has been eliminated. The spectral titration curves may then be examined as a function of protein concentration in

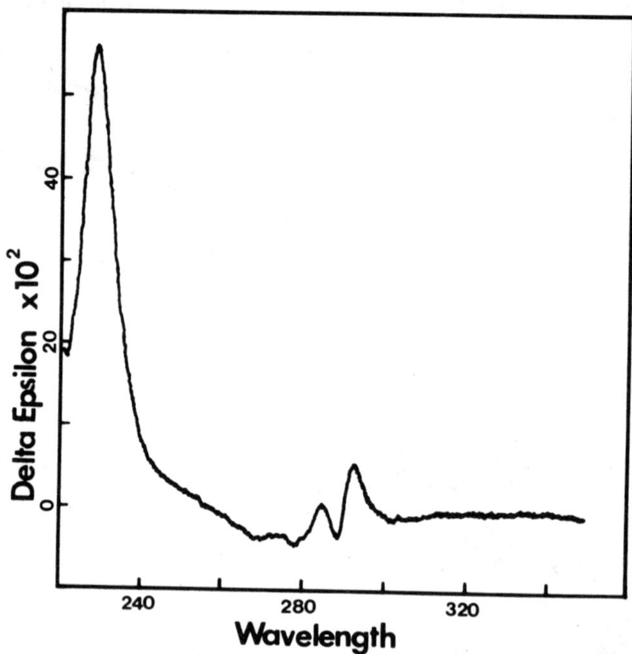

FIGURE 3. Ultraviolet difference spectra of prothrombin fragment 1 in the presence and absence of calcium. Absorption spectra for fragment 1 in the presence and absence of calcium were obtained on a Cary 219 spectrophotometer (Varian) and transferred directly to a PDP 11/34 computer (Digital Equipment Corp.). The subtraction of the spectra, fragment 1 with calcium minus fragment 1 alone, was done using the computer.

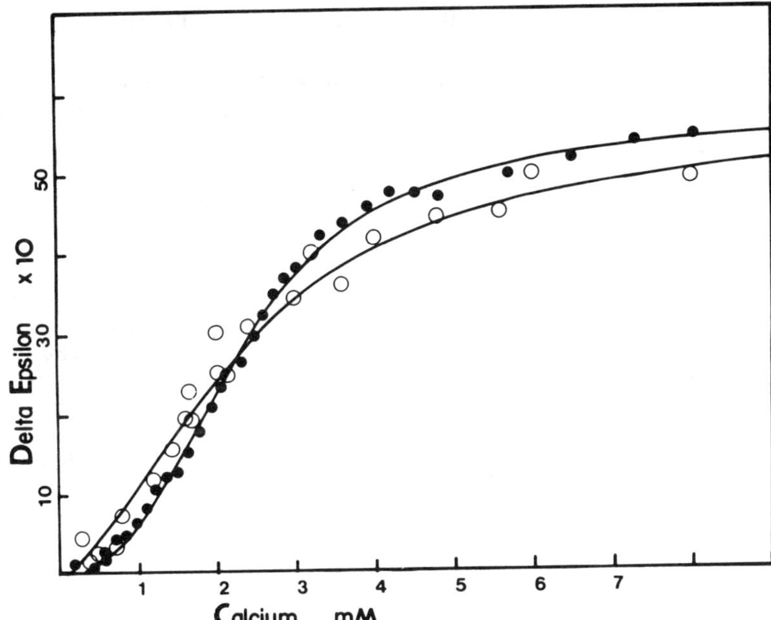

FIGURE 4. Ultraviolet difference spectral titration curves of fragment 1 at 0.89 mg/ml (●), and 0.03 mg/ml (○). Delta epsilon represents the change in the molar absorptivity at 292 nm. Data were collected as outlined in FIGURE 3.

order to determine whether the calcium-induced dimerization which clearly alters calcium binding also alters the spectral behavior. Second, in a multisite system, it is not known whether the occupation of each binding site contributes equally to the total spectral shift. It may be that some sites do not contribute at all.[33] Using the calcium binding data, it was found that only three or four of the binding sites contribute to the spectral response.

The maximum spectral response was found to be independent of protein concentration, indicating that the same final state is reached at all protein concentrations. However, the calcium concentration at which the half maximal spectral response is obtained does vary with protein concentration (FIGURE 4), decreasing from 0.28 mM at 2 mg/ml fragment 1 to 0.14–0.16 mM at 0.02–0.03 mg/ml. Using the calcium binding data, it is possible to examine the spectral perturbation as a function of average site occupancy. The average number of sites that must be filled for maximum spectral response decreases from 7 to 3 as the protein concentration is lowered, indicating that the degree of spectral response is different for different sites and that the order in which the sites are filled is a function of protein concentration. The sigmoidicity in the spectral titration curves also decreases at lower protein concentration (FIGURE 4). It is clear from these results that the spectral response to calcium binding also reflects the effects of calcium-mediated dimerization observed directly in the Hummel-Dreyer column experiments.

The Nature of the Calcium-induced Spectral Perturbations

As presented above, the fluorescence and difference spectral perturbations are due mainly to perturbation of tryptophan. From comparison with ion- and solvent-induced perturbations of model indole compounds, the divalent-ion-induced difference spectrum of fragment 1 appears to be due to alteration of the electrostatic environment in the vicinity of the tryptophan indole ring(s).[34, 35] This interpretation is supported by the fact that high concentrations of monovalent ions induce difference spectra that are very similar to the divalent ion induced spectra,[24] indicating that the spectral behavior may be due to general ionic strength effects rather than a specific divalent ion induced protein transition. The ion-induced perturbations have also been monitored by fluorescence quenching. At 1.25 M NaCl the fluorescence is quenched by about 10% and at 4.5 M LiCl the quenching reaches 20–30%. Calcium at 10 mM induces 35–40% quenching. Fragment 1 has three tryptophan residues (residues 42, 90, and 126) and it is unclear whether all three or only a single tryptophan is being perturbed by calcium binding. Chymotrypsin has been shown to cleave bonds 45–46 (tyrosyl-serine) and 42–43 (tryptophanyl-alanine) in fragment 1 leaving residues 46–156 (F1(-GD)) and 1–42 (fragment 1 Gla domain).[23, 36] The spectral behavior of these peptides in the presence of monovalent ions (Na and Li) and Mg has been examined. Calcium has not been used as this causes the Gla domain peptide to precipitate. Both peptides are perturbed upon addition of monovalent or divalent ions, indicating that the spectral response in intact fragment 1 is most likely due to the perturbation of more than one tryptophan.

Nature of the Circular Dichroism (CD) Spectral Response to Calcium Ions and Other Perturbants

The far ultraviolet circular dichroism spectra of prothrombin and prothrombin fragment 1 have been investigated in a number of laboratories as this technique provides an opportunity for measurement of gross changes in secondary structure.[21-23, 37, 38] The binding of calcium, magnesium, or manganese ions to fragment 1 has been shown to cause small changes in its far ultraviolet CD spectrum;[21, 23, 37] this observation has been interpreted as support for the hypothesis that changes in the fluorescence and absorption spectra in the near ultraviolet reflect a conformational change during divalent metal ion binding.[21] This change has been estimated to correspond to an increase of 6–10% in the helix and 6% in the beta sheet content of fragment 1.[21, 38] In addition to peptide backbone chromophores, however, nonpeptide chromophores such as aromatic side chains, disulfides, and oligosaccharide also can contribute to CD in the far ultraviolet.[39, 40] Indeed, curve-fitting procedures reveal relatively poor correspondence of the fragment 1 spectrum to the several sets of model spectra for helix, beta sheet, and nonrepetitive structure used to obtain estimates of secondary structure.[41-43] Such a result would be expected if nonpeptide contributions to the far ultraviolet CD spectrum were significant. Similar changes in the far ultraviolet CD spectra are observed when the NaCl concentration is raised from 0.1 to 1 M, demonstrating that, like the fluorescence and absorption spectral changes, this phenomenon is not specific for divalent metal ions alone. Decreasing the pH from 7.5 to 5 or below has similar effects on the far ultraviolet CD spectrum,[23, 37, 38] with the exception that larger changes near 230 nm are observed than in the case of calcium.

The quite strong near ultraviolet CD signal of fragment 1 near 280–290 nm resembles that of tryptophan and is decreased in intensity by the addition of calcium.[21, 23, 37] F1(-GD), residues 46–156, was found to retain a large part of the tryptophan-like CD signal of fragment 1,[23] suggesting that tryptophans 90 and/or 126 contribute much of the near ultraviolet CD spectrum of fragment 1. F1(-GD) also contributes an intense positive peak at 230 nm, corresponding to the positive shoulder seen near this wavelength in intact fragment 1.[23] In both F1(-GD) and in intact fragment 1, the tryptophan signal near 280 nm and the peak near 230 nm are greatly diminished at low pH. The parallel disappearance of these two signals, together with the comparable changes at 230 and 280–290 nm in the calcium-induced ultraviolet difference spectrum (FIGURE 3), suggest that the 230 nm CD peak is largely due to tryptophan indole contributions. This is also consistent with the known CD of tryptophan derivatives.[39, 40]

The pH-induced CD difference spectrum of F1(-GD) (neutral minus low pH) was used as a first approximation to such side-chain contributions to the CD spectrum of fragment 1. In order to examine its effect on the estimates of secondary structure obtained by curve-fitting to sets of model spectra, it was included as a fourth reference spectrum in the sets of Greenfield and Fasman[41] and of Chen, Yang, and Chau.[42] The resulting unconstrained least squares best fits were markedly closer to the fragment 1 spectrum, and in addition gave total amounts of peptide which were physically more reasonable (near 100%). This is especially true of the polylysine-based reference spectra of Greenfield and Fasman, which contain no aromatic side chain contribution at all (FIGURE 5). The resulting estimates of secondary structure (comparing unconstrained fits to the Chen, Yang, and Chau spectra with or without the "side chain" estimate) change from 11% to 24% for helix, from 40% to 4% for beta sheet, and from 98% to 78% for nonrepetitive structure. The sum of these fractions changes from 150% to the more reasonable value of 107%. The unconstrained fit of the CD spectrum of fragment 1 in 10 mM Ca²⁺ to this augmented set of spectra gives a slight (3%) increase in helix and larger increases in beta sheet and nonrepetitive structure, but the fit still overestimates the amount of peptide present by 40%. It thus appears that fragment 1 may contain more helix and less beta sheet than previously estimated. Much of the calcium-induced change in the CD spectrum near 230 nm appears to be due to non-peptide backbone chromophores. The changes below 220 nm probably do in fact reflect increases in ordered secondary structure due to calcium binding, but some features of this spectrum are still poorly matched by the model reference spectra. Estimates of the extent of change involved must therefore remain tentative.

SUMMARY

1. The protein concentration dependence observed in the calcium binding to fragment 1 indicates that calcium-mediated dimerization is responsible for the cooperative calcium binding behavior usually observed. "Unusual" fragment 1, which exhibits negative cooperativity (the type of binding behavior

expected for ions interacting with a charged protein) at high concentration, also exhibits altered self-association behavior.

2. The calcium-induced spectral perturbations that are observed by fluorescence and ultraviolet difference spectroscopy are influenced by calcium-mediated dimerization. Similar spectral perturbations may also be induced by other divalent, trivalent, and monovalent ions, as well as changes in pH. Because this is a multi-site system, only limited interpretation of the spectral data is possible without calcium binding data.

3. Although strong side chain CD signals make estimation of fragment 1 secondary structure ambiguous, the CD data do indicate small changes in

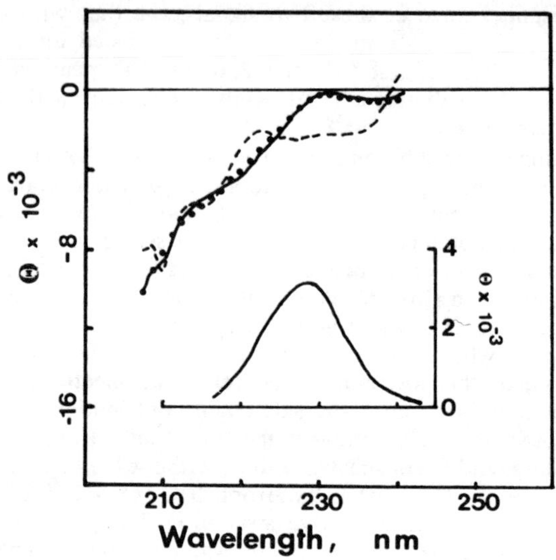

FIGURE 5. Best fits of the far ultraviolet circular dichroism spectrum of bovine prothrombin fragment 1 to secondary structure reference spectra. The points represent the average of a number of spectra of bovine prothrombin fragment 1 in 0.1 M NaCl, 0.01 M Tris, pH 7.5. Mean residue ellipticity (deg cm²/dmol) is presented on the ordinate. The broken line represents the best fit by unconstrained least squares of the three reference spectra for helix, beta sheet, and nonregular secondary structure of Greenfield and Fasman.[60] The unbroken line shows the effect on this fit of including the pH-induced circular dichroism difference spectrum of fragment 1 residues 46–156 (shown in the inset) as a fourth "reference" spectrum.

structure during calcium binding. Similar changes are observed upon addition of monovalent ions at high concentration or after lowering the pH. No coupling between changes in conformation and the cooperative calcium binding behavior has yet been observed to exist.

REFERENCES

1. NELSESTUEN, G. L., M. BRODERIUS, T. H. ZYTKOVICZ & J. B. HOWARD. 1976. On the role of gamma-carboxyglutamic acid in calcium and phospholipid binding. Biochem. Biophys. Res. Commun. **65:** 233–240.

2. BENSON, B. J. & D. J. HANAHAN. 1975. Structural studies on bovine prothrombin. Isolation and partial characterization of the Ca2+ binding and carbohydrate containing peptides of the N-terminus region. Biochemistry **14:** 3265–3277.

3. NELSESTUEN, G. L. & J. W. SUTTIE. 1972. Mode of action of vitamin K. Calcium binding properties of bovine prothrombin. Biochemistry **11:** 4961–4964.

4. HENRIKSEN, R. A. & C. M. JACKSON. 1975. Cooperative calcium binding by the phospholipid binding region of bovine prothrombin: A requirement for intact disulfide bridges. Arch. Biochem. Biophys. **170:** 149–159.

5. PRENDERGAST, F. G. & K. G. MANN. 1977. Differentiation of metal ion-induced transitions of Prothrombin Fragment 1. J. Biol. Chem. **252:** 840–850.

6. BENAROUS, R., J. ELION & D. LABIE. 1976. Ca⁺⁺ binding properties of human prothrombin. Biochemie **58:** 391–394.

7. BAJAJ, S. P., R. J. BUTKOWSKI & K. G. MANN. 1975. Prothrombin fragments. Ca2⁺ binding and activation kinetics. J. Biol. Chem. **250:** 2150–2156.

8. BENSON, B. J., W. KISIEL & D. J. HANAHAN. 1973. Calcium binding and other characteristics of bovine Factor II and its activation intermediates. Biochim. Biophys. Acta **329:** 81–87.

9. STENFLO, J. & P. O. GANROT. 1973. Binding of Ca2⁺ to normal and Dicoumarol-induced prothrombin. Biochem. Biophys. Res. Commun. **50:** 98–104.

10. FURIE, B. C., K. G. MANN & B. FURIE. 1976. Substitution of lanthanide ions for calcium ions in the activation of bovine prothrombin by activated Factor X. High affinity metal-binding sites of prothrombin and the derivatives of prothrombin activation. J. Biol. Chem. **251:** 3235–3241.

11. BAJAJ, S. P., T. NOWAK & F. J. CASTELLINO. 1976. Interaction of manganese with bovine prothrombin and its thrombin-mediated cleavage products. J. Biol. Chem. **251:** 6294–6298.

12. NELSESTUEN, G. L. 1975. Prothrombin's calcium ion binding site. Carbon-13 nuclear magnetic resonance studies. Thromb. Res. **7:** 871–877.

13. NELSESTUEN, G. L. 1976. Role of gamma-carboxyglutamic acid. An unusual protein transition required for the calcium-dependent binding of prothrombin to phospholipid. J. Biol. Chem. **251:** 5648–5656.

14. TANFORD C. 1961. Physical Chemistry of Macromolecules. pp. 457–586. John Wiley and Sons, New York.

15. JACKSON, C. M. & G. M. BRENCKLE. 1980. Divalent ion binding to bovine Prothrombin Fragment-1 and its consequences. *In* The Regulation of Coagulation. Developments in Biochemistry. K. G. Mann & F. B. Taylor, Eds. Vol. **8:** 11–19. Elsevier North Holland. New York.

16. JACKSON, C. M. 1980. Cooperativity of calcium ion binding to bovine prothrombin, Prothrombin Fragment 1 and Factor X. An alternative to conformational changes for explaining such behavior in Vitamin K Metabolism and Vitamin K Dependent Proteins. J. W. Suttie, Ed. pp. 54–57. University Park Press. Baltimore, MD.

17. PRENDERGAST, F. G., J. BLOOM, M. R. DOWNING & K. G. MANN. 1979. Correlation of metal ion-induced fluorescence transitions with conformational changes in Prothrombin Fragment 1. *In* Vitamin K Metabolism and Vitamin K Dependent Proteins. J. W. Suttie, Ed. pp. 39–48. University Park Press. Baltimore, MD.

18. MANN, K. G., F. K. PRENDERGAST & J. W. BLOOM. 1980. The metal ion and phospholipid interactions of the vitamin-K dependent factors. *In* The Regulation of Coagulation. Developments in Biochemistry. K. G. Mann & F. B. Taylor, Jr., Eds. Vol. **8:** 3–10. Elsevier North-Holland, New York.

19. SCOTT, M. E., K. A. KOEHLER & R. G. HISKEY. 1979. The effects of calcium

ions and pH on bovine Prothrombin Fragment 1. Intrinsic fluorescence studies. Biochem. J. **177:** 879–886.

20. NELSESTUEN, G. L., M. BRODERIUS & G. MARTIN. 1976. Role of gamma-carboxyglutamic acid. Cation specificity of prothrombin and Factor X phospholipid binding. J. Biol. Chem. **251:** 6886–6893.

21. BLOOM, J. W. & K. G. MANN. 1978. Metal ion induced conformational transitions of prothrombin and Prothrombin Fragment 1. Biochemistry **17:** 4430–4438.

22. BJORK, I. & J. STENFLO. 1973. A conformational study of normal and dicoumarol-induced prothrombin. FEBS Lett. **32:** 343–346.

23. CARLISLE, T. L., T. MORITA & C. M. JACKSON. 1980. Gla-region secondary structure in prothrombin and Factor X. *In* Vitamin K Metabolism and Vitamin K Dependent Proteins, J. W. Suttie, Ed., pp. 58–61. University Park Press. Baltimore, MD.

24. BRENCKLE, G. M., C. W. PENG & C. M. JACKSON. 1979. Calcium binding to Prothrombin Fragment-1 by ultraviolet difference spectroscopy. *In* Vitamin K Metabolism and Vitamin K Dependent Proteins. J. W. Suttie, Ed. pp. 16–27. University Park Press. Baltimore, MD.

25. BENAROUS, R., G. GACON, M. J. RABIET & D. LABIE. 1979. Calcium induced conformational change in human prothrombin. *In* Vitamin K Metabolism and Vitamin K Dependent Proteins. J. W. Suttie, Ed. pp. 49–53. University Park Press. Baltimore, MD.

26. JACKSON, C. M., C. W. PENG, G. M. BRENCKLE, A. JONAS & J. STENFLO. 1979. Multiple modes of association in bovine prothrombin and its proteolysis products. J. Biol. Chem. **254:** 5020–5026.

27. NICHOL, L. W. & D. J. WINZOR. 1976. Ligand induced self association. Biochemistry **15:** 3015–3019.

28. LEVITSKI, A. & J. SCHLESSINGER. 1974. Cooperativity in associating proteins. Monomer-dimer equilibrium coupled to ligand binding. Biochemistry **13:** 5214–5218.

29. NICHOL, L. W. 1980. The interplay between ligand binding and protein acceptor association. *In* The Regulation of Coagulation. Developments in Biochem. K. G. Mann & F. B. Taylor, Jr., Eds. Vol. **8:** 43–66. Elsevier North-Holland. New York.

30. CANN, J. R. 1978. Ligand-binding by associating systems. Methods Enzymol. **48:** 299–307.

31. HUMMEL, J. P. & W. J. DREYER. 1962. Measurement of protein-binding phenomena by gel-filtration. Biochim. Biophys. Acta **63:** 530–532.

32. CANN, J. R. & N. D. HINMAN. 1976. Hummel Dreyer gel chromatographic procedure as applied to ligand mediated association. Biochem. **15:** 4614–4622.

33. DERANLEAU, D. A. 1969. Theory of the measurement of weak molecular complexes II consequences of multiple equilibria. J. Am. Chem. Soc. **91:** 4050–4054.

34. STRICKLAND, E. H., C. BILLUPS & E. KAY. 1972. Effects of hydrogen bonding and solvents upon the tryptophanyl 1La absorption band. Studies using 2,3-dimethylindole. Biochemistry **11:** 3657–3662.

35. ANDREWS, L. J. & L. S. FORSTER. 1972. Protein difference spectra. Effect of solvent and charge on tryptophan. Biochemistry **11:** 1857–1879.

36. MORITA, T. & C. M. JACKSON. 1980. Structural and functional characteristics of a proteolytically modified "gla domain-less" bovine Factor X and Xa (des light chain residues 1–44). *In* Vitamin K Metabolism and Vitamin K Dependent Proteins, J. W. Suttie, Ed. pp. 124–128. University Park Press, Baltimore, MD.

37. GABRIEL, D. A., D. J. SCHAEFER, H. R. ROBERTS, D. L. ARONSON & K. A. KOEHLER. 1975. Prothrombin profragment-1 optical rotatory dispersion and circular dichroism. Thromb. Res. **7:** 839–846.

38. MARSH, H. C., P. ROBERTSON, JR., M. E. SCOTT, K. A. KOEHLER, & R. G. HISKEY. 1979. Magnesium and calcium binding to bovine Prothrombin Fragment 1. A circular dichroism, fluorescence, and $^{45}Ca^{2+}$ and $^{25}Mg^{2+}$ nuclear magnetic resonance study. J. Biol. Chem. **254:** 10268–10275.
39. SEARS, D. W. & S. BEYCHOK. 1973. Circular dichroism. *In* Physical Principles and Techniques of Protein Chemistry. S. J. Leach, Ed. Part C: 445–593. Academic Press. New York, N.Y.
40. WOODY, R. W. 1978. Aromatic side-chain contributions to the far ultraviolet circular dichroism of peptides and proteins. Biopolymers **17:** 1451–1467.
41. GREENFIELD, N. & G. D. FASMAN. 1969. Computed circular dichroism spectra for the evaluation of protein conformation. Biochemistry **8:** 4108–4115.
42. CHEN, Y. H., J. T. YANG & K. H. CHAU. 1974. Determination of the helix and beta form of proteins in aqueous solution by circular dichroism. Biochemistry **13:** 3350–3359.
43. CHANG, C. T., C. S. C. WU & J. T. YANG. T. 1978. Circular dichroic analysis of protein conformation: Inclusion of the beta-turns. Anal. Biochem. **91:** 13–31.

THE ROLE OF FACTOR V IN THE ASSEMBLY OF THE PROTHROMBINASE COMPLEX *

Kenneth G. Mann, Michael E. Nesheim,† Lyndon S. Hibbard,†
and Paula B. Tracy †

Hematology Research Section
Mayo Clinic/Foundation
Rochester, Minnesota 55901

INTRODUCTION

In 1943, Owren,[1] observed a patient with a congenital lack of a factor essential in the conversion of prothrombin to thrombin. In subsequent work, Owren,[2] Ware and Seegers,[3] and Murphy and Seegers [4] established that this component, named factor V, was one of the essential components required for the rapid conversion of prothrombin to thrombin. These earlier workers also applied the term "labile factor" in discussions of factor V because of the extreme instability of the protein during manipulation and storage. Because of this instability problem, factor V proved difficult to isolate. The first practical preparations of factor V were provided by Esnouf and Jobin,[5] and Barton and Hanahan,[6] and studies of preparations at this level of purity provided a great deal of insight into the function of factor V in the prothrombinase complex.[7, 8] Numerous additional reports of factor V purification have appeared in the literature;[9-14] however, until recently, no preparations were reported which met the usual criteria associated with homogeneous protein preparations.

Recently, our laboratory,[15] and that of Esmon,[16] have described preparations of factor V for which the usual criteria of homogeneity can be applied, such as a single component when analyzed by gel electrophoresis.

The protein prepared in our laboratory has also been evaluated immunochemically [17] using burro antisera raised against the isolated protein. FIGURE 1 presents an immunodiffusion experiment which compares the antigen present in plasma with purified factor V. By this method of analysis, only a single antigenic species is observed in plasma, and this antigenic species is identical to the isolated protein when evaluated by this technique. In addition, the factor V antigen present in plasma, and in platelets, has been compared using a radioimmunoassay toward bovine factor V established in our laboratory. Using these criteria as well, factor V present in plasma and in platelets is immunochemically indistinguishable from the factor V isolated by the procedure of Nesheim, *et al.*[15]

We have used a variety of physical and chemical techniques to establish the relative homogeneity and gross physical properties of the factor V isolated in our laboratory. These properties are summarized in TABLE 1.

The molecular weight of factor V was determined by the sedimentation

* This research was supported by Grant HL-16150 and HL-17430D and the Mayo Foundation.

† Supported by Blood Banking and Hemostasis Training Program Grant HL-07069.

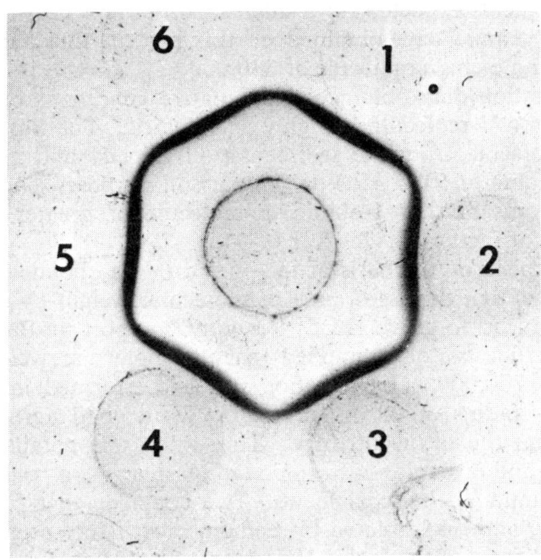

FIGURE 1. Double immunodiffusion in agar analysis of burro anti-bovine factor V antibody. The center well contained the antiserum raised against bovine factor V. Wells 1 to 3 contained purified bovine factor V and wells 4 to 6 contained whole bovine plasma. (From Tracy *et al.*[24] Used with permission.)

equilibrium technique in dilute aqueous solvents which presumably represents native conditions, and in 6 M guanidinium chloride after disulfide bond reduction. In all cases, a molecular weight consistent with a value of 330,000 was obtained, which strongly suggested, as did electrophoresis in sodium dodecylsulfate, that unactivated factor V is a large, single-chain protein with no complex subunit structure. In view of the extraordinarily large single-chain length of this protein (approximately 2700 amino acid residues) we also evaluated the molecular weight by assessing the random coil sedimentation

TABLE 1

GROSS PHYSICAL PROPERTIES OF BOVINE FACTOR V

Molecular weight	330,000
S^0_{20w} (sec^{-1})	9.19
Stokes radius (Å)	91.2
f/fmin	2.01
$\bar{v}$ (cc/gm)	0.712
Axial ratio	25:1
$E^{1\%}_{280}$	9.6
NH$_2$ terminal	ALA

velocity in 6 M guanidinium chloride. Reduced factor V in 6 M guanidinium chloride sedimentated at a rate expected for a random coil containing the number of amino acids expected for a single chain of molecular weight 330,000. Thus, all hydrodynamic data obtained on this protein thus far are consistent with its being a single-chain molecule of 330,000.

The sedimentation data obtained under native conditions of factor V indicate that the factor V molecule is highly asymmetric. The Stokes radius computed for the molecule from the sedimentation velocity and molecular weight data indicate a value of 91.2 Å. For comparison purposes, similar calculation of the Stokes radius of thyroglobulin, a molecule of greater than twice the molecular weight of factor V, is 89 Å.

One would expect, on the basis of the physical data obtained for factor V in the ultracentrifuge, that the assessment of molecular weight by gel filtration for this protein could lead to grave error. Recently, a report by Bartlett et al.[18] on gel filtration of crude factor V implied that the molecular weight of factor V was greater than 700,000. Gel filtration studies performed in our laboratory indicate a Stokes radius of 93 Å for factor V, in good agreement with the physical data from the ultracentrifuge. This value was obtained both on the purified factor V and on factor V in inhibited plasma. As a result of the above, and based upon immunochemical identity, we conclude that factor V isolated in our laboratory, and that isolated by Esmon, most likely represent the undegraded circulating form of the factor V molecule.

Factor V Is a Procofactor

Factor V is typically assayed by its ability to shorten the clot time of factor V-deficient plasma. The factor V obtained by our isolation procedure, when measured in a factor V deficient plasma assay, typically increases in activity approximately 80-fold upon exposure to catalytic amounts of thrombin. The protein isolated by our procedure represents a "pro" cofactor form of factor V. Indeed, the realization of the significance of the procofactor state of plasmatic factor V was key to the development of our isolation procedure. FIGURE 2 represents the alterations in the detergent gel electrophoretic patterns when factor V is subjected to catalytic amounts of thrombin. In the particular experiment presented in FIGURE 2, factor V was treated with thrombin at a molar ratio of about 30:1 (weight ratio, 300:1). The gels depicted in FIGURE 2 correspond to the sample taken before thrombin addition, and at 10, 20, 60 and 180 sec after the addition of thrombin. A variety of components can be seen in this experiment, and by virtue of this, and similar, experiments [19, 20] one can identify seven components which are produced as a consequence of the conversion of the factor V procofactor to the factor Va cofactor.

Two of these components, B and C, with apparent molecular weights 205,000 and 150,000, can be clearly identified as intermediates in the process of conversion to ultimate end products, since they appear, and disappear, as a consequence of the activation process. The increased biological activity in the factor V deficient plasma assay is observed coincident with the cleavage which results in the product (D) of molecular weight 94,000 when analyzed by SDS gel electrophoresis.[19]

A variety of studies are ongoing regarding the mechanism of activation of factor V to factor Va. These studies have included, in addition to gel electrophoresis, isolation of the fragments produced during activation, NH_2-terminal sequence, amino acid composition, and activity reconstitution following dissociation in the presence of chelators. All results obtained thus far are consistent with the model posed in FIGURE 3. In this model, the factor V procofactor single polypeptide chain (A, 330,000) is cleaved by thrombin (IIa) to yield initially two components, but no measurable activity. These components are identified as C (150,000) and B (205,000). Subsequently component C is cleaved leading to the appearance of component D (94,000) concurrent with an increase in activity. In addition, component B is subsequently cleaved with some increase in activity.

Dissociation and reconstitution experiments using EDTA and Ca^{++} to effect factor Va subunit dissociation and reversal, respectively, suggest that complexes

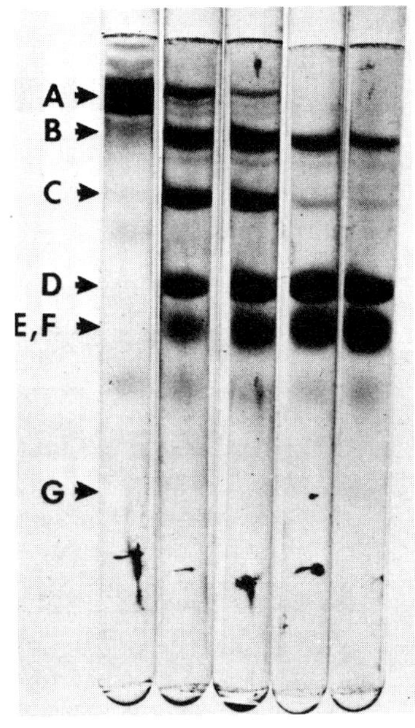

FIGURE 2. $DodSO_4$-5% polyacrylamide gel analysis of the rapid activation of factor V. The gels from left to right are of samples taken at 0,10,20,60 and 180 s., respectively, after the addition of thrombin $(1.9 \times 10^{-8} M)$ to a solution of factor V $(7.0 \times 10^{-7} M)$ at 37°C in 0.02 M imidazole/HCl, 0.15 M NaCl, pH 7.4. Reactions were stopped with the thrombin inhibitor DAPA. The molecular weight of component A was found by sedimentation equilibrium to be 330,000. Apparent molecular weights of the remaining components were deduced from electrophoretic mobilities, and were found to be: B, 205,000; C, 150,000; D, 94,000; E. 74,000; F, 71,000, and G, 31,000. (From Nesheim and Mann.[19] Used with permission.)

composed of components D and B, or components D and E, are sufficient to provide activity in the bioassay. This observation is similar to that reported by Esmon, who was able to isolate two activation peptides that probably correspond to components D and E. When these two peptides are reconstituted in the presence of calcium ion, bioactivity is restored.

The cleavage of factor V by activated protein C has also been studied in our laboratory in collaboration with Dr. Walter Kisiel and coworkers at the University of Washington.[21] These studies indicate that catalytic amounts of activated protein C rapidly inactivate factor Va, and more slowly inactivate factor V. The inactivation process, like the thrombin-catalyzed activation process, is accompanied by discrete proteolysis which can be observed on sodium dodecyl sulfate electrophoresis. While a number of cleavages have been observed as a consequence of activated protein C treatment of factor Va, it is interesting to note that the cleavage of component D can be associated with loss of activity. The inactivation of factor V by activated protein C is Ca^{++} and phospholipid dependent. Furthermore, factor Xa (which binds tightly to factor Va) protects the molecule from inactivation by activated protein C. In contrast, the substrate of the prothrombinase complex, prothrombin, is incapable of protecting factor Va from activated protein C cleavage.

THE INTERACTION OF FACTOR VA WITH OTHER COMPONENTS IN THE PROTHROMBINASE COMPLEX

The prothrombinase complex, which is thought to be responsible for the biologically significant conversion of the zymogen to thrombin, is composed of

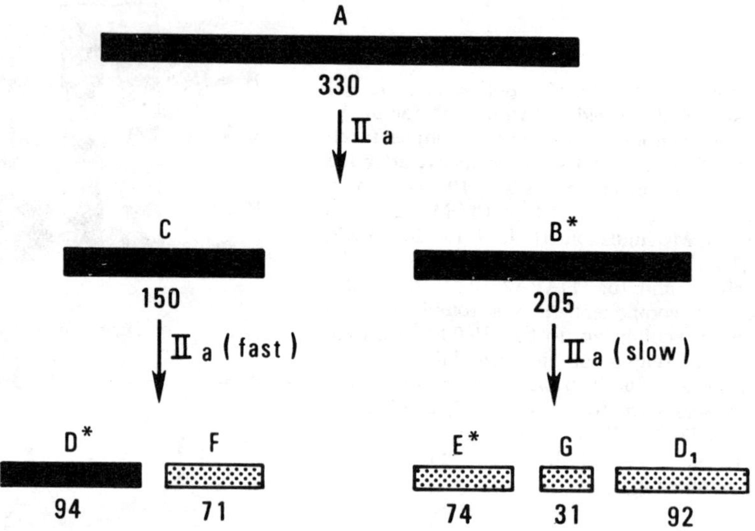

FIGURE 3. Model proposed for the thrombin-catalyzed activation of bovine factor V. The majority of procoagulant activity corresponds temporally with the cleavage of component C. (From Neheim et al.[20] and Nesheim and Mann.[19] Used with permission.)

the enzyme factor Xa, the cofactor, factor V(Va), Ca^{++} and phospholipid (or its equivalent). A comparison of the activation rate of prothrombin in the presence of the complete prothrombinase complex to the rate when any one component is absent has been conducted. The accessory components of the prothrombinase complex provide for a 10^5-fold increase in the rate of prothrombin activation when compared to the rate with factor Xa alone. The deletion of factor Va from the otherwise complete complex results in a 10,000-fold decrease in rate, while the deletion of phospholipid from the reaction mixture with all other components present results in a 1000-fold decrease in the rate. Ca^{++} is required for virtually all interactions as expressed by kinetic parameters in the assembly of the prothrombinase complex.

We have examined directly the binding of factor V and factor Va to some of the components of the prothrombinase complex, and these may be summarized as follows:

CALCIUM ION BINDING

Factor V has unique Ca^{++} binding properties.[22] Equilibrium dialysis studies conducted in our laboratory indicate that the factor V molecule possesses two exchangeable binding sites with $K_d = 5.9 \times 10^{-5}$ M. In addition, there exists a high affinity binding site in the factor V molecule from which Ca^{++} can be removed under native conditions only by strong chelators. Atomic absorption analysis of factor V after exhaustive dialysis *versus* buffers with endogenous Ca^{++} concentrations of approximately 10^{-8} M indicated that one mole of Ca^{++} is tightly bound per mole of factor V.

LIPID BINDING PARAMETERS

The binding of factor V and factor Va to phospholipid vesicles was studied by light scattering.[23] These studies indicate that both factor V and factor Va bind to phospholipid vesicles, and that the binding of the protein is dependent upon the presence of acidic phospholipid in the vesicle. In contrast, the affinity of the protein for phospholipid vesicles is independent of the ionic strength of the medium in the range from 0.15 to 1 ionic strength. Although the binding of factor V to the lipid vesicles increased as the phosphatidylserine content of the vesicle increased, the overall interaction was independent of Ca^{++}. This is in marked contrast to the binding of prothrombin and factor X to the same vesicles. The affinity of factor V and factor Va for these acidic phospholipid vesicles was from 10 to 100 times greater than the affinity of factor X and prothrombin for the same vesicles.

FACTOR V/VA PLATELET BINDING

The binding of factor V and factor Va to washed bovine platelets has been studied in our laboratory using radioiodinated proteins and an oil centrifugation technique.[17, 24] The results of this study indicate that both factor V and factor Va bind to platelets rather tightly. The binding of both procofactor and activated cofactor did not require prior activation of the platelet, and, in fact, activation of the platelet had no influence on the binding isotherms for the protein. The platelet binding results are summarized in TABLE 2. Since the plasma concentration of factor V by both radioimmunoassay and specific activity is approximately 10^{-7} M, one can infer from the dissociation constants presented in TABLE 2 that the circulating platelet factor V binding sites are saturated with factor V at plasma concentrations of this protein.

COMPONENT-COMPLEX INTERACTIONS

We have inferred the dissociation constant for any single component of the prothrombinase complex for the other components of the complex by

TABLE 2

PROPERTIES OF FACTOR V AND FACTOR VA BINDING TO PLATELETS

	High Affinity Sites		Low Affinity Sites	
	K_d ($\times 10^{10}$ M)	n	K_d ($\times 10^{10}$ M)	n
Factor Va				
Nonactivated platelets	4.0 ± 2.1	837 ± 48	3.6 ± 0.8	3403 ± 30
Thrombin-activated platelets	3.4 ± 1.7	827 ± 230	2.9 ± 1.3	3946 ± 104
Factor V				
Nonactivated platelets	——— none ———		2.8 ± 1.5	816 ± 92
Thrombin-activated platelets	——— none ———		3.6 ± 2.4	919 ± 283

analysis of kinetic data for thrombin production using the fluorescent probe DAPA.[25, 26] These experiments were conducted by holding all components of the complex but one fixed, and titrating the complex activity with the remaining varied component. The hyperbolic saturation curves obtained for each titration were then analyzed as assumed binding isotherms. The double reciprocal plots obtained from the data in each case were linear and from these plots apparent dissociation constants for the presumed binding of the varied component to the remainder of the complex were calculated. The values obtained by these analyses are contained within TABLE 3. Also contained within TABLE 3 are the bimolecular data obtained for some of the complex components using light scattering measurements.

Inspection of TABLE 3 leads to the following observations. First, the value obtained when prothrombin was varied with other components fixed, 1×10^{-6} M, is very similar to the value obtained for prothrombin binding to the same

TABLE 3

BINDING INTERACTIONS OF PROTHROMBINASE COMPONENTS

Varied Components	Fixed Components	K_d (M)	Stoichiometry
II	PCPS, Va, Xa	1.03×10^{-6} *	
V	II, PCPS, Xa	2.9×10^{-9} *	0.95 §
Va	II, PCPS, Xa	7.3×10^{-10} *	0.87 §
Xa	II, PCPS, Va	7.1×10^{-10} *	0.61 §
PCPS	II, Xa, Va	7.3×10^{-7} *	
Va	PCPS	5.4×10^{-7} †	
X	PCPS	2.6×10^{-6} †	
II	PCPS	2.5×10^{-6} †	
Va	Platelets	4×10^{-10} †	
Xa	Platelets (Va)	1.9×10^{-10} ‡	

* Apparent K_d determined using kinetics.
† Equilibrium value.
‡ Dahlbäck, B. & J. Stenflo. 1978. Biochemistry **17:** 4938–4945.
§ Expressed as Xa/Va, or Va/Xa.

vesicles using light scattering. The values obtained when V, Va or Xa were varied suggest equivalent cofactor-enzyme stoichiometry, and these values appear to reflect the association between these two proteins. The apparent dissociation constant obtained when phospholipid was varied is difficult to interpret rigorously. However, the value is extremely similar to that obtained by light scattering for factor Va binding to the same phospholipid vesicles.

The collection of data presented in TABLE 3 suggests that the principle property reflected by the concentration dependence of prothrombin as a substrate for the prothrombinase complex is the affinity of the substrate toward the phospholipid vesicle itself. In contrast, the data for phospholipid dependence and for factor Va-Xa interdependence, suggests that factor Va is the vehicle which maintains factor Xa on the phospholipid vesicle.

The collected data suggest that one substantial contribution of complex assembly is the condensation of substrate (by virtue of phospholipid binding) and the enzyme (by virtue of cofactor (factor Va) binding) on the phospholipid surface. Under the conditions used in our experimental studies, each of the proteins in the prothrombinase complex are near, or at, plasma concentration. At these concentrations one would conclude that in the course of the prothrombin conversion reaction, 95% of the enzyme is bound to the phospholipid vesicle, while 99% of the substrate is in solution. However, the amount of substrate bound on the vesicle, by virtue of its phospholipid association, would lead to approximately two substrate (prothrombin) molecules bound for every enzyme molecule (factor Xa) bound.

A summary of this conclusion is presented in FIGURE 4. Here the phospholipid surface is represented as the now traditional, bilayer model. The hydrophobic factor Va molecule is imbedded in the bilayer, while factor Xa is bound to the embedded factor Va molecule. The substrate prothrombin, represented as a three-domain structure, is shown both in solution and on the vesicle surface. The phospholipid binding of the substrate is represented to occur *via* Ca^{++} bridging to the γ-carboxyglutamic acid residues present in the NH_2-terminal fragment 1 region. A prothrombin dimer, also formed by Ca^{++} bridging, as proposed by Bloom and Mann,[27] is represented in solution. In the catalytic complex, prothrombin is depicted as interacting through its fragment 2 domain with factor Va, an inference drawn from previous kinetic studies of prothrombin activation.[28]

SIGNIFICANCE TO BLOOD COAGULATION PROCESSES

The hemostatic event occurs in what can be defined as an open system. The blood vessel lesion at which coagulation occurs is constantly being bathed in, and supplied with, fresh reagents. The remarkable property of the blood coagulation reaction is that (most frequently) the reaction can be turned on rapidly, is localized, and ordinarily does not become systemic. Membrane binding of factor V(Va) at the platelet surface provides a vehicle to explain the mechanical fixation of this blood coagulation reaction at the locus of the blood vessel lesion. Thus, factor Xa would be fixed at the site of platelet adhesion and aggregation by virtue of its interaction with factor Va, and the factor Va interaction with the membrane surface.

A number of other blood coagulation reactions are similar to prothrombinase complex formation, in that they involve a vitamin-K dependent protein

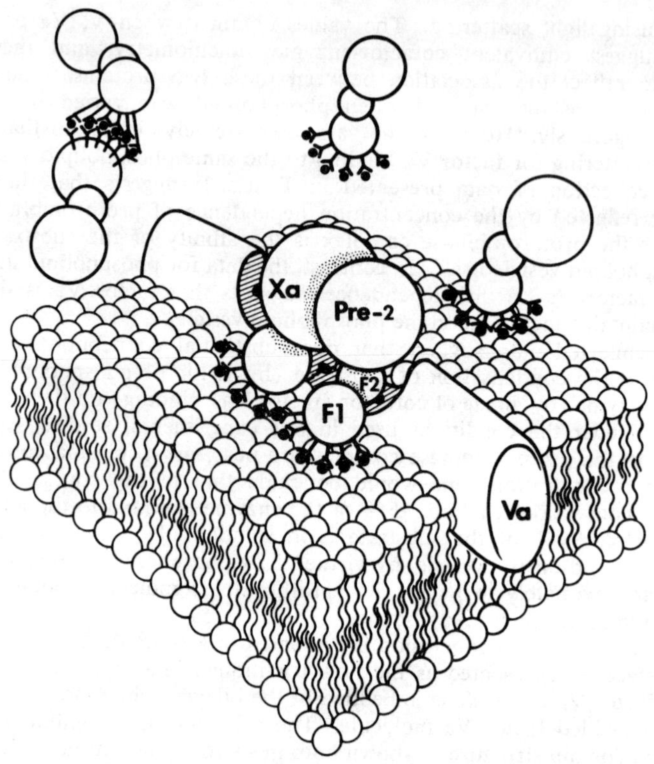

FIGURE 4. Model of the activation of prothrombin as catalyzed by the prothrombinase complex. (From Nesheim *et al.*[20] Used with permission.)

TABLE 4

COFACTOR COMPARISON

Factor V	Factor VIII
1. Plays a cofactor role with factor Xa, Ca^{++} and phospholipid to activate prothrombin	Plays a cofactor role with factor IXa, Ca^{++} and phospholipid to activate factor X
2. Activated by thrombin	Activated by thrombin
3. Inactivated by activated protein C	Inactivated by activated protein C
4. $S^0_{20w} = 9.19$	Coagulant activity $S^0_{20w} = 9.2$
5. Binds to QAE cellulose and octyl-Sepharose	Binds to QAE cellulose and octyl-Sepharose

with lipid binding capacity and a cofactor protein of substantial molecular dimensions. One of these, for which we have only limited information, is the assembly of the factor VIII-dependent factor X converting activity involving factor IXa as enzyme. The molecular structure of factor VIII procoagulant activity has not yet been adequately described. However, many properties of this cofactor molecule suggest it is very similar to factor V. These properties are outlined in TABLE 5. In addition to the properties related in TABLE 5, the

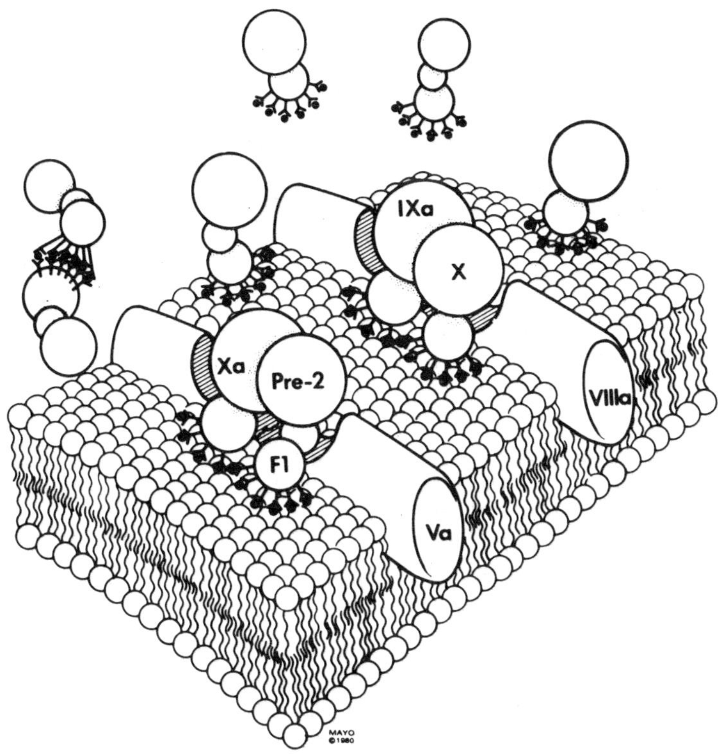

FIGURE 5. Model of two collected blood coagulation reactions: conversion of factor X to factor Xa; conversion of prothrombin to thrombin. Their respective catalysts are bound adjacent to one another on their respective cofactors on the platelet membrane.

recent report by Vehar and Davie [29] of factor VIII procoagulant isolation suggest properties similar to some of the fragments of factor V. In view of these similarities, it is tempting to speculate that just as factor Va is the vehicle fixing factor Xa to the platelet surface, factor VIIIa may provide a similar function, fixing factor IXa at the platelet surface. In such a model, depicted in FIGURE 5, factor X could be converted to factor Xa in a complex of factor IXa-VIIIa in a manner completely analogous with complexation to factor Va to form a prothrombin converting activity.

REFERENCES

1. OWREN, P. A.   1947.   Lancet **1:** 446–448.
2. OWREN, P. A.   1947.   Acta Med. Scand. Suppl. **194:** 1–316.
3. WARE, A. G. & W. H. SEEGERS.   1948.   Am. J. Physiol. **152:** 699–705.
4. MURPHY, R. C. & W. H. SEEGERS.   1948.   Am. J. Physiol. **154:** 134–139.
5. ESNOUF, M. P. & F. JOBIN.   1967.   Biochem. J. **102:** 660–665.
6. BARTON, P. G. & D. J. HANAHAN.   1967.   Biochim. Biophys. Acta **133:** 506–518.
7. MANN, K. G.   1976.   Prothrombin. Methods in Enzymol. **45:** 123–156.
8. SUTTIE, J. W. & C. M. JACKSON.   1977.   Physiol. Rev. **57:** 1–70.
9. COLMAN, R. W.   1969.   Biochemistry **8:** 1438–1445.
10. DOMBROSE, F. A. & W. H. SEEGERS.   1974.   Thromb. Diath. Haemorrh. **57** (Suppl): 241–254.
11. CHULKOVA, T. & G. HERNANDEZ.   1975.   Clin. Chem. Acta **62:** 21–28.
12. DAY, W. C.   1975.   Biochim. Biophys. Acta **386:** 352–361.
13. SMITH, C. M. & D. J. HANAHAN.   1976.   Biochemistry **15:** 1830–1838.
14. SARASWATHI, S., R. RAWALA & R. W. COLMAN.   1978.   J. Biol. Chem. **253:** 1024–1029.
15. NESHEIM, M. E., K. H. MYRMEL, L. S. HIBBARD & K. G. MANN.   1978.   Fed. Proc. **37**(6): 1750.
16. ESMON, C. G.   1979.   J. Biol. Chem. **254:** 964–973.
17. TRACY, P. B., J. M. PETERSON, M. E. NESHEIM, F. C. McDUFFIE & K. G. MANN.   1979.   J. Biol. Chem. **254:** 10354–10361.
18. BARTLETT, S., P. LATSON & D. J. HANAHAN.   1980.   Biochemistry **19:** 273–277.
19. NESHEIM, M. E. & K. G. MANN.   1979.   J. Biol. Chem. **254:** 1326–1334.
20. NESHEIM, M. E., L. S. HIBBARD, P. B. TRACY, J. W. BLOOM, K. H. MYRMEL & K. G. MANN.   1980.   Participation of Factor Va in Prothrombinase. *In* The Regulation of Coagulation, K. Mann & F. Taylor, Jr., Eds.: 145–159. Elsevier-North Holland. New York.
21. CANFIELD, W., M. E. NESHEIM, W. KISIEL & K. G. MANN.   1978.   Circulation (Part II) **58** (4): No. 816.
22. HIBBARD, L. S. & K. G. MANN.   1980.   J. Biol. Chem. **255:** 638–645.
23. BLOOM, J. W., M. E. NESHEIM & K. G. MANN.   1979.   Biochemistry **18:** 4419–4425.
24. TRACY, P. B., J. M. PETERSON, M. E. NESHEIM, F. C. McDUFFIE & K. G. MANN.   1980.   Platelet Interaction with Bovine Coagulation Factor V and Factor Va. *In* The Regulation of Coagulation, K. Mann & F. Taylor, Jr., Eds., 237–243. Elsevier-North Holland, New York.
25. NESHEIM, M. E., F. G. PRENDERGAST & K. G. MANN.   1979.   Biochemistry **18:** 996–1003.
26. NESHEIM, M. E., J. B. TASWELL & K. G. MANN.   J. Biol. Chem. **254:** 10952–10983.
27. BLOOM, J. W. & K. G. MANN.   1978.   Biochemistry **17:** 4430–4438.
28. BAJAJ, S. P., R. W. BUTKOWSKI & K. G. MANN.   1975.   J. Biol. Chem. **250:** 2150–2156.
29. VEHAR, G. A. & E. W. DAVIE.   1980.   Biochemistry **19:** 401–410.

APPROACHES TO THE STUDY OF PROTHROMBIN CONFORMATION AND ACTIVATION IN BIOLOGICAL FLUIDS *

Barbara C. Furie,† Mindy M. Tai, Marie-Josèphe Rabiet,‡
and Bruce Furie §

*Division of Hematology-Oncology
Department of Medicine
Tufts-New England Medical Center
Boston, Massachusetts 02111*

*Department of Biochemistry and Pharmacology
Tufts University School of Medicine
Boston, Massachusetts 02111*

Over the past decade our understanding of the nature of the plasma proteins involved in blood coagulation and their interactions has been vastly expanded. In particular, those plasma proteins whose syntheses are vitamin K dependent and for which a well-defined role in coagulation has been established—factor VII, factor IX, factor X, and prothrombin—have been isolated and well characterized. A unique amino acid, γ-carboxyglutamic acid, has been identified in these proteins and its role in metal ion binding explored.[1,2] The amino acid sequences of bovine factors IX and X and human and bovine prothrombin are known[3-8] as are the sequences of the carbohydrate moieties on prothrombin and factor X.[9-11] The positions of the proteolytic cleavages that occur concomitant with and subsequent to zymogen activation of factor IX, factor X, and prothrombin have been identified (References 1 & 2 and references cited therein). For some of these proteins spectroscopic studies have demonstrated conformational changes occurring when ligands are bound[12-15] or when zymogen activation occurs.[16] All of this information has been accumulated in studies using purified protein solutions or reaction mixtures made by recombining purified proteins and cofactors. The physiologic relevance of proteolytic cleavage products and conformational changes observed *in vitro* must somehow be assessed in biological systems. We have taken two different approaches to this kind of assessment. One involves the use of conformation-specific antibodies to study protein tertiary structure. The other employs purified radiolabeled coagulation zymogens supplemented to plasma. The changes in primary structure associated with zymogen conversion can be monitored in biologic fluid. Both approaches will be illustrated with studies carried out on prothrombin.

* This research was supported by Grants HL-21543 and HL-18834 from the National Institutes of Health. A portion of these studies was performed by M. M. Tai in partial fulfillment of the requirement for the degree of Doctor of Philosophy from Tufts University.

† Recipient of a Research Career Development Award from the National Institutes of Health.

‡ Recipient of awards from Foundation pour la Recherche Medicale Francaise, Paris, France and the Philippe Foundation, Paris, France.

§ Established Investigator of the American Heart Association and its Massachusetts affiliate.

389

Bovine prothrombin is a glycoprotein with a molecular weight of about 70,000 and contains 10 γ-carboxyglutamic acids.[1] Its amino acid sequence has been determined [6-8] and the sites of proteolysis *in vitro* of the zymogen by the enzymes factor Xa and thrombin have been identified (FIGURE 1).[1, 2] Fragment 1 and prethrombin 1 are generated by thrombin cleavage of the Arg 156–Ser 157 bond. Alternatively thrombin can cleave fragment 1·2 at the same bond to release fragment 1 and fragment 2. Fragment 1·2 and prethrombin 2 are produced when factor Xa cleaves the Arg 274–Thr 275 bond in prothrombin. Finally factor Xa cleaves the Arg 323–Ileu 324 bond in prethrombin 2 to yield the A and B chain of α-thrombin. Human prothrombin, similarly a glycoprotein containing 10 γ-carboxyglutamic acid residues, has a molecular weight of about 70,000.[1] In addition to the proteolytic cleavages defined for bovine prothrombin in purified protein systems human prothrombin can be cleaved between Arg 287 and Thr 288 to release a 13 residue peptide.[17, 18] Although cleavage of the bond between Arg 156 and Ser 157 to give either fragment 1 and prethrombin 1 or fragment 1 and fragment 2 had been attributed to thrombin for bovine prothrombin, evidence exists for cleavage of that bond as well as the Arg 287–Thr 288 bond by either thrombin or factor Xa in the human protein.[19, 20] Furthermore evidence suggests that in human blood, free fragment 1 is not produced.[21-24] In order to determine the pathways and kinetics of activation of human prothrombin in plasma and ultimately in

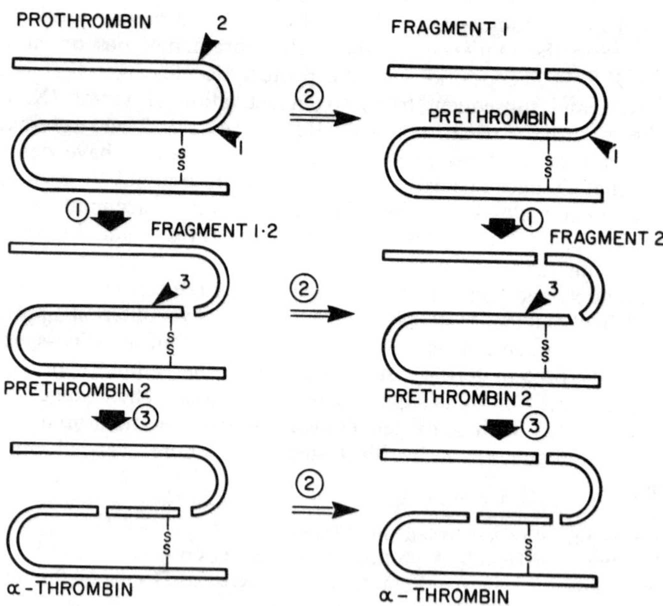

FIGURE 1. Established pathways of prothrombin cleavage *in vitro*. When bovine prothrombin is the substrate reactions 1 and 3 are catalyzed by activated factor X. Reaction 2 is catalyzed by thrombin. When human prothrombin is the substrate reaction 2 may be catalyzed by activated factor X as well. Products and intermediates of prothrombin (M_r, 70,000) activation include prethrombin 1 (M_r, 51,000), prethrombin 2 (M_r, 35,000), fragment 1 (M_r, 23,000), and fragment 2 (M_r, 13,000).

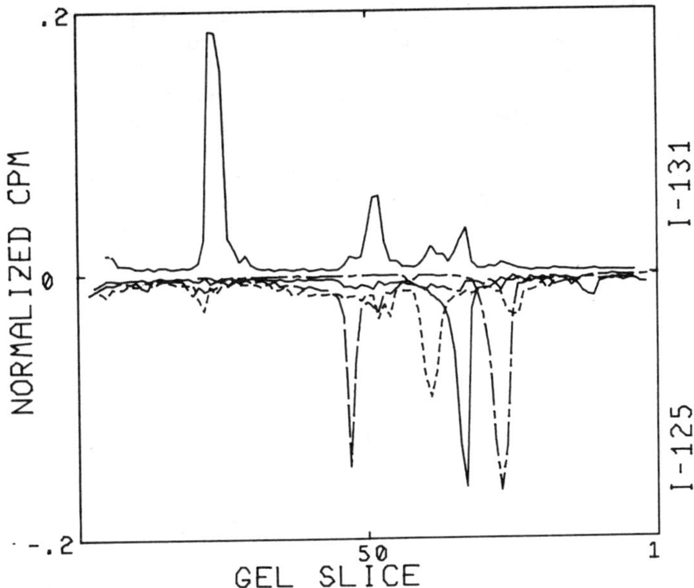

FIGURE 2. Dodecyl sulfate-polyacrylamide gel electrophoresis of ^{125}I-labeled human prothrombin fragments (lower panel) and clotted plasma containing ^{131}I-labeled human prothrombin (upper panel). Lower panel: (- — - —) fragment 1; (————) thrombin B chain; (- - - -) prethrombin 2; and (— — —) prethrombin 1.

clotting blood we have developed a method for studying the products of prothrombin activation and the rate of their appearance using polyacrylamide gel electrophoresis in the presence of dodecyl sulfate and radiolabeled prothrombin as a tracer (FIGURE 2).

Human prothrombin radiolabeled with ^{131}I by the Chloramine T method [25] was added to plasma. Clotting was initiated with kaolin and calcium using the conditions described in the legend to FIGURE 3. The plasma was sampled at various times before and after clot formation. Reactions were terminated by adding aliquots of the reaction mixture to solutions containing sodium dodecyl sulfate, 2-mercaptoethanol, and EDTA at 80° C. Products of the plasma activation were separated in polyacrylamide gels containing dodecyl sulfate. The polyacrylamide gels were divided into 1-mm segments and the segments assayed for [131]I. The identity of the activation products was established by comparing their migrations in the polyacrylamide gels with standards of independently isolated proteolytic products of human prothrombin labeled with [125]I. In order to maximize resolution of prethrombin 1, fragment 1·2, prethrombin 2, and the B chain of thrombin, the polyacrylamide gels were subjected to electrophoreses for extended periods of time. The extended electrophoreses times result in migration of fragment 2 and the A chain of thrombin from the gel.

Prothrombin, prethrombin 2, thrombin B chain, and, several minutes after clot formation, fragment 1 are observed in the electrophoretograms. One major product of prothrombin proteolysis visible in the electrophoretograms cannot be identified by comparison to the migration of previously identified prothrombin proteolysis products. This product is smaller than prethrombin 1, larger than prethrombin 2, and, as can be seen in FIGURE 3, is slightly larger than fragment 1·2. Its migration in polyacrylamide gels in the absence of 2-mercaptoethanol is also different from that of prothrombin and its known proteolysis products. We have established conditions for generating and isolating this unidentified activation product from reaction mixtures containing nonradiolabeled prothrombin, activated factor X, brain phospholipid, and CaCl$_2$. We are currently characterizing the activation product. Preliminary

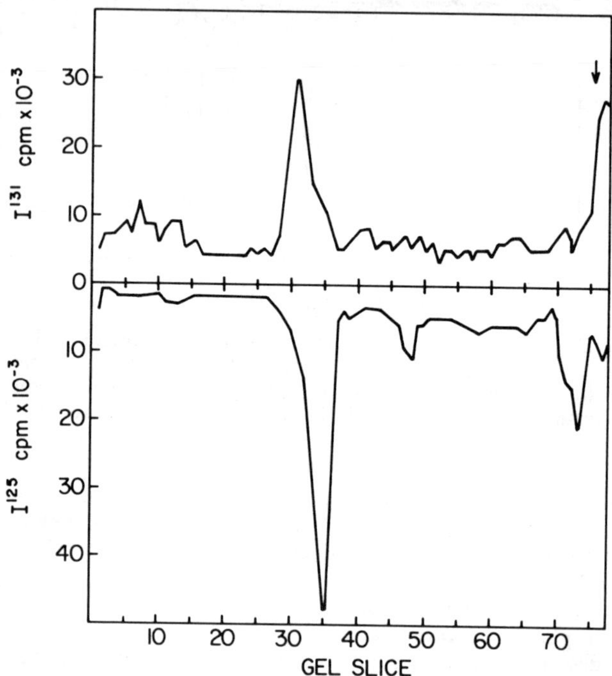

FIGURE 3. Dodecyl sulfate-polyacrylamide gel electrophoresis of ^{125}I-labeled human prothrombin fragment 1·2 (lower panel) and clotted plasma containing ^{131}I-labeled human prothrombin (upper panel). ^{131}I-labeled prothrombin (50 μg) was added to 0.4 ml of plasma at 37° C. Clot formation was initiated by simultaneous addition of 40 μl of kaolin/cephalin and 0.4 ml of 0.025 M CaCl$_2$.

evidence indicates that this activation product binds tightly to barium salts, shares the same NH$_2$-terminus as prothrombin, is a single polypeptide chain, and contains fragment 1 and fragment 2 within its structure.

From earlier studies on the products of prothrombin activation in artificial activation systems it is clear that the products obtained depended markedly on the components of the activation mixture. Kisiel and Hanahan [26] have demonstrated that when human prothrombin is activated at room temperature in the presence of activated factor X, CaCl$_2$, and hirudin (a specific thrombin inhibitor), no thrombin is generated and no fragment 1 or prethrombin 1 appears.

However, Rosenberg, Beeler, and Rosenberg activated human prothrombin in the presence of factor V and cephalin as well as activated factor X, $CaCl_2$, and hirudin at 37° C. While no thrombin activity was generated, they found that fragment 1 and prethrombin 1 did appear.[12, 20] It is clear from these results and our own results described above that, whereas *in vitro* studies of zymogen activation of plasma coagulation factors can identify what reactions may occur, activation studies performed in the native milieu, clotting blood, are required to identify what can occur during physiologic coagulation. Indeed, *in vivo* experiments may be required to account for contributions to coagulation by substances not found in circulating blood, but contributed by the surfaces or contents of cells within the circulation or the vessel walls.

Optical spectroscopic methods for studying protein conformational change are limited in application to purified protein systems. A solution must be essentially transparent except for the interaction of radiation with the protein of interest. Furthermore it is difficult to assign specific conformational changes in the protein to spectroscopic perturbations observed, i.e., where within a protein a conformational change occurs. Using conformation-specific antibodies to protein antigens, we have developed approaches that circumvent these problems. Conformation-specific antibodies have been used to study many phenomena involving protein conformation alterations. For example, conformation-specific antibodies were employed to evaluate protein flexibility and conformational equilibria in staph nuclease[27] and to determine differential degrees of flexibility in regions of the sperm whale myoglobin polypeptide chain close to the heme group and those regions remote from the heme group.[29] A similar approach was used to demonstrate that the conformation of the carboxy-terminal end of the hemoglobin β chain was significantly affected by the presence or absence of ligand.[28] We have used conformation-specific antibodies to further study the conformational alteration observed spectroscopically when prothrombin binds metal ions.[2, 12–15]

Rabbits were immunized with bovine prothrombin. Anti-prothrombin antibodies were purified by affinity chromatography on columns of prothrombin-agarose in the presence of calcium ions. Anti-prothrombin antibodies were eluted with 4 *M* guanidine·HCl. These antibodies were rechromatographed on columns of prothrombin-agarose in the presence of calcium ions. Antibodies specific for the conformation of prothrombin bound to Ca^{2+}, anti-prothrombin-Ca^{2+} antibodies, were eluted with EDTA. The remainder of the anti-prothrombin antibodies were again eluted with 4 *M* guanidine·HCl.[30]

To demonstrate the specificity of the anti-prothrombin-Ca^{2+} antibodies, their binding to prothrombin in the presence and absence of Ca^{2+} ions was studied.[30] In FIGURE 4 it can be observed that the binding of this antibody subpopulation to prothrombin is almost entirely Ca^{2+}-dependent and only minimal binding is observed in the presence of EDTA. Similar results are obtained when metal-free reagents are used in place of the chelating agent EDTA. The Ca^{2+} dependence of the interaction of the anti-prothrombin-Ca^{2+} antibodies was explored by studying the dependence of the antibody–prothrombin interaction on calcium ion concentration. Half maximal binding of antibody to prothrombin is achieved at 0.2 mM Ca^{2+}. In parallel studies the interaction of a metal-ion-dependent antibody population against the region of bovine prothrombin from residues 12–44 (containing 8 of 10 γ-carboxyglutamic acids in prothrombin) was characterized with respect to its dependence on a variety of metal ions.[31, 32] The results of these studies are presented in TABLE 1, corre-

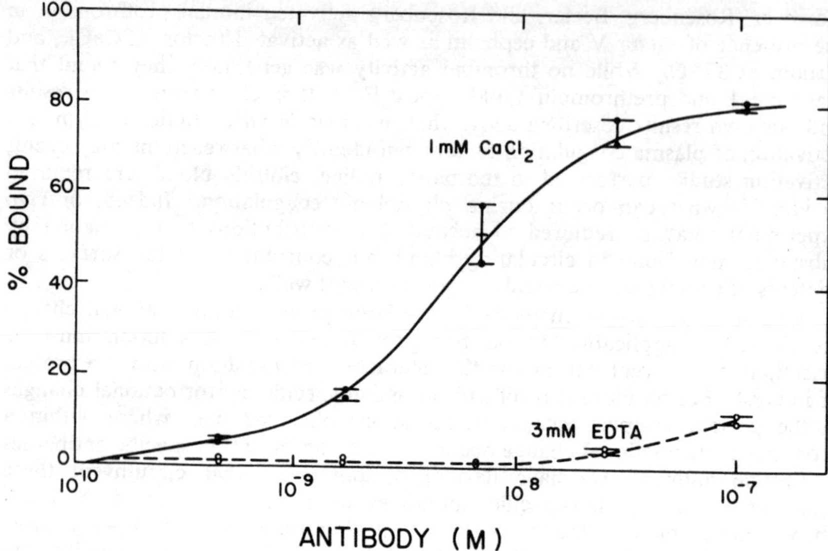

FIGURE 4. Interaction of anti-prothrombin-Ca^{2+} antibodies with prothrombin in the presence of $CaCl_2$ or EDTA. The incubation mixture (300 μl) contained ^{125}I-labeled prothrombin (9.4×10^{-10} M), anti-prothrombin-Ca^{2+} antibody, albumin (100 μg), and $CaCl_2$ (1 mM) (●—●) or EDTA (3 mM) (○ - - - ○). From reference 30.

TABLE 1
IMMUNOCHEMICAL ASSAY OF CONFORMATIONAL TRANSITIONS (T_m) IN THE
γ-CARBOXYGLUTAMIC ACID-RICH REGION OF PROTHROMBIN *

		K_D High Affinity Site	Immuno-chemical T_m	CD † T_m	Fluorescence ‡ T_m	Fluorescence § T_m
Ca^{2+}	PT	0.31 mM ¶	0.2 mM	0.18 mM		0.40 mM
	F1	0.63 mM ¶		0.20 mM	0.35 mM	0.40 mM
Mg^{2+}	PT		0.2 mM			0.40 mM
	F1			0.21 mM	0.45 mM	0.43 mM
Mn^{2+}	PT	12 μM ‖	20 μM			<50 μM
	F1	22 μM		22.8 μM	12.6 μM	
Gd^{3+}	PT	0.75 μM #	0.1 μM			
	F1	0.16 μM			5.3 μM	

* Comparison with equilibrium measurements of metal binding and metal-induced fluorescence and circular dichroism changes in prothrombin and prothrombin Fragment 1. Prothrombin (PT); prothrombin Fragment 1 (F1).
 † Reference 15.
 ‡ Reference 13.
 § Reference 14.
 ‖ Reference 34.
 # Reference 35.
 ¶ Reference 33.

lated with the dissociation constants for these metal ions with prothrombin or prothrombin fragment 1. The concentration of various metal ions required to induce half maximal binding of anti-$(12–44)_N$ antibodies are also compared to half maximal transitions observed spectroscopically for either prothrombin or prothrombin fragment 1 when titrated with the same metal ions. The data in TABLE 1 indicate that the metal-induced conformational transition in prothrombin measured immunologically in solutions containing high concentrations of albumin is the same conformational alteration observed by various spectroscopic techniques.

To localize the regions of prothrombin that undergo a conformational change upon metal binding, the interaction of anti-prothrombin-Ca^{2+} antibodies with fragment 1 and prethrombin 1 was studied (FIGURE 5). In the presence

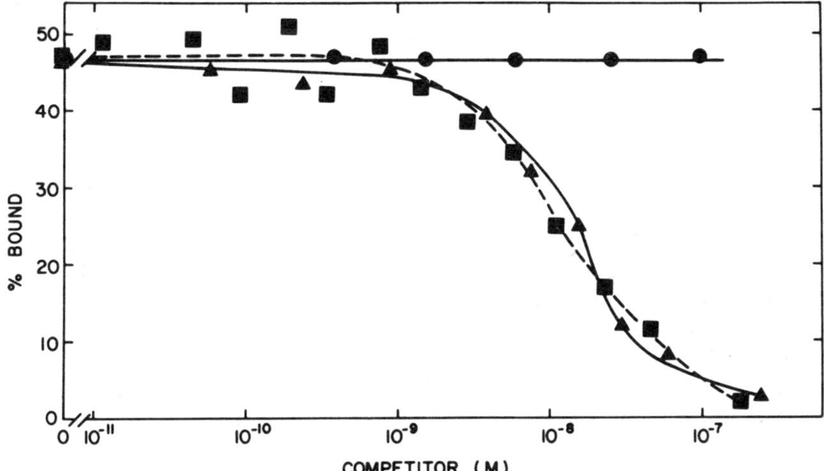

FIGURE 5. Specificity of anti-prothrombin-Ca^{2+} antibodies. The specificity of the antibody population was determined by assessing the ability of fragments of prothrombin to displace ^{125}I-labeled prothrombin from the antibody. Incubation mixtures (300 μl) contained ^{125}I-labeled prothrombin (7.3 × 10⁻⁹M), antibody (7.6 × 10⁻⁹M), albumin (100 μg), and unlabeled antigen as indicated Prothrombin (■ - - - ■); fragment 1 (▲—▲); and prethrombin 1 (●—●). From reference 30.

of Ca^{2+}, fragment 1 can displace prothrombin completely from anti-prothrombin-Ca^{2+} antibodies while prethrombin 1 causes no displacement of prothrombin. We conclude that all the antigenic determinants to which the anti-prothrombin-Ca^{2+} antibodies bind are located in the fragment 1 region of prothrombin. Recent studies with a CNBr fragment of fragment 1, fragment 1–72, indicate that most, if not all, of the antigenic determinants reside in the first 72 residues of prothrombin. Efforts are underway to define these determinants further. Conformation specific antibodies such as the anti-prothrombin-Ca^{2+} antibodies described here may prove useful for exploring conformational alterations in proteins occurring in clotting blood in response to alterations in ligand concentration.

The study of hemostasis has passed through several phases during the past 50 years. Initially, major advances were based upon the correlation of clinical observations with the *in vitro* clotting of blood. Investigation of patients with congenital bleeding disorders, in particular, led to the identification of components involved in hemostasis. More recently, these identified components have been purified and extensively characterized at the molecular level. The structural correlates of activation of blood coagulation are in the process of being carefully defined. However, from our recent experience and the experience of others, it is clear that the biochemical events that take place in plasma may be somewhat different from those observed in systems reconstituted with purified components. It would appear that to understand hemostasis in its physiological context, it will be necessary to evaluate blood coagulation in whole clotting blood or in living animals. Such studies, appropriately based on existing biochemical data, will require new conceptual and technological approaches. Our studies using conformation-specific antibodies and tracer proteins in plasma to monitor changes in protein structure offer two examples of methods that can be developed to examine blood coagulation in complex biological fluids.

REFERENCES

1. DAVIE, E. W. & D. J. HANAHAN. 1977. *In* The Plasma Proteins. F. W. Putnam, Ed. Vol. **3:** 421–544. Academic Press, New York, N.Y.
2. NEMERSON, Y. & B. FURIE. 1980. CRC Crit. Rev. Biochem. **9:** 45–85.
3. KATAYAMA, K., L. H. ERICSSON, D. ENFIELD, K. A. WALSH, H. NEURATH, E. W. DAVIE & K. TITANI. 1979. Proc. Natl. Acad. Sci. (USA) **76:** 4990.
4. ENFIELD, D. L., L. H. ERICSSON, K. FUJIKAWA, K. A. WALSH, H. NEURATH & K. TITANI. 1980. Biochem. **19:** 659–667.
5. TITANI, K., K. FUJIKAWA, D. L. ENFIELD, L. H. ERICSSON, K. A. WALSH & H. NEURATH. 1975. Proc. Natl. Acad. Sci. (USA) **72:** 3082–3086.
6. MAGNUSSON, S., T. E. PETERSON, L. JENSON-SOTTRUP & H. CLAEYS. 1975. *In* Proteases and Biological Control. E. Reich, D. B. Rifkin, and W. Shaw, Eds. p. 123 Cold Spring Harbor, N.Y.
7. WALZ, D. A., D. HEWETT-EMMETT & W. H. SEEGERS. 1977. Proc. Natl. Acad. Sci. USA **74:** 1969.
8. BUTKOWSKI, R. J., J. ELION, M. R. DOWNING & K. G. MANN. 1977. J. Biol. Chem. **252:** 4942.
9. NELSESTUEN, G. L. & J. W. SUTTIE. 1972. J. Biol. Chem. **247:** 6096–6102.
10. MIZOUCHI, T., K. YAMASHITA, K. FUJIKAWA, W. KISIEL & A. KOBATA. 1979. J. Biol. Chem. **254:** 6419.
11. MIZOUCHI, T., K. YAMASHITA, K. FUJIKAWA, K. TITANI & A. KOBATA. 1980. J. Biol. Chem. **255:** 3526–3531.
12. NELSESTUEN, G. L. 1976. J. Biol. Chem. **252:** 5648.
13. PRENDERGAST, F. C. & K. G. MANN. 1977. J. Biol. Chem. **252:** 840–850.
14. NELSESTUEN, G. L., M. BRODERIUS & G. MARTIN. 1976. J. Biol. Chem. **251:** 6886.
15. BLOOM, J. W. & K. G. MANN. 1978. Biochem. **17:** 4430–4438.
16. FURIE, B. & B. C. FURIE. 1976. J. Biol. Chem. **251:** 6807.
17. WALZ, D. A. & W. H. SEEGERS. 1974. Biochem. Biophys. Res. Commun. **60:** 717–722.
18. DOWNING, M. R., R. J. BUTKOWSKI, M. M. CLARK & K. G. MANN. 1975. J. Biol. Chem. **250:** 8897–8906.

19. ROSENBERG, J. S., D. L. BEELER & R. D. ROSENBERG. 1975. J. Biol. Chem. **250:** 1607–1617.
20. LAU, H. K., J. S. ROSENBERG, D. L. BEELER & R. D. ROSENBERG. 1979. J. Biol. Chem. **254:** 8751–8761.
21. ARONSON, D. L., L. STEVAN, A. P. BALL, B. R. FRANZA, JR. & J. S. FINLAYSON. 1977. J. Clin. Invest. **60:** 1410–1418.
22. WALZ, D. A., J. N. LOVE, W. H. SEEGERS & T. R. BROWN. 1981. Ann. N.Y. Acad. Sci. This volume.
23. FURIE, B. C., E. GREENE & B. FURIE. 1977. Blood **51** (Suppl.): 266.
24. FURIE, B. C., E. GREENE, L. VOO & B. FURIE. 1979. Thrombosis and Haemostasis **42:** 209.
25. HUNTER, W. M. & F. C. GREENWOOD. 1962. Nature **194:** 495–496.
26. KISIEL, W. & D. J. HANAHAN. 1973. Biochim. Biophys. Acta **304:** 103–113.
27. FURIE, B., A. N. SCHECHTER, D. H. SACHS & C. B. ANFINSEN. 1975. J. Mol. Biol. **92:** 497–506.
28. DEAN, J. & A. N. SCHECTER. 1979. J. Biol. Chem. **254:** 9185–9193.
29. HURRELL, J. G. R., J. A. SMITH & S. J. LEACH. 1977. Biochem. **16:** 175–185.
30. TAI, M., B. C. FURIE & B. FURIE. 1980. J. Biol. Chem. **255:** 2790–2795.
31. FURIE, B., K. L PROVOST, R. A. BLANCHARD & B. C. FURIE. 1978. J. Biol. Chem. **253:** 8980–8987.
32. FURIE, B. & B. C. FURIE. 1979. J. Biol. Chem. **254:** 9766–9771.
33. BAJAJ, S. P., R. J. BUTKOWSKI & K. G. MANN. 1975. J. Biol. Chem. **250:** 2150–2156.
34. BAJAJ, S. P., T. NOWAK & F. J. CASTELLINO. 1976. J. Biol. Chem. **251:** 6294–6299.
35. FURIE, B. C., K. G. MANN & B. FURIE. 1976. J. Biol. Chem. **251:** 3235–3241.

RADIOIMMUNOASSAYS FOR
HUMAN PROTHROMBIN FRAGMENTS:
DEVELOPMENT AND IMPLEMENTATION *

Daniel A. Walz,† Jeffrey N. Love,† Walter H. Seegers,† and
Thomas R. Brown ‡

*† Department of Physiology, and
‡ Hutzel Hospital Medical Unit
Wayne State University School of Medicine
Detroit, Michigan 48201*

The interrelationship between the vessel wall, platelets, and the plasma blood coagulation proteins, a collective control mechanism called hemostasis, has long been recognized as a fundamental example of homeostasis. Other aspects of this text have or will address the complexity of the individual components of both the cellular and micellar reactions in hemostasis. This paper attempts to examine narrowly the quantitation of the penultimate amplification reaction of clot formation, namely, the conversion of human prothrombin to the active enzyme thrombin, and the nature and fate of the activation products, fragments 1 and 2. Whereas certain aspects of these activation mechanisms of coagulation have been thoroughly reviewed,[1-3] selected features of the human prothrombin protein are described herein by way of introduction to the accompanying research.

Human prothrombin is a vitamin K-dependent, single-chained glycoprotein found in plasma at a concentration of approximately 1.5 μM.[4] The activation of purified human prothrombin has been examined by a number of investigators who have variously monitored the appearance of new amino-terminal residues upon activation,[5] the chromatographic behavior of the activated molecule,[6] the changes apparent upon thrombin hydrolysis of prothrombin,[7] and the molecular weight of the activation products determined by SDS electrophoresis.[8-13] Each of these activation products is similar to the bovine counterparts. Indeed, the entire human prothrombin amino acid sequence is now known.[14-18] In purified form, human prothrombin is proteolytically cleaved by factor Xa, giving rise to a combined fragment 1·2 (F 1·2) and thrombin.[8, 11, 13] In addition, and as purified material, thrombin will proteolytically hydrolyze prothrombin, generating fragment 1 (F 1) and prethrombin 1; thrombin will also cleave F 1·2 to yield the distinct fragments, F 1 and fragment 2 (F 2). Human thrombin, isolated as a purified protein, contains an A chain shortened by 13 residues when compared with the similar bovine A chain.[14] This 13-residue peptide, designated fragment 3 (F 3), is autocatalytically removed from thrombin during its preparative isolation.[19, 20]

An immunochemical evaluation of human prothrombin activation has not been systematically undertaken. Shapiro[21] was one of the earliest investigators to monitor prothrombin conversion to thrombin by immunochemical techniques and he found that gel-filtered serum contained essentially two predominant

* This work was supported by Grant-in-Aid 79–891 from the American Heart Association and by funds contributed in part by the Michigan Heart Association.

components, one equivalent to thrombin and the other of a similar molecular size (and now recognized as F 1·2). Aronson and coworkers[22] subsequently monitored the conversion of prothrombin to thrombin by recalcification of plasma in the presence of Russell's viper venom (RVV) and concluded that the principal, if not exclusive, end product of this reaction was thrombin and F 1·2, despite the fact that less than 10 units per milliliter of thrombin were detected by bioassays. A radioimmunoassay (RIA) for human thrombin has been developed[23] that was specific for thrombin in that it failed to detect thrombin complexed with antithrombin. A radioimmunoassay for human prothrombin has also been developed[24] and quantifies the plasma prothrombin at 86 μg/ml. Human prothrombin fragment antisera have also been utilized to probe the appearance of specific fragments upon activation of the purified components.[25, 26] McDuffie, Mann, and coworkers[27] have reported on the use of an RIA for human prethrombin 1 and its use in disseminated intravascular coagulation, noting that no appreciable prethrombin 1 was detected in such plasma. An alternate approach for evaluating prothrombin activation by means of cross-immunoelectrophoresis of urine samples[28] has demonstrated the presence of F 1 in normal human urine.

We have undertaken the systematic development and evaluation of RIAs for human prothrombin and each of its activation components and report our preliminary observations here.

MATERIALS AND METHODS

Antigens

Human fragment material (supplied by J. W. Fenton) was concentrated with an Amicon UM-2 membrane. It was then applied to a DEAE-Sephadex® column and eluted with a linear gradient (0.1–0.6 NaCl) which separated F 1 and F 2 from other activation products. Gel filtration with Sephadex G-75 clearly resolved F 1 from F 2. The purity of these products was determined with SDS polyacrylamide gel electrophoresis.[17] Thrombin was donated by J. W. Fenton, while F 3 was commercially synthesized (Bachem Fine Chemicals, Inc., Torrence, CA). Prothrombin was purified from plasma according to the method of Novoa *et al.*[29] Prethrombin 1 was produced from controlled digestion of purified prothrombin with thrombin. The digestion products were added to a DEAE-Sephadex column, which resolved prethrombin 1 from F 1.

Antisera

Female New Zealand white rabbits were immunized with F 1 and F 2 according to the method of Vaitukaitis *et al.*[30] The initial immunization dose consisted of 0.5 ml attenuated pertussis vaccine, 0.72 mg purified protein dissolved in 1.2 ml of physiological saline solution, and homogenization with an equal volume of complete Freund's adjuvant until the mixture was fully emulsified. Fifteen to twenty sites were injected intradermally on the dorsal aspect of the rabbit's thorax/abdomen. Three months after initial immunization a booster was given of 0.3 mg purified protein dissolved in 0.6 ml of saline solution and emulsified in an equal volume of Freund's incomplete adjuvant.

A volume of 50 ml of whole blood was collected from the proximal vein of the rabbit's ear 1 week after "boosting." The resulting serum was stored at 4° C until use with a final concentration of 0.1 percent added sodium azide.

Production of Preprecipitated Goat Anti-Rabbit Antiserum

Second antibody, used in the precipitation of antiserum-antigen complexes, was produced in the goat according to the procedure of Brown *et al.*[31] Goats were initially immunized with 25 mg of rabbit immunoglobulins (Rabbit Gamma Globulins, F II, Miles Laboratories) emulsified in Freund's complete adjuvant. A booster injection of 10 mg rabbit immunoglobulins emulsified in Freund's incomplete adjuvant followed the initial immunization by 3 months. One week after boosting, 300 ml of whole blood was drawn from the goat's jugular vein. The resulting serum was fractioned three times with ammonium sulfate (1.4 M) and dialyzed against PBS with 0.01 percent sodium azide. An aliquot of the goat anti-rabbit serum was then titrated against rabbit immunoglobulins to determine that proportion between the two that would bind the greatest percentage of added radioactive tracer. The rabbit immunoglobulins and goat anti-rabbit serum were then stored individually at −70° C. Twenty-four hours before use, the two were mixed at the previously determined optimal proportions and stored at 4° C to allow complete formation of preprecipitated second antibody.

Labeled Antigens

Labeled antigen was prepared by the chloramine-T method of Hunter and Greenwood,[32] with several modifications. The reaction mixture consisted of 10 μl of sodium iodide (^{125}I) in NaOH solution (100 mCi/ml, Amersham Corporation), 10 μl of analytical grade chloramine-T (1 mg/ml 0.05 M PBS), and 10 μl of purified antigen (1 μg/4 μl 0.5 M PBS, pH 7.5). After 20 to 60 seconds, the reaction was quenched with 400 μl of freshly made sodium metabisulfide (4 mg/10 ml 0.05 M PBS). The reaction mixture was then "gel-filtered" over a Sephadex G-10 column (10 cm × 1 cm) that had been pre-equilibrated with 2 to 3 ml of 2 gm percent BSA/0.05 M PBS, pH 7.5, and fractions of 0.9 ml were collected into 0.1-ml 2 gm percent BSA/0.05 M PBS. The iodinated protein peak was detected with a Searle model 1185 gamma counter. The fractions containing this peak were pooled, "vortexed," divided into aliquots of approximately 200 μl, and stored at −70° C until use.

Prothrombin Fragment 1 and 2 Standards

An initial stock of both F 1 and F 2 was prepared in 0.05 M PBS/0.1 gm percent BSA at a concentration of 100 μg/ml. From this initial stock three more stock solutions were prepared, each representing a onefold dilution of the stock from which it was made. From each of the four stock solutions four standards were prepared, each representing a 25 percent greater dilution of the stock than the preceding standard. Standards at protein concentrations giving greater than 90 percent or less than 10 percent of the value for optimal binding of iodinated protein were dropped, resulting in a standard curve made up of approximately 10 concentrations. For F 1, concentrations ranged from 25 μg/ml–100 ng/ml and for F 2 from 25 μg/ml–25 ng/ml. Prothrombin, thrombin, prethrombin 1, and F 3 standards to be used in specificity studies were prepared in a manner similar to that for F 1 and F 2.

Assay Procedure

The RIAs for both F 1 and F 2 were done under the same assay conditions. Preparatory studies indicated that optimal conditions (timing and temperature) for each incubation period were the same as those determined for F 3.[33] The initial assay mixture consisted of the following components: 100 μl of protein standard or sample biological fluid, 100 μl of iodinated protein (which provided approximately 10,000 cpm), 100 μl of antiserum (at the dilution that gives titer), and 700 μl 2.0 gm percent BSA/0.05 M PBS, pH 7.5. To increase precision, all of the aforementioned volumes were delivered with an automatic pipettor (Micromedic model #25004) and all determinations were done in triplicate. Total-count tubes (100 μl of tracer only), nonspecific binding tubes (initial assay mixture minus antiserum), and B_0 tubes (initial assay mixture minus protein sample) were a part of each assay.

Once placed in polystyrene test tubes (Sarstedt, 5 ml) the initial assay mixture was vortexed and incubated at 37° C for 30 minutes to reach an equilibrium, followed by 45 minutes in an icewater bath at 4° C. To separate bound from free antigen, 300 μl pre-precipitated goat anti-rabbit antiserum was added and the tubes were vortexed and placed in an icewater bath for another 45 minutes. A 3-ml wash of 0.05 M PBS, pH 7.5, was added to each test tube and followed by centrifugation for 30 minutes at 1200 $\times$ g and 4° C. The supernatant was then decanted and the precipitate was counted.

The standard curve was generated and unknowns were calculated with the use of a computer program (Hewlett-Packard RIA computer program #09839–75329).

Blood-drawing Procedure and Sample Preparation

Using a double-syringe venipuncture with a 19-gauge needle, whole blood was drawn from the antecubital fossae of human subjects. The first 3 ml of blood were drawn into a 5 ml syringe and discarded. The subsequent syringes were used in plasma and serum production. Plasma was prepared by mixing nine parts of whole blood and one part potassium oxalate (1.85 percent). Once blood was collected in the anticoagulant, they were mixed well and centrifuged at 1200 $\times$ g and 4° C for 30 minutes. The plasma was then separated from the cells. Plasma samples were always assayed on the day of collection and never stored frozen. For serum formation, blood was drawn in a manner similar to that for plasma. Once drawn, this whole blood was placed in sterile glass tubes at 37° C for 30 minutes. This was followed by centrifugation at 1200 $\times$ g at 4° C for 30 minutes, after which the serum was removed from the formed elements.

In timed studies of whole blood's conversion to serum, a five-component anticoagulant was used to inhibit further coagulation cascade activation at the desired time. One milliliter of this anticoagulant consisted of: 0.3 ml of EDTA (Mallinckrodt, 10 gm/dl in 0.05 M PBS), 0.3 ml of theophylline (Sigma, 340 mg/dl in 0.05 M PBS), 0.3 ml of PGE_1 (Upjohn, 1 μg/ml in 20 mg/ml sodium bicarbonate), 0.05 ml of heparin sodium (Chromalloy Pharmaceutical, 1,000 USP units/ml), and 0.05 ml of benzamidine-HCl (1.0 M). One part anticoagulant was used for every nine parts of whole blood. To assure equal distribution of the anticoagulant, a circular mixing board was used for 5 minutes after manual agitation. Mixing was followed by centrifugation for 60 minutes at 1200 $\times$ g and 4° C. As with serum, the volume of sample assayed for each RIA was 5 μl for F 1 and 25 μl for F 2.

Barium Carbonate Adsorption

Washed barium carbonate has been used throughout these studies for the removal of proteins containing γ-carboxyglutamic acid residues (prothrombin, F 1, F 1·2). In our experience, the most effective single barium carbonate adsorption occurred at concentrations of 200 mg/ml of fluid. Adsorption took place in 20 minutes on a circular mixing board followed by centrifugation at 1200 $\times$ g for 10 minutes. The supernatant was then removed from the insoluble barium.

RESULTS

RIA Development

The specificity of the F 1 antiserum in purified systems can be found in FIGURE 1. In this system, F 1 antiserum was no more specific for F 1 than for prothrombin, although it was 100 times more effective in its recognition of these substrates than towards F 2 or prethrombin 1. In biological fluids such as plasma, the ability of F 1 antiserum to recognize prothrombin decreased by 25 percent, while no corresponding decrease was noted in F 1 detection.

In a manner similar to that of F 1 antiserum, that for F 2 demonstrated approximately equal specificity for F 2 and prethrombin 1, with reduced specificity for F 1 and prothrombin, which were again similarly recognized (FIG. 2). In purified systems, F 2 and prethrombin 1 were two orders of magnitude more effective at displacing radiolabeled F 2 from F 2 antiserum than either F 1 or prothrombin. Also similar to other antisera tested was antiF 2's demonstrated increased specificity in biological fluids, such as plasma.

Antiserum Sensitivity

The sensitivity of an antiserum refers to the minimal concentration of unlabeled antigen that can be detected by the RIA. By definition, sensitivity is that concentration of unlabeled antigen that decreases radiolabeled antigen binding to 90 percent of B_0. The specificity of the F 2 antiserum was approximately 25 ng/ml (1.79 pmol/ml) (FIG. 2), which was slightly more sensitive than the lower limit of the F 1 antiserum, 100 ng/ml (4.54 pmol/ml) (FIG. 1).

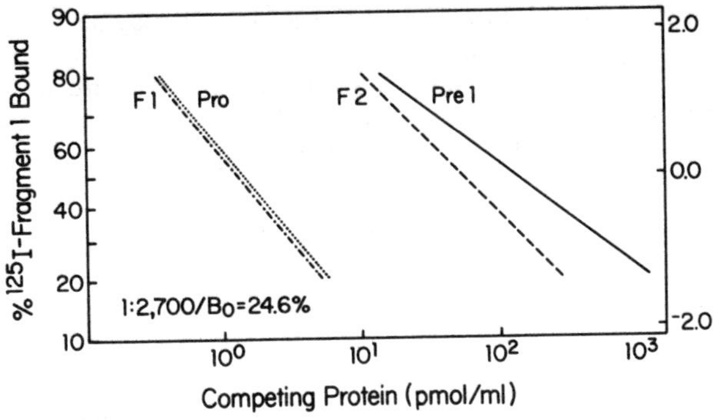

FIGURE 1. Individual standards for fragment 1 (F 1) (-·····-), prothrombin (Pro) (·····), fragment 2 (F 2) (− − −), and prethrombin 1 (Pre1) (———) were dissolved in 0.05 *M* PBS/0.1 percent BSA and triplicate tubes run over a 10-point range from 0.5–1000 pmol/ml. Iodinated F 1 (100 μl) was added to each assay tube and 100 μl of 1:2700 diluted F 1 antisera was also added. Assay conditions were as described in the text. After the counting procedure, background and nonspecific binding values were subtracted from all tubes, and each point for the Pro, F 2, and Pre 1 were computer-calculated and plotted on the basis of the F 1 standard curve. Assay sensitivity was determined to be 4.5 pmol for F 1.

Recoveries and Precision

A known amount of unlabeled antigen was added to each fluid and the RIA was used to calculate experimentally the corresponding increase in antigen concentration. The calculated value for antigen addition was then expressed as a percentage of the known value (TABLE 1). When the criterion for an acceptable RIA recovery was judged to be 100 ± 10 percent, then only the F 2 assay in urine failed to demonstrate satisfactory recovery.

Intra-assay variation was determined in seven normal serum samples as-

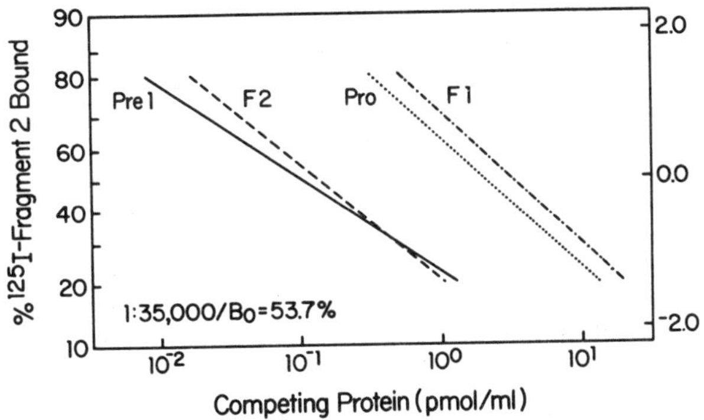

FIGURE 2. Individual standards for fragment 2 (F 2) (− − −), prethrombin 1 (Pre) 1) (———), prothrombin (Pro) (·····), and fragment 1 (F 1) (-·····-) were prepared as described for FIGURE 1, except that 100 μl of a 1:35,000 diluted F 2 antisera was added to each tube. Data processing was similar that of F 1. This assay sensitivity was determined to be 1.8 pmol at the 90 percent intercept for F 2.

sayed in quadruplicate with the F 1 and F 2 RIAs. Employing freshly iodinated products which required different antisera titers, the intra-assay procedure was repeated. The results were compared with those for the previous intra-assay study to determine the interassay variation (TABLE 1). The results of both variation studies for each RIA fell within acceptable limits.

Prothrombin Fragment Studies in Plasma

As previously mentioned, although F 1 immunoreactive material was found in plasma (283 pmol/ml), no corresponding F 2 could be detected. It appeared unlikely that free F 1 (or F 1·2) could exist at substantial levels in plasma when F 2 immunoreactive material (F 2, F 1·2, prethrombin 1) could not be detected at a concentration of at least 1.79 pmol/ml (sensitivity limits of the assay). This led us to conclude that the F 1 immunoreactive material in plasma was cross-reacting prothrombin.

Prothrombin Fragment Studies in Urine

Quantitation of prothrombin fragment levels in urine began with the collection of early morning urine specimens from normal individuals. The concentrations of prothrombin fragments in these samples, as determined by RIA, can be observed in TABLE 2. The usefulness of the F 1 levels from these random specimens is limited without a knowledge of the accompanying urinary output and some standardization of collection. For this reason, 24-hour urinary output was collected from four volunteers. At the end of collection, the total urinary outputs were measured, as were the F 1 concentrations, and excretion rates per 24 hours were determined from these (TABLE 3). Similar calculations for F 2 were not undertaken because of the poor recovery performance of F 2 antiserum in urine.

Prothrombin Fragment Studies in Serum

RIAs for F 1 and F 2 were performed on serum samples from normal volunteers. These serum samples were used to establish the normal concentration of fragments in sera at 23.2 µg/ml for F 1 and 14.1 µg/ml for F 2 (TABLE 4). Using these serum values for F 1 and F 2, and calculating the percentage of the entire prothrombin mass represented respectively by F 1 and F 2, and assuming quantitative conversion of prothrombin to the fragments and their complete recovery, we used these values to calculate a plasma prothrombin concentration of 77.0 µg/ml (using F 1 data) and 74.7 µg/ml (using F 2 data). Furthermore, several normal serum samples and a serum pool, consisting of the specimens used to establish normal values, were treated with *Echis carinatus* venom to determine the amount of remaining thrombin precursor (TABLE 5). Significant concentrations of residual prothrombin or prethrombin were not detected.

A clinical condition found to be associated with abnormal bioactive prothrombin levels in plasma is that caused by coumarin therapy. In studies with serum from recipients of dicumarol, a highly significant decrease ($p < 0.005$)

TABLE 1

PROTHROMBIN FRAGMENT RECOVERIES IN BIOLOGICAL FLUIDS

Biological Fluid	Fragment 1 Recovery	Fragment 2 Recovery
Serum	108.9%	101.8%
Plasma	92.8%	96.2%
Urine	92.7%	65.6%
Serum		
Intra-assay variance	5.55%	4.63%
Interassay variance	11.01%	9.31%

TABLE 2

PROTHROMBIN FRAGMENTS IN RANDOM EARLY-MORNING URINE SAMPLES

Sample No.	Fragment 1 Concentration (nmol/ml)*	Fragment 2 Concentration (nmol/ml)*
1	0.022	ND †
2	0.032	0.006
3	0.015	0.004
4	0.009	ND
5	0.009	ND
6	0.022	ND
7	0.026	ND
8	0.004	ND
9	0.007	ND
10	0.019	0.006
11	0.003	ND
12	0.022	ND
13	0.004	ND
14	0.018	ND
15	0.009	ND
16	0.019	ND
17	0.020	ND
18	0.004	ND
19	0.019	ND
20	0.021	ND
21	0.034	0.021
22	0.019	ND
23	0.026	ND
24	0.009	ND
25	0.014	ND
26	0.014	ND
27	0.013	ND
28	0.029	ND
29	0.034	0.002

* No correction has been made for the individual urinary volumes.
† In these samples, no detectable quantity of fragment 2 was noted.

TABLE 3

24-HOUR URINARY EXCRETION OF FRAGMENT 1

Subject	24-Hour Output	Fragment 1 Concentration	Fragment 1 24-Hour Output
1	755 ml	16.36 pmol/ml	12.68 nmol
2	1060 ml	5.45 pmol/ml	5.78 nmol
3	1035 ml	7.73 pmol/ml	8.00 nmol
4	895 ml	18.64 pmol/ml	16.68 nmol

TABLE 4

NORMAL PROTHROMBIN FRAGMENT LEVELS IN SERUM

Prothrombin Fragment	N *	Mean Serum Concentration	Standard Deviation	Standard Error of the Mean
F 1	22	23.20 μg/ml	5.47	1.17
F 2	35	14.09 μg/ml	3.08	0.52

* The number of individual serum samples used to determine the fragment concentrations.

TABLE 5

PROTHROMBIN FRAGMENT 2 CONCENTRATION IN HUMAN SERUM
BEFORE AND AFTER
TREATMENT WITH *Echis carinatus* VENOM

Sample	F 2 Concentration Before *E. carinatus* Treatment	F 2 Concentration After *E. carinatus* Treatment *
#1	10.22 μg/ml	10.83 μg/ml
#2	10.83 μg/ml	11.73 μg/ml
#3	11.65 μg/ml	12.81 μg/ml
#4	10.90 μg/ml	9.63 μg/ml
#5	11.93 μg/ml	12.78 μg/ml
#6	11.28 μg/ml	11.97 μg/ml
Pooled Serum	11.14 μg/ml	11.75 μg/ml

* Individual serum samples were incubated at 37° C for 60 minutes in the presence of 50 μg/ml crude venom and 0.025 M CaCl$_2$. Control (pretreatment) samples were incubated with a similar amount of RVV and calcium.

was found in F 2 concentrations (TABLE 6). The extent of this decrease was found to have no correlation with the degree of prothrombin time (PT) prolongation (Pearson's r not significant at 0.05), the clinical means whereby coumarin's effectiveness as an anticoagulant is monitored.

Prothrombin Fragment Generation in Whole Blood's Conversion to Serum

By means of the F 2 RIA before and after barium carbonate adsorption, F 2 and F 1·2 were monitored during the conversion of whole blood to serum

TABLE 6

A COMPARISON OF PROTHROMBIN TIME AND SERUM FRAGMENT 2 LEVELS
IN PATIENTS RECEIVING DICUMAROL

| Patient | Prothrombin Time Determination | | F 2 Concentration (μg/ml) |
	Value for Patient	Standard Normal Plasma	
1	26.0	11.0	2.61
2	22.0	11.1	3.12
3	15.0	11.6	3.25
4	25.6	11.1	3.60
5	23.3	11.3	3.84
6	15.2	10.9	4.63
7	21.0	10.9	4.81
8	22.2	11.1	5.13
9	25.0	11.2	5.22
10	25.7	11.5	5.46
11	19.7	11.7	5.48
12	23.1	11.2	5.69
13	11.4	11.4	6.08
14	30.5	10.9	6.28
15	17.3	11.3	6.37
16	14.2	11.0	6.61
17	31.5	11.4	6.96
18	19.4	11.3	7.10
19	15.6	12.0	7.77
20	25.1	11.2	8.63
21	11.5	10.9	8.86
22	15.0	12.0	9.44
23	11.8	11.4	12.80

(FIG. 3). Simultaneously, platelet release was followed by means of an RIA for the release protein β-thromboglobulin (β-TG).[34]

The only nonthrombin fragment noted prior to clot formation was F 1·2, whose levels were found to appear and increase between 0 and 9 minutes. Concurrently, a detectable increase in platelet release of β-TG was first observed between 2 and 4 minutes after the blood was drawn. These levels continued to rise for the following 4 to 6 minutes, at which point the concentration of platelet release protein became greater than we were prepared to measure.

Clot formation took place at 9 minutes after the blood was drawn. If we assume a normal plasma prothrombin concentration of 75 μg/ml, F 1·2 levels at 9 minutes represent only 9.86 percent of total prothrombin concentration activated in initiating clot formation. This percentage is consistent with the findings from similar studies performed in this laboratory.

Free F 2 levels (nonadsorbed by barium carbonate) were first detected at 1 minute after clot formation and they increased for the remainder of the study. F 1·2 levels continued to increase after clot formation until 20 minutes after the blood was drawn, at which point a decrease in concentration over the next 5 minutes was observed. Thus, from 20 to 25 minutes after the blood was drawn, free F 2 levels increased, F 1·2 decreased, and the molar concentration of prothrombin fragment 2 immunoreactive material did not significantly change.

That the F 2 immunoreactive material removed by barium adsorption was F 1·2 was determined by the addition of saline solution (control), thrombin, or factor Xa to serum samples (TABLE 7). Addition was followed by incubation at 37° C for 30 minutes. The barium-adsorbable F 2 immunoreactive material of the control sample was no longer adsorbed upon pretreatment of the serum with excess thrombin. Furthermore, addition of factor Xa to serum had no effect on this same pool of F 2 immunoreactive material, in disagreement with the findings of other reports.[25, 26]

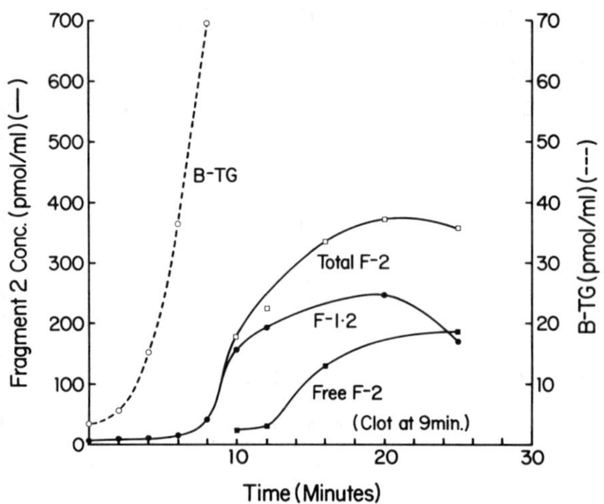

FIGURE 3. Human blood was placed in glass test tubes at 37° C. Measurements made were for β-thromboglobulin (β-TG), total prothrombin fragment 2 immunoreactive material, and prothrombin fragment 2 immunoreactive material after adsorbing serum with barium carbonate (free F 2). Subtracting the free F 2 value from total F 2 value gave the curve for F 1·2. It is likely that the effects of thrombin were in the given order: (a) release of β-thromboglobulin; (b) formation of fibrin; and (c) cleavage of F 1·2 and/or prothrombin to form free F 2 substance (F 2 or prethrombin 1). Free F 2 and prethrombin 1 do not form before clotting.

TABLE 7

CHARACTERIZATION OF SERUM PROTHROMBIN FRAGMENT 2
IMMUNOREACTIVE MATERIAL

| | BaCO$_3$ Adsorption | |
Conditions	Before *	After †
Serum + saline solution	1.217 nmol/ml	0.122 nmol/ml
Serum + factor Xa	1.193 nmol/ml	0.125 nmol/ml
Serum + thrombin	1.231 nmol/ml	1.114 nmol/ml

* The concentration of fragment 2 in fresh serum immediately prior to a 5-minute mix with solid barium carbonate.

† Incubation of fresh serum for 30 minutes at 37° C with saline solution, factor Xa (final concentration, 20 u/ml), or thrombin (10 u/ml) prior to barium adsorption. Net decrease after adsorption indicates that fragment 2 is present as F1·2 and not the free fragment.

DISCUSSION

It was necessary to establish normal F 1 and F 2 concentrations before attempting to isolate clinical conditions in which there are significant deviations from normal serum levels. The established normal serum F 1 and F 2 concentrations appear reliable in that the treatment of normal serum samples and a serum pool (consisting of those specimens used in the establishment of normal values) with *Echis carinatus* venom failed to increase significantly prothrombin fragment levels. It was therefore concluded that complete prothrombin consumption occurred in the formation of the serum samples used to establish normal values. The reliability of normal serum F 1 and F 2 concentrations is further supported by the fact that both represent a plasma prothrombin concentration of approximately 75 μg/ml.

The reduction in serum prothrombin fragments found in persons receiving dicumerol was a result of decreased pathway effectiveness in prothrombin activation as well as a decreased activational ability of the prothrombin substrate. The former will occur before the latter because of the shorter plasma half-life of factors VII, IX and X compared with that of factor II. Regardless of the varying plasma half-lives of vitamin K-dependent factors, a negative correlation between serum F 2 reductions and prothrombin time prolongation would be expected in persons receiving dicumerol if prothrombin was the rate-limiting zymogen in prothrombin time determination. That no such correlation was found suggests that one of the other clotting factors is rate-limiting. Secondly, in TABLE 6 samples 1 and 6 were drawn from the same patient (patient #1) at different times, while samples 17 and 18 were drawn from a different individual (patient #2). The two prothrombin time determinations for each individual differed considerably from one another, while the serum F 2 levels were quite consistent. Concurrently, in spite of both patients' having similar prothrombin times (patient #2's were slightly more prolonged), patient #1's F 2 levels (<33 percent of normal) were lower than patient #2's levels (approximately 50 percent of normal). One possible interpretation of this and similar data from this laboratory suggests that the degree to which dicumerol affects the different vitamin K-dependent proteins varies from person to person.

Timed studies of prothrombin fragment generation in whole blood's conversion to serum provided information from which several conclusions were drawn regarding normal prothrombin activation. An important point noted in these studies was that the only nonthrombin fragment detected prior to clot formation was F 1·2, which appeared and increased in concentration over the time period from 0 to 9 minutes after the blood was drawn. This was interpreted to indicate that low concentrations of thrombin were present prior to clot formation and were at least partially responsible for the platelet release noted. Through its action on fibrinogen, thrombin was responsible for the clot formation that follows platelet release, and through its action on prothrombin and/or F 1·2, it was solely responsible for the generation of the free F 2 which followed clot formation. Thus, we have some evidence from thrombin affinities in this system: platelet > fibrinogen > prothrombin and/or F 1·2. This finding is supported by studies which have established the same order of thrombin affinities in purified systems.[19, 20] Increased circulating levels of platelet release proteins have been cited in the literature as an early indication of hypercoagulable states.[34–36] By contrast, there is lack of such findings in the case of free prothrombin fragments in plasma. In consideration of this and the aforementioned thrombin affinities, it appears that an increase in circulating platelet release proteins is a more sensitive indicator of the early presence of thrombin in plasma than are assays for prothrombin fragments.

Since F 1·2 was the only nonthrombin fragment found prior to clot formation, we can conclude that the alternate pathway of thrombin formation from prothrombin (with prethrombin 1 as an intermediate) plays no role in initiating or controlling clot formation.

Finally, free prothrombin fragment 2 was not detected until 1 minute after clot formation, then it increased for the remainder of the study. The fact that F 1·2 levels decreased from 20 to 25 minutes after the initial drawing of blood while the concentration of F 2 immunoreactive material did not change led to the conclusion that F 1·2 hydrolysis by thrombin was the sole source of free F 2. In light of our data, it is interesting to note that Aronson et al.[22] concluded that hydrolysis of prothrombin by thrombin was slower in purified systems relative to similar hydrolysis of F 1·2.

Studies on the possible existence of prothrombin fragments in plasma required an understanding of the assay's performance in order to determine that no proof for a normal prothrombin metabolism through activation could be found. If such a postulated type of metabolism normally exists, the inability to detect prothrombin fragments in plasma by RIA could be interpreted to suggest a basal rate of prothrombin activation too slow to produce detectable levels of prothrombin fragments (<1.79 pmol/ml). Further understanding of possible normal prothrombin metabolism through activation came from studies of urinary prothrombin fragments.

In both 24-hour and randomly collected urine specimens, small but quantifiable concentrations of F 1 immunoreactive material were found. In view of the poor glomerular filtration of a molecule the size of prothrombin and the fact that investigators employing different techniques have failed to detect prothrombin in urine,[37] it appears unlikely that F 1 immunoreactive material in urine represents prothrombin.

Plasma prothrombin has a normal half-life of 55 to 80 hours.[37] The F 1 immunoreactive material that we have detected in urine thus represents approximately 0.76 to 2.00 percent of normal prothrombin consumption. There are several interpretations of these data. First, it may be that the larger number of instances of prothrombin degradation occur in such a way that the generated fragments, if found in urine, are not immunologically recognizable as F 1 or F 2. This concept may be supported by studies in which it has been concluded that activation plays a minor role in normal prothrombin metabolism.[37] In these same studies no circulating levels of prothrombin catabolic products could be found. Thus, it appears likely that most prothrombin metabolism occurs in a limited location, which prevents circulatory release of catabolic products. Shapiro and Martinez[37] have found, after the introduction of radiolabeled prothrombin to the circulation of normal subjects, that radioactivity appeared in the urine at the same rate that iodinated prothrombin was cleared from plasma. Another interpretation of our detection of such low levels of F 1 and F 2 in urine is possible in view of such a finding. It is conceivable that the isotope was stripped from prothrombin and excreted through normal kidney function, whereas prothrombin degradation products, which may or may not be immunologically recognized as F 1 and F 2, were dealt with in another manner.

Unlike F 1, urinary F 2 immunoreactive material only appears to exist in some specimens. Poor F 2 recoveries in urine make it difficult to quantitate these levels, much less to understand the circumstances under which they may be detected. Consequently, only the F 1 RIA could be employed to screen randomly selected urine specimens. In such preliminary studies, diuretics and physical exercise appeared effective at increasing urinary F 1 levels.

ACKNOWLEDGMENTS

The expert assistance of June Snow and Debra McKinley is gratefully acknowledged.

REFERENCES

1. SEEGERS, W. H., H. I. HASSOUNA, D. HEWETT-EMMETT & D. A. WALZ. 1975. Prothrombin and thrombin. Selected aspects of thrombin formation, properties, inhibition and immunology. Semin. Thromb. Hemostas. **1:** 211–283.
2. DAVIE, E. W. & K. FUJIKAWA. 1975. Basic mechanisms in blood coagulation. Ann. Rev. Biochem. **44:** 799–829.
3. SUTTIE, J. W. & C. M. JACKSON. 1977. Prothrombin structure, activation, and biosynthesis. Physiol. Rev. **57:** 1–70.
4. ARONSON, D. L. & D. MENACHE. 1966. Chromatographic analysis of the activation of human prothrombin with human thrombokinase. Biochemistry **8:** 2635–2640.
5. ARONSON, D. L. 1965. N-terminal amino acids formed during the activation of prothrombin. Nature **194:** 475–476.
6. ARONSON, D. L. 1966. Chromatographic differentiation of human prothrombin. Thromb. Diath. Haemorrh. **16:** 491–496.
7. LANCHANTIN, G. F., J. A. FRIEDMANN & D. W. HART. 1968. On the occurrence of polymorphic human prothrombin. Electrophoretic and chromatographic alterations of the molecule due to the action of thrombin. J. Biol. Chem. **243:** 476–486.
8. DOWNING, M. R., R. J. BUTKOWSKI, M. M. CLARK & K. G. MANN. 1975. Human prothrombin activation. J. Biol. Chem. **250:** 8897–8906.

9. KISIEL, W. & D. J. HANAHAN. 1973. Purification and characterization of human Factor II. Biochim. Biophys. Acta **304:** 103–113.

10. KISIEL, W. & D. J. HANAHAN. 1973. The action of Factor Xa, thrombin, and trypsin on human Factor II. Biochim. Biophys. Acta **329:** 221–232.

11. KISIEL, W. & D. J. HANAHAN. 1974. Proteolysis of human Factor II by Factor Xa in the presence of hirudin. Biochem. Biophys. Res. Commun. **59:** 570–577.

12. LANCHANTIN, G. F., J. A. FRIEDMAN & D. W. HART. 1969. Interaction of soybean trypsin inhibitor with thrombin and its effect on prothrombin activation. J. Biol. Chem. **244:** 865–875.

13. ROSENBERG, J. S., D. L. BEELER & R. D. ROSENBERG. 1975. Activation of human prothrombin by highly purified human Factors V and Xa in the presence of human antithrombin. J. Biol. Chem. **250:** 1607–1617.

14. WALZ, D. A. & W. H. SEEGERS. 1974. Amino acid sequence of human thrombin A chain. Biochem. Biophys. Res. Commun. **60:** 717–722.

15. WALZ, D. A., D. HEWETT-EMMETT, J. REUTERBY & W. H. SEEGERS. 1976. Human thrombin: Amino acid sequence of the autocatalytically removed 13 residue A 1 peptide. Thromb. Res. **9:** 289–292.

16. WALZ, D. A., D. HEWETT-EMMETT & W. H. SEEGERS. 1977. Primary structure of the amino-terminal (vitamin K-dependent) region of human prothrombin. Life Sci. **20:** 79–84.

17. WALZ, D. A., D. HEWETT-EMMETT & W. H. SEEGERS. 1977. Amino acid sequence of human prothrombin fragments 1 and 2. Proc. Natl. Acad. Sci. USA **74:** 1969–1972.

18. BUTKOWSKI, R. J., J. ELION, M. R. DOWNING & K. G. MANN. 1977. The primary structure of human prethrombin 2 and α-thrombin. J. Biol. Chem. **252:** 4942–4957.

19. FENTON, J. W., B. H. LANDIS, D. A. WALZ & J. S. FINLAYSON. 1977. Human thrombins. *In* Chemistry and Biology of Thrombin. R. L. Lundblad, J. W. Fenton and K. G. Mann, Eds.: 43–70. Ann Arbor Science. Ann Arbor, MI.

20. FENTON, J. W., B. H. LANDIS, D. A. WALZ, D. H. BING, R. D. FEINMAN, M. P. ZABINSKI, S. A. SONDER, L. J. BERLINER & J. S. FINLAYSON. 1979. Human thrombin: Preparative evaluation, structural properties, and enzyme specificity. *In* The Chemistry and Physiology of Human Plasma Proteins. D. H. Bing, Ed.: 151–184. Pergamon Press. New York.

21. SHAPIRO, S. S. & J. COOPER. 1968. Biological activation of radioactive human prothrombin. Fed. Proc. **27:** 628.

22. ARONSON, D. L., L. STEVAN, A. P. BALL, B. R. FRANZA & J. S. FINLAYSON. 1977. Generation of the combined prothrombin activation peptide (F 1·2) during the clotting of blood and plasma. J. Clin. Invest. **60:** 1410–1418.

23. SHUMAN, M. A. & P. W. MAJERUS. 1976. The measurement of thrombin activity in clotting blood by radioimmunoassay. J. Clin. Invest. **58:** 1249–1258.

24. LOX, C. D., G. H. STROHM & J. J. CORRIGAN. 1978. Radioimmunoassay of human prothrombin: The quantitation of plasma factor II antigen. Am. J. Hematol. **4:** 261–268.

25. LAU, H. K., J. S. ROSENBERG, D. L. BEELER & R. D. ROSENBERG. 1979. The isolation and characterization of a specific antibody population directed against the prothrombin activation fragments F 2 and F 1·2. J. Biol. Chem. **254:** 8751–8761.

26. ROSENBERG, R. D. This conference.

27. MCDUFFIE, F. C., C. GRIFFIN, R. NIEDRINGHAUS, K. G. MANN, C. A OWEN, E. J. W. BOWIE, J. PETERSON, G. CLARK & G. G. HUNDER. 1979. Prothrombin, thrombin and prothrombin fragments in plasma of normal individuals and of patients with laboratory evidence of disseminated intravascular coagulation. Thromb. Res. **16:** 759–774.

28. BEZEAUD, A., D. L. ARONSON, D. MENACHE & M. C. GUILLIN. 1978. Identifica-

tion of a prothrombin derivative in human urine. Thromb. Res. **13:** 551–556.

29. NOVOA, E., W. H. SEEGERS & H. I. HASSOUNA. 1976. Improved procedures for the purification of selected vitamin K-dependent proteins. Prep. Biochem. **6:** 307–338.

30. VAITUKAITIS, J., J. B. ROBBINS, E. NIESCHLAG & G. T. ROSS. 1971. A method for producing specific antisera with small doses of immunogen. J. Clin. Endocrinol. Metab. **33:** 988–991.

31. BROWN, T. R., N. BAGCHI, T. T. S. HO & R. E. MACK. 1980. Preprecipitated and solid-phase second antibody compared in radioimmunoassays. Clin. Chem. **26:** 503–507.

32. HUNTER, W. M. & F. C. GREENWOOD. 1962. Preparation of iodine-131 labeled human growth hormone of high specific activity. Nature **194:** 495–496.

33. WALZ, D. A. & T. R. BROWN. 1980. Human prothrombin activation: Radioimmunoassay of fragment 3. *In* Vitamin K Metabolism and Vitamin K-Dependent Proteins. J. W. Suttie, Ed.: 116–120. University Park Press. Baltimore, MD.

34. BROWN, T. R., T. T. S. HO & D. A. WALZ. 1980. Improved radioimmunoassay of platelet factor 4 and β-thromboglobulin in plasma. Clin. Chim. Acta **101:** 225–233.

35. KAPLAN, K. L., M. J. BROEKMAN, A. CHERNOFF, G. R. LESNIK & M. DRILLINGS. 1979. Platelet α-granule proteins: Studies on release and subcellular localization. Blood **53:** 604–618.

36. GERRARD, J. M., D. R. PHILLIPS, G. H. R. RAO, E. F. PLOW, D. A. WALZ, R. ROSS, L. A. HARKER & J. G. WHITE. 1980. Biochemical studies of two patients with the gray platelet syndrome: Selective deficiency of platelet alpha granules. J. Clin. Invest. **66:** 102–109.

37. SHAPIRO, S. S. & J. MARTINEZ. 1969. Human prothrombin metabolism in normal man and in hypercoagulable subjects. J. Clin. Invest. **48:** 1292–1298.

CHARACTERIZATION OF A VARIANT OF HUMAN PROTHROMBIN: PROTHROMBIN MADRID

Marie-Claude Guillin and Annie Bezeaud

Service Central d'Immunologie et Hématologie
Hôpital Beaujon
92110, Clichy, France
Departement d'Hématologie
Faculté Xavier Bichat
75018, Paris, France

INTRODUCTION

Under physiological conditions, conversion of human prothrombin to thrombin is catalyzed by a proteolytic enzyme, activated factor X (Xa). Factor Xa is responsible for two cleavages,[1-3] which are, as for bovine prothrombin,[4] both necessary and sufficient for thrombin formation: the first cleavage at Arg^{274}-Thr splits prothrombin into fragment 1·2 and prethrombin 2; the second cleavage at Arg^{323}-Ile yields enzymatically active thrombin, constituted of two disulfide-bridged polypeptide chains (A and B chains). Three other peptide bond cleavages are due to autoproteolysis of prothrombin (and/or its activation products) by thrombin; cleavage at Arg^{156}-Ser splits off the amino terminal fragment, fragment 1;[1-3] cleavage at Arg^{287}-Thr splits off a 13 amino acid fragment, fragment 3;[3] an unidentified peptide bond is cleaved on fragment 1, yielding the two polypeptide chains fragment 1'.[5] However, the physiological importance of these thrombin-induced cleavages is questionable since it has been reported that the reaction does not occur to an appreciable extent in whole blood.[6,7] Cleavage of prothrombin by factor Xa alone proceeds very slowly but is dramatically accelerated through the binding of both prothrombin and Xa to phospholipids [8-10] and to factor Va.[11-13] Two regions of prothrombin are involved in the acceleration of factor Xa action by these accessory factors: the fragment 1 region functions in the binding of prothrombin of phospholipids via calcium ions;[14,15] the fragment 2 region is necessary for prothrombin binding to factor Va.[12,16]

Nine variants of human prothrombin [17-27] have been reported. Although in none of the cases the structural defect is known, the functional defect has been related in one case [26] to an abnormality in the active site of the zymogen, and, in another case [27] to an impairment of factor Xa enzymatic action at the bond linking the propart of the molecule and the thrombin moiety. We have previously reported [25] a case of congenital abnormality of prothrombin, designated prothrombin Madrid, detected in a Spanish family, the propositus being homozygote and her parents heterozygotes. Conversion of prothrombin Madrid by physiological activators or Taïpan snake venom was shown to proceed slowly whereas both functional activity assayed with either *Echis carinatus* or *Dispholidus typus* venoms, and immunological reactivity were found to be normal. Molecular weight of prothrombin Madrid did not appear to be significantly different from normal as assessed by SDS polyacrylamide gel electrophoresis. The present report deals with further characterization of the

414

functional defect of prothrombin Madrid and the attempts made for locating the structural abnormality.

MATERIAL AND METHODS

Prothrombin was isolated as previously described [25] from fresh frozen acid citrate dextrose plasma obtained by plasmapheresis from a normal donor and the propositus. Specific activity of prothrombin preparations, when determined using a two-stage assay with *Dispholidus typus* venom as activator,[28] was in the range of 750 to 850 US units/mg. When determined using a two-stage assay with physiological activators,[25] the range of specific activity of these preparations was 1,100 to 1,300 US units/mg for normal prothrombin and 120 to 130 US units/mg for prothrombin Madrid.

Prothrombin activation was studied using the following material: purified bovine factor Xa, purified bovine factor Va (both were supplied by C. M. Jackson, Washington University, School of Medicine, Saint Louis, MO), crude human brain cephalin, prepared according to Bell and Alton,[29] *Oxyuranus scutellatus scutellatus* (Taïpan snake) venom (crude venom from Sigma Chemical Co., Saint Louis, MO) and the coagulant principle isolated from *Dispholidus typus* venom as previously described.[28]

Thrombin clotting activity was determined by the enzyme ability to clot human purified fibrinogen and expressed as US thrombin units, using human thrombin (lot B3, supplied by Dr. D. L. Aronson, Bureau of Biologics, Food and Drug Administration, Bethesda, MD) for the calibration curve. Amidolytic activity of thrombin and thrombin-like enzymes was determined spectrophotometrically using the chromogenic substrate S 2238 (Kabi Diagnostica, Stockholm, Sweden) according to the instructions of the manufacturer.

Gel electrophoresis in the presence of sodium dodecyl sulfate was performed according to Weber and Osborn [30] in 10% w/v acrylamide 0.1% w/v SDS. A current of 8 mA per gel was applied for 3 hours. Gels were stained with Coomassie blue and destained electrophoretically. Each gel was scanned at 540 nm in a Gilford Model 240 Spectrophotometer equiped with a Model 2410 linear transport accessory. Mobility of each protein was determined from the densitometry tracing and its molecular weight (mol. wt.) calculated from a linear semi-logarithmic plot of molecular weight versus mobility, drawn with six standard proteins purchased from Sigma Chemical Co., Saint Louis, MO (bovine serum albumin, fumarase, carboxypeptidase A, soybean trypsin inhibitor, myoglobin, lysosyme).

EXPERIMENTS AND RESULTS

In order to determine if the functional defect of prothrombin Madrid was related to an impairment of factor Xa enzymatic action or to a lack of acceleration of the reaction by accessory components, normal prothrombin and prothrombin Madrid have been activated with factor Xa, in the presence of calcium ions, and either in the absence or presence of phospholipids or phospholipids plus factor Va (TABLE 1). The reaction rate was determined by assaying thrombin clotting activity at 5-min intervals for 60 min when the activator consisted of either factor Xa and calcium (experiment 1), or factor Xa, calcium and phospholipids (experiment 2), and at 1-min intervals for 8 min when the activator consisted of factor Xa, calcium, phospholipids and factor Va (experiment 3). Under the conditions used, linearity of the thrombin generation rate over a period of 30 min in experiment 1, 15 min in experiment 2, and 5 min in experiment 3, permitted determination of the initial reaction rates in each case. The enhancement of the reaction rate by phospholipids (experiment 2) or phospholipids plus factor Va (experiment 3) was calculated as the initial rate in experiments 2 or 3 divided by the initial rate in experiment 1. Results obtained showed that upon the addition of factor Xa, prothrombin Madrid activation was slower than normal. When prothrombin Madrid activation by factor Xa proceeded in the additional presence of phospholipids or phospholipids plus factor Va, the reaction rate was persistently slower than normal, but the rate

TABLE 1

PROTHROMBIN ACTIVATION BY FACTOR XA

(Initial reaction rate and acceleration of the reaction by phospholipids (PL) and factor Va)

Experiment Reactants	1 Xa, Ca^{2+}	2 Xa, Ca^{2+}, PL	3 Xa, Ca^{2+}, PL, Va
Initial reaction rate (US units/mg/mn)			
Normal prothrombin	0.300	3,30	2 100
Prothrombin Madrid	0.023	0.32	207
Rate enhancement			
Normal prothrombin	1	11	7 000
Prothrombin Madrid	1	14	9 000

Normal or abnormal prothrombin (1 mg in 1 ml 0.05 M NaCl 0.01 M $CaCl_2$/0.02 M Tris HCl, pH 7.5) was incubated at 20°C with Xa (6.5 μg in experiments 1 and 2, 0.65 μg in experiment 3), human brain cephalin (50 μg) in experiments 2 and 3, Va (16 U) in experiment 3. The number obtained in experiment 3 had to be multiplied by 10 as the proteolytic enzyme concentration was 10-fold less than in experiments 1 and 2. (This was required so that the rate of thrombin production was sufficiently slowed to permit sequential analysis by manual sampling and clotting times measurements).

enhancement by either phospholipids or phospholipids plus factor Va was normal.

Determination of amidolytic activity generation was performed in parallel with the determination of clotting activity generation during the incubation course of prothrombin with various activators (FIG. 1). Upon the action of either factor Xa (FIG. 1a, d) or Taïpan snake venom (FIG. 1b, e), the rate of amidolytic activity production by prothrombin Madrid was grossly similar to that obtained with normal prothrombin, while the rate of clotting activity production was much slower. In contrast, when prothrombin Madrid was activated by *Dispholidus typus* venom (FIG. 1c, f) the appearance rate of both clotting activity and amidolytic activity was normal.

The activation products obtained from prothrombin Madrid upon the action of factor Xa, were analyzed by SDS polyacrylamide gel electrophoresis and

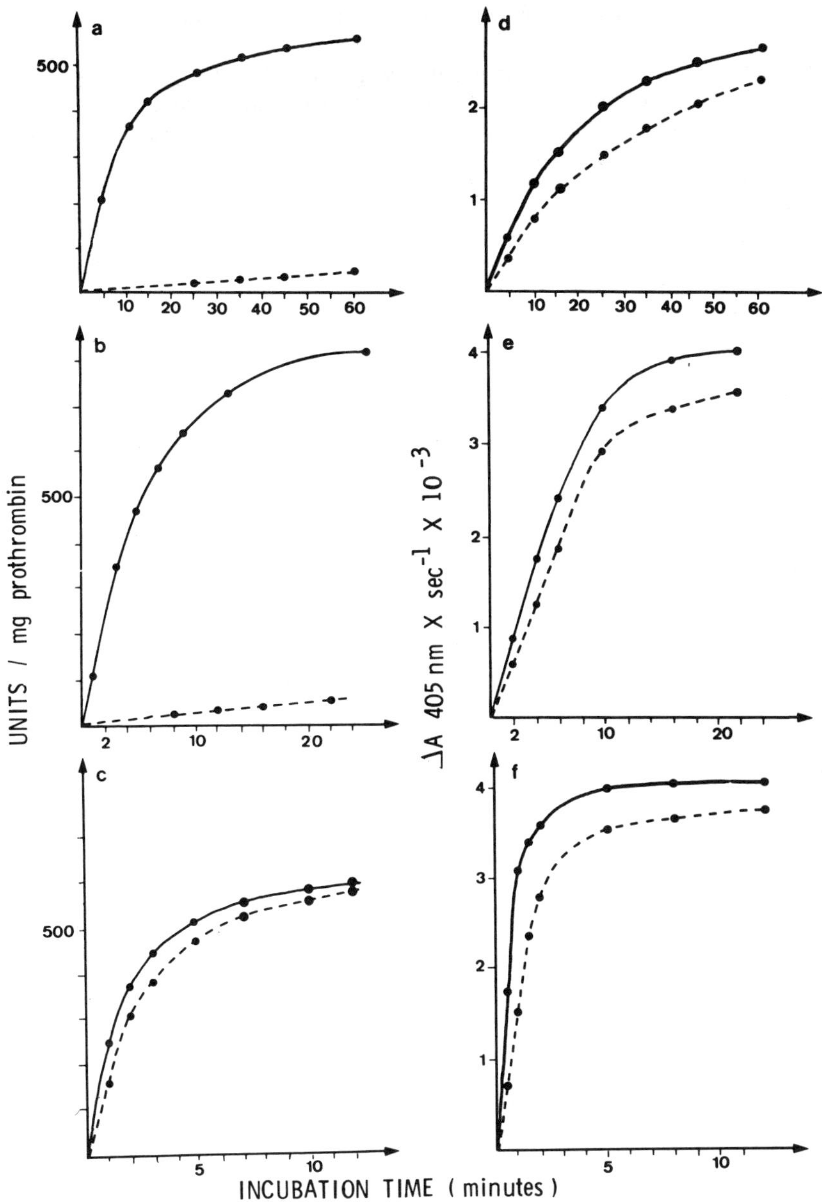

FIGURE 1. Generation of clotting activity and amidolytic activity upon the action of various prothrombin activators. *Upper panel* (**a** and **d**); 10 μg prothrombin were incubated with 0.1 unit factor Xa, and 50 μg human brain cephalin in one ml 0.05 M NaCl 0.01 M $CaCl_2$/0.02 M Tris-HCl, pH 7.5. *Middle panel* (**b** and **e**): 10 μg prothrombin were incubated with 0.1 μg Taïpan snake venom and 50 μg cephalin in one ml 0.05 M NaCl 0.01 M $CaCl_2$/0.02 M Tris-HCl, pH 7.5. *Lower panel* (**c** and **f**) : 10 μg prothrombin were incubated with 0.01 μg *Dispholidus typus* venom in one ml 0.05 M NaCl/0.02 M Tris-HCl, pH 7.5. **a**, **b** and **c**:clotting activity. **d**, **e** and **f** : amidolytic activity, assayed using the chromogenic substrate S 2238. ———— Normal prothrombin. – – – –, prothrombin Madrid.

identified according to their molecular weight and their behavior upon disulfide bonds reduction (FIG. 2). After 8 hours incubation with factor Xa in the presence of calcium and phospholipids, normal prothrombin was fully activated, giving rise to thrombin (mol. wt. 38,000, composed of chain B, mol. wt. 32,000, and chain A, not visible on the gel), fragment 1 (mol. wt. 28,000, one polypeptide chain), fragment 1' (mol. wt. 28,000, composed of subfragment β, mol. wt. 21,000, and subfragment α, not visible on the gel), and fragment 2 (mol. wt. 17,000, one polypeptide chain). Under the same experimental conditions, prothrombin Madrid yielded 30% of the thrombin clotting activity

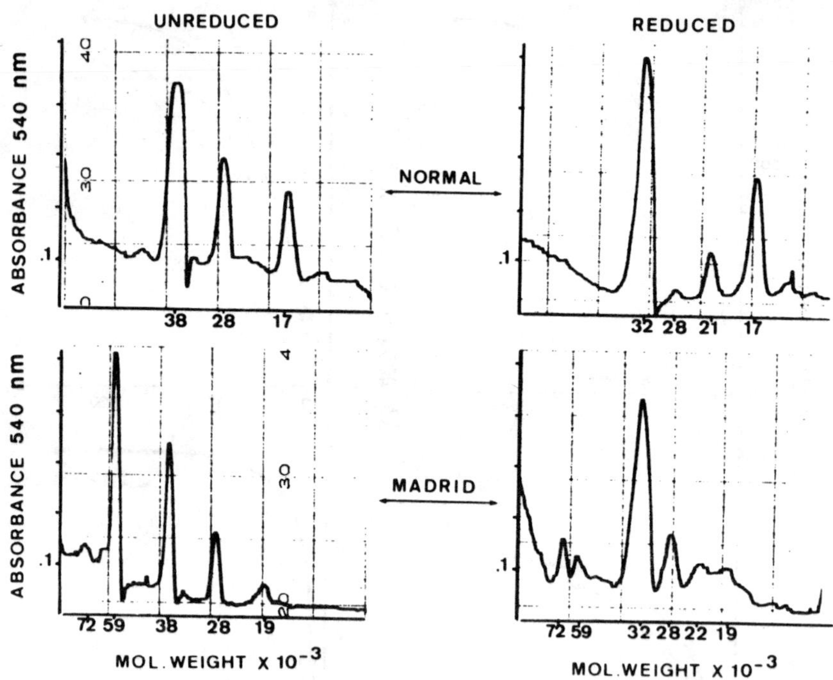

FIGURE 2. Prothrombin activation by factor Xa : densitometric scan of SDS gels. 100 μg of normal prothrombin (*top*) or prothrombin Madrid (*bottom*) were incubated at 20°C with 1 unit Xa and 5 μg human brain cephalin in 100 μl 0.05 M NaCl 0.01 M CaCl₂/0.02 M Tris-HCl, pH 7.5, for 8 hours, then diluted in 0.01 M sodium phosphate, pH 7, 1% SDS (unreduced samples) or in 0.01 M sodium phosphate, pH 7, 1% SDS 1% 2-mercaptoethanol (reduced samples) and submitted to gel electrophoresis.

generated by normal prothrombin. In addition to thrombin and fragment 1, a major proteolysis product of molecular weight 59,000 was obtained (FIG. 2). Since upon reduction the 59,000-dalton band disappeared almost completely, while on the one hand, the intensity of the 32,000-dalton band was more than expected from the amount of thrombin formed and, on the other hand, a 22,000-dalton band appeared (this molecular weight corresponding to the sum of the molecular weights of fragment 2 and thrombin A chain), it could be concluded that the 59,000-dalton species obtained from prothrombin Madrid corresponded only in part to prethrombin 1 but mostly to meïzothrombin (des fragment 1). Whereas no fragment 1' and no fragment 2 (mol. wt. 17,000) was detected on the gel, small amounts of a 19,000-dalton species were produced. Prolongation for 20 hours of prothrombin Madrid incubation with factor Xa, calcium, and phospholipids resulted in the decrease of the 59,000-dalton band intensity with a concomitant increase in the intensity of both the 38,000 and 19,000 bands (TABLE 2), suggesting that the latter species arose from the nonthrombin part of meïzothrombin (des fragment 1): consequently the 19,000-dalton species will be designated fragment 2 Madrid.

When incubated for 30 min with Taïpan snake venom in the presence of calcium and phospholipids, normal prothrombin yielded 80% of maximum thrombin clotting activity. The major proteolysis products formed (FIG. 3) were thrombin, fragment 1, fragment 1' and fragment 2; incomplete activation was evidenced by the persistence of early intermediate products: prethrombin 1 (mol. wt. 59,000, one polypeptide chain) and prethrombin 2 (mol. wt. 38,000, one polypeptide chain). Under the same experimental conditions, prothrombin Madrid yielded 10% of the thrombin clotting activity generated by normal prothrombin. The proteolysis products formed at this time were identified (FIG. 3) as prethrombin 1 (in trace amounts), thrombin, fragment 1 and fragment 2 Madrid (in trace amounts) but mostly as the same product as occurring upon factor Xa action i.e. meïzothrombin (des fragment 1). A faint band migrating slightly slower than the thrombin B chain is visible on FIGURE 3, gel 2 (reduced sample); this band could correspond to prethrombin 2 although migrating slightly faster (mol. wt. 36,000) than normal prethrombin 2 (mol. wt. 38,000), as shown on gel 1 (reduced sample).

Although prothrombin Madrid activation by *Dispholidus typus* venom appeared to proceed normally since the generation of clotting and amidolytic activities was found to be normal (FIG. 1), analysis of the proteolysis products obtained after 5, 30, 60, 90, and 120 minutes was performed using SDS gel electrophoresis of unreduced and reduced samples. As expected, the appearance

TABLE 2

PROTHROMBIN ACTIVATION BY XA

(Relative percentage of proteolysis products obtained after various incubation times)

	8 hr. incubation		20 hr. incubation	
	Normal	Madrid	Normal	Madrid
Prothrombin	–	5	–	2
Meïzothrombin (des F1) or prethrombin 1	–	43	–	18
Thrombin	45	18	44	34
F1	33	30	33	31
F2	22	–	23	–
F2 Madrid	–	4	–	17

Prothrombin (100 μg) was incubated with factor Xa (1 unit), human brain cephalin (5 μg) in 100 μl 0.05 M NaCl 0.01 M CaCl$_2$/0.02 M Tris-HCl pH 7.5. After 8 or 20 hours incubation, unreduced and reduced samples have been submitted to SDS gel electrophoresis, and the percentage of proteolysis products formed has been calculated by scanning of the gels and determination of the peaks surfaces.

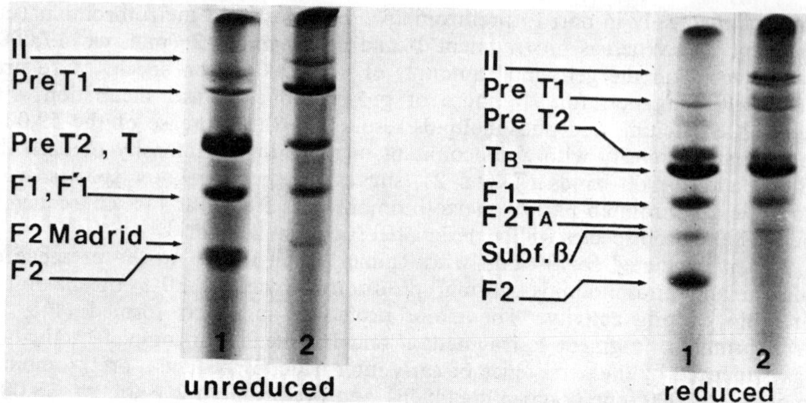

FIGURE 3. Prothrombin activation by Taïpan snake venom : SDS gel electrophoresis analysis of the activation products. 100 µg of normal prothrombin (gel 1) or prothrombin Madrid (gel 2) were incubated at 20°C with 1 µg Taïpan snake venom and 5 µg cephalin in 100 µl 0.05 M NaCl 0.01 M CaCl₂/0.02 M Tris-HCl, pH 7.5, for 30 minutes, then diluted in 0.01 M sodium phosphate, pH 7, 1% SDS (unreduced samples) or in 0.01 M sodium phosphate, pH 7, 1% SDS 1% 2-mercaptoethanol (reduced samples) and submitted to gel electrophoresis.

rate of both the early product meïzothrombin (des fragment 1) and the final products thrombin, fragment 1 and fragment 2 was found to be normal. The only abnormal feature (FIG. 4, gel 4) was the production of fragment 2 Madrid, characterized by a mobility different from that of normal fragment 2, accounting for a 2,000-dalton difference in molecular weight. The abnormal mobility of fragment 2 Madrid was obvious from the early stage of production until full prothrombin activation (FIG. 5, gel b). But, when prothrombin was incubated with *Dispholidus typus* venom for a longer period (72 hours), the mobility of fragment 2 obtained from prothrombin Madrid was found to be similar to that of normal fragment 2 (FIG. 5, gel c). Incubation of prothrombin Madrid with the venom for 20 hours resulted in the production of two fragment 2 populations of respective molecular weights 19,000 and 17,000 (FIG. 6, gel b). The mobility of normal fragment 2 did not change whatever the incubation period of prothrombin with the venom. Fragment 2 Madrid proteolysis could be related to the enzymatic action of the thrombin generated since, when the experiment was repeated in the presence of hirudin (2,000 antithrombin units/mg prothrombin), the only proteolytic cleavage (even after 72 hours of incubation) was that of the bond linking the A and B chains of thrombin, as already described for normal prothrombin.[28]

DISCUSSION

A functional defect of the prothrombin molecule may be related to an abnormality of the zymogen active site (as reported [26] for prothrombin Quick and suggested [23] for prothrombin Metz), or to an impairment of the enzymatic action of Xa (as reported [27] for prothrombin Barcelona), or to a lack of acceleration of the reaction by calcium ions and phospholipids (as demonstrated [10] for descarboxyprothrombin) and/or to the lack of acceleration of the reaction by factor Va. The catalytic site of prothrombin Madrid appears to be functionally normal since the abnormal molecule is able to generate clotting activity upon *Echis carinatus* or *Dispholidus typus* venom action, in the same manner as normal prothrombin. Although upon factor Xa action, generation of clotting activity by prothrombin Madrid is very slow, the reaction rate is accelerated in the presence of calcium and phospholipids, or calcium, phospholipids and factor Va, with a rate enhancement coefficient similar to that determined for normal prothrombin, suggesting that the functional abnormality is related to an impairment of factor Xa enzymatic action and not to a defect in prothrombin binding to phospholipids or factor Va.

Whereas a weak clotting activity was slowly produced upon prothrombin Madrid incubation with factor Xa, the generation of amidolytic activity was

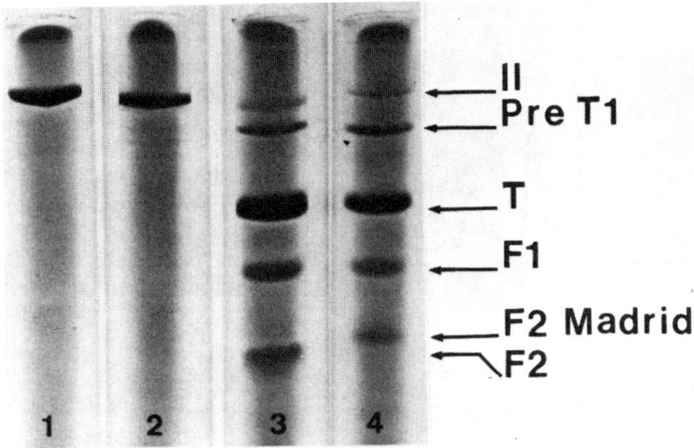

FIGURE 4. Prothrombin activation by *Dispholidus typus* venom : SDS gel electrophoresis of the activation products. 100 μg of normal prothrombin (gel 3) or prothrombin Madrid (gel 4) were incubated at 20°C with 0.1 μg *Dispholidus typus* venom in 100 μl 0.05 M NaCl/0.02 M Tris-HCl, pH 7.5, for 90 minutes, then diluted in 0.01 M sodium phosphate, pH 7, 1% SDS and submitted to gel electrophoresis. Uncleaved prothrombin is shown on gel 1 (normal prothrombin) and gel 2 (prothrombin Madrid). Identification of the activation products was based on SDS gel electrophoresis analysis of reduced samples (not shown).

grossly normal, indicating that factor Xa was responsible for unmasking the active site of the zymogen. Gel electrophoresis analysis of the products obtained allow us to state that prothrombin Madrid proteolysis occurred upon factor Xa action. But, whereas in normal prothrombin, factor Xa splits (FIGURE 7) first bond 2, giving rise to prethrombin 2 and then bond 3, yielding thrombin, proteolysis of prothrombin Madrid by factor Xa leads to the appearance of meïzothrombin (des fragment 1) which corresponds to the prethrombin 1 region of prothrombin, cleaved at the bond linking the A and B chains of thrombin. This product has been demonstrated to occur upon normal prothrombin activation by either *Echis carinatus* [5, 31, 32] or *Dispholidus typus* venom,[28] but has never been observed during the course of normal prothrombin activation by factor Xa. Therefore the functional defect of prothrombin Madrid appears to be very similar to that reported for prothrombin Barcelona.[27]

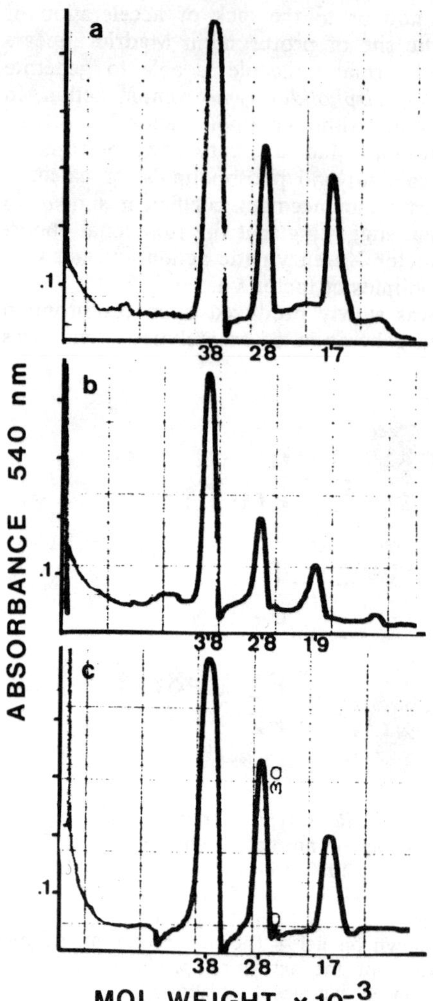

FIGURE 5. Modification of fragment 2 Madrid mobility upon prolonged incubation of prothrombin with *Dispholidus typus* venom : densitometric scan of SDS gels. 100 μg of normal prothrombin (a) or prothrombin Madrid (b, c) were incubated with 0.1 μg *Dispholidus typus* venom in 100 μl 0.05 M NaCl/0.02 M Tris-HCl pH 7.5 for 3 hours (a and b) or 72 hours (c), then diluted in 0.01 M sodium phosphate, pH 7, 1% SDS and submitted to gel electrophoresis.

The two variants are characterized by an impairment of bond 2 cleavage by factor Xa, whereas accessibility of bond 3 is preserved, resulting in a change in the order for bond cleavages: exposition of the active site, due to a first cleavage by factor Xa at bond 3, would be responsible for fast cleavage at bond 1 and production of meïzothrombin (des fragment 1). Inasmuch as bond 2′ is known to be thrombin-sensitive,[3] it is proposed that slow production of thrombin could be related to the cleavage of this bond, due to the thrombin-like enzymes formed; proteolysis of bond 2′ would therefore account for the production of fragment 2 Madrid (mol. wt. 19,000) composed of fragment 2 (mol. wt. 17,000) plus the 13 amino acid residues peptide fragment 3 attached to it.

Owen and Jackson[33] have reported that the mechanism of bovine prothrombin activation by Taïpan snake venom is indistinguishable from factor

Xa-catalyzed prothrombin activation. As expected, the order of bond cleavages during the course of prothrombin Madrid proteolysis by Taïpan snake venom appeared to be similar to that previously observed with factor Xa. Production, among the activation intermediates of a 36,000-dalton species composed of one polypeptide chain, is on behalf of the proposed scheme (FIG. 7) for prothrombin Madrid activation by either factor Xa or Taïpan snake venom: this intermediate could correspond to prethrombin 2 (des fragment 3) originating from prothrombin or prethrombin 1 Madrid by proteolysis at bond 2′ due to the thrombin-like enzymes formed.

Impairment of bond 2 proteolysis is not restricted to factor Xa or Taïpan snake venom enzymatic action: bond 2 proteolysis by thrombin or thrombin-like enzymes is apparently also impeded since upon *Dispholidus typus* venom action, prothrombin Madrid activation leads to the production of fragment 2 Madrid (mol. wt. 19,000). In contrast, either susceptibility of bond 3 to the

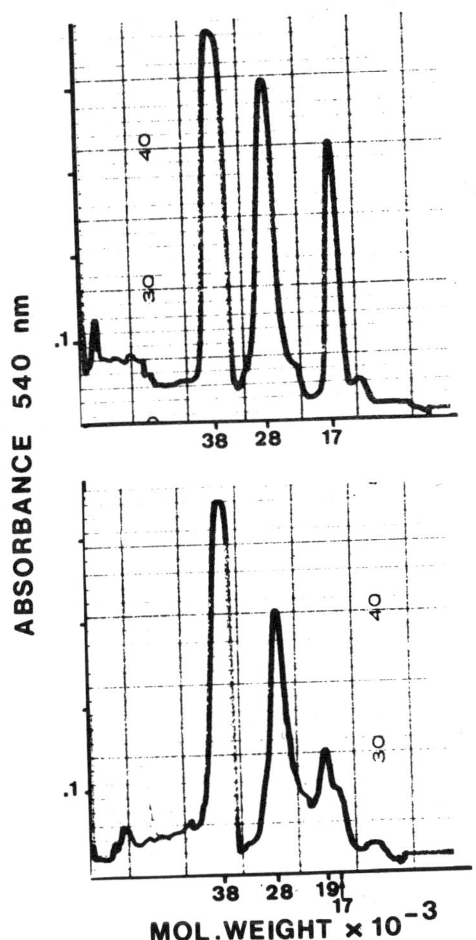

FIGURE 6. Production of two populations of fragment 2 upon 20 hours incubation of prothrombin Madrid with *Dispholidus typus* venom : densitometric scan of SDS gels. Conditions are the same as in FIGURE 5, except for the incubation time (20 hours). Top: activated normal prothrombin. Bottom: activated prothrombin Madrid.

proteolytic action of *Dispholidus typus* venom or susceptibility of bond 1 to the proteolytic action of thrombin or thrombin-like enzymes are both normal.

It has been observed during the course of prothrombin Madrid incubation with *Dispholidus typus* venom, in the absence of thrombin inhibitors, a decrease in molecular weight of fragment 2 Madrid, the 19,000-dalton species giving rise to a 17,000-dalton fragment. The proteolysis is not observed in the presence of hirudin and may therefore be ascribed to the enzymatic action of thrombin, suggesting that bond 2 proteolysis by thrombin is not completely impeded, but only dramatically slowed down.

The impairment of bond 2 cleavage either upon factor Xa or Taïpan snake action or upon thrombin action may be related to an amino acid substitution at bond 2, or, more likely, in the vicinity of this bond.

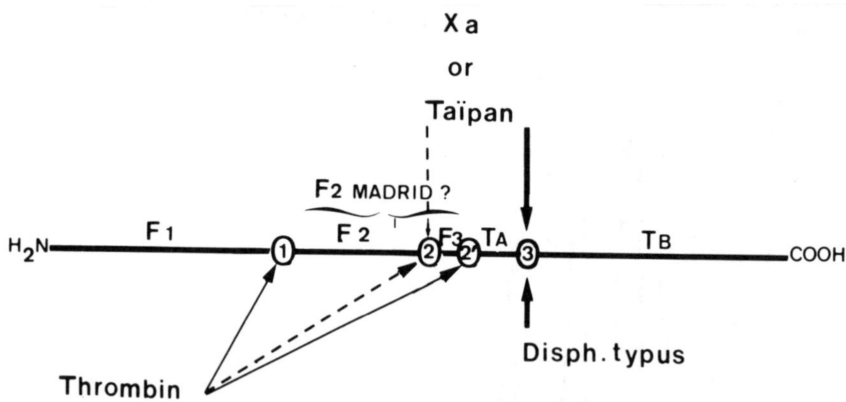

FIGURE 7. Proposed model for prothrombin Madrid activation. Functional defect of prothrombin Madrid is characterized by the impairment of bond 2 proteolysis by factor Xa, Taïpan snake venom or thrombin. Proteolysis of bond 3 by factor Xa, Taïpan snake venom or *Dispholidus typus* venom unmasks the active site and is followed by autocatalytic proteolysis of bond 1, yielding meïzothrombin (des fragment 1) and fragment 1, and proteolysis of bond 2', yielding thrombin and fragment 2 Madrid (mol. wt. 19,000), which could consist of fragment 2 (mol. wt. 17,000) plus the 13 amino acid residues peptide fragment 3 attached to it.

ACKNOWLEDGMENTS

This work was supported by grants from Institut National de la Santé et de la Recherche Médicale, CRL n° 78 2 103 1, and from Faculté Xavier Bichat, Université Paris VII, Paris, France.

The authors are indebted to Drs. F. Olmeda, M. Quintana and N. Gomez, Instituto Nacional de Hematologia y Hemotherapia, Madrid (Spain) for having kindly provided the plasma of the propositus. They are grateful to Ms. Joëlle Crick and Ms. Martine Vincent for skillful secretarial assistance.

REFERENCES

1. KISIEL, W. & D. J. HANAHAN. 1973. Biochim. Biophys. Acta **329:** 221–232.
2. KISIEL, W. & D. J. HANAHAN. 1974. Biochem. Biophys. Res. Commun. **59:** 570–577.

3. DOWNING, M. R., R. J. BUTKOWSKI, M. M. CLARK & K. G. MANN. 1975. J. Biol. Chem. **250:** 8897–8906.
4. ESMON, C. T. & C. M. JACKSON. 1974. J. Biol. Chem. **249:** 7782–7790.
5. FRANZA, B. R., D. L. ARONSON & J. S. FINLAYSON. 1975. J. Biol. Chem. **250:** 7057–7068.
6. ARONSON, D. L., L. STEEVAN, A. P. BALL, B. R. FRANZA & J. S. FINLAYSON. 1977. J. Clin. Invest. **60:** 1410–1418.
7. WALZ, D. A. & T. R. BROWN. 1979. *In* Vitamin K Metabolism and Vitamin K-Dependent Proteins, J. W. Suttie, Ed.: 116–119. University Park Press, Baltimore, MD.
8. BARTON, P. G. & D. J. HANAHAN. 1969. Biochim. Biophys. Acta **187:** 319–327.
9. BULL, R. K., S. JEVONS & P. G. BARTON. 1972. J. Biol. Chem. **247:** 2747–2754.
10. ESMON, C. T., J. W. SUTTIE & C. M. JACKSON. 1975. J. Biol. Chem. **250:** 4095–4099.
11. ESMON, C. T., W. G. OWEN, D. L. DUIGUID & C. M. JACKSON. 1973. Biochim. Biophys. Acta **310:** 289–294.
12. BAJAJ, S. P., R. J. BUTKOWSKI & K. G. MANN. 1975. J. Biol. Chem. **250:** 2150–2156.
13. SEEGERS, W. H., E. NOVOA, D. A. WALZ, T. J. ANDARY & H. I. HASSOUNA. 1976. Thromb. Res. **8:** 83–97.
14. BENSON, B. J., W. KISIEL & D. J. HANAHAN. 1973. Biochim. Biophys. Acta **329:** 81–87.
15. GITEL, S. N., W. G. OWEN, C. T. ESMON & C. M. JACKSON. 1973. Proc. Natl. Acad. Sci. USA **70:** 1344–1348.
16. ESMON, C. T. & C. M. JACKSON. 1974. J. Biol. Chem. **249:** 7791–7797.
17. SHAPIRO, S. S., J. MARTINEZ & R. R. HOLBURN. 1969. J. Clin. Invest. **48:** 2251–2259.
18. JOSSO, F., J. MONASTERIO DE SANCHEZ, J. M. LAVERGNE, D. MENACHE & J. P. SOULIER. 1971. Blood **38:** 9–16.
19. GIROLAMI, A., G. BAREGGI, A. BRUNETTI & A. STICCHI. 1974. J. Lab. Clin. Med. **84:** 654–666.
20. KAHN, M. J. P. & A. GOVAERTS. 1974. Thromb. Res. **5:** 141–156.
21. SHAPIRO, S. S. 1975. *In* Prothrombin and related factors, Hemker, H. C. & J. J. Veltkamp, Eds.: 205–212. Leiden University Press.
22. GIROLAMI, A., S. COCCHERI, C. PALARETI, M. POGGI, A. BURUL & G. CAPPELLATO. 1978. Blood **52:** 115–125.
23. JOSSO, F., Y. RIO & S. BEGUIN. 1978. XVIIth Cong. Int. Soc. Hemat. and XVth Cong. Int. Soc. Blood Transf. Paris. Abst. book, p. 860.
24. OWEN, C. A., R. A. HENRIKSEN, F. C. MCDUFFIE & K. G. MANN. 1978. Mayo Clin. Proc. **53:** 29–33.
25. BEZEAUD, A., M. C. GUILLIN, F. OLMEDA, M. QUINTANA & N. GOMEZ. 1979. Thromb. Res. **16:** 47–58.
26. HENRIKSEN, R. A., W. G. OWEN, M. E. NESHEIM & K. G. MANN. 1979. Thromb. Haemostas. **42:** 57; Abst. 125.
27. RABIET, M. J., J. ELION, R. BENAROUS, D. LABIE & F. JOSSO. 1979. Biochim. Biophys. Acta **584:** 66–75.
28. GUILLIN, M. C., A. BEZEAUD & MÉNACHÉ. 1978. Biochim Biophys. Acta. **537:** 160–168.
29. BELL, W. N. & H. G. ALTON. 1954. Nature. **174:** 880–881.
30. WEBER, K. & M. OSBORN. 1969. J. Biol. Chem. **244:** 4406–4412.
31. KORNALIK, F. & B. BLOMBÄCK. 1975. Thromb. Res. **6:** 53–63.
32. MORITA, T., S. IWANAGA & T. SUZUKI. 1976. J. Biochem. **79:** 1089–1108.
33. OWEN, W. G. & C. M. JACKSON. 1973. Thromb. Res. **3:** 705–714.

DICOUMAROL-INDUCED PROTHROMBINS

Om P. Malhotra

Medical Research Service
Veterans Administration Medical Center
Cleveland, Ohio 44106

Institute of Pathology
Case Western Reserve University
Cleveland, Ohio 44106

Prothrombin is a vitamin K-dependent zymogen of thrombin, the enzyme that participates in the final stages of blood coagulation by converting fibrinogen to fibrin (clot). Dicoumarol or dicoumarol-like drugs are antagonists of vitamin K; therefore, these drugs are of therapeutic value against thromboembolic disease as they decrease the bioactivity of vitamin K-dependent factors, *viz.*, prothrombin and factors VII, IX, and X. Early studies, performed two or three decades ago, suggested that the effect of dicoumarol was due to the synthesis of altered prothrombin molecules.[1-4] In general, however, inhibition of prothrombin synthesis was accepted as the cause of reduced plasma prothrombin activity produced by dicoumarol.

Because of the isolation of dicoumarol-induced prothrombin by several investigators [5-14] during the early seventies, it is now unquestionably established that dicoumarol does induce the production of abnormal molecules which are lacking in their ability to bind calcium—the divalent ion necessary for the physiological generation of thrombin from prothrombin. The difference in calcium-binding was shown to reside in the amino-terminal fragment, prothrombin fragment 1 (F_1), the non-thrombin portion of the molecule. Thus, the atypical prothrombins reported earlier were found to yield thrombin comparable to normal protein in the presence of 25% sodium citrate,[15] trypsin,[8] snake venoms,[8, 16-18] or staphylocoagulase [9]—the reactions that do not depend upon Ca^{2+}. Continued efforts have since resulted in the discovery of a new amino acid, γ-carboxyglutamic acid (Gla),[19-21] which provides the prothrombin molecule with its Ca^{2+}-binding ability. The ten glutamyl residues present in the 33-residue NH_2-terminal sequence of normal prothrombin [21] are carboxylated at the γ-carbon atoms to yield Gla.

By adapting our procedures used in the purification of normal bovine prothrombin,[22] we isolated and purified dicoumarolized prothrombin from the plasma of dicoumarol-treated steers.[5] These initial dicoumarolized preparations were found to contain an admixture of normal and abnormal molecules which were later successfully separated from each other. In 1972, we then reported the isolation of multiple forms of dicoumarol-induced atypical prothrombins.[6, 7] In contrast to normal (10-Gla) prothrombin, the atypical prothrombins contained 7-, 5-, and 2-Gla's, and were adsorbable, respectively, onto barium citrate but not onto barium oxalate, barium oxalate but not onto alumina gel, and alumina gel but not onto the insoluble barium salts.[16-18] In addition to these variants, we have further isolated two more variants both adsorbable onto alumina gel and containing 1- and 0-Gla.

Thrombin cleaves the Arg^{156}–Ser peptide bond of prothrombin to generate

426

Gla-containing amino-terminal prothrombin fragment 1 (F_1, residues 1 to 156) and prethrombin 1 (P_1), the remaining 426 amino acid residues of the molecule.[23] The P_1 portion contains the thrombin potential of the prothrombin molecule. In this paper, we shall describe some of the properties, not only of the normal and various atypical prothrombins but also of their F_1's and P_1's.

EXPERIMENTAL

Physiological activity was determined by a modified version[24] of the two-stage assay procedure of Ware and Seegers.[25] For nonphysiological activity, *Echis carinatus* (EC) venom was used to generate thrombin.[16] Ouchterlony double diffusion analysis was performed in 1% agarose in 0.075 M sodium barbital buffer (pH 8.6) containing either 2.5 mM calcium lactate or 2.0 mM EDTA. Rocket electrophoresis,[26] sodium dodecyl sulfate gel electrophoresis,[27] and gel electrofocusing[28] were performed as described previously.[18, 29] Calcium binding ability was determined by the ultrafiltration method as described before.[15, 16]

Highly purified bovine preparations of normal (10-Gla), 7-, 5-, and 2-Gla prothrombins[16-18, 22] were prepared by methods detailed previously. Briefly, for the isolation of dicoumarol-induced atypical prothrombin, plasma containing about 17% of normal bioactivity was treated with barium citrate. After removing the barium citrate with adsorbed normal and 7-Gla prothrombins, the supernatant was treated with barium oxalate, which adsorbs prothrombin molecules containing 5 Gla's. From the barium oxalate-extracted plasma, then the remaining atypical variants were removed by adsorption onto alumina C γ-gel (Bio-Rad), as shown schematically in FIGURE 1.

After centrifugation, each of the resultant precipitates with their adsorbed prothrombins, *viz.*, barium citrate, barium oxalate, and alumina gel, was washed separately with a solution consisting of 0.15 M NaCl, 3.1 mM sodium citrate, and 1 mM benzamidine hydrochloride. The adsorbed prothrombins were then eluted from their respective precipitates with 0.2 M sodium citrate in 0.15 M NaCl and 10 mM benzamidine-HCl, pH 7.4. The eluates were next subjected to $(NH_4)_2SO_4$ fractionation. From the 50 to 67% $(NH_4)_2SO_4$ saturation fraction of each of the eluates from barium citrate, barium oxalate, and alumina gel, precipitates were obtained at pH 4.6 by isoelectric precipitation, and, respectively, contained 7-Gla (admixed with 10-Gla, normal), 5-Gla, and 2-Gla prothrombins. The 7-Gla variant was freed from its normal molecules by first treating the preparation, containing 0.04 M sodium oxalate, with barium sulfate (which adsorbs normal protein preferentially) followed by DEAE-cellulose chromatography. The 5- and 2-Gla variants were further purified by preparatory polyacrylamide-gel electrophoresis, alone or in conjunction with heparin-agarose chromatography. Finally, the 0- and 1-Gla atypical prothrombins were obtained in contrast from the 40 to 50% $(NH_4)_2SO_4$ saturation fraction and precipitated out at pH 6.0 and pH 5.4, respectively, during isoelectric precipitation. The purified proteins were then purified as described for the 2-Gla variant. The 0-Gla preparation usually contained up to 0.6 mole of Gla per mole of protein.

For the generation of F_1's and P_1's, normal and atypical prothrombins were digested with thrombin with a wt/wt ratio of 36:1, as described elsewhere,[30] for 4 hr for 10-, 7-, and 5-Gla prothrombins, and 6 hr for 2-Gla protein. The

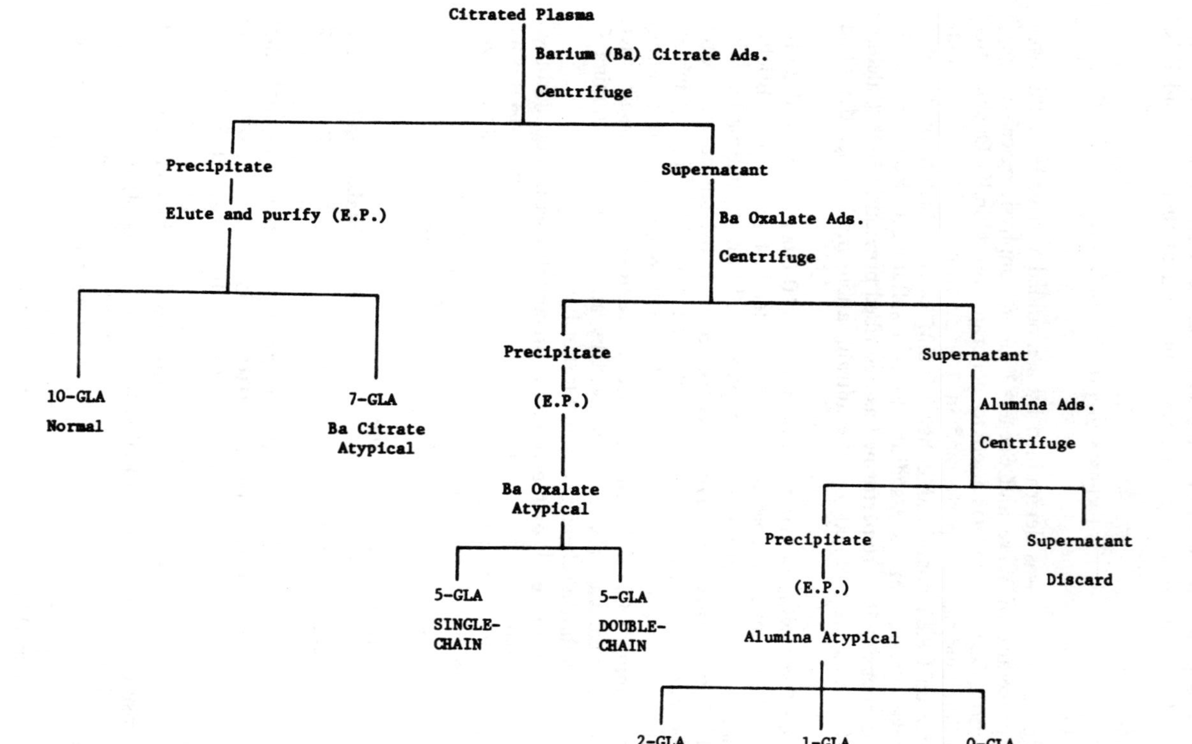

FIGURE 1. Schematic isolation of normal and dicoumarol-induced prothrombins. Bovine plasma containing 17% normal bioactivity, after treatment with barium citrate which adsorbs normal (10-) and 7-Gla prothrombins, was treated with barium oxalate which adsorbs 5-Gla variant. Subsequently, the barium oxalate-extracted plasma was treated with alumina gel which adsorbs the remaining 2-, 1-, and 0-Gla atypical proteins. The prothrombins were purified as described briefly in the text and detailed elsewhere.[16-18, 22]

digested materials were concentrated at 4° C by ultrafiltration through PM-10 membranes (Amicon). After dialysis (using 0.25 inch diameter dialysis bags) for 2 to 3 hr and against 0.05 M sodium phosphate buffer, pH 7.0, the materials were applied on a DEAE-cellulose column equilibrated with the same sodium phosphate buffer (FIGURE 2). Thrombin fractions came through first, immediately followed by P_1 and lastly F_1. The P_1 and F_1 fractions were separately pooled, concentrated, and, respectively, subjected to Sephadex G-100 (FIGURE 3) and G-75. The purified materials so obtained showed a single component by sodium dodecyl sulfate–gel electrophoresis.

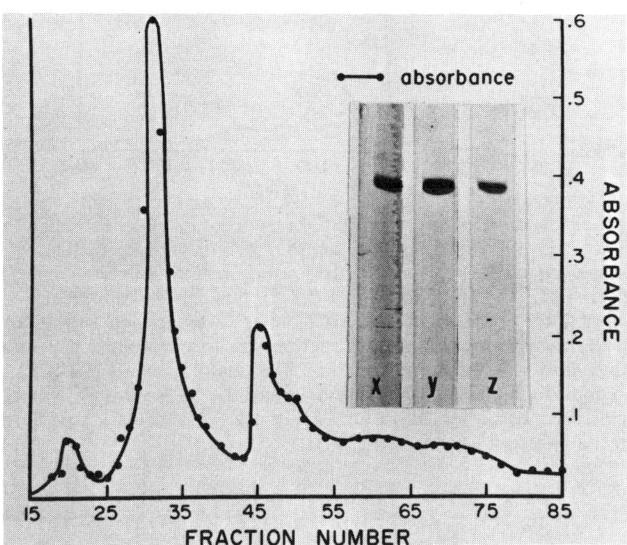

FIGURE 2. DEAE-cellulose (cellex D; Bio-Rad) chromatography of 2-Gla, pH 4.6, alumina atypical prothrombin treated with thrombin. The concentrated sample, approximately 2.3 ml (approximately 10 mg), in 0.05 M sodium phosphate buffer, pH 7.0, was applied to the cellulose column (1.6 cm × 54 cm) which had already been equilibrated with the same buffer. At tube 6 the buffer was changed to 0.05 M sodium phosphate buffer with 0.07 M NaCl, and at tube 24 the elution was continued with an increasing salt gradient, generated by allowing 400 ml of 0.4 M NaCl in 0.05 M sodium phosphate buffer, pH 7.0, to flow into a mixing chamber containing 400 ml of 0.13 M NaCl in the same phosphate buffer. The small peak was centered at tube 20 and contained thrombin activity, followed by the major peak centered at tube 31 and containing prethrombin 1. Pictured with the graph are SDS gels, x, y, and z, which represent, respectively, fractions 29, 31, and 35.

RESULTS

Normal (10-Gla) and each of the atypical prothrombins, *viz.*, 7-, 5-, 2-, 1-, and 0-Gla prothrombins, consisted of a single polypeptide chain with a molecular mass of 70,000 daltons and showed a single component by SDS-gel electrophoresis (FIGURE 4). Each of the prothrombins contained essentially the designated number of Gla's except for the 0-Gla variant which usually contained 0.6 Gla's. By rocket electrophoresis, the atypical variants were found to contain 100% of normal antigenic activity (FIGURE 5).

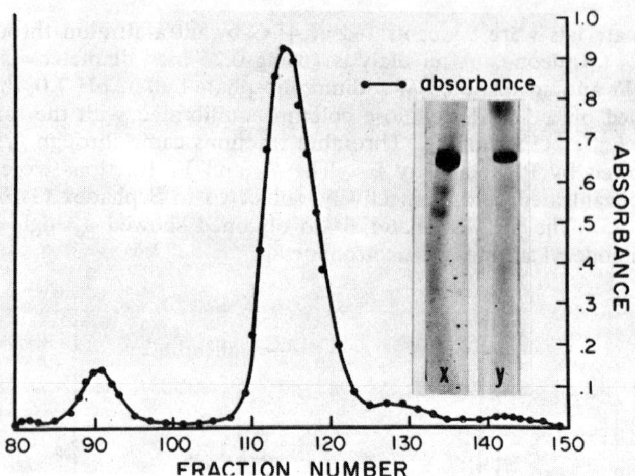

FIGURE 3. Gel filtration of prethrombin 1 (from 2-Gla prothrombin) fractions 29 to 37 plus P_1 fractions 14 to 32 (from another similar DEAE-cellulose chromatography run) on a superfine Sephadex G-100 column (2.6 cm × 90 cm), equilibrated with 0.02 M Tris-HCl buffer (pH 7.4) in 0.1 M NaCl. The sample (approximately 10 mg protein in 2 ml of the same Tris-HCl buffer) was applied to the column from the bottom using a two-way stopcock. Fractions of approximately 1.9 ml each were collected with a flow rate of 8.5 ml per hr. The major protein peak from fractions 110 to 122 contained highly purified prethrombin 1. SDS gel (x) was run using a control sample taken before gel filtration, while gel (y) reflects a sample of material obtained after gel filtration.

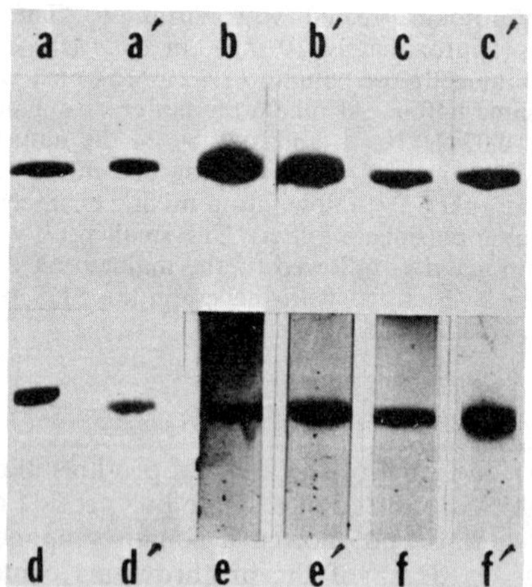

FIGURE 4. Sodium dodecyl sulfate-(SDS-)gel electrophoresis of 10-Gla (a,a'), 7-Gla (b,b'), 5-Gla (c,c'), 2-Gla (d,d'), 1-Gla (e,e'), and 0-Gla (f,f') prothrombins. Samples $a,b,c,d,e,$ and f were reduced with mercaptoethanol.

The physiological activation characteristics of dicoumarol-induced prothrombins more or less followed the general pattern of normal protein being activated in the absence of factor X, *i.e.* the activation time is long, 35 min (vs 6 to 8 min) and the amount of thrombin generation is low, 70% (FIGURE 6) as compared to when activated in the presence of factor X. The 1-Gla variant, even in the presence of factor X, took 4 to 6 hr and generated thrombin on an average of 19% of normal protein, compared to 52, 35, and 22% for the 7-, 5-, and 2-Gla prothrombins. These results confirmed our earlier observations that the time required for activation and the amount of thrombin generated correlate directly with the number of Gla's, and thereby, indirectly with the Ca^{2+}-binding ability of the molecules. Consequently, the P_1's (non-Gla, but containing the thrombin portion of prothrombin) derived from the 10-, 7-, 5-, and 2-Gla variants and exhibiting comparable antigenic activity, each generated approximately similar amounts of thrombin, 1563 U per mg of protein, equivalent to 40% normal prothrombin on a molar basis. The time required for thrombin generation was 5 hr. These results concur with our earlier observations for normal and atypical prothrombins; that is, if the major defect of the atypical proteins is related to their Ca^{2+}-binding abilities, and if these sites are located in the F_1 portion of the molecule, then the atypical prothrombins should have some bioactivity and their bioactivation times should indeed be long.[31, 32] Therefore, when the activation reaction does not require Ca^{2+}, e.g. in the presence of EC venom, then normal and the various atypical prothrombins generated comparable amounts of thrombin.

Electrophoretic mobilities of the 2- to 10-Gla prothrombins and their fragments, F_1's and P_1's, also relate to the number of Gla's. The prethrombin,

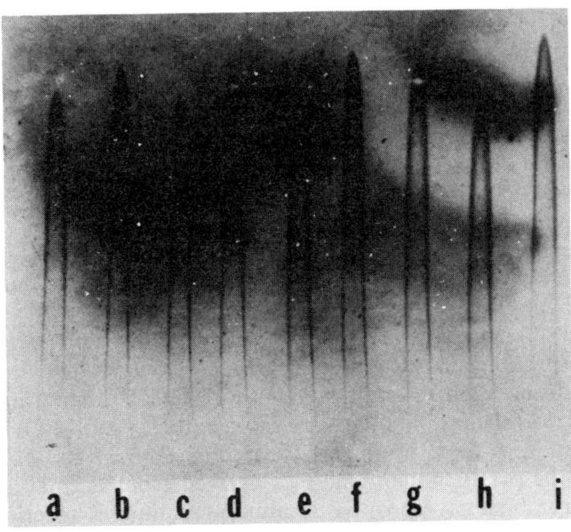

FIGURE 5. Rocket immunoelectrophoresis of prothrombins in 1% agarose containing 5% antiprothrombin serum. The electrophoresis was performed in 0.075 *M* sodium barbital buffer with 2.0 m*M* EDTA at a field strength of about 15 V per cm. Samples of 5 µl (containing 0.35 µg) each were applied using double constriction pipets. Pictured are 7-Gla (*a,i*), 5-Gla (*b*), 2-Gla (*c*), 1-Gla (*d,h*), 0-Gla (*e,g*), and 10-Gla prothrombins (*f*). The antigenic activities of the atypical proteins were comparable to that of normal prothrombin.

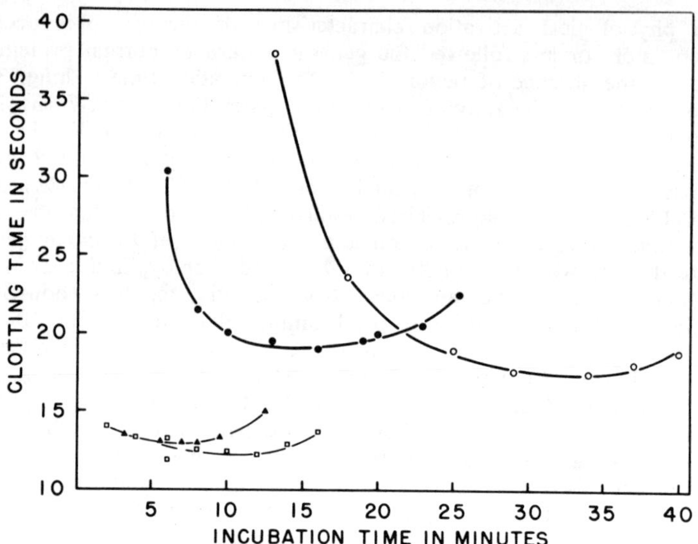

FIGURE 6. Activation of normal, purified and plasma (naturally deficient in factor X) prothrombins in the presence or absence of factor X. The activation mixture contained thromboplastin, factor V, and Ca^{2+}, as employed in the two-stage procedure. Shown are purified prothrombin, with (□—□) and without (○—○) factor X, and plasma prothrombin, in the presence (▲—▲) or absence (●—●) of factor X. Prothrombin activates slowly and generates less thrombin in the absence of factor X.

non-Gla portion of the molecule, derived from various prothrombins did not show any differences in mobility, whether or not Ca^{2+} was present. On the other hand, when the electrophoresis was performed in the presence of 2.5 mM EDTA, 10-Gla prothrombin and its (10-Gla) F_1 were the most mobile, followed by 7-Gla, then 5-Gla and lastly, the 2-Gla variant and its F_1. In the presence of Ca^{2+}, however, 10-Gla prothrombin and its F_1, with their high capacities to bind the divalent Ca^{2+} ions, showed the greatest decreases in mobility, while the 2-Gla counterparts' mobilities were affected the least.[29]

The differences among the various F_1's are noticeably more pronounced than among their parent prothrombins. For example, the 10- and 7-Gla prothrombins could not be separated by the electrofocusing technique because each of these proteins focused at pH 4.55.[16] However, their respective F_1's were easily differentiated (FIGURE 7), with 10-Gla F_1 exhibiting a pI of 3.58 versus 3.79 for 7-Gla F_1. Similarly, a mixture of 5- and 2-Gla F_1's was seen to yield two bands, as these fragments focused at pH 3.97 and 4.29, respectively.

Similar to the prothrombins, the P_1's derived from normal and each of the atypical prothrombins gave positive immunoprecipitation reactions against anti (normal) prothrombin serum, both in the presence of Ca^{2+} or EDTA (FIGURE 8). On the other hand, in the presence EDTA, none of the F_1's gave a positive reaction, although in the presence of Ca^{2+} they all gave positive reactions. However, the intensity of the immunoprecipitate related to the number of Gla's, because the 10-Gla F_1 gave a good antigen–antibody precipitation reaction, followed by 7- and 5- and lastly 2-Gla F_1, where the immunoprecipitate was essentially imperceptible (FIGURE 8).

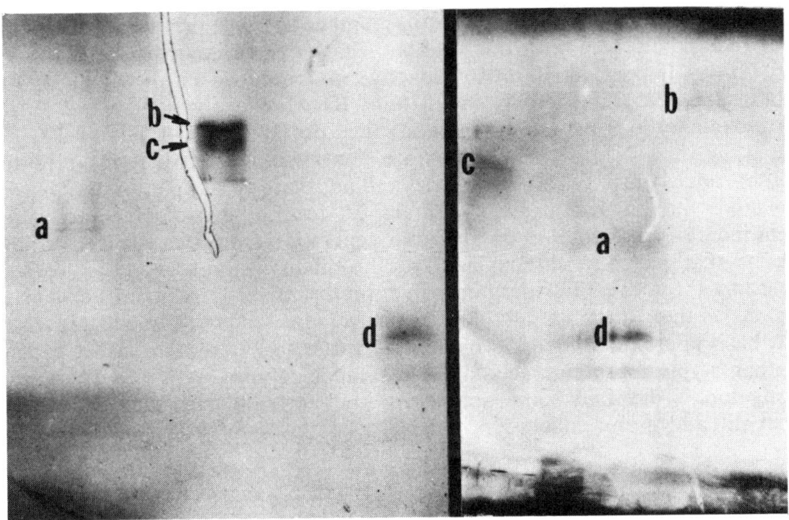

FIGURE 7. Electrofocusing of prothrombin fragments 1 from normal and atypical prothrombins in a thin layer of polyacrylamide gel in pH 3 to 5. Illustrated are the prothrombin fragments 1 from each of two separate runs (left and right), *viz.* 5-Gla F_1 (*a*), 10-Gla F_1 (*b*), 7-Gla F_1 (*c*), and 2-Gla F_1 (*d*). The pH values at which 10-, 7-, 5-, and 2-Gla F_1's focused were 3.58, 3.79, 3.97, and 4.29, respectively.

DISCUSSION

For the generation of thrombin, prothrombin undergoes two cleavages by activated factor X (factor Xa), one at the Arg^{274}–Thr peptide bond to generate prothrombin fragment 1·2 and prethrombin 2 (P_2), and another at the Arg^{323}–Ile bond. The latter cleavage transforms single-chain P_2 into the physiologically active 2-chain molecule, thrombin.[33, 34] Calcium is necessary for the two cleavages because of its capacity to bind to the two high affinity metal-binding sites provided by 2 of the 10 Gla's present in normal prothrombin, resulting in a conformational transition of the prothrombin molecule.[35–39] When thrombin is generated by factor X_a in the presence of factor V, this conformational change is essential for the Ca^{2+}-mediated protein–phospholipid interaction,[36] which occurs via the lower affinity metal-binding sites, formed by single or paired adjacent Gla residues.[40] Dicoumarol-induced prothrombins generally do not undergo such conformational transition;[35, 39] therefore, they should be physiologically relatively inactive.

Phospholipid in the presence of Ca^{2+} enhances the generation of thrombin because of its ability to bind to prothrombins through Ca^{2+} bridges formed between the phospholipid micelles and Gla residues of the protein. Binding of partially acarboxylated prothrombins to phospholipid micelles should relate to the number of Gla's. In fact, this hypothesis has been employed[41] to isolate atypical prothrombins. Consequently, the physiological activity and the rate of thrombin generation should relate to the number of Gla's present. This theory agrees remarkably well with our results. That is to say, normal prothrombin with 10 Gla's is considered 100% bioactive in 7 min; Ba citrate atypical with 7 Gla's shows 52% bioactivity in 90 min; Ba oxalate atypical with 5 Gla's, 30% bioactivity in 3 hr; and alumina atypical prothrombin with 1- or 2-Gla's, 18 to 25% in 4–7 hr. These values are, however, higher than the reported value of approximately 3%.[8-10] Our finding that by supplying the newly-discovered vitamin K-dependent protein M to the physiological activation system increased the amount of thrombin generation from the atypical variants indicates that partially carboxylated prothrombins will, to a certain extent, convert to thrombin. Furthermore, that prethrombin 1, which is devoid of Gla's, generates thrombin and has a physiological activity calculated on a molar basis approximating 40% of normal, further supports our earlier conclusion that atypical proteins should have some biological activity. That some investigators [41] did find some activity in the partially carboxylated variants further still affirms our conclusion.

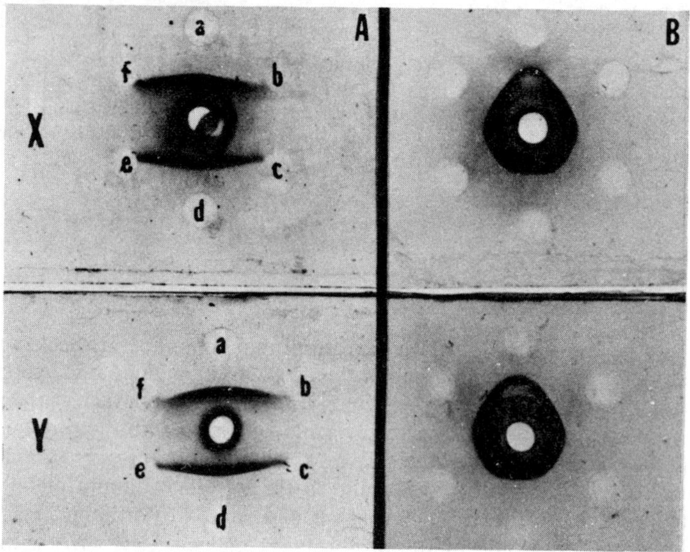

FIGURE 8. Ouchterlony double diffusion analysis of prothrombin fragment 1 (A) and prethrombin 1 (B) derived from normal and various atypical prothrombins in the presence of 2.5 mM calcium lactate (X) or 2.0 mM EDTA (Y). The central well in each case contained 10 μl of normal prothrombin antisera. (A) Normal prothrombin (a,d), 10-Gla F$_1$ (b), 7-Gla F$_1$ (c), 5-Gla F$_1$ (e), and 2-Gla F$_1$ (f). (B) Clockwise starting at the top of each pattern normal prothrombin, P$_1$'s derived from each of normal (10-Gla), 7-Gla, 5-Gla, 2-, and 0-Gla prothrombins. Except for prothrombin, each of the wells contained 0.7 μg of designated material. Prethrombins gave positive immunoprecipitation reactions both in the presence of Ca^{2+} or EDTA and showed no immunochemical differences. On the other hand, none of the F$_1$'s gave positive reactions in the presence of EDTA. However, when Ca^{2+} was present, the F$_1$'s gave a positive reaction but the intensity of the immunoprecipitates related to the number of Gla's with normal (10-Gla) F$_1$ giving the most and 2-Gla F$_1$, the least intense reaction.

Our observations show that normal (10-Gla) and three groups of atypical (*viz.*, 7-, 5-, and 2- or less Gla) prothrombins can be differentiated by physiological activation. However, in living plasma (or blood), the bioactivity of atypical variants, we feel, is of no consequence because of their long activation times and the presence of inhibitors like antithrombin III, which inactivate several clotting factors including thrombin and factor X_a, amid the existing decrease in the other vitamin K-dependent clotting factors X, IX, and VII during dicoumarol regimen.

The Gla's appear to affect the immunochemical reaction as we found that antigen–antibody precipitation, in the presence of Ca^{2+}, related directly to the number of Gla's. For example, normal (10-Gla) F_1, which binds the most Ca^{2+}, gave a good immunoprecipitate, while 2-Gla F_1 gave a negative reaction. For the same reason, 7-Gla gave a faint reaction, while 5-Gla F_1 was so faint that the immunoprecipitate was essentially imperceptible. The fact that none of the F_1's, in the presence of EDTA, gave positive antigen–antibody reactions further suggests that the Ca^{2+} induced some configurational changes in the 10-Gla F_1, and to a lesser degree in 7-Gla F_1 to make its antigenic determinants available to (some population of) antibodies raised against normal prothrombin. The fact that Ca^{2+} induces conformational transition in normal prothrombin but not in dicoumarol-induced prothrombin supports the above hypothesis.

The above observation, together with the facts that each of the P_1's (derived from the various atypical prothrombins) gives a positive immunoprecipitation reaction both in the presence of Ca^{2+} or EDTA, and shows complete immunological identity with each other, indicates that two major classes of antibodies are produced against (normal) prothrombin. One class of antibody is against that portion of the prothrombin molecule which does not interact with Ca^{2+}, while the second is against the Gla-containing portion of the molecule which does. Apparently, when the antibodies are being raised, prothrombin in Freund's adjuvant after injection picks up Ca^{2+} from extracellular fluid to assume the Ca^{2+}-dependent conformation *in vivo*. This hypothesis is supported by the fact that protein immunogen in Freund's adjuvant does not undergo any detectable conformational change,[42] and an immunogen(s), e.g., copolymer of glutamic acid, alanine, and tyrosine was reported to yield antibodies directed against a conformation of the immunogen as if it were stabilized in the presence of Ca^{2+}.[43] As a matter of fact, antibodies directed against the prothrombin specific to its conformation stabilized in Ca^{2+} have been obtained recently.[44]

Since we did not find any differences among the P_1's derived from normal and various atypical proteins, and since the properties of the F_1's as well as of their parent molecules follow the same trends, relating directly (or indirectly through Ca^{2+}-binding ability) to the number of Gla's further emphasizes that the defect exclusively resides in the lack (or decrease) of carboxylation of the glutamyl-residues present in the amino-portion of the prothrombin molecule.

REFERENCES

1. LEIN, J. & P. S. LEIN. 1948. Altered prothrombin produced by dicoumarol-treated rabbits. Amer. J. Physiol. **155:** 394–401.
2. SHANBERGE, J. N. 1956. The effect of dicoumarol on certain factors of blood coagulation. J. Lab. Clin. Med. **48:** 218–222.

3. CARTER, J. R., C. V. NORDSCHOW, E. D. WARNER & A. T. LUND. 1961. The *in vivo* synthesis of defective prothrombin molecules. Thromb. Diathes. Haemorrh. (Stuttg.) **5**: 598.

4. HEMKER, H. C., J. J. VELTKAMP, A. HENSEN & E. A. LOELIGER. 1963. Nature of prothrombin biosynthesis: Preprothrombinemia in vitamin K deficiency. Nature **200**: 589–590.

5. MALHOTRA, O. P. & J. R. CARTER. 1971. Isolation and purification of prothrombin from dicoumarolized steers. J. Biol. Chem. **246**: 2665–2671.

6. MALHOTRA, O. P. 1972. Atypical prothrombin in purified preparations from dicoumarol-treated steers. Life Sci. **11**(Part II): 901–907.

7. MALHOTRA, O. P. 1972. Atypical prothrombins induced by dicoumarol. Nature New Biol. **239**: 59–60.

8. NELSESTUEN, G. L. & J. W. SUTTIE. 1972. The purification and properties of an abnormal prothrombin protein produced by dicoumarol-treated cows. (A comparison to normal prothrombin). J. Biol. Chem. **247**: 8176–8182.

9. CESBRON, N., C. BOYER, M. C. GUILLIN & D. MÉNACHÉ. 1973. Human coumarin prothrombin chromatographic, coagulation and immunologic studies. Thromb. Diathes. Haemorrh. **30**: 437–450.

10. STENFLO, J. & P. O. GANROT. 1972. Vitamin K and the biosynthesis of prothrombin I. Identification and purification of a dicoumarol-induced abnormal prothrombin from bovine plasma. J. Biol. Chem. **247**: 8160–8166.

11. STENFLO, J. 1972. Vitamin K and the biosynthesis of prothrombin II. Structural comparison of normal and dicoumarol-induced bovine prothrombin. J. Biol. Chem. **247**: 8167–8175.

12. MORRISON, S. A. & M. P. ESNOUF. 1973. The nature of heterogeneity of prothrombin during dicoumarol therapy. Nature New Biol. **242**: 92–94.

13. HEMKER, H. C. & P. P. M. REEKERS. 1974. Isolation and purification of proteins induced by vitamin K absence. Thromb. Diathes. Haemorrh. Suppl. **57**: 83–85.

14. MALHOTRA, O. P. 1974. Purification and properties of normal and abnormal prothrombins. Thromb. Diathes. Haemorrh. Suppl. **59**: 27–43.

15. MALHOTRA, O. P. & J. R. CARTER. 1972. Biological and nonbiological activation of normal and dicoumarol-treated prothrombin. Life Sci. **11** (Part II): 445–454.

16. MALHOTRA, O. P. 1979. Purification and characterization of dicoumarol-induced prothrombins. I. Barium citrate atypical (7-Gla) prothrombin. Thromb. Res. **15**: 427–437.

17. MALHOTRA, O. P. 1979. Purification and characterization of dicoumarol-induced prothrombin. II. Barium oxalate atypical (5-Gla) variant. Thromb. Res. **15**: 439–448.

18. MALHOTRA, O. P. 1979. Purification and characterization of dicoumarol-induced prothrombins. III. Alumina pH 4.6 atypical (2-Gla) variant. Thromb. Res. **15**: 449–463.

19. NELSESTUEN, G., T. H. ZYTKOVICZ & J. B. HOWARD. 1974. The mode of action of vitamin K. Identification of γ-carboxyglutamic acid as a component of prothrombin. J. Biol. Chem. **249**: 6347–6350.

20. STENFLO, J., P. FERNLUND, W. EGAN & P. ROEPSTORFF. 1974. Vitamin K-dependent part of prothrombin. Proc. Natl. Acad. Sci. USA **71**: 2730–2733.

21. MAGNUSSON, S., L. SOTTRUP-JENSEN, T. E. PETERSEN, H. R. MORRIS & A. DELL. 1974. Primary structure of the vitamin K-dependent part of prothrombin. Fed. European Biochem. Soc. Letters **44**: 189–193.

22. MALHOTRA, O. P. & J. R. CARTER. 1968. Modified method for the preparation of purified bovine prothrombin of high specific activity. Thromb. Diathes. Haemorrh. **19**: 178–185.

23. KISIEL, W. & D. J. HANAHAN. 1973. The action of factor X_a, thrombin, and trypsin on human factor II. Biochim. Biophys. Acta **329**: 221–232.

24. MALHOTRA, O. P. & J. R. CARTER. 1965. Modification of two-stage assay of purified or plasma prothrombin. Fed. Proc. **24:** 154.
25. WARE, A. G. & W. H. SEEGERS. 1949. Two-stage procedure for the quantitative determination of prothrombin concentration. Amer. J. Clin. Pathol. **19:** 471–482.
26. LAURELL, C. B. 1966. Quantitative estimation of proteins by electrophoresis in agarose gel containing antibodies. Anal. Biochem. **15:** 45–52.
27. WEBER, K. & M. OSBORN. 1969. The reliability of molecular weight determination by dodecyl sulfate-polyacrylamide gel electrophoresis. J. Biol. Chem. **244:** 4406–4412.
28. VESTERBERG, O. & H. SVENSSON. 1966. Isoelectric fractionation, analysis, and characterization of ampholytes in natural pH gradients. IV. Further studies on the resolving power in connection with separation of myoglobins. Acta Chem. Scand. **20:** 820–834.
29. MALHOTRA, O. P. 1981. Purification and characterization of prothrombin fragment 1 from various dicoumarol-induced prothrombins. (Submitted for publication.)
30. MALHOTRA, O. P. 1981. Degradation of normal and dicoumarol-induced prothrombins with thrombin. Ann. N.Y. Acad. Sci. **370.** This volume.
31. MALHOTRA, O. P. 1975. Bioactivity of dicoumarol-induced prothrombins. Fed. Proc. **34:** 221.
32. MALHOTRA, O. P. 1975. Activation of dicoumarol-induced atypical prothrombin. Thromb. Diathes. Haemorrh. **34:** 592.
33. ESMON, C. T. & C. M. JACKSON. 1974. The conversion of prothrombin to thrombin. III. The factor X_a-catalyzed activation of prothrombin. J. Biol. Chem. **249:** 7782–7790.
34. SEEGERS, W. H., D. A. WALZ, J. REUTERBY & L. E. McCOY. 1974. Isolation and properties of thrombin E and other prothrombin derivatives. Thromb. Res. **4:** 829–860.
35. BJÖRK, G. & J. STENFLO. 1973. A conformational study of normal and dicoumarol-induced prothrombin. FEBS Lett. **32:** 343–346.
36. NELSESTUEN, G. L., M. BRODERIUS & G. MARTIN. 1976. Role of γ-carboxyglutamic acid. Cation specificity of prothrombin and factor X-phospholipid binding. J. Biol. Chem. **251:** 6886–6893.
37. PRENDERGAST, F. G. & K. G. MANN. 1977. Differentiation of metal ion-induced transition of prothrombin fragment 1. J. Biol. Chem. **252:** 840–850.
38. BLOOM, J. W. & K. G. MANN. 1978. Metal ion induced conformational transitions of prothrombin and prothrombin fragment 1. Biochemistry **17:** 4430–4438.
39. MALHOTRA, O. P., W. B. RIPPON, D. D. SOLOMON & A. G. WALTON. 1979. Structural and physiological relationships in blood clotting proteins: Thrombin and prothrombin. Internat. J. Biol. Macromol. **1:** 137–143.
40. FURIE, B. C., M. BLUMENSTEIN & B. FURIE. 1979. Metal binding sites of a γ-carboxyglutamic acid-rich fragment of bovine prothrombin. J. Biol. Chem. **254:** 12521–12530.
41. FRIEDMAN, P. A., R. D. ROSENBERG, P. V. HAUSCHKA & A. FITZ-JAMES. 1977. A spectrum of partially carboxylated prothrombins in the plasmas of coumarin-treated patients. Biochem. Biophys. Acta **494:** 271–276.
42. BERZOFSKY, J. A., A. N. SCHECTER & H. KON. 1976. Does Freund's adjuvant denature protein antigens? EPR studies of emulsified hemoglobin. J. Immunol. **116:** 270–272.
43. LIBERTI, P. A., P. H. MAURER & L. G. CLARK. 1971. Antigenicity of polypeptides (poly-alpha-amino acids). Physiochemical studies of calcium-dependent antigen–antibody reaction. Biochemistry **10:** 1632–1639.
44. BLANCHARD, R. A., B. C. FURIE & B. FURIE. 1979. Antibodies specific for bovine abnormal (des-γ-carboxy-)prothrombin. J. Biol. Chem. **254:** 12513–12520.

DEGRADATION OF NORMAL AND
DICOUMAROL-INDUCED
PROTHROMBINS WITH THROMBIN *

Om P. Malhotra

Medical Research Service
Veterans Administration Medical Center
Cleveland, Ohio 44106

Institute of Pathology
Case Western Reserve University
Cleveland, Ohio 44106

Prothrombin is a glycoprotein, consisting of a single polypeptide chain with a molecular weight of about 70,000. This protein plays a pivotal role in blood coagulation; therefore, its purification, characterization, kinetics of activation, and biosynthesis continue to be studied intensively. The amino-terminal portion of normal prothrombin contains 10 γ-carboxyglutamyl residues (Gla)[1, 2] which provide the ability of the molecule to bind Ca^{2+}, the divalent ions necessary for the activation of prothrombin. Two of the 10 Gla's are the high affinity metal-binding sites, and upon exposure to Ca^{2+}, the normal prothrombin undergoes conformational transition as observed by circular dichroism and fluorescence spectroscopy.[3-7] This transition is essential for the Ca^{2+}-mediated protein–phospholipid interaction[4] for the generation of thrombin by activated factor X (factor X_a) in the presence of factor V. During the formation of thrombin, prothrombin is first cleaved at the Arg^{274}-Thr peptide bond to generate prothrombin fragment $1 \cdot 2$ ($F_{1 \cdot 2}$) and prethrombin 2 (P_2). The single-chain P_2 is then transformed into the physiologically active 2-chain molecule, thrombin, after another cleavage by factor X_a at the Arg^{323}-Ile bond.[8, 9]

Vitamin K is required for the carboxylation of the γ-carbon atoms of the 10 glutamyl residues; therefore, during its deficiency, whether dietary or induced by its antagonists (e.g. warfarin or dicoumarol), abnormal prothrombin molecules are produced that are (partially) acarboxylated. Three such varieties of atypical prothrombins, induced by dicoumarol, have been isolated by us. These prothrombins, viz., the barium citrate (7-Gla), barium oxalate (5-Gla), and pH 4.6 alumina (2-Gla) variants, originally given designations according to their adsorptive properties[10-12] are more recently referred to by their Gla contents[13-15] as well. Dicoumarol-induced prothrombins, isolated by Björk and Stenflo[3] and by us (unpublished data), have shown that these variants do not undergo Ca^{2+}-mediated transition. It is perhaps for this reason that the atypical prothrombin(s) are relatively physiologically inactive. As a matter of fact, our prothrombin activation studies have shown that the time and the amount of thrombin generation by physiological means correlated with their number of Gla's or indirectly with their Ca^{2+}-binding capacities.[13-15] Understandably then, in systems where Ca^{2+} is not required, e.g. in the presence of

* This work was supported by the Medical Research Service of the Veterans Administration.

snake venom from *Echis carinatus*[15-17] or *Dispholidus typus*,[16] staphylocoagulase,[17] 25% sodium citrate with some factor X_a,[18] and trypsin,[16] each of the prothrombins, normal and atypical, generated similar amounts of thrombin. In other words, the rate of hydrolysis of the two peptide bonds, Arg^{274}-Thr and Arg^{323}-Ile in normal and atypical protein(s) is similar.

Prothrombin, after undergoing cleavage at the Arg^{156}-Ser peptide bond by thrombin, generates Gla-containing amino-terminal prothrombin fragment 1 (F_1) and prethrombin 1 (P_1), the remaining 426 amino acid residues.[19, 20] If, however, the reaction is prolonged, we have found that thrombin also cleaves the Arg^{52}-Asn peptide bond of F_1, thus converting single-chain F_1 to a double-chain F_1 molecule. In this paper, we describe how in normal and in each of our atypical prothrombins, the rates of generation of P_1 and F_1 and the conversion of single-chain F_1 to a double-chain molecule by thrombin are affected by the Gla's, without the mediation of Ca^{2+}.

MATERIAL AND METHODS

Prothrombin, Thrombin, and Antithrombin III

The preparation of normal, 10-Gla,[21] 7-Gla,[10, 13] 5-Gla,[14] and 2-Gla[15] prothrombins has been previously described. Bovine thrombin was purified from commercial topical thrombin (Parke-Davis) by DEAE-cellulose and subsequently by cationic Sephadex C-50 (Pharmacia) chromatography (O. P. Malhotra, unpublished observations). The specific bioactivity of the thrombin approximated $3,850 \pm 525$ units (U) (or $2,200 \pm 300$ NIH U) per mg protein and consisted primarily of α-thrombin admixed with some β-thrombin. Antithrombin III was obtained during the purification of alumina (2-Gla) prothrombin by heparin-agarose chromatography.

Determination of Thrombin and Antithrombin Activities

Thrombin activity was determined by the two-stage procedure for prothrombin[22] except that serum, a source of factors V, VII, and X, was not added to the activation mixture, and the clotting time determined, as originally reported by Ware and Seegers.[23] For antithrombin determination, the methods of Abildgaard *et al.*[24] and Yue *et al.*[25] were incorporated into the assay procedure as described below. Before performing the test, one tube of thrombin (Parke-Davis) containing 100 NIH U per ml was diluted 25-fold with a freshly prepared solution containing 0.12 M NaCl, 0.024 M $CaCl_2$, 0.05 M imidazole-HCl buffer (pH 7.3), and 10 mg per ml bovine serum albumin (crystallized and lyophilized, Sigma). This thrombin solution was kept cold (4° C) in a Falcon tube. (Siliconized glassware and/or plastic pipets and Falcon tubes were used).

Four-tenths ml of thrombin solution warmed to 25° C was mixed with 0.1 ml of appropriately diluted test sample (or defibrinogenated plasma) and kept at room temperature. Immediately after mixing (zero time) and at 15 min (sometimes also at 20 and 30 min), 0.1 ml of the mixture was transferred to a plastic cup containing 0.2 ml of 0.25% fibrinogen (65% clottable, Miles Laboratories, Inc.), and clotting time was determined using a fibrometer

(Baltimore Biological Laboratories). The assays were performed at least in triplicate, utilizing concurrently the test samples as well as the defibrinogenated plasma. The antithrombin activity of the test sample was determined by comparing clotting times as described in TABLE 1.

Sodium Dodecyl Sulfate-Gel Electrophoresis

Electrophoresis carried out in 5×125 mm columns with gel heights of 10 cm each was performed according to the technique of Weber and Osborn.[26] Samples were prepared by a) adding SDS-reaction mixture to a small aliquot of the protein solution; b) heating the sample in boiling H_2O for 1 min; and

TABLE 1

ESTIMATION OF ANTITHROMBIN ACTIVITY FROM COMPARATIVE THROMBIN TIMES

Date	Sample	Dilution	Clotting time in sec	
			Reaction time	
			0 time	15 min
1st trial	Normal prothrombin to which antithrombin was added (A)	1:4	18.3	22.4
	Plasma	1:5	17.0	24.0
	Buffer control	1:10	16.8	21.0
		1:20	17.4	20.4
			18.8	19.8
2nd trial	Test sample A	1:4	18.4	23.0
		1:4	17.9	22.9
	Plasma	1:5	18.3	24.9
		1:10	18.3	21.8
		1:20	16.3	18.9
	Buffer control	1:20	21.9	22.0

NOTE: From the data above, it appears that 25 μl of the sample (1:4 dilution) contained as much antithrombin activity as did approximately 14 μl of plasma (between 1:5 and 1:10 dilution). From these data, it was estimated that the test sample contained about 56% of plasma antithrombin activity.

c) incubating the sample at $37°$ C for 2 h. For the preparation of reduced samples, the protein solution was mixed with an SDS-reaction mixture containing 1% (vol/vol) mercaptoethanol. Gels, after the electrophoresis, were stained with a Coomassie Brilliant Blue staining solution and destained by the method of Fairbanks et al.[27] in the Bio-Rad Diffusion-Destainer (Model 172).

Digestion

Normal and each of the three atypical prothrombins in buffered saline (0.02 M Tris-HCl plus 0.1 M NaCl, pH 7.4) and each at concentrations of approximately 1.85 mg per ml were transferred to small Falcon tubes. A calculated amount of thrombin (containing about 25,000 U per ml) was added to achieve a final thrombin concentration of approximately 200 U per ml, with a w/w ratio of 36:1. Two small aliquots were taken just after the addition and mixing of thrombin with prothrombin (zero time), 5 min later, and every 30 or 60 min thereafter for approximately 6 h, to monitor fragmentation by SDS-gel electrophoresis and to determine thrombin activity.

RESULTS

The proteolytic effect of thrombin on prothrombin is described schematically in FIGURE 1. The amount of thrombin activity present in the different prothrombin samples at zero time (just after the addition of thrombin) and at various time intervals is given in TABLE 2. Thrombin activity in the preparations devoid of antithrombin remained reasonably constant for 4 or more hours. In such cases, more than 65% of normal prothrombin was degraded to form profragment 1 (F_1) and prethrombin 1 (P_1) almost immediately after the addition of thrombin (FIGURE 2). Under similar conditions, approximately 50% Ba citrate, 30 to 50% Ba oxalate, and only 30% of pH 4.6 alumina atypical prothrombins were degraded.

The conversion of normal (10-Gla) protein to F_1 and P_1 was almost complete within 30 min. Completion of the reaction for 7-gla and 5-gla variants took 2.5 (or 3) h, while the 2-gla prothrombin took approximately 5 h. Moreover, within the initial period of 5 h, F_1 generated from 10-Gla and 7-Gla prothrombins began to convert from a single-chain to a double-chain molecule, as evidenced by the appearance of a heavy chain of the latter molecule at the expense of single-chain F_1 (FIGURES 2, 3 Y). Within another 5 to 12 h, almost all the F_1 (from 10- and 7-Gla prothrombins) consisted of double polypeptide chains. The light chain was visible when SDS-gel electrophoresis was performed in 15% polyacrylamide gels (FIGURE 3 X). The total molecular mass of either the single- or double-chain F_1 approximated 24,000 daltons, while the heavy and light chains of the double-chain F_1 had molecular weights of approximately 19,000 and 5,000, respectively. Profragment 1 from both Ba oxalate and pH 4.6 alumina variants did not undergo such a transformation from a single-chain to a double-chain molecule for at least 24 h. However, conversion of 5- and 2-Gla variants to a double-chain molecule was indicated by the appearance of the heavy chain of the double-chain fragment within 40 h. Within 3 days the conversion was complete (FIGURE 4).

Effect of Antithrombin

Antithrombin inactivates thrombin; therefore, a prothrombin solution containing antithrombin should require more than the calculated amount of thrombin to maintain thrombin activity at 200 U per ml. To demonstrate that the rates of the two cleavages at Arg^{156}-Ser and at Arg^{52}-Asn in normal prothrombin are faster than in the atypical variants, we studied the degradation patterns of normal and 2-Gla prothrombins, to which antithrombin III had been added to contain 56% and 45% normal plasma antithrombin activity, respectively. Soon after the addition of thrombin, each sample was found to contain 170 U of thrombin per ml (TABLE 2). However, approximately 60 to 70% of normal prothrombin was degraded, compared to only 20 to 30% of the alumina variant (FIGURE 5, X-b, Y-b). The normal protein appeared to be degrading

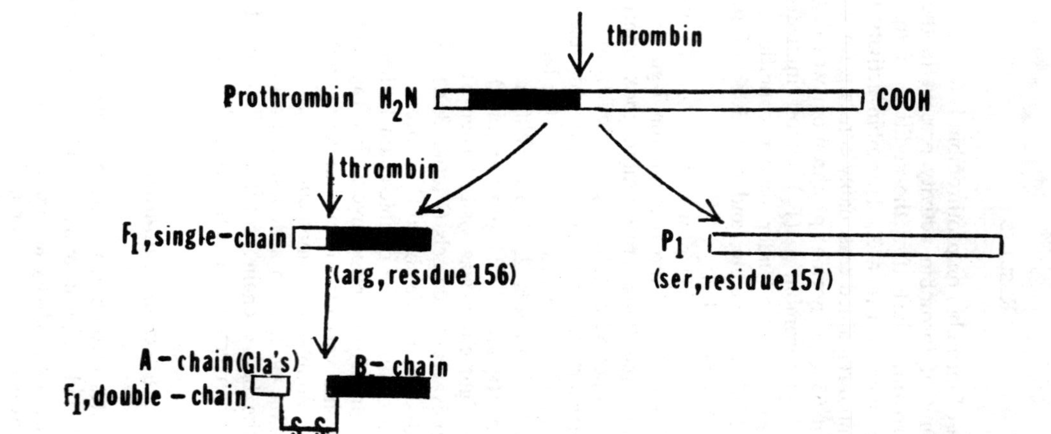

FIGURE 1. Degradation of prothrombin with thrombin. The enzyme thrombin at first generates prothrombin fragment 1 (F_1) and prethrombin 1 (P_1) by splitting the arginyl-serine (residues 156 and 157) bond; it subsequently converts the single-chain F_1 to a double-chain molecule by breaking the peptide bond between Arg (residue 52) and Asn (residue 53).

Table 2

Relative Thrombin Activity Used to Generate Prethrombin 1 and Prothrombin Fragment 1 From Normal and Atypical Prothrombins

Prothrombin	Thrombin Bioactivity (units per ml) at Different Time Intervals											
	0 time	5 min	30 min	1 h	2 h	3 h	4 h	5 h	6 h	7.5 h	16 h	18 h
Normal	220		215	227		242		237				
Ba citrate	180		200									
Ba oxalate atypical	230		230	220				180				
pH 4.6 alumina atypical	210		188	185		232	226					
pH 4.6 alumina * atypical plus antithrombin III	170		121	64	50	51	48	300 †	300	262		240
Normal plus * antithrombin III	170	40	5	‡			182 †	64	32	260 †	255	

Note: Normal (10-Gla), barium (Ba) citrate (7-Gla), Ba oxalate (5-Gla), and pH 4.6 alumina atypical (2-Gla) prothrombin (1.85 ± 0.25 mg per ml) with and without antithrombin were digested with thrombin to achieve a final concentration of approximately 200 U of thrombin per ml. Soon after mixing, and at various succeeding time intervals, small aliquots were taken for SDS-gel electrophoresis (Figures 1, 3, 4) and for assay of thrombin activity. For the samples containing antithrombin, extra thrombin was added (†) to raise its activity. Whenever thrombin activity remained stable for an hour or two, its activity generally did not deteriorate for at least 24 h. To minimize the variables, these studies were carried out concurrently. A slight time variation does exist, in that the zero times for thrombin addition to each of the prothrombin samples were staggered at approximately 10 min intervals.

* Normal and pH 4.6 alumina atypical prothrombins, respectively, contained per ml 56% and 45% plasma antithrombin-III activity.

† Extra thrombin was added to raise its activity.

‡ Very little, if any.

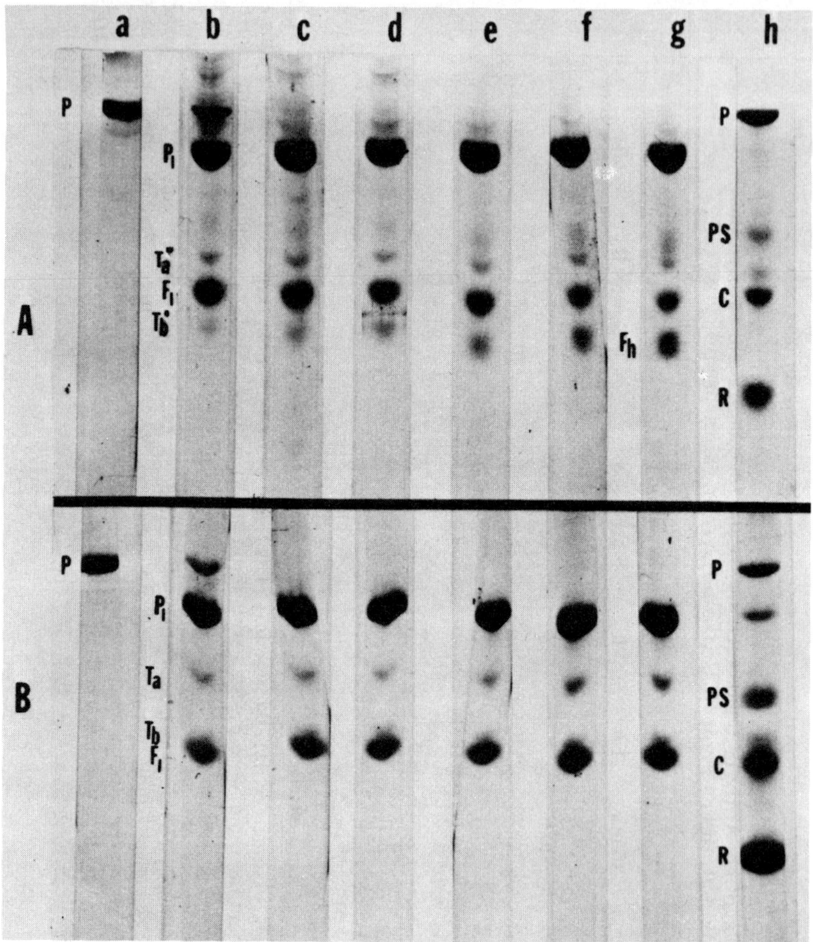

FIGURE 2. Time-course digestion of normal (10-Gla) prothrombin (P) with thrombin (α-thrombin, T_a, admixed with some β-thrombin, T_b). Prothrombin (1.64 mg per ml) was fragmented with thrombin (200 U per ml). Sodium dodecyl sulfate-gel electrophoretic patterns of aliquots taken out at different time intervals, after reduction with (A) and without (B) mercaptoethanol are shown: control prothrombin (a), soon after the addition of thrombin (b), after 35 min (c), 1 h (d), 2 h (e), 3.25 h (f), 5.25 h (g), and standard (h). Standards used for (A) and (B) were prothrombin, 70,000; pepsin, 35,000; chymotrypsinogen, 25,000; and ribonuclease, 13,700. More than 65% prothrombin was digested to give prethrombin 1 (P_1) and profragment 1 (F_1), and within 2 h all of the prothrombin had disappeared. Within 3.25 h, the F_1 band (tube f in A) heavy chain (F_h) of F_1 with double-chains began to appear.

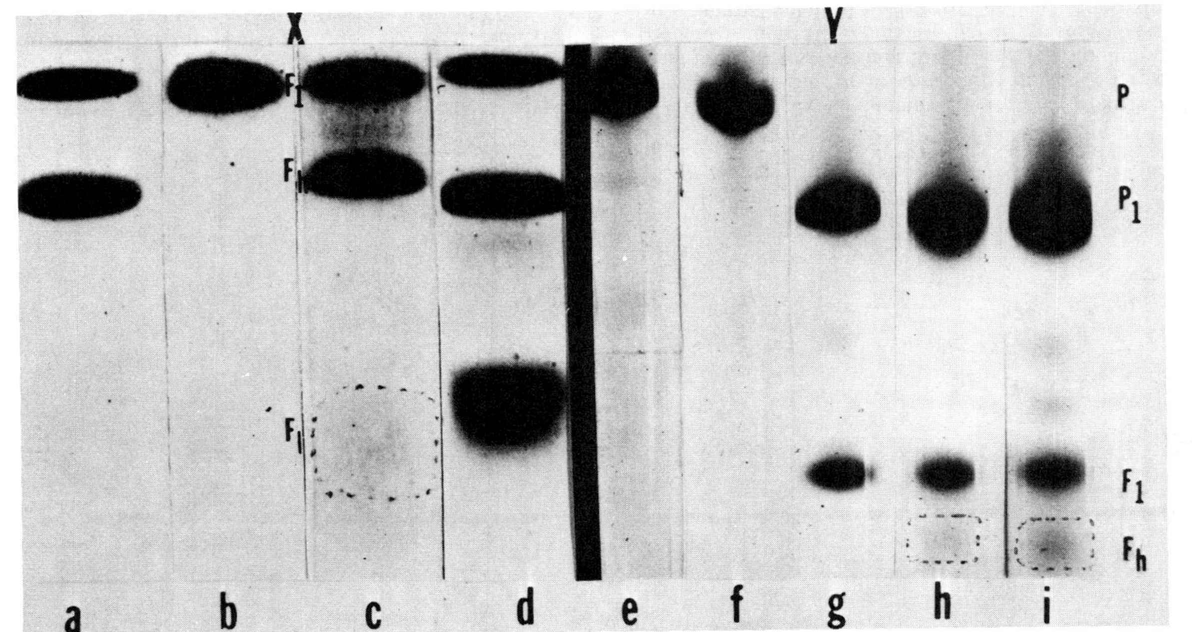

FIGURE 3. Sodium dodecyl sulfate-gel electrophoresis of normal (10-Gla) F_1 in 15% polyacrylamide gel (X), and 10-Gla and 7-Gla (Ba citrate atypical) prothrombin (1.8 mg per ml) in 10% gel after having been digested with thrombin (200 U per ml) for 6 h (Y). Samples used were either nonreduced (a,b,e,g) or reduced (c,d,h,i). X: Single-chain F_1 (b) had a molecular weight of 24,000 (moving in the vicinity of chymotrypsinogen), while the heavy (F_h) and light chains (F_1) of F_1 revealed respective molecular weights of approximately 19,000 and 5,000. Standards used (in a,d) were chymotrypsinogen (25,000), myoglobin (17,800), and bovine trypsin inhibitor (6,100, used only in standard d). Y: 7-Gla prothrombin (e,f) digested with thrombin showed evidence of a heavy chain (F_h) of F_1 in 5 h (h). The 10-Gla prothrombin, digested under similar conditions, also showed F_h (i), but the 5-Gla prothrombin did not (not shown).

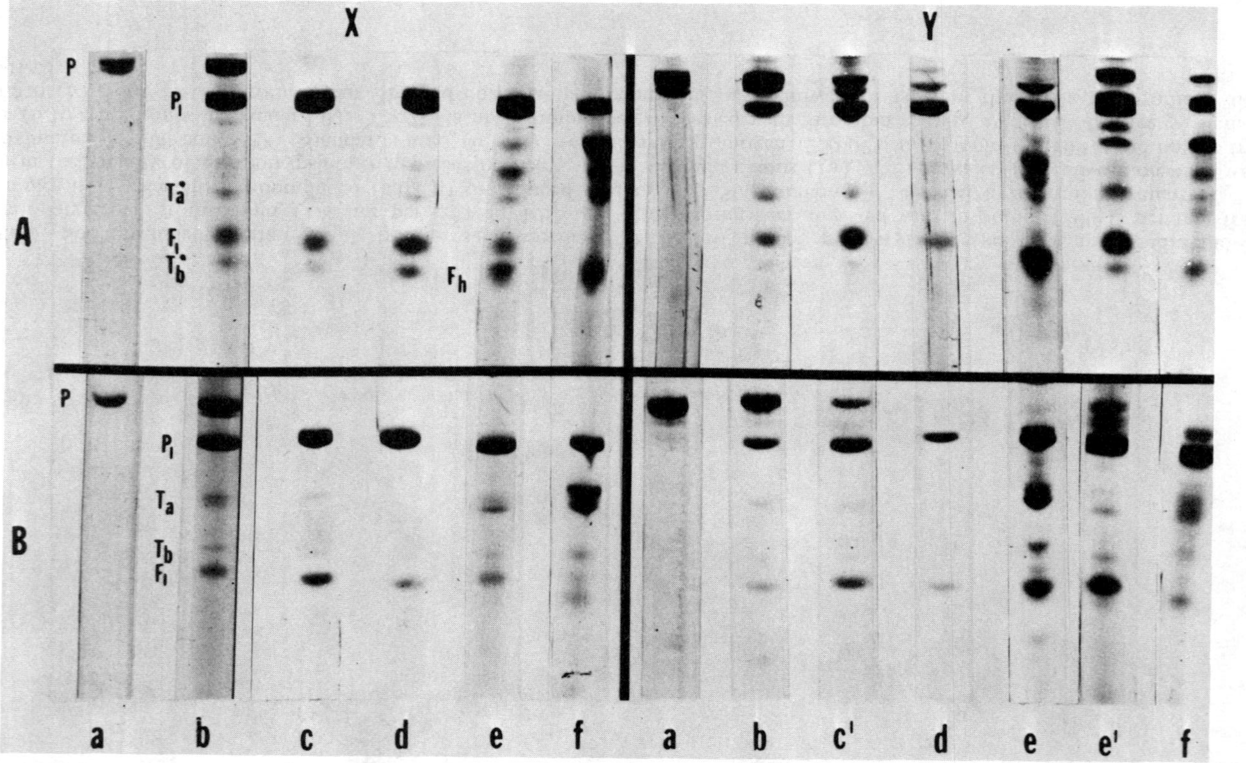

FIGURE 4. Time-course digestion of 5-Gla (barium oxalate atypical) (X), and 2-Gla (pH 4.6 alumina atypical) (Y) prothrombins with thrombin (T_a, α-thrombin; T_b, β-thrombin). Soon after the addition of thrombin, each of the two prothrombin samples (approximately 1.8 mg per ml) contained 210 ± 10 U per ml of thrombin activity that remained more or less constant for at least 4 h. Sodium dodecyl sulfate-gel electrophoresis at different time intervals, after reduction with (A) and without (B) mercaptoethanol are shown: control atypical variant (a), soon after the addition of thrombin (b), 30 min (c'), 2.5 h (c), approximately 4 to 5 h (d), 40 h (e), approximately 40 h (e'), and 3 days (f). The 5-Gla and, to a certain extent, 2-Gla F_1's showed some signs of conversion to double-chain molecules as evidenced by the appearance of the heavy chain in 40 h (F_h). Conversion was complete within 3 days.

faster than the alumina variant. Despite the fact that thrombin activity in the 10-Gla protein deteriorated at a rapid rate and at 30 min only traces remained, almost 90% of the normal prothrombin had degraded. On the other hand, the 2-Gla variant, in which thrombin activity remained as high as 121 U (vs. zero for normal) per ml at 30 min (TABLE 2), underwent only 50% degradation (FIGURE 5, X-c, Y-c). These results unequivocally confirm our observation that the Arg^{156}-Ser bond split at a significantly more accelerated rate for normal prothrombin than for the (partially) decarboxylated prothrombin.

Extra amounts of thrombin were added, once to the 2-Gla after 4.5 h and twice to the normal (10-Gla) preparation, first at 3.5 h and again at 7.5 h, to replenish the loss of thrombin (TABLE 2). As compared to normal sample, thrombin activity was well maintained in the 2-Gla sample during the initial period of 7 h. It was the 10-Gla rather than the 2-Gla protein that showed the appearance of double-chain F_1 at 7 h (FIGURE 5, X-f, Y-f). The F_1 from the 2-Gla variant containing 240 thrombin U per ml at 23 h did not even give the indication of the appearance of a double-chain molecule, while the 10-Gla material had been completely converted to double-chain F_1 (FIGURE 5, X-g, Y-g), again reinforcing our observations that Gla's also do indeed affect the rate of cleavage of the Arg^{52}-Asn peptide bond.

DISCUSSION

The difference between the normal and the atypical prothrombins can be related solely to the extent of carboxylation of the 10 glutamyl residues (Gla) present in the amino portion of the molecule, directly or indirectly through their Ca^{2+}-binding ability. For example, physiological activation criteria of the proteins depend upon their capacities to bind Ca^{2+}, which in turn relate to the number of Gla's present in the molecule. The differences in pI's of the proteins also relate directly to the negative charges contributed by the Gla's, with similar but more pronounced pI differences observed in the F_1's.

The degradation studies which were conducted in the absence of Ca^{2+}, however, reveal some conformational differences because the normal (10-Gla), and to a certain extent the 7-Gla protein, generated F_1 and P_1 at a much faster rate than the 5-Gla and 2-Gla materials.

Apparently the three Gla's in the normal protein, but missing from Ba citrate atypical prothrombin, induce some configurational changes in the molecule such that the peptide bond between Arg (residue 156) and Ser (residue 157) is readily available to thrombin. The two Gla's responsible for the difference between the Ba citrate (7-Gla) and Ba oxalate (5-Gla) variants probably play a very small role in the reaction, because the difference in the rate of prothrombin cleavage between the two variants was not significant. The three Gla's, the difference between the 5-Gla and the 2-Gla prothrombins, affected the rate of generation of P_1 and F_1 to a certain extent because the cleavage of the 2-Gla variant was the slowest. The observation that the F_1 from dicoumarol-induced abnormal prothrombin when digested with trypsin produced more peptides than did normal F_1,[28] supports our contention that Gla's do influence the availability of certain peptide bonds to the enzyme(s).

Profragment 1 generated from normal and Ba citrate atypical prothrombins, respectively, contains all of the 10 and 7 carboxylated glutamyl residues.[29] These two fragments were converted from a single-chain to a double-chain

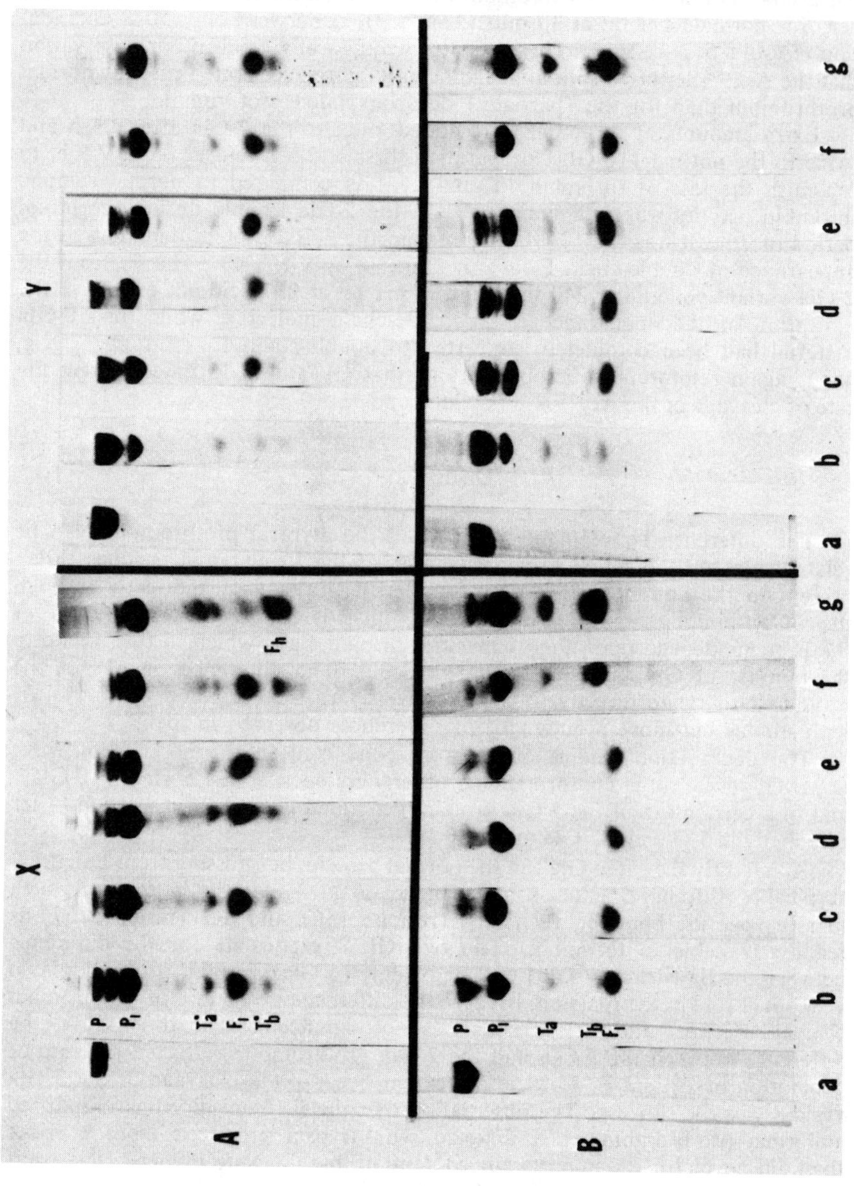

FIGURE 5. Time course digestion of 10-Gla normal (X) and 2-Gla (pH 4.6 alumina atypical) (Y) prothrombins with thrombin (T_a, α-thrombin; T_b, β-thrombin). Normal (1.72 mg per ml) and alumina (1.57 mg per ml) prothrombins, respectively, contained 56 and 45% normal plasma antithrombin activity. Soon after the addition of thrombin, each of the two samples contained 170 U of thrombin per ml. Sodium dodecyl sulfate-gel electrophoretic patterns of aliquots taken at different time intervals, after reduction with (A) and without (B) mercaptoethanol are shown: control prothrombin samples containing antithrombin III (a), soon after the addition of thrombin (b), 30 min (c), 1 h (d), 2 h (e), 7 h (f), and 23 h (g). Although the thrombin activity in the 10-Gla material (X) deteriorated at a rapid pace as shown by the very little or no activity left after 5 to 30 min, the 2-Gla preparation (Y) contained 121 U per ml at 30 min and about 50 U at 2 to 3 h (see TABLE 2). Approximately 60 to 70% of normal (X) compared to only 20 to 30% of the alumina (Y) preparation had been degraded soon after the addition of thrombin (b) to generate prethrombin 1 (P_1) and profragment 1 (F_1). Almost all the 10-Gla prothrombin, compared to a little more than 50% of the 2-Gla variant, was digested in 30 min (c), showing that 10-Gla (normal) prothrombin in the presence of thrombin generates P_1 and F_1 more rapidly than does the 2-Gla variant.

Extra amounts of thrombin were added both to the 2-Gla variant (after 4.5 h) and to the normal preparation (4 and 7.5 h) to raise their thrombin activity to about 275 U per ml. Despite the fact that the next morning (g) both the samples contained about 240 U of thrombin per ml, almost all the F_1 generated from 10-Gla normal prothrombin had been converted to a double-chain molecule, while no such conversion was observed in F_1 obtained from the 2-Gla prothrombin.

molecule by thrombin within 5 to 6 h. No such conversion was observed in F_1 from both 5- and 2-Gla variants for at least 24 h. At 40 h or more, however, F_1 from the two variants converted to a double-chain molecule. Assuming that carboxylation of the glutamyl residues is not random but specific, as may be the case since the amino acid residue adjacent to a glutamyl residue can influence its carboxylation,[30] the following hypotheses are made: a) the extra carboxyl groups, which are common to both 7- and 5-Gla prothrombins, play some although not a very significant role in the splitting of the peptide bond between Arg (residue 52) and Asn (residue 53) to convert single-chain F_1 to a double-chain molecule; b) the extra carboxyl groups present in the Ba citrate atypical (7-Gla) molecule but missing in the Ba oxalate (5-Gla) atypical variant do not influence the generation of F_1 and P_1 from the Ba citrate variant, although they do significantly augment the conversion of single-chain F_1 to a double-chain molecule; c) the extra carboxyl groups present in the normal (10-Gla) prothrombin but absent in the Ba citrate atypical (7-Gal) protein, which makes the Arg-Ser peptide bond readily available for the generation of F_1 and P_1, do not play a significant role in the conversion of single-chain F_1 to a double-chain molecule by thrombin; and d) the light chain of double-chain F_1 is from the amino portion of the molecule, because our preliminary data show that the mobility of the light chain depends upon Ca^{2+}. The light chain perhaps represents the first 52 residues of the parent prothrombin molecule.[31]

ACKNOWLEDGMENTS

This work was supported by the Medical Research Service of the Veterans Administration. The author is deeply indebted to Dr. J. R. Carter for his interest and counsel, and Dr. M. Levine for reviewing the manuscript. The technical assistance of Mrs. Peggy Mendelson is also greatly appreciated.

REFERENCES

1. MAGNUSSON, S., L. SOTTRUP-JENSEN, T. E. PETERSEN, H. R. MORRIS & A. DELL. 1974. Primary structure of the vitamin K-dependent part of prothrombin. FEBS Lett. **44:** 189–193.
2. FERNLUND, P., J. STENFLO, P. ROEPSTORFF & J. THOMSEN. 1975. Vitamin K and the biosynthesis of prothrombin. V. γ-carboxyglutamic acids, the vitamin K-dependent structures in prothrombin. J. Biol. Chem. **250:** 6125–6133.
3. BJÖRK, G. & J. STENFLO. 1973. A conformational study of normal and dicoumarol-induced prothrombin. FEBS Lett. **32:** 343–346.
4. NELSESTUEN, G. L., M. BRODERIUS & G. MARTIN. 1976. Role of γ-carboxyglutamic acid. Cation specificity of prothrombin and factor X-phospholipid binding. J. Biol. Chem. **251:** 6886–6893.
5. PRENDERGAST, F. G. & K. G. MANN. 1977. Differentiation of metal ion-induced transitions of prothrombin fragment 1. J. Biol. Chem. **252:** 840–850.
6. BLOOM, J. W. & K. G. MANN. 1978. Metal ion induced conformational transitions of prothrombin and prothrombin fragment 1. Biochemistry **17:** 4430–4438.
7. MALHOTRA, O. P., W. B. RIPPON, D. D. SOLOMON & A. G. WALTON. 1979. Structural and physiological relationships in blood clotting proteins: thrombin and prothrombin. Intl. J. Biol. Macromol. **1:** 137–143.
8. ESMON, C. T. & C. M. JACKSON. 1974. The conversion of prothrombin to

thrombin. III. The factor X_a-catalyzed activation of prothrombin. J. Biol. Chem. **249:** 7782–7790.

9. SEEGERS, W. H. & T. ANDARY. 1974. Formation of prethrombin-E, thrombin, and thrombin-E and their inhibition with antithrombin and enzyme inhibitors. Thromb. Res. **4:** 869–874.

10. MALHOTRA, O. P. 1972. Atypical prothrombin in purified preparations from dicoumarol-treated steers. Life Sciences **11:** 901–907.

11. MALHOTRA, O. P. 1972. Atypical prothrombins induced by dicoumarol. Nature New Biology **239:** 59–60.

12. MALHOTRA, O. P. 1974. Purification and properties of normal and abnormal prothrombin. Thrombos. Diathes. Haemorrh. Suppl. **59:** 27–43.

13. MALHOTRA, O. P. 1979. Purification and characterization of dicoumarol-induced prothrombins. I. Barium citrate atypical (7-Gla) prothrombin. Thromb. Res. **15:** 427–437.

14. MALHOTRA, O. P. 1979. Purification and characterization of dicoumarol-induced prothrombins. II. Barium oxalate atypical (5-Gla) variant. Thromb. Res. **15:** 438–448.

15. MALHOTRA, O. P. 1979. Purification and characterization of dicoumarol-induced prothrombins. III. Alumina pH 4.6 atypical (2-Gla) variant. Thromb. Res. **15:** 449–463.

16. NELSESTUEN, G. L. & J. W. SUTTIE. 1972. The purification and properties of an abnormal prothrombin protein produced by dicoumarol-treated cows (A comparison to normal prothrombin). J. Biol. Chem. **247:** 8176–8182.

17. CESBRON, N., C. BOYER, M. C. GUILLIN & D. MÉNACHÉ. 1973. Human coumarin prothrombin-chromatographic, coagulation and immunologic studies. Thrombos. Diathes. Haemorrh. **30:** 437–450.

18. MALHOTRA, O. P. & J. R. CARTER. 1972. Biological and nonbiological activation of normal and dicoumarol-treated prothrombin. Life Sciences **11:** 445–454.

19. STENFLO, J. 1973. Vitamin K and biosynthesis of prothrombin. III. Structural comparison of an amino terminal fragment from normal and from dicoumarol-induced bovine prothrombin. J. Biol. Chem. **248:** 6325–6332.

20. KISIEL, W. & D. J. HANAHAN. 1973. The action of factor X_a, thrombin and trypsin on human factor II. Biochim. Biophys. Acta **329:** 221–232.

21. MALHOTRA, O. P. & J. R. CARTER. 1968. Modified method for the preparation of purified bovine prothrombin of high specific activity. Thrombos. Diathes. Haemorrh. **19:** 178–185.

22. MALHOTRA, O. P. & J. R. CARTER. 1965. Modification of two-stage assay of purified or plasma prothrombin. Fed. Proc. **24:** 154.

23. WARE, A. G. & W. H. SEEGERS. 1949. Two-stage procedure for the quantitative determination of prothrombin concentration. Am. J. Clin. Pathol. **19:** 471–482.

24. ABIDGAARD, U., K. GRAVEM & H. C. GODAL. 1970. Assay of progressive antithrombin in plasma. Thrombos. Diathes. Haemorrh. **24:** 224–229.

25. YUE, R. H., T. STARR & M. GERTLER. 1973. Quantitative determination of total antithrombin III in plasma. Thrombos. Diathes. Haemorrh. **30:** 84–92.

26. WEBER, K. & M. OSBORN. 1969. The reliability of molecular weight determinations by dodecyl sulfate—polyacrylamide gel electrophoresis. J. Biol. Chem. **244:** 4406–4412.

27. FAIRBANKS, G., T. L. STECK & D. F. H. WALLACH. 1971. Electrophoretic analysis of the major polypeptides of the human erythrocyte membrane. Biochemistry **10:** 2606–2617.

28. STENFLO, J. 1974. Vitamin K and the biosynthesis of prothrombin. IV. Isolation of peptides containing prosthetic groups from normal prothrombin and the corresponding peptides from dicoumarol-induced prothrombin. J. Biol. Chem. **249:** 5527–5535.

29. ESNOUF, M. P. & C. V. PROWSE. 1977. The γ-carboxyglutamic acid content of human and bovine prothrombin following warfarin treatment. Biochim. Biophys. Acta **490:** 471–476.
30. RICH, D. H., S. R. LEHRMAN, J. M. HAGEMAN & J. W. SUTTIE. 1977. Vitamin K-dependent carboxylase: synthesis and activity of peptides substrates. Fed. Proc. **36:** 1081.
31. WALZ, D. A., D. HEWETT-EMMETT & W. H. SEEGERS. 1977. Primary structure of the amino-terminal (Vitamin K-dependent) region of human prothrombin. Life Sci. **20:** 79–84.

THREE ASPECTS OF PROTHROMBIN ACTIVATION RELATED TO PROTEIN M, ECARIN, ACUTIN, MEIZOTHROMBIN 1 AND PRETHROMBIN 2 *

Walter H. Seegers, Che-Ming Teng, Abha Ghosh,
and Eduardo Novoa

*Department of Physiology
Wayne State University School of Medicine
Detroit, Michigan 48201*

INTRODUCTION

The need to obtain purified proteins from plasma, platelets, and tissues continues to be at the forefront. The conservative, systematic fractionation of blood is one of the topics considered in this report. One of the components, protein M, has only recently been obtained in purified form and more information is needed about its function and properties. Earlier, prethrombin 2 was obtained in concentrated form but mixed with thrombin.[1,2] We have now found a way to obtain it easily as a single component and have studied requirements for its conversion to α-thrombin. The method for purification was made possible by the limited digestion of purified prothrombin with acutin, a thrombin-like enzyme recently isolated[3,4] from the venom of *Agkistrodon acutus.*

In like manner, snake venom is useful for the purification of another prothrombin derivative; namely, meizothrombin 1.[5,6] Ecarin is obtained as the prothrombin activating principle of *Echis carinatus* venom.[7,8] Using this enzyme it was possible to produce and isolate meizothrombin 1. Its esterolytic activity was found to be 14.5 times greater than the proteolytic activity. The two activities of meizothrombin 1; namely, esterase and fibrinogen clotting were brought to a one-to-one ratio by adding purified factor Xa, purified factor V, phospholipids, and calcium ions.

MATERIALS AND METHODS

Fractionation of Bovine Blood

In the interest of conservation, the maximum amount of useful material is wanted from a blood collection and a system has been evolving in this laboratory that goes a great distance toward that goal.[9] At the outset, the choice of anticoagulant(s) is of importance. Oxalates, citrates, EDTA, heparin, and combinations thereof are commonly used. For some purposes, soybean trypsin

* This work was supported by grants HLB-03424-22, HLB-18435-03 from the National Heart, Lung and Blood Institute, National Institutes of Health, U.S. Public Health Service, and the Skillman Foundation. Che-Ming Teng was recipient of a Fogarty International Research Fellowship (TW-02743-01). We are indebted to Daniel Walz of this laboratory and F. Kornalik (Prague) for Ecarin supplies.

453

inhibitor, benzamidine, and even diisopropylfluorophosphate (DFP) alone or together are added to the anticoagulant.

A useful approach to the fractionation of anticoagulated blood for products of interest for blood coagulation studies is outlined (FIGURE 1). Platelet-rich anticoagulated plasma is first obtained by slow centrifugation. The platelets can be harvested by centrifugation of the plasma. Freezing and thawing the plasma yields a cryoprecipitate containing fibrinogen and antihemophilic factor. Washed barium carbonate or barium sulfate added to the plasma adsorbs the vitamin K-dependent proteins, which can be eluted and the eluate is commonly called prothrombin complex. The adsorbed plasma is useful for isolating either antithrombin III or Ac-globulin.

Fractionation of Prothrombin Complex

In our fractionation procedure we used a DEAE-Sephadex A-50 column and eluted with a salt gradient.[10] This has now been modified by using a stepwise elution series with salt.[11, 12] The main fractions and subfractions obtained are outlined (TABLE 1). The important purified proteins for the discussion below are prothrombin, factor VII, factor X and with 0.30 M salt fraction 1 plus protein M.

Activity of Protein M

Purified protein M shortened the prothrombin time of plasma from dicumarol-treated steers, as well as that of factor VII-deficient human plasma. The activated partial thromboplastin time of factor VIII- and IX-deficient plasma was also shortened by protein M. It functioned with thromboplastin in the conversion of factor X to factor Xa. For various reasons, however, we

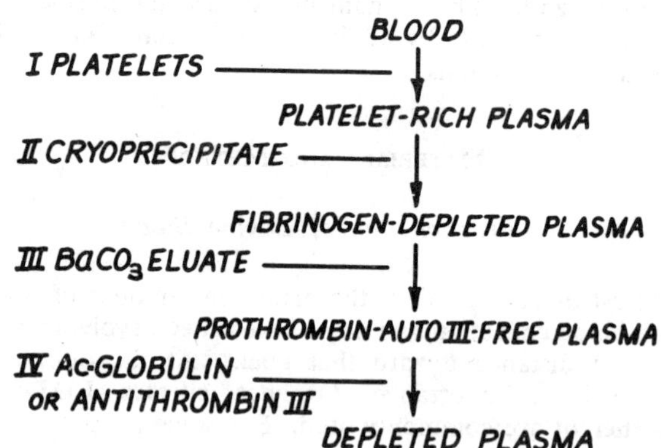

FIGURE 1. Fractionation of bovine anticoagulated blood. Slow-speed centrifugation separates platelet-rich plasma as a source of platelets obtained by further centrifugation. Freezing and thawing yields a fibrinogen-rich cryoprecipitate that can be collected by centrifugation. Addition of barium carbonate to the remaining plasma adsorbs prothrombin complex proteins. The depleted plasma is a source for either Ac-globulin or antithrombin III.

TABLE 1

FRACTIONATION OF BOVINE PROTHROMBIN COMPLEX ON
DEAE-SEPHADEX A-50 COLUMN (2.5 × 15 cm)

Molar NaCl	Eluted Material *	Remarks
0.15	Factor VII +Unknown Components	Resolved on Sephadex G-100 column (2.5 × 180 cm) to obtain clean Factor VII
0.20	Multiple Components	No activity identified
0.25	Prothrombin + Protein M-2 +F-IX+Trace Protein M +Unknown Component	Resolved on heparin-Sepharose column (1.5 × 18 cm) to obtain pure Prothrombin, F-IX and nearly pure Protein M-2 †
0.30	Fraction 1+Protein C, +Protein M+Inhibitor +Protein D	Resolved on Sephadex G-100 column (2.5 × 180 cm) four fractions ‡
0.50	F-X+Inactive Material	Resolved on Sephadex G-100 column (2.5 × 180 cm) §

* In all cases a single symmetrical elution curve.

† Some protein is removed from this protein M-2 fraction on Sephadex G-100 column (2.5 × 180 cm). Protein M-2 modifies the initial velocity of thrombin generation from purified prothrombin when Ac-globulin is left out of the five-component system.

‡ The second fraction was passed through a heparin-Sepharose column. Protein C did not bind, and the second protein eluted with 0.25 *M* salt solution. We call this protein D. It seems to be different from other known vitamin K-dependent proteins. The content of basic amino acids was found to be high; and the neutral sugar content was near 7.7%. It contained glucosamine and γ-carboxyglutamic acid. No procoagulant or anticoagulant activity was found. It is a single-chain protein and when mixed with protein C a single band was observed by polyacrylamide gel electrophoresis under non-reducing medium.

§ F-X is obtained as a single component. The inactive material is also pure, with amino acid composition and with some other properties similar to factor X.

eventually ruled out its possible identity with factor VII. This was especially evident by its acceleration of thrombin formation under conditions where factor VII had no effect. Two main effects of protein M are summarized:

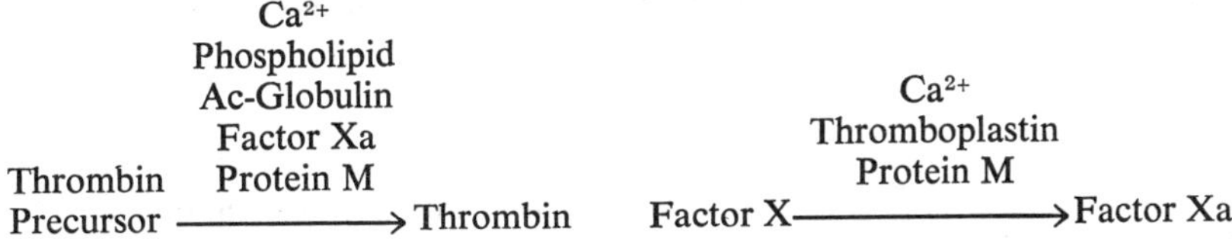

In the generation of thrombin by the above five-component systems, the activation mixture was composed of the following: 0.1 ml thrombin zymogen (12,000 U/ml); 0.1 ml crude "cephalin" (0.3% suspension); 0.1 ml factor Xa (300 U/ml); 0.1 ml Ac-globulin (factor V, 120 U/ml); 0.1 ml calcium chloride (0.1 *M*); and 0.5 ml imidazole buffer (pH 7.2). Samples were repeatedly taken from the mixture for thrombin analysis to follow the time course of the activation.

In the above combination of procoagulants, protein M had a synergistic effect when the thrombin precursor was purified prothrombin, purified prethrombin 1, purified prethrombin 2, and three kinds of atypical prothrombin molecules isolated from plasma of steers given dicumarol; namely, 2-Gla prothrombin, 5-Gla prothrombin, and 7-Gla prothrombin.[12, 13] An example of the activation, typical for the zymogens mentioned above, is given (FIGURE 2) for prethrombin 1. With the data now available there is no evident way to interpret, at the structural level, the mechanisms by which protein M functions. Under several conditions it functions as a procoagulant, and generates factor Xa activity from factor X in the presence of thromboplastin and calcium ions. One might speculate that protein M is the procoagulant that accounts for the short prothrombin time observed when vitamin K is given to reverse the effects of dicumarol. Under those conditions the prothrombin time is short when the

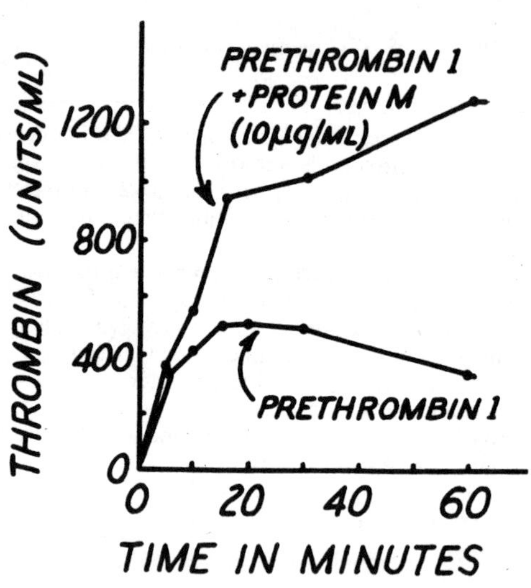

FIGURE 2. The generation of thrombin from purified prethrombin 1 in the system outlined in text. Activation mixture consisted of prethrombin 1, factor V, phospholipid, factor Xa, and calcium chloride. Complete activation required addition of protein M. All purified components of bovine origin.

concentrations of prothrombin and factor X are still low.[14] The same is true for the plasma of newborn human beings.[15] Another possibility is that protein M is the main effective component in prothrombin complex preparations found to have therapeutic value for hemophiliac patients with inhibitors.[16–18]

PROPERTIES OF PROTEIN M

At the outset it seemed likely that protein M might be a form of factor VII. Unexpectedly, however, the similarity is with prethrombin 1. This is true with respect to molecular weight as measured by SDS-polyacrylamide gel electrophoresis, amino acid composition, H_2N-terminal amino acid sequence, and carbohydrate content. Both precursor proteins have Gla amino acid residues; namely, prothrombin and fraction 1 (TABLE 1).

The differences between protein M and prethrombin 1 include the procoagulant properties of protein M discussed above. Prethrombin 1 does not have these properties. Protein M and its precursor are eluted from DEAE-Sephadex A-50 column with 0.3 M salt whereas prethrombin 1 is eluted with 0.1 M salt and its precursor with 0.25 M salt (TABLE 1). The precursor of protein M undergoes spontaneous activation on standing at 4° C for two or three days to give protein M and another protein with inhibitor activity. This does not happen with prothrombin as precursor of prethrombin 1 and pro-thrombin fragment 1.

The highest specific activity of protein M precursor obtained was 55 pro-thrombin units/mg. On standing at $-70°$ C for a week or at 4° C for a couple of days, this specific activity approximately doubled and at the same time protein M procoagulant properties developed. On SDS polyacrylamide gel electrophoresis, two new bands were observed in place of purified protein M precursor. Our prothrombin preparations usually had a specific activity ranging from 3,500 to 4,200 prothrombin units/mg. This kind of prothrombin prepara-tion did not show increased specific activity upon standing either at $-70°$ C or at 4° C.

One purified sample of protein M preparation had the highest specific activation; namely, 380 prothrombin units/mg. By comparison, a prethrombin 1 preparation was 3,000. Twenty μg of this protein M preparation as accessory procoagulant generated thrombin to 100% either from prothrombin or pre-thrombin 1 zymogen when tested in the five-component assay system. When the same quantity or the same number of units of prethrombin 1 were substi-tuted for protein M in the five-component assay, using either prothrombin or prethrombin 1 as zymogen, no such enhancement in rate or yield of thrombin was observed.

Factor X is converted to factor Xa to an extent of 40% in the presence of thromboplastin and calcium ions by protein M. An increase in the quantity of protein M did not help further. Prethrombin 1 does not convert factor X to factor Xa under the same experimental conditions.

Protein M precursor (1 mg/ml), on digestion with thrombin (60 U/ml for 30 min), gave rise to bands corresponding to protein M and inhibitor protein on SDS-polyacrylamide gel electrophoresis. If the digestion was continued, a new band in the molecular weight region of 38,000 appeared. The appearance of a new component is due to the attack of thrombin on protein M. Pro-thrombin, under similar conditions, gave rise to only two bands even if the digestion was continued for three hours. Thrombin digestion products of prothrombin always moved comparatively slower than those of protein M precursor on SDS-polyacrylamide gel electrophoresis. On polyacrylamide gel electrophoresis in Tris-glycine buffer, protein M migrated more slowly than prethrombin 1.

In agar double-diffusion experiments, the antibodies against protein M precursor recognized protein M and inhibitor protein but did not recognize prethrombin 1 though different concentrations of prethrombin 1 were tried. In a similar experiment, antibody to purified prothrombin was used. A line of identity was observed for prethrombin 1, a very faint line of recognition for protein M, but nothing appeared for protein M precursor and inhibitor during 18 hours of incubation. These relationships are outlined in TABLE 2.

A combined solution of protein M precursor, protein M, inhibitor, and protein C are easily separated in a 2.5 × 180 cm Sephadex G-100 column.[12] By contrast, when gel filtration is repeated with a solution containing pro-

TABLE 2

RECOGNITION OF ANTIBODY TO PROTEIN M PRECURSOR OR PROTHROMBIN

Antibody	Recognition	No Recognition
Protein M Precursor	1. Protein M 2. Inhibitor 3. Itself	1. Prethrombin 1
Prothrombin	1. Prethrombin 1 2. Protein M 3. Itself	1. Protein M precursor 2. Inhibitor

thrombin, prethrombin 1, prothrombin fragment 1, and protein C, no clear separation takes place. From this it does not appear that Protein M precursor is the same as prothrombin, nor that protein M is the same as prethrombin 1, nor that inhibitor is the same as prothrombin fragment 1.

α-THROMBIN, β-THROMBIN-E, ECARIN, AND MEIZOTHROMBIN 1

Historical

It was observed many years ago that the esterase activity predominates when prothrombin is converted to thrombin and that the full proteolytic activity as measured on fibrinogen develops later.[19-22] Prior to this observation esterase and protease activities of an enzyme were believed to be controlled by the same active site of the enzyme. The two functions seemed to be inseparable. They were repeatedly found to be inhibited or activated simultaneously and to the same extent. In addition to showing that esterase activity develops first it was also found that thrombin deteriorates on standing. Esterase activity is retained while fibrinogen-clotting activity declines and nearly vanishes. Twelve years after these discoveries the activities were separated in trypsin.[23] These facts are not covered in a recent review on prothrombin structure, activation, and biosynthesis.[24] With purified ecarin, isolated from *Echis carinatus* venom, prethrombin 1 was converted to meizothrombin 1. This involved only the splitting of the Arg-Ile bond that corresponds to H_2N-terminal Ile residue to the heavy chain of thrombin and the Arg HOOC-terminal residue of the light chain of thrombin.

Meizothrombin 1 Purification

A method was developed to purify meizothrombin 1, and it was found to have 14.5 times greater esterase activity than proteolytic activity. The main problem was to prevent α-thrombin formation by autolysis. Our starting material was 50 mg prethrombin 1 in 0.05 M phosphate buffer, pH 6.5, plus 0.01 M benzamidine. To this was added 0.1 mg pure ecarin. Volume was 50 ml, and kept at 37° C. Activation was complete in two hours (FIGURE 3). This mixture was applied to a DEAE-Sephadex A-50 column (2.5×10 cm) equilibrated to match the activation medium. The column was washed with starting buffer and the meizothrombin 1 was eluted with salt. The meizothrombin 1 was concentrated to 5 ml by ultrafiltration (Amicon, PM-10). By successive dilutions and reconcentration, the solution was converted to 0.05 *M* phosphate buffer pH 6.5 and 0.001 *M* benzamidine. To this an equal volume of glycerol was added. The product was stored at −20° C.

Formation of Thrombin

The conversion of meizothrombin 1 to α-thrombin by purified factor Xa required factor V, phospholipid, and calcium ions; however, without calcium ions or phospholipid the yield was more than when prothrombin was the substrate in the same system (FIGURE 4). The results are shown in TABLE 3.

Autolysis of Thrombin

The α-thrombin that was derived from meizothrombin 1 was purified and allowed to undergo autolysis in 0.2 *M* ammonium bicarbonate solution pH 8 at 4° C. The B1 chain[25] consisting of 73 amino acid residues from the H_2N-terminal end of the B chain remained bound to the parent molecule and most likely supplied the active His residue needed for the charge-relay activation reactions. To summarize the changes due to Ecarin, factor Xa, and autolysis, FIGURE 5 is presented, and the associated activities are as follows:

	Predominantly	Esterase and	Primarily
Prethrombin 1 →	Esterase →	Proteolytic →	Esterase

PREPARATION OF PRETHROMBIN 2

In earlier purification procedures the prethrombin 2 yield was low and much α-thrombin was in the products.[1, 2] We found that the thrombin-like enzyme

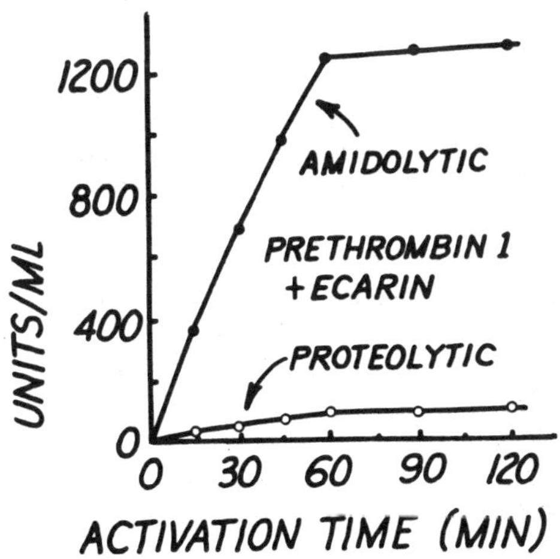

FIGURE 3. Activation of purified prethrombin 1 with ecarin at 500 to 1 (w/w) in 0.05 *M* phosphate buffer at pH 6.5, 0.001 *M* benzamidine, at 37° C. Note 14.5 times greater development of amidolytic, as compared with clotting activity. Meizothrombin 1 is obtained from the activation mixture as a single component by chromatography on a DEAE-Sephadex A-50 column.

TABLE 3

CONVERSION OF MEIZOTHROMBIN 1 TO THROMBIN WITH FACTOR XA, PHOSPHOLIPID, FACTOR V, AND CALCIUM IONS

Components	α-Thrombin
All present	100%
No factor V added	none
No factor Xa added	none
No calcium ions added	55%
No phospholipid added	55%

isolated from *Agkistrodon acutus*[3,4] degrades either prothrombin or prethrombin 1 to prethrombin 2 and no further degradation occurs.[26] The thrombin-like enzyme was called Acutin.

With an activation mixture consisting of 80 to 1 (w/w) prethrombin 1 and Acutin, all of the prethrombin 1 was converted to prethrombin 2 and prothrombin fragment 2. The components were easily separated by using a DEAE-Sephadex A-50 fractionation column.[26] The thrombin content of the prethrombin 2 preparation was less than 1% on the basis of U/U. We were able to dry prethrombin 2 from the frozen state without loss of activity. Before drying the solution was made salt-free by dialyzing against distilled water.

ACTIVATION OF PRETHROMBIN 2

To achieve the conversion of prethrombin 2 to α-thrombin it was only necessary to break the Arg^{49}-Ile^{50} bond of the molecule.[6] To study this the

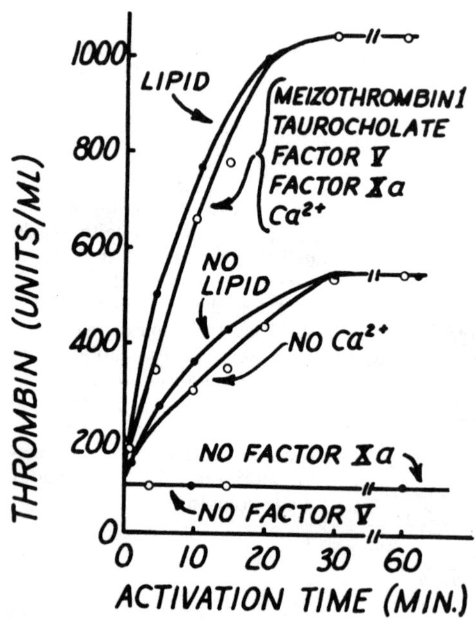

FIGURE 4. Conversion of meizothrombin 1 to α-thrombin and prothrombin fragment 2 in a five-component system consisting of meizothrombin 1, factor Xa, factor V, calcium ions, and phospholipid, or sodium taurocholate.

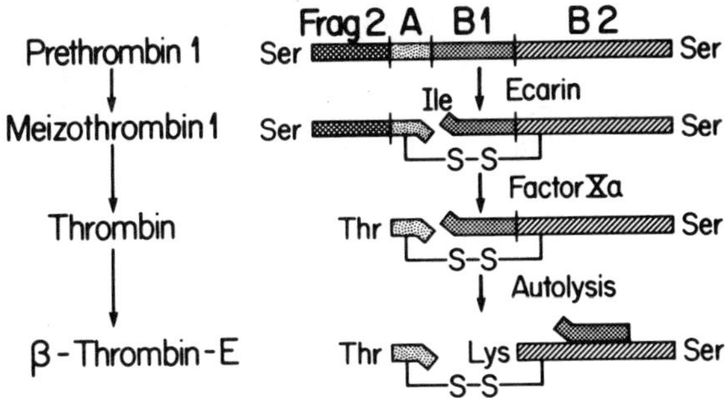

FIGURE 5. Prethrombin 1 drawn to scale as disulfide-bond reduced single chain. ecarin, in presence of benzamidine, opens a bond corresponding to $\text{Arg}^{49}\text{-Ile}^{50}$ in thrombin. The resulting meizothrombin 1 is converted to α-thrombin by Factor Xa plus Ac-globulin plus phospholipid and calcium ions. By slow autolysis of α-thrombin the $\text{Arg}^{73}\text{-Lys}^{74}$ bond of the B chain is split forming β-thrombin-E consisting of 49 amino acid residues for the light chain connected by a disulfide bond to B2 chain having 186 amino acid residues. To supply the function of the active His (His 43 of the B1 chain, or residue number 366 of prothrombin), it is assumed that the B1 chain functions in the noncovalent state. Thus far it has only been removed by denaturing agents.[25]

following arrangement was set up: 0.1 ml prethrombin 2 (8,000 U/ml); 0.1 ml crude "cephalin" (0.3% suspension); 0.1 ml factor Xa (200 U/ml); 0.1 ml Ac-globulin (factor V, 500 U/ml); 0.1 ml calcium chloride (0.1 M); and 0.5 ml imidazole buffer (pH 7.2).†

The yield of α-thrombin in the above activation mixture was about 10% (FIGURE 6). Adding purified prothrombin fragment 2 helped improve the yield a little and the same was true for the addition of prothrombin fragment 1. The two fragments together were sufficient to increase the yield to 100%. Both fragments were necessary. This does not confirm the observations of Esmon, Owen, and Jackson [27] who stated that both fragments were not sufficient, and that fragment 1·2 was necessary. Furthermore we observed that prothrombin, at the level of only 50 units, served as a supplement to the activation mixture. This was not true when purified prethrombin 1 was used, and that is explained on the basis that it contains only prothrombin fragment 2 and not fragment 1. The activation of prethrombin 2 can then be summarized as follows:

Calcium ions
Phospholipid
Ac-Globulin
Prothrombin fragment 1
Prothrombin fragment 2
Factor Xa

Prethrombin 2———————————————→α-thrombin

Since the term prothrombinase was introduced many years ago, its meaning has not changed; namely, it is the prothrombin activating complex. We can redefine the ingredients as consisting of the procoagulants listed above, and write as follows:

† Other materials incorporated according to plan of study.

$$\text{Prethrombin 2} \xrightarrow{\text{Prothrombinase}} \alpha\text{-thrombin}$$

Prothrombinase is not the only system with the capacity to generate α-thrombin from prethrombin 2 as the substrate. Protein M can be substituted for prothrombin fragment 1 and prothrombin fragment 2. In the particular experiment illustrated (FIGURE 7), 500 units of prethrombin 2 served as substrate. The yield with the five-component system was increased to 100% with only 76 μg of purified protein M. This procoagulant effect is similar to that which occurs with other substrates such as prethrombin 1 or the atypical pro-thrombins induced in steers with dicumarol.[11, 13] The maximum amount of potential thrombin in the 76 μg of purified protein M measured by our standard prethrombin assay was 22 units, and thus could not be the source of the much greater amount of thrombin that was generated.

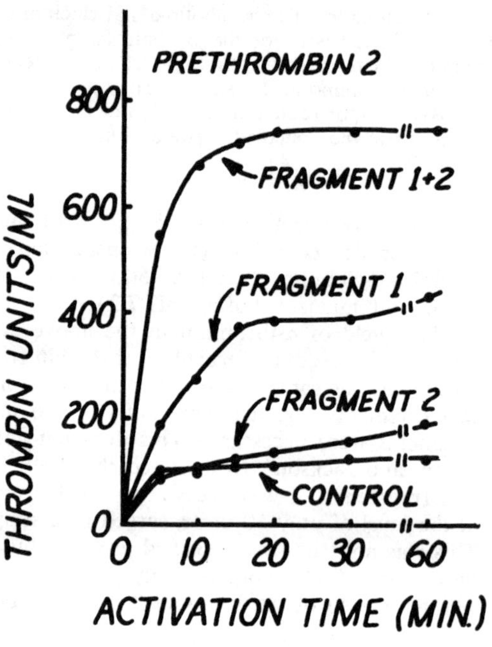

FIGURE 6. The conversion of prethrombin 2 to α-thrombin. The control activation mixture consisted of factor Xa, factor V, phospholipid, calcium ions, and the substrate. Adding either prothrombin fragment 1 or pro-thrombin fragment 2 alone was not sufficient for obtaining α-thrombin. Both fragments were needed. Both fragments could also be supplied when covalently connected as in prothrombin.

Some of the structural changes for prothrombin following the use of Acutin and prothrombinase are outlined (FIGURE 8).

PROTHROMBIN ACTIVATION SEQUENCE

For the generation of α-thrombin from prothrombin it is only necessary to break two polypeptide bonds; namely, at Arg^{274}-Thr^{275} and Arg^{323}-Ile^{324}. This yields prothrombin fragment 1·2 and α-thrombin consisting of two polypeptide chains. One is the A chain with 49 residues and the other is the B chain with 259 residues. It has been suggested on the basis of extensive data[28] that the first event consists of breaking the Arg-Thr bond followed by cleavage of the Arg-Ile bond. That conclusion, however, does not account for the fact that

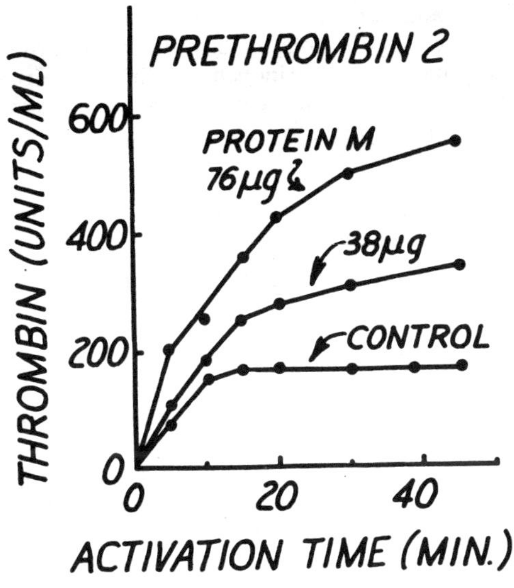

FIGURE 7. The control or basic activation mixture contained 500 U/ml prethrombin 2 with factor V, phospholipid, factor Xa, and calcium ions (see text). This mixture yielded only 30% of the thrombin. The addition of protein M brought the yield to 100%.

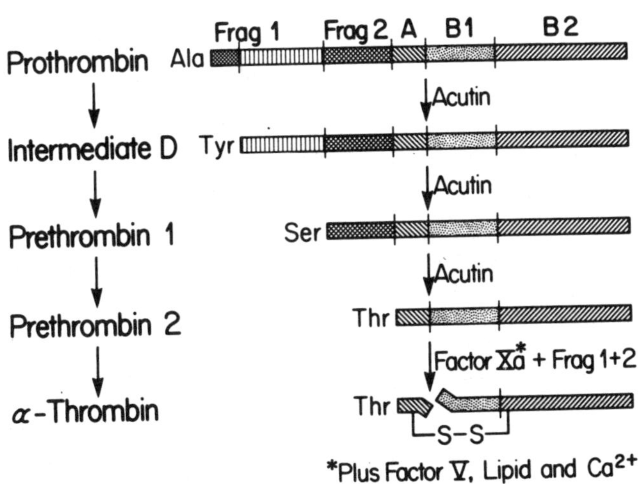

FIGURE 8. Single chain prothrombin molecule drawn to scale. Disulfide bonds reduced. Acutin breaks bond between Lys^{44}-Tyr^{45}. Intermediate D is formed. Further degradation produces prethrombin 1 as intermediate and finally prethrombin 2 where the degradation stops. To produce α-thrombin prothrombinase is required.

esterase activity can first predominate and then become equal to fibrinogen clotting activity.[29] By first breaking the Arg-Ile bond, meizothrombin forms with predominantly esterase activity and weak fibrinogen clotting activity. Then by cleavage of the Arg-Thr bond α-thrombin forms with far greater clotting activity than meizothrombin. This sequence is outlined as follows:

$$\text{Prothrombin} \xrightarrow{\text{Prothrombinase}} \text{Meizothrombin}$$

$$\text{Meizothrombin} \xrightarrow{\text{Prothrombinase}} \alpha\text{-Thrombin} + \text{Prothrombin Fragment } 1 \cdot 2$$

Prethrombin 2, Ecarin, and Prothrombin Fragment 1

As stated earlier in this paper, ecarin is the enzyme that generates α-thrombin from prothrombin, and that it breaks the peptide bond corresponding to Arg^{49}-Ile^{50} of prethrombin 2. In a ratio of (w/w) of 500 to 1 very little thrombin activity developed. The yield of α-thrombin was, however, 100% when prothrombin fragment 2 was added (FIGURE 9). This fragment is associated with the binding of factor V, but with ecarin it has an important role without factor V.

Summary

A procoagulant called protein M has been purified from bovine plasma. It is derived from a precursor that has Gla amino acid residues. Protein M accelerates the generation of α-thrombin in a five-component system consisting of thrombin zymogen, factor Xa, Ac-globulin, phospholipid, and calcium ions. In this system the zymogen can be purified prothrombin, purified prethrombin 1 or 2, or purified dicumarol-induced atypical prothrombins as isolated by Om Malhotra. Protein M shortens the prothrombin time of plasma from steers given dicumarol and of factor VII-deficient plasma. The activated partial thromboplastin time of factor VIII- and IX-deficient human plasma was shortened, as well as plasma from dicumarol-treated persons. Protein M functions with thromboplastin and calcium ions in the generation of factor Xa from factor X. The precursor of protein M is in many respects similar to prothrombin and protein M is similar to prethrombin 1. There are, however, distinct differences.

Purified ecarin from *Echis carinatus* venom converted purified bovine prethrombin 1 to meizothrombin 1. This involved only the breaking of an Arg-Ile bond. Meizothrombin 1 was purified. It was free of α-thrombin and was a single component by polyacrylamide gel electrophoresis. It had 14.5 times more esterase activity than proteolytic activity on fibrinogen. Like α-thrombin it degraded purified prothrombin to prethrombin 1. Meizothrombin 1 itself converted to α-thrombin plus prothrombin fragment 2 by autolysis, and also with purified factor Xa. In the latter case, factor V plus phospholipids or sodium taurocholate plus calcium ions accelerated the reaction. A likely sequence for thrombin formation by factor Xa as enzyme begins with the production of meizothrombin possessing strong esterase and weak coagulant activity. Next, meizothrombin is converted to α-thrombin plus prothrombin fragment $1 \cdot 2$. Ecarin generated very little α-thrombin from prethrombin 2, but the yield was 100% when purified prothrombin fragment 2 was also added. Optimum conditions were a molar ratio of 1-to-1 for prethrombin 2 and prothrombin fragment 2.

The thrombin-like enzyme isolated from *Agkistrodon acutus* venom has been called acutin. It degrades purified bovine prothrombin in several steps. A bond at Lys⁴⁴-Tyr⁴⁵ is broken with formation of prothrombin intermediate D plus a predicted 44-residue peptide formerly called P fragment.[30] Then pre-thrombin 1 forms from intermediate D followed by prethrombin 2. The digestion stops at the level of prethrombin 2. The latter is then easily isolated. By activating prethrombin 2 with factor Xa alone at a 40:1 molar ratio very little α-thrombin forms. To obtain α-thrombin from prethrombin 2 it is necessary to supply an enzyme system consisting of factor Xa, phospholipid, calcium ions, Ac-globulin, and in addition prothrombin fragment 1 and pro-

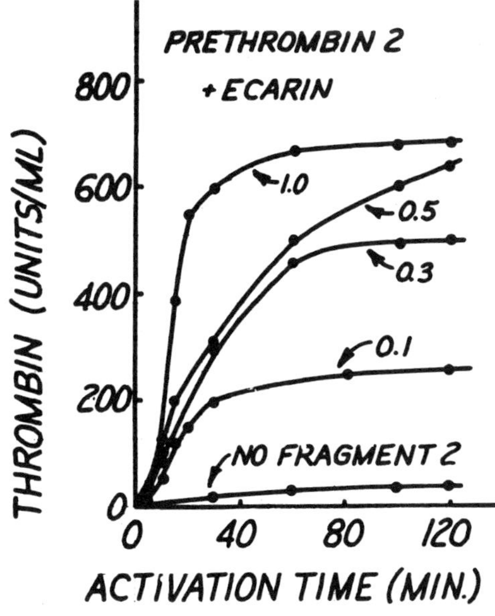

FIGURE 9. In the generation of α-thrombin from prethrombin from prethrombin 2 ecarin splits the Arg⁴⁹-Ile⁵⁰ bond of prethrombin 2. Prothrombin fragment 2 is required as a cofactor, at an optimum concentration of a one-to-one molar ratio with respect to prethrombin 2. Decreasing the concentration of fragment 2 gave a proportionately lower yield of thrombin. No calcium ions added.

thrombin fragment 2. It is proposed that this enzyme system be called *pro-thrombinase*. The amount of fragments 1 and 2 can be much less than the proportion that naturally occurs in prothrombin. Under conditions where one or more of the procoagulants is present in suboptimal amounts, protein M can compensate for the deficiency.

Another protein was separated from the fraction used to purify protein C. It contained γ-carboxyglutamic acid and is called protein D. It seems to be different from any previously recognized vitamin K-dependent proteins.

REFERENCES

1. HELDEBRANT, C. M., R. J. BUTKOWSKI, S. P. BAJAJ & K. G. MANN. 1973. The activation of prothrombin. II. Partial reactions, physical and chemical characteristics of the intermediates of activation. J. Biol. Chem. **248:** 7149–7163.

2. OWEN, W. G., C. T. ESMON & C. M. JACKSON. 1974. The conversion of prothrombin to thrombin. I. Characterization of the reaction products formed during the activation of bovine prothrombin. J. Biol. Chem. **249:** 594–605.
3. OUYANG, C., J. S. HONG & C. M. TENG. 1971. Purification and properties of the thron oin-like principle of *Agkistrodon acutus* venom and its comparison with bovine thrombin. Thromb. Diath. Haemorrh. **26:** 224–234.
4. OUYANG, C., Y. C. CHEN & C. M. TENG. 1979. The clotting activity of the thrombin-like enzyme of *Agkistrodon acutus* (hundred-pace snake) venom. Toxicon **17:** 313–316.
5. KORNALÍK, F. & B. BLOMBÄCK. 1975. Prothrombin activation induced by Ecarin. A prothrombin converting enzyme from *Echis carinatus* venom. Thromb. Res. **6:** 53–63.
6. MORITA, T., S. IWANAGA & T. SUZUKI. 1976. The mechanism of activation of bovine prothrombin by an activator isolated from *Echis carinatus* venom and characterization of the new active intermediates. J. Biochem. **79:** 1089–1108.
7. SCHIECK, A., F. KORNALÍK & E. HABERMANN. 1972. The prothrombin activating principle from *Echis carinatus* venom. I. Preparation and biochemical properties. Naunyn-Schmiedebergs Arch. Pharmacol. **272:** 402–416.
8. SCHIECK, A., E. HABERMANN & F. KORNALÍK. 1972. The prothrombin activating principle from *Echis carinatus* venom. II. Coagulation studies in vitro and in vivo. Naunyn-Schmiedebergs Arch. Pharmacol. **274:** 7–17.
9. SEEGERS, W. H. 1974. Systematic fractionation of blood with special reference to blood coagulation. Thromb. Diath. Haemorrh. Suppl. **57:** 7–11.
10. NOVOA, E., W. H. SEEGERS & H. I. HASSOUNA. 1976. Improved procedures for the purification of selected vitamin K-dependent proteins. Prep. Biochem. **6:** 307–338.
11. SEEGERS, W. H., A. GHOS.i & V. Y. WU. 1980. Function of previously unrecognized plasma protein M in thrombin generation. *In* Vitamin K Metabolism and Vitamin K-Dependent Proteins. J. W. Suttie, Ed.: 96–101. University Park Press. Baltimore, Md.
12. SEEGERS, W. H. & A. GHOSH. 1980. Activation of prothrombin and Factor X: Function of previously unrecognized plasma protein. Thromb. Res. **17:** 71–81.
13. SEEGERS, W. H., A. GHOSH & O. MALHOTRA. 1980. Protein M and the activation of dicoumarol induced atypical prothrombin. Thromb. Res. **18:** 131–137.
14. RENO, R. S. & W. H. SEEGERS. 1967. Two-stage procedure for the quantitative determination of autoprothrombin III concentration and some applications. Thromb. Diath. Haemorrh. **18:** 198–210.
15. OWEN, C. A., G. R. HOFFMAN, S. E. ZIFFREN & H. P. SMITH. 1939. Blood coagulation during infancy. Proc. Soc. Exp. Biol. Med. **41:** 81–83.
16. FEKETE, L. F., S. L. HOLST, F. PETOOM & L. L. DEVEBER. 1972. "Auto" Factor IX concentrate: A new therapeutic approach to treatment of hemophilia and patients with inhibitors. *In* Abstracts, 14th Intl. Congress of Hematology. Abstract No. 295. San Paulo.
17. KURCZYNSKI, E. M. & J. A. PENNER. 1974. Activated prothrombin concentrate for patients with factor VIII inhibitors. New Eng. J. Med. **291:** 164–167.
18. PENNER, J. A. & P. E. KELLY. 1975. Management of patients with Factor VIII or IX inhibitors. Semin. Thromb. Hemost. **1:** 386–398.
19. LANDABURU, R. H. & W. H. SEEGERS. 1957. Further studies of prothrombin derivatives. Proc. Soc. Exp. Biol. Med. **94:** 708–710.
20. SEEGERS, W. H. & R. H. LANDABURU. 1957. Esterase and clotting activity derived from purified prothrombin. Am. J. Physiol. **191:** 167–173.
21. SEEGERS, W. H., R. H. LANDABURU & J. F. JOHNSON. 1960. Significance of thrombin-E in the prothrombin activation sequence. Nature **185:** 930–931.

22. LANDABURU, R. H. & W. H. SEEGERS.   1959.   Generation of proteolytic activity during activation of prothrombin. Am. J. Physiol. **197:** 1178–1180.

23. COLETTI-PREVIERO, M. A., A. PREVIERO & E. ZUCKERKANDL.   1969.   Separation of the proteolytic and esterase activities of trypsin by reversible structural modifications. J. Mol. Biol. **39:** 493–501.

24. SUTTIE, J. W. & C. M. JACKSON.   1977.   Prothrombin structure, activation and biosynthesis. Physiol. Rev. **57:** 1–70.

25. SEEGERS, W. H., J. REUTERBY, G. MURANO, L. E. McCOY & B. B. L. AGRAWAL.   1971.   Studies on the nature of thrombin. Thromb. Diath. Haemorrh. Suppl. **47:** 325–337.

26. SEEGERS, W. H., C. M. TENG & E. NOVOA.   1980.   Preparation of bovine prethrombin 2: Use of acutin and activation with prothrombinase or ecarin. Thromb. Res. **19:** 11–20.

27. ESMON, C. T., W. G. OWEN & C. M. JACKSON.   1974.   The conversion of prothrombin to thrombin: V. The activation of prothrombin by Factor Xa in the presence of phospholipid. J. Biol. Chem. **249:** 7798–7807.

28. ESMON, C. T., W. G. OWEN & C. M. JACKSON.   1974.   A plausible mechanism for prothrombin activation by Factor Xa, phospholipid, and calcium ions. J. Biol. Chem. **249:** 8045–8047.

29. NOVOA, E. & W. H. SEEGERS.   1980.   Mechanisms of α-thrombin and β-thrombin-E formation: Use of ecarin for isolation of meizothrombin 1. Thromb. Res. **18:** 657–668.

30. SEEGERS, W. H., D. A. WALZ, J. REUTERBY & L. E. McCOY.   1974.   Isolation and some properties of thrombin-E and other prothrombin derivatives. Thromb. Res. **4:** 829–859.

THROMBIN SPECIFICITY *

John W. Fenton II

*Division of Laboratories and Research
New York State Department of Health
Albany, New York 12201*

INTRODUCTION

Procoagulant α-thrombin is the central bioregulatory enzyme in hemostasis.[1–4] Hemostasis is the containment of circulating blood necessary for supplying essential substances and eliminating wastes from dependent tissues. Vascular control of blood flow occurs at three levels: 1) the stationary vessel wall; 2) the circulating blood cells; and 3) the fluid-phase plasma components. The various functions of α-thrombin (FIGURE 1) include those at all three levels of hemostatic control (TABLE 1). The severity of tissue injury and circulatory complications determines the extent to which this enzyme participates in thrombotic events. Underscoring its central functions and importance, human disabilities and deaths attributed to hemostatic disorders (coronary thrombosis, pulmonary embolism, stroke, etc.) exceed those caused by cancer and constitute one of the foremost problems of health/medical economic concerns in our society. It is a tribute to Dr. Walter H. Seegers that his pioneering studies, begun over four decades ago, have formed the foundation for much of our current understanding of thrombin functions and hemostasis.

THROMBIN REGULATION

Physiologic functions of α-thrombin appear to follow concentration relationships, in which its concentration is regulated by prothrombin activation and by offsetting consumptive processes. Like most plasma proteins, prothrombin is synthesized in the parenchymal cells of the liver.[5, 6] It is, unlike most plasma proteins, a vitamin K-dependent protein, as also are the coagulation factors VII, IX, and X, as well as lesser known proteins. Vitamin K antagonists (e.g., coumarin compounds) inhibit the biosynthetic completion of these factors required for their physiological activation.[7, 8] The antagonist sodium warfarin is not only the hemorrhagic ingredient of rat poison but also is administered to patients with thrombotic tendencies and is one of the most widely used pharmaceuticals today.[9]

Prothrombin circulates in blood as a single-chain protein consisting of three domains [10]: fragment F1, fragment F2, and the thrombin moiety (pre-thrombin-2). The 10 vitamin K-dependent γ-carboxyglutamate residues [11, 12] are located in the NH_2-terminus of the F1 domain (FIGURE 2). During physiologic activation the γ-carboxyglutamate residues are believed to form Ca^{2+} salt bridges joining the F1 domain with phospholipid micelles, while activated factor V (factor V′) is thought to associate with the F2 domain to enhance

* Supported by the National Heart, Lung, and Blood Institute Grant HL 13160.

468

activation by factor Xa in the prothrombin activation complex (FIGURE 1).
Since factor Xa also binds Ca^{2+} and is believed to be bound to the same phospholipid micellar surface as prothrombin, how these two micellar bound proteins interact with one another is not clear. However, factor Xa proteolytically cleaves prothrombin, first between its NH_2-terminal F1·2 and CO_2H-terminal thrombin (prethrombin-2) halves, and then it cleaves the latter half to produce the A and B chains of α-thrombin.[7, 8] Because the first cleavage produces two noncovalent fragments (F1·2 and prethrombin-2; FIGURE 2), the intermediate proenzyme, prethrombin-2, must be noncovalently retained for the second cleavage to occur in the generation of the active enzyme, α-thrombin.

Although blood coagulation is usually thought of as enzyme cascades,[13] activation complexes such as that for prothrombin activation appear to occur redundantly in the blood-coagulation pathways (FIGURE 1). These complexes consist of a high M_r nonenzymic protein and an active protease (e.g., factors V' and Xa, respectively, in the prothrombin activation complex). The majority require Ca^{2+}, and several also require phospholipids. The classical "intrinsic" pathway simplifies to four complexes (the collagen/factor XIIa, the high M_r kininogen/factor XIa, the factor VIII'/factor IXa, and the factor V'/factor Xa complexes) while the thromboplastin "extrinsic" pathway reduces to two (the tissue factor/factor VIIa and the factor V'/factor Xa complexes).

Membrane surfaces of stimulated platelets (and perhaps of other cells) constitute a third system for prothrombin activation.[14, 15] Stimulated platelets excrete Ca^{2+}, phospholipids (platelet factor 3), and other substances (e.g., platelet factor 4, which binds heparin and retards its enhancement of antithrombin III); such excreted products assist in the fluid-phase pathways. The interrelations of the plasma-protein systems and those of platelet membranes suggest that the plasma-protein complexes have evolved from cell-membrane systems of more primitive origins. The complexity of the pathways appears to have grown to regulate the common terminal product, α-thrombin.[3, 4]

Human plasma contains sufficient prothrombin to generate an α-thrombin concentration of 130–160 U.S. "NIH" clotting units/ml.[1, 16] However, during the clotting of whole blood the concentrations do not exceed 7–10 units/ml despite activation of over three-fourths of the prothrombin[16] because of thrombin consumption processes (see below). The activation fragment F1·2 of prothrombin (FIGURE 2) is not degraded[16, 17] and the 13-residue F3 peptide does not appear to be autolytically removed from the NH_2-termini of the thrombin A chain.[18] In contrast, preparative activation of human prothrombin concentrates produces high α-thrombin concentrations (500–1,000 units/ml), and F3 is cleaved from the enzyme to produce the isolable form of human α-thrombin.[1-3] Under these conditions, F1·2 is cleaved to F1 and F2, and F1 is further degraded to the disulfide-linked product F1αβ.[19] Although the isolable form of human α-thrombin seems to differ from the physiologic form in its loss of F3, it nevertheless possesses high procoagulant activity (~3,000 units/mg protein) and all other thrombin-ascribed activities.[1-4]

Thrombin consumption reactions include: 1) α-thrombin binding to platelets, endothelial cells, and possibly other cells at sites of vascular damage; 2) active incorporation of α-thrombin into fibrin clots, where it becomes partitioned from blood; and 3) inactivation of the enzyme by reactions with plasma protease inhibitors, antithrombin III, $α_2$-macroglobulin, and perhaps $α_1$-antitrypsin. Since α-thrombin binds with high affinities to platelets, endothelial

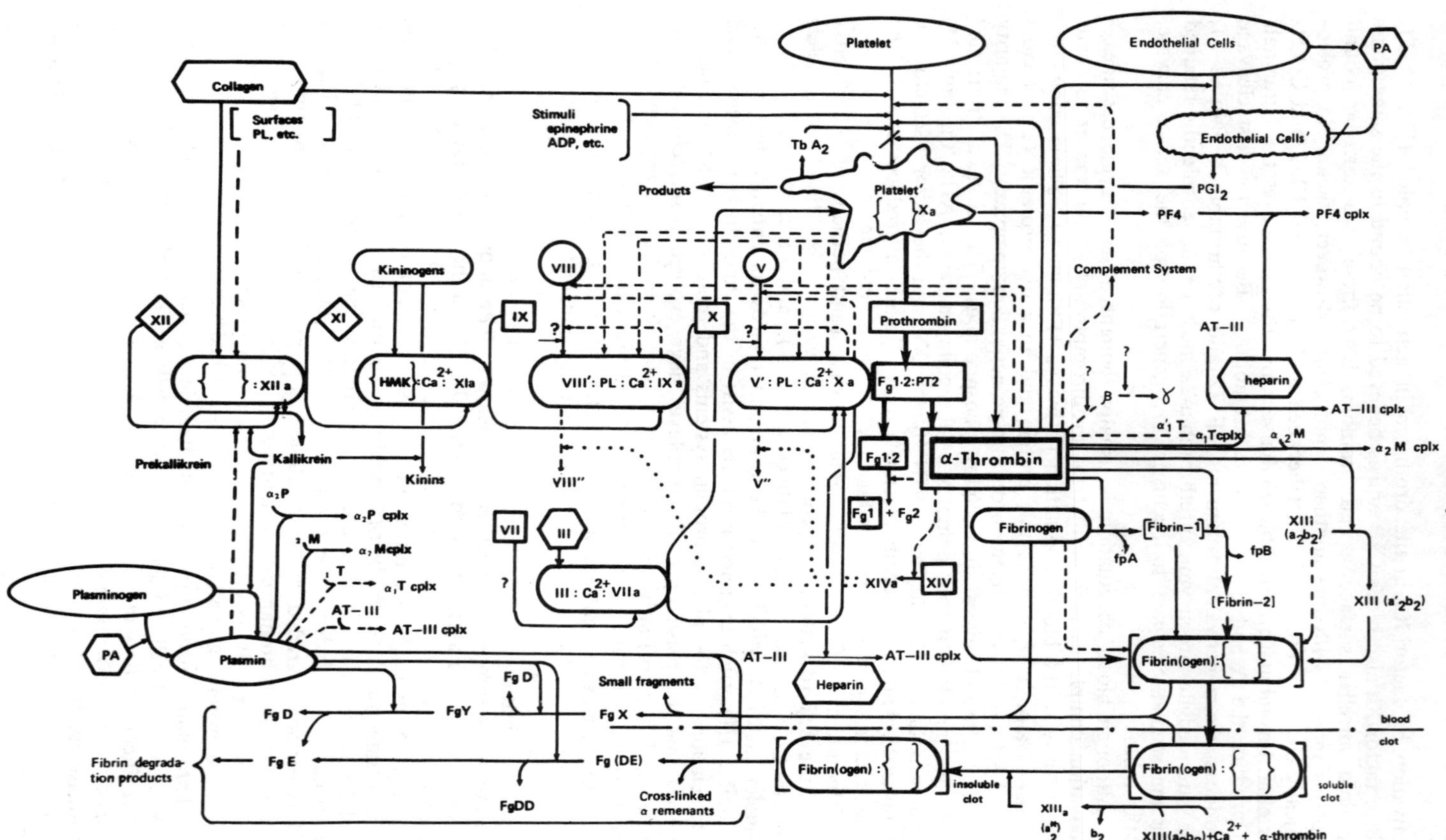

Platelet
Endothelial Cells
PA
Collagen
Surfaces PL, etc.
Stimuli epinephrine ADP, etc.
Tb A2
Endothelial Cells'
Products
Platelet'
Xa
PGI2
PF4
PF4 cplx
Complement System
Kininogens
VIII
V
Prothrombin
AT-III
XII
XI
IX
X
?
?
heparin
AT-III cplx
HMK : Ca2+ : XIa
VIII' : PL : Ca2+ : IXa
V' : PL : Ca2+ : Xa
Fg 1·2 : PT2
α'1 T
α1 Tcplx
α2 M
α2 M cplx
Prekallikrein
Kallikrein
Kinins
VIII''
V''
Fg1·2
α-Thrombin
β
γ
α2 P
α2 P cplx
2 M
α2 Mcplx
T
α1 T cplx
Fg1 + Fg2
Fibrinogen
Fibrin-1
fpA
fpB
XIII (a2 b2)
VII
III
?
Plasminogen
AT-III
AT-III cplx
III : Ca2+ : VIIa
XIVa
XIV
Fibrin-2
XIII (a'2 b2)
PA
Plasmin
AT-III
AT-III cplx
Heparin
Fibrin(ogen) :
Fg D
Small fragments
Fg X
blood
clot
Fg D
FgY
Fg E
Fg (DE)
FgDD
Fibrin degradation products
Cross-linked α remenants
Fibrin(ogen) :
insoluble clot
Fibrin(ogen) :
soluble clot
XIIIa (a2M) 2
b2
XIII(a'2b2)+Ca2+ + α-thrombin

FIGURE 1. Activation pathways for generating procoagulant α-thrombin and its functions in hemostasis. Ellipsoids denote high-M_r proteins and their complexes (see text); brackets, components that may not be obligatory within complexes; hexagons, substances of nonplatelet cellular origins; diamonds, non-vitamin K-dependent proenzymes. Blood coagulation factors are represented by their accepted Roman numerals, whereas "III'" stands for tissue factor (thromboplastin), "XIII" (a_2b_2) for the plasma fibrin-stabilizing factor, and "XIV" for protein C or S. Other abbreviations: AT-III, anti-thrombin III (heparin cofactor); F_g, fragment; f_p, fibrino-peptide; HMK, high-M_r kininogen; PA, plasminogen activation; PF4, platelet factor 4; PGI_2, prostaglandin I_2; PL, phospholipid; PT2, prethrombin-2; TbA_2 thromboxane A_2; α_1T, α_1-antitrypsin; α_2M, α_2-macroglobulin; and α_2P, α_2-antiplasmin. References for α-thrombin functions are given in the text and TABLE 1; those for its activation are found elsewhere (e.g. references 5, 7, 8, 13). This diagram is drawn to the best of the author's knowledge and may therefore contain errors, omissions, and/or oversimplifications. It is an attempt to illustrate the redundant theme of semimembrane complexes involving coagulation enzymes and the diverse central functions of α-thrombin in hemostasis.

TABLE 1

CIRCULATORY CONTROL LEVELS AND FUNCTIONS OF α-THROMBIN IN HEMOSTASIS

Control Level	Cell or Protein	α-Thrombin Function

Level I: Stationary phase	Vessel wall	1) Endothelial cells of vessel lining
		  a) Selectively binds to cells.[71]
		  b) Stimulates prostacyclin (PGI$_2$) synthesis.[72]
		  c) Inhibits plasminogen activator.[73]
		  d) Could have other functions.
		2) Other cells exposed by vascular injury
		  a) Could bind to cells analogous to fibroblasts.[59]
		  b) Could initiate cell division in wound healing processes.[74]

Level II: Particulate phase	Blood cells	1) Platelets
		  a) Binds to saturable and nonsaturable sites.[57, 75]
		  b) Stimulates excretion of Ca^{2+}, platelet factor 3 (phospholipids), platelet factor 4 (heparin inhibitor), β-thromboglobulin, platelet mitogen, and other substances.[76]
		  e) Initiates factor Xa binding.[14, 15]
		  d) Stimulates thromboxane A$_2$ synthesis.[78, 79]
		  e) Initiates factor Xa binding.[14, 15]
		  f) Causes morphologic transformations.[76]
		2) Erythrocytes
		  a) Incorporates into fibrin gels deposited on erythrocytes surfaces.[21]
		3) Lymphocytes
		  a) Might interact with components of the complement system to affect lymphocytes.[80]

Level III: Fluid phase	Plasma proteins	1) Fibrinogen and Fibrin
		  a) Cleaves fibrinopeptide A to convert fibrinogen into clottable fibrin.[43]
		  b) Secondarily cleaves fibrinopeptide B.[43, 61]
		  c) Actively incorporates in fibrin clots during polymerization.[20, 21]
		2) Factor XIII (fibrin stabilizing factor)
		  a) Cleaves it to form factor XIIIa'b, which converts to factor XIIIa in the presence of Ca^{2+}.[81]
		3) Factor VIII (antihemophilic factor)
		  a) Activates the procoagulant component, presumably by proteolytic cleavage to factor VIII'.[27]

TABLE 1 (Continued)

Control Level	Cell or Protein	α-Thrombin Function
		b) Might participate in the presumably proteolytic inactivation of factor VIII'.[27]
		4) Factor V (accelerator globulin)
		a) Activates by proteolytic cleavage to factor V'.[28]
		b) Might proteolytically inactivate factor V'.[28]
		5) Factor XIV (proteins C or S)
		a) Activates to factor XIVa, which is believed to be responsible for inactivating factors V' and VIII'.[29–30]
		6) Antithrombin III (heparin cofactor)
		a) Causes a proteolytic cleavage in forming a stable inhibitor complex.[50]
		b) Inactivation is accelerated non-stoichiometrically by heparin, more so than factor Xa, and not plasmin.[22]
		c) Several plasma proteases are inhibited.[22]
		d) Reacts similarly with pro- and noncoagulant thrombins.[23, 24]
		7) α₂-Macroglobulin
		a) Forms stable apparent-covalent complexes.[22]
		b) Several plasma proteases are inhibited.[22]
		c) Pro- and noncoagulant thrombins appear to react similarly.[25]
		8) α₁-Antitrypsin
		a) Forms stable apparent-covalent complexes.[82, 83]
		b) Several plasma proteases are inhibited.[82, 83]
		9) Complement Component Proteins
		a) Cleaves C3 to generate C3a-like fragments.[80]
		b) Cleaves C5 to generate C5a-like fragments.[80]
		c) Pro- and noncoagulant thrombins have factor $\bar{D}$-like activities in the alternative complement pathway.[84]
		d) Causes platelet-mediated activation of complement system.[85]
		10) Other Proteins
		a) Will cleave prothrombin F1·2 to F1 and F2 and subsequently degrade F1.[16, 19]
		b) Can cleave F1 from prothrombin.[16]
		c) Does not activate plasminogen to plasmin.[2, 3]

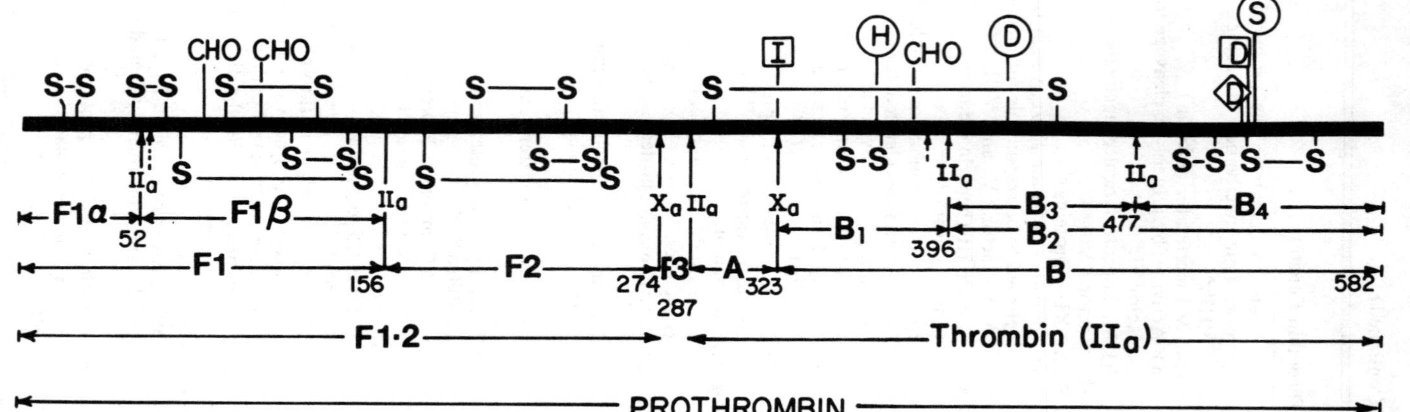

FIGURE 2. Gross structures of human prothrombin, fragments, and thrombin forms. Structures are based on amino acid sequences for human fragment F1·2 [90] and thrombin.[91] Residue numbering corresponds to the sequence for bovine prothrombin,[11] in which the position 4 of human prothrombin is deleted.[19, 90] Factor Xa-activation cleavages (Xa) and thrombin-postactivation cleavages (IIa) are shown. In the human, but not the bovine, enzyme the 13-residue fragment F3 is autolytically removed to form the isolable form of human α-thrombin (see text). This form consists of a 36-residue A chain covalently joined to the midportion of the larger 259-residue B chain. Human β-thrombin arises autolytically or by tryptic cleavage of the B chain to produce the noncovalent B₁ chain and the B₂ chain, which is covalently attached to the A chain.[2] A secondary tryptic cleavage within the B₁ chain [3] is indicated by a dotted arrow. Human γ-thrombin subsequently arises through cleavage of the B₂ chain into the B₃ chain (with the attached A chain) and the noncovalent B₄ chain. This form thus has three noncovalent B chain fragments (B₁, B₃, and B₄) separating its functional residues. The functional histidine (H) aspartic acid (D) and serine (S) triad are circled; the isoleucine (I) and aspartic acid (D) of the activation salt bridge are boxed; and the aspartic acid (D) of the counterion in the arginine side-chain pocket is enclosed by a diamond.

Cleavage products of the activation fragment F1·2 produced by α-thrombin are F1, F2, and the disulfide-joined products F1α and F1β, (in which a secondary cleavage occurs, 16, 19, indicated by a dotted arrow). Positions of disulfide-bridge (-S-S-) and carbohydrate attachments (CHO) are extrapolated from those in bovine prothrombin.[11] The three structural domains of the proenzyme correspond to F1, F2, and the thrombin moiety (prethrombin-2 or F3+α-thrombin, see text). (From Fenton & Landis,[4] Figure 1. With permission of Pergamon Press, Inc.)

cells, and various other cells, its cellular consumption should occur in the early stages of thrombin generation (K_ds 10^{-7} to 10^{-9} M; TABLE 2). However, the cellular binding capacity appears to be relatively limited, and with continued generation, α-thrombin should become available to carry out lower-affinity reactions, such as the conversion of fibrinogen to clottable fibrin monomers ($K_m \sim 10^{-6}$ M for clotting[3]). The capacity of clotting fibrin to incorporate the enzyme appears contrastingly high.[20, 21] This may explain why α-thrombin concentrations decline rapidly with the onset of clotting and why its concentrations do not exceed $\sim$5% of its potential from prothrombin during activation in the clotting of whole human blood.[16, 20] Since fibrin-incorporated α-thrombin is enzymically active,[21] it can potentially leach from the clot or be released during fibrinolysis. The plasma protease inhibitors, except for antithrombin III in the presence of heparin, probably function by consuming enzyme overloads when other systems become saturated. This may explain why depressed antithrombin III levels in plasma are indicative of chronic hemostatic disorders and thrombotic tendencies.[22]

To date no evidence exists for physiologic degradation of procoagulant α-thrombin into noncoagulant β- and γ-thrombins as a regulatory mechanism. These forms do not incorporate into fibrin clots[21] and should therefore be free to circulate. However, since antithrombin III and α_2-macroglobulin readily inactivate them,[23-25] they may be cleared from circulation by the plasma protease inhibitors. The most likely agent, plasmin, does not rapidly convert α-thrombin into noncoagulant forms[2, 3] but does inactivate prothrombin by cleaving an F1-like fragment[26] a possible thrombin-generation control during fibrinolysis.

THROMBIN FUNCTIONS

Abnormalities in thrombin generation result in bleeding tendencies, although α-thrombin may not be necessary for certain hemostatic processes (e.g., collagen stimulation of platelets; FIGURE 1). Prothrombin circulates at higher concentrations ($\sim$0.1 mg protein/ml plasma, or $\sim$1.5 μM proenzyme[2-4]) than the preceding coagulation factors in its activation pathways. Its activation product, α-thrombin, in contrast to other activated coagulation factors, is the terminal enzyme of the pathways and has several important biological functions (FIGURE 1). Despite the seemingly high prothrombin content of human plasma and its extensive activation during whole-blood clotting, α-thrombin does not exceed 0.06 to 0.09 μM concentrations (2–3 μg/ml, or 7–10 clotting units/ml), because of the consumptive processes already discussed. Physiologic concentrations of α-thrombin generated at any given time are, furthermore, believed to be below this range and perhaps may be quite low, with dilution occurring as the consequence of blood circulation.

As initially generated, α-thrombin at very low concentrations is believed to stimulate platelets, interact with vascular endothelial cells, and perhaps interact with other cells exposed at sites of vascular injury (e.g., initiate cellular responses like those caused in tissue culture). Such cells have high-affinity binding sites or receptors for the enzyme and can respond to very low α-thrombin concentrations (e.g., concentrations 1 to 3 orders of magnitude lower than generated during clotting; TABLE 2). Their response requires the catalytically active enzyme. The wide variation in the response time (4–5 sec for

TABLE 2

CELLULAR RESPONSES TO α-THROMBIN

Cell	Property	α-Thrombin Concentration	Time	Binding Affinity K_d	Reference
Human platelets (washed)	Binding of [^{125}I]α-thrombin	0.2 to 1 nM	<15 sec	~2 nM	75
		1 to 10 nM	<15 sec	~10 nM	75
	Half-maximum stimulation	1 to 4 nM	4 to 5 sec		62
Human umbilical vein endothelial cells (cultured)	Binding of [^{125}I]α-thrombin	0.005 units/ml	<1 min (37° C)	~0.1 nM	71
	Half-maximum stimulation of PGI$_2$	0.1 to 0.5 units/ml	1–2 min (37° C)		72
Bovine vascular endothelial cells (cultured)	Half-maximum inhibition of plasminogen activator	0.1 nM	<30 min		73
Bovine corneal endothelial cells (cultured)	Binding	<1.25 μg/ml	<15 sec (37° C)	~0.3 nM	86
Chick embryo cells (cultured)	Binding	~0.3 nM	~30 min (37° C)	~1.2 nM	60
	Half-doubling of cells	~100 ng/ml	24 to 48 hours (37° C)		64
Mouse embryo cells (cultured)	Binding	4–2,000 ng/ml	~2 hours (22° C)	~1 nM	87
	Half-doubling of cells	~0.3 nM	~30 min (37° C)	~1.4 nM	60
		~100 ng/ml	24 to 48 hours (37° C)		64

half-maximum platelet stimulation vs. ~30 min for half-maximum inhibition of plasminogen activator in endothelial cells vs. 24–48 h for doubling of cultured fibroblasts; TABLE 2) suggests that it may constitute an important regulatory mechanism in the sequence of thrombin functions. It presumably arises from the complexities of multistep events in various cellular processes.

As increasing concentrations are generated, α-thrombin initiates clotting by converting fibrinogen into clottable fibrin monomers. It then activates factor XIII, which stabilizes the clot (FIGURE 1). In the fluid phase of blood it is also thought at low concentrations (below those required for clotting) to activate factor VIII[27] and at higher concentrations to activate factor V.[28] (Where other enzymes may perform such functions *in vivo* is unclear.) Both of these activated factors (factors VIII′ and V′) are thought to be destroyed by one or more thrombin-activated proteases (factor XIVa or activated proteins C and S)—a possible terminating mechanism in thrombin generation.[29–31]

Unlike the cellular systems with varying response times, α-thrombin functions involving plasma proteins are relatively simple enzymic processes that appear to differ from one another by their individual concentration dependencies (e.g., binding affinities, as well as the availability of enzyme and substrate). These processes should sequentially follow one another as increasing α-thrombin concentrations generated prior to the maximum concentration at the onset of clotting. The extent to which α-thrombin incorporated into fibrin clots (see above) may carry out functions in fibrin gel matrices, independent of its functions in the fluid phase of blood, is not known.

The discrete, yet diverse biologic functions of α-thrombin suggest that it has a restricted, but not an absolute, enzyme specificity. As would be predicted for a proteolytic function of the enzyme,[32] events catalyzed by it are characteristically irreversible; in the cleavage of fibrinopeptide A and B from fibrinogen, activation of factor XIII, and hydrolysis of other known thrombin-susceptible bonds in proteins, it is clearly a protease (TABLE 3). How it initiates cellular processes, however, can only be speculated from what is known about its proteolytic functions in better-defined systems.

PROTEOLYTIC SPECIFICITY

The larger thrombin B chain arises from the CO_2H-terminal half of prothrombin (FIGURE 2), and its amino acid sequence is homologous to those of the pancreatic serine proteases.[11] This chain contains the functional residues of the catalytic triad (charge-relay system), those of the activation salt bridge, and those implicated as contact residues adjacent to the catalytic site. An aspartic acid residue in the thrombin B chain corresponds to that which serves as the counteranionic residue at the base of the arginine side-chain binding pocket of trypsin.[11] Unlike the pancreatic enzyme, however, thrombin B chain contains insertions, has a carbohydrate attachment, and lacks a disulfide bridge adjacent to the catalytic serine. This bridge is replaced by the disulfide bridge from the middle of the B chain, which joins the smaller thrombin A chain.

The proximity of the A chain to the catalytic site of thrombin has been shown by affinity-labeling techniques,[33] it appears to contribute to exosite regions of lesser specificity importance than those involved in fibrinogen recognition (see below). It is also believed to contribute to the stability of the thrombin catalytic site, since the B chain attachment of the A chain disulfide

TABLE 3

HUMAN PROTEIN WITH IDENTIFIED THROMBIN-SUSCEPTIBLE BONDS *

Protein	Major Cleavage	Amino Acid Sequence	Ref.
Fibrinogen †	Aα 16–17	...Asp-Phe-Leu-Ala-Glu-Gly-Gly-Gly-Val-Arg-Gly-Pro-Arg-Val-Val-Glu-Arg-His-Gln-Ser-...	88
	Bβ 18–19	...Asp-Asn-Glu-Glu-Gly-Phe-Phe-Ser-Ala-Arg-Gly-His-Arg-Pro-Leu-Asp-...	88
Factor XIII	36–37	...Pro-Thr-Val-Glu-Leu-Gln-Gly-Val-Pro-Arg-Gly-Val-Asx-Leu-Glx-Glx-...	89
Prothrombin	F1·2 155–156	...Asp-Gly-Val-Thr-Val-Met-Val-Thr-Pro-Arg-Ser-Glu-Gly-Ser-Ser-Val-Asn-Leu-Ser-Pro-...	90
	F1 51–52	...Ala-Lys-Tyr-Thr-Ala-Cys-Glu-Thr-Ala-Arg-Thr-Pro-Arg-Asp-Lys-Leu-Ala-Ala-Cys-Leu...	19, 90
Thrombin	A-chain 13–14	...Ser-Glu-Tyr-Gln-Thr-Phe-Phe-Asn-Pro-Arg-Thr-Phe-Gly-Ser-Gly-Glu-Ala-Asp-Cys-Gly...	91, 92
Antithrombin III	385–386	...Ala-Ser-Thr-Ala-Val-Val-Ile-Ala-Gly-Arg-Ser-Leu-Asn-Pro-Asn-Arg-Val-Thr-Phe-Lys-...	50, 93
Complement C3a	69–70	...Ile-Thr-Glu-Leu-Arg-Arg-Gln-His-Ala-Arg-Ala-Ser-His-Leu-Gly-Leu-Ala-Arg-CO_2H	80
Pituitary growth hormone ‡	134–135	...Gly-Arg-Glu-Leu-Glu-Asp-Gly-Ser-Pro-Arg-Thr-Gly-Gln-Ile-Phe-Lys-Gln-Thr-Tyr-Asp...	45
Apolipoprotein CIII	40–41	...Gln-Ser-Gln-Gln-Val-Ala-Ala-Gln-Gln-Arg-Gly-Trp-Val-Thr-Asp-Gly-Phe-Ser-Ser-Leu...	94

* Major cleavages are aligned and are shown by arrows (↑). Minor cleavages are indicated by dotted arrows (⇡).

† Fibrinopeptide A is more rapidly released by α-thrombin cleavage at the Aα side than fibrinopeptide B at the Bβ site.[43, 61] This may or may not be due to the influences of contiguous amino acid residues.

‡ Human pituitary growth hormone is relatively resistant to thrombin digestion, while the bovine hormone is slowly digested the ovine hormone is moderately sensitive to thrombin digestion. These differ by the 131–139 corresponding sequences of . . .Gly-*Thr*-Pro-Arg-*Ala*-Gly-Gln-Ile-*Leu* . . . for the bovine hormone and. . . *Val*-*Thr*-Pro-Arg-*Ala*-Gly-Gln-Ile-*Leu* . . . for the ovine hormone, where residue substitutions are italicized.[45]

bridge should, by homology to trypsin, be located near the catalytic serine. The absence of the "serine disulfide loop" found in trypsin may partially explain why α-thrombin is more prone to denaturation (e.g., pH < 5 [1,2]).

Like trypsin, α-thrombin preferentially cleaves peptide or protein substrates at arginine bonds, although it is also capable of doing so at lysine or S-amino-ethylcysteine bonds.[34] However, its proteolytic capabilities are rather limited, compared to those of the pancreatic enzyme, which carries out digestive functions in the gastrointestinal tract. Nor does the blood-coagulation enzyme generally cleave synthetic substrates as readily. Its arginine side-chain pocket appears to have a more limited bulk tolerance than does that of trypsin,[35] and acylation rather than binding (k_2 vs. k_1/k_{-1} in FIGURE 3) may become limiting for α-thrombin.[36] This suggests not only that α-thrombin lacks the substrate adaptivity of trypsin but also that such substrate adaptivity has evolved to extend the proteolytic capabilities of the digestive enzyme. On the other hand, a few synthetic substrates,[37] particularly the tripeptide chromogenic substrates,[38-40] have been found to be more sensitive to thrombin than to the related serine proteases. The thrombin-sensitive tripeptide substrates have either an aromatic blocking group or a hydrophobic D-amino acid residue at their NH_2-termini, and the more specific substrates have a proline (or its analog, pipecolic acid) adjacent to their CO_2H-terminal arginines.[39] The specificity of these substrates is believed to result from an apolar binding site adjacent to and to the left of the catalytic site in thrombin (FIGURE 4 and 5; see below). It is of interest that the tripeptide substrates have evolved through trial and error to where they no longer correspond to the residue sequences of thrombin-susceptible bonds in proteins.[4]

Examination of amino acid sequences on either side of thrombin-susceptible bonds in proteins (see TABLE 1 [39] and TABLE 10 [41]) has revealed no unique requirements for contiguous residues, even when sequence data are analyzed for predicted secondary peptide structures.[42] Tabulation of sequence data for susceptible bonds in human proteins (TABLE 3) illustrates the lack of individual residue requirements and unique patterns. While these examples include only examples of susceptible arginine bonds, autolytic cleavage for formation of human γ-thrombin (see below) is believed to occur at a lysine.[2]

Although the human protein examples indicate a high incidence of proline immediately preceding the susceptible arginine, such prolines do not make certain bonds more susceptible than others (e.g., the Arg-Gly vs. the Arg-Val bond in the fibrinogen Aα chain in TABLE 3). However, residues immediately to the left of susceptible arginines are generally hydrophobic (like the thrombin-sensitive tripeptide-chromogenic substrates, see above). Negatively charged residues (as found at the factor-Xa cleavage sites for prothrombin activation) two positions to the left of thrombin-susceptible arginines are apparently absent. Nevertheless, thrombin will cleave at such sites in prothrombin when the disulfide bridges have been disrupted by performic acid oxidation.[41] It will also hydrolyze the tripeptide chromogenic substrate for factor Xa, but only very slowly.[38-40]

One of the major problems in attempting to extract information from protein-sequence data is that little is known, except on a qualitative basis, about the relative thrombin susceptibilities of various bonds. For fibrinogen it is well established that α-thrombin releases fibrinopeptide A more rapidly than fibrinopeptide B.[43] The release of fibrinopeptide B is believed to be more rapid than factor XIII activation and much more rapid than prothrombin F1$\cdot$2

$$E + S \underset{k_{-1}}{\overset{k_1}{\rightleftharpoons}} ES \xrightarrow[P_1]{k_2} ES' \xrightarrow{k_3} P_2 + E$$

$k_2 \longrightarrow 0$

Compounds: simple competitive inhibitors
(e.g., benzamidine)

Proteins: hirudin; possibly fibropeptides and fibrin;
receptor binding of inactivated enzyme

$k_3 \longrightarrow 0$

Compounds: active-site titrants (e.g., NPGB);
affinity-labeling reagents (e.g., TLCK)

Proteins: antithrombin III; most likely α_2-macroglobulin and
α_1-antitrypsin; possibly receptor-enzyme complexes

non-limiting

Compounds: turnover substrates (e.g., BzArgoEt, tripeptide
chromogenic substrates)

Proteins: fibrinogen, Factor XIII, etc.

FIGURE 3. Examples of enzymic reactions of α-thrombin (E) with synthetic and protein substances (S). The equilibrium complex (ES) gives rise to the first product (P_1) and the acyl intermediate (ES'), and this intermediate produces the second product (P_2) in the regeneration of the enzyme.

fragmentation.[44] The serine and the threonine at two positions to the left of the arginines in the fibrinogen B chain and in prothrombin F1·2, respectively, might retard cleavage (e.g., at the apolar binding site; see below), but factor-XIII activation should precede fibrinopeptide-A release if the left-hand adjacent residues predominantly determine thrombin susceptibility.

Human pituitary growth hormone should perhaps not be included with other thrombin-susceptible proteins, since it is only slightly cleaved after 30-h incubation, while the bovine hormone is partially cleaved after 8 h, and the ovine hormone is completely cleaved within 2 h.[45] The ovine hormone differs from the bovine only in having a single residue at the fourth position to the left of the arginine, while it differs from the human hormone by this residue plus two other substitutions to the right of the arginine (footnote ‡ in TABLE 3). Since these differences are very minor compared to the variance in thrombin susceptibility among the three hormones, other protein structural factors appear determinant; for instance, accessibility of susceptible peptide bonds to the enzyme and protein binding interactions with the enzyme.[2-4]

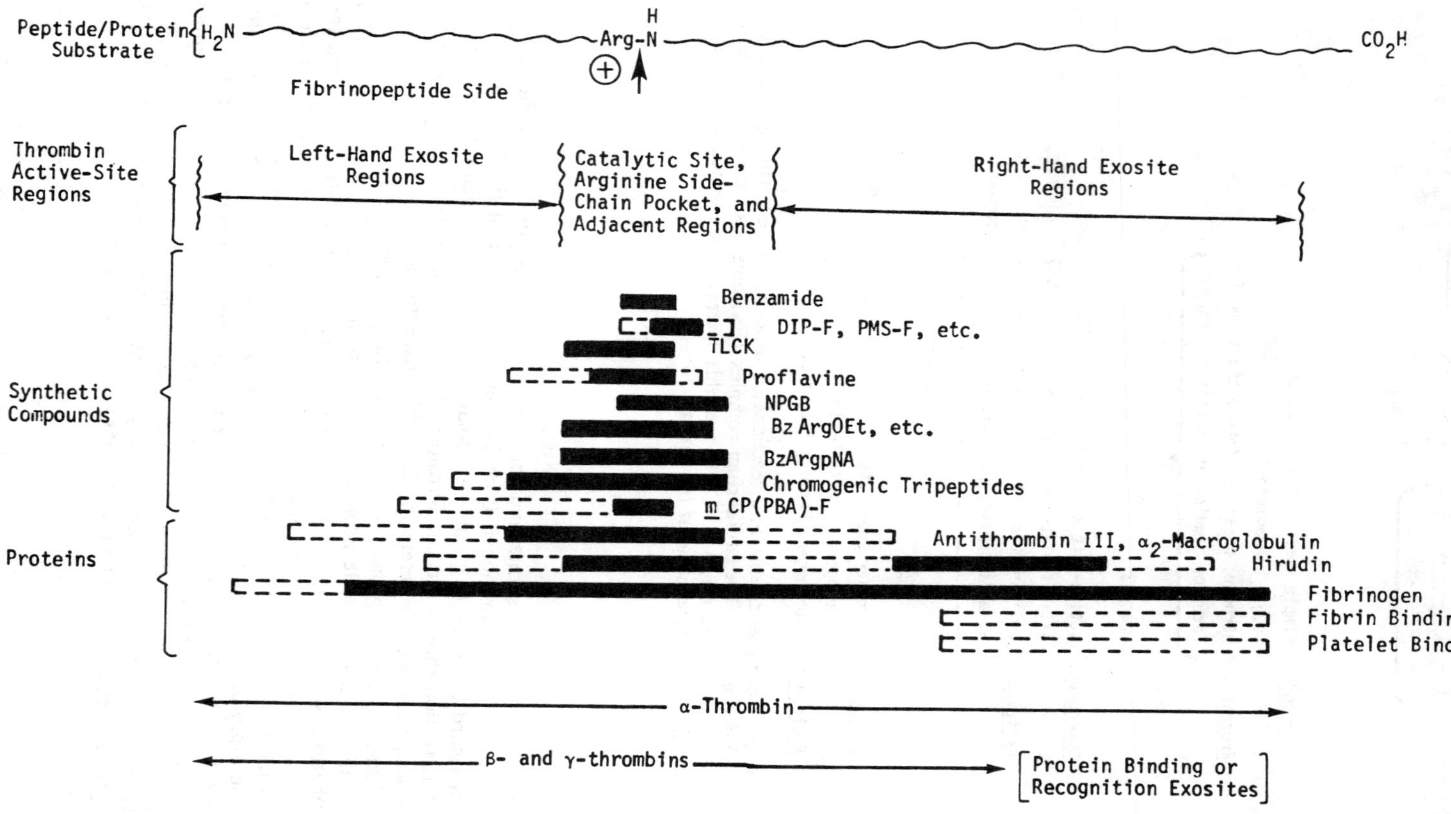

Peptide/Protein Substrate
H2N
Arg-N
H
CO2H
Fibrinopeptide Side
Thrombin Active-Site Regions
Left-Hand Exosite Regions
Catalytic Site, Arginine Side-Chain Pocket, and Adjacent Regions
Right-Hand Exosite Regions
Synthetic Compounds
Benzamide
DIP-F, PMS-F, etc.
TLCK
Proflavine
NPGB
BzArgOEt, etc.
BzArgpNA
Chromogenic Tripeptides
m CP(PBA)-F
Proteins
Antithrombin III, α2-Macroglobulin
Hirudin
Fibrinogen
Fibrin Binding
Platelet Binding
α-Thrombin
β- and γ-thrombins
Protein Binding or Recognition Exosites

FIGURE 4. A schematic two-dimensional map of thrombin active-site regions. Evidence for the positioning of interactions of various compounds and proteins is given in text. Relative distances are shown to the best of the author's knowledge, where uncertainties are indicated by dotted lines. Abbreviations used are: BzArgOEt, $N\alpha$-benzoyl-L-arginine ethyl ester; BzArgpNA, $N\alpha$benzoyl-L-arginine p-nitroanalide; mCP(PBA)-F, m-[o-(2-chloro-5-fluorosulfonylphenylureido)phenoxylbutoxy]benzamidine; DIP-F, diisopropylphosphoro-fluoridate; NPGB, p-nitrophenyl-p'-guanidino-benzoate; PMS-F phenylmethyl sulfonyl fluoride; and TLCK, $N\alpha$-tosyl-L-lysine chloromethyl ketone.

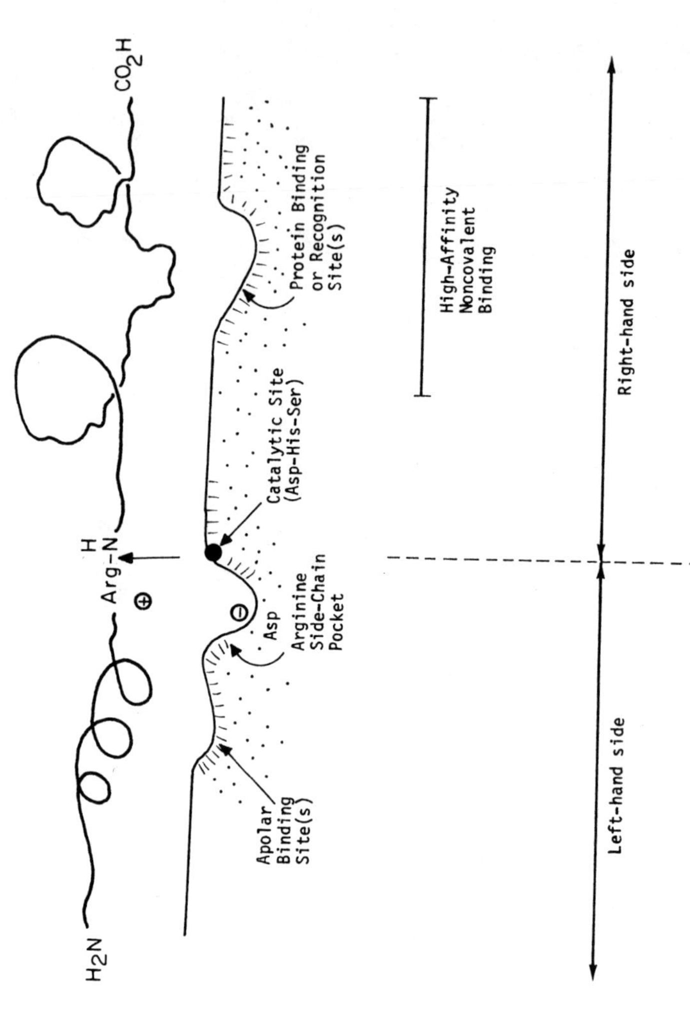

FIGURE 5. A schematic diagram depicting a peptide or protein segment with a thrombin susceptible arginine bond and corresponding regions of the α-thrombin active site. See FIGURE 4 and text.

ACTIVE-SITE REGIONS

The additive contributions of residues in extented peptide segments have been inferred from the increasing rates of thrombin cleavage with increasing chain length of synthetic peptide analogs and fibrinogen Aα chain fragments.[46] Such peptides define a point of cleavage and two directions on either side of the susceptible bond (FIGURES 4 and 5). Within the enzyme the susceptible bond aligns with the catalytic site that consists of the functional residues of the catalytic triad (His[43], Asp[99], and Ser[205] of the thrombin B chain). The arginine (or lysine) residue binds in the arginine side-chain pocket, as do simple competitive inhibitors (e.g., benzamidine). This pocket has a negatively charged counterion (Asp[204] of the B chain) and a hydrophobic lining that enhances binding. In general, good inhibitor ligands are not good substrate ligands, and vice versa, because the orientations of the ligand are critical for efficient catalysis (i.e., k_2-limiting substrates [3, 36]).

Immediately to the left of the pocket is believed to be a second hydrophobic or apolar binding region important in thrombin specificity. Such an apolar binding region (FIGURE 5) is inferred from the occurrence of such residues to the left of susceptible bonds in tripeptide chromogenic substrates and in proteins (see above). This region (FIGURE 4) is believed to be where proflavine binds,[47] since plasmin does not bind proflavine,[36] the region may account for certain specificity differences between the fibrinogen-clotting and fibrinolytic enzymes. Furthermore, since noncoagulant γ-thrombin (see below) binds proflavine similarly to procoagulant α-thrombin,[23] this apolar binding region appears to be independent of a major region required for fibrin(ogen) recognition (see below). The large extended-chain exosite affinity-labeling reagent mCP(PBA)-F (see FIGURE 4 for abbreviations) also reacts similarly with pro- and noncoagulant thrombins,[33] and three-dimensional model based on the structure of trypsin suggests that this reagent binds to the left of the catalytic site.[48]

Interactions with the plasma protease inhibitors, antithrombin III (±heparin) and α_2-macroglobulin, seem mainly to involve regions to the left of the thrombin catalytic sites, since these inhibitors react independently of clotting activity.[23-25] Both form stable, apparently covalent complexes with a variety of proteases, although they inactivate some more rapidly than others.[22] The heparin rate-enhancement effect on antithrombin III is, for example, greatest for thrombin, greater than for factor Xa, and is less for other proteases.[49] Thrombin has recently been shown to cleave an M_r ~5,000 disulfide-retained peptide from the CO_2H-terminus of antithrombin III.[50] The residues to the left of this cleavage site are notably hydrophobic (TABLE 3), suggesting that heparin may induce a conformational change in antithrombin III [51, 52] to increase the exposure of the hydrophobic peptide segment and to promote thrombin reactivity. Since heparin enhances the inactivation of pro- and noncoagulant thrombins similarly,[23, 24] its enhancement of antithrombin III reactivity does not appear to involve thrombin active-site regions for fibrin(ogen) recognition.

Studies with fibrinogen fragments containing the intact fibrinopeptide A suggest that peptide segments to the right of the Aα-cleavage site are of major importance to thrombin specificity.[43] Human α-thrombin with high clotting activity will convert autolytically or by trypsin to noncoagulant β- and subsequently γ-thrombin.[2] These forms arise from the proteolytic fragmentation of the thrombin B chain approximately one-third and two-thirds of the distance from its NH_2-terminus, producing noncovalent fragments (FIGURE 2). Because these forms retain the synthetic-substrate activities of the parent α-thrombin form, and because the B chain fragments contribute the functional residues of the catalytic triad, the fragments must be retained noncovalently in their enzymically active states. Furthermore, since formation of β-thrombin precedes that of γ-thrombin, a conformational change, which correlates with the loss of clotting activity, presumably occurs with the first cleavage to expose the second cleavage site.[1-4] Because of the retention of esterase and related activities is ascribed to active-site regions to the left of the catalytic site (see above), conformational changes, which cause loss of clotting activity, must affect fibrinogen recognition site(s) to the right of the catalytic site (FIGURES 4 and 5). Human γ-thrombin, which lacks clotting activity, cannot interact with either fibrinogen or the polymerizing fibrin monomer; it does not incorporate into clotting fibrin,[21] and fibrinogen does not compete with the tripeptide-chromogenic substrate activity of this thrombin form.[23]

Related to these lost activities with fibrin(ogen), γ-thrombin has an affinity for hirudin two to three orders of magnitude less than α-thrombin.[3, 4, 53] Unlike the plasma protease inhibitors (see above), hirudin, which is a low M_r protein derived from leech salivary glands, is a highly specific thrombin inhibitor.[54] It forms a noncovalent complex with α-thrombin, yet essentially irreversibly inactivates the enzyme through its exceedingly high binding affinity (i.e., $K_i = 6.3 \times 10^{-11}\ M$ [3]). Although hirudin prevents incorporation of DIP-F at the active-site serine, it complexes with active-site serine spin-labeled α-thrombin. This causes very pronounced immobilization of the spin label, which demonstrates that an intact catalytic apparatus is not necessary for complex formation.[3, 53] Thrombin complexing is believed to involve the . . .Pro^{46}-Lys^{47}-Pro^{48}-. . . segment of hirudin, and the Lys-Pro bonds should resist proteolysis.[55] The synthetic peptide homolog of this segment, however, is not an effective thrombin inhibitor,[56] and the inhibitory capability of hirudin is destroyed by disruption of its three disulfide bridges.[55] These observations clearly implicate noncontiguous binding residues, and they show the importance of the three-dimensional structure of hirudin in its interaction with high-affinity protein-binding or recognition sites removed from the catalytic site of α-thrombin (TABLE 4).

The existence of protein-binding or recognition sites to the right of the catalytic site accounts for other unique properties of α-thrombin. Although the active-site serine-conjugated enzyme does not cause clotting either [^{125}I]DIP- or [^{125}I]PMS-α-thrombin, in presence of trace amounts of unlabeled enzyme, incorporates into fibrin clots to a similar extent as does [^{125}I]α-thrombin; neither [^{125}I]γ-thrombin nor the hirudin complex of [^{125}I]α-thrombin incorporates into clots under the same conditions.[21] These data demonstrate that α-thrombin incorporation into fibrin clots involves active-site regions that are independent of the catalytic site and are either not present in γ-thrombin or are masked by hirudin. Likewise, the serine-inactivated enzyme does not stimulate platelets, but [^{125}I]DIP- or [^{125}I]PMS-α-thrombin binds to platelet receptors in the same manner as does [^{125}I]α-thrombin.[57, 58] Hirudin competes for receptor binding and rapidly displaces [^{125}I]PMS-α-thrombin from platelets. However, it displaces biphasically [^{125}I]α-thrombin, suggesting that the functional enzyme participates in events other than those of a simple equilibrium process.[58]

Analogously to platelet interactions, mitogenically responsive cells require the catalytically functional enzyme to initiate cell division, and they specifically bind [^{125}I]α-thrombin to cell-surface receptors.[59] Certain, but not all, cell types will bind [^{125}I]DIP-α-thrombin similarly to the active enzyme.[60]

RECOGNITION COUPLING

The high specificity with which α-thrombin releases fibrinopeptide A requires complementarity of the enzyme active site with fibrinogen (see above). The finding that this enzyme cleaves the fibrinopeptide more rapidly than does trypsin [61] suggests that the Aα-cleavage site is not readily accessible for proteolytic cleavage. If, on the other hand, α-thrombin initially binds to a recognition site on fibrinogen, a high local concentration of the two reactants is achieved. The bound enzyme might also induce a conformational change in fibrinogen to increase the accessibility of the susceptible bond and thus enable more efficient catalysis. Such catalytic enhancement due to protein binding at recognition sites can be considered a recognition-coupled reaction.

Recognition-coupled reactions appear also to occur for cellular receptors (TABLE 4). The initial combining of the enzyme with a recognition site is an equilibrium process and will localize the enzyme at (or within) the receptor (FIGURE 6). Alignment of the enzyme for the performance of its catalytic function may or may not be dependent on other events, and the efficiency with which the enzyme performs its catalytic function will determine the degree of coupling. Chymotryptic treatment of platelets causes uncoupling of binding and stimulation, which makes α-thrombin behave more like γ-thrombin or trypsin.[62]

Unlike typical enzyme-catalyzed reactions, the extent of stimulation of either platelets or mitogenically responsive cells is dependent on the initial concentration of enzyme.[63, 64] This dose relationship suggests that the enzyme does not turn over, or turns over only slowly, in the performance of its catalytic function. If thrombin has a proteolytic function, it will cleave a peptide bond, whose first product corresponds to the CO_2H-terminus of the protein substrate (FIGURE 4). This product, which is presumably the biologic signal (FIGURE 6), could be a newly formed enzyme (e.g., from the CO_2H-terminus of its proenzyme) or perhaps a biologically active peptide.[32] Alternatively, a proteolytic cleavage could cause a conformational rearrangement and perturb membrane processes. Regardless of the precise mechanism, the isolation of stable [^{125}I]α-thrombin receptor complexes from mitogenically responsive cells, from endothelial cells, and in trace amounts from platelets provides evidence for enzyme intermediates [65–67] in the performance of membrane-surface proteolytic functions.[57, 62, 68–70] Coupled interactions with protein-binding or recognition sites might both assist in stabilization of such intermediates and retard enzyme turnover.

GENERAL CONCLUSIONS

Procoagulant α-thrombin is not only the central bioregulatory enzyme in hemostasis but is also the most extensively studied regulatory protease to date. Methods originating from those of Dr. Kent D. Miller while in Albany, New

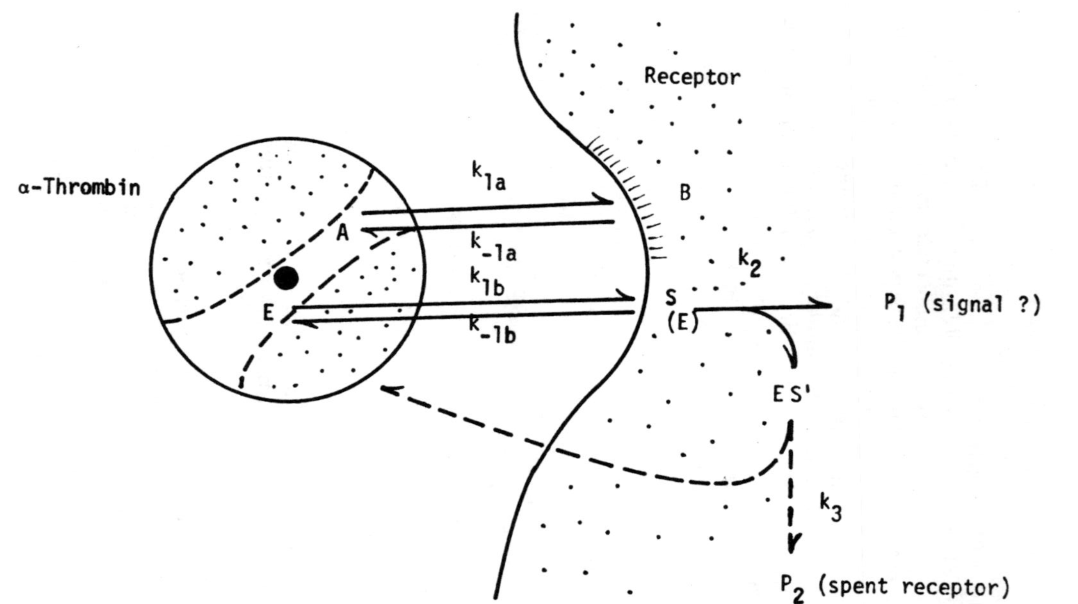

FIGURE 6. A model for an α-thrombin high-affinity receptor on a cellular surface. In this model, the initial complex is formed by high-affinity interaction of a protein binding or recognition exosite (A) in α-thrombin with a complementary noncovalent binding exosite (B) in the receptor. Subsequently, the enzyme catalytic site (E) aligns to interact with the substrate cleavage site (S) in the receptor, as a recognition-coupled reaction (see text). Proteolytic cleavage generates the first product (P_1), which is presumably the biological signal. Degradation of the enzyme intermediate (ES') yields the second product (P_2) or spent receptor and regenerates the enzyme. The regenerated enzyme, however, may not be readily released due to its affinity for the receptor high-affinity binding (A-B binding). Slow turnover of the enzyme intermediate (ES') would also cause a dosage dependency on the enzyme concentration initially added (see text).

TABLE 4

EVIDENCE FOR PROTEIN-BINDING OR RECOGNITION EXOSITES IN α-THROMBIN

Protein or Cell	Evidence
1) Fibrinogen	a) Only α-thrombin has significant clotting activity, whereas β- and γ-thrombins retain activities with synthetic substrates and inhibitors.[1-4] b) Fibrinogen does not compete with the tripeptide chromogenic substrate or antithrombin-III activities of γ-thrombin.[23] c) Unlike the generally more capable protease trypsin, α-thrombin cleaves fibrinopeptide A readily.[61] d) Amino acid sequences on either side of the Aα-cleavage site are unrelated to those for other thrombin-susceptible bonds in proteins (TABLE 3). e) Fibrinogen fragments with the intact fibrinopeptide A are more rapidly hydrolyzed than synthetic oligopeptide analogs.[43, 46]
2) Hirudin	a) Hirudin complexes with active-site–serine spin-labeled α-thrombin, causing pronounced immobilization of the spin label.[3, 4, 53] b) Loss of clotting activity correlates with reduced hirudin affinity: low-affinity inhibition of γ-thrombin is competitive and reversible, while high-affinity inhibition of α-thrombin is noncompetitive and essentially irreversible.[e, 4, 53]
3) Fibrin	a) In the presence of unlabeled α-thrombin, [^{125}I]DIP- or [^{125}I]PMS-α-thrombin incorporates into fibrin clots similar to [^{125}I]α-thrombin.[21] b) Neither [^{125}I]γ-thrombin nor the hirudin complex of [^{125}I]α-thrombin incorporate into fibrin clots in the presence of unlabeled α-thrombin.[21]
4) Platelets	a) Procoagulant α-thrombin is a more potent stimulus than noncoagulant γ-thrombin or trypsin.[62] b) Although [^{125}I]DIP- or [^{125}I]PMS-α-thrombin does stimulate, both forms bind similarly to [^{125}I]α-thrombin.[57, 58] c) Hirudin inhibits saturable binding of [^{125}I]PMS-α-thrombin.[58]
5) Mitogenically responsive cells	a) Depending on cell types, γ-thrombin is a poor or non-stimulus in contrast to α-thrombin.[60] b) Only certain cell types bind [^{125}I]DIP-α-thrombin similarly to [^{125}I]α-thrombin.[60]

York, and dating back to his graduate studies under Dr. Seegers in Detroit, Michigan, have enabled the preparation of gram amounts of the human enzyme and have permitted numerous investigations over the past decade.[1-4] This enzyme may best be classified as a "weak serine protease" with a preferential arginine specificity. Its high-affinity protein-binding or recognition sites, which are independent of its catalytic site, account for its exceptional biologic specificity.

Only relatively low concentrations of α-thrombin exist in blood because of various consumptive processes. The physiologic functions of the enzyme appear to be initially at the cellular level and subsequently, with increasing enzyme concentrations, at the fluid-phase level in blood. The events seem to be separated at the cellular level by their response times, whereas in the fluid phase reactant-concentration dependencies appear to regulate thrombin interactions with the plasma proteins. Regardless of their regulation, such events are irreversible, which indicates a proteolytic function for the enzyme. Proteolytic cleavage clearly occurs with the plasma-protein substrates and also appears to be required for cellular stimulation. Coupling of protein-binding or recognition interactions with those for proteolysis evidently has evolved to perfect the physiologic specificity of α-thrombin.

ACKNOWLEDGMENTS

I am indebted to numerous colleagues with whom I have had the privilege to work over the past ten years and who have contributed enormously to my understanding of thrombin functions in hemostasis. In particular, I would like to thank Dr. John S. Finlayson and Dr. Andrei F. Budzynski for their comments incorporated in Figure 1. I would also like to thank Ms. Nancy Massaroni for her assistance in the preparation of this manuscript.

REFERENCES

1. FENTON, J. W., II, M. J. FASCO, A. B. STACKROW, D. L. ARONSON, A. M. YOUNG & J. S. FINLAYSON. 1977. Human thrombins. Production, evaluation, and properties of α-thrombin. J. Biol. Chem. **252:** 3587–3598.
2. FENTON, J. W., II, B. H. LANDIS, D. A. WALZ, & J. S. FINLAYSON. 1977. Human thrombins. *In* Chemistry and Biology of Thrombin. R. L. Lundblad, J. W. Fenton II & K. G. Mann, Eds.: 43–70. Ann Arbor Science Publishers. Ann Arbor, Michigan.
3. FENTON, J. W., II, B. H. LANDIS, D. A. WALZ, D. H. BING, R. D. FEINMAN, M. P. ZABINSKI, S. A. SONDER, L. J. BERLINER & J. S. FINLAYSON. 1979. Human thrombin: preparative evaluation, structural properties and enzymic specificity. *In* The Chemistry and Physiology of Human Plasma Proteins. D. H. Bing, Ed.: 151–183. Pergamon Press. New York.
4. FENTON, J. W., II & B. H. LANDIS. 1980. Prothrombin and thrombin transformations: bioregulations and functions. *In* Perspectives in Hemostasis. J. Fareed, H. L. Messmore, J. W. Fenton II & K. M. Brinkhous, Eds. Pergamon Press. New York. In press.
5. BIGGS, R. 1976. Human Blood Coagulation, Hemostasis and Thrombosis. R. Biggs, Ed. 2nd edit. Blackwell Scientific Publications. Oxford.

6. RATNOFF, O. D. 1977. The hemostatic defects of liver disease. *In* Hemostasis: Biochemistry, Physiology and Pathology. D. Ogston & B. Bennett, Eds.: 446–466. John Wiley and Sons. London.

7. JACKSON, C. M. & J. W. SUTTIE. 1977. Recent developments in understanding the mechanism of vitamin K and vitamin K-antagonist drug action and the consequences of vitamin K action in blood circulation. Prog. Hematol. **10**: 333–359.

8. SUTTIE, J. W. & C. M. JACKSON. 1977. Prothrombin structure, activation, and biosynthesis. Physiol. Rev. **57**: 1–70.

9. O'REILLY, R. A. 1976. Vitamin K and the oral anticoagulant drugs. Ann. Rev. Med. **27**: 245–261.

10. BLOOM, J. W. & K. G. MANN. 1979. Prothrombin domains: circular dichroic evidence for a lack of cooperativity. Biochemistry **18**: 1957–1961.

11. MAGNUSSON, S., T. E. PETERSEN, L. SOTTRUP-JENSEN & H. CLAEYS. 1975. Complete primary structure of prothrombin: isolation, structure, and reactivity of ten carboxylated glutamic acid residues and regulation of prothrombin activation by thrombin. *In* Proteases and Biological Control. E. Reich, D. B. Rifkin & E. Shaw, Eds.: 123–149. Cold Spring Harbor Laboratory. Cold Spring Harbor, N. Y.

12. STENFLO, J. & J. W. SUTTIE. 1977. Vitamin K-dependent formation of γ-carboxyglutamic acid. Ann. Rev. Biochem. **46**: 157–172.

13. DAVIE, E. W., K. FUJKAWA, K. KURACHI & W. KISIEL. 1979. The role of serine proteases in the blood coagulation cascade. Adv. Enzymol. **48**: 277–318.

14. DAHLBACK, B. & J. STENFLO. 1978. Binding of bovine coagulation Factor Xa to platelets. Biochemistry **17**: 4938–4945.

15. MILETICH, J. P., C. M. JACKSON & P. W. MAJERUS. 1978. Properties of the Factor Xa binding site on human platelets. J. Biol. Chem. **253**: 6908–6916.

16. ARONSON, D. L., L. STEVAN, A. P. BALL, B. R. FRANZA, JR. & J. S. FINLAYSON. 1977. Generation of the combined prothrombin activation peptide (F1·2) during the clotting of blood and plasma. J. Clin. Invest. **60**: 1410–1418.

17. FURIE, B. C., E. GREENE, L. VOO & B. FURIE. 1979. Pathways and kinetics of prothrombin activation in human plasma. Thromb. Haemostas. (Stuttg.) **42**: 209.

18. WALZ, D. A. & T. R. BROWN. 1979. Human prothrombin activation: determination of plasma and serum levels of prothrombin fragment 3 by radioimmunoassay. Thromb. Haemostas. (Stuttg.) **42**: 56.

19. ARONSON, D. L., A. P. BALL, R. B. FRANZA, T. E. HUGLI & J. W. FENTON II. 1980. Human prothrombin fragments F1($\alpha\beta$) and F2: preparation and characterization of structural and biological properties. Thromb. Res. **20**: 239–253.

20. LIU, C. Y., H. L. NOSSEL & K. L. KAPLAN. 1979. The binding of thrombin by fibrin. J. Biol. Chem. **254**: 10421–10425.

21. WILNER, G. D., M. P. DANITZ, J. W. FENTON II & M. S. MUDD. 1979. Selective immobilization of thrombin by surface-bound fibrin. Clin. Res. **27**: 642A.

22. HARPEL, P. C. & R. D. ROSENBERG. 1976. α_2-Macroglobulin and antithrombin-heparin cofactor: modulators of hemostatic and inflammatory reactions. Prog. Hemostasis Thromb. **3**: 145–189.

23. CHANG, T.-L., R. D. FEINMAN, B. H. LANDIS & J. W. FENTON II. 1979. Antithrombin reactions with α- and γ-thrombins. Biochemistry **18**: 113–119.

24. MESSMORE, H. L., J. FAREED, M. P. ZABINSKI, P. ORFEI, J. KNIFFIN & J. W. FENTON II. 1979. Quantitation of antithrombin III(AT-III) with various molecular forms of human thrombins. Fed. Proc. **38**: 758.

25. BOWER, M. S., P. C. HARPEL, M. B. HAYES & J. W. FENTON II. 1979. α_2-Macroglobulin interaction with β-trypsin, α- and γ-thrombins Blood **54**: 272A.

26. BALL, A. P., R. B. FRANZA & D. L. ARONSON. 1976. The effect of plasmin on prothrombin structure and activity. Fed. Proc. **35**: 805.

492　　　　Annals New York Academy of Sciences

27. RICK, M. E. & L. W. HOYER. 1978. Thrombin activation of Factor VIII. II. A comparison of purified Factor VIII and the low molecular weight Factor VIII procoagulant. Brit. J. Haematol. **38:** 107–119.
28. NESHEIM, M. E. & K. G. MANN. 1979. Thrombin-catalyzed activation of single chain bovine Factor V. J. Biol. Chem. **254:** 1326–1334.
29. SEEGERS, W. H., E. NOVOA, R. L. HENRY & H. I. HASSOUNA. 1976. Relationship of "new" vitamin K-dependent protein C and "old" autoprothrombin II-A. Thromb. Res. **8:** 543–552.
30. KISIEL, W., W. M. CANFIELD, L. H. ERICSSON & E. W. DAVIE. 1977. Anticoagulant properties of bovine plasma protein C following activation by thrombin. Biochemistry **16:** 5824–5831.
31. VEHAR, G. A. & E. W. DAVIE. 1980. Preparation and properties of bovine Factor VIII (antihemophilic factor). Biochemistry **19:** 401–410.
32. NEURATH, H. & K. A. WALSH. 1976. Role of proteolytic enzymes in biological regulation (a review). Proc. Natl. Acad. Sci. USA **73:** 3825–3832.
33. BING, D. H., M. CORY & J. W. FENTON II. 1977. Exo-site affinity labeling of human thrombins. Similar labeling of the A chain and B chain/fragments of clotting α- and nonclotting γ/β-thrombins. J. Biol. Chem. **252:** 8027–8034.
34. ELMORE, D. T. 1973. The enzymic properties of thrombin and Factor Xa. Biochem. Soc. Trans. **1:** 1191–1194.
35. FASCO, M. J. & J. W. FENTON II. 1973. Specificity of thrombin. I. Esterolytic properties of thrombin, plasmin, trypsin, and chymotrypsin with N_β-substituted guanidino derivatives of p-nitrophenyl-p'-guanidinobenzoate. Arch. Biochem. Biophys. **152:** 802–812.
36. RYAN, T. J., J. W. FENTON II, T-L. CHANG & R. D. FEINMAN. 1976. Specificity of thrombin: evidence for selectivity in acylation rather than binding for p-nitrophenyl-α-amino-p'-toluate. Biochemistry **15:** 1337–1341.
37. WONG, S-C. & SHAW, E. 1976. Inactivation of trypsin-like proteases by active-site–directed sulfonylation. Ability of departing group to confer selectivity. Arch. Biochem. Biophys. **176:** 113–118.
38. BANG, N. U. & L. E. MATTLER. 1977. Thrombin sensitivity and specificity of three chromogenic peptide substrates. *In* Chemistry and Biology of Thrombin. R. L. Lundblad, J. W. Fenton II & K. G. Mann, Eds.: 305–310. Ann Arbor Science Publishers. Ann Arbor, Michigan.
39. BLOMBÄCK, B., B. HESSEL, D. HOGG & G. CLAESON. 1977. Substrate specificity of thrombin on proteins and synthetic substrates. *In* Chemistry and Biology of Thrombin. R. L. Lundblad, J. W. Fenton II & K. G. Mann, Eds.: 275–290. Ann Arbor Science Publishers. Ann Arbor, Michigan.
40. CLAESON, G., L. AURELL, G. KARLSON & P. FRIBERGER. 1977. Substrate structure and activity relationship. *In* New Methods for the Analysis of Coagulation Using Chromogenic Substrates. I. Witt, Ed.: 39–54. Walter de Gruyter. Berlin.
41. SEEGERS, W. H., H. I. HASSONNA, D. HEWETT-EMMETT, D. A. WALZ & T. J. ANDARY. 1975. Prothrombin and thrombin. Selected aspects of thrombin formation, properties, inhibition, and immunology. Semin. Thromb. Hemostasis **1:** 211–283.
42. MARLAR, R. A., D. A. WALZ, J. W. FENTON II & W. H. SEEGERS. 1977. The secondary structure requirements for thrombin susceptible bonds. Am. Chem. Soc., Div. Biol. Chem., 174th Natl. Mtg. Abst. 99.
43. BLOMBÄCK, B., B. HESSEL, D. HOGG & L. THERLSIDLSEN. 1978. A two-step fibrogen-fibrin transition in blood coagulation. Nature **275:** 501–505.
44. ARONSON, D. L. 1976. Comparison of the actions of thrombin and the thrombin-like venom enzymes ancrod and bathraboxin. Thromb. Haemostas. (Stuttg.) **36:** 9–13.

45. GRÁF, L., E. BARÁT, J. BORVENDÉG, I. HERMANN & A. PATTLEY. 1976. Action of thrombin on ovine, bovine and human pituitary growth hormones. Eur. J. Biochem. **64:** 333–340.

46. SCHERAGA, H. A. 1977. Action site mapping of thrombin. *In* Chemistry and Biology of Thrombin. R. L. Lundblad, J. W. Fenton II & K. G. Mann, Eds.: 145–158. Ann Arbor Science Publishers. Ann Arbor, Michigan.

47. BERLINER, L. J. & Y. Y. L. SHEN. 1977. Physical evidence for an apolar binding site near the catalytic center of human α-thrombin. Biochemistry **16:** 4622–4626.

48. FELDMANN, R. J., D. H. BING, B. C. FURIE & B. FURIE. 1978. Interactive-computer surface graphics approach to study of the active site of bovine trypsin. Proc. Natl. Acad. Sci. USA **75:** 5409–5412.

49. ABILDGAARD, U. 1979. A review of antithrombin III. *In* The Physiological Inhibitors of Blood Coagulation and Fibrinolysis. D. Collen, B. Wiman, & M. Verstraete, Eds., 19–29. Elsevier/North-Holland Biomedical Press. Amsterdam.

50. JÖRNVAL, H., W. W. FISH & I. BJÖRK. 1979. The thrombin cleavage site in bovine antithrombin. FEBS Lett. **106:** 358–362.

51. ROSENBERG, R. D. & P. S. DAMUS. 1973. The purification and mechanism of action of human antithrombin-heparin cofactor. J. Biol. Chem. **248:** 6490–6505.

52. VILLANUEVA, G. & I. DANISHEFSKY. 1979. Conformational changes accompanying the binding of antithrombin III to thrombin. Biochemistry **18:** 810–817.

53. LANDIS, B. H., M. P. ZAMBINSKI, G. J. M. LAFLEUR, D. H. BING & J. W. FENTON II. 1978. Human α- and γ-thrombin differential inhibition with hirudin. Fed. Proc. **37:** 1445.

54. MARKWARDT, F. 1970. Hirudin as an inhibitor of thrombin. Methods Enzymol. **19:** 924–932.

55. BAGDY, D., E. BARBAS, L. GRAF, T. E. PETERSEN & S. MAGNUSSON. 1976. Hirudin. Methods Enzymol. **45:** 669–678.

56. MAGNUSSON, S., L. SOTTRUP-JENSEN, T. E. PETERSEN, G. DUDEK-WOJCIECHOWSKA & H. CLAEYS. 1976. Homologous "krinkle" structures common to plasminogen and prothrombin. Substrate specificity of enzymes activating prothrombin and plasminogen. *In* Proteolysis and Physiological Regulation. D. W. Ribbons & K. Brew, Eds.: **2:** 203–238. Miami Winter Symposia. Academic Press, Inc. New York.

55. TOLLEFSEN, D. M., J. R. FEAGLER & P. M. MAJERUS. 1974. The binding of thrombin to the surface of human platelets. J. Biol. Chem. **249:** 2646–2651.

58. TAM, S. W., J. W. FENTON II & T. C. DETURLER. 1979. Dissociation of thrombin from platelets by hirudin. Evidence for receptor processing. J. Biol. Chem. **254:** 8723–8725.

59. CUNNINGHAM, D. D., D. H. CARNEY & K. C. GLENN. 1979. A cell-surface component involved in thrombin-stimulated cell division. *In* Hormones and Cell Culture. G. H. Stato & R. Ross, Eds.: 199–215. Cold Spring Harbor Laboratory. Cold Spring Harbor, New York.

60. GLENN, K. C., D. H. CARNEY, J. W. FENTON II & D. D. CUNNINGHAM. 1980. Thrombin active-site regions required for fibroblast receptor binding and initiation of cell division. J. Biol. Chem. **255:** 6609–6616.

61. BILEZIKIAN, S. B., H. L. NOSSEL, V. P. BUTLER & R. E. CANFIELD. 1975. Radioimmunoassay of human fibrinopeptide B and kinetics of fibrinopeptide cleavage by different enzymes. J. Clin. Invest. **56:** 438–445.

62. TAM, S. W., J. W. FENTON II & T. C. DETWILER. 1980. Platelet thrombin receptors: binding of thrombin is coupled to signal generation by a chymotrypsin-sensitive mechanism. J. Biol. Chem. **255:** 6626–6632.

63. DETWILER, T. C. & R. D. FEINMAN. 1973. Kinetics of the thrombin-induced release of calcium $(++)$ by platelets. Biochemistry **12:** 282–289.
64. CARNEY, D. H., K. C. GLENN & D. D. CUNNINGHAM. 1978. Conditions which affect initiation of animal cell division by trypsin and thrombin. J. Cell Physiol. **95:** 13–22.
65. BAKER, J. B., R. L. SIMMER, K. C. GLENN & D. D. CUNNINGHAM. 1979. Thrombin and epidermal growth factor become linked to cell surface receptors during mitogenic stimulation. Nature **278:** 743–745.
66. CARNEY, D. H., K. C. GLENN, D. D. CUNNINGHAM, M. DAS, C. F. FOX & J. W. FENTON II. 1979. Photoaffinity labeling of a single receptor for α-thrombin on mouse embryo cells. J. Biol. Chem. **254:** 6244–6247.
67. ISAACS, J. D., N. SAVION, J. W. FENTON II & M. A. SHUMAN. 1979. Thrombin binds to a specific site on endothelial cells. Blood **54:** 284a.
68. PHILLIPS, D. R. & P. P. AGIN. 1977. Platelet plasma membrane glycoproteins. Identification of a proteolytic substrate for thrombin. Biochem. Biophys. Res. Commun. **75:** 940–947.
69. GLENN, K. C. & D. D. CUNNINGHAM. 1979. Thrombin-stimulated cell division involves proteolysis of its cell surface receptor. Nature **278:** 711–714.
70. MOSHER, D. F., A. VAHERI, J. J. CHOATE & C. G. GAHMBERG. 1979. Action of thrombin on surface glycoproteins of human platelets. Blood **53:** 437–445.
71. AWBREY, B. J., J. C. HOAK & W. G. OWEN. 1979. Binding of human thrombin to culture human endothelial cells. J. Biol. Chem. **254:** 4092–4095.
72. WEKSLER, B. B., C. W. LEY & E. A. JAFFE. 1978. Stimulation of endothelial cell prostacyclin (PGI₂) production by thrombin, trypsin, and the ionophore A 23187. J. Clin Invest. **62:** 923–930.
73. LOSKUTOFF, D. 1979. Effect of thrombin on the fibrinolytic activity of cultured bovine endothelial cells. J. Clin. Invest. **64:** 329–332.
74. BUCHANAN, J. M., L. B. CHEN & B. R. ZETTER. 1976. Protease-related effects in normal and transformed cells. Cancer Enzymology. J. Schultz & F. Ahmad, Eds. **12:** 1–24. Miami Winter Symposia. Academic Press, Inc. New York.
75. MARTIN, B. M., W. W. WASIEWSKI, J. W. FENTON II & T. C. DETWILER. 1976. Equilibrium binding of thrombin to platelets. Biochemistry **15:** 4886–4893.
76. HOLMSEN, H., L. SALGANICOFF & M. H. FUKAMI. 1977. Platelet behavior and biochemistry. *In* Hemostasis: Biochemistry, Physiology and Pathology. D. Ogston & B. Bennett, Eds.: 239–319. John Wiley & Sons. London.
77. LYONS, R. M. & R. M. ATHERTON. 1979. Characterization of a platelet protein phosphorylated during the thrombin release reaction. Biochemistry **18:** 544–552.
78. MARCUS, A. J. 1978. The role of lipids in platelet function. J. Lipid Res. **19:** 793–826.
79. BURCH, J. W. & P. W. MAJERUS. 1979. The role of prostaglandis in platelet function. Semin. Hemotaol. **16:** 196–207.
80. HUGLI, T. C. 1977. Complement factors in inflammation: Effects of α-thrombin on components C3 and C5. *In* Chemistry and Biology of Thrombin. R. L. Lundblad, J. W. Fenton II & K. G. Mann, Eds.: 345–360. Ann Arbor Science Publishers. Ann Arbor, Michigan.
81. LORAND, L. 1975. Controls in the clotting of fibrinogen. *In* Proteases and Biological Control. E. Reich, D. B. Rigkin & E. Shaw, Eds.: 79–84. Cold Spring Harbor Laboratory. Cold Spring Harbor, New York.
82. MATHESON, N. R. & J. TRAVIS. 1976. Inactivation of human thrombin in the presence of human α₁-proteinase inhibition. Biochem. J. **159:** 495–502.
83. DOWNING, M. R., J. W. BLOOM & K. G. MANN. 1977. α₁-Antitrypsin inhibition of thrombin. *In* Chemistry and Biology of Thrombin. R. L. Lundblad, J. W. Fenton II & K. G. Mann, Eds.: 441–450. Ann Arbor Science Publishers. Ann Arbor, Michigan.

84. DAVIS, A. E., III, C. ZALUT, F. S. ROSEN & C. A. ALPER. 1979. Human Factor $\bar{D}$ of the alternative complement pathway. Physiochemical characteristics and N-terminal amino acid sequence. Biochemistry 18: 5082–5087.
85. POLLEY, M. J. & R. NACHMAN. 1978. The human complement system in thrombin-mediated platelet function. J. Exp. Med. 147: 1713–1726.
86. ISAACS, J. O., N. SAVION, N. GASPODAROWICZ, J. W. FENTON II & M. A. SHUMAN. 1980. Covalent binding of thrombin to corneal endothelial cells. Biochemistry. In press.
87. CARNEY, D. H. & D. D. CUNNINGHAM. 1978. Role of specific cell surface receptors in thrombin-stimulated cell division. Cell 15: 1341–1349.
88. BLOMBÄCK, B., M. BLOMBÄCK, B. HESSEL & S. IWANAGA. 1967. Structure of N-terminal fragments of fibrinogen and specificity of thrombin. Nature 215: 1445–1448.
89. TAKAGI, T. & R. F. DOOLITTLE. 1974. Amino acid sequence studies on Factor XIII and the peptide released during its activation by thrombin. Biochemistry 13: 750–756.
90. WALZ, D. A., D. HEWETT-EMMETT & W. H. SEEGERS. 1977. Amino acid sequence of human prothrombin fragments 1 and 2. Proc. Natl. Acad. Sci. USA 74: 1969–1972.
91. BUTKOWSKI, R. J., J. ELION, M. R. DOWNING & K. G. MANN. 1977. The primary structure of human prethrombin 2 and α-thrombin. J. Biol. Chem. 252: 4942–4957.
92. THOMPSON, A. R., D. L. ENFIELD, L. H. ERICSSON, M. E. LEGAZ & J. W. FENTON II. 1977. Human thrombin partial primary structure. Arch. Biochem. Biophys. 178: 356–367.
93. PETERSON, T. E., G. DUDEK-WOJCIECHOWSLEA, L. SOTTRUP-JENSEN & S. MAGNUSSON. 1979. Primary structure of antithrombin-III (heparin cofactor). Partial homology between α_1-antitrypsin and antithrombin III. In The Physiological Inhibitors of Blood Coagulation and Fibrinolysis. D. Collen, W. Wiman & M. Verstraete, Eds.: 43–54. Elsevier/North-Holland Biomedical Press. Amsterdam.
94. SPARROW, J. T., H. J. POWNALL, F-J. HSU, L. D. BLUMENTHAL, A. R. CULWELL & A. M. GOTTO. 1977. Lipid binding by fragments of apolipoprotein C-III-1 obtained by thrombin cleavage. Biochemistry 16: 5427–5431.

A COMPUTER-GENERATED THREE-DIMENSIONAL MODEL OF THE B CHAIN OF BOVINE α-THROMBIN *

David H. Bing † and Richard Laura

Center for Blood Research
Boston, Massachusetts 02115

David J. Robison, Bruce Furie,† and Barbara C. Furie †

Tufts New England Medical Center and
Tufts University School of Medicine
Boston, Massachusetts 02111

Richard J. Feldmann

Division of Computer Research and Technology
National Institutes of Health
Bethesda, Maryland 20205

INTRODUCTION

The study of enzyme function has been greatly facilitated by the availability of three-dimensional representations of the protein structure based upon X-ray crystallographic, diffraction data. These models of protein structure can be utilized to aid in the design of experiments that use chemical and physical techniques to evaluate the solution structure of the protein. The availability of these models has led to proposed relationships between structure and function, either directly or in concert with information obtained through other methods. A major example of the usefulness of three-dimensional models of enzymes has been the elucidation of the mechanisms of action of the serine proteases, chymotrypsin, trypsin, and elastase.[1-3] A comparison of these structures, of substrate and inhibitor kinetic data, and of spectral data as well as data obtained through other investigations of the structures of these enzymes has delineated features of each which represent common functional characteristics and differences that account for the unique substrate specificity and biological role of each enzyme.[4] These enzymes demonstrate significant primary, secondary, and tertiary structural homologies. However, the basic structure of these enzymes demonstrates a greater similarity than consideration of their primary sequence homology would predict. In spite of significant differences in primary structures, these three enzymes maintain similar secondary and tertiary structural features.[5]

We have begun to develop a method for generating three-dimensional representations of proteins that share considerable homology with the pancreatic

* This work was supported by grants from the Burroughs-Wellcome Company (Research Triangle Park, North Carolina), Merck, Sharp and Dohme (Rahway, New Jersey), and the National Institutes of Health (grants AM 17351, HL 25066, and HL 21543).

† D.H.B. and B.F. are Established Investigators of the American Heart Association. B.C.F. is the recipient of a Research Career Development Award from the National Institutes of Health.

496

serine proteases but that have not yet been crystallized or for which X-ray diffraction studies have not yet been performed. The plasma serine protease, bovine thrombin, shares primary structure homology with the pancreatic enzymes chymotrypsin, elastase, and trypsin.[6-8] ‡ The homology between thrombin and trypsin and chymotrypsin is particularly high in the region of the active site (69% for thrombin vs. trypsin and 66% for thrombin vs. chymotrypsin). The 32,000 molecular weight B chain of thrombin contains the active-site catalytic triad of serine 195, histidine 57, and aspartate 102, as well as the amino acids that form the substrate binding pocket, which determines enzyme specificity.[7, 8] Thrombin substrate specificity for arginine residues resembles that of trypsin but is restricted with respect to its possible protein substrates.[9, 10] Unlike trypsin, thrombin contains a 4,600 molecular weight A chain covalently bonded through a disulfide bridge to cysteine 122,§ near the middle of the B chain.

There is precedence for the construction of three-dimensional models of homologous proteins based upon knowledge of the three-dimensional structure of one protein in the group. Trypsin demonstrates a 44–50% primary structural homology with chymotrypsin.[11] This observation led Kiel *et al.* in 1968 to construct a three-dimensional model of trypsin by substituting the trypsin sequence onto the, then newly described, structure of *N*-tosyl-α-chymotrypsin.[12] A comparison of trypsin with chymotrypsin reveals specific amino acid substitutions that are responsible, in part, for trypsin's preference for the cationic side chains of lysine and arginine. Changes in the vicinity of the primary binding pocket, specifically, the substitution in trypsin of an aspartate at position 189 for the serine found in chymotrypsin, relate directly to trypsin substrate specificity.[5, 13, 14] Subsequent independent crystallographic studies showed striking similarities between the structures of these two enzymes.[1, 2, 15-18] Both are globular molecules in which the secondary structure is characterized by the presence of extensive β structure and little α-helix. This internal β structure is organized into two, six-stranded β-barrels composed of a high percentage of hydrophobic amino acids. In addition, chymotrypsin and trypsin are homologous with respect to the positions of the interchain disulfide bridges. Although there are six disulfide bonds in trypsin and five in chymotrypsin, four disulfide bonds are found in identical positions in both enzymes. The remaining two disulfide bonds join the two β-barrels of trypsin in a manner that is consistent with the three-dimensional structure of chymotrypsin. Trypsin also differs from chymotrypsin in that its active form is a single polypeptide chain while the active form of chymotrypsin consists of three polypeptide chains. Finally, trypsin is shorter than chymotrypsin, missing a single amino acid at three positions, two amino acids at two positions, and four amino acids at a single position relative to chymotrypsin. These structural features are summarized in FIGURE 1.[19]

It is now accepted that homology between the primary structures of two

‡ Elastase is omitted from this portion of the discussion. Elastase demonstrates a lower degree of primary sequence homology with thrombin than either trypsin or chymotrypsin. The active-site histidine 57 is located on a separate polypeptide chain from serine 195 and aspartate 102, and the highly conserved residue tryptophan 215 is replaced by phenylalanine. In spite of these differences there is no question, however, that elastase retains many of the structural features of trypsin and chymotrypsin.[3]

§ The numbering system is based on the amino acid sequence of bovine chymotrypsin.

proteins suggests secondary and tertiary structural similarities. A more striking observation, however, is the retention in related proteins of similar secondary and tertiary structural elements despite significant differences in portions of the amino acid sequence.[21–23] We have employed these principles in the development of a model of the thrombin B chain by maintaining the secondary and tertiary elements found in chymotrypsin. We are using this model to investigate possible surface structural features that may contribute to the known functional characteristics of α-thrombin. Magnusson *et al.* reported the construction of a partial model of the B chain of thrombin based on the structure of α-chymotrypsin.[24] We have now constructed a complete model of the thrombin B chain based on the published three-dimensional structure chymotrypsin.[15–18] Chymotrypsin was chosen as the basis for this model due to the greater degree of homology with respect to the number and positions of the disulfide bonds than is found with trypsin. Where possible, the homologous primary sequence was maintained. Because of the importance of the β-barrels to the structure of all known serine proteases,‖ insertions and deletions which occurred in the thrombin sequence were placed, wherever possible, outside those portions of the polypeptide chain which, by analogy with chymotrypsin, would form the β-barrel structure of thrombin. This aspect of the model is presented in FIGURE 1. We found that all insertions and deletions occurred outside the intrachain disulfide loops in thrombin except for a two amino acid insertion between residues 204 and 205. The homology of the primary sequence between the model of thrombin B chain and α-chymotrypsin is presented in FIGURE 2 and has been calculated to be 36%. The present report details the steps used in the construction of this model and the initial tests of the model that have been made by an examination of the fit of models of two small synthetic inhibitors into the active site of the thrombin model.

MATERIAL AND METHODS

Use of the Molecular Graphics Display

The model of thrombin B chain was constructed at the Macromolecular Graphics Display facility at the National Institutes of Health, Bethesda, Maryland as previously described.[25] In this system,# computer-generated protein structures are displayed as molecular surfaces composed of component spheres, each representing atoms in the protein. The atoms are presented as nondeformable spheres with diameters proportional to the first approximations of the electron density of individual atoms. Each atom type has a characteristic van der Waals radius, and the molecular surface may be considered an approximation of the van der Waals surface of the protein. As emphasized by Richards,[26] this description of protein structure remains arbitrary, within limits, with regard to the representation of molecular structure. Proteins are represented as static structures, although in solution they exhibit conformational motility.[27, 28] Like space-filling models, however, these constructs emphasize useful concepts of covalent and three-dimensional structure.

‖ The bacterial serine proteases that have arisen as the result of parallel evolutionary changes also demonstrate extensive β structure.

Programs used to construct the models are available through R.J.F. at the Division of Computer Research and Technology, National Institutes of Health, Bethesda, Maryland.

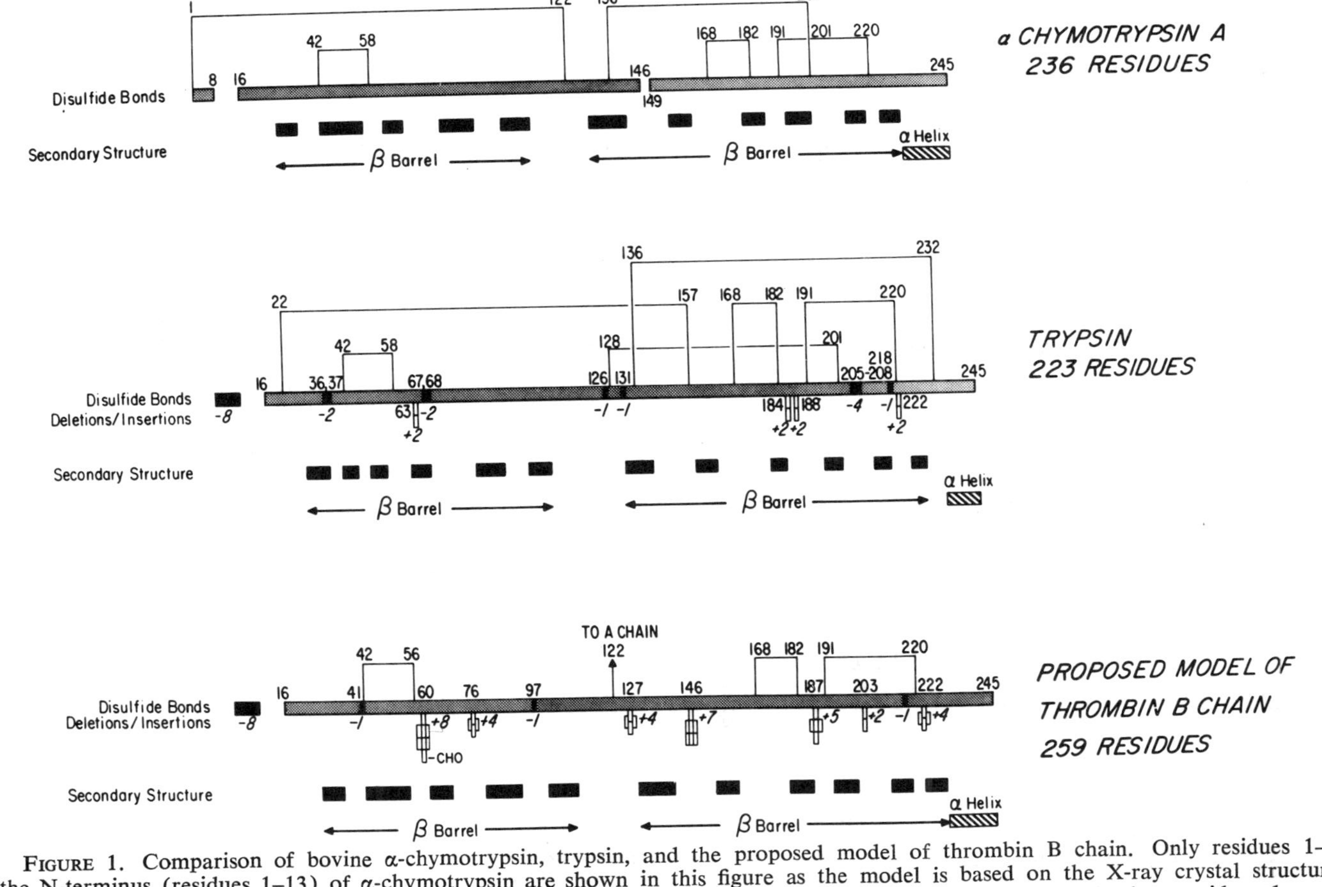

FIGURE 1. Comparison of bovine α-chymotrypsin, trypsin, and the proposed model of thrombin B chain. Only residues 1–8 of the N-terminus (residues 1–13) of α-chymotrypsin are shown in this figure as the model is based on the X-ray crystal structure of α-chymotrypsin. No resolution of residues 9–13 is found in the X-ray crystallographic analysis. As a result, these residues do not appear in the three-dimensional representation of α-chymotrypsin.

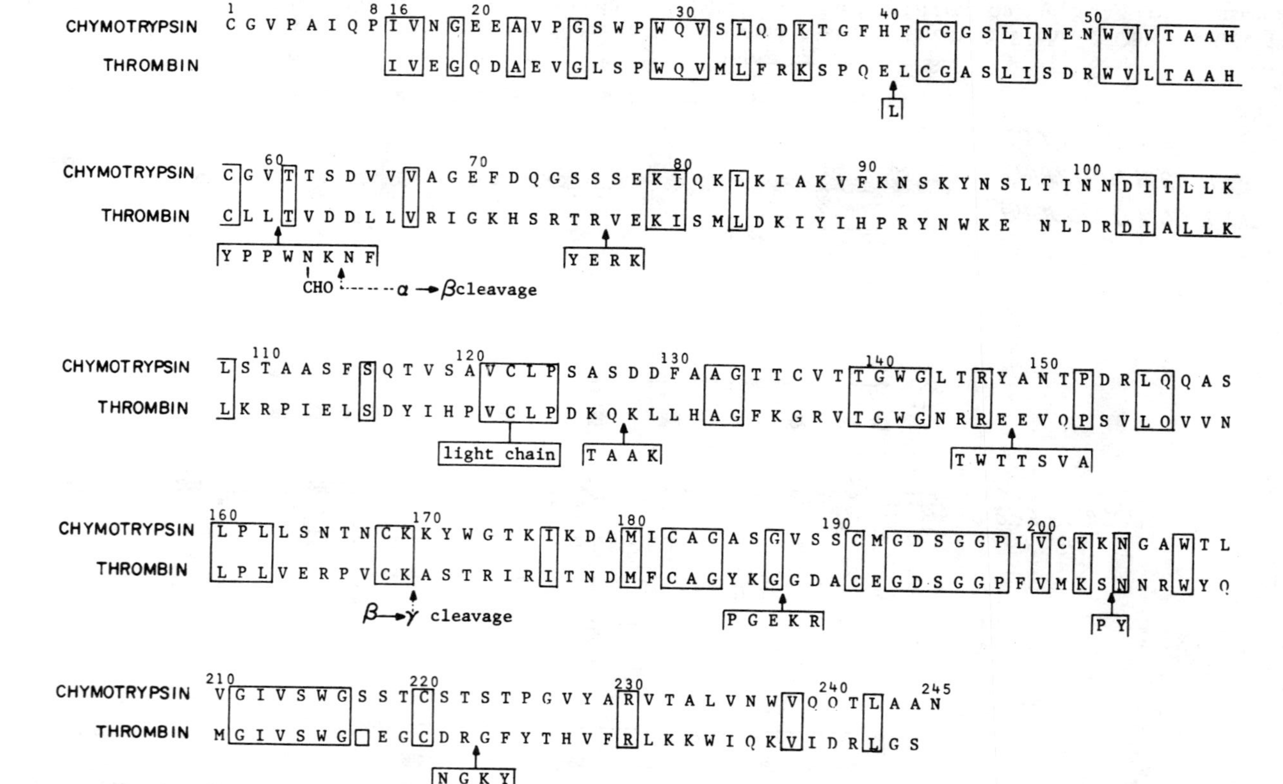

FIGURE 2. Sequence homology between bovine α-chymotrypsin and the thrombin B chain model. Insertions are indicated by arrows. The single letter amino acid code is used for this table. CHO is the carbohydrate.

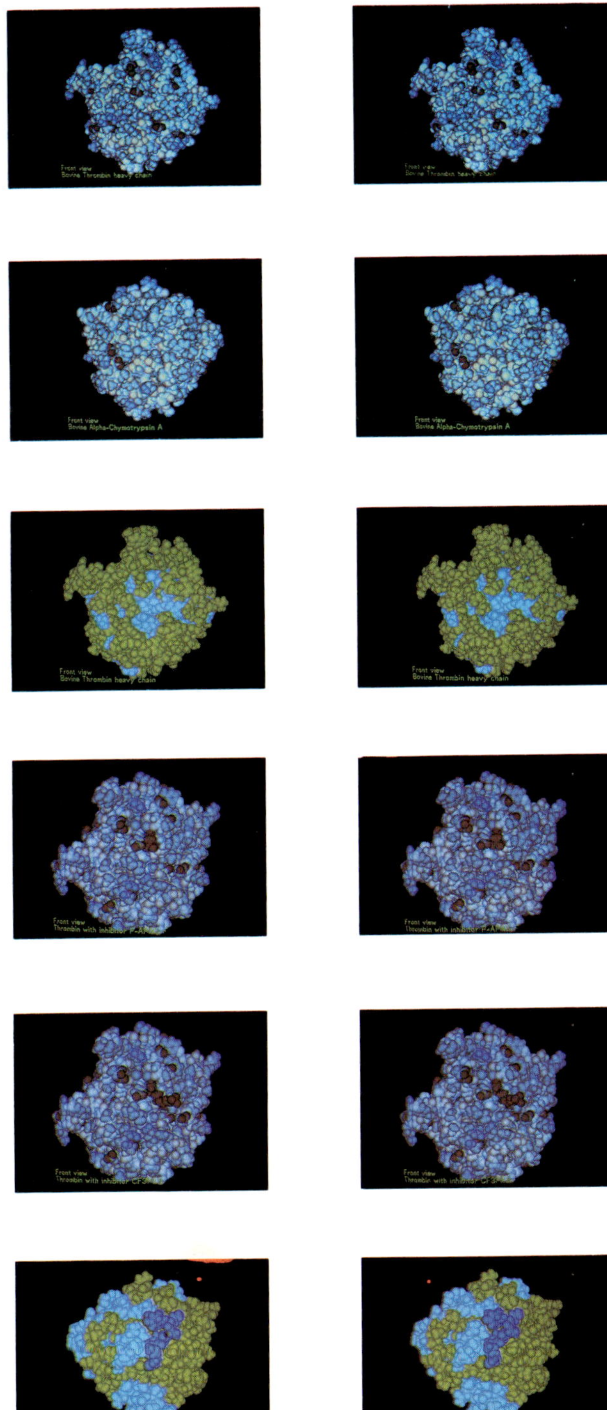

Front view
Bovine Thrombin heavy chain
Front view
Bovine Thrombin heavy chain
Front view
Bovine Alpha-Chymotrypsin A
Front view
Bovine Alpha-Chymotrypsin A
Front view
Bovine Thrombin heavy chain
Front view
Bovine Thrombin heavy chain
Front view
Thrombin with inhibitor P-APMSF
Front view
Thrombin with inhibitor P-APMSF
Front view
Thrombin with inhibitor CF3A
Front view
Thrombin with inhibitor CF3A
Back view
Bovine Alpha-Chymotrypsin A
Back view
Bovine Alpha-Chymotrypsin A

FIGURE 4. *Reading top to bottom:* (A) Stereo pair thrombin B chain model in functional coloring code, centered on active site. Hydrophobic residues, black; neutral, white; positively charged, blue; negatively charged, red; electropositive, light blue; electronegative, pink. (B) Stereo pair α-chymotrypsin in functional coloring code centered on active site. (C) Stereo pair thrombin B chain model in special coloring code. Altered or inserted amino acids are yellow; conserved amino acids are light blue. (D) Stereo pair *p*-APMS-F in red inserted into active site of thrombin B chain model in functional coloring code. Centered on active site. (E) Stereo pair CF_3 PPB in red inserted into active site of thrombin B chain model in functional coloring code. Centered on active site. (F) Stereo pair α-chymotrypsin residues 1–8 blue, 16–146 yellow and 149–245 light blue; view at site of binding of the A chain (residues 1–8) to B chain (residues 16–146).

The computer display system includes a DEC system 10 computer, a DEC PDP 11/70 computer, an Evans and Sutherland picture system 2 vector display, a frame buffer color display, and camera station. In the macromolecular display system,[29] protein structures are presented on the vector displays as an array of points (representing atoms) connected by lines to represent the covalent connectivity. The position of each atom except hydrogen is defined by the atomic coordinates determined by X-ray crystallography. Hydrogens have been added to carbon, oxygen, and nitrogen atoms of the protein structure by using known average bond angles and bond lengths. A view of these displays is translated into a molecular surface on the frame buffer color display. The displayed molecular structure is a two-dimensional projection of a three-dimensional array of points. By a recently developed algorithm,[30] each point is the center of a shaded, colored sphere. Intersection of the surface of the spheres yields a surface topography that characterizes the molecular surface of the protein. Features of the surface can be color-coded to facilitate representation of specific amino acid residues, atoms, or chemical and physical features of the spheres as desired. Photographs were obtained directly from the color display screen with a Nikon 35 mm camera. The surface of the protein may also be color-coded to identify regions of hydrophobicity, hydrophilicity, and charge (functional color code). Hydrophobic atoms are indicated by black, hydrophilic uncharged atoms by white, positively charged atoms by blue, and negatively charged atoms by red. Intermediate shades of black, blue, and red indicate intermediate degrees of hydrophobicity, electropositivity, or electronegativity, respectively. In this way, the color scheme provides a description of the chemical nature of the surface.

Programs used in the development of the thrombin models included XRAY, RESSUB and BIG. The steps in the construction of the model are summarized as follows: The primary sequence of thrombin B chain [24, 31] was matched for maximum homology with the primary sequence of α-chymotrypsin [19, 32, 33] and altered residues substituted for the chymotrypsin sequence. Comparison of the primary structure of the partially constructed model revealed that deletions and insertions would have to occur to accommodate all the changes between thrombin B chain and α-chymotrypsin. However, no insertions or deletions were allowed to occur in the model in any area that corresponded to a strand of a β-barrel in chymotrypsin. The results of matching homology while keeping β-barrel strands intact are shown in FIGURE 1. Amino acid residues were removed from the chymotrypsin structure at the sites of deletions. The inserted sequences were modeled on the vector display by altering the backbone conformation of the sequence to eliminate conformations that interfere with the pre-existing structure derived from chymotrypsin. The distance between the broken ends of inserted sequences in the peptide backbone was always adjusted to .15 to .18 nm, the approximate bond length of the peptide bond. All break points in the model were then rejoined. The amino acid side chains (including hydrogens) were added to the peptide chain, and the model was subjected to a computational annealing process, in which the amino acid side chains were rotated to minimize van der Waals contacts.

Computer programs available in the NIH PROPHET computer system were used to construct models of the inhibitors *p*-amidinophenylmethyl-sulfonyl-fluoride (*p*-APMS-F) and *m*-[*m*-(trifluoromethyl)phenoxypropoxy]-benzamidine (CF$_3$PPB). These structures were inserted into the active site of the thrombin B chain model on the vector display. Noncovalent bonding distances were based on similar structures observed in the reported X-ray crystal structure of benzamidine inhibited trypsin.[2, 15–18]

Human α-thrombin was generously provided by Dr. John W. Fenton, II, New York State Laboratories, Albany, New York. It was 97% α-thrombin, had 2.54 NIH units/μg and was 88% active by p'-nitrophenyl-p-guanidino benzoate titration.[35] The inhibitors p-APMS-F and tritiated [³H]CF₃PPB were synthesized as previously described.[36, 37] The inhibition of α-thrombin by p-APMS-F and determination of the K_i were performed as described by Laura et $al.$[36] following the method originally described by Rakitzis.[38] Equilibrium dialysis with [³H]CF₃PPB was performed in 100 μl Lucite dialysis chambers for 2 days at 23° C in 100 mM Tris-HCl buffer, pH 7.4, containing 0.5 M NaCl. The α-thrombin was 17.5 μM and [³H]CF₃PPB was 20.3 to 203 μM. The data for the binding of [³H]CF₃PPB to thrombin was subjected to Scatchard analysis.[39]

Collectively, these experiments confirm the previously reported trypsin-like specificity of α-thrombin for arginine residues. Benzamidine is a suitable model for the side chains of arginine and lysine and has been used as an inhibitor to distinguish trypsin-like serine proteases from enzymes with chymotrypsin- or elastase-like specificity.[9, 10, 40] It should be emphasized that thrombin is readily distinguishable from trypsin with respect to the quantitative differences in the interactions with substituted benzamidines,[41] with peptide chloromethylketone inhibitors,[42] and with respect to differences in the reactivity of active site titrants such as p-nitrophenyl-p'-amidinophenylmethyl-sulfonate.[43]

Description of the Model of Thrombin B Chain and Experimental Results

The primary sequence of the thrombin B chain model has 36% homology with α-chymotrypsin. By analogy to the region of the activation domain of trypsin described by Huber and Bode [2] (residues 16–19, 142–145, 194–193, and 216–223) thrombin demonstrates only 26.8% homology with this region of chymotrypsin as a result of two large insertions (7 and 5 amino acids, respectively), and one deletion (1 residue). The sequence homology in the vicinity of the charge-relay triad and the residues that form the specificity binding pocket (189–201, 211–220, 55–60, and 99–104) is much higher (66%) emphasizing the similarity of the active site of the serine proteases. Between residues 211 and 220, which contribute to the secondary binding site for protein substrates, there is 86% homology. This is one of the most highly conserved areas observed in the thrombin B chain model. A front view of the thrombin active site and the positions of some of the residues are indicated in FIGURE 3.

Three deletions (one of eight residues and two single residues), occur in thrombin B chain as compared to α-chymotrypsin. Eight insertions were required to accommodate the additional amino acids found in the thrombin B chain as compared to α-chymotrypsin. These insertions were placed at position 41, 60, 76, 127, 146, 187, 204, and 222 (FIGURES 1 and 2). The largest (8 residues) includes the carbohydrate attachment site of thrombin and the α- to β-cleavage site, which results during autolysis of α-thrombin.[44] The insertion at residue 146 occurs at the position that corresponds to the N-terminus of the third polypeptide (C) chain in α-chymotrypsin. The insertion at 222 is found in all known mammalian serine proteases, including trypsin, and is necessary to accommodate an apparent change in the position of cysteine 220. The insertion of 5 amino acids at residue 187 is near the active site. The insertion at position 76 is in the middle of the region in which trypsin binds Ca^{2+}. Thus, 5 of the 7 insertions occur in areas of the thrombin:chymotrypsin sequence that can be identified as structural features of functional importance.

The resulting thrombin B chain (FIGURE 4A) reveals a globular protein that retains the separate segments constituting the β-barrel structures found in α-chymotrypsin. Comparison of the surfaces of chymotrypsin and the thrombin model displayed in the functional coloring code reveals an increase in charged and hydrophilic groups on the surface (see FIGURE 4A vs. FIGURE 4B) relative to chymotrypsin. FIGURE 4C is the thrombin B chain model shown in FIGURE 4A but the altered residues have been colored yellow and the conserved residues

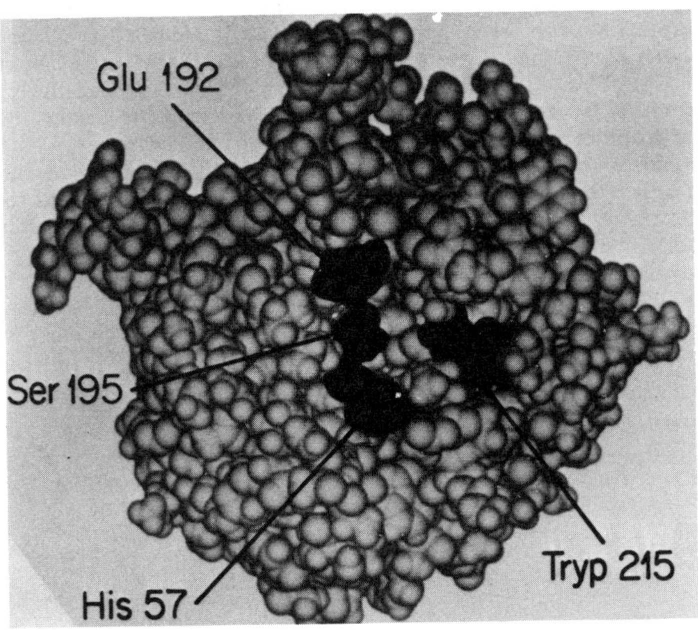

FIGURE 3. Computer-generated model of thrombin B chain (front). Selected residues (His 57, Asp 189, Glu 192, Ser 195, Trp 215) have been highlighted in grey, remaining residues white.

light blue. With the exception of two residues in the binding pocket, all of the changes appear on the surface. The structural core of the protein as found in chymotrypsin is conserved. This is true for the insertions as well as those residues that are altered (FIGURE 4C).

Although the geometry of the charge relay system and specificity binding pocket is conserved in the thrombin B chain model, several changes occur in the area of the active site. The change from serine to aspartate at position 189 at the rear of the specificity binding pocket is consistent with the trypsin-like specificity of thrombin. Two other changes found in this area of the thrombin B chain are a serine to alanine at position 190 and a threonine to glycine at 219. In trypsin, these two residues (serine 190 and glycine 219) are hydrogen bonded to the positively charged group of a substrate or inhibitor. The change to alanine would eliminate one of these hydrogen bonds and may contribute to the observed higher inhibition constant of benzamidine for thrombin (173 μM for thrombin as compared to 16 μM for trypsin). To demonstrate more completely the unique geometry of this aspect of the active site of thrombin, we have inserted a model of the inhibitor p-APMS-F (FIGURE 5A) into the active site of the thrombin B chain model. This inhibitor is a highly reactive irreversible inhibitor of thrombin and other trypsin-like serine proteases. Its reactivity results from the combination of the specificity of the benzamidine group with the unique reactivity of a sulfonylfluoride. The K_i of p-APMS-F for thrombin is 1.27 μM (FIGURE 6), the pseudo-first-order inactivation constant, exceeds 10^{-2} sec^{-1}.[36] A representation of the complex of thrombin with p-APMS-F (FIGURE 4D) demonstrates that the stereochemistry of the active site of the serine proteases is conserved in the thrombin B chain model.

Another change near the active site is that of a methionine to glutamate at position 192. This results (FIGURE 4A) in the placement of a negatively charged residue within 0.5 nm of the binding pocket and catalytic center. This carboxylate group may influence residues adjacent to the newly formed C-terminal amino acid of thrombin substrates. It is notable that in all known thrombin protein substrates, the new N-terminus, which would be aligned next to residue 192, contains a glycine, threonine, or serine residue. These amino amino acids can readily hydrogen bond to carbonyl oxygens. Interaction with the glutamate 192 may stabilize the enzyme–substrate complex. The highly conserved area near residue 215 is hydrophobic in character (FIGURE 4A). It is known that a variety of hydrophobic compounds including proflavins,[45] chromogenic pep-

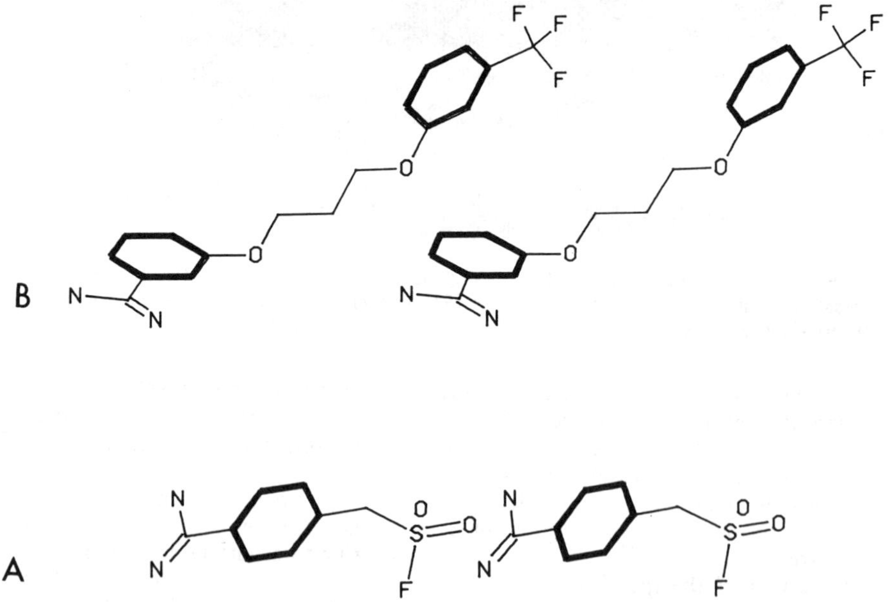

FIGURE 5. (A) Stereo-pair Drieding model of p-APMS-F. (B) Stereo-pair Drieding model of CF$_3$PPB.

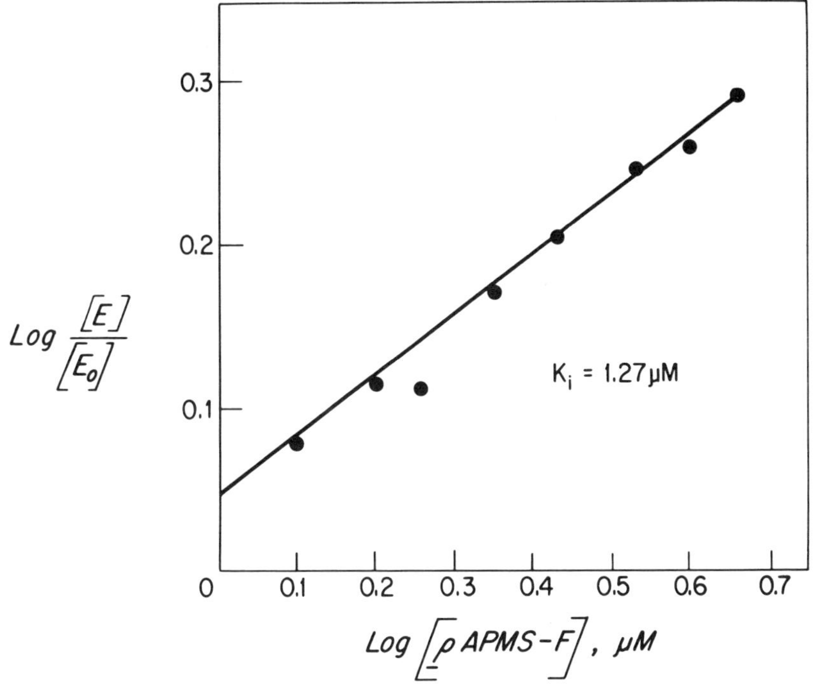

FIGURE 6. Determination of K_i of *p*-APMS-F for α-thrombin.

tides,[46] and extended benzamidine inhibitors, such as the affinity label *m*-[*o*-(2-chloro-5-fluorosulfonylphenylureido)phenoxybutoxy]-benzamidine,[10]   react with the active site of thrombin. CF_3PPB, an extended benzamidine derivative (FIGURE 5B) which contains the hydrophobic trifluoromethyl group attached to the benzamidine via a propoxyphenoxy bridging group, is an excellent inhibitor of thrombin. Analysis of the interaction of CF_3PPB with α-thrombin by equilibrium dialysis demonstrates a K_D of 2.7 µM and 1.03 moles bound/mole of thrombin active sites (FIGURE 7). When a model of CF_3PPB was inserted into the model of the active site of the thrombin B chain, it was found that the hydrophobic portion of the inhibitor could be placed within the environment of tryptophan 215 with the trifluoromethyl group oriented toward a hydrophobic area containing tyrosine and phenylalanine (FIGURE 4E).

DISCUSSION

We have constructed a computer generated model of the B chain of bovine thrombin based on the previously published three-dimensional structure of bovine α-chymotrypsin. The construction of this model was based on the observation that the pancreatic serine proteases are quite similar in three-dimensional structure despite significant differences in primary structure. We conclude that the secondary and tertiary features of these enzymes may be conserved, independent of alterations in primary structure. For this reason, a model of the B chain of thrombin may be derived from the backbone of chymotrypsin and used both in the design of experiments as well as in the interpretation of previous data on the reactivity of thrombin.

A major consideration in the construction of such a model is that of defining criteria for the placement of amino acid insertions into the chymotrypsin peptide backbone.[24] Since the β-barrel structures are major features of the structures of the serine proteases, we have chosen to conserve these features in the construction of the thrombin B chain model. All insertions and deletions have been placed at points which, by analogy with α-chymotrypsin, would be between the strands of the β-barrel structures. As a first step, amino acid homology was maximized. No insertions or deletions were permitted in the portion of the thrombin sequence analogous to the α-helical portion of the

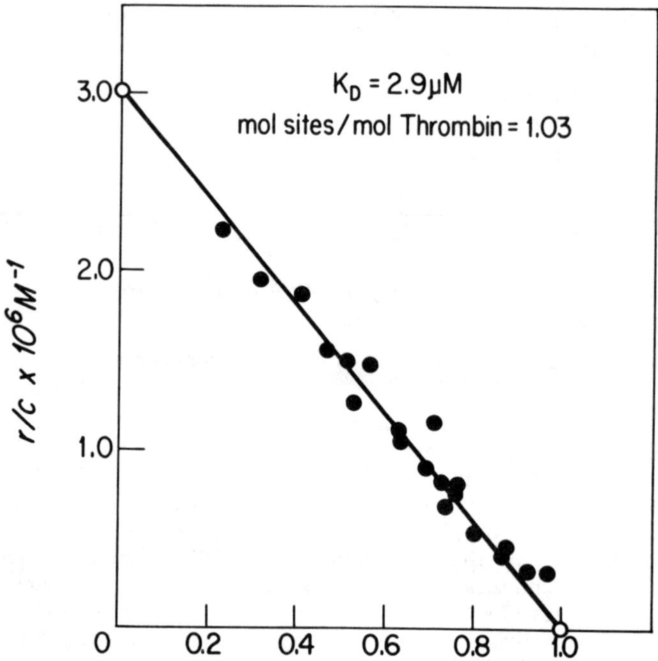

FIGURE 7. Scatchard analysis of the interaction of [³H]CFCF₃PPB with α-thrombin.

C-terminal of chymotrypsin (FIGURE 1). Virtually all changes in the resulting model occur on the surface of the protein, preserving the core and general shape of chymotrypsin. The model retains four of the five disulfide bonds found in chymotrypsin, assuming that the disulfide bond that connects the B chain to the A chain corresponds to the cysteine 122 to cysteine 1 bond in chymotrypsin. Thus, we have observed in the model the conservation of tertiary structure that has been demonstrated empirically by comparisons of other series of homologous proteins such as cytochrome c,[47] myoglobin,[22] lysozyme,[48] the NADH binding site of dehydrogenases,[49] and the pancreatic serine proteases.[5]

Lesk and Chothia [23] describe in detail the conservation of the secondary and tertiary structures of nine globins that share as little as 16% primary structural homology. They suggest a mechanism of protein evolution that allows complementary modifications in secondary structural features that result in the preservation of the functional structures of the proteins. They have verified and extended other investigations that have identified a specific domain of hydrophobic residues that forms a common nucleus or core of these proteins. These residues are located in interior positions and are highly conserved between globins of different species. It is tempting to speculate that this mechanism may provide a general model for protein evolution and apply equally well to other comparisons of related proteins. This point is dramatically demonstrated in FIGURE 4C in which the conserved "core" of hydrophobic residues common to both thrombin and chymotrypsin are colored blue while those regions that have been altered in the construction of the model are colored yellow. This conservation of a central core of hydrophobic amino acids is demonstrated equally well when one compares trypsin with chymotrypsin, thrombin with trypsin, or any of a series of serine proteases with either trypsin or chymotrypsin.

The model of the thrombin B chain finds great utility as a three-dimensional map of the positions of residues that may directly influence the function and activity of this protein. Within the specificity binding pocket, changes are observed that are consistent with the differences in binding specificity. The change to an aspartate at position 189 explains the trypsin-like substrate specificity but the presence of an alanine at 190 eliminates the possibility for hydrogen bonding with positively charged amino, amidino, or guanidino groups and predicts a lower binding affinity of thrombin as compared to trypsin for benzamidine. The glutamate at position 192 may affect the type of residue that is allowed adjacent to the arginine of peptide substrates. The observation that all known thrombin protein substrates have neutral residues at this position is consistent with the assumed role of this group with respect to the observed limited substrate specificity. Also, in the thrombin B chain model we observe a hydrophobic area adjacent to the active site that includes tryptophan 215 and represents, we believe, an extended or secondary binding site for substrates and inhibitors. Examination of models of two benzamidine-derived inhibitors inserted into the active site of the thrombin model provides evidence that the geometry of residues in this area of the protein is maintained and emphasizes the importance of this area to the catalytic function of thrombin.

This model also suggests a structural basis for other enzymic properties of thrombin outside the immediate vicinity of the active site. α-Thrombin undergoes a rapid, self-mediated, limited proteolysis that converts the B chain from a molecular weight of 32,000 to 28,000. The resulting species, termed β-thrombin, has no clotting activity. The α- to β-cleavage is known to occur within a region we have identified as an insertion, exposed on the surface. The slower autolytic conversion of β- to γ-thrombin (the B chain molecular weight reduces from 28,000 to 15,000) occurs at a site that lies within the model in a less exposed, more highly conserved region.

This model also raises significant questions that relate to the structure of the entire α-thrombin molecule and its relationship to α-chymotrypsin. For example, where does the A chain of thrombin lie on the surface of the B chain? There is structural homology of the A chain with the region of chymotrypsinogen, which is cleaved during its activation to chymotrypsin, as well as with the amino terminal peptide (residues 1 to 13) of chymotrypsin, which is disulfide-linked to cysteine 122. Examination of the molecular graphics display of chymotrypsin reveals that the peptide is attached on the opposite side of the protein from the active site and runs up towards the top of the molecule (FIGURE 4F). As noted by Magnusson *et al.*,[24] by analogy the A chain may lie in a similar position. It may be found that the A chain is situated near the cleft seen in the upper left of the front view of the thrombin model (FIGURE 4A). This may explain why the A chain is essential for activity. Located in this area, it would serve the same function as does the A chain (residues 1 to 13) in chymotrypsin, namely, to allow the N-terminal isoleucine to form a salt bridge with aspartate 194 and stabilize the active site.[2,3]

The placement of insertions in the sequence has been guided by the rules described above. Conformations of peptide backbone alterations and insertions, however, have been arbitrarily chosen to permit fitting of these structures to the new ends of the peptide backbone at the insertion site. We wish to emphasize that this model of thrombin B chain in no way purports to be a true representation of the actual thrombin structure. Sufficient similarities noted to exist between trypsin and chymotrypsin resulted in a trypsin model that was quite similar to the structure of trypsin as elucidated by X-ray diffraction techniques. In this regard, the utility of the thrombin B chain model may be realized with respect to the design of experiments that may prove or disprove aspects of it and as an aid to the interpretation of substrate and inhibitor binding and kinetic data, spectroscopic data, and other investigations of thrombin structure and function.

SUMMARY

A computer graphic molecular display system has been used to construct a three-dimensional model of the B chain of bovine thrombin. The model is derived from the bovine α-chymotrypsin structure as determined by X-ray crystallographic studies. The amino acid sequence of bovine thrombin has been substituted for that of α-chymotrypsin, preserving the β-barrel structure and maximizing homology of the amino acid sequence of the two proteins. With the exception of an area in the vicinity of the specificity binding pocket, most of the changes observed in thrombin occur on the surface of the molecule. The most notable changes observed in the model are the increases on the surface of positively charged (arginine and lysine) and negatively charged (glutamate and aspartate) residues. A glutamate replaces methionine 192 near the entrance to the specificity binding pocket. The nature of this site was further altered by the substitution of an aspartate for serine 189 and an alanine for serine 190. The structure of the resulting specificity binding pocket is consistent with that of serine proteases, which have trypsin-like substrate specificity. The computer graphics molecular display system has been used to insert models of synthetic thrombin inhibitors into the active site of the thrombin B chain model. With the model, it has been possible to correlate the interaction of thrombin with the observed binding constants of two inhibitors of trypsin-like serine proteases, p-amidinophenylmethylsulfonylfluoride ($K_i = 1.27 \times 10^{-6}$ M) and m-[m-(trifluoromethyl)phenoxypropoxy]benzamidine ($K_D = 2.9 \times 10^{-6}$ M).

ACKNOWLEDGMENT

We would like to acknowledge the secretarial assistance of Rachelle Rosenbaum in typing this manuscript.

REFERENCES

1. BLOW, D. M. 1976. Accts. Chem. Res. **9:** 145–152.
2. HUBER, R. & P. BODE. 1978. Accts. Chem. Res. **11:** 114–122.
3. WALSH, K. A. 1975. Unifying concepts among proteases. *In* Proteases and Biological Control. E. Reich, D. Rifkin & E. Shaw, Eds.: 1–12. Cold Spring Harbor Laboratory. Cold Spring Harbor, N. Y.
4. STROUD, R. M., M. KREIGER, R. E. KOEPPE, A. A. KOSSIAKOFF & J. L. CHAMBERS. 1975. Structure-function relationships in the serine proteases. *In* Proteases and Biological Control. E. Reich, D. Rifkin & E. Shaw, Eds.: 13–32. Cold Spring Harbor Laboratory. Cold Spring Harbor, N.Y.
5. NEURATH, H. 1975. Limited proteolysis and zymogen activation. *In* Proteases and Biological Control. E. Reich, D. Rifkin & E. Shaw, Eds.: 51–64. Cold Spring Harbor Laboratory. Cold Spring Harbor, N.Y.
6. MAGNUSSON, S. 1970. Structural aspects of thrombin and prothrombin. *In* Structure-Function Relationships of Proteolytic Enzymes. P. Desnuella, H. Neurath & M. Ottesen, Eds.: 138–143. Academic Press, Inc. New York, N.Y.
7. MAGNUSSON, S., J. L. SOTTRUP, T. E. PETERSEN & H. CLAEYS. 1975. The primary structure of prothrombin, the role of vitamin K in blood coagulation and a thrombin-catalyzed "negative feed-back" control mechanism for limiting the activation of prothrombin. *In* Prothrombin and Related Coagulation Coagulation Factors. H. C. Hemker & J. Veltkamp, Eds.: 25–46. Leiden Universitaire. Pers, Leiden, The Netherlands.
8. ELION, J., M. R. DOWNING, R. J. BUTKOWSKI & K. G. MANN. 1977. Structure of human thrombin: Comparison with other serine proteases. *In* Chemistry and Biology of Thrombin. R. L. Lundblad, J. W. Fenton, II & K. G. Mann, Eds.: 97–112. Ann Arbor Press. Ann Arbor, Michigan.
9. FENTON, J. W., II. 1981. Thrombin specificity. Ann. N.Y. Acad. Sci. **370:** This volume.
10. FENTON, J. W., B. H. LANDIS, D. A. WALZ, D. H. BING, R. D. FEINMAN, P. ZABINSKI, S. A. SONDER, L. J. BERLINER & J. S. FINLAYSON. 1979. Human thrombin: Preparative evaluation, structural properties, and enzymic specificity. *In* The Chemistry and Physiology of the Human Plasma Proteins. D. H. Bing, Ed.: 151–184. Pergamon Press. New York, N.Y.
11. KEIL, B. P., V. COUHÁ, V. HOLEYŠUVSKÝ & F. SORM. 1968. Coll. Czech. Chem. Commun. **33:** 2307–2315.
12. KEIL, B. 1970. Structural aspects of interaction of trypsin with macromolecular inhibitors. *In* Structure-Function Relationships of Proteolytic Enzymes. P. Desnuella, H. Neurath & M. Ottesen, Eds.: 102–112. Academic Press, Inc. New York, N.Y.
13. NEURATH, H. & K. A. WALSH. 1976. The role of proteases in biological regulation. *In* Proteolysis and Physiological Regulation. D. W. Ribbons & K. Brew, Eds. Miami Winter Symposia Vol. 11: 29–42. Academic Press, Inc. New York, N.Y.
14. NEURATH, H., K. A. WALSH & W. P. WINTER. 1967. Science **158:** 1638–1644.
15. KREIGER, M., L. M. KAY & R. M. STROUD. 1974. J. Mol. Biol. **83:** 209–230.
16. STROUD, R. M., L. M. KAY & R. E. DICKERSON. 1974. J. Mol. Biol. **83:** 185–208.
17. HUBER, R., D. KUKLA, W. BODE, P. SCHWAGER, K. BARTELS, J. DEISENHOFER & W. STERGMANN. 1974. J. Mol. Biol. **89:** 73–101.
18. BODE, W. & P. SCHWAGER. 1975. J. Mol. Biol. **98:** 693–717.
19. FELDMANN, R. J. 1976. Atlas of Macromolecular Structure on Microfiche. Vol. 1: 638–641. Tracor Jitco. Rockville, Md.
20. HOOD, L. E., J. H. WILSON & W. B. WOOD, Eds. 1975. Molecular evolution. *In* Molecular Biology of Eucaryotic Cells. 265–285. W. A. Benjamin, Inc. Reading, Mass.

21. PAULING, L. & E. ZUCKER-KANDL. 1963. Acta Chem. Scand. **17:** S9–S30.
22. LOVE, W. E., P. A. KLOCK, F. E. LATTMAN, E. A. PADLOU & K. B. S. WARD. 1971. Cold Spring Harbor Symp. Quant. Biol. **36:** 349–357.
23. LESK, A. M. & C. CHOTHIA. 1980. J. Mol. Biol. **136:** 225–270.
24. MAGNUSSON, S., T. E. PETERSEN, L. SOTTRUP-JENSEN & H. CLAEYS. 1975. Complete primary structure of prothrombin: Isolation, structure and reactivity of ten carboxylated glutamic acid residues and regulation of prothrombin activation by thrombin. *In* Proteases and Biological Control. E. Reich, D. Rifkin & E. Shaw, Eds.: 123–150. Cold Spring Harbor Laboratory. Cold Spring Harbor, N. Y.
25. FELDMANN, R. J., D. H. BING, B. C. FURIE & B. FURIE. 1978. Proc. Natl. Acad. Sci. USA **75:** 5409–5412.
26. RICHARDS, F. F. 1977. Ann Rev. Biophys. Bioeng. **6:** 151–176.
27. GURD, F. R. N. & T. M. ROTHGEB. 1979. Adv. Prot. Chem. **33:** 73–165.
28. FURIE, B., A. N. SCHECTER, D. H. SACHS & C. B. ANFINSEN. 1975. J. Mol. Biol. **92:** 497–506.
29. FELDMANN, R. J. 1976. Ann. Rev. Biophys. Bioeng. **5:** 477–509.
30. PORTER, T. K. 1978. Abstract, SIGGRAPH.
31. DAYHOFF, M. O. 1976. Atlas of Protein Sequence and Structure **5:** 95.
32. TULINSKY, A., R. L. VANDLER, C. M. MORIMOTO, N. V. MANI & L. H. WEIGHT. 1973. Biochemistry **12:** 4185–4192.
33. TULINSKY, A., N. V. MANI, C. N. MORIMOTO & R. L. VANDLER. 1973. Acta Cryst. **329:** 1309–1322.
34. THE PROPHET System. 1973. Fed. Proc. **32:** 1744.
35. CHASE, T., JR. & E. SHAW. 1969. Biochemistry **8:** 2212–2224.
36. LAURA, R., D. J. ROBISON & D. H. BING. 1980. Biochemistry. In press.
37. CORY, M., J. M. ANDREWS & D. H. BING. 1977. Design of exo affinity labeling reagents. Methods Enzymol. **46:** 115–130.
38. RAKITZIS, E. T. 1974. Biochem. J. **141:** 601–603.
39. SCATCHARD, G. 1949. Ann. N.Y. Acad. Sci. **51:** 660–672.
40. MARES-GUIA, M. & E. SHAW. 1965. J. Biol. Chem. **240:** 1579–1585.
41. ANDREWS, J. M., D. P. ROMAN, JR., D. H. BING & M. CORY. 1979. J. Med. Chem. **21:** 1202–1207.
42. KETTNER, C. & E. SHAW. 1979. Thromb. Res. **14:** 969–973.
43. WONG, S. C. & E. SHAW. 1974. Arch. Biochem. Biophys. **161:** 536–543.
44. KINGDON, H. S., C. M. NOYES & R. L. LUNDBLAD. 1977. Some aspects of the primary structure of bovine alpha, beta, and gamma thrombins. *In* Chemistry and Biology of Thrombin. R. L. Lundblad, J. W. Fenton, II & K. G. Mann, Eds.: 91–96. Ann Arbor Press. Ann Arbor, Michigan.
45. KOEHLER, K. A. & S. MAGNUSSON. 1974. Arch. Biochem. Biophys. **160:** 175–184.
46. BANG, N. U. & L. E. MATTLER. 1977. Thrombin sensitivity and specificity of three chromogenic peptide substrates. *In* Chemistry and Biology of Thrombin. R. L. Lundblad, J. W. Fenton, II & K. G. Mann, Eds.: 305–310. Ann Arbor Press. Ann Arbor, Michigan.
47. DAYHOFF, M. O. & W. C. BAKER. 1976. Atlas of Protein Structure **5:** 25–51.
48. MATTHEWS, B. W. & S. J. REMMINGTON. 1974. Proc. Natl. Acad. Sci. USA **71:** 4178–4182.
49. ROSSMAN, M. G., A. LILJAS, C.-I. BRÄNDÉN & L. J. BANASZAK. 1975. Evolutionary and structural relationships among dehydrogenases. *In* The Enzymes. P. D. Boyer, Ed. **11:** 61–102. Academic Press, Inc. New York, N. Y.

THE EVOLUTIONARY RELATIONSHIPS OF THE ENZYMES INVOLVED IN BLOOD COAGULATION AND HEMOSTASIS *

David Hewett-Emmett

*Department of Human Genetics
University of Michigan Medical School
Ann Arbor, Michigan 48109*

John Czelusniak and Morris Goodman

*Department of Anatomy
Wayne State University School of Medicine
Detroit, Michigan 48201*

INTRODUCTION

Many of the blood coagulation factors circulate in the plasma as inactive precursors (zymogens), which upon activation by limited proteolysis become proteolytic enzymes with a high degree of substrate specificity.[1-3] Like the pancreatic digestive enzymes, the blood coagulation factors are serine proteases possessing an Asp, Ser, His at their active site.[1,2] Unlike the pancreatic enzymes, most of the blood coagulation factors, upon activation, retain a large polypeptide chain linked by a disulfide-bridge to the chain containing the active site. Although crystals of thrombin have been grown,[4] no three-dimensional structure has yet been adduced, but it seems clear that the blood coagulation serine proteases will share many of the active-site features revealed by X-ray crystallography of the pancreatic enzymes, chymotrypsin A, trypsin, and elastase. Such studies have explained the difference in specificity of these enzymes [5,6] however in their case almost all of the peptide bonds of the required specificity are cleaved; in the case of the blood coagulation factors only a few of the many arginyl bonds are cleaved.[1-3] In spite of the dearth of three-dimensional structures, amino acid sequence data are providing clues to understanding the diversity of this enzyme family.

Several investigators [7-9] have built gene phylogenies (genealogies) of the serine proteases using data sets of limited sizes. De Haën *et al.*[7] concluded that the presence of disulfide bridges and deletions/insertions might prove better phylogenetic markers than the sequences themselves. However, the recent publication of several new amino acid sequences provides us with an opportunity to shed some light on serine protease evolution by using the maximum parsimony method and extending earlier studies.[8,9] The maximum parsimony approach assumes that evolution has taken the shortest course to reach the present array of diversity: it has been used effectively on such protein families as the hemoglobins,[10] intracellular calcium-binding proteins,[11] and carbonic anhydrase isozymes.[12] In this preliminary report, we describe the tree of lowest nucleotide replacement length that we found for each of the data sets used and draw some general conclusions about the evolution of the blood coagulation factors.

* This work was supported by National Science Foundation Grant DEB-7810717.

511

Materials and Methods

The available amino acid sequences (Table 1) were grouped into four data sets and aligned to maximize homology, a procedure that even when computerized contains a large subjective input. To test whether aligned sequences showed significant homology with each other, an alignment statistic was used.[13] The aligned data sets created were:

1) SP—16 enzyme chain sequences which are more than 95% complete. For alignment, using the one-letter amino acid code (see Table 2). 2) SPIN-COMPL—The above 16 sequences with an additional 13 partial sequences. Since these align straightforwardly with the 16 complete sequences, the alignment for this data set is not illustrated, 3) VIT K—9 sequences (5 complete) representing the NH_2-terminal regions of the vitamin K-dependent blood coagulation factor zymogens. 4) KRINGLE—9 kringle loop structures of prothrombin and plasminogen aligned with 4 regions of putative homology in factor X, factor IX, protein C, and haptoglobin α chain.

For each data set, the maximum parsimony method was used to construct the tree that requires the fewest nucleotide replacements to explain the descent of extant sequences.[10, 11] Proteins are grouped so as to maximize the number of shared derived nucleotide replacements. Using a branch-swapping algorithm, many thousands of alternative trees are tested. No assumptions of constancy of rate of evolution are needed to construct genealogical trees by this method. The trees produced can be "rooted" subjectively (i.e. given a time dimension); however, inclusion of a bacterial serine protease enables the root to be placed on the branch to the eukaryotic serine proteases (see discussion [44]).

Results and Discussion

Tree Derived for 16 Serine Proteases (SP)

After testing many trees, that with the lowest nucleotide replacement length (1936 NR) is shown in Figure 1. The main features of the tree are:

1. The close grouping of the factors involved in fibrin-clot formation, supporting the view that blood coagulation was once a simple process involving perhaps a single thrombin-like enzyme that clotted a fibrinogen-like material.

2. The distant separation of plasmin from these blood coagulation factors. This was tested by submitting several alternative trees with widely different positions for plasmin. In all cases, plasmin was successively moved by the branch-swapping algorithm to its final position in the tree illustrated.

3. The finding that protein C was the first of the vitamin K-dependent factors to become a separate lineage, before the duplications that resulted in the factor IX and factor X lineages.

Haptoglobin is closely related to the blood coagulation factors. Like them, it is of hepatic origin, but during evolution it has lost the active-site His and Ser residues and its present role seems to be to bind hemoglobin virtually irreversibly.[9] Our tree is compatible with that of Kurosky *et al.,*[9] if they were to place the root of their tree in the same position as ours.

TABLE 1

AMINO ACID SEQUENCE DATA USED *

Protein	Species	Non-Enzyme Region	Enzyme Chain	References
Prothrombin	Human	322 (100%)	259 (100%)	14–16
	Ox	323 (100%)	259 (100%)	17–20
	Chicken	45 (14%)	0 (0%)	21
Factor X	Ox	191 (100%)	256 (100%)	22,23
Factor IX	Ox	181 (100%)	235 (100%)	24
Protein C	Ox	169 (100%)	242 (99%)	25
Factor VII	Ox	13 (?)	25 ($\sim$10%)	26
Protein S	Human	13 (?)	0 (0%)	27
	Ox	13 (?)	0 (0%)	27
Factor XI	Ox, Human	--------	36 ($\sim$14%)	28,29
Factor XII	Ox	--------	40 ($\sim$16%)	30
Plasminogen	Human	560 (100%)	230 (100%)	31,32
Haptoglobin	Human	83 (100%)	245 (100%)	9,33,34
	Rat	0 (0%)	40 (16%)	34
	Rabbit	0 (0%)	40 (16%)	34
	Dog	0 (0%)	40 (16%)	34
Kallikrein	Pig (pancreas)	--------	233 (96%)	35
Trypsinogen	Ox	--------	223 (100%)	cf. 7,36
	Pig	--------	223 (100%)	cf. 7
	Dogfish	--------	222 (100%)	cf. 7
Trypsinogen B	African lung fish	--------	147 (66%)	cf. 7
Cocoonase	Silkmoth	--------	30 ($\sim$12%)	37
RVV-V activator	Russell's viper	--------	14 ($\sim$6%)	38
Crotalase	Rattlesnake	--------	45 ($\sim$18%)	39
Complement CIr	Human	--------	20 ($\sim$8%)	40
Complement CIs	Human	--------	20 ($\sim$8%)	40
Complement Factor D	Human	--------	50 ($\sim$20%)	41
Group Specific Protease	Rat (intestine)	--------	224 (100%)	42
Chymotrypsinogen A	Ox	--------	230 (100%)	cf. 7,36
Chymotrypsinogen B	Ox	--------	230 (100%)	cf. 7,36
Proelastase B	Pig	--------	240 (100%)	cf. 7,36
Bacterial trypsin	*Streptomyces griseus*	--------	221 (100%)	43

* In the case of some zymogens, the non-enzyme chain region has been sequenced, but is not used in this presentation.

TABLE 2

ALIGNMENT OF DATA SET SP (16 SERINE PROTEASES, >95% COMPLETE) *

```
          16   20 22  27 30 32        40 42      50     57 60              70        80        90       100
HUMAN THROMBIN        IVEGSNAEIGMSPWQVMLFRKSPQ—ELLCGASLISNRWVLTAAHCLLYPPWNKNFTENDLLVRIGKHSRTRYERNIEKISMLEKIYIHPRYNWRENLD—
BOVINE THROMBIN       IVEGQDAEVGLSPWQVMLFRKSPQ—ELLCGASLISDRWVLTAAHCLLYPPWBKNFTVDDLLVRIGKHSRTRYERKVEKISMLDKIYIHPRYNWKENLD—
FACTOR Xa             IVGGRDCAEGECPWQALLVNEEN—EGFCGGTILNEFYVLTAAHCLHQAKR—FT—VRVG—DRNTQEGDEEMAHEVEMTVKHSRFV—KETYD—
FACTOR IXa            VVGGEDAERGQFPWQVLLHGEI—AAFCGGSIVNEKWVVTAAHCIKPGVK—IT—VVAGEHNTEKPEPTEQKRN—VIRAIPYHSYNASIN—K
PROTEIN C             IVDGQEAGWGESPWQAVLLDSKK—KLVCGAVLIHVSWVLTVAHCXRKKLI—VRLGEYDMRRWESWEVDLD—IKEVIIHPNYTKSYSDN—
PLASMIN               VVGGCVAHPHSWPWQVSLRTRFG—MHFCGGTLISPEWVLTAAHCLEKSPRPSSYK—VILGAHQEVNLEPHVQEIE—VSRLFLEP—TRK—
HAPTOGLOBIN           ILGGHLDAKGSFPWQAKMVSHH—NLTTGATLINEQWLLTTAKNLFLNHSENAT—AKDIAPTLTLYVGKKQLVE—IEKVVLHPNYSQV—
OX TRYPSIN            IVGGYTCGANTVPYQVSLN—SG—YHFCGGSLINSQWVVSAAHCYKSGIQ—VRLGQDNINVVEGNQQFIS—ASKSIVHPSYNSNTLNN—
PIG TRYPSIN           IVGGYTCAANSIPYQVSLN—SG—SHFCGGSLINSQWVVSAAHCYKSRIQ—VRLGEHNIDVLEGNEQFIN—AAKIITHPNFNGNTLDN—
DOGFISH TRYPSIN       IVGGYECPKHAAPWTVSLN—VG—YHFCGGSLIAPGWVVSAAHCYQRRIQ—VRLGEHDISANEGDETYID—SSMVIRHPNYSGYDLDN—
CHYMOTRYPSIN A        IVNGEEAVPGSWPWQVSLQDKTG—FHFCGGSLINENWVVTAAHCGVTTSD—VVVAGEFDQGSSSEKIQKLK—IAKVFKNSKYNSLTINN—
CHYMOTRYPSIN B        IVNGEDAVPGSWPWQVSLQDSTG—FHFCGGSLISEDWVVTAAHCGVTTSD—VVVAGEFDQGLETEDTQVLK—IGKVFKNPKFSILTVRN—
ELASTASE              VVGGTEAQRNSWPSQISLQYRSGSSWAHTCGGTLIRQNWVMTAAHCVDRELT—FR—VVVGEHNLNQNNGTEQYVG—VQKIVVHPYWNTDDVAA—
KALLIKREIN (GLAND.)   IIGGRECEKNSHPWQVAIYHYS—SFQCGGVLVNPKWVLTAAHCKNDNYE—VGWLRHNLFENENTAQFFG—VTADFPHPGFNLSADGKD
GROUP Sp. PROTEASE    IIGGVESIPHSRPYMAHLDIVTEKGLRVICGGFLISRQFVLTAAHCKGREIT—VILGAHDVRKRESTQQKIK—VEKQIIHESYNSVPNL—
BACTERIAL TRYPSIN     VVGGTRAAQGEFPFMVRL—SMG—CGGALYAQDIVLTAAHCVSGSGN—NT—SITATGGVVDLQSAVKVLRSTKVLQAPGYNGTGK—
```

```
                 102      110    120 122 127   130     136 140              150     157 160     168 170       180    180G
HUMAN THROMBIN       --RDIALMKLKKPVAFSDYIHPVCLPNRETAAS-LLGAGYKGRVTGYGNLKSTVTADVGKGQPSVLQVVNLALVQRPVCKDS-TRI-RITDNM--
BOVINE THROMBIN      --RDIALLKLKRPIELSDYIHPVCLPDKQTAAK-LLHAGFKGRVTGWGNRRETWTTSVAEVQPSVLQVVNLPLVERPVCKAS-TRI-RITNDM--
FACTOR XA            --FDIAVLRLKTPIRF-RNVAPACLPEKDWAAE-TLQTKT-GIVSGFGR----TH-EKGRLSSTLKMLEVPYVDRSTCKLS-SSF-TITPNM--
FACTOR IXA           YSHDIALLELDEPLELNSYVTPICIADRDY----TNIF-SKFGYGYVSGWGKVFNRGRSASILQYLKVPLVDRATCLRS-TKF-SIYSHM--
PROTEIN C            --DIALLRLAKPATLSQTIVPICLPDSGLSERKLTQVGQETVVTGWGYRDE----TKRNRTFVLSFIKVPVVPYXACVHA-MEN-KISENM--
PLASMIN             --DIALLKLSSPAVITDKVIPACLPSPNY----VVADRTECFITGWGE----TQ--GTFGAGLLKEAQLPVIENKVCNRYEFLNGRVQSTE--
HAPTOGLOBIN          --DIGLIKLKQKVSVNERVMPICLPSKDYA----EVGRVGYVSGWGR----NA-NFKFTDHLKYVMLPVADQDQCIRH-YEGSTVPEKKTPKSPVG
OX TRYPSIN           --DIMLIKLKSAASLNSRVASISLPTSCA----SAGTQCLISGWGN----TKSSGTSYPDVLKCLKAPILSNSSCKSA-YPG-QITSNM--
PIG TRYPSIN          --DIMLIKLSSPATLNSRVATVSLPRSCA----AAGTECLISGWGN----TKSSGSSYPSLLQCLKAPVLSDSSCKSS-YPG-QITGNM--
DOGFISH TRYPSIN      --DIMLIKLSKPAALNRNVDLISLPTGCA----YAGEMCLISGWGN----TM-DGAVSGDQLQCLDAPVLSDAECKGA-YPG-MITNNM--
CHYMOTRYPSIN A       --DITLLKLSTAASFSQTVSAVCLPSASD----DFAAGTTCVTTGWGL----TRYTNANTPDRLQQASLPLLSNTNCKK-YWGTKIKDAM--
CHYMOTRYPSIN B       --DITLLKLATPAQFSETVSAVCLPSADE----DFPAGMLCATTGWGK----TKYNALKTPDKLQQATLPIVSNTDCRK-YWGSRVTDVM--
ELASTASE            -GYDIALLRLAQSVTLNSYVQLGVLPRAGT----ILANNSPCYITGWGL----TR-TNGQLAQTLQQAYLPTVDYAICSSSSYWGSTVKNSM--
KALLIKREIN (GLAND.)  YSHDLMLLRLQSPAKITDAVKVLELPTQEP----ELGSTCEASGWGSI--EPGPDDFEFPDEIQCVQLTLLQNTFCAHA-BPB-KVTESM--
GROUP SP. PROTEASE   --HDIMLLKLEKKVELTPAVNVVPLPSPSD----FIHPGAMCWAAGWGK----TG-VRDPTSYTLREVELRIMDEKACVDYRYYEYKF---Q--
BACTERIAL TRYPSIN    --DWALIKLAQPIN----QP-TLKIATT----TAYNQGT-FTVAGWGA----NR-EGGSQQRYLLKANVPFVSDAACRSA-YGNELVANEE--
```

Table 2 (continued)

```
                                182          189 191  195   200 201        210 214 216   220        226       232         240   245
Human thrombin      ——————————FCAGYKPDEGKRGDACEGDSGGPFVMKSPFNNRWYQMGIVSWGE—GCDRDGKYGFYTHVFRLKKWI—QKVIDQFGE
Bovine thrombin     ——————————FCAGYKPGEGKRGDACEGDSGGPFVMKSPYNNRWYQMGIVSWGE—GCDRNGKYGFYTHVFRLKKWI—QKVIDRLGS
Factor Xa           ——————————FCAGY—DTQPE–DACQGDSGGPHV—TRFKDTYFVTGIVSWGE—GCARKGKFGVYTKVSNFLKWI–DKIMKARAGAAGSRGHSEAPATW
Factor IXa          ——————————FCAGY—HEGGK–DSCQGDSGGPHV—TEVEGTSFLTGIISWGE—ECAMKGKYGIYTKVSRYVNWIKEKTKLT–
Protein C           ——————————LCAGI—LGDPR–DACEGDSGGPMV—TFFRGTHFLVGLVSWGE—GCGRLYNYGVYTKVSRYLDWIYGHIKAQEAPLESQVP
Plasmin             ——————————LCAGH—LAGGT–DSCQGDSGGPLV—CFEKDKQILQGVTSWGL—GCARPNKPGVYVRVSRFVTWI—EGVMRNN
Haptoglobin         VQPILNEHTFCAGM—SKYQE–DTCYGDAGSAFAVHDLEENTWYATGILSFDK——CSAVAEYGVYVKVTSIQNWV–QKTIAEN
Ox trypsin          ——————————FCAGY—LEGGK–DSCQGDSGGPVV—CSGK——LQGIVSWGS—GCAQKNKPGVYTKVCNYVSWI–KQTIASN
Pig trypsin         ——————————ICVGF—LEGGK–DSCQGDSGGPVV—CNGQ——LQGIVSWGY—GCAQKNKPGVYTKVCNYVNWI–QQTIAAN
Dogfish trypsin     ——————————MCVGY—MEGGK–DSCQGDSGGPVV—CNGM——LQGIVSWGY—GCAERDHPGVYTRVCHYVSWI–HETIASV
Chymotrypsin A      ——————————ICAG——ASGV—SSCMGDSGGPLV—CKKNGAWTLVGIVSWGSS-TCS–TSTPGVYARVTALVNWV–QQTLAAN
Chymotrypsin B      ——————————ICAG——ASGV—SSCMGDSGGPLV—CQKNGAWTLAGIVSWGSS-TCS–TSTPAVYARVTALMPWV–QETLAAN
Elastase            ——————————VCAG——GNGVR–SGCQGDSGGPLH—CLVNGQYAVHGVTSFVSRLGCNVTRKPTVFTRVSAYISWI–NNVIASN
Kallikrein (gland.) ——————————LCAGY—LPGGK–DTCMGDSGGPLI—CNGM——WQGITSWGHT–PCGSANKPSIYTKLIFYLDWI–BBTITENP
Group Sp. protease  ——————————VCVGS—PTTLR–AAFMGDSGGPLL—CAGV——AHGIVSYGH—PDAKP—PAIFTRVSTYVPTI–NAVIN——
Bacterial trypsin   ——————————ICAGY–PDTGGV–DTCQGDSGGPMFRKDNADE–WIQVGIVSWGY—GCARPGYPGVYTEVSTFASAI–ASAARTL
```

* Numbering based on chymotrypsin A. X=residue not identified.
——— = residue/region deleted.

Tree Derived for 29 Serine Proteases (*SPINCOMPL*)

After testing many trees, that with lowest nucleotide replacement length (2076 NR) is shown in FIGURE 2. The main features are:

1. The addition of 13 partial sequences has altered the arrangement of the pancreatic enzymes (trypsin, chymotrypsin, elastase, kallikrein) and the rela-

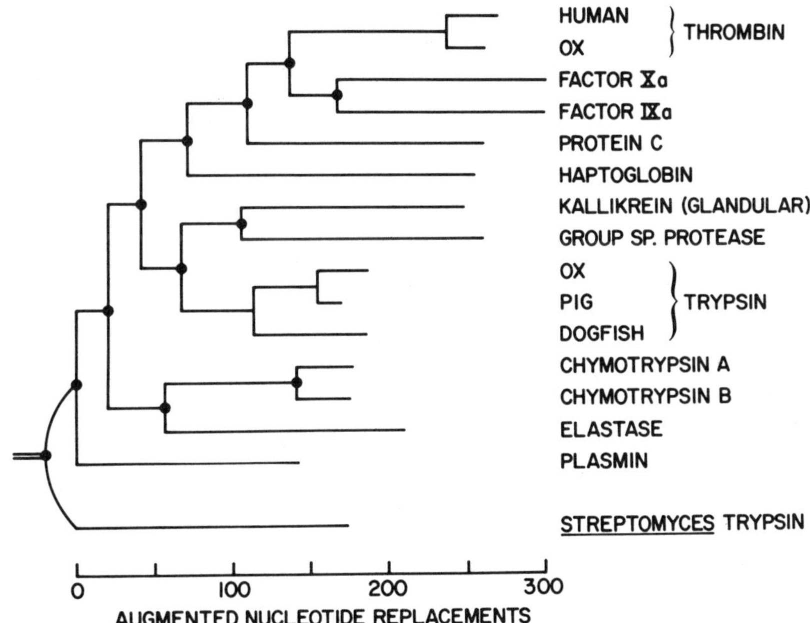

FIGURE 1. Genealogy of serine proteases based on data set SP (16 sequences more than 95% complete: TABLE 2). This tree has a nucleotide replacement length of 1936, the lowest found for this data set. The tree was "rooted" by use of the bacterial (*Streptomyces griseus*) trypsin. It should be noted that Hartley [45, 46] continues to believe that this gene is not of bacterial origin, having been inserted into the bacterial genome. It still seems to be the most distantly related of all the serine proteases examined in this data set. Other bacterial serine proteases, e.g. *Streptomyces griseus* protease B,[47] are clearly homologous to these proteases but many more insertions and deletions are required to align them. In earlier work (R. A. Marlar and D. Hewett-Emmett, 1976, unpublished), we included protease B and found that the "rooting" of the tree was identical, although plasmin was not available for inclusion at that time. Branch lengths are augmented to compensate for undetected multiple mutations in long separate lineages.[11] The branches are drawn to scale, their lengths being the augmented nucleotide replacements per enzyme chain. ● represent gene duplications.

tionship of plasmin. At an intermediate stage of the work, before complement factor D and crotalase were added to the data set, plasmin still represented the earliest ancestral eukaryotic branch. It may well be that the addition of a complete complement factor sequence will be necessary to resolve the true position of plasmin in the genealogy. In general, experience with the hemoglobins has shown that additional sequences iron out discordances.[10]

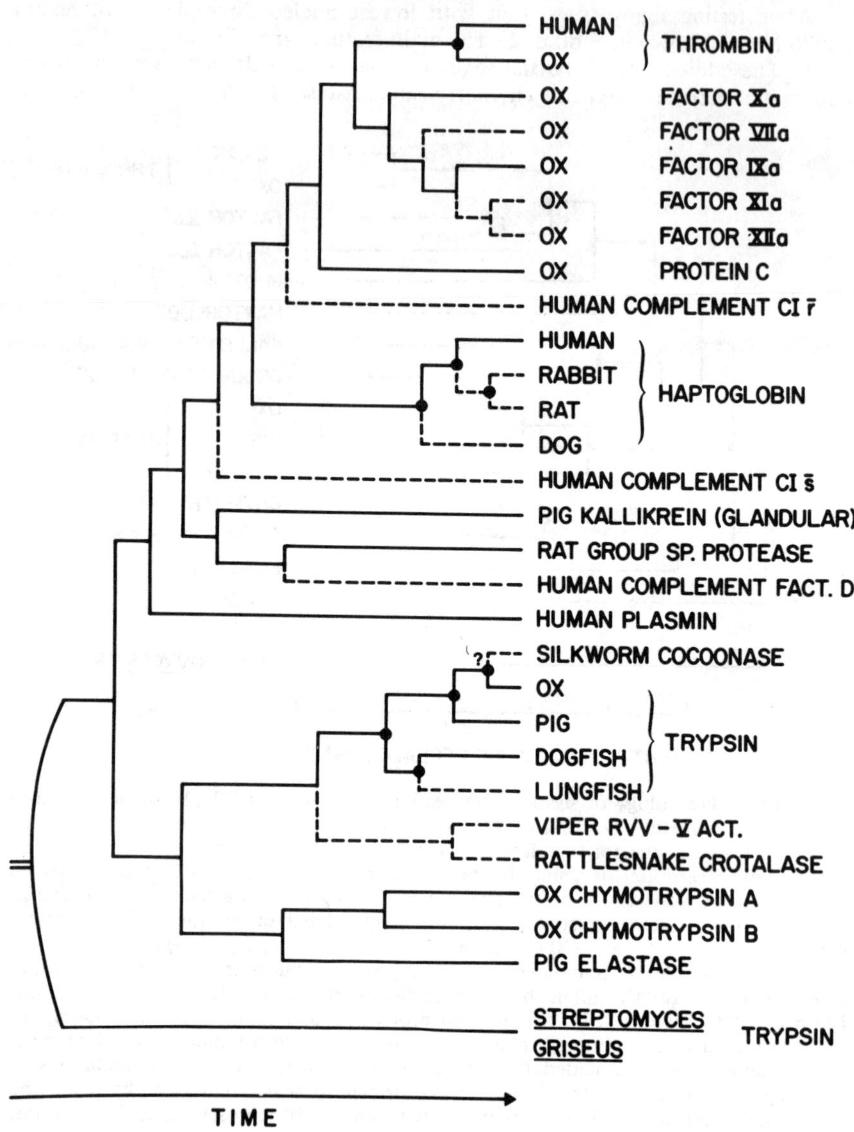

FIGURE 2. Genealogy of serine protease based on data set SPINCOMPL. This tree has a nucleotide replacement length of 2076, the lowest found for this data set. As in FIGURE 1, the tree was rooted by use of *S. griseus* trypsin. Broken lines indicate the 13 partial sequences whose positions in the tree are necessarily much less reliable. ● represent species divergencies; remaining bifurcations in the tree are gene duplications.

2. From the small stretches of sequence available, clotting factors VII, XI and XII show most affinity for factor IX. However, as with the complement factors, complete sequences will be needed to decide whether or not this is true. Factor XIIa probably possesses a disulfide bridge (residues 136–202) not present in the vitamin K-dependent coagulation factors.[30]

3. The snake venom proteases are clearly trypsin-like and not thrombin-like in their evolutionary relationship. This is supported by the probable presence of a disulfide bridge (residues 22–157 in TABLE 2) that is absent in all the hepatic serine proteases.[38, 39]

4. From the available data, it seems that the complement factors may not form a single grouping. It has been pointed out that factor D shows most similarity to the pancreatic serine proteases,[41] and in our tree it clusters with group-specific protease and kallikrein.

5. The relationship of haptoglobin to the blood coagulation factors is unaltered by the addition of the 13 partial sequences.

Tree Derived for NH$_2$-Terminal Regions of Vitamin K-Dependent Factors (VIT K)

After testing many trees, two with equal nucleotide replacement lengths (112 NR) were found. One tree split up the two partial protein S sequences and so the other tree is considered more likely to represent the true genealogy and is illustrated in FIGURE 3. The main features are:

1. The branching pattern is similar to that in FIGURES 1 and 2. However, the limited factor VII data indicate that it diverged earlier than was indicated in FIGURE 2. Until the full sequence is known this discrepancy cannot be resolved.

2. Based on equally weak evidence, protein S seems to be most closely related to factor X. Its function is not presently known.

Tree Derived for Kringle and Homologous Regions (KRINGLE)

The tree illustrated in FIGURE 4 is that with lowest nucleotide replacement length (504 NR). In this case, we know the order of the kringle regions on the plasminogen gene. Fitch[48] has pointed out that some phylogenies are incompatible with simple unequal crossover events. We have illustrated a mechanism involving unequal crossover events and gene deletions (7 events) whereby the observed kringle order can be derived. We disagree with Fitch[48] inasmuch as he does not allow gene deletion events in his scheme. It is of interest that the trees proposed by Young *et al.*[8] and Kurosky *et al.*[9] require at least 10 extra nucleotide replacements, although they require only 3 gene duplication events instead of 7 unequal crossover events in the scheme we advocate. The main features of the tree are:

1. The plasminogen kringle loops are most closely related to prothrombin kringle 1. It has been noted previously that prothrombin kringle 1 has been more conserved than kringle 2 or the vitamin K-dependent Ca^{2+}-binding region of prothrombin during mammalian evolution.[49, 50] No function has yet been ascribed to this region of either prothrombin or plasminogen however.

2. The branching pattern differs from those of FIGURES 1–3 inasmuch as factors X and IX do not share a period of evolution with prothrombin, assuming of course that the root has been placed correctly.

3. The putative kringle loops of factor X, factor IX, protein C, and haptoglobin are only weakly homologous with those of prothrombin and plasminogen using the Moore and Goodman [13] test. It is notable that on a less permissive visual test used previously,[50] factor X showed no detectable homology with either prothrombin kringle. Clearly if they are truly homologous, the kringle loops of protein C, factor X, and factor IX have diverged considerably while retaining significant homology to each other.

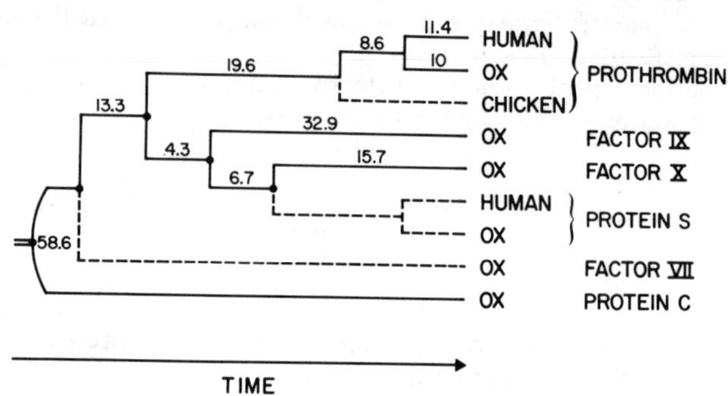

FIGURE 3. Genealogy of data set VIT K, representing regions homologous to residues 1–65 of bovine prothrombin (TABLE 3). This tree has a nucleotide replacement length of 112 and is one of two found with that length; the other split up the two protein S partial sequences and was considered less likely to represent the true genealogy. The tree was rooted using information derived from FIGURES 1 and 2, i.e. that protein C was the first separate lineage of those represented. This is supported by divergence data; protein C represents the longest branch. Broken lines indicate the 4 partial sequences. Branches have a time dimension and are *not* drawn to scale. The figures on the branches representing complete sequences are augmented nucleotide replacements per 100 codons. ● represent gene duplications.

CONCLUSIONS

This section will describe general conclusions based on the trees in FIGURES 1–3.

1. The order of gene duplication among the serine proteases involved in blood coagulation seems to be as follows:

Trypsin→*Trypsin–Plasmin*→*Trypsin–Thrombin*–Plasmin→
Trypsin–*Thrombin–Protein C*–Plasmin→
Trypsin–*Thrombin–Factor X*–Protein C–Plasmin→
Trypsin–Snake Venom Protease–Thrombin–*Factor X–Factor IX*–Protein C–Plasmin

The true place of factors VII, XI, XII, and the complement factors must await completion of their amino acid sequences.

2. The kringle loop structure regions provide strong evidence that plasminogen may be a hybrid gene, with kringle loops derived from prothrombin kringle 1 coding region having been fused to the plasmin light-chain coding region

TABLE 3

ALIGNMENT OF DATA SET VIT K, THE NH$_2$-TERMINAL REGIONS OF THE VITAMIN K-DEPENDENT BLOOD COAGULATION FACTOR *

```
                          1        10        20        30        40              50          60    65
Human    Prothrombin      ANT-FLEE-VRKGNLERECVEETCSYEEAFEALESSTATDVFWAKYTA — CETARTPRDKLAACLE-GN

Ox       Prothrombin      ANKGFLEE-VRKGNLERECLEEPCSREEAFEALESLSATDAFWAKYTA — CESARNPREKLNECLE-GN

Chicken  Prothrombin      ANKGFLEE-MIKGNLERECLEETCNYEEAFEALESTVDTDAFWAKY

Ox       Factor X         ANS-FLEE-VKQGNLERECLEEACSLEEAREVFEDAEQTDEFWSKYKDGDQCEG ——————— HPCLNQGH

Ox       Factor IX        YNSGKLEEFVR-GNLERECKEEKCSFEEAREVFENTEKTTEFWKQYVDGDQCES ——————— NPCLNGGM

Ox       Protein C        ANS-FLEE-LRPGNVERECSEEVCEFEEAREIFQNTEDTMAFWSKYSDGEQCEDRPSGSPCDLPCCGRGK

Ox       Factor VII       AN-GFLEELL-PGSL

Human    Protein S        ANS-LLEE-XKQGNL

Ox       Protein S        ANT-LLEE-TKKGNL
```

* Numbering based on bovine profragment 1.
——— = residue/region deleted.

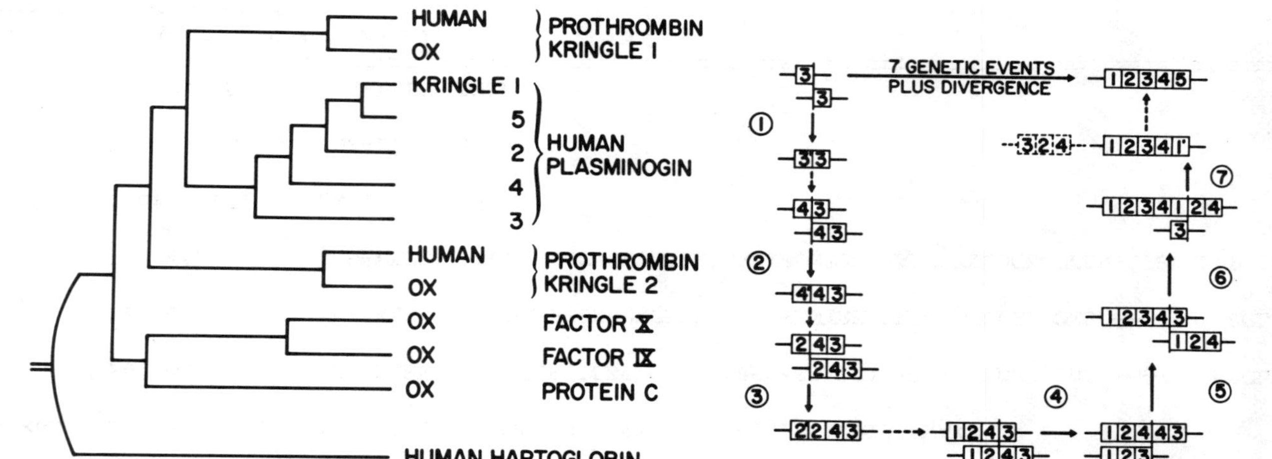

FIGURE 4. Hypothetical genealogy of the kringle structures of prothrombin and plasminogen and regions of putative homology in other serine protease zymogens (data set KRINGLE, TABLE 4). This tree has a nucleotide replacement length of 504, the lowest found for this data set. However at least 6 and probably 7 genetic events (unequal crossovers, etc.) are required to assemble the plasminogen kringles in the correct order on the chromosome. Alternative trees suggested elsewhere [9, 9] require at least 10 additional nucleotide replacements. The root of the tree is placed by assuming that haptoglobin represents the earliest ancestral branch. Since the homology of haptoglobin, factor X, factor IX, and protein C with the kringles of prothrombin and plasminogen is equivocal, this tree should be treated with caution with regard to genealogical conclusions. Branches are not drawn to scale although they have a time dimension.

Table 4

Alignment of "Kringle" Regions of Prothrombin and Plasminogen with Putative "Kringle" Regions
of Other Serine Protease Zymogens *

	1 10 20 30 34A 40 50 60 70 79
Pro Kr 1 (H)	CAEGLGTNYRGNVSITRSGIECQLWRSRYPHKPE–INSTTHPGADLQENFCRNPDSSITGPWCYTTDPTA–RRQEC —— STPV–C
(B)	CAEGVGMNYRGNVSVTRSGIECQLWRSRYPHKPE–INSTTHPGADLRENFCRNPDGSITGPWCYTTSPTL–RREEC —— SVPV–C
Pro Kr 2 (H)	CVPDRGQQYQGRLAVTTHGLPCLAWASAQAKALS–KHQDFNSAVQLVENFCRNPDGDEEGVWCYVAGKPG–DFGYC —— DLNY–C
(B)	CFPDRGREYRGRLAVTTSGSRCLAWSSEQAKALS–KDQDFNPAVPLAENFCRNPDGDEEGAWCYVADQPG–DFEYC —— DLNY–C
Plas Kr 1	CKTGDGKNYRGTMSKTKNGITCQKWSSTSPHRPR–FSPATHPSEGLEENYCRNPDNDPQGPWCYTTDPEK–RYDYC —— DILE–C
Kr 2	CMHCSGENYDGKISKTMSGLECQAWDSQSPHAHG–YIPSKFPNKNLKKNYCRNPDREL–RPWCFTTDPNK–RWELC —— DIPR–C
Kr 3	CLKGTGENYRGNVAVTVSGHTCQHWSAQTPHTHN–TRPENFPCKNLDENYCRNPDGKR–APWCHTTNSQV–RWEYC —— KIPS–C
Kr 4	CYHGDGQSYRGTSSTTTTGKKCQSWSSMTPHRHQ–KTPENYPNAGLTMNYCRNPDADK–GPWCFTTDPSV–RWEYC —— NLKK–C
Kr 5	CMFGNGKGYRGKRATTVTGTPCQDWAAQEPHRHS IFTPETNPRAGLEKNYCRNPDGDVGGPWCYTTNPRK–LYDYC —— DVPQ–C
Factor X	CKNGIG–DYTCTCAEGFEGKNCEFSTREI ————— CSLDNGGCDQFC–REERSEVRCSCAHGYVLGDDSKSCVS — TERFPC
Factor IX	CKTDIN–SYECWCQAGFEGTNCELDAT ————— CSIKNGRCKQFCKRDTDNKVVCSCTDGYRLAEDQKSCEP — AVPFPC
Protein C	CIHGLG–GFRCDCAEGWEGRFCLHEVRFS ————— NCSAEBGGCAHYC–MEEEGRRHCSCAPGYRLEDDHQLCVS — KVTFPC
Haptoglobin	VDSGNDVTDIADDGCPK–PPQIAHGYV–EHSVRYQC —— KNYYKLR–TEGDGV — YTLNNEK–QWINKAVGDKLPE–C

* Numbering based on bovine prothrombin kringle 1.
—— = residue/region deleted.

much later in time than the gene duplication generating the plasmin and thrombin lineages.

3. It seems clear that haptoglobin was once a hepatic serine protease that lost its proteolytic activity.[9] Our trees (FIGURES 1 and 2) are compatible with those of Kurosky et al.[9] provided that they alter the root of their tree. By contrast, the tree suggested by Doolittle[51] underestimates how closely related haptoglobin is to the hepatic serine proteases and, in particular, the blood coagulation factors.

ACKNOWLEDGMENTS

We appreciate the participation, at an earlier stage of the work, of Dr. Richard A. Marlar and the encouragement of Dr. Walter H. Seegers. We are particularly grateful to Dr. Alex Kurosky for providing us with a preprint of his work on haptoglobin and for discussion of his and our findings.

[**Note added in proof:** Since the meeting, several relevant amino acid sequences of serine proteases have been published. In particular, Bradshaw et al.[52] describe a chymotrypsin-like collagenase from the hepato-pancreas of the fiddler crab and a trypsin-like protease that comprises the γ-subunit of mouse nerve growth factor. Brunisholz et al.[53] provide substantial structural data on bovine and porcine plasminogen, which further emphasize the conservative nature of the kringle structure. Mole and Nieman[54] have partially sequenced human complement factor B, which is a novel serine protease and shows most similarity with plasminogen and rat intestine group-specific protease; as stated in the text, the addition of complement sequences may be necessary to identify the true phylogenetic relationships of plasminogen. Group-specific protease is now known to derive from atypical mast cells of the intestine and, in an excellent minireview on this topic, Woodbury and Neurath[55] describe a different but homologous protease from rat peritoneum and skeletal muscle mast cells. Interestingly, atypical mast cells do not contain heparin which is known to interact with lysine residues and the atypical mast cell protease contains almost 50% less lysine than the mast cell protease. Finally, Petersen et al.[56] have determined the amino-terminal sequence of protein Z from bovine plasma whose homology with the other vitamin K-dependent plasma clotting factors was previously inferred but not firmly proved by Prowse and Esnouf.[57] Protein Z contains γ-carboxyglutamic acid, but seems only distantly related to the other vitamin K-dependent factors.]

REFERENCES

1. SEEGERS, W. H., H. I. HASSOUNA, D. HEWETT-EMMETT, D. A. WALZ & T. J. ANDARY. 1975. Prothrombin and thrombin. Selected aspects of thrombin formation, properties, inhibition and immunology. Sem. Thromb. Hemost. **1:** 211–283.
2. DAVIE, E. W. & K. FUJIKAWA. 1975. Basic mechanisms in blood coagulation. Ann. Rev. Biochem. **44:** 799–829.
3. SUTTIE, J. W. & C. M. JACKSON. 1977. Prothrombin structure, activation and biosynthesis. Physiol. Rev. **57:** 1–70.
4. TSERNOGLOU, D., D. A. WALZ, L. E. McCOY & W. H. SEEGERS. 1974. An X-ray crystallographic study of thrombin. J. Biol. Chem. **249:** 999.

5. SEGAL, D. M., J. C. POWERS, G. H. COHEN, D. R. DAVIES & P. E. WILCOX. 1971. Substrate binding site in chymotrypsin A$_\gamma$. Biochemistry **10:** 3728–3738.

6. STROUD, R. M. 1974. A family of protein-cutting proteins. Sci. Am. **231:** 74–88.

7. DE HAËN, C., H. NEURATH & D. C. TELLER. 1975. The phylogeny of trypsin-related serine proteases and their zymogens. New methods for the investigation of distant evolutionary relationships. J. Mol. Biol. **92:** 225–259.

8. YOUNG, C. L., W. C. BARKER, C. M. TOMASELLI & M. O. DAYHOFF. 1978. Serine proteases. *In* Atlas of Protein Sequence and Structure. M. O. Dayhoff, Ed. Vol. 5 (Suppl. 3): 73–89. National Biomedical Research Foundation. Washington, D.C.

9. KUROSKY, A., D. R. BARNETT, T.-H. LEE, B. TOUCHSTONE, R. E. HAY, M. S. ARNOTT, B. H. BOWMAN & W. M. FITCH. 1980. Covalent structure of human haptoglobin: A serine protease homolog. Proc. Natl. Acad. Sci. USA **77:** 3388–3392.

10. GOODMAN, M., J. CZELUSNIAK, G. W. MOORE, A. E. ROMERO-HERRERA & G. MATSUDA. 1979. Fitting the gene linkage into its species linkage, a parsimony strategy illustrated by cladograms constructed from globin sequences. Syst. Zool. **28:** 132–163.

11. GOODMAN, M., J.-F. PECHÈRE, J. HAIECH & J. G. DEMAILLE. 1979. Evolutionary diversification of structure and function in the family of intracellular calcium-binding proteins. J. Mol. Evol. **13:** 331–352.

12. TASHIAN, R. E., D. HEWETT-EMMETT & M. GOODMAN. Evolutionary diversity in the structure and activity of carbonic anhydrase. *In* Protides of the Biological Fluids. Colloquium No. 28. H. Peeters, Ed.: 153–156. Pergamon Press. Oxford.

13. MOORE, G. W. & M. GOODMAN. 1977. Alignment statistic for identifying related protein sequences. J. Mol. Evol. **9:** 121–130.

14. WALZ, D. A., D. HEWETT-EMMETT & W. H. SEEGERS. 1977. Amino acid sequence of human prothrombin fragments 1 and 2. Proc. Natl. Acad. Sci. USA **74:** 1969–1972.

15. BUTKOWSKI, R. J., J. ELION, M. R. DOWNING & K. G. MANN. 1977. Primary structure of human prethrombin 2 and α-thrombin. J. Biol. Chem. **252:** 4942–4957.

16. THOMPSON, A. R., D. L. ENFIELD, L. H. ERICSSON, M. E. LEGAZ & J. W. FENTON II. 1977. Human thrombin: Partial primary structure. Arch. Biochem. Biophys. **178:** 356–367.

17. REUTERBY, J., D. A. WALZ, L. E. MCCOY & W. H. SEEGERS. 1974. Amino acid sequence of O fragment of bovine prothrombin. Thromb. Res. **4:** 885–890.

18. HEWETT-EMMETT, D., L. E. MCCOY, H. I. HASSOUNA, J. REUTERBY, D. A. WALZ & W. H. SEEGERS. 1974. A partial gene duplication in the evolution of prothrombin? Thromb. Res. **5:** 421–430.

19. HEWETT-EMMETT, D., D. A. WALZ, J. REUTERBY, L. E. MCCOY & W. H. SEEGERS. 1975. The amino acid sequence of PR fragment (NH$_2$-terminal fragment) of bovine prothrombin. Thromb. Res. **7:** 227–234.

20. MAGNUSSON, S., T. E. PETERSEN, L. SOTTRUP-JENSEN & H. CLAEYS. 1975. Complete primary structure of prothrombin. *In* Proteases and Biological Control. E. Reich, D. B. Rifkin & E. Shaw, Eds.: 123–149. Cold Spring Harbor Laboratory. Cold Spring Harbor, N. Y.

21. WALZ, D. A. 1978. Comparative aspects of prothrombin activation. Bibliotheca Haemat. **44:** 8–14.

22. TITANI, K., K. FUJIKAWA, D. L. ENFIELD, L. H. ERICSSON, K. A. WALSH & H. NEURATH. 1975. Bovine factor X (Stuart factor): Amino acid sequence of heavy chain. Proc. Natl. Acad. Sci. USA **72:** 3082–3086.

23. ENFIELD, D. L., L. H. ERICSSON, K. FUJIKAWA, K. A. WALSH, H. NEURATH & K. TITANI. 1979. Amino acid sequence of the light chain of bovine factor X, (Stuart factor). Biochemistry **19:** 659–667.

24. KATAYAMA, K., L. H. ERICSSON, D. L. ENFIELD, K. A. WALSH, H. NEURATH, E. W. DAVIE & K. TITANI. 1979. Comparison of amino acid sequence of bovine coagulation factor IX (Christmas factor) with that of other vitamin K-dependent plasma proteins. Proc. Natl. Acad. Sci. USA **76:** 4990–4994.

25. FERNLUND, P. & J. STENFLO. 1980. Amino acid sequence of bovine protein C. *In* Vitamin K Metabolism and Vitamin K-dependent Proteins. J. W. Suttie, Ed.: 84–88. University Park Press. Baltimore, Md.

26. KISIEL, W., K. FUJIKAWA & E. W. DAVIE. 1977. Activation of bovine factor VII (proconvertin) by factor XIIa (activated Hageman factor). Biochemistry **16:** 4189–4194.

27. DISCIPIO, R. G. & E. W. DAVIE. 1979. Characterization of protein S, a γ-carboxyglutamic acid containing protein from bovine and human plasma. Biochemistry **18:** 899–904.

28. KOIDE, T., M. A. HERMODSON & E. W. DAVIE. 1977. Active site of bovine factor XI (plasma thromboplastin antecedent). Nature **266:** 729–730.

29. KURACHI, K. & E. W. DAVIE. 1977. Activation of human factor XI (plasma thromboplastin antecedent) by factor XIIa (activated Hageman factor). Biochemistry **16:** 5831–5839.

30. FUJIKAWA, K., K. KURACHI & E. W. DAVIE. 1977. Characterization of bovine factor XIIa (activated Hageman factor). Biochemistry **16:** 4182–4188.

31. WIMAN, B. 1977. Primary structure of the β-chain of human plasmin. Eur. J. Biochem. **76:** 129–137.

32. SOTTRUP-JENSEN, L., H. CLAEYS, M. ZAJDEL, T. E. PETERSEN & S. MAGNUSSON. 1978. The primary structure of human plasminogen isolation of two lysine-binding fragments and one "mini"-plasminogen (MW, 38,000) by elastase-catalysed-specific limited proteolysis. *In* Progress in Chemical Fibrinolysis and Thrombolysis. J. F. Davidson, R. M. Rowan, M. M. Samama & P. C. Desnogens, Eds. Vol. 3: 191–209. Raven Press. New York.

33. KUROSKY, A., D. R. BARNETT, M. A. RASCO, T.-H. LEE & B. H. BOWMAN. 1974. Evidence of homology between the β-chain of human haptoglobin and the chymotrypsin family of serine proteases. Biochem. Genet. **11:** 279–293.

34. KUROSKY, A., H.-H. KIM & B. TOUCHSTONE. 1976. Comparative sequence analysis of the N-terminal region of rat, rabbit and dog haptoglobin β-chains. Comp. Biochem. Physiol. **55:** 453–459.

35. TSCHESCHE, H., G. MAIR, G. GODEC, F. FIEDLER, W. EHRET, C. HIRSCHAUER, M. LEMON & H. FRITZ. 1979. The primary structure of porcine glandular kallikrein. Adv. Exp. Med. & Biol. **120:** 245–260.

36. DAYHOFF, M. O. 1972. Proteases related to trypsin. *In* Atlas of Protein Sequence and Structure. M. O. Dayhoff, Ed. Vol. **5:** D99–D111. National Biomedical Research Foundation. Washington, D.C.

37. KRAMER, K. J., R. L. FELSTED & J. H. LAW. 1973. Cocoonase. V. Structural studies on an insect serine protease. J. Biol. Chem. **248:** 3021–3028.

38. KISIEL, W. 1979. Molecular properties of the factor V-activating enzyme from Russell's viper venom. J. Biol. Chem. **254:** 12230–12234.

39. BAUMGARTNER, R., T. FLETCHER, I. THEODOR, S. S. BAJWA, F. S. MARKLAND & H. PIRKLE. 1980. Amino acid sequences in crotolase, a thrombin-like enzyme from the venom of *Crotalus adamanteus.* Fed. Proc. **39:** 1027 (Abst #4001).

40. SIM, R. B., R. R. PORTER, K. B. M. REID & I. GIGLI. 1977. The structure and enzymatic activities of the C1r and C1s subcomponents of C1, the first component of human serum complement. Biochem. J. **163:** 219–227.

41. VOLANAKIS, J. E., A. S. BHOWN, J. C. BENNETT & J. E. MOLE. 1980. Partial

amino acid sequence of human factor D: Homology with serine proteases. Proc. Natl. Acad. Sci. USA **77:** 1116–1119.

42. WOODBURY, R. G., N. KATUNUMA, K. KOBAYASHI, K. TITANI & H. NEURATH. 1978. Covalent structure of a group-specific protease from rat small intestine. Biochemistry **17:** 811–819.

43. OLAFSON, R. W., L. JURÁSEK, M. R. CARPENTER & L. B. SMILLIE. 1975. Amino acid sequence of *Streptomyces griseus* trypsin. Biochemistry **14:** 1168–1177.

44. COOK, C. N. & D. HEWETT-EMMETT. 1974. The uses of protein sequence data in systematics. *In* Prosimian Biology. R. D. Martin, G. A. Doyle & A. C. Walker, Eds.: 937–958. Duckworth. London.

45. HARTLEY, B. S. 1970. Homologies in serine proteinases. Phil. Trans. Royal Soc. London B **257:** 77–87.

46. HARTLEY, B. S. 1979. Evolution of enzyme structure. Proc. Royal Soc. London B **205:** 443–452.

47. JOHNSON, P. & L. B. SMILLIE. 1974. The amino acid sequence and predicted structure of *Streptomyces griseus* protease B. FEBS Lett. **47:** 1–6.

48. FITCH, W. M. 1977. Phylogenies constrained by the crossover process as illustrated by human hemoglobins and a thirteen-cycle, eleven-amino-acid repeat in human apolipoprotein A-1. Genetics **86:** 632–644.

49. HEWETT-EMMETT, D., D. A. WALZ & W. H. SEEGERS. 1977. Evolutionary and functional observations on the primary structure of the non-thrombin region (residues 1–273) of human prothrombin. Biochem. Soc. Trans. (UK) **5:** 1452–1455.

50. HEWETT-EMMETT, D. 1978. Amino acid sequence homology and the vitamin K-dependent proteins. Bibliotheca Haemat. **44:** 94–104.

51. DOOLITTLE, R. F. 1979. 3rd Edit. Protein evolution. *In* The Proteins. H. Neurath & R. L. Hill, Eds.: 1–118. Academic Press, Inc. New York.

52. BRADSHAW, R. A., G. A. GRANT, K. A. THOMAS & A. Z. EISEN. 1980. Mouse NGF γ subunit and crab collagenase: Two serine proteases of unusual function. *In* Protides of the Biological Fluids. Colloquium No. 28. H. Peeters, Ed.: 119–122. Pergamon Press. Oxford.

53. BRUNISHOLZ, R., P. MOSER, J. SCHALLER & E. RICKLI. 1980. Partial sequence comparison between human, bovine and porcine plasminogen. *In* Protides of the Biological Fluids. Colloquium No. 28. H. Peeters, Ed.: 103–106. Pergamon Press. Oxford.

54. MOLE, J. E. & M. NIEMANN. 1980. Structural evidence that complement factor B constitutes a novel class of serine protease. J. Biol. Chem. **255:** 8472–8476.

55. WOODBURY, R. G. & H. NEURATH. 1980. Structure, specificity and localization of the serine proteases of connective tissue. FEBS Lett. **114:** 189–196.

56. PETERSEN, T. E., H. C. THØGERSEN, L. SOTTRUP-JENSEN, S. MAGNUSSON & H. JORNVALL. 1980. Isolation and *N*-terminal sequence of protein Z, a.γ-carboxyglutamic acid containing protein from bovine plasma. FEBS Lett. **114:** 278–282.

57. PROWSE, C. W. & M. P. ESNOUF. 1977. The isolation of a new warfarin-sensitive protein from bovine plasma. Biochem. Soc. Trans. (UK) **5:** 255–256.

IMMUNOLOGY OF FIBRINOGEN: COMPARISON OF SEROLOGIC AND CELLULAR IMMUNE RESPONSES TO HUMAN FIBRINOPEPTIDE B (hFPB) *

George D. Wilner, Kun-hwa Hsieh, and David W. Thomas

*Department of Pathology
The Jewish Hospital and
Washington University School of Medicine
St. Louis, Missouri 63110*

INTRODUCTION

The course of fibrin clot formation and dissolution *in vivo* is believed to be associated with the activities of at least three enzymes for which fibrinogen or fibrin represents the primary substrate: thrombin, whose action catalyzes the conversion of fibrinogen to fibrin; factor XIII, which introduces cross-links into the fibrin clot; and plasmin, which digests both fibrinogen and fibrin.[1–4] The activities of each of these three enzymes associated with detectable changes in either the chemical or physical properties of fibrinogen, rendering it distinguishable from the native protein. Furthermore, the action of thrombin or plasmin on fibrinogen results in the release of soluble, specific proteolytic fragments whose measurement, in theory, may be used as indices of *in vivo* enzymatic activity.[5]

With the recent report by Doolittle and associates on the complete primary structure of the human fibrinogen Aα chain,[6, 7] studies on the sequence of human fibrinogen have at last been completed. Since the structure of any fibrinogen proteolytic fragment can now be expressed with precision, a critical problem in the development of clinical tests to detect proteolytically modified fibrinogen and fibrin is the specificity of the methods used. Technological advances in the areas of peptide synthesis, affinity chromatography, as well as immunochemistry and cellular immunology have made possible the development of extremely specific serologic and cellular immune probes capable of recognizing limited characteristic sequences in proteolyzed fibrinogen.

A theoretical and experimental basis for the use of immunological probes in recognizing proteolytically modified fibrin and fibrinogen is a result of the elegant studies of Plow, Edgington, and co-workers.[8, 9] In studies on the neoantigenic expression of fragment E derived from fibrinogenolysis by plasmin, these workers have demonstrated that the major epitopic site recognized by heterogeneous rabbit antisera specific for fragment E is localized to a limited sequence within the γ-chain (γ 36–53). These findings demonstrate that neoantigenic determinants characteristic of proteolytically altered fibrinogen or fibrin may be contained within relatively small limited sequences within the larger proteolytic fragment. Furthermore, studies on the immunochemistry

* This work was supported by Grants HL-22642 and IA-14226 from the National Institutes of Health. Dr. Thomas is recipient of Research Career Development Award AI-00352 from the National Institute of Allergy and Infectious Diseases, National Institutes of Health.

528

of human fibrinopeptides A and B clearly show that populations of antibodies that are specific for the fibrinopeptides can recognize the parent protein molecule to varying extents, which in turn is dependent upon the epitopic responses of these particular sera.[10-12] On the basis of these experimental findings, a hypothesis has been advanced that immune probes that are highly specific for neoantigenic determinants characteristic of proteolyzed fibrinogen and fibrin may be prepared by using small peptides containing the characteristic neoantigenic determinants as immunogens. The use of such small antigens as immunogens offers the potential advantage of restricting the immune response, thereby increasing the specificity of these immune probes by limiting its response to relevant epitopes. However, an unfortunate consequence of limiting antigen size is generally a concomitant loss in antigenicity as indicated by antibody production. Small peptides (~10 residues) are poor antigens for eliciting antibodies, and even peptides conjugated to carrier proteins often require prolonged hyperimmunization to raise detectable antibodies. We have recently shown that it is possible to obtain a primary T-cell immune response in guinea pigs within 2 weeks following immunization of unconjugated peptide antigens as small as octapeptides.[13, 14] While this immune response in guinea pigs to the peptides studied thus far appears to be exclusively a T-cell response, (i.e., no detectable antibodies are produced), it has been possible to directly compare the specificity of this cellular response to peptide antigens with that of antibodies directed toward the same antigen elicited in other animals. The intent of this paper is to review our recent work contrasting the serologic with the cellular immune response to human fibrinopeptide B (hFPB) as part of an overall series of studies aimed at developing immune probes specific for limited homologous sequences within the fibrinogen molecule.

Serologic Immune Response to Human Fibrinopeptide B

The primary structure of hFPB is shown in TABLE 1.[15] This peptide as well as its COOH-terminal sequential homologues and related analogues were prepared synthetically using Merrifield's solid-phase methodology.[12]

The antibodies studied, generously provided by Dr. H. L. Nossel, were prepared by hyperimmunization of outbred rabbits with peptide-albumin conjugates as previously described.[16] A total of 7 different antisera were examined using a competitive binding radioimmunoassay system to assess antibody function. Specificity of these sera were compared in terms of the molar amounts of hFPB or its related homologues required for displacement of 50% of bound ^{125}I-Tyr-hFPB analogue, which served as tracer. TABLE 2 summarizes the characteristics of these different hFPB-specific antisera. Our studies indicated that major immunoreactive sites in hFPB appear to be localized to the COOH-terminal 8–10 residues of this molecule. (TABLE 2, FIGURE 1). Furthermore, isoelectric focusing experiments carried out using the technique of Briles and Davie [17] showed that the antigen binding by each serum was limited to 8–10 discrete antibody bands, indicating that a restricted clonal antibody response was associated with limited structural heterogeneity of the peptide antigen.

Cellular Immune Response to Human Fibrinopeptide B

The cellular immune responsiveness to hFPB and its sequential homologues was studied using a T-cell proliferative immunoassay as diagrammed in FIG-

TABLE 1

HUMAN FIBRINOPEPTIDE B (hFPB, Bβ 1–14) AND RELATED SEQUENCES

| Residue * |
| 1 2 3 4 5 6 7 8 9 10 11 12 13 14 |

PCA-Gly-Val-Asn-Asp-Asn-Glu-Glu-Gly-Phe-Phe-Ser-Ala-Arg-OH (I)
H-Asp-Asn-Glu-Glu-Gly-Phe-Phe-Ser-Ala-Arg-OH (II)
H-Glu-Glu-Gly-Phe-Phe-Ser-Ala-Arg-OH (III)
H-Gly-Phe-Phe-Ser-Ala-Arg-OH (IV)
H-Asp-Asn-Glu-Glu-Gly-Phe-Tyr-Ser-Ala-Arg-OH (V)
H-Asp-Asn-Glu-Glu-Gly-Tyr-Phe-Ser-Ala-Arg-OH (VI)

* Primary structure of hFPB (I) is shown, as elucidated by Blombäck *et al.*[15] Peptides II–IV are COOH-terminal sequential hFPB homologues, while peptides V and VI are analogues of the Bβ 5–14 sequence containing Phe→Tyr substitutions. Peptides were synthesized by a modification of Merrifield's solid-phase procedure as described.[12]

URE 2.[13] In this system, strain 2 guinea pigs were immunized with unconjugated hFPB or a homologue: 2–4 weeks following immunization, peritoneal exudate cells (PEL) were harvested, and enriched for T-cells by passage through rayon weel columns. T-cells were then cultured with the peptide antigens, and stimulation assessed by the incorporation of tritiated thymidine (^{3}H-TdR) into newly synthesized DNA. FIGURE 3 shows the proliferative response of hFPB-immune strain 2 guinea pig T-lymphocytes when challenged in culture with either hFPB or one of its sequential homologues. These data indicate that progressively greater incorporation of tritiated thymidine occurred as a function of increasing antigen size. We interpret these data as suggesting that differing clones or subpopulations of T-lymphocytes were responding to relatively limited sets of determinants within the total hFPB sequence, and as the size of the challenging peptides was increased, progressively more and more of these responsive T-cell populations were recruited. To test this hy-

TABLE 2

CHARACTERISTICS OF RABBIT ANTI-hFPB ANTISERA

Antiserum	Assay Dilution *	hFPB, (I) 50% (pmol) †	Bβ 5–14, (II) 50% (pmol) †	Bβ 7–14, (III) 50% (pmol) †
R22	1:2000	0.45	1.4	>10⁴
R24	1:3000	0.41	1.1	560
R30	1:2500	0.50	1.3	1900
R28	1:5000	0.38	0.42	1.7
R31	1:4000	0.38	0.91	3.3
R29	1:1500	0.46	1.4	40
R23	1:1000	0.52	3.5	48

* Value represents initial antiserum dilution added to assay mixture.

† Each value represents the quantity (picamoles) of unlabeled peptide required for displacement of 50% of bound radiolabeled tracer at the given assay dilution. Roman numerals refer to structures shown in TABLE 1.

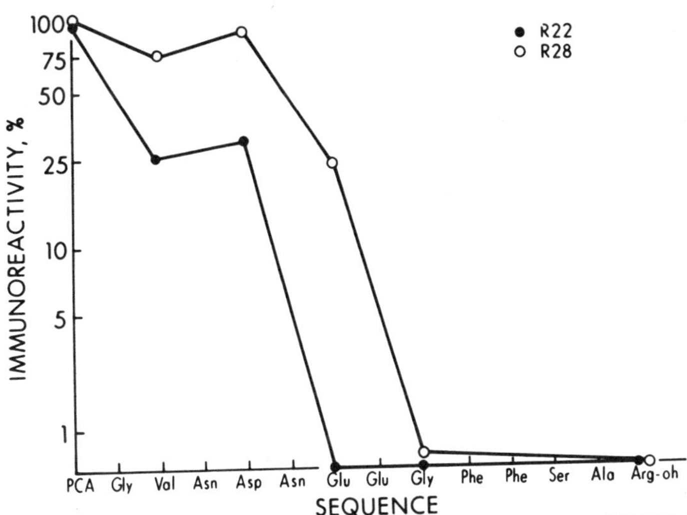

FIGURE 1. The ability of sequential COOH-terminal homologues of hFPB (human fibrinopeptide B) to displace 50% of ^{125}I-Tyr-hFPB bound to rabbit anti-hFPB antisera R22 (●) and R28 (○). Percentage immunoreactivity is calculated from normalized molar ratios, assuming 100% reactivity for intact hFPB.

pothesis, we employed the technique of clonal elimination of T-cell responsiveness to different antigenic determinants present in hFPB using bromodeoxyuridine (BUdR) and light elimination of stimulated lymphocytes, as schematically shown in FIGURE 4.[18] A population of T-cells in culture which are immune to two different antigens (A and B) are challenged with antigen A and the immune cells responsive to antigen A begin to proliferate, incorporate BUdR, and in the presence of light, will be eliminated due to cross-linking of the BUdR-DNA. The remaining T-cells that are immune to antigen B are retained by this procedure and can be tested for their responsiveness to antigen B. In the case

FIGURE 2. Schematic diagram of cellular proliferative immunoassay used to assess T-cell immune responsiveness to hFPB and related peptides.[18]

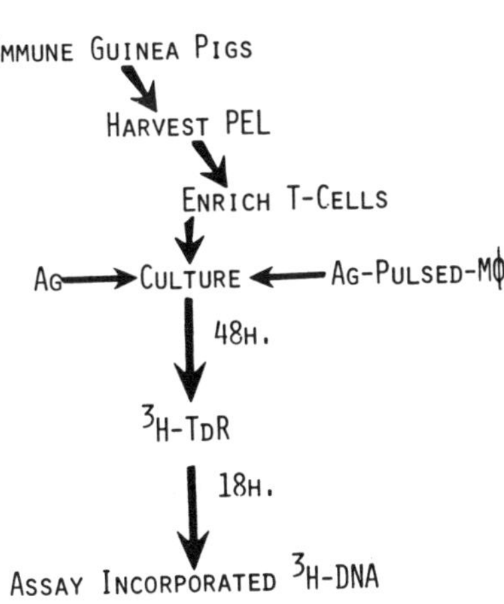

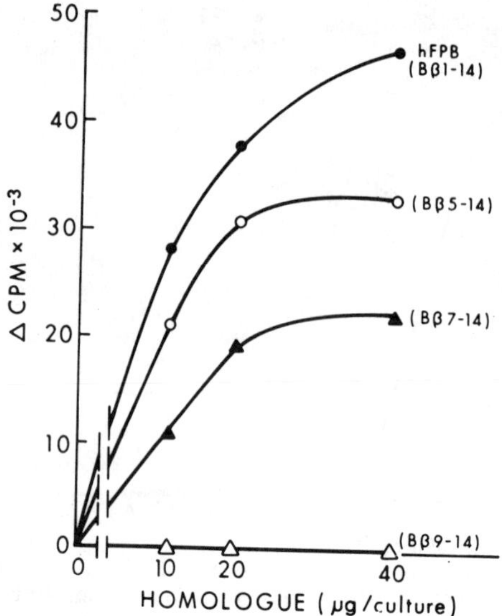

FIGURE 3. Proliferative response of hFPB-immune strain 2 guinea pig T-cells to varying amounts of hFPB (I), Bβ 5–14 (II), Bβ 7–14 (III), and Bβ 9–14 (IV). Roman numerals refer to structures shown in TABLE 1. Ordinate represents antigen-specific counts per minute incorporated.

of our studies, hFPB-immune T-lymphocytes were challenged in culture with sequential homologues of hFPB, and following BUdR and light treatment, restimulated in a second culture with hFPB or the homologues and the proliferative response assessed after further culture (FIGURE 5). Our data with the strain 2 immune T-cell response to hFPB indicates that 50–60% of the immune response may be localized to the COOH-terminal octapeptide sequence Bβ 7–14; an additional 20–30% of the activity is expressed in the COOH-terminal decapeptide Bβ 5–14, with the remaining 20% contained in epitopes localized to the NH_2-terminal sequences of the fibrinopeptide.

COMPARATIVE SPECIFICITIES OF THE SEROLOGICAL VERSUS CELLULAR IMMUNE RESPONSES

Initial studies were begun comparing the relative specificities of antibodies versus T-cell immune probes in terms of their abilities to distinguish subtle differences in these small sequential antigens. For these experiments, analogues of the COOH-terminal decapeptide sequence of hFPB were prepared containing single residue (Phe → Tyr) substitutions in positions 10 and 11. (TABLE 1, Peptides V and VI) Substitutions involving these aromatic residues, while judged a relatively conservative modification of this particular sequence, were

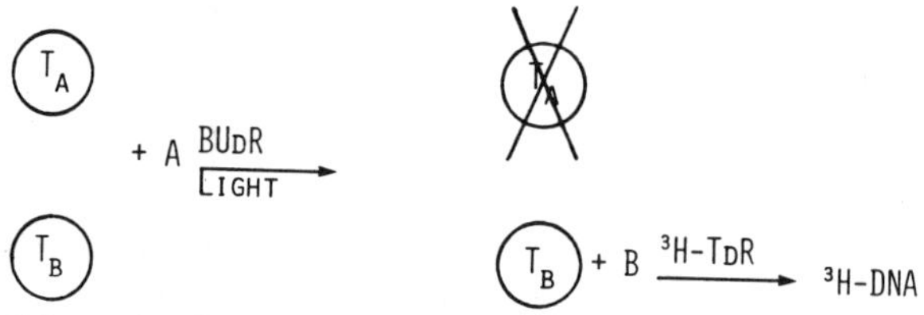

FIGURE 4. Schematic diagram of immune T-cell clonal elimination technique employing bromodeoxyuridine (BUdR) and light.[18]

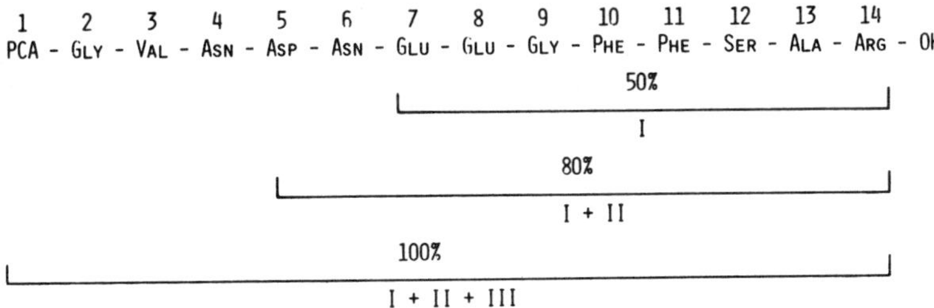

FIGURE 5. Clonal response of hFPB-immune T-cells to different regions in hFPB, as determined by the BUdR and light elimination technique described earlier.

thought sufficient to alter the physical properties of this peptide in solution and therefore represent a reasonable yardstick for comparing these two classes of immune probes. FIGURE 6 compares the reactivity of one particular anti-hFPB antiserum (R22) with the intact decapeptide (Bβ 5–14) versus the two phenylalanine-substituted analogues in a competitive binding radioimmuno-assay system using ^{125}I-hFPB analogue as tracer. While there was little or no cross-reactivity between Bβ 5–14 and the Tyr^{10} analogue, the antiserum was incapable of distinguishing the Tyr^{11} analogue from the intact Bβ 5–14 sequence.

By contrast, cellular immune probes appeared capable of distinguishing both tyrosyl analogues from the intact Bβ 5–14 sequence. As shown in TABLE 3, the Phe → Tyr substitutions result in the formation of unique antigenic species that do not cross react with the unmodified Bβ 5–14 sequence. Of further interest is the fact that substitution of Tyr for Phe in position 11 is not only unreactive with T-cells that respond to the unmodified sequence, but is also nonimmunogenic as well (TABLE 3). These data suggest that T-cell immune probes that are responsive to a particular sequence in fibrinogen are capable of specificities that are at least equal to that obtainable using antisera. However, a precise definition of the relative specificities of cellular versus serologic probes awaits comparison of both immune responses in the same animal species.

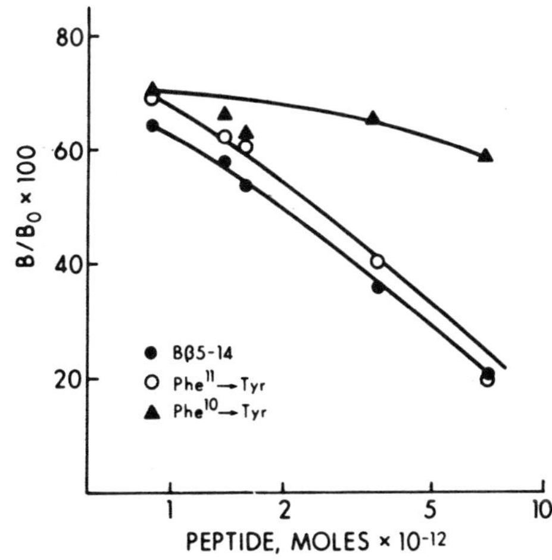

FIGURE 6. The comparative abilities of Bβ 5–14 (II) (●) Bβ 5–14 (Phe^{11}→Tyr) (V) (○), and Bβ 5–14 (Phe^{10}→Tyr) (VI) (▲) to inhibit binding of ^{125}I-Tyr-hFPB tracer to rabbit anti-hFPB antiserum R22. Roman numerals refer to structures shown in TABLE 1. Assays were performed using a competitive binding radioimmunoassay procedure as previously described.[12]

SUMMARY AND CONCLUSIONS

As was mentioned earlier, a body of evidence has emerged supporting measurement of proteolytically altered fibrin and fibrinogen as *in vivo* indices of the activities of specific enzymes. The critical problem limiting advancement of work in this area has been the specificity of the immune probes employed by various investigators. It has become increasingly evident that dramatic chemical alterations in the fibrinogen-to-fibrin transformation are unassociated with significant immunochemical alterations using conventional immunological approaches. The failure of immune probes in many cases to discriminate between intact and altered species of the fibrin(ogen) molecule suggests that the majority of epitopes recognized by these probes involve determinants that are unaltered by the specific enzymatic events that one wishes to characterize. One approach for developing highly specific immune probes involves restricting the antigen size to a limited pertinent sequence in the fibrin(ogen) molecule in the vicinity of a particular enzymatic event.

TABLE 3

CELLULAR IMMUNE RESPONSE TO AROMATIC ANALOGUES OF THE COOH-TERMINAL
DECAPEPTIDE SEQUENCE OF hFPB

Immunized [†]	Antigen in Culture *		
	Bβ 5–14	Bβ 5–14 Phe^{10}→Tyr	Bβ 5–14 Phe^{11}→Tyr
Bβ 1–14 (I)	+++	−	−
Bβ 5–14 (Phe^{10}→Tyr) (VI)	−	+++	−
Bβ 5–14 (Phe^{11}→Tyr) (V)	−	−	−

* Peritoneal exudate T-cells from strain 2 guinea pigs immunized with 400 μg of either hPPB (I) or one of the Bβ 5–14 tyrosyl analogues (V, VI) in complete Freund's adjuvant, were cultured with 40 μg per culture as indicated, and ^{3}H-TdR counts per minute were determined on the third day of culture. The stimulation index (SI) was determined by dividing the mean cpm from cultures with antigen by the mean cpm from cultures without antigen: +++, SI > 5; −, SI ≤ 1.

[†] Roman numerals refer to structures shown in TABLE 1.

All preliminary data suggests that immune T-cells may possess significant advantages over immunoglobulins in terms of recognizing subtle neoantigen expression in such restricted sequences. One potential advantage lies in the fact that an immune T-cell response may be induced following primary immunization with an unconjugated peptide representing the particular homologous sequence that one wishes to measure, whereas antibody production requires extensive hyperimmunization with peptide–protein conjugates. Since most conjugating procedures involve some chemical modification of active group side chains in residues present in the peptide, these modified groups may no longer be recognizable by the probe when challenged with the intact, unmodified sequence. Furthermore, conjugation may confer a ridgity or alteration in the peptide shape which is different from the free peptide in solution or from the peptide attached to its parent molecule. For these reasons, T-cells may prove to be a valuable alternative to antibodies in recognizing neoantigenic expression in limited sequences in fibrin(ogen) structure.

References

1. MURANO, G. 1974. The molecular structure of fibrinogen. Sem. Thromb. Hemostas. **1:** 1–31.
2. DOOLITTLE, R. F. 1975. Fibrinogen and fibrin. *In* The Plasma Proteins. F. W. Putnam, Ed. Vol. **2:** 109–161. Academic Press, New York, N.Y.
3. MOSESSON, M. W. & J. S. FINLAYSON. 1976. The search for the structure of fibrinogen. *In* Progress in Hemostasis and Thrombosis. T. H. Spaet, Ed. Vol. **3:** 61–107. Grune and Stratton, New York, N.Y.
4. BLOMBÄCK, B., D. H. HOGG, B. GÅRDLUND, B. HESSEL & B. KUDRYK. 1976. Fibrinogen and fibrin formation. Thromb. Res. **8** (Suppl. 2): 329–346.
5. WILNER, G. D. 1978. Molecular basis for measurement of circulating fibrinogen derivatives. *In* Progress in Hemostasis and Thrombosis. T. H. Spaet, Ed. Vol. **4:** 211–248. Grune and Stratton, New York, N.Y.
6. DOOLITTLE, R. F., K. W. K. WATT, B. A. COTTRELL, D. D. STRONG & M. RILEY. 1979. The amino acid sequence of the α-chain of human fibrinogen. Nature **280:** 464–468.
7. WATT, K. W. K., B. A. COTTRELL, D. D. STRONG & R. F. DOOLITTLE. 1979. Amino acid sequence studies of the α-chain of human fibrinogen. Overlapping sequences providing the complete sequence. Biochemistry **24:** 5410–5416.
8. PLOW, E. F. & T. S. EDGINGTON. 1975. A cleavage-associated neoantigenic marker for a γ chain site in the NH$_2$-terminal aspect of the fibrinogen molecule. J. Biol. Chem. **250:** 3386–3392.
9. PLOW, E. F. & T. S. EDGINGTON. 1977. Localization and characterization of the cleavage-associated neoantigen in the E domain of fibrinogen. Thromb. Hemostas. **38:** 27.
10. CANFIELD, R. E., J. DEAN, H. L. NOSSEL, V. P. BUTLER, JR. & G. D. WILNER. 1976. Reactivity of fibrinogen and fibrinopeptide A containing fibrinogen fragments with antisera to fibrinopeptide A. Biochemistry **15:** 1203–1209.
11. WILNER, G. D., H. L. NOSSEL, R. E. CANFIELD & V. P. BUTLER, JR. 1976. Immunochemical studies of human fibrinopeptide A using synthetic peptide homologues. Biochemistry **15:** 1209–1213.
12. WILNER, G. D., D. W. THOMAS, H. L. NOSSEL, P. F. ROBBINS & M. S. MUDD. 1979. Immunochemical analysis of rabbit anti-human fibrinopeptide B antibodies. Biochemistry **18:** 5078–5082.
13. THOMAS, D. W., S. K. MELTZ & G. D. WILNER. 1979. Nature of T lymphocyte recognition of macrophage-associated antigens. I. Response of guinea pig T cells to human fibrinopeptide B. J. Immunol. **123:** 759–764.
14. THOMAS, D. W. & G. D. WILNER. 1980. Macrophage regulation of guinea pig T lymphocyte responses to human fibrinopeptide B. *In* Macrophage regulation of Immunity. E. R. Unanue & A. S. Rosenthal, Eds. pp. 47–58. Academic Press, New York, N.Y.
15. BLOMBÄCK, B., M. BLOMBÄCK, P. EDMAN & B. HESSEL. 1966. Human fibrinopeptides, isolation, characterization and structure. Biochim. Biophys. Acta **115:** 371–396.
16. BILEZEKIAN, S. B., H. L. NOSSEL, V. P. BUTLER, JR. & R. E. CANFIELD. 1975. Radioimmunoassay of human fibrinopeptide B and kinetics of fibrinopeptide cleavage by different enzymes. J. Clin. Invest. **56:** 438–445.
17. BRILES, D. E. & J. M. DAVIE. 1975. Detection of isoelectric focused antibody by autoradiography and hemolysis of antigen-coated erythrocytes. A comparison of methods. J. Immunol. Meth. **8:** 363–372.
18. THOMAS, D. W. & E. M. SHEVACH. 1978. Nature of the antigenic complex recognized by T lymphocytes. V. Genetic predisposition of independent F$_1$ T cell subpopulations responsive to antigen-pulsed parental macrophages. J. Immunol. **120:** 638–640.

MECHANISM OF FIBRIN FORMATION
AND ITS REGULATION *

B. Blombäck, B. Hessel, M. Okada, and N. Egberg

*Department of Blood Coagulation Research
Karolinska Institute
Stockholm, Sweden*

*New York Blood Center
New York, New York 10021*

In the following we will present some data and thoughts concerning the structure of fibrinogen, its activation by thrombin, and the subsequent polymerization reaction. We will also consider ways by which the fibrin formation may be physiologically regulated.

The primary structure of fibrinogen has by now been almost completely elucidated.[1-10] Fibrinogen is built up by two identical halves, combined in the N-terminal end by symmetrical disulfide bridges with 2-fold symmetry.[3, 11] The half-molecules each consist of three polypeptide chains (Aα, Bβ, γ), which are held together by disulphide bonds. The interchain disulfides occur in two clusters in the molecule; one in the N-terminal part (N-DSK region)[3, 10] and a similar cluster in a more C-terminal part (fragment D region). Intrachain disulfide loops occur in C-terminal portions of all three chains.[1-3]

The shape of fibrinogen has been much discussed but no agreement has been reached. We believe that the electron-microscopic picture deduced by Bachmann *et al.*[12] may represent the shape of the hydrated molecule as it circulates in blood. These authors deduced the most likely molecular form as a rod-like particle with a length of 45 nm and a width of 9 nm. Stryer *et al.*[13] found in X-ray diffraction studies of hydrated fibrinogen and fibrin that the axial repeat in both specimens was 22.6 nm. This may represent the length of the half-molecule. This would mean that, since the half-molecules are joined at the N-terminal ends by symmetrical disulfides, these half-molecules must protrude from the point of linkage in opposite directions in space. The symmetry demands[4] that the two half-molecules of fibrinogen do not lie on the same plane and that they are joined in such a manner that, on observing the molecule from any one projection, we see one side of one half-molecule and an opposite side of the other. The overall shape of the molecule may then look something like the model we have depicted in FIGURE 1. In this model the N-terminal symmetrical disulfides are in the center.

Our previous studies have suggested that, in regard to polymerization, the functional domains are located in two different domains of the molecule.[2, 14, 15] One domain, N-DSK, is in the N-terminal part. This contains a polymerization site (A), which is activated by release of fibrinopeptide A (FPA). After activation with thrombin this domain acquires affinity for a C-terminal domain (a) located in the fragment D region of the molecule. The location of these

* This research work was supported by grants from the Swedish Medical Research Council (B81–13X–02475–14A), the U.S. National Institutes of Health (HL 07379–15 and HL 09011), and The Bank of Sweden Tercentenary Foundation.

sites is indicated in FIGURE 1. Interaction between these sites (A and a) of neighboring molecules leads to formation of a linear polymer. How such a polymer may be formed is shown in FIGURE 2A–B.

We have recently obtained evidence for the occurrence of a second set of polymerization sites (B and b) in fibrinogen.[16] After activation of the B site by release of fibrinopeptide B (FPB), this site can interact with a complementary site, b. The location of this set of sites has not yet been determined with certainty. However, the fact that FPB is part of N-DSK and also the results of binding experiments [15] suggest that at least the B site is also located in N-DSK. The location of these sites has also been tentatively indicated in FIGURE 1. Since the release of FPB by thrombin is initially much slower than that of FPA, it is likely that the second set of polymerization sites (B and b) becomes operative only after the linear polymer (fibrin I) has formed. We therefore assume that the interactions between the B and b sites occur predominantly on fibrin I as it grows. The interaction between the B and b sites may also result in formation of a linear polymer. However, depending on the

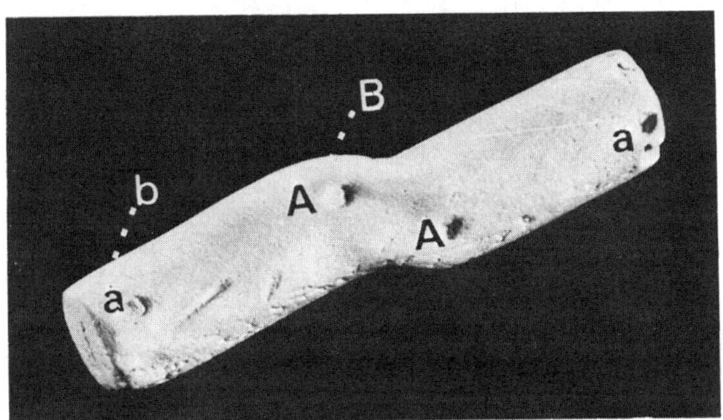

FIGURE 1. Plaster model of fibrinogen. Model made of plaster. Axial ratio about 1:5. The two half-molecules, combined in the center have one 2-fold axis of symmetry (perpendicular to the plane of the surface). Polymerization sites are denoted A, a, B, b.

geometry of association, it provides for branching of the fiber as is illustrated in FIGURE 2C–D. The branch formed by B:b interactions has on its outside A and a sites and these may serve as nuclei for formation of new fibrin I strands.

Eventually a highly branched compact structure is formed. This is called fibrin II. The formation of fibrin II is initially very slow depending on the slow release of FPB. The release of FPB is greatly accelerated as a result of gel formation.[16] We believe that this accelerated release of FPB is a consequence of interaction between B and b sites, which may lead to conformational changes in the molecule that make still nonactivated B sites more susceptible to thrombin action. Olexa *et al.*[17] have recently also obtained evidence for the occurrence of a second set of polymerization sites in fibrinogen, most likely the B:b set of sites. Interestingly, these authors claim that this set of sites was fully operative only in cross-linked fibrin.

The models of the different fibrins that are shown in FIGURE 2 are of course speculative. The model for fibrin I agrees with that proposed by Ferry.[18]

However, there is strong evidence that different types of fibrin form on release of FPA and FPB, respectively. Thus Laurent and Blombäck[19] showed by viscosity and light-scattering measurements that fibrin formed in the presence of bathroxobin (FPA release) was different from the polymer formed on release of both FPA and FPB by thrombin. We have in recent preliminary experiments by calorimetric measurements[20] shown that the total heat production during polymerization in the presence of bathroxobin is roughly half of that produced in the presence of thrombin (TABLE 1). More research must, however, be done for an accurate interpretation of these calorimetric data. Nonetheless, they do suggest that major differences, apart from cleavage of

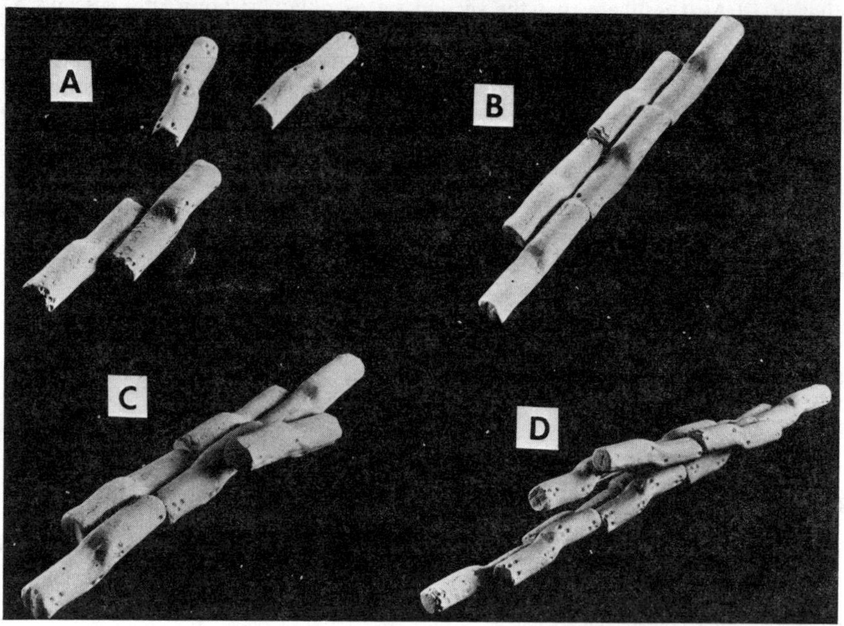

FIGURE 2. Model of formation of a linear fibrin polymer. (A–B) Through interaction between the sites A and a (FIGURE 1) of neighboring molecules a linear polymer is built up. (C–D) Fibrinogen units interact with the linear polymer through interaction between sites B and b (FIGURE 1). A branched structure is eventually formed.

peptide bonds, exist in the fibrinogen–fibrin transitions induced by bathroxobin and thrombin, respectively.

Formation of fibrin II during clotting may have both physiological and pathophysiological consequences. At a site of a lesion in the vessel wall, fibrin II is most likely quickly formed. Extensive formation of fibrin II away from the lesion may be an important factor in thrombosis. In a previous study[16] we presented preliminary experiments showing that in whole blood that was allowed to clot, the formation of fibrin II was relatively slow. This conclusion was based only on N-terminal analysis of clots formed in blood allowed to stand for a long time at 37° C. In recent experiments we have been unable to confirm

TABLE 1

CALORIMETRIC MEASUREMENT DURING FIBRINOGEN–FIBRIN TRANSITION

Exp.	Cell I	Cell II	Heat * (mJ)
1	2 ml tris buffer, pH 7.2 4 ml 0.3% fibrinogen	2 ml thrombin conc. 15 E/ml 4 ml 0.3% fibrinogen	+16.293
2	2 ml tris buffer, pH 7.2 4 ml 0.3% fibrinogen	2 ml reptilase conc. 15 E/ml 4 ml 0.3% fibrinogen	+10.227
3	1.75 ml reptilase, 15 E/ml 3 ml 0.3% fibrinogen	1.75 ml thrombin 15 E/ml 3 ml 0.3% fibrinogen	+ 4.323
4	2 ml tris buffer, pH 7.2 4 ml 0.3% fibrinogen	2 ml thrombin conc. 15 E/ml 4 ml 0.3% fibrinogen	+18.750
5	2 ml tris buffer, pH 7.2 4 ml 0.3% fibrinogen	2 ml reptilase conc. 15 E/ml 4 ml 0.3% fibrinogen	+10.430
6	2 ml thrombin conc. 15 E/ml 4 ml 0.3% fibrinogen	2 ml reptilase conc. 30 E/ml 4 ml 0.2% fibrinogen	− 5.831

* Plus sign signifies exothermic reaction in Cell II. Analysis performed by I. Pettersson at LKB AB, Stockholm.

this conclusion. Rather, we are now convinced that in whole blood and platelet-rich plasma, where prothrombin consumption is fast (meaning fast thrombin formation), fibrin II is formed extremely quickly (FIGURE 3b–c); in fact, by the time a visible clot occurs the fibrin appears to be mainly type II. This conclusion was based on determination of FPA and FPB [21, 22] during clotting and was confirmed by N-terminal analysis of the clots formed. However, in platelet-poor plasma where prothrombin consumption is slow (and consequently

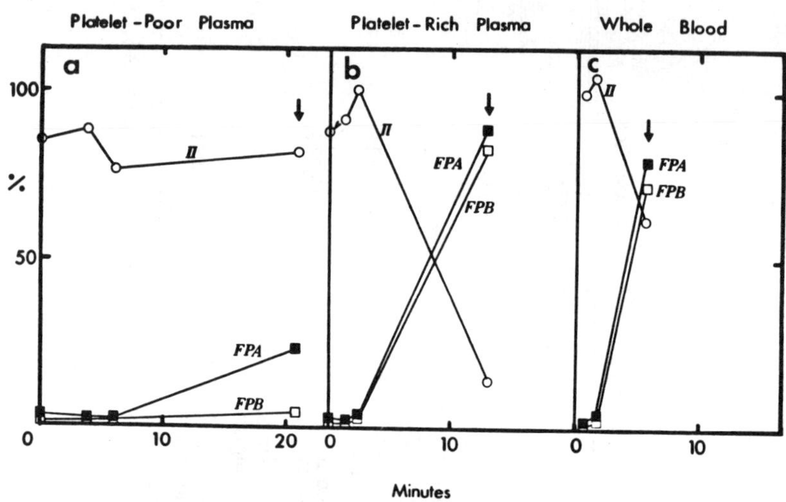

FIGURE 3. Fibrin formation and prothrombin consumption in whole blood and platelet-rich plasma (PRP) and platelet-poor plasma (PPP). *Whole blood:* Aliquots of 30 ml of blood were collected in glass tubes and allowed to clot at 37° C. At different times before clotting (clotting time marked with an arrow in the figure) 0.6 ml of 0.13 M EDTA containing 375 AT units of hirudin was added to an aliquot. The samples were centrifuged at 1000g for 20 min. The plasma was used for assay of FPA and FPB according to Nossel *et al.*[21, 22] and for prothrombin determination using the two-stage procedure of Noren.[26] *PRP:* 50 ml of blood were collected in citrate (1 part 3.8% citrate, 9 parts of blood) containing Trasylol (8000 KIE) and 0.4 g of EACA. PRP was obtained by centrifugation 100 g for 20 minutes. Clotting was initiated by adding CaCl₂ (200 μl, 1 M) to 10 ml Portions of PRP. At different times before clotting, 200 μl 0.13 M EDTA containing 125 AT units of Hirudin was added. These additions blocked prothrombin conversions and thrombin activity in the sample. Analysis of FPA and FPB was as described for whole blood. *PPP:* Blood was collected in citrate as described for PRP. Centrifugation at 2000 g for 30 min. Otherwise the procedure is the same for PRP and whole blood.

also thrombin formation), fibrin I may possibly be the main product at the onset of clotting (FIGURE 3a). These experiments show that the concentration of thrombin (in whole blood 7–20 NIH units per ml at the onset of clotting *in vitro*) is an important factor in determining which type of fibrin is formed.

Are there regulatory mechanisms for fibrin II formation? Theoretically antithrombin and plasmin could influence the amount of fibrin II formed. Also, factors influencing the speed of prothrombin conversion might be of importance. Nossel *et al.*[11] have recently presented an interesting hypothesis on the regulatory role of plasmin in fibrin II formation. These authors found that a fragment of the Bβ chain (Bβ 1–42) is highly susceptible to release by plasmin. However, at least in plasma, fibrin I rather than fibrinogen appears to be the preferred substrate for plasmin. Nossel *et al.* postulates that by release of the Bβ 1–42 fragment, which also contains FPB, subsequent activation of the second set of polymerization sites would be abolished or hampered. Nossel *et al.* base this hypothesis on clinical studies on the occurrence of thrombosis in patients after surgical or other interventions.[23, 24] The possibility was discussed that in those patients developing thrombosis the ratio between free FPA and Bβ 1–42 is high, whereas in those not developing thrombosis the ratio is low. We have in recent *in vitro* studies obtained some evidence that may be in favor of this concept. Fibrinogen was treated with small amounts of trypsin and the polymerization activity of fibrinogen was followed at different incubation times (1–5 minutes). This was done by adding thrombin and determining the increase by optical density at 450 nm (TABLE 2). In parallel samples fibrinogen was at different time periods precipitated by adding ethanol to a concentration of 50%. The Bβ 15–42 fragment was determined in the supernatant using a radioimmunoassay procedure.[25] The precipitated fibrinogen was redissolved in urea and subjected to SDS-gel electrophoresis on 7% gels before and after reduction. We found that during the incubation with trypsin there was a dramatic decrease in polymerization activity, and, parallel with this release of Bβ 15–42 occurred (TABLE 2). No appreciable degradation of the fibrinogen occurred during the digestion, as judged by SDS-gel electrophoresis of unreduced samples, and the Bβ and γ chains appeared to be normal as judged by SDS-gel electrophoresis of reduced samples. Release of Bβ 1–42 would, however, not be expected to significantly influence the mobility of the

TABLE 2

CORRELATION BETWEEN LOSS OF POLYMERIZATION ACTIVITY AND RELEASE OF
Bβ 15–42 Fragment During Tryptic Digestion *

Time	Inactive Fibrinogen (nmole/ml)	Bβ 15–42 (nmole/ml)
0	0	0
1	0.72	0.20
2	1.40	0.37
5	2.70	0.97

* Purified fibrinogen (97–100% coagulability) was digested with trypsin (0–5 min) in 0.15 M tris-NaCl buffer, pH 7.2, containing calcium ions (20 mM) at an enzyme: protein ratio (wt/wt) of 1:1000. The reaction was stopped by adding soybean trypsin inhibitor (SBTI). The ratio SBTI: trypsin was 4:1. In the 0-time sample, SBTI was added before trypsin. In the control SBTI and trypsin were replaced by saline. The control sample gave almost the same result as the 0-time samples. After incubation thrombin was added to the samples to a final concentration of 1 NIH-unit/ml. Polymerization was judged by the increase in light absorbance at 450 nm after addition of thrombin. The reaction was followed until the absorbance readings approached plateau values. Deduction of inactive fibrinogen is based on the difference in absorbance between control sample and that of a trypsin-treated sample.

Bβ chain. The Aα chain band appeared to decrease slightly in the course of the digestion. The failure to detect degradation products in the unreduced gels suggests that the degradation of the Aα-chain has not occurred at the C-terminal end by release of PL-1.[4] This experiment thus suggests that subtle changes in fibrinogen including changes in the N-terminal part of the Bβ chain may be responsible for the decrease in polymerization activity.

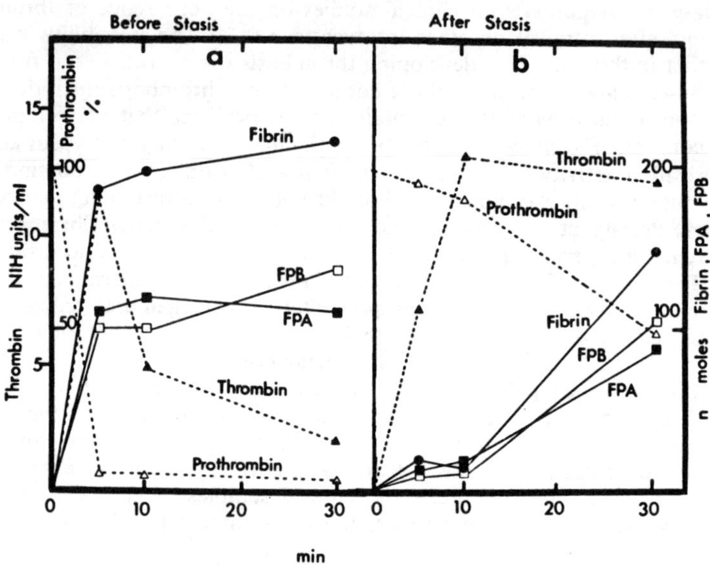

FIGURE 4. Influence of venous stasis on fibrin formation, prothrombin consumption and thrombin formation. Aliquots of 10 ml blood was collected from an antecubital vein before and after venous stasis (using a blood-pressure cuff at a pressure of approximately 100 mm Hg). The blood samples were incubated at 37° C. At different incubation times samples for assay of factors IIa were quickly withdrawn, centrifuged for 15 sec in Beckman Microfuge and 10 μl samples of plasma immediately assayed according to procedures described.[27, 28] To the rest of the aliquot was added 0.2 ml of 0.13 M EDTA (no change in pH occurred) and 0.5 ml of Trasylol (10 000 KIE/ml and 100 μl of hirudin (150 ATU). Fibrin that had formed during incubation was removed by filtering through gauze and washed as described.[16] The rest of the blood was centrifuged and the plasma used for assay of the following components: fibrinopeptide (FPA and FPB) and prothrombin.[21, 22, 26] Hemoconcentration was assessed by analysis of hematocrit, total protein and albumin. For assessment of the fibrinolytic potential in the blood the euglobulinlysis test [27] was performed on a separate aliquot of blood collected in citrate before and immediately after stasis.

Some preliminary studies we have performed suggest that other factors may also participate in the regulation of fibrin formation. We studied fibrin formation in samples of whole blood from 10 individuals taken before and after venous stasis (10 min with a blood pressure cuff at 100 mm Hg). The blood samples, collected in glass tubes, were allowed to clot for various times. Appearance of activators of plasminogen in the blood was assessed by performing the euglobulin lysis test on citrated plasma samples taken before and after stasis. Interesting changes were noted in the individuals (6 out of 10) who showed a positive euglobulin lysis test. These changes are demonstrated in FIGURE 4a–b. After venous stasis in those individuals there is a delay in fibrin formation, which correlates well with a delay in release of FPA and FPB. The amount of fibrin eventually formed in static blood is only slightly less than that in blood before stasis. There was no obvious change in chain structure of this fibrin as judged by SDS-gel electrophoresis before and after reduction. However, radioimmunoassay of clot supernatants revealed small amounts of Bβ 15–42 fragments. As is seen in FIGURE 4, prothrombin consumption was greatly delayed after stasis and thrombin formation was also delayed. The conclusion we draw from these experiments is that the delay in fibrin formation is not so much dependent on degradation of fibrinogen but rather due to an impaired prothrombin utilization. This impairment may be due to impaired platelet activation in the static blood or to the presence of inhibitors influencing the activation of blood coagulation.

The finding that the effect is only seen in blood showing a positive euglobulin lysis test would suggest that the causative agent (not necessarily plasminogen activators) is a substance (or substances) released from the vessel wall during stasis. Is PGI_2 or adenosine involved? It is not likely that the effect is caused by the hemoconcentration occurring during stasis (about 20–30% increase in cell volume and plasma proteins) since individuals showing no anticoagulant effect showed the same hemoconcentration as those with delayed fibrin formation. Whatever the explanation may be, the results demonstrate that the regulation of fibrin formation may depend not only on plasmin, but also on one or several other mechanisms that may come into play *in vivo*.

REFERENCES

1. BLOMBÄCK, B., M. BLOMBÄCK, A. HENSCHEN, B. HESSEL, S. IWANAGA & K. R. WOODS. 1968. Nature **218:** 130–134.
2. BLOMBÄCK, B. & M. BLOMBÄCK. 1972. Ann. N.Y. Acad. Sci. **202:** 77–97.
3. BLOMBÄCK, B., B. HESSEL & D. HOGG. 1976. Thromb. Res. **8:** 639–658.
4. GÅRDLUND, B., B. HESSEL, G. MARGUERIE, G. MURANO & B. BLOMBÄCK. 1977. European J. Biochem. **77:** 595–610.
5. HENSCHEN, A., F. LOTTSPEICH, T. SEKITA & R. WARBINEK. 1976. Hoppe-Seyler's Z. Physiol. Chem. **357:** 605–608.
6. HENSCHEN, A. & F. LOTTSPEICH. 1977. Hoppe-Seyler's Z. Physiol. Chem. **358:** 1643–1646.
7. HENSCHEN, A., F. LOTTSPEICH & B. HESSEL. 1979. Hoppe-Seyler's Z. Physiol. Chem. **360:** 1951–1956.
8. TAKAGI, T. & R. F. DOOLITTLE. 1975. Biochim. Biophys. Acta **386:** 617–622.
9. WATT, K. W. K., T. TAKAGI & R. F. DOOLITTLE. 1979. Biochemistry **18:** 68–76.
10. DOOLITTLE, R. F., K. W. K. WATT, B. A. COTTRELL, D. D. STRONG & M. RILEY. 1979. Nature **280:** 464–468.
11. BLOMBÄCK, B., D. H. HOGG, B. GÅRDLUND, B. HESSEL & B. KUDRYK. 1976. Thromb. Res. **8** (Suppl. 2): 329–345.
12. BACHMANN, L., W. W. SCHMITT-FUMIAN, R. HAMMEL & K. LEDERER. 1975. Macromol. Chem. **176:** 2603–2618.
13. STRYER, L., C. COHEN & R. LANGRIDGE. 1963. Nature **197:** 793–794.
14. KUDRYK, B. J., D. COLLEN, K. R. WOODS & B. BLOMBÄCK. 1974. J. Biol. Chem. **249:** 3322–3325.

15. York, L. & B. Blombäck. 1976. Thromb. Res. **8:** 607–618.
16. Blombäck, B., B. Hessel, D. H. Hogg & L. Therkildsen. 1978. Nature **251:** 501–505.
17. Olexa, S. A. & A. Z. Budzynski. 1980. Proc. Natl. Acad. Sci. USA **77:** 1374–1378.
18. Ferry, J. D. 1954. Physiol. Rev. **34:** 753–760.
19. Laurent, T. C. & B. Blombäck. 1958. Acta Chem. Scand. **12:** 1875–1877.
20. Blombäck, B., S. Söderman & M. Söderberg. 1980. In preparation.
21. Nossel, H. L., I. Yudelman, R. E. Canfield, V. P. Butler, Jr., K. Spanondis, K. D. Wilner & G. D. Qureshi. 1974. J. Clin. Invest. **54:** 43–53.
22. Bilezikian, S. B., H. L. Nossel, V. P. Butler, Jr. & R. E. Canfield. 1975. J. Clin. Invest. **56:** 438–445.
23. Nossel, H. L., Y. Wasser, K. L. Kaplan, K. S. Lagamma., I. Yudelman & R. E. Canfield. 1979. J. Clin. Invest. **64:** 1371–1378.
24. Nossel, H. L. 1979. Thromb. Haemostas. **42:** (Abstr. 0823) 245.
25. Kudryk, B. 1980. In preparation.
26. Noren, I. 1970. Scand. J. Clin. Lab. Invest. **25:** 47–58.
27. Noren, I., G. Ramström & P. Wallen. 1975. Haemostasis **4:** 110–124.

MECHANISM OF
THROMBIN BINDING BY FIBRIN *

Chung Yuan Liu

Department of Medicine
College of Physicians & Surgeons
Columbia University
New York, New York 10032

INTRODUCTION

Thrombin (EC 3.4.21.5) is a serine protease generated from prothrombin by factor Xa. The principal function of thrombin is to convert fibrinogen to fibrin, activate factors V, VIII, and XIII, and cause platelet aggregation and release of granular contents. It was observed in a bovine system [1] that after thrombin clotted fibrinogen, the thrombin was adsorbed from the fluid by the fibrin (FIGURE 1, inset). These data were further analyzed by Seegers [2] with the Freundlich equation. [3] If the Freundlich equation could be applied to these data, a straight line would result when the logarithm of thrombin remaining in solution was plotted against the logarithm of thrombin adsorbed by fibrin. However, a curved line resulted. No comprehensive reaction mechanism could be inferred from this analysis. It is the purpose of the present paper to suggest an alternative interpretation of the data and to discuss the physiological significance of the thrombin adsorption by fibrin.

METHODS

Scatchard analysis, Steck-Wallach plot, and Sips analysis were described previously. [4,5] Briefly, the Scatchard equation has the form:

$$\frac{r}{(T)_f} = K_a (n - r),$$

where $(T)_f$ = molar concentration of free thrombin in solution, $r = (T)_b / (F)$ = (total number of moles of thrombin bound)/(total number of moles of fibrin), $(T)_b$ = molar concentration of bound thrombin in clot, (F) = molar concentration of total fibrin in clot, n = maximum number of thrombin-binding sites per fibrin molecule or maximum molar binding ratio between thrombin and fibrin, and K_a = association constant (M^{-1}).

The Steck-Wallach equation is written:

$$\frac{1}{r} = \frac{1}{n \cdot Ka} \cdot \frac{1}{(T)_f} + \frac{1}{n}.$$

For definitions of r, n, K_a, and $(T)_f$, see the Scatchard equation.

* This work was supported by National Institutes of Health Grants HL-15486 and HL-15596.

545

And the Sips equation can be expressed as:

$$\log\left(\frac{r}{n-r}\right) = a \log K_a + a \log (T)_f,$$

where a is the index for the heterogeneity of binding sites with respect to K_a. For definitions of r, n, K_a, and $(T)_f$, see the Scatchard equation.

RESULTS AND DISCUSSION

Thrombin adsorption by fibrin increased with increasing thrombin concentration, as previously reported by Seegers *et al.* in a bovine system (FIGURE 1, inset).[1] Since this curve has the appearance of an adsorption isotherm but cannot be well described by the Freundlich equation, it was analyzed by the Scatchard plot (FIGURE 1).[4] Linearity is apparent in this plot, suggesting the existence of equilibrium binding of thrombin by fibrin. This curve (FIGURE 1, inset) was further analyzed by the Steck-Wallach plot [4] and linearity is again obtained, confirming the results from the Scatchard analysis. Only a single class of binding sites was suggested by these analyses (TABLE 1).

In order to examine the heterogeneity of the binding sites with respect to the association constant, the Sips plot (FIGURE 2) [4] was carried out. A straight line was observed in this plot, of which the value of index a for heterogeneity was 0.92, indicating a high degree of homogeneity of these binding sites and further confirming the existence of equilibrium binding between thrombin and fibrin. Since no exception was made for the description of the existing data (FIGURE 1, inset) by the Scatchard analysis and the Steck-Wallach analysis, while exceptions were required when the Freundlich plot was used,[2] the data are better described by the Scatchard and the Steck-Wallach equations than by the Freundlich equation. Such a mechanism is compatible with product inhibition of thrombin by fibrin, consistent with the observation that fibrin acts like an antithrombin,[6] indicating a physiological significance for this reaction.

The adsorption of thrombin by fibrin was also observed by Liu, Nossel, and Kaplan in a human system (FIGURE 3 A & B).[5] The results in the bovine system appear to resemble those for the higher affinity binding site in the human system (TABLE 1). These observations indicate that there are similarities and also differences between the human and bovine systems, possibly resulting from the similarities and also differences in the molecular structures of thrombin and fibrin between these two systems.[7, 8]

Fibrin can instantaneously and reversibly adsorb thrombin, and can further immobilize thrombin by fibrin polymerization,[5] limiting and localizing thrombin action to the location where it is generated. On the other hand, antithrombin III and heparin can strongly bind and inactivate thrombin. It is intriguing to speculate that the reactions of fibrin together with those of antithrombin III and heparin may be regarded as a cooperative defense mechanism against excessive thrombin activity generated in the circulation as a response to injury. Accordingly, blood clotting is not only a primary defense mechanism against hemorrhagic trauma but also a well-organized defense mechanism against excessive clotting activity in circulation. In addition, the adsorption of thrombin by fibrin also provides an explanation for the thrombin source required for factor XIII activation in the fibrin clot.

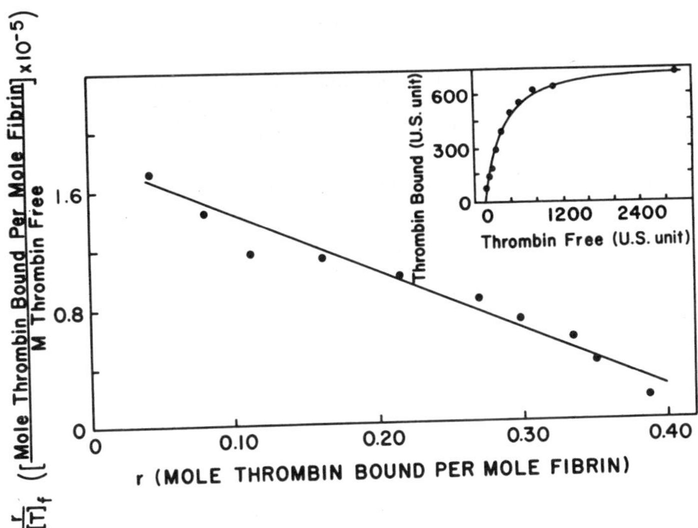

FIGURE 1. Scatchard plot of thrombin binding by fibrin. For detailed experimental conditions and original thrombin-binding data, see Seegers et al.[1] The curve shown in the inset is the original data obtained from this paper. 1 ml of fibrinogen solution (10 mg/ml of 0.9% NaCl solution) was added to 1 ml of thrombin solution (various concentrations) in such a way as to produce virtually instantaneous mixing. After 10 min. the fibrin was removed with a glass rod and the remaining thrombin was measured quantitatively by clotting assay, reaction temperature 25° C. The Scatchard plot of the original data was performed according to the Scatchard equation as described previously.[4] The correlation coefficient was −0.93. The maximum molar binding ratio of thrombin to fibrin and the association constant of the thrombin-fibrin binding estimated from this plot are shown in TABLE 1.

TABLE 1

SUMMARY OF APPARENT ASSOCIATION CONSTANTS AND MAXIMUM MOLAR
RATIOS OF THROMBIN BINDING TO FIBRIN *

Material and Method	Max. Molar Binding Ratio, n (Thrombin/Fibrin)	Association Constant, K_a (M⁻¹)
Bovine system		
Scatchard plot	0.47	4.0×10^5
Steck-Wallach plot	0.46	4.0×10^5
Sips plot †	0.5	3.9×10^5
Human system		
High affinity binding	0.39	5.8×10^5
Low affinity binding	1.6	6.8×10^4

* Calculations were based on the results from the Scatchard plot, the Steck-Wallach plot, and the Sips plot (FIGURES 1–3) (See METHODS). For experimental conditions see the original papers.[4, 5]

† The value of index a of heterogeneity is 0.92 estimated by this plot.

SUMMARY

Seegers *et al.* observed in a bovine system that after thrombin clotted fibrinogen, the thrombin was adsorbed from the fluid by the fibrin. These data were further analyzed with the Freudlich equation in which (1) an exception has to be assumed for the interpretation of the thrombin adsorption by fibrin at higher concentrations of thrombin, and (2) no comprehensive reaction mechanism between thrombin and fibrin is further indicated by this suggestion. Existing data were shown to suggest an alternative interpretation since these data can be described by the Scatchard equation and the Steck-Wallach equa-

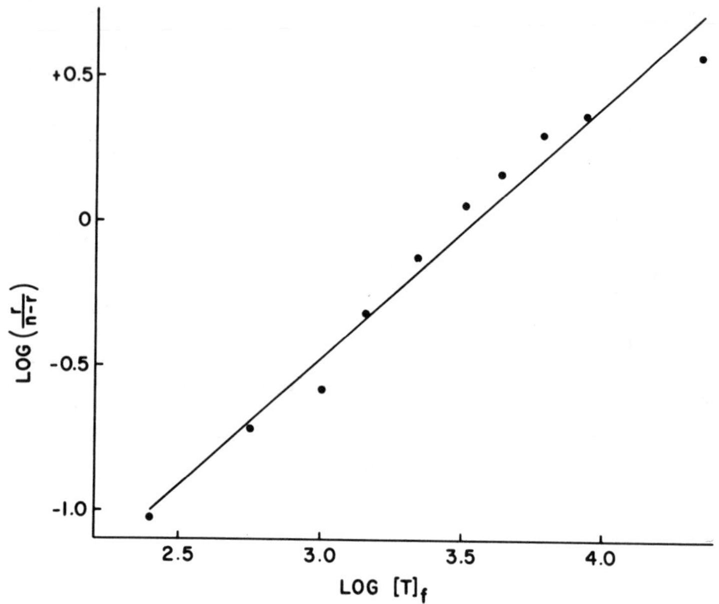

FIGURE 2. Sips plot of thrombin binding by fibrin. For experimental procedures see FIGURE 1. The Sips plot of the original data (FIGURE 1, inset) was performed according to the Sips equation as described previously [4] assuming that the maximum molar binding ratio was 0.5, which was an approximate value obtained from the Scatchard and Steck-Wallach plots (TABLE 1). The correlation coefficient was 0.95. The association constant of the binding and the index value for heterogeneity of the binding sites with respect to the association constant are shown in TABLE 1. The concentration $(T)_f$ is shown in nanomolar units.

tion without exception. A single class of equilibrium binding sites was suggested by the analyses with a maximum molar binding ratio between thrombin and fibrin about one to two, and an association constant of 4.0×10^5 M^{-1}. These results are further confirmed by a Sips plot with a value of index for heterogeneity 0.92, indicating a high degree of homogeneity of these binding sites. Such a mechanism is compatible with product inhibition of thrombin by fibrin, indicating a physiological significance for this reaction. The adsorption of thrombin by fibrin was also observed in a human system by Liu, Nossel, and Kaplan. The results in the bovine system appear to resemble those for the

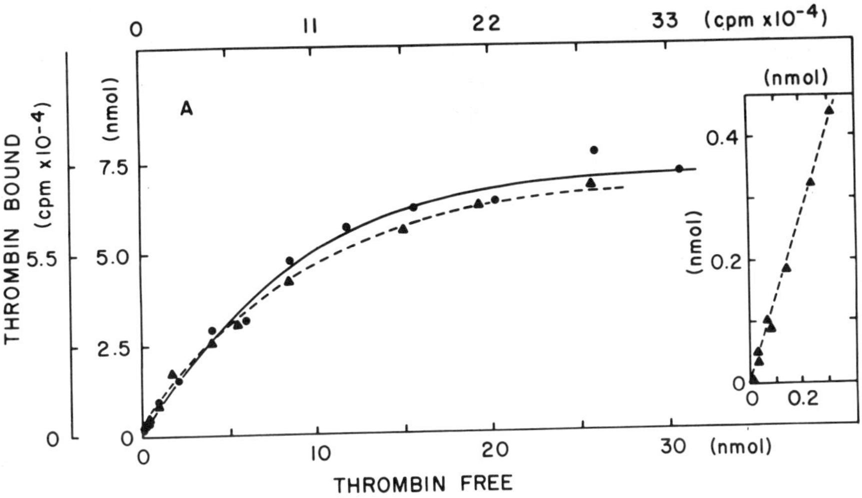

FIGURE 3. Binding of thrombin to fibrin as a function of thrombin concentration. For detailed experimental procedures see the original paper by Liu *et al.*[5] (A) Increasing amounts of thrombin solution were added to separate tubes with constant amounts of fibrinogen (2 mg) in barbital buffer at 25° C, final reaction volume 0.7 ml. Non-cross-linked fibrin clots were formed: (●—●) thrombin by clotting activity; (▲- - -▲) ^{125}I-thrombin by radioactivity. (B) A Scatchard plot of ^{125}I-thrombin binding by fibrin. The plot was similar when thrombin clotting activity was measured.

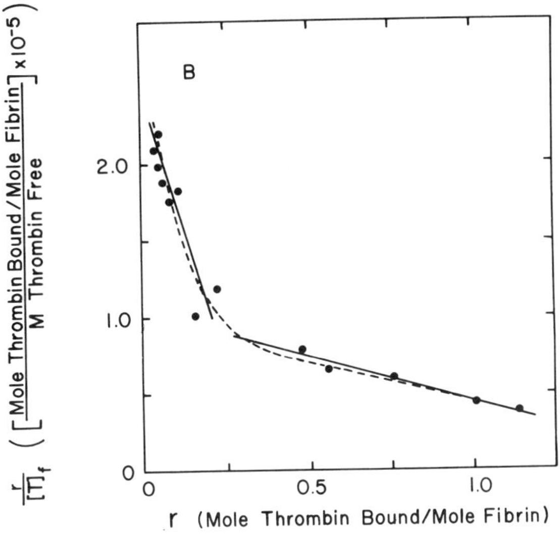

higher affinity binding site in the human system. Fibrin can instantaneously and reversibly adsorb thrombin and further immobilize thrombin by fibrin polymerization, limiting and localizing thrombin action to the location where it is generated. It is intriguing to speculate that the reactions of fibrin together with those of antithrombin III and heparin may be regarded as a cooperative defense mechanism against excessive clotting activity generated in the circulation as a response to injury.

ACKNOWLEDGMENTS

The author wishes to express his deep appreciation to Drs. Hymie L. Nossel and Karen L. Kaplan for their thoughtful comments, encouragement, and support. Without them this work could not have been done.

REFERENCES

1. SEEGERS, W., M. NIEFT & E. C. LOOMIS. 1945. Note on the adsorption of thrombin on fibrin. Science **101:** 520–521.
2. SEEGERS, W. 1947. Multiple protein interactions as exhibited by the blood-clotting mechanism. J. Phys. Colloid Chem. **51:** 198–206.
3. JIRGENSONS, B. & M. E. STRAUMANIS. 1962. Colloid Chemistry. 2nd edit., pp. 88–91. Macmillan, New York, N.Y.
4. LIU, C. Y. 1980. Mechanism of the reaction of thrombin with fibrin in a bovine system. Enzyme **25:** 64–68.
5. LIU, C. Y., H. L. NOSSEL & K. L. KAPLAN. 1979. The binding of thrombin by fibrin. J. Biol. Chem. **254:** 10421–10425.
6. SEEGERS, W. 1962. Prothrombin. pp. 285–287. Harvard Univ. Press, Cambridge, Mass.
7. ELION, J., M. R. DOWNING, R. J. BUTKOWSKI & K. G. MANN. 1977. Structure of human thrombin: Comparison with other serine proteases. *In* Chemistry and Biology of Thrombin. Lundblad, Fenton, and Mann, Eds. pp. 97–111. Ann Arbor Science Publishers, Ann Arbor, Mich.
8. MURANO, G. 1974. The molecular structure of fibrinogen. Sem. Thromb. Hemostas. **1:** 1–31.

MOLECULAR ASPECTS OF FIBRINOLYSIS

Patrick J. Gaffney

*National Institute for Biological Standards and Control
Holly Hill, London NW3 6RB, England*

INTRODUCTION

The purpose of these introductory remarks is to limit the scope of the broad intention that may be inferred from the title. Herein it is proposed to discuss the subunit interactions that underlie the hydrolysis of fibrinogen and fibrin by plasmin. One hastens to add that "the molecular aspects of fibrinolysis" should include a discussion of the interactions that take place between plasminogen and fibrin and between plasmin and α_2-antiplasmin (for a recent review, see reference 1), since aspects of these reactions have been proposed as a plausible explanation of a controlled fibrinolytic mechanism *in vivo*.[2] However, only the molecular aspects of fibrinolysis associated with the interactions of plasmin with fibrinogen and fibrin are discussed here. Indeed, since a number of recent reviews have outlined the major interactions between fibrinogen and plasmin,[3-6] only brief mention will be made of this topic. Fibrin-plasmin interactions and their possible clinical relevance will form the main subject for review, prominence being given to the details of the more recent data. It would also be well to point out that this discussion is limited to the interaction of fibrin with plasmin, the latter being the major terminal expression of the fibrinolytic "cascade" system; this in spite of the growing interest in the roles which a variety of proteolytic enzymes of cellular origin may play in thrombolysis.[7-9]

Moroz and Gilmore have suggested that enzymes having their origin in the cellular components of blood may play a far more important role than plasmin in the lysis of established thrombi.[9] However, there is little doubt that the fibrinolytic system, which involves plasminogen to plasmin conversion, plays a major protective role against fibrin deposition *in vivo*. Perusal of this type of fibrinolysis has preoccupied workers for some time and possibly the first "molecular" comment in the literature may be attributed to Seegers and his colleagues in 1945, when they showed that plasmin-digested fibrinogen consisted of two major electrophoretic fragments, which they called α-fibrinogen and β-fibrinogen.[10] There was little advance in the subject until, in 1961, Nussenzweig *et al.* fractionated digested fibrinogen into five major chromatographic fractions.[11] They called these A, B, C, D, and E, following the order in which they were eluted from an ion exchange column; the fractions labeled D and E were the α- and β-fibrinogens of Seegers *et al.*,[10] while the A, B, and C fractions were peptide material of a variety of sizes. While the work of Nussenzweig *et al.* indicated that fibrinogen fragments D and E were plasmin-resistant 'core' domains of the parent fibrinogen molecule, they also observed plasmin-labile intermediate degradation products,[11] which were subsequently named X and Y fragments by other workers.[12] The major molecular events that explain the interactions of plasmin with fibrinogen will only be outlined briefly below and used mainly as a background against which we can more effectively discuss the lysis of fibrin by plasmin. The details of the precise points of lysis of the

551

individual chains of the fibrinogen molecule by plasmin have been reviewed recently elsewhere.[6] After all, there is a reasonable consensus that physiological fibrinogenolysis is a rare event and that most of the fibrinogen-fibrin degradation products (FDP) in plasma emanate from fibrin formed during systemic or localized hypercoagulability. These opinions echo those of Astrup concerning the physiological state of balance between the coagulation and fibrinolytic systems.[13]

FIBRINOGEN-PLASMIN INTERACTIONS

Examination of the polypeptide chain composition of the various fragments derived from timed digests of fibrinogen with plasmin, together with carbohydrate staining and thrombin susceptibility analyses of their individual peptide chains, has allowed a number of schemes of fragmentation, which have some common features, to be developed.[14–18] FIGURE 1 shows the major features of

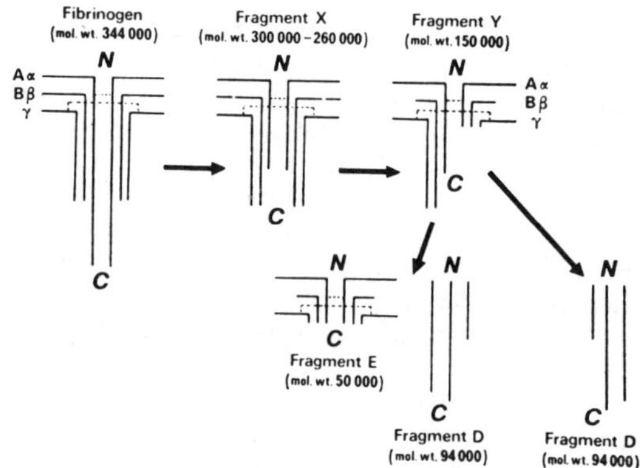

FIGURE 1. A schematic representation of the plasmin-mediated conversion of fibrinogen to its core fragments D and E, showing the intermediate fragments X and Y. The scheme is constructed such that the polypeptide chain origin of the constituent subunits of each type of fragment can be related to the polypeptide chains of the originating fibrinogen molecules (Aα, Bβ, or γ). N and C denote the NH_2- and COOH-terminal ends of these molecules. (From Gaffney.[4])

the sequence of digestive reactions with which most workers in the field would now concur. The conservation of both NH_2-terminal amino acids of the Aα chain remnants in the earliest digestion products (designated X in FIGURE 1)[19, 20] indicates that the initial lysis of these chains removes peptide material from the carboxy ends. Peptides of about 40,000 molecular weight are released rapidly, leaving the NH_2-terminal remnants of the Aα chains disulfide-bonded to the intact Bβ and γ chains. The next reactions involve the removal of peptides (MW 6000) from the NH_2-terminal ends of the Bβ chains,[20-23] followed by the asymmetric splitting of the three chains at one side of the partly-degraded dimer. These latter cleavages release fragment D and, thus, all lysis points of the three chains must be adjacent to the NH_2-terminal ends of the chains, on the assumption that fragment D is located at the approximate carboxy end of each of the subunits of fibrinogen.[24] The remaining fragment is called Y and the subsequent lysis of its Aα, Bβ, and γ chain remnants generates a second D fragment and a fragment E. Thus the terminal or "core" fragments D are made up of three disulfide-bonded remnants of the fibrinogen chains, namely: Aα' (MW 12,000), Bβ' (MW 43,000), γ' (MW 39,000), having an overall molecular weight of 94,000.[25, 26] Much of the reported electrophoretic heterogeneity of the D fragment[27] is mediated by further digestion of the γ chain remnant.[25, 28] The "core" fragment E is a dimer containing disulphide-bonded subunits, each subunit containing remnants of all three fibrinogen chains, namely: Aα' (MW 10,000), Bβ' (MW 7,000), and γ (MW 9,000).[29] Thus, the dimeric E molecule has an overall molecular weight of 52,000. The amino acids at which much of the above described lysis takes place have been elaborated in a number of laboratories and have been reviewed recently by Furlan.[6]

The above asymmetric scheme of fibrinogen degradation was first proposed by Marder and his colleagues[12] and, since then, further support has been added. The release of fragment D as a monomeric entity having the NH$_2$-terminal amino acids aspartic, methionine, and valine has supported the notion that D comes from the carboxy end of each fibrinogen subunit, while, during the fragmentation sequence, the maintenance of the fibrinogen Aα and γ chain amino-terminals (alanine and tyrosine, respectively) in fragments X, Y, and E has been demonstrated.[30] Furthermore, it has been shown that fragment Y contains 2 M fibrinopeptide A and a set each of heavy and light chains,[23] explaining the asymmetric structure proposed in FIGURE 1.

This brief appraisal of the reactions occurring during the degradation of fibrinogen by plasmin is intended to aid the reader in understanding the mechanisms involved in the more clinically relevant fibrin-plasmin interactions.

FIBRIN-PLASMIN INTERACTIONS

The thrombin-mediated reactions that accompany the conversion of fibrinogen to fibrin and the activation of the plasma transglutaminase (factor XIII) have been adequately discussed elsewhere in this volume (B. Blombäck's contribution). Here we will only summarize those features which affect the kinetics and mechanisms of fibrin lysis. Fibrin formation is initiated by the cleavage of the fibrinopeptides A and B from fibrinogen (Aα_2, Bβ_2, γ_2) by thrombin.[31] The resultant fibrin monomer (α_2, β_2, γ_2) can polymerize to nonstabilized polymers (α_2, β_2, γ_2)p, which can subsequently be crosslinked in the presence of calcium and Factor XIII (activated by thrombin) to form stabilized fibrin.[32] The glutamyl-lysyl crosslinks form rapidly in an intermolecular fashion between the γ chains to form γ dimers[33, 34] and it is now established that this reaction occurs when fibrin polymers are still in the so-called soluble state in blood.[35] The α-chain crosslinks form more slowly to form rather complex aggregates (α^p) of molecular weights in excess of 400,000.[36] There is a degree of interdependence between these reactions in that, generally, the formation of fibrin is necessary for the γ chain crosslinks to occur and the insertion of γ chain crosslinks allows the subsequent slowly-forming α chain crosslinks to occur.[37] Thus, it seems that at least three major forms of fibrin could be present *in vivo*: (1) noncrosslinked fibrin (NXL-FN), (2) partly crosslinked fibrin (PXL-FN), and (3) totally crosslinked fibrin (TXL-FN). Part of the diagram in FIGURE 2 shows these fibrin molecules with the approximate locations of the Factor XIII crosslinks. The α chain crosslinks have been located near the carboxy termini for ease of presentation, though we now know that they are located near the mid-section of the α chains.[38]

Since NXL-FN is chemically quite similar to fibrinogen, only lacking fibrinopeptides A and B, it is not surprising to find that its interaction with

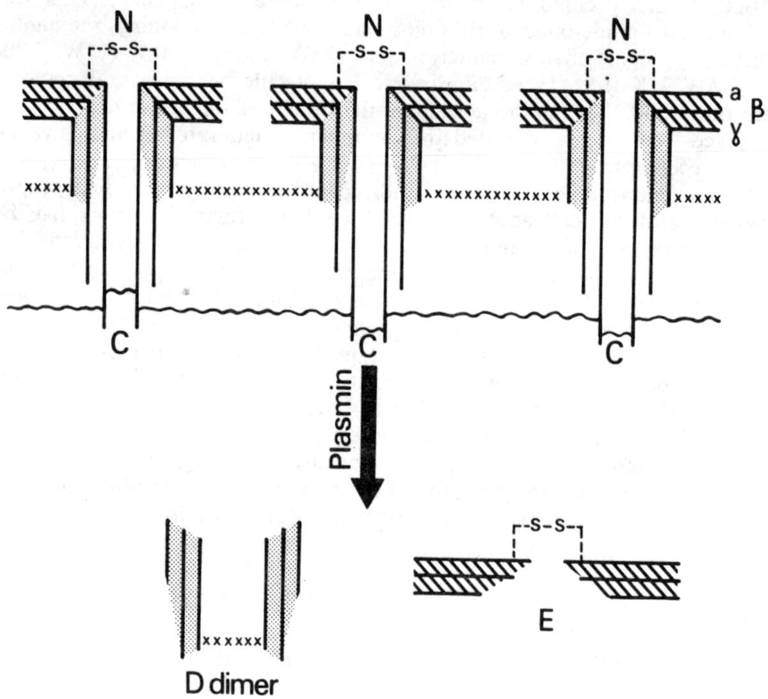

FIGURE 2. A schematic representation of the polypeptide chains of crosslinked (XL) fibrin and its plasmin-mediated degradation products D dimer and E. The crosslinked γ chain dimers (×××), the crosslinked α chain polymers (∼), and the uncrosslinked β chains are here related to each other schematically. Disulphide (s-s) bonds (not shown here except for one s-s bond joining the amino (N)-terminal ends of the two subunits of each fibrin molecule) link the individual chains of all the structures shown. Noncovalent bonds hold the units of the fibrin polymer together at the polymerization sites, but these are not shown, in order to simplify the diagram and highlight the bonds that are involved in the generation of the D dimer and E fragments from XL fibrin. The intermolecular nature of the γ chain crosslinks indicates that D dimer is made up of two D domains from adjacent fibrin molecules. The antigenically-distinct D and E domains in fibrin are represented by diagonally lined and shaded areas, respectively. (From Gaffney et al.[58])

plasmin yields an array of fragments similar in molecular weight to those obtained from fibrinogen.[39] It is, of course, obvious that the X, Y, and E fragments derived from fibrinogen will at least differ from those fragments obtained from NXL-FN in that the former contain fibrinopeptide A while the latter do not; other structural differences exist between the respective fragments from fibrinogen and NXL-FN that can be detected by radioimmunoassay using appropriate antisera.[40]

Information concerning the lysis of fibrin containing γ chain crosslinks (PXL-FN and TXL-FN) has been acquired gradually and we will highlight only the major events. It is obvious from FIGURE 2 that crosslinked D dimer fragments will be formed during the digestion of crosslinked fibrin (XL-FN); this was observed by three groups of workers at about the same time.[41–43] The D dimer was shown to be held together by the factor XIII–mediated crosslinks originating in the XL-FN.[42, 43] Thus, as shown in FIGURE 2, XL-FN degrades to D dimer and E fragments and a variety of peptides, some of which (from the α chains of the fibrin) are crosslinked. Later, it was found that some D dimer and E molecules were present in digestion mixtures as electrophoretically stable but noncovalent complexes.[44, 45] Subsequent experiments (FIGURE 3), in which the lysis of XL-FN was performed in serum containing plasmin inhibitors, indicated that all the D dimer and E molecules were present as a stoichiometrically satisfied complex having the formula $(D - D)E$,[46, 47] while the complex could be disrupted by 8 M urea and reformed upon removal of the detergent.[48] Lysis of XL-FN in the presence of trasylol (FIGURE 3) also yielded the D dimer–E complex. Olexa and Budzynski have reported that the complex is made up of a 1:1 molar mixture of D dimer and E and the same workers have shown that the conversion of the complex to free D dimer and E fragments is mediated by the digestion of the E domain.[47] Since the two major polymerizing sites in fibrin are located in the D and E domains of fibrin,[48] it seems that the D dimer–E complex is held together by the fibrin polymerization sites and that the complex is made up of domains from each of three distinct fibrin subunits (FIGURE 4). That this should be useful in gleaning further information about fibrin polymerization is quite feasible.

Specific antigenic markers have been recognized in the D dimer and the D dimer–E complex,[49] but, since these crosslink-related epitopes represent only a very small proportion of the total antigenicity of the D dimer species, it is difficult to devise a useful specific test for these fragments *in vivo*.

During experiments in which radiolabeled XL-FN was digested under physiological conditions in serum, it was observed that very large molecular weight complexes eluted near the void volume (V_0 in FIGURE 5) of a Sepharose chromatographic column. These labeled high molecular weight complexes have already been observed by other workers.[50, 51] In an effort to reproduce the formation of similar complexes during the digestion of purified XL-FN, a variety of digestion procedures was used, employing SK, UK, and plasminogen in differing regimens. At 50% and 100% lysis, the various regimens yielded digestion mixtures containing different amounts of electrophoretically free fragment E. Also, one particular form of digestion (50% lysis of plasminogen-enriched fibrin in SK solution, e.g., plgn $\rightarrow$ SK) yielded a large amount of high molecular weight (HMW) fragments, together with fragments similar in mobility to fragments X and the D dimer. This type and duration of digestion contained no free fragment E, since the E domain was complexed with D dimer and remained incorporated in the other higher molecular weight material. The Sepharose 4B chromatographic profiles of this type of digest (FIGURE 6a) compared well with that obtained when XL-FN was digested in serum (FIGURE 5); thus, the partial (50%) lysis of XL-FN in streptokinase solutions acts as a satisfactory model for the study of the mechanisms involved under more physio-

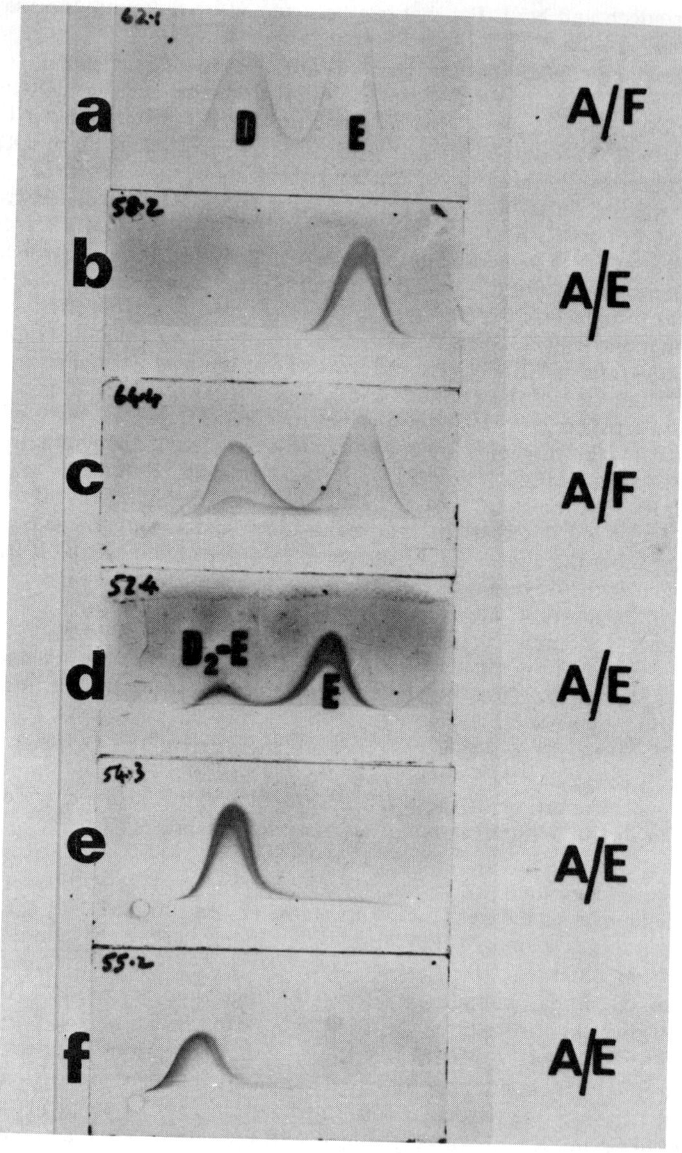

FIGURE 3. Two-dimensional immunoelectrophoretic patterns of plasmin-mediated digests of crosslinked (XL) fibrins. The digests shown in panels c and d were made in buffered solutions, while those in panels e and f were made in human serum and trasylol, respectively. Panels a and b show marker fragments D and E, using antisera to whole human fibrinogen (A/F), and fibrinogen fragment E (A/E) in the second dimension. This fibrinogen digest marker mixture of D and E demonstrates the specificity of the antisera used and the presence of the E domain as a pure or complexed fragment in the other digests. (From Gaffney and Joe.[46])

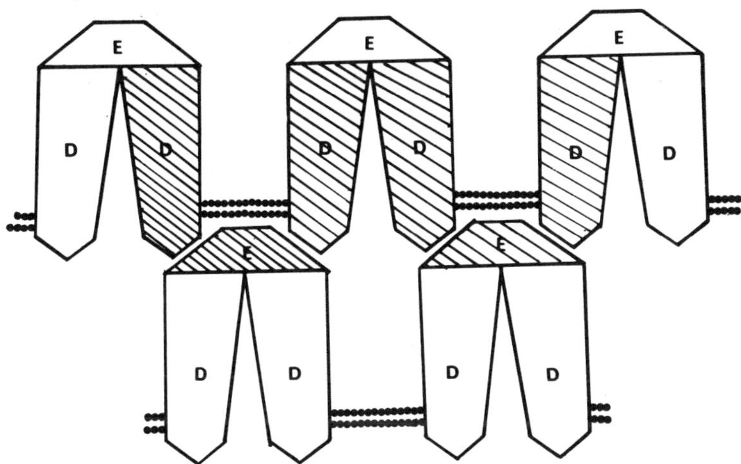

FIGURE 4. A suggested scheme showing the most probable relative locations of the domains (hatched areas) making up the D dimer–E complex. The γ chain crosslinks joining the various fibrin units together are denoted by a dotted line. This diagram is based on the evidence of Doolittle *et al.*,[60] which shows that the γ chain crosslinks are all intermolecular, and the report of Kudryk *et al.*, which demonstrates the locations of the D and E polymerization sites. (From Gaffney and Joe.[46]

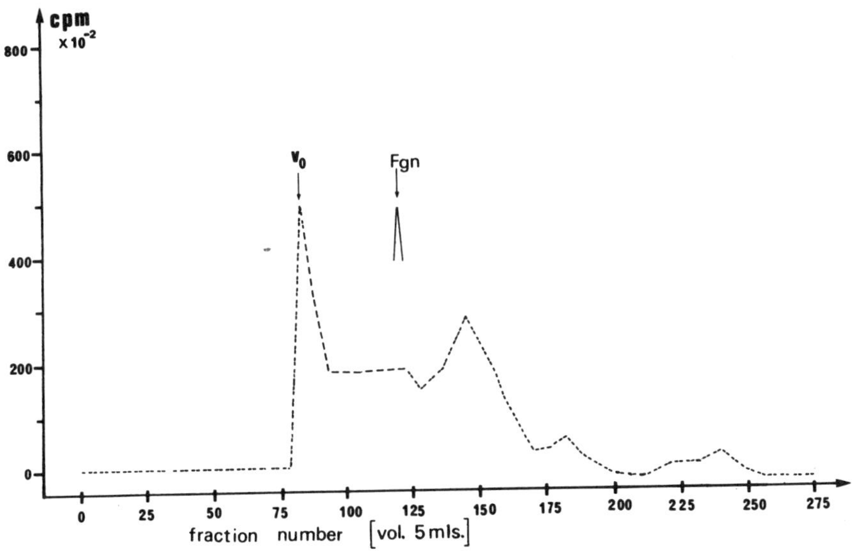

FIGURE 5. Sepharose 4B chromatographic profile (^{125}I counts) of a crosslinked fibrin digest made in human serum. High levels of radioactivity near the void volume (V₀) suggest the presence of many large fibrin fragments, while the expected D dimer–E complex is eluted after the elution point of fibrinogen (Fgn).

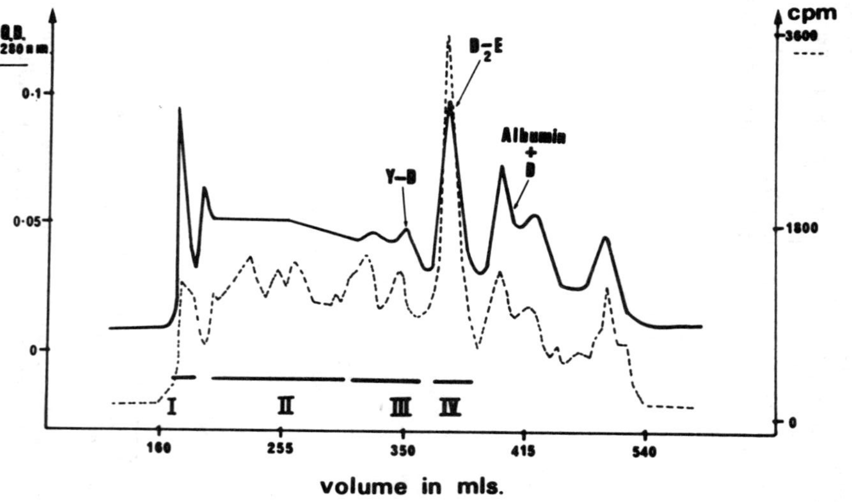

FIGURE 6A. Sepharose 4B chromatographic profiles (^{125}I counts and protein) of XL-fibrin digest containing a large proportion of high molecular weight (HMW) fragments. The identities of some of the fractions are marked; this information is assessed mainly from the data in FIGURE 6B. Fractions I, II, III, and IV were concentrated by perevaporation and stored as concentrated solutions in liquid N_2.

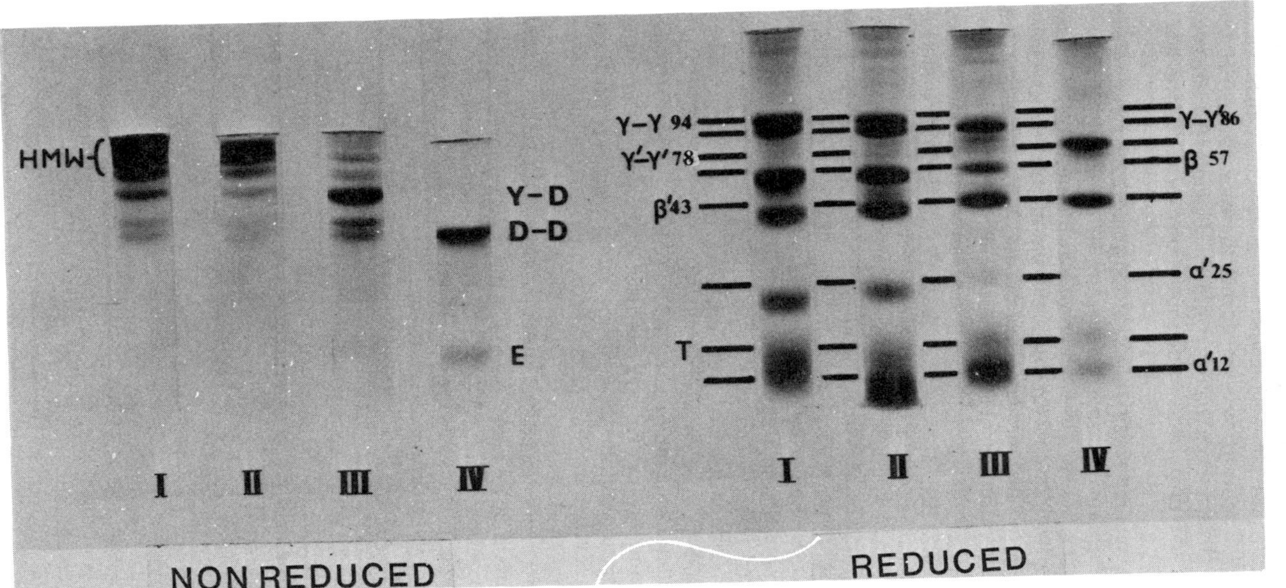

FIGURE 6B. Fractions from Sepharose 4B separation on SDS–polyacrylamide gel electrophoresis. The whole fragments and their reduced subunits were analyzed. The identities of subunits were judged by known marker mixtures of polypeptide chains, carbohydrate staining, and ^{125}I counting of the relevant gel slices. The naming of the subunits was based on the fibrin chain origin and the molecular weight (e.g., γ-γ′ 86 describes an intact γ chain of MW 47,000 crosslinked with a γ chain remnant of MW 39,000). (From Gaffney et al.[59])

logical conditions. It seems that, while the D dimer–E complex is the physiological condition of the D dimer fragment and has been found in patient plasma,[52] high molecular weight aggregates (of molecular weight range 1–10×10^6) are the first fragments released during the lysis of XL-FN; indeed, such fragments have already been reported during disseminated intravascular coagulation (DIC)[51] and in patients with thrombosis, both before and after thrombolytic therapy.[53]

With a view to developing sensitive assays for the HMW fraction and the D dimer–E complex in human plasma, Sepharose 4B column chromatography was employed to separate the various fractions, as in FIGURE 6a. The detergent gel electrophoretic analyses of the various fractions of interest are shown in FIGURE 6b and highly purified preparations of the X-like fragment (subsequently identified as a crosslinked Y-D complex) and the D dimer–E complex were achieved. It was surprising to observe that, even in the most carefully prepared HMW fractions, e.g., fraction I, an impurity of the Y-D and D dimer fragments was present, as observed through detergent-gel electrophoresis. This can be explained by the hypothesis that cleavages occurred in the HMW fraction that allow the release of crosslinked Y-D and D dimer complexes in detergent but not in aqueous solution. Examination of the HMW fraction, following reduction of its disulfide bonds, on detergent-gel electrophoresis indicated a polypeptide chain composition as follows: α' 25,000 MW, intact β chains MW 56,000, and crosslinked intact γ chains MW 94,000 (FIGURE 7). Considering the polypeptide chain composition of fibrinogen fragment X (Aα' ~ 25,000 MW, Bβ chains 58,000 MW, γ chains 47,000 MW; see FIGURE 1) and the elution volume of material on Sepharose 4B, identifying these HMW fragments as crosslinked X-oligomers is justified and has already been suggested by Graeff and colleagues in order to describe the high molecular weight fibrin fragments found in patients with severe abruptio placenta.[51]

It was observed that the homogenous peak (fraction IV) in FIGURE 6a, that contains the D dimer–E complex, shows the separated domains by electrophoresis in detergent (FIGURE 6b). Thus, our analytical electrophoretic procedures dissociate the polymerization sites holding the D dimer and E domains together. Similarly, the HMW and Y-D fractions are involved in polymerization-mediated aggregates of considerably greater molecular size than suggested by the detergent-gel electrophoresis shown in FIGURE 6b. The size of these X-oligomer aggregates remains unknown, but may be as high as 10×10^6 in molecular weight. Thus, FIGURE 7, which shows the subunits of the various fragments prepared from the digestion of XL-fibrin under physiological conditions, suggests aggregated extensions of all these structures via the D and E polymerizing domains.

CONCLUDING REMARKS

Since fibrinogen-plasmin interactions have been recently reviewed,[3–6] the above discussion has concentrated mostly on fibrin fragmentation, indeed on the more recent work suggesting that high molecular weight crosslinked X-oligomers are the major products of the physiological degradation of preformed crosslinked fibrin. While the report of Francis *et al.* describing γ-γ chain crosslinked aggregates in patients with thrombosis could be readily predicted,[53] it is far more difficult to visualize how the crosslinked X-oligomers described by Graeff and colleagues[51] and by Whitaker *et al.*[52] can be formed *in vivo*. These crosslinked aggregates have been isolated from patient plasma and their polypeptide chain composition was shown to include the essential subunits of the crosslinked X-oligomers described above, namely crosslinked intact γ chain dimers, intact β chains, and α chain remnants of about 25,000 molecular weight ($\alpha'25$).[51] FIGURE 8 shows a number of pathways by which these crosslinked high molecular weight X-oligomers might be formed during the competitive interactions of thrombin and plasmin for fibrinogen in DIC; at this stage, no one particular pathway is favored. Indeed, all the pathways suggested may apply or each type of DIC may involve a particular pathway. Also, in FIGURE 9, the formation of crosslinked X-oligomers is predicted from the XL-fibrin in thrombi and it is evident from the above that this can take place through the action of plasmin alone. It is here suggested that the presence of crosslinked X-oligomers (probably in conjunction with crosslinked Y-D and D-D) may be important markers present in blood both before and after various forms of thrombosis. Efforts to design a solid phase sensitive radioimmunometric assay specific for these crosslinked fragments have not met with success to date. However, antisera to the purified X-oligomers prepared in rabbits, following adsorption with fibrinogen, have been shown to interact avidly with the X-oligomers, poorly with a standard preparation of fibrinogen and fibrin degradation products (FDP-X, Y, D, and E), and not at all with fibrinogen (FIGURE 9). As the competitive interactions between FDP fractions and crosslinked X-oligomers for the antisera in solution did not reflect the data in FIGURE 9, a specific assay procedure still awaits development. Efforts are continuing in the author's laboratory to achieve such an assay, since it may be of useful in diagnosing the onset and progression of the thrombotic state. While the release of fibrinopeptide A has also been proposed as such a diagnostic test, it can be argued that transient raised levels of fibrinopeptide A may not be clinically relevant, while the formation of crosslinked fragments, representing a more advanced hypercoagulable state, may more readily reflect thrombosis. Indeed, the crosslinked X-oligomers may be regarded as soluble foci for thrombus formation.[51]

Initially, it may be surprising that aggregates of crosslinked fibrin fragments, associated by factor XIII–mediated covalent bonds and the native polymerization sites of fibrin and having molecular weights as high as 10×10^6, can remain soluble in plasma; however, Henry *et al.* suggest that, during coagulation, fibrin polymers of about twenty units long can exist in solution before insolubilization occurs[55] and, thus, it would seem reasonable that large fibrin aggregates could be solubilized from XL-fibrin. The so-called soluble fibrin monomer complexes (SFMC) of fibrinogen and fibrin, which are normally a feature of the hypercoagulable state, can exist in solution as long as they do not exceed the threshold state (i.e., $\sim 30\%$) of the total fibrinogen present.[56] It is unlikely that there are monomolecular complexes of fibrinogen and fibrin (for a review, see reference 57). The role of fibrinogen as a chelating agent for fibrin as it is formed would argue that the complexes must be made up of two fibrinogen molecules for each fibrin molecule (see FIGURES 4 and 7, which suggest that the polymerization site in the E domain is divalent). This supports the ideas of Shainoff and Page concerning the "threshold state" of fibrin with respect to residual fibrinogen in plasma.[56]

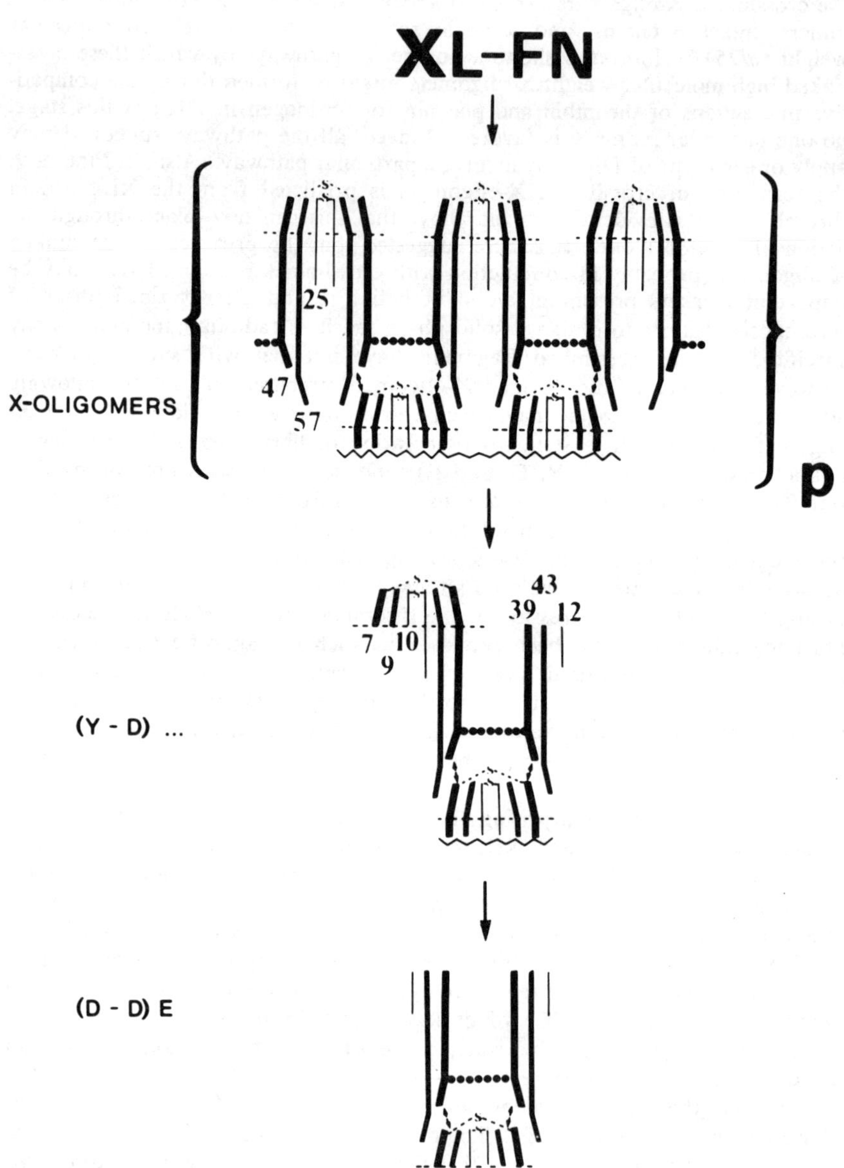
XL-FN
X-OLIGOMERS
25
47
57
p
43
39 12
7 10
9
(Y - D) ...
(D - D) E

FIGURE 7. A schematic representation of the various molecular complexes formed during the degradation of crosslinked fibrin (XL-FN) by plasmin. The polypeptide subunits making up each molecular complex are joined by many disulfide bonds (s-s), but only those joining the dimeric NH_2-terminals are shown. The thickness of the line denoting the polypeptide chain designates the fibrin chain origin, i.e., thin line = α, medium line = β chain, and thick line γ chain. The molecular weight ($\times 10^{-3}$) of each composite subunit chain is shown only once, although these chains are repeated a number of times throughout the scheme. The broken line denotes the demarcation between the E and D domains in the fibrin fragment structures, while the zig-zag line indicates molecular extensions of an indefinite nature. The scheme suggests that crosslinked fibrin (XL-FN) degrades to X-oligomers P subunits long, while polymerization sites ($\leftrightarrow$) allow extensions of the γ chain crosslinked (. . . .) X units into quite large aggregates. The aggregated X oligomers digest further to complexes described as Y-D and (D-D)E. (From Gaffney et al.[59])

DIC

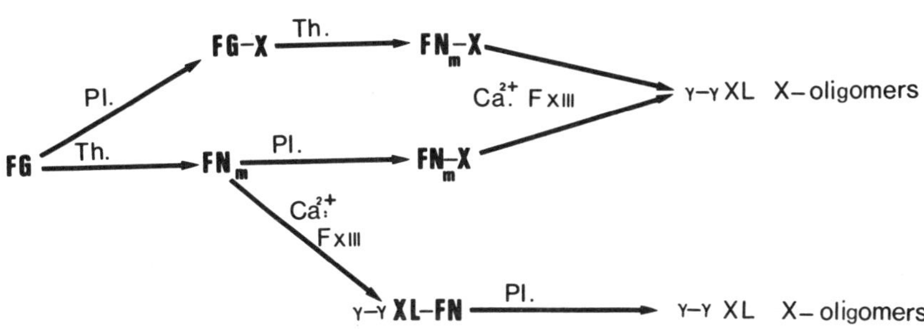

Thrombolysis

FIGURE 8. Suggested alternative pathways through which plasmin (PL) and thrombin (Th) can compete for fibrinogen (FG) to form γ chain crosslinked (γ-γXL) X-oligomers during disseminated intravascular coagulation (DIC). Calcium (Ca^{2+}), factor XIII (FXIII), fibrin monomer (FN_m), and fibrin polymer (FN) are included in this scheme. The formation of similar crosslinked X oligomers during thrombolysis is suggested by direct fibrinolytic atack on the XL-FN in thrombi. (From Gaffney et al.[59])

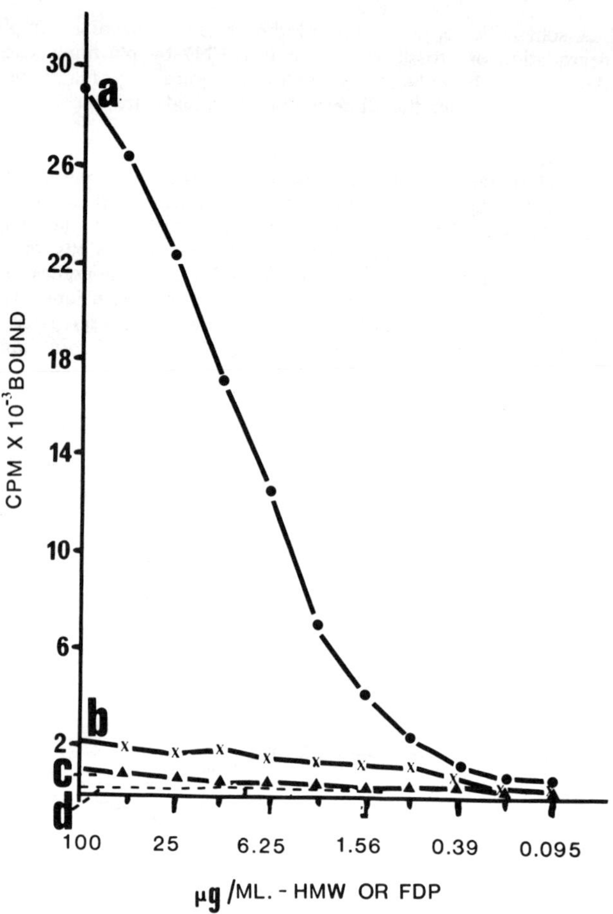

FIGURE 9. The binding curves of an absorbed rabbit antiserum to X-oligomers (HMW). Various concentrations of X-oligomers, a; fibrinogen fragments X-Y-D-E, b; fibrin degradation products X-Y-D-E, c; and fibrinogen, d, were immobilized on polyvinyl plates and the antiserum (1/1000 dilution) was allowed to interact. The amount of the antibody binding at each specific antigen concentration is shown as cpm bound, measured by a labeled second antibody to rabbit IgG. It can be seen that, on a weight basis, the antiserum has a far greater affinity for the X-oligomers.

REFERENCES

1. COLLEN, D. 1980. On the regulation and control of fibrinolysis. Thromb. Haemos. **43:** 77–89.
2. WIMAN, B. & D. COLLEN. 1978. Molecular mechanism of physiological fibrinolysis. Nature (London) **272:** 549–550.
3. GAFFNEY, P. J. 1977. The biochemistry of fibrinogen and fibrin degradation products. *In* The Biochemistry, Physiology and Pathology of Haemostasis. D. Ogston & B. Bennett, Eds.: 105–108. John Wiley and Sons. New York.

4. GAFFNEY, P. J. 1977. Fibrin(ogen) interactions with plasmin. Haemostasis **6:** 2–25.

5. GAFFNEY, P. J. 1977. Structure of fibrinogen and degradation products of fibrinogen and degradation products of fibrinogen and fibrin. Brit. Med. Bull. **33:** 245–252.

6. FURLAN, M. 1978. Features of the interaction of plasmin with fibrinogen. *In* Fibrinolysis: Current Clinical and Fundamental Concepts. P. J. Gaffney & S. Balkuv-Ulutin, Eds.: 97–108. Academic Press. London.

7. LATALLO, Z. S., E. TEISSEYRE, W. ARDELT, Z. WEGRZYNOWICZ & M. KOPEC. 1978. Fibrino(geno)lysis by enzymes other than plasmin. *In* Fibrinolysis: Current Clinical and Fundamental Concepts. P. J. Gaffney & S. Balkuv-Ulutin, Eds.: 129–136. Academic Press. London.

8. PLOW, E. & T. S. EDGINGTON. 1975. An alternative pathway for fibrinolysis. I. The cleavage of fibrinogen by leucocyte protease at physiologic pH. J. Clin Invest. **56:** 30–38.

9. MOROZ, C. A. & N. J. GILMORE. 1976. Fibrinolysis in normal plasma and blood; evidence for significant mechanisms independent of the plasminogen-plasmin system. Blood **48:** 531–545.

10. SEEGERS, W. H., M. L. NIEFT & J. M. VANDENVELT. 1945. Decomposition products of fibrinogen and fibrin. Arch. Biochem. **7:** 15–19.

11. NUSSENZWEIG, V., M. SELGMAN, J. PELMONT & P. GRABAR. 1961. Les produits de degradation du fibrinogene humain par la plasmine. I. Separation et proprietes physicochimiques. Ann. Inst. Pasteur Paris **100:** 377–387.

12. MARDER, V. J., N. R. SHULMAN & W. R. CARROLL. 1969. High molecular weight derivatives of human fibrinogen produced by plasmin. I. Physico-chemical and immunological characterization. J. Biol. Chem. **244:** 2111–2119.

13. ASTRUP, T. 1956. The biological significance of fibrinolysis. Lancet **2:** 565–568.

14. PIZZO, S. V., M. L. SCHWARTZ, R. L. HILL & P. A. McKEE. 1972. The effect of plasmin on the subunit structure of human fibrinogen. J. Biol. Chem. **242:** 636–645.

15. MILLS, D. & S. KARPATKIN. 1972. The initial macromolecular derivatives of human fibrinogen produced by plasmin. Biochim. Biophys. Acta **271:** 163–173.

16. MILLS, D. A. 1972. A molecular model for the proteolysis of human fibrinogen by plasmin. Biochem. Biophys. Acta **263:** 619–630.

17. FURLAN, M. & E. A. BECK. 1972. Plasmin degradation of human fibrinogen. I. Structural characterization of degradation products. Biochim. Biophys. Acta **263:** 631–644.

18. MOSESSON, M. W., J. S. FINLAYSON & D. K. GALANAKIS. 1973. The essential covalent structure of human fibrinogen evidenced by analysis of derivatives formed during plasmic hydrolysis. J. Biol. Chem. **248:** 7913–7929.

19. SHERMAN, L. A., M. W. MOSESSON & S. SHERRY. 1969. Isolation and characterization of the clottable low molecular weight fibrinogen derived by limited plasmin hydrolysis of human fraction I-4. Biochemistry **8:** 1515–1523.

20. MOSESSON, M. W., J. S. FINLAYSON, R. A. UMFLEET & D. GALANAKIS. 1972. Human fibrinogen heterogeneities. I. Structural and related studies of plasma fibrinogens which are high solubility catabolic intermediates. J. Biol. Chem. **247:** 5210–5219.

21. SHAINOFF, J. R., B. LAHIRI & F. M. BUMPUS. 1970. Ultracentrifuge studies on the reaction between thrombin and plasminized fibrinogen. Thromb. Diath. Haemorrh. Suppl. **39:** 203–217.

22. KIERULF, P. 1972. N-terminal analysis of 'fibrins' from plasmin hydrolysed fibrinogen—evidence for lack of fibrinopeptide B. Thromb. Res. **1:** 527–532.

23. BUDZYNSKI, A. Z., V. J. MARDER & J. R. SHAINOFF. 1974. Structure of

plasmic degradation products of human fibrinogen. Fibrinopeptide and polypeptide chain analysis. J. Biol. Chem. **249:** 2294–2302.

24. GAFFNEY, P. J. 1972. Localization of carbohydrate in the subunits of human fibrinogen and its plasmin induced fragments. Biochim. Biophys. Acta **263:** 453–458.

25. GAFFNEY, P. J. & P. DOBOS. 1971. A structural aspect of human fibrinogen suggested by its plasmin degradation. FEBS Lett. **15:** 13–16.

26. PIZZO, S. V., M. L. SCHWARTZ, R. L. HILL & P. A. MCKEE. 1972. The effect of plasmin on the subunit structure of human fibrinogen. J. Biol. Chem. **247:** 636–645.

27. JAMIESON, G. A. & P. J. GAFFNEY. 1966. Heterogeneity of fibrin polymerization inhibitor. Biochim. Biophys. Acta **121:** 217–220.

28. GAFFNEY, P. J. 1975. Molecular pathology of the multiple forms of fibrinogen and its fragments. *In* Isozymes: Physiological Function, Vol. 2, C. L. Markert, Ed.: 343–368. Academic Press. New York.

29. KOWALSKA-LOTH, B., H. GARLUND, M. EGEBERG & B. BLOMBÄCK. 1973. Plasmic degradation products of human fibrinogen. II. Chemical and immunological relation between fragment E and N-DSK. Thromb. Res. **2:** 423–450.

30. MARDER, V. J., A. Z. BUDZYNSKI & H. L. JAMES. 1972. High molecular weight derivatives of human fibrinogen produced by plasmin. III. Their NH$_2$-terminal amino acids and comparison with the "NH$_2$-terminal disulfide knot." J. Biol. Chem. **247:** 4775–4781.

31. BETTELHEIM, F. R. & K. BAILEY. 1952. The products of the action of thrombin on fibrinogen. Biochim. Biophys. Acta **9:** 578–579.

32. LORAND, L. & K. KONISHI. 1964. Activation of the fibrin stabilizing factor of plasma by thrombin. Arch. Biochem. Biophys. **105:** 58–67.

33. MATACIC, S. & A. G. LOWEY. 1968. The identification of isopeptide crosslinks in insoluble fibrin. Biochem. Biophys. Res. Commun. **30:** 356–362.

34. PISANO, J. J., J. S. FINLAYSON, M. P. PEYTON & Y. NAGAI. 1971. ϵ-(γ-Glutamyl) lysine in fibrin: Lack of crosslink formation in factor XIII deficiency. Proc. Natl. Acad. Sci. USA **68:** 770–772.

35. LY, B., P. KIERULF & E. JAKOBSEN. 1974. Stabilization of soluble fibrin/fibrinogen complexes by fibrin stabilizing factor (FSF). Thromb. Res. **4:** 509–522.

36. MCKEE, P. A., P. MATTOCK & R. L. HILL. 1970. Subunit structure of human fibrinogen, soluble fibrin and crosslinked insoluble fibrin. Proc. Natl. Acad. Sci. USA **66:** 738–744.

37. GAFFNEY, P. J. 1978. Fibrinolysis by plasmin and brinase: In vitro and in vivo observations. *In* Progress in Chemical Fibrinolysis and Thrombolysis, vol. 3. J. F. Davidson, R. M. Rowan, M. M. Samama & P. C. Desnoyers, Eds.: 349–372. Raven Press. New York.

38. FINLAYSON, J. S. & M. W. MOSESSON. 1973. Crosslinking of α chain remnants in human fibrin. Thromb. Res. **2:** 467–478.

39. GAFFNEY, P. J. 1973. Subunit relationships between fibrinogen and fibrin degradation products. Thromb. Res. **2:** 201-218.

40. EDGINGTON, T. W. & E. PLOW. 1975. Conformational and structural modulation of the NH$_2$-terminal regions of fibrinogen and fibrin associated with plasmin cleavage. J. Biol. Chem. **250:** 3393–3398.

41. KOPEC, M., E. TEISSEYRE, G. DUDEK-WOJCIECHOWSKA, M. KLOCEWIAK, A. PANKIEWICZ & Z. S. LATALLO. 1973. Studies on the "double D" fragment from stabilized bovine fibrin. Thromb. Res. **2:** 283–291.

42. GAFFNEY, P. J. & M. BRASHER. 1973. Subunit structure of the plasmin-induced degradation products of crosslinked fibrin. Biochim. Biophys. Acta **295:** 308–313.

43. PIZZO, S. V., L. M. TAYLOR, M. L. SCHWARTZ, R. L. HILL & P. A. MCKEE. 1973. Subunit structure of fragment D from fibrinogen and crosslinked fibrin. J. Biol. Chem. **248:** 4584–4590.

44. HUDRY-CLERGEON, G., L. PATURAL & M. SUSCILLON. 1974. Identification d'un complexe (D-D). . .E dans les produits de degradation de la fibrin bovine stabilisee par le factor XIII. Pathol. Biol. Suppl. **22:** 47–52.

45. GAFFNEY, P. J., D. A. LANE, V. V. KAKKAR & M. BRASHER. 1975. Characterization of a soluble D dimer-E complex in crosslinked fibrin digests. Thromb. Res. **7:** 89–99.

46. GAFFNEY, P. J. & F. JOE. 1979. The lysis of crosslinked human fibrin by plasmin yields initially a single molecular complex, D dimer-E. Thromb. Res. **15:** 673–687.

47. OLEXA, S. A. & BUDZYNSKI, A. Z. 1979. Primary soluble plasmic degradation products of crosslinked human fibrin. Isolation and stoichiometry of the (DD)E complex. Biochemistry **18:** 991–995.

48. KUDRYK, B. J., D. COLLEN, K. R. WOODS & B. BLOMBÄCK. 1974. Evidence for localization of polymerization sites in fibrinogen. J. Biol. Chem. **249:** 3322–3325.

49. BUDZYNSKI, A. Z., V. J. MARDER, M. E. PARKER, P. SHAMES, B. S. BRIZUELA & S. A. OLEXA. 1979. Antigenic markers of fragment D-D, a unique plasmic derivative of human crosslinked fibrin. Blood **54:** 794–804.

50. ALKJAERSIG, N., A. DAVIES & A. P. FLETCHER. 1977. Fibrin and fibrinogen proteolysis products: comparison between gel filtration and SDS polyacrylamide electrophoresis analysis. Thromb. Haemos. **38:** 524–535.

51. GRAEFF, H., R. HAFTER & L. BACHMANN. 1979. Subunit and macromolecular structure of circulating fibrin from obstetric patients with intravascular coagulation. Thromb. Res. **16:** 313–328.

52. WHITAKER, A. N., E. A. ROWE, P. MASCI & P. J. GAFFNEY. 1979. Identification of D dimer-E complex in disseminated intravascular coagulation (DIC). Thromb. Haemos. **42:** 274 (abstr.); Thromb. Res. 1980. **18:** 453–459.

53. FRANCIS, C. W., V. J. MARDER & S. E. MARTIN. 1979. Detection of circulating crosslinked fibrin derivatives by a heat extraction-SDS gradient gel electrophoretic technique. Blood **54:** 1282–1295.

54. NOSSEL, H. L., M. TI, K. L. KAPLAN, K. SPANONDIS, T. SOLAND & V. P. BUTLER, JR. 1976. The generation of fibrinopeptide A in clinical blood samples. Evidence for thrombin activity. J. Clin. Invest. **58:** 1136–1144.

55. HENRY, F., M. NESTLER & J. D. FERRY. 1977. Identification of fibrin oligomers in sonicated fibrin clots. Biophys. Chem. **6:** 161–165.

56. SHAINOFF, J. R. & I. H. PAGE. 1962. Significance of cryoprofibrin in fibrinogen-fibrin conversion. J. Exp. Med. **116:** 687–707.

57. BANG, N. U. & M. L. CHANG. 1974. Soluble fibrin complexes. Sem. Thrombos. Haemos. **1:** 91–128.

58. GAFFNEY, P. J., M. BRASHER, K. LORD, C. J. L. STRACHAN, A. R. WILKINSON, V. V. KAKKAR & M. F. SCULLY. 1976. Fibrin subunits in venous and arterial thromboembolism. Cardiovasc. Res. **10:** 421–426.

59. GAFFNEY, P. J., F. JOE & M. MAHMOUD. 1980. Giant fibrin fragments derived from crosslinked fibrin: structure and clinical implication. Thromb. Res. **20:** 647–662.

60. DOOLITTLE, R. F., R. CHEN & F. LAU. 1971. Hybrid fibrin proof of the intermolecular nature of the γ-γ crosslinking limits. Biochem. Biophys. Res. Commun. **44:** 94–100.

MONOCYTE/MACROPHAGE-MEDIATED CATABOLISM
OF FIBRINOGEN AND FIBRIN

N. U. Bang, M. L. Chang, L. E. Mattler, P. J. Burck,
R. M. Van Frank, R. E. Zimmerman, C. A. Marks, and L. J. Boxer

Lilly Research Laboratories
and
Departments of Medicine, Pathology, and Pediatrics
Indiana University School of Medicine
Indianapolis, Indiana 46202

INTRODUCTION

Traditionally, studies on fibrinogen and fibrin catabolism have focused on the humoral plasmin-mediated pathway. However, additional enzyme systems of considerable pathophysiological importance in the catabolism of fibrin deposits, as well as circulating soluble fibrin complexes, are located in cells of phagocytic potential, the polymorphonuclear leukocytes, and the monocytes-macrophages of the reticuloendothelial system. Soluble fibrin complexes (SFC) formed through either thrombin-fibrinogen interactions or limited proteolysis of noncrosslinked fibrin have been shown in several laboratories, including our own, to be removed from the circulation mainly by monocytes-macrophages of the reticuloendothelial system in the liver and spleen.[1-4] Our longstanding interest in SFC, which is demonstrable in large quantities in the circulation in clinical and experimental thrombotic states,[5] led us to the systematic exploration of the degradation of these macromolecules by intact macrophages and macrophage enzymes reported below.

MATERIALS AND METHODS

Proteins

Human fibrinogen, rabbit fibrinogen, plasminogen, and plasmin were purified and characterized as previously reported.[3, 6] SFC formed through limited plasmin proteolysis of noncrosslinked fibrin, "late fibrin degradation products," and "early and late fibrinogen degradation products" were prepared and characterized as previously reported.[3] Human thrombin was the generous gift of Dr. J. W. Fenton II, New York State Board of Health Laboratories, Albany, New York. Trasylol, 10,000 kallikrein inhibitor units (KIU)/ml, was purchased from FBA Pharmaceutical Company, New York, New York. Pepstatin A and elastin were purchased from Sigma, St. Louis, Missouri and leupeptin was obtained from the Protein Research Foundation, Osaka, Japan.

Synthetic Substrates

Benzoyl (Bz)-Arg-para-nitroanilide (pNA) and Acetyl-Tyr-ethyl ester (Ac-TyrOEt) were purchased from Sigma. Succinyl (Succ)-Ala$_3$-pNA was

568

purchased from Calbiochem. Bz-Arg-Gly-Phe-4-methoxy-β-naphthylamide (MNA), Bz-Ala-Arg-Arg-MNA and H_2N-Lys-Ala-MNA were synthesized and kindly supplied by Dr. E. L. Smithwick of the Lilly Research Laboratories. All other chemicals were of the highest purity available, usually reagent grade.

1. ^{125}I-labeled fibrinogen was prepared by the iodine monochloride technique.[7] The labeled product incorporated 0.5 atoms of iodine per molecule of protein. The final products contained 92–98% clottable radioiodine and contained no radiolabeled macromolecular aggregates, as determined by gel exclusion chromatography.

2. Gel exclusion chromatography was performed on Bio-Gel A5M (Bio-Rad) according to the method of Sachs and Painter,[8] as previously described.[3]

3. Sodium dodecyl sulphate polyacrylamide gel electrophoresis (SDS PAGE) was performed according to Weber and Osborn[9] or Laemli[10] under reducing and nonreducing conditions. Typically, in experiments to assess fibrinogen and fibrin degradation, ^{125}I-labeled fibrinogen was subjected to SDS PAGE. The gels were cut into segments according to the band patterns after completion of electrophoresis, staining, and electrical destaining. The radioactivity of each segment was expressed as a percentage of total gel radioactivity.

Animal Experiments

Male and female white rabbits weighing 2–2.5 kg were used. The general protocol has been reported previously.[3] Groups of six rabbits were given 100 mg (20 μCi) of ^{125}I-labeled soluble fibrin complexes at time 0 and individual groups were sacrificed at 1, 2½, 5, 12, 18, and 24 hr. After the rapid removal of the liver and spleen, nonextractable protein deposited in these organs was quantified by the method of Busch and Saldeen,[11] modified as previously reported.[3]

Intact Macrophage Studies

Rabbit alveolar macrophages were harvested from rabbits 2–3 weeks after the intravenous injection of 1 ml of complete Freund's adjuvant.[12, 13] The resulting preparations contain an almost pure preparation of monocytes-macrophages with only 1–3% contamination of PMN leukocytes and remain 92–97% viable at 24 hours, as determined by trypan blue exclusion.

SFC Adhesion to and Internalization by Macrophages

Immediately after harvesting, alveolar macrophages were washed twice in 1 cc ice cold saline and resuspended to 10^7 cells/ml in medium 199 with 20% fetal calf serum. ^{125}I-labeled SFC, fibrinogen, or fibrinogen-fibrin degradation products prepared and characterized as above were added to 1 ml aliquots of cells and mixtures incubated at 37° C for up to four hours. After incubation, one aliquot of cells was washed twice in ice cold saline and the cell pellet counted for residual radioactivity. Another aliquot of cells was centrifuged, the supernatant discarded, and the cell pellet resuspended in 1 ml of tissue culture medium containing 2 mg of trypsin and 2 mg of ribonuclease. After

30 min incubation at 37° C, the trypsinized cells were washed in two volumes of ice cold saline and the cell pellet was counted for radioactivity. In all experiments, blank tubes containing the appropriate ^{125}I-labeled proteins were incubated in 1 ml of tissue culture medium 199 plus 20% fetal calf serum without cells, washed, centrifuged, and counted in parallel with cell-containing tubes. Blank values representing nonspecific protein precipitation and/or adhesion were subtracted in all experiments.

Catabolism of SFC by Intact Macrophages

Freshly harvested rabbit alveolar macrophages (RAM) were washed twice in 1 cc ice cold saline and resuspended to 10^7 cells/cc in medium 199 with 20% fetal calf serum. One cubic centimeter cell aliquots were incubated with 100 μg ^{125}I-labeled SFC for 2 hr at 37° C to ensure maximal adhesion of SFC to rabbit alveolar macrophages. At 2 hr, the cells were washed twice in saline and resuspended in tissue culture medium 199—20% fetal calf serum. At this time, ^{125}I-labeled SFC adhering to the cells was quantified. Aliquots of cells were centrifuged and the supernatants analyzed at 2 hr plus 10 min, 1, 4, 16, 18, and 24 hr. The experiments compared macrophage catabolism of SFC in plasminogen-rich and plasminogen-free systems. In the plasminogen-rich system, SFC was prepared from rabbit plasminogen-rich fibrinogen.[14] In the plasminogen-free system, SFC were prepared from fibrinogen made plasminogen-free by lysine sepharose affinity chromatography.[15] Fetal calf serum, which contributes substantial quantities of plasminogen, was made plasminogen-free by the same technique. In a few experiments, fibrinogen was freed of factor XIII using the method of Mosesson and Finlayson.[16]

Cell-free supernatants were assayed for trichloroacetic acid soluble radiolabel. Bovine serum albumin was added to 5 mg/ml as a carrier, followed by equal volumes of 15% trichloroacetic acid. The distribution of cell-free supernatant radiolabel by molecular weight was analyzed by Bio-Gel A5M gel exclusion chromatography.[3] Results were expressed as a percentage of the total radiolabel applied to the columns appearing in individual fractions.

Subcellular Fractionation of Macrophages

Freshly harvested rabbit alveolar macrophages were washed and resuspended in Krebs-Ringer phosphate buffer to approximately 10^8 cells/cc. The cells were disrupted mechanically or through compression under nitrogen and rapid decompression. Subcellular fractions were obtained through differential centrifugation or sucrose gradient zonal centrifugation,[17] the latter procedure providing the highest yield and the highest purity of lysosomal granules. Macrophage lysosomes were disrupted through seven-fold freezing and thawing.

Characterization of Macrophage Lysosomal Fibrinolytic Activity

In standard experiments, 1 mg of plasminogen-free ^{125}I-labeled fibrinogen was incubated with lysosomal protein equivalent to 10^8 cells in 1 cc volumes. Plasminogen-free noncrosslinked fibrin was prepared by the addition of 10 units of highly purified thrombin to fibrinogen lysosomal incubation mixtures at time 0. Fibrinogen or fibrin-lysosome mixtures were incubated for up to 24 hr at 37° C and hydrolysis was monitored by SDS polyacrylamide gel electrophoresis under nonreducing and reducing conditions.[10] The use of ^{125}I labeled fibrinogen and fibrin made it possible to distinguish fibrinogen-derived proteins from lysosomal proteins and to arrive at semiquantitative estimates of hydrolysis rates. Fibrinogen coagulability of the incubation mixtures was estimated by thrombin clotting times. Thrombin (0.5 NIH units) was added to 0.5 ml of incubation mixture in both the absence and the presence of an additional 1.5 mg of purified fibrinogen.

Initial Purification of Macrophage Proteolytic Enzymes

Since the fibrinolytic activity upon subcellular fractionation was found to be not exclusive to the lysosomal fractions, the starting material for the purification of macrophage fibrinolytic enzymes was crude macrophage protein. Freshly harvested macrophages were suspended in 0.05 molar [2-(N-morpholino) ethanesulfonic acid], pH 5.3, 1 mM dithiothreitol (DTT), 1 mM ethylene (dinitrilo)tetraacetic acid (EDTA), and 0.2% triton X-100 and disrupted through freezing-thawing $\times$ 5. After centrifugation at 48,000 $\times$ g for 30 min, 50 ml of supernatant representing 1.7 g protein (as estimated by OD$_{280/260\,nm}$ measurements) was applied to a 5 $\times$ 100 cm Sephadex G-150 column equilibrated with the same buffer used for suspension of the macrophages, omitting only the triton X-100. Chromatography was performed at +4° C at a 60 ml/hr flow rate; 12 ml fractions were collected.

Fractions appearing between the second and third protein peak containing fibrinolytic activity (see Results) were pooled and dialyzed against 0.025 M acetate buffer, pH 4.6, containing 1 mM DTT and 1 mM EDTA, and applied to a 0.9 $\times$ 30 cm SP-Sephadex column equilibrated with the same buffer. The column was developed with starting buffer until OD$_{280}$ was 0, at which time 0.025 M acetate, 0.2 M NaCl, pH 4.6, containing DTT and EDTA, as above, was added. The two partially resolved peaks containing fibrinolytic activity (see Results) were further separated by gradient elution. The combined peaks were dialyzed against 0.05 M acetate buffer, pH 4.0, containing 1 mM EDTA and DTT, and applied to a 0.7 $\times$ 10 cm SP-Sephadex column equilibrated with the same buffer. The column was first developed with the starting buffer and when OD$_{280}$ readings had reached 0, a linear gradient was established using 150 ml of 0.05 M acetate buffer, pH 4.0, in one chamber and 150 ml of 0.05 M acetate, 0.4 M sodium chloride in the second chamber. Both buffers contained DTT and EDTA to 1 mM. Additional steps, which resulted in the complete separation of these two enzyme activities, will be reported elsewhere.

Fibrinolytic Assay for the Quantification of Macrophage Proteases

[125]I-labeled fibrinogen, 1.0 mg/ml, 0.3 ml, was incubated with 0.1 ml of fraction and the trichloroacetic acid (TCA)-soluble radiolabel was determined after the addition of 0.4 ml 15% TCA at time 0 and after 60 min of incubation. We defined here arbitrarily one fibrinolytic unit as 1% increase in TCA solubility over the one hour incubation period. For comparison, 1 international unit (IU) of plasmin equals 385 fibrinolytic units in this system.

Bovine pancreatic cathepsin B was purified and characterized by R. M. Van Frank.[18]

Assays for the Characterization of Macrophage Proteases

Casein plate assays for nonspecific protease activity and elastin plate assays for elastase-like activity were performed according to Schumacher and Schill.[19]

Neutral, trypsin-like activity was quantified with the synthetic substrate Bz-Arg-pNA, pH 7.8, according to Fritz *et al.*[20]

Chymotrypsin-like activity was determined against AcTyrOEt, pH 7.8, according to Schwert and Takanaka[21] or against substrate Bz-Arg-Gly-Phe-MNA, pH 7.8.[22]

Elastase-like activity was determined using the substrate Succ-Ala$_3$-pNA, pH 7.8, according to Bieth *et al.*[23]

Plasminogen activator activity was quantified using purified plasminogen and substrate S-2251 (Kabi, Mölndal, Sweden) as previously reported.[24]

Cathepsin D semiquantitative estimates were made using the casein plate technique[19] at pH 3.0 and was defined as that activity which caused hydrolysis at pH 3.0 and which was completely inhibited by pepstatin, 1 mg/ml. Cathepsin B was quantified using either the casein plate technique[19] at pH 6.0 or the synthetic substrate Bz-Ala-Arg-Arg-MNA at pH 6.0.[25]

Dipeptidyl aminopeptidase II and neutral aminopeptidases were quantified using the substrate H$_2$N-Lys-Ala-MNA at pH 5.0 and 7.8, respectively.[26]

RESULTS

The experiments depicted in FIGURE 1 demonstrate the *in vivo* spleen and liver uptake and release of ^{125}I-labeled SFC administered intravenously to rabbits. There is a sharp increase in the uptake of radiolabeled SFC up to 5–6 hours and a falloff thereafter, with essentially no radiolabel being demonstrable in either the liver or the spleen at 24 hr. These experiments suggest not only that the liver and spleen monocytes-macrophages are capable of effectively removing SFC from the circulation, as has previously been pointed out through a variety of experimental approaches,[1-4] but also that these phagocytic cells are capable of releasing these macromolecules, presumably in an extensively degraded form. To prove these points, our subsequent work involved the use of isolated rabbit alveolar macrophages. When standard quantities of ^{125}I-labeled SFC were incubated with a fixed number of freshly harvested rabbit alveolar macrophages and the cells were subsequently washed extensively and centrifuged at the designated time intervals, radiolabel firmly associated with the cells substantially increased with time for up to 4 hr, reaching peak values of 2.3 μg/10^7 cells (FIGURE 2). The lower part of FIGURE 2 depicts results for cells trypsinized subsequent to incubation with radiolabeled SFC. About 10% of the total cell-associated radiolabel or 200 ng/10^7 cells can be considered pinocytized and internalized after 4 hr incubation, since this much radiolabel was not removable by trypsin treatment. As illustrated in the experiments summarized in FIGURE 3, radiolabeled SFC adhered to and was pinocytized by rabbit alveolar macrophages to a significantly greater extent than either fibrinogen or a variety of well-characterized degradation products of fibrinogen and fibrin.

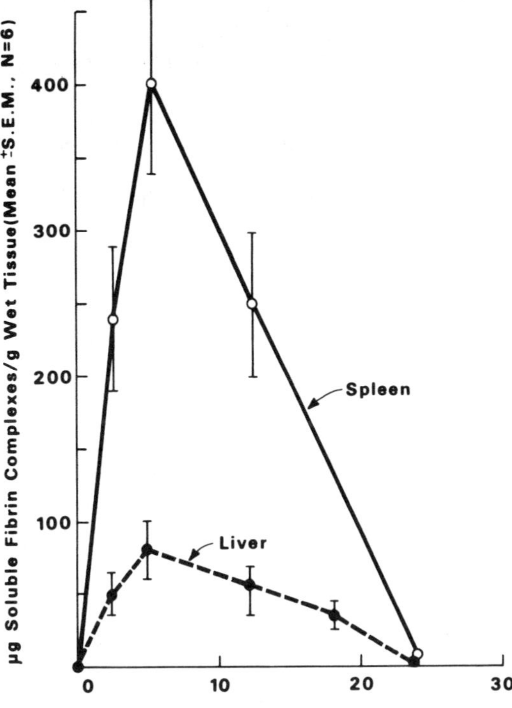

FIGURE 1. Spleen and liver uptake and clearance of ^{125}I SFC administered IV to rabbits. Each data point represents mean ± SEM of six rabbit experiments.

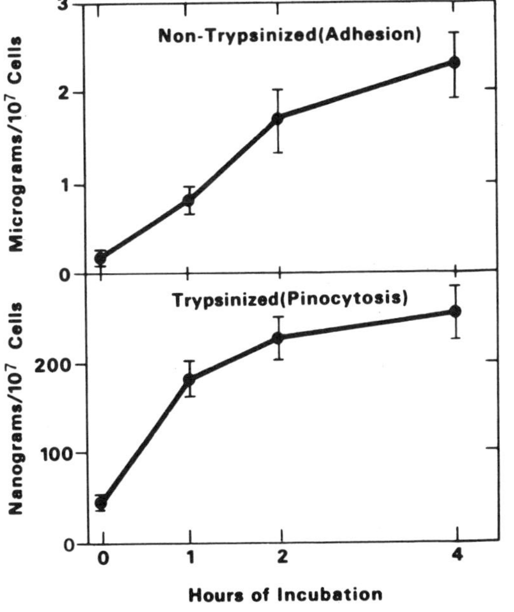

FIGURE 2. ^{125}I SFC adhering to and internalized by rabbit alveolar macrophages for up to 4 hr incubation.

We next addressed the question, are viable intact macrophages capable of digesting SFC and, if so, what would be the major enzymatic mechanisms? Unkeless and colleagues published data concluding that stimulated mouse peritoneal macrophages were capable of digesting fibrinogen and fibrin through the elaboration of plasminogen activator.[27] The following experiments aimed at testing this hypothesis. In the experiments illustrated in FIGURE 4, SFC was incubated with rabbit alveolar macrophages for 2 hr, at which time the cells were extensively washed to free them from radioactive protein not adhering to and not internalized by the cells. After resuspension of the cells in medium 199–20% fetal calf serum, at the designated time intervals up to 24 hr, aliquots of cells were centrifuged and cell-free supernatants analyzed for released radiolabel. One series of experiments studied a plasminogen-rich system and a second series of plasminogen-free system. The release of radio-

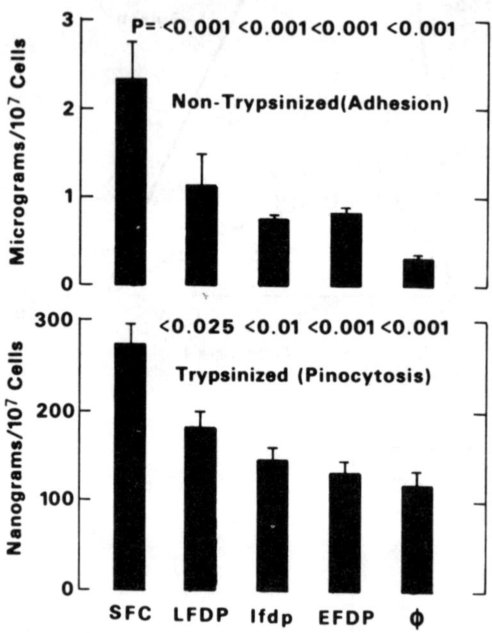

FIGURE 3. The adhesion to and internalization of soluble fibrin complexes (SFC), fibrinogen (ϕ), "early and late" fibrinogen degradation products (EFDP and LFDP), and "late" fibrin degradation products (lfdp) by rabbit alveolar macrophages.

label into the supernatant increases with time of incubation, reaching a maximum of 80–90% of the initial radiolabel adhering to the cells at 24 hr in both systems, plasminogen-rich and plasminogen-free. The rate of release of radiolabel from the macrophages does not differ significantly between plasminogen-rich and plasminogen-free systems.

The release of ^{125}I-labeled soluble fibrin complexes from rabbit alveolar macrophages was completely blocked by 1 mM iodacetamide for up to 4 hr, the time during which the cells remain >70% viable in the milieu of this metabolic inhibitor (FIGURE 5).

To further characterize the degradation products released during macrophage hydrolysis of SFC, we studied the trichloroacetic acid solubility and gel filtration behavior of the radiolabel of cell-free supernatants obtained after different periods of incubation. In the montage of Bio-Gel A5M chromato-

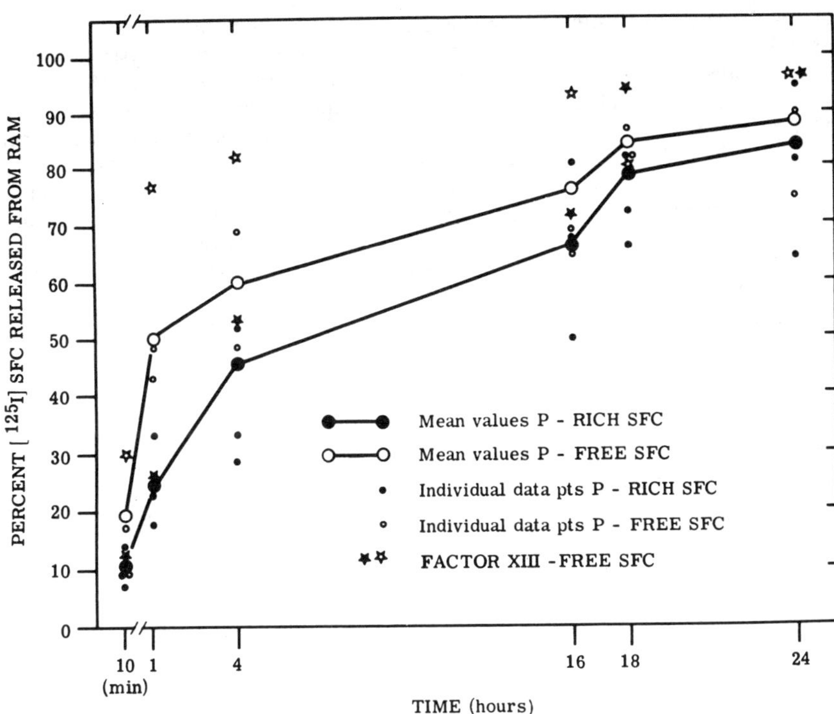

FIGURE 4. The release of radiolabel from [125I] SFC adhering to or internalized by macrophages. The figure compares the rate of release in plasminogen-rich and plasminogen-free systems.

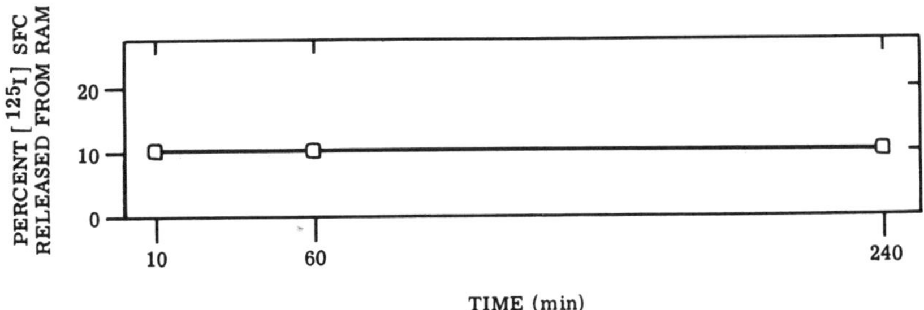

FIGURE 5. The inhibition of release of 125I-labeled SFC from rabbit alveolar macrophages by 1 mM iodoacetamide.

grams depicted in FIGURE 6, there is clear evidence that the increasing release of ^{125}I-radiolabel with time illustrated in FIGURE 4 reflects hydrolysis. Whereas SFC applied to rabbit alveolar macrophages is approximately 25% TCA soluble, the radiolabel released into the cell supernatant is 60% TCA soluble. The majority of the radiolabel elutes after the V_E for purified fibrinogen fragment E (M_r = approximately 40,000), irrespective of the total time of incubation. There appears to be no significant difference in the molecular weight distribution between SFC hydrolysis products in plasminogen-rich and plasminogen-free systems. In other experiments not shown here, gel chromatography on Sephadex G-100 showed these released degradation products to possess molecular weights of $\leq$20,000 daltons.

From these experiments, we concluded that plasminogen activator, although it may be present in stimulated rabbit alveolar macrophages, contributes little, if any, to macrophage catabolism of soluble fibrin. For these reasons, we entered the final phase of our work, which was aimed at fully characterizing the non-plasmin-mediated catabolic pathways of fibrinogen and noncrosslinked fibrin by macrophages. Initial experiments examining subcellular fractions of rabbit alveolar macrophages demonstrated that the fibrinogenolytic activity was concentrated in the lysosomal fractions, although significant activity was also present in the 400 × g pellet and 16,000 × g supernatant. Plasminogen-free fibrinogen (97–99% clottable) was used in all subsequent experiments. FIGURE 7 demonstrates an experiment in which 1 mg of fibrinogen was incubated with lysosomal protein equivalent to 10^7 cells. Thrombin clotting times were

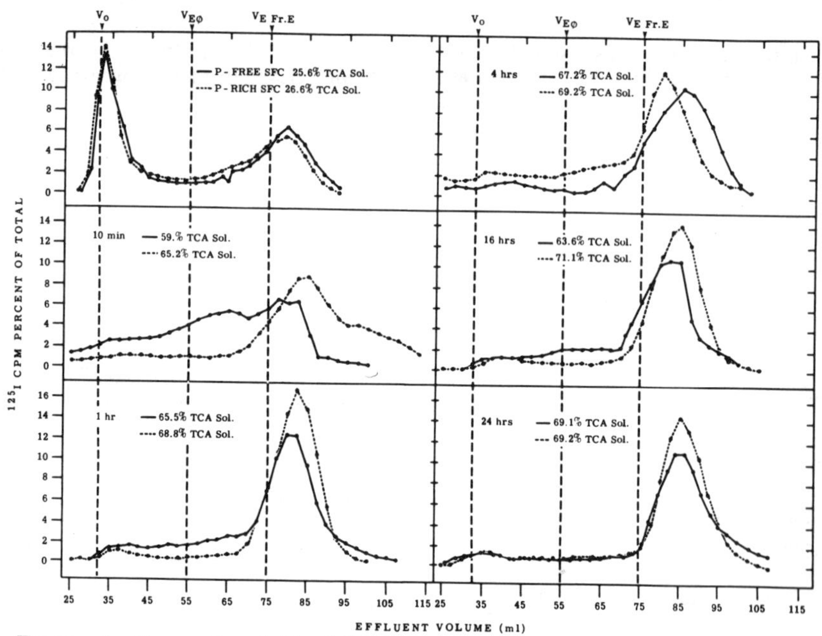

FIGURE 6. Composite of Bio-Gel A5M chromatograms of cell-free supernatants representing degraded [^{125}I] SFC released with time from rabbit alveolar macrophages.

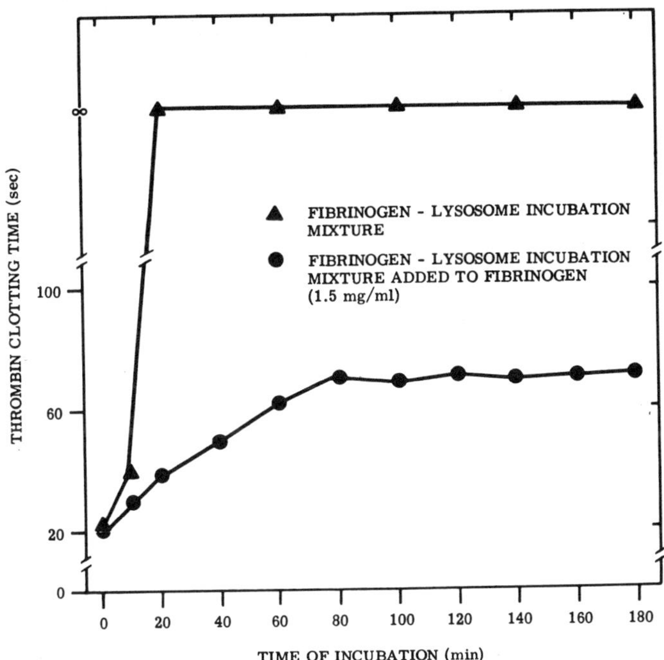

FIGURE 7. Thrombin clottability and anticoagulant activity of fibrinogen (1 mg/ml) incubated with crude macrophage lysosomal protein, pH 7.3, 37° C.

performed in the absence and presence of additional purified fibrinogen at the stated time intervals. Fibrinogen lysosome incubation mixtures became incoagulable after 20 min and progressively inhibited normal fibrinogen to fibrin conversion, reaching a plateau of inhibitory activity after 80 min incubation.

To further characterize this fibrinogenolytic activity, ^{125}I-labeled fibrinogen or noncrosslinked fibrin was incubated with lysosomal protein for 3 hr at pH 7.3 or 6.0 (FIGURE 8). Incubation mixtures were electrophoresed on 6% SDS polyacrylamide gels and the distribution of radioactivity was assessed after sectioning the gels. Radiolabeled protein, indicated by the stars in FIGURE 8, was found almost exclusively in the high molecular weight regions of the gels, accounting in all instances for 95% of the total gel radioactivity. The heavy bands labeled A in the first four gels represent unlabeled albumin added in some experiments for stabilization of radiolabeled fibrinogen. At pH 7.3, there was only a modest reduction in staining intensity and molecular weight of fibrinogen and fibrin after 3 and 24 hr incubation (not shown); there was no further reduction in the staining intensity or molecular size of fibrinogen or fibrin degradation products. At pH 7.3, after 3 hr, the radiolabel of high molecular weight bands represented approximately 60% of the original time 0 high molecular weight radiolabel. In contrast, at pH 6.0 after 3 hr incubation, residual radiolabel of faintly staining residual high molecular weight bands was 14% for fibrinogen and 27% for fibrin compared to the time 0 radiolabel. Thus, macrophage lysosomal enzymes hydrolyze fibrinogen and fibrin more effectively at pH 6.0 than at 7.3.

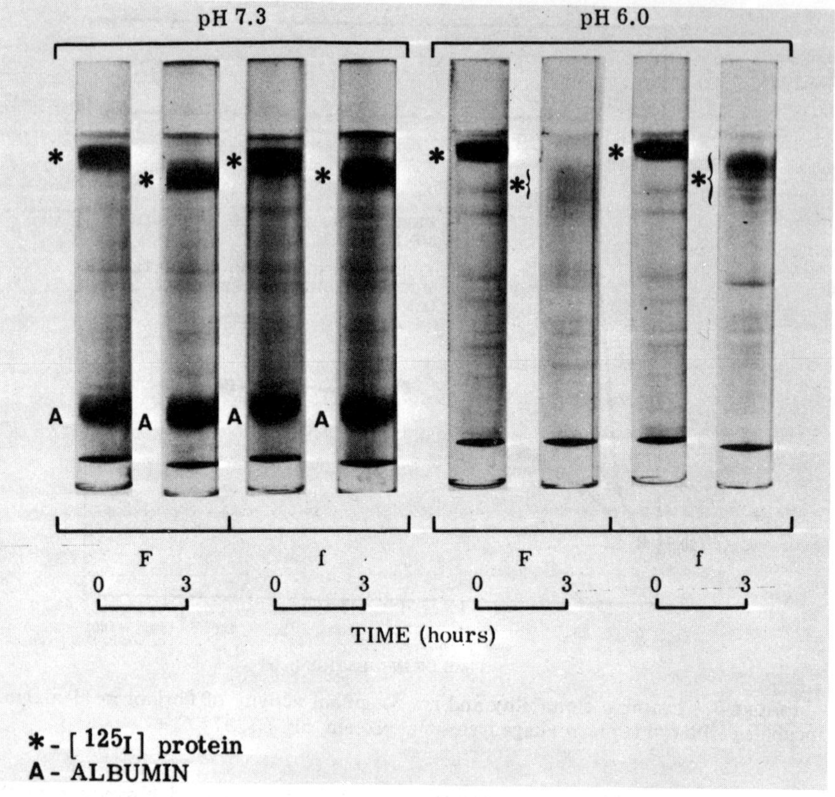

FIGURE 8. SDS PAGE (6% nonreducing conditions) of mixtures of ^{125}I-labeled fibrinogen or noncrosslinked fibrin with macrophage lysosomal protein for 3 hr at pH 7.3 and 6.0. For details, see text.

Hydrolysis of fibrinogen and fibrin was further enhanced in the presence of 1 m*M* DTT and 4 m*M* EDTA (FIGURE 9). Shown in this figure are the SDS gels of mixtures of fibrinogen and lysosomal enzymes incubated for up to 3 hr at pH 6.0 in the presence of DTT and EDTA. Residual radiolabel of the faint high molecular weight bands after 2 hr was 30% of time 0 radiolabel; after 3 hr, no radiolabel was demonstrable in any area of the gel except the band corresponding to the tracking dye. Thus, macrophage lysosomal enzymes hydrolyze fibrinogen and fibrin into peptides too small for detection on 6% SDS gels. The control gel shown represents fibrinogen incubated with DTT and EDTA. The single sharp band in this nonreduced gel indicates that DTT at this low concentration does not cause cleavage of fibrinogen through reduction of disulfide bonds.

TABLE I briefly summarizes a survey of the enzyme activities of rabbit alveolar macrophage lysosomal proteases, as estimated in standard natural and synthetic substrate assays. Macrophage lysosomes contain only trace neutral protease, trypsin-like, chymotrypsin-like, or elastase-like activities. Plasminogen activator activity was not demonstrable. As expected because of the ubiquitous nature of this protease, cathepsin D was demonstrable in significant quantities.

The most striking activity resided in a protease with a pH optimum of 6.0, which showed extremely high activity against the synthetic substrate Bz-Ala-Arg-Arg-MNA, which increased an additional ten-fold in the presence of DTT and EDTA and which was completely blocked by iodoacetamide and by leupeptin. Synthetic substrate assays also revealed the presence of at least two aminopeptidases, dipeptidyl aminopeptidase II with a pH optimum 5.0 and neutral aminopeptidase activity. The characteristics of the major macrophage enzyme, its pH optimum of 6.0, its high activity against the synthetic substrate Bz-Ala-Arg-Arg-MNA, the enhancement of its activity by thiol compounds and chelators of divalent cations, and the inhibition profile for the crude lysosomal enzyme are all identical to the properties of purified cathepsin B reported by Barrett and coworkers, among others.[28] In addition, we purified cathepsin B to homogeneity from bovine pancreas [18] and found that this purified enzyme degraded fibrinogen almost as effectively as did the lysosomal protease mixture. We therefore initially decided to purify and characterize macrophage cathepsin B.

An initial and very effective purification step was Sephadex G-150 gel filtration of crude macrophage protein (FIGURE 10). Fibrinolytic activity was found in the initial peak eluting with the void volume for the column and was

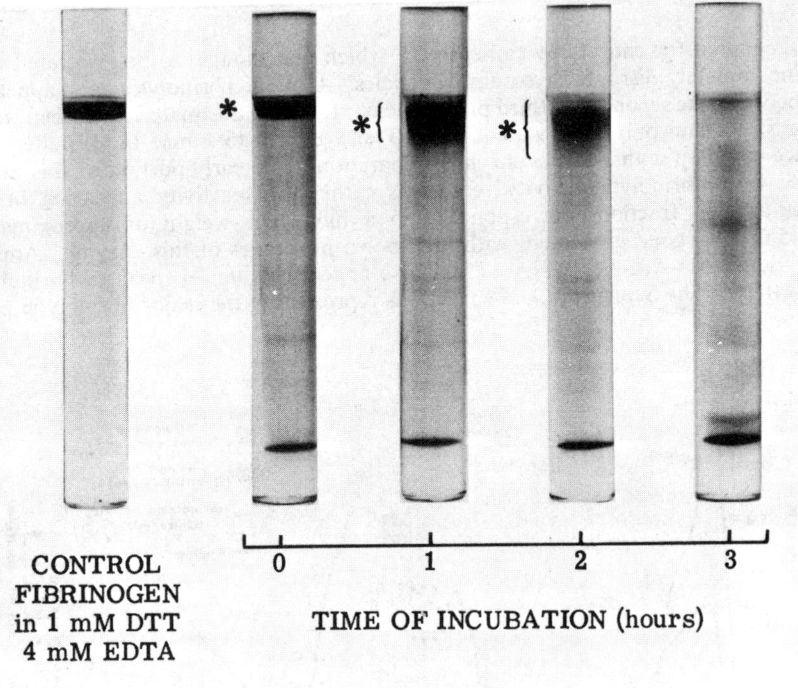

FIGURE 9. Enhancement of hydrolysis of fibrinogen and fibrin at pH 6.0 in the presence of 1 mM DTT and 4 mM EDTA. For details, see text.

TABLE 1

CHARACTERIZATION OF MACROPHAGE LYSOSOMAL PROTEASES

Enzyme Activity		Substrates
Trypsin-like	0	Casein plate, pH 7.6
	+	Bz-Arg-pNA, pH 7.8
Chymotrypsin-like	0	Ac-TyrOEt, pH 7.8
	+	Bz-Arg-Gly-Phe-MNA, pH 7.8
Elastase	0	Elastin, pH 7.8
	±	Succ-Ala$_3$-pNA, pH 7.8
Plasminogen activator	0	Plasminogen
Cathepsin D	++	Casein plate, pH 3.0
Cathepsin B	+++	Casein plate, pH 6.0
		Bz-Ala-Arg-Arg-MNA, pH 6.0
Dipeptidyl aminopeptidase II	++	H$_2$N-Lys-Ala-MNA, pH 5.0
Aminopeptidases	+++	H$_2$N-Lys-Ala-MNA, pH 7.0, 7.8, & 8.5

accounted for entirely by cathepsin D, which was thought to be associated with incompletely disrupted lysosomal particles. A major fibrinolytic peak appeared between the second and third protein peak. Initially, this material was extremely unstable and only after we added DTT and EDTA to 1 mM to all buffers did we come up with a stable enzyme preparation. The early portion of this major peak of fibrinolytic activity represents cathepsin D activity appearing in the effluent in fractions corresponding to a molecular weight of approximately 45,000, in good agreement with the known properties of this enzyme. Amidolytic Bz-Ala-Arg-Arg-MNA activity also appears within this peak of fibrinolytic activity. The Sephadex G-150 fractions representing the major fibrinolytic peak

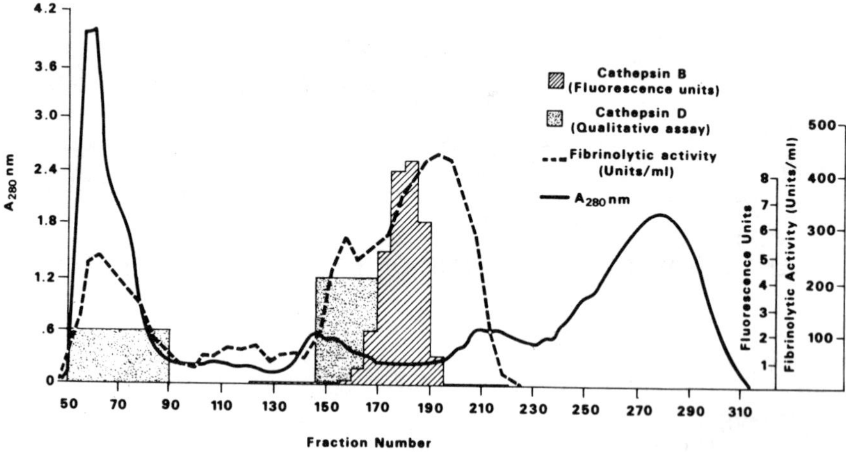

FIGURE 10. Sephadex G-150 gel filtration of crude macrophage protein, pH 5.3, 0.15 M. For details, see text.

were pooled and subjected to batch chromatography on SP-Sephadex (FIGURE 11). At 0.2 *M* ionic strength, the bulk of the protein came off in a sharply defined peak, but the fibrinolytic activity emerged in two partially resolved peaks.

Further resolution was obtained on SP-Sephadex, using a linear ionic strength gradient at pH 4.0 (FIGURE 12). The amidolytic activity against Bz-Ala-Arg-Arg-MNA characteristic of cathepsin B emerges with the protein

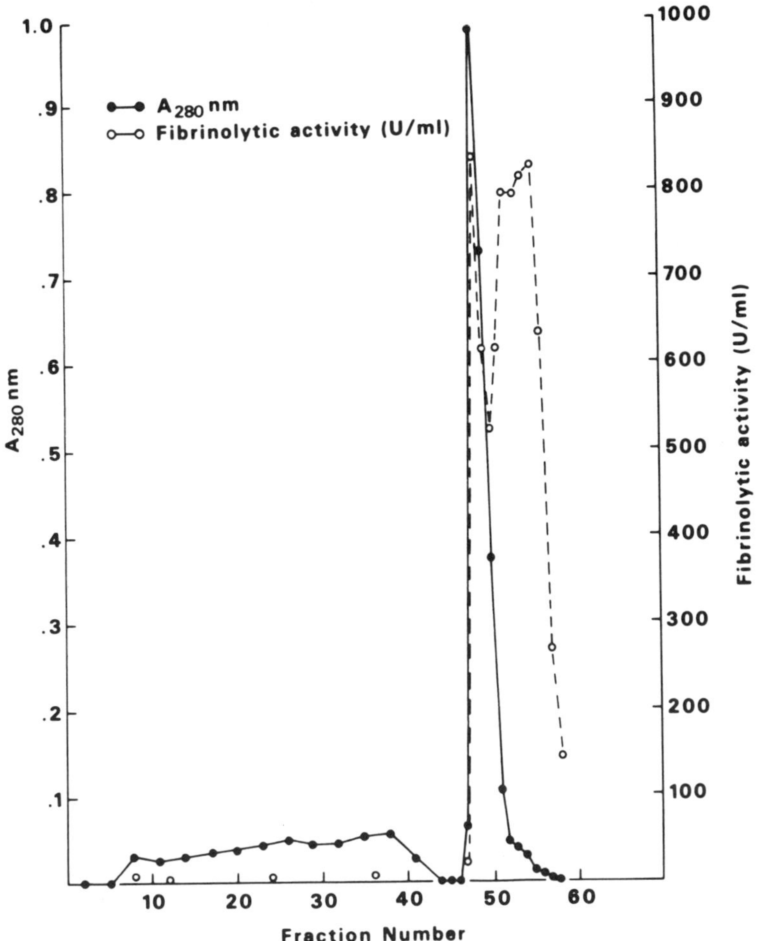

FIGURE 11. Batch chromatography, pH 4.6, on SP-Sephadex of the major fibrinolytic peak obtained from Sephadex G-150 gel filtration.

peak, which also exhibits substantial fibrinolytic activity. However, the major peak of fibrinolytic activity appears at the tail end of the protein and amidolytic activity peak. After additional steps (to be published), these two enzymes were completely separated. TABLE II summarizes the data for the two enzymes that we have collected to this point; we are sure that one of the enzymes represents cathepsin B and we have named the other macrophage protease X (MPX)

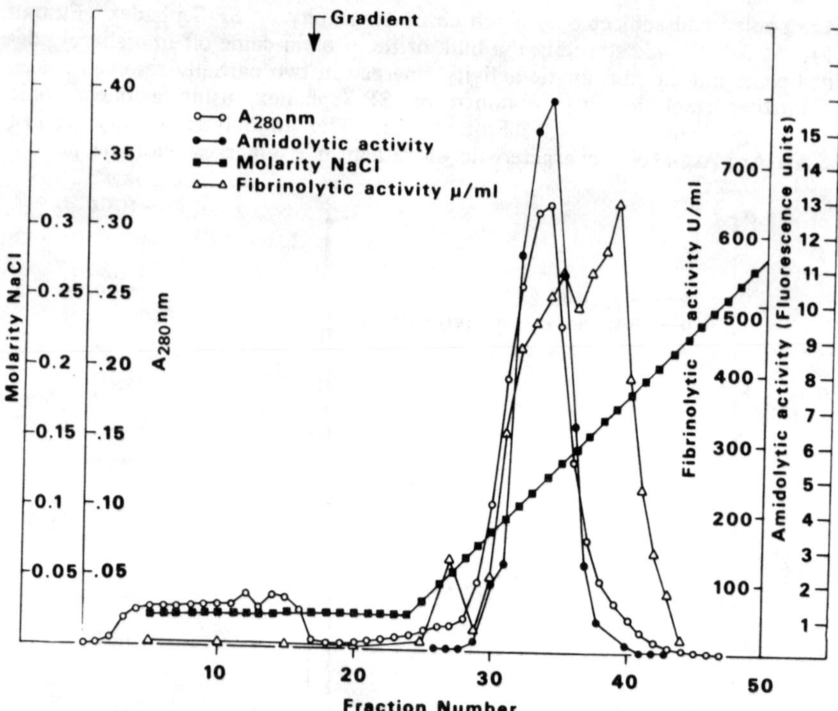

FIGURE 12. SP-Sephadex gradient (0.05–0.4 M NaCl) elution, pH 4.0, for further separating cathepsin B from MPX.

TABLE 2

PARTIAL CHARACTERIZATION OF MACROPHAGE CATHEPSIN B AND MPX

	Cathepsin B	MPX
M_R	26,000	24,000
pH optimum	6.5	5.5
Amidolytic activity against Bz-Ala-Arg-Arg-MNA	Yes	No
Activity enhanced by reducing and chelating agents	Yes	No
Inhibition of fibrinolytic activity by:		
DFP (10^{-3} M)	5%	4%
Trasylol (100 KIU)	11%	4%
εACA (10^{-3} M)	2%	4%
Leupeptin (1 mg/ml)	98%	97%
Pepstatin (1 mg/ml)	24%	27%
Iodoacetamide (10^{-3} M)	99%	100%

for lack of a better name at present. Their molecular weights are similar, 26,000 for cathepsin B and 24,000 for the unidentified protease. Their pH optima are slightly different, pH 6.5 for cathepsin B and 5.5 for MPX. Cathepsin B has potent amidolytic activity against Ala-Arg-Arg-MNA, while the unidentified protease has no amidolytic activity against this substrate. In all other respects, the two enzymes are similar, behaving like typical sulfhydryl proteases. Reducing agents and chelators of divalent cations are necessary for full expression of activity for both enzymes. They are inhibited only slightly by typical serine protease inhibitors such as diisopropyl fluorophosphate (DFP) and trasylol. They are both strongly inhibited by leupeptin, only minimally inhibited by pepstatin, and completely inhibited by iodoacetamide, a typical sulfhydryl inhibitor. Finally, neither enzyme has plasminogen activator activity, nor are they inhibited by ϵ-aminocaproic acid (ϵACA). The specific activity of the unidentified enzyme is 44,000 fibrinolytic units/mg protein, corresponding to approximately 112 plasmin CTA units. In the experiments depicted in FIGURE 13, 1 mg of fibrinogen was digested by 50 units of either enzyme and, at the designated time intervals, the digest mixtures were subjected

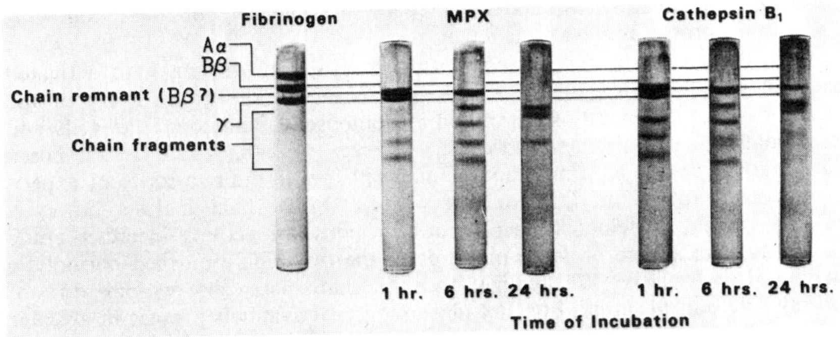

FIGURE 13. SDS PAGE (10% reducing conditions) of fibrinogen incubated for 1, 6, and 24 hr with purified cathepsin B and purified MPX. For details, see text.

to SDS gel electrophoresis under reducing conditions. Both enzymes extensively degrade fibrinogen according to very similar patterns. After 1 hr incubation, there were no intact A chains left, the Bβ chain was partly converted into a lower molecular weight chain fragment approximately 6,000 daltons lighter than the normal Bβ chain, and the staining intensity of the γ chain was sharply reduced, indicating significant proteolysis of that part of the fibrinogen molecule early in the game. After 6 and 24 hr, there were no demonstrable intact chains left and the only discrete band was the Bβ chain remnant observed early during proteolysis.

DISCUSSION

Not only did our initial *in vivo* observations confirm older reports showing that monocytes-macrophages of the reticuloendothelial system of the spleen and liver readily remove SFC from the circulation, but they also added new quantitative information regarding the rapid rate of catabolism of SFC by macrophages. We next noted that SFC readily adhere to and are pinocytized by macrophages and that they are effectively catabolized in those cell systems which hydrolyze these macromolecular aggregates into low molecular weight degradation products. Our observations differed markedly from the findings reported by Unkeless et al.,[27] in that our experiments demonstrated no role for plasminogen activator, which, according to Unkeless and colleagues, represents the major macrophage fibrin-degrading mechanism. The differences between these two series and observation are not completely explained, although several theoretical possibilities can be raised. It is possible that alveolar and peritoneal macrophages could possess different proteolytic enzyme spectra. It is well known that alveolar and peritoneal macrophages differ metabolically, the former cell deriving most of its energy from aerobic and the latter from anaerobic metabolism. To the best of our knowledge, however, no systematic analysis of the lysosomal proteases of these two cell systems has been performed to date. Unkeless et al. observed that plasminogen activator was elaborated by stimulated but not by unstimulated macrophages. The difference between the stimulated and the completely unstimulated state of macrophages is difficult to establish. We presume that the macrophage population harvested in our experiments was significantly stimulated, since these cells were obtained following the IV injection of Freund's adjuvant.

In indirect support for the contention that we are dealing with activated macrophages, we can point to histological observations of the lungs of the rabbits which showed diffuse granulomas composed of mononuclear cells and occasionally giant multinucleated cells. However, we cannot rule out the possibility that the degree of stimulation of macrophages in the two series of experiments could explain the different observations. In the final analysis, however, we were unable to demonstrate plasminogen activator activity in either crude lysosomal macrophage protease mixtures or the two highly purified fibrinolytic enzyme preparations. We realize, though, that these observations do not entirely rule out the possibility that plasminogen activator is present in alveolar macrophage lysosomal granules. Plasminogen activator could be present, but other enzymes capable of degrading and inactivating plasminogen used in the assay system could obscure the presence of plasminogen activators. In very recent experiments, to be published elsewhere, we found no plasminogen activator activity using the synthetic substrate S-2444 (L-Pyroglu-Gly-Arg-pNA, HCl). Thus, our final conclusion at this time is that the macrophage preparations used in our experiments contained undetectable levels of plasminogen activator.

Our attempts at purifying cathepsin B resulted in two surprising discoveries. First, it was unexpected that cathepsin B would remain stable only after the addition of DTT and EDTA to all buffers employed during purification. These observations are in sharp contrast to the observations made by Barrett, which indicate that cathepsin B, in the course of purification, becomes unstable in the presence of thiol reagents, presumably as a consequence of self-degradation.[28] The differences between Barrett's and our own observations are not clear at this time. Second, we made the unexpected discovery that macrophages contain, in addition to cathepsin B, another sulfhydryl enzyme closely related to but not identical with cathepsin B. That the unidentified enzyme of very high fibrinolytic activity is not an isozyme of cathepsin B is clearly established by the observation that the unidentified enzyme possesses no amidolytic activity against the substrate Bz-Ala-Arg-Arg-MNA. The unidentified enzyme has characteristics in common with and could be identical with a sulfhydryl protease described by Kirschke *et al.* and termed cathepsin L.[29] Cathepsin L was described by these authors as being strongly inhibited by leupeptin, like the unidentified protease in our studies. It is an exceptionally potent protease against natural substrates like azo-casein and glucagon but possesses no significant amidolytic activity against Bz-DL-Arg-2-naphthylamide or Bz-Arg-OEt. However, the final proof of the identity of our macrophage derived enzyme with cathepsin L purified from rat liver lysosomes is not available at this time.

Our studies conclusively show that rabbit alveolar macrophage lysosomal enzymes, most notably two closely related sulfhydryl proteases, are capable of degrading fibrinogen and fibrin via a unique, non-plasmin-mediated pathway. Degradation of fibrinogen and fibrin by macrophage enzymes is distinct and different from that reported for granulocytes by Plow and Edgington as being mediated by chymotrypsin-like and elastase-like neutral proteases.[30] Cellular catabolism of fibrin and SFC following different pathways in monocytes-macrophages and PMN leukocytes supplement, and may be as relevant in physiology and pathophysiology as, the classical humoral plasmin-mediated pathway. The quantitative contribution of cellular, as opposed to humoral, fibrinogen-fibrin catabolism clearly needs to be established.

SUMMARY

Intravenously administered [^{125}I] soluble fibrin complexes arising either from limited thrombin proteolysis of fibrinogen (F) or limited plasmin proteolysis of noncrosslinked fibrin (f) rapidly accumulate in the reticuloendothelial systems of the spleen and liver in rabbits. However, after 24 hr, the radiolabel was no longer demonstrable in those organs. [^{125}I] SFC adhered to and was pinocytized by rabbit alveolar macrophages (RAM) to a significantly greater extent than F and plasmin hydrolysis products of F or f. Incubation of [^{125}I] SFC adhering to intact RAM resulted in the liberation of fragments of $M_r \leq$ 20,000. SFC hydrolysis in these systems was progressive with time and 80–90% complete in 24 hr. The rate of SFC hydrolysis by intact RAM was no different in plasminogen-rich and plasminogen-free systems. Thus, under our experimental conditions, we were unable to confirm the observations by Unkeless *et al.* that stimulated macrophages hydrolyze F and f through the elaboration of plasminogen activator. RAM fibrinolytic activity was concentrated in the lysosomal fraction. Crude RAM lysosomal protein readily digested F and f at pH 6.0 but not at pH 7.3. The activity was enhanced by EDTA and DTT was inhibited by iodoacetamide and leupeptin but not by diisopropylfluorophosphate, pepstatin, trasylol, or ε-aminocaproic acid. Fractionation of crude RAM protein, using 1 mM DTT and 1 mM EDTA in all buffers, by Sephadex G-150 gel filtration followed by stepwise and gradient elution SP-Sephadex chromatography at pH 4.6 and 4.0 respectively, as the major steps resulted in the purification of two enzymes, one that had all the characteristics of cathepsin B and one that differed from cathepsin B in that it did not possess the characteristic amidolytic activity of this enzyme. The unidentified cathepsin B–like sulfhydryl protease was of high specific activity (approximately 112 plasmin IU/mg). Thus, macrophage lysosomal enzymes degrade F and f via a unique nonplasmin-mediated pathway involving, most prominently, cathepsin B and a cathepsin B–like enzyme. Macrophage catabolism of F and f is different from that of PMN leukocytes reported to be mediated by chymotrypsin-like and elastase-like neutral proteases. Cellular, particularly macrophage, catabolism of F and f supplement, and may be as relevant in pathophysiology as, the classical plasmin-mediated humoral pathway.

REFERENCES

1. LEE, L. 1962. Reticuloendothelial clearance of circulating fibrin in the pathogenesis of the generalized Schwartzman reaction. J. Exp. Med. **115:** 1065.
2. LEE, L. & R. T. MCCLUSKEY. 1962. Immunohistochemical demonstration of the reticuloendothelial clearance of circulating fibrin aggregates. J. Exp. Med. **116:** 611.
3. GUREWICH, V., R. WETMORE, A. NOWAK, et al. 1974. The fate of soluble fibrin monomer in relation to intravascular fibrin formation and degradation in rabbits. Blood **44:** 723.
4. CHANG, M. L. & N. U. BANG. 1977. Biological behavior of higher molecular weight products of fibrinolysis. J. Lab. Clin. Med. **90:** 216.
5. BANG, N. U. & M. L. CHANG. 1974. Soluble fibrin complexes. Sem. Thromb. Hemostas. **1:** 91.
6. HANSEN, M. S., N. U. BANG, R. D. BARTON & L. E. MATTLER. 1975. Enhancement of blood coagulation by soluble fibrin complexes. J. Exp. Med. **141:** 944.
7. IZZO, J. L., W. F. BALE, M. J. IZZO, et al. 1964. High specific activity labeling of insulin with ^{125}I. J. Biol. Chem. **239:** 3743.
8. SACHS, D. H. & E. PAINTER. 1972. Improved flow rates with porous sephadex gels. Science **175:** 781.
9. WEBER, K. & M. OSBORN. 1969. The reliability of molecular weight determinations by dodecyl sulfate polyacrylamide gel electrophoresis. J. Biol. Chem. **244:** 4406.
10. LAEMLI, M. K. 1970. Cleavage of structural proteins during the assembly of the head of bacteriophage T4. Nature (London) **227:** 680.
11. BUSCH, C. & T. SALDEEN. 1973. Amount of fibrin in different organs after intravenous, intraportal, and intraaortal injection of thrombin in the rat. Thromb. Diath. Haemorrh. **29:** 87.
12. MOORE, R. D. & M. D. SCHOENBERG. 1964. The response of histiocytes and macrophages in the lungs of rabbits injected with Freund's adjuvant. Brit. J. Exp. Pathol. **45:** 488.
13. MYRVIK, O. N., E. S. LEAKE & B. FARISS. 1967. Studies on pulmonary alveolar macrophages from the normal rabbit: a technique to procure them in a high state of purity. J. Immunol. **86:** 128.
14. REGOECZI, E. & B. A. STANNARD. 1969. In vivo behavior of frozen and freeze-dried fibrinogen and of that prepared from outdated blood. Biochim. Biophys. Acta **181:** 287.
15. SUMMARIA, L., L. ARZADIN, P. BERNABE & K. C. ROBINS. 1973. Studies on the isolation of the multiple molecular forms of human plasminogen and plasmin by isoelectric focusing methods. J. Biol. Chem. **248:** 2984.
16. MOSESSON, M. W. & J. S. FINLAYSON. 1963. Biochemical and chromatographic studies of certain activities associated with human fibrinogen preparations. J. Clin. Invest. **42:** 747.
17. VAN FRANK, R. M. & I. S. JOHNSON. 1972. Fractionation by zonal centrifugation of brains of normal rats and rats treated with morphine. Life Sci. **11:** 365.
18. VAN FRANK, R. M. To be published.
19. SCHUMACHER, G. F. V. & W.-B. SCHILL. 1972. Radial diffusion in gel for micro determination of enzymes. II. Plasminogen activator, elastase and nonspecific proteases. Anal. Biochem. **48:** 9.

20. FRITZ, H., G. HARTWICH & E. WERLE. 1966. Über Proteaseinhibitoren, I. Isolierung und Charakterisierung des Trypsininhibitors aus Pankreasgewebe und Pankreasseikret vom Hund. Hoppe-Seyler's Z. Physiol. Chem. **345:** 150.
21. SCHWERT, G. W. & Y. TAKANAKA. 1955. A spectrophotometric determination of trypsin and chymotrypsin. Biochem. Biophys. Acta **16:** 570.
22. BURCK, P. J. & E. L. SMITHWICK. To be published.
23. BIETH, J., B. SPEISS & C. G. WERMUTH. 1974. The synthesis and analytical use of a highly sensitive and convenient substrate of elastase. Biochem. Med. **11:** 350.
24. MATTLER, L. E. & N. U. BANG. 1977. Serine protease specificity for peptide chromogenic substrates. Thromb. Haemost. **38:** 776.
25. SMITH, R. E. & R. M. VAN FRANK. 1975. The use of amino acid derivatives of 4-methoxy-β-naphthylamine for assay and subcellular localization of tissue proteinases. *In.* Lysosomes in Biology and Pathology. J. T. Dingle & R. T. Dean, Eds. Vol. 4. North-Holland Publishing Company. Amsterdam, New York, Oxford.
26. MCDONALD, J. K., F. H. LEIBACK, R. E. GINDELAND & S. ELLIS. 1968. Purification of dipeptidyl aminopeptidase II (dipeptidyl aryl amindase II) of the anterior pituitary gland. Peptidase and dipeptide esterase activities. J. Biol. Chem. **243:** 4143.
27. UNKELESS, J. C., S. GORDON & E. REICH. 1974. Secretion of plasminogen activator by stimulated macrophages. J. Exp. Med. **139:** 834.
28. BARRETT, A. J. 1977. Cathepsin B and other thiol proteinases. *In.* Proteinases in Mammalian Cells and Tissues. A. J. Barrett, Ed. North-Holland Publishing Company. Amsterdam, New York, Oxford.
29. KIRSCHKE, H., J. LANGNER, B. WIEDERANDERS, S. ANSORGE, P. BOHLEY & U. BROGHAMMER. 1976. Intrazellularer Proteinabbau. VII. Kathepsin L und H: Zwei neue Proteinasen aus Rattenleberlysosomen. Acta Biol. Med. Ger. **35:** 285.
30. PLOW, E. F. & T. S. EDGINGTON. 1975. An alternative pathway for fibrinolysis. I. The cleavage of fibrinogen by leukocyte proteases at physiologic pH. J. Clin. Invest. **56:** 30.

PLASMIN AND PLASMINOGEN ACTIVATORS: KINETICS, AND KINETICS OF PLASMINOGEN ACTIVATION

Kenneth C. Robbins, Robert C. Wohl, and Louis Summaria

Michael Reese Research Foundation
Chicago, Illinois 60616

Departments of Medicine and Pathology
Pritzker School of Medicine
University of Chicago
Chicago, Illinois 60637

INTRODUCTION

The human blood fibrinolytic system *in vivo* is regulated primarily by activation of plasminogen, a circulating plasma zymogen, to plasmin by one or more activators found in the plasma and the vascular endothelium. Plasmin, a proteolytic enzyme, is regulated in the blood by its interaction with the plasma α_2-plasmin inhibitor to form enzymatically inactive, irreversible, complexes that are rapidly eliminated. Fibrin and thrombus formation probably accelerate plasminogen activation. The naturally occurring plasminogen activators found in plasma and tissues appear to be serine proteases and will activate plasminogen to plasmin by peptide-bond cleavage. A single molecular event is involved in the activation of plasminogen to plasmin, and, in isolated systems, it is the primary cleavage of the Arg_{560}-Val peptide bond in the enzymatically inactive zymogen monomer to form an active two-chain enzyme with two interchain disulfide bonds. Since enzymatic reactions in plasma operate by kinetic principles, it is essential that we understand the kinetic behavior of plasmin and plasminogen activators, and the kinetic parameters of plasminogen activation both in isolated systems and in the plasma milieu. Since native plasma and vascular endothelial cell plasminogen activators are not readily available, we have used highly purified human urinary urokinase(s) and streptokinase, obtained from culture filtrates of hemolytic streptococci, to develop the methodology to study plasminogen activation. Other types of activators were also studied to develop the concept of physiological activation in soluble systems.

PLASMIN KINETICS

Various forms of human plasmin can be prepared and have been isolated and studied. They are Glu_1-plasmin, Lys_{77}-plasmin, Val_{442}-plasmin, and the plasmin-derived Val_{561}-light(B) chain (Val_{561}-plasmin). The active center is found in the COOH-terminal light(B) chain portion of the enzyme. The form of plasmin generated in purified activation mixtures will depend upon the nature of the zymogen form, the ratio of zymogen to activator, the pH, temperature, the presence or absence of glycerol, the presence and concentration of lysine and/or ϵ-aminocaproic acid, and the presence or absence of a plasmin inhibitor and its relative effectiveness and reversibility.

588

Plasmin is a serine protease with trypsinlike specificity. It cleaves proteins and peptides at arginyl and lysyl peptide bonds and basic amino acid esters and amides. The enzyme has a preference for lysyl peptide bonds. The active site can be readily titrated with *p*-nitrophenyl-*p'*-guanidinobenzoate to determine molarity of enzyme in solution. One can also use inhibitors like Trasylol, or the basic pancreatic trypsin inhibitor, or the α_2-plasmin inhibitor, to titrate active enzyme in solution.

In our studies on the steady-state kinetic parameters of plasmin, N^α-Cbz-L-lysine-*p*-nitrophenyl ester was used as a substrate at pH 6.0 and 30° C,[1] and H-D-valyl-L-leucyl-L-lysyl-*p*-nitroanilide was used as a substrate at pH 7.4 and 37° C.[2] At pH 6.0 and 30° C, Glu_1-plasmin and Lys_{77}-plasmin gave similar apparent Michaelis constants, K_m, ~14 μM, and similar catalytic rate constants, k_{cat}, ~22 s^{-1}. At pH 7.4 and 37° C, these two enzyme species, and Val_{442}-plasmin, also gave similar K_m values, ~250 μM, and k_{cat} values, ~25 s^{-1}; the K_m values being more than 20-fold higher at pH 7.4 when compared to pH 6.0, but with different substrates and also different temperatures. Val_{561}-plasmin gave K_m values of ~83 μM and ~1260 μM, and k_{cat} values of ~2 s^{-1} and ~15 s^{-1}, at pH 6.0 and pH 7.4, respectively.

PLASMINOGEN ACTIVATOR KINETICS

Streptokinase

The interaction of the various plasminogen and plasmin species with stoichiometric amounts of streptokinase (SK) generates equimolar complexes that are now plasminogen activators. At pH 6.0 and 30° C, on the ester substrate,[1] the zymogen-SK and enzyme-SK activator species gave different K_m values of ~19 μM and ~33 μM, respectively, but similar k_{cat} values of about 22 s^{-1}. At pH 7.4 and 37° C on the amide substrate,[2] these same zymogen-SK and enzyme-SK activator species gave different K_m values, ~320 μM and ~780 μM, respectively, and different k_{cat} values, ~39 s^{-1} and ~52 s^{-1}, respectively. Also, at pH 7.4 and 37° C, Val_{442}-plasminogen-SK, Val_{442}-plasmin-SK, and Val_{561}-plasmin-SK gave K_m values of ~210 μM, ~370 μM, and ~520 μM, respectively, with k_{cat} values of ~29 s^{-1}, ~43 s^{-1}, and ~36 s^{-1}, respectively. Although steady-state kinetic parameter differences between the various streptokinase activator species have been found, all of these enzyme species are nearly equivalent, at pH 7.4 and 37° C, in their catalytic efficiencies, or second-order rate constants, k_{cat}/K_m, ~0.1 $\mu M^{-1} s^{-1}$.

Urokinase

Urokinase activator species (UK) can be prepared and isolated from both human urine and human kidney tissue culture systems, in both high molecular weight forms (UK-HMW), ~54,000 daltons, and low molecular weight forms (UK-LMW), ~32,000 daltons. The UK-LMW form is derived from the UK-HMW form by limited proteolysis. At pH 7.4 and 37° C, the steady-state kinetic parameters of the highly purified UK-HMW and UK-LMW forms, with H-L-glutamyl-glycyl-L-arginyl-*p*-nitroanilide as a substrate, were similar, with K_m values of ~200 μM and ~270 μM, respectively, and k_{cat} values of ~21 s^{-1} and

~ 16 s^{-1}, respectively, with catalytic efficiencies, or k_{cat}/K_m values, of ~ 0.1 μM^{-1} s^{-1},[2] the same as that found for the streptokinase activator species.

Urokinase preparations have been used as thrombolytic agents in human subjects with pulmonary embolism, deep-vein thrombosis and cerebral thrombosis. These clinical preparations vary in their specific activities, with purities ranging from 30% to 50%. Each clinical preparation is assayed against a World Health Organization reference preparation, and the vial contains a stated amount of International Units (I.U.). Each preparation can contain either the HMW form or the LMW form, or a mixture of the two forms. The activator preparation can be titrated with p-nitrophenyl-p'-guanidinobenzoate to determine the enzyme active-site concentration, and from the I.U. value of the preparation, the molar concentration of UK can be determined. Pure UK-HMW and UK-LMW have specific activities of $\sim 100,000$ I.U./mg protein and $\sim 220,000$ I.U./mg protein, respectively. The clinical UK preparations that we have studied gave similar amidase activities at pH 7.4 and 37° C; the V_{max} per 500 I.U. was determined to be ~ 1 μM s^{-1}.[3]

PLASMINOGEN ACTIVATION KINETICS IN PURIFIED SYSTEMS

Mathematic models for studying plasminogen activation kinetics have been developed;[2, 4] the general equations will accommodate all activator species. Steady-state kinetic measurements were carried out under physiological conditions at pH 7.4 and 37° C with the human Glu$_1$-plasminogen, Lys$_{77}$-plasminogen, and Val$_{442}$-plasminogen forms, the latter two being the plasmin-degraded and elastase-degraded forms, respectively. The various SK and UK activator species described above were used in these studies. The plasmin generated was measured with a tripeptide p-nitroanilide substrate.

For the SK activator species, the apparent Michaelis constants of activation, K_{plg}, were similar for the Glu$_1$-, Lys$_{77}$-, and Val$_{442}$-zymogens, ~ 0.1 to 0.3 μM, but, the catalytic rate constants, k_{plg}, varied with both the zymogen form and the SK activator species. With Val$_{561}$-plasmin-SK, the degraded zymogens, Lys$_{77}$-plasminogen and Val$_{442}$-plasminogen, gave k_{plg} values of ~ 55 min^{-1} and ~ 64 min^{-1}, respectively, compared to ~ 25 min^{-1} for the native Glu$_1$-plasminogen zymogen. With SK (Glu$_1$-plasminogen-SK), the k_{plg} values for the Glu$_1$-, and Lys$_{77}$-zymogens were ~ 9 min^{-1} and ~ 52 min^{-1}, respectively. The highest catalytic efficiency of activation (the k_{plg}/K_{plg} value) for Glu$_1$-plasminogen was with the Val$_{561}$-plasmin-SK activator complex, namely ~ 169 μM^{-1} min^{-1}. Higher catalytic efficiencies were obtained for Lys$_{77}$-plasminogen and Val$_{442}$-plasminogen with the same activator species, namely ~ 424 μM^{-1} min^{-1} and ~ 321 μM^{-1} min^{-1}, respectively. The highest catalytic efficiency of activation was obtained with the Lys$_{77}$-plasminogen substrate and the Glu-plasminogen-SK activator complex, namely ~ 476 μM^{-1} min^{-1}.

For the pure UK activator species, UK-HMW and UK-LMW, the K_{plg} values were similar for the Glu$_1$-, Lys$_{77}$-, and Val$_{442}$-zymogens, ~ 1 to 2 μM. But, the k_{plg} values varied somewhat with the zymogen and the molecular weight of the UK. For UK-HMW, the k_{plg} values for the Glu$_1$-, Lys$_{77}$-, and Val$_{442}$-zymogens were ~ 47 min^{-1}, ~ 50 min^{-1}, and ~ 22 min^{-1}, respectively, whereas for the UK-LMW, the k_{plg} values for the Glu$_1$- and Lys$_{77}$-zymogens were ~ 63 min^{-1} and ~ 23 min^{-1}, respectively. The catalytic efficiencies of activation with Glu_1-plasminogen for both UK-HMW and UK-LMW were $\sim 27 \ \mu M^{-1}$ min^{-1} and $\sim 24 \ \mu M^{-1}$ min^{-1}, respectively.

A comparison was also made between the UK clinical preparations, both HMW and LMW, from both urine and tissue culture sources.[3] The K_{plg} values varied between $\sim 1 \ \mu M$ and $\sim 7 \ \mu M$ with Glu_1-plasminogen, and between $\sim 3 \ \mu M$ and $\sim 6 \ \mu M$ with Lys_{77}-plasminogen; and the k_{plg} values varied between ~ 29 min^{-1} and ~ 66 min^{-1} with Glu_1-plasminogen, and ~ 42 min^{-1} and ~ 79 min^{-1} with Lys_{77}-plasminogen. The catalytic efficiencies of activation varied between $\sim 9 \ \mu M^{-1}$ min^{-1} and $\sim 47 \ \mu M^{-1}$ min^{-1} for the Glu_1-zymogen and between $\sim 12 \ \mu M^{-1}$ min^{-1} and $\sim 78 \ \mu M^{-1}$ min^{-1}, for the Lys_{77}-zymogen. The highest catalytic efficiencies were obtained with a urine UK-HMW tissue-culture preparation. There are substantial differences between clinical UK preparations, all having essentially the same I.U. values, when determined in a fibrin-clot lysis assay. A World Health Organization UK reference preparation is used in the determination of functional activity in the assay. It is obvious from these data that when SK and UK preparations are used for both *in vitro* and *in vivo* studies, they must be carefully defined by quantitative physical, chemical, and functional measurements.

We have studied other types of plasminogen activators in these systems. Trypsin, with Glu_1-plasminogen, has a K_{plg} value similar to UK, but a k_{plg} value 200-fold lower. Staphylokinase, with Glu_1-plasminogen, has a K_{plg} value similar to the SK activator species but a k_{plg} value 500-fold lower. Kallikrein, human plasmin, and thrombin do not give measurable activation rates in this system. The SK, UK, and staphylokinase species have second-order rate constants of activation of 2.5×10^5 to 2.8×10^6 M^{-1} s^{-1}; the lower limit of our activation measurements is about 1.5×10^2 M^{-1} s^{-1}. On this scale, kallikrein and maybe Hageman factor, both described as plasminogen activators, would have at least 1,000-fold lower second-order rate constants for plasminogen activation in solution than either SK or UK. This class of plasminogen activators probably requires a different mechanism and different sets of conditions for activation, probably fibrin surfaces.

References

1. WOHL, R. C., L. ARZADON, L. SUMMARIA & K. C. ROBBINS. 1977. Comparison of the esterase and human plasminogen activator activities of various activated forms of human plasminogen and their equimolar streptokinase complexes. J. Biol. Chem. **252:** 1141–1147.
2. WOHL, R. C., L. SUMMARIA & K. C. ROBBINS. 1980. Kinetics of activation of human plasminogen by different activator species at pH 7.4 and 37° C. J. Biol. Chem. **255:** 2005–2013.
3. ROBBINS, K. C., R. C. WOHL & L. SUMMARIA. 1979. Activation of human plasminogen in both purified systems and plasma by streptokinase and urokinase activator species. *In* Progress in Chemical Fibrinolysis and Thrombolysis. J. F. Davidson, V. Cepelak, M. M. Samama & P. C. Desnoyers, Eds. IV: 330–338. Churchill Livingstone. Edinburgh.
4. WOHL, R. C., L. SUMMARIA, L. ARZADON & K. C. ROBBINS. 1978. Steady state kinetics of activation of human and bovine plasminogens by streptokinase and its equimolar complexes with various activated forms of human plasminogen. J. Biol. Chem. **253:** 1402–1407.

PRODUCTION BY HUMAN TISSUES IN CULTURE OF IMMUNOLOGICALLY DISTINCT, MULTIPLE MOLECULAR WEIGHT FORMS OF PLASMINOGEN ACTIVATORS *

Maria B. Bernik, G. Wijngaards and D. C. Rijken

Section of Nephrology-Hypertension
Department of Medicine
Northwestern University Medical School and
Northwestern Memorial Hospital
Chicago, Illinois 60611
and
Gaubius Institute
Health Research Organization TNO
Leiden, the Netherlands

INTRODUCTION

Plasminogen activators are widely distributed in the human organism. They are usually named according to the source from which they are isolated: blood (or plasma) activators present in the circulation, tissue activator isolated from tissue homogenates, vascular activator released from vessel walls, and urokinase present in urine. Until recently only urokinase had been highly purified and characterized, and specific antibodies obtained for immunoassays. The recent development, however, of a purified plasminogen-activator preparation from human uterine tissue and of specific antiserum to this preparation has permitted biochemical characterization of human tissue activator,[1] and study of the immunologic relationship to other activators of human origin.[2-4] Quenching assays with this antiserum showed that tissue activator from uteri or other sources (lung, heart, spleen, kidney, intestine) is immunologically distinct from urokinase but related to vascular activator released by vessel walls during perfusion or venous occlusion.[2-4]

Observations of living tissues and cells in cultures have provided information on the origin and production of plasminogen activator, not readily accessible to studies *in vivo*. These observations have shown that the kidney is a rich source of activator in urine, urokinase,[5] and that immunologically similar activators may be produced in other tissues throughout the body.[6, 7] These studies also indicated that urokinase may be produced in tissues in an inactive form (activatable by trypsin and other serine proteinases), and representing presumably a precursor form of the enzyme.[7] Such form was isolated from lung[8] and, more recently, by Nolan *et al.*[9] from fetal kidney cultures.

* This research was supported by the Praeventiefonds, Projectnr, 28–443, by a NATO Research Grant, Nr. RG 018.80, and partly by O.S.A. Sprague Foundation, Kidney Research Fund, and Nephrology Education Fund of Northwestern Memorial Hospital. Some material utilized for this study was obtained from patients admitted to the Clinical Research Center, which is supported by grant RR-48, Division of Research Resources, National Institutes of Health.

Lung and other cultures, however, also yielded activities not quenched by antibodies to urokinase,[6, 8] suggesting the production and release of more than one immunologic type of activator. Further evidence to this effect was obtained by an immunoassay that combined quenching of the biologic activity by anti-urokinase serum with electrophoresis on polyacrylamide gel in the presence of sodium dodecyl sulfate (SDS-PAGE).[10] This study, however, was hampered in part by lack of antibodies to activators other than urokinase. Subsequent observations with specific antiserum to tissue activator as well as antisera to urinary and tissue-culture urokinase demonstrated the production in several human tissues of two immunologically distinct plasminogen activators.[11] Similar approaches are used in the present experiments to examine the immunologic identity and some of the characteristics of plasminogen activators produced in cultures of various human tissues.

METHODS

Tissue Culture

Cells from normal tissues were from adult and fetal lung, fetal heart, adult intestine, adult and fetal kidney, and fetal liver, all grown as monolayers in plastic flasks. Adult lung, obtained surgically from six individuals, was studied in primary cultures and up to five subcultures. Fetal lung consisted of primary cultures and of Wi38 diploid cell line obtained on the 30th passage (Flow Laboratories, Rockville, Md.). Fetal heart and liver were obtained in primary culture (International Scientific Industries, Cary, Ill.) and studied up to 6 subcultures. Intestine consisted of subcultures from a biopsy specimen of small intestine. Adult kidney tissue was from surgical nephrectomies or cadaver donors and was studied for up to 6 passages. Fetal kidney, obtained commercially as primary culture (Flow Laboratories or International Scientific Industries), was also subcultured for 5–7 passages. Growth medium consisted of Eagle's Basal Medium (BME) with 10% calf serum. When cells in primary cultures or subcultures were nearly confluent, they were fed chemically defined, serum-free medium BME, containing 0.5% lactalbumin hydrolysate. Accumulation of plasminogen activator in the medium was monitored by assaying samples of the medium on fibrin plates. The medium was harvested after varying intervals, cultures fed again, and additional harvests obtained. The harvested medium was assayed for activator content, pooled and concentrated, and studied by SDS-PAGE with or without prior chromatography on Sephadex or Sephacryl columns.

Additional samples of plasminogen activator were from cultures of adult spleen and thyroid and fetal ureter examined previously [6, 7] and kept frozen at −20° or −70° C. Also from previous studies were supernatants from cultures of a heteroploid cell line from fetal kidney (Human embryonic kidney cell line, Baltimore Biol. Co., Baltimore, Md.).[6] Not examined previously were harvests from fetal intestine (colon) grown in primary culture.

Cultures from tumor tissue, trypsinized and grown as monolayers in flasks, were obtained from carcinoma of the thyroid (two individuals), carcinoma of the kidney (two individuals), and SV$_3$ clone of HeLa cells (Grand Island Biol. Co., Grand Island, N.Y.), a cell line derived from human cervical carcinoma. Also examined were cultures from a carcinoma of the prostate and several surgical specimens from benign prostatic hypertrophy, grown as monolayers or as primary explants.

Antisera

Antibodies to tissue activator, raised in a rabbit against purified activator from human uteri, consisted of IgG fractions used previously.[2-4] Antiserum to high molecular weight urokinase (M_r 54,000) from urine was raised in a rabbit with urokinase obtained as a gift of Choay, (Paris, France). Antisera to low molecular weight urokinase (M_r 35,000) provided by Abbott Laboratories (North Chicago, Ill.) were identical to those used previously [8, 10, 11] and consisted of a γ-globulin fraction from antiserum to the $5S_1$ urokinase of White et al.[12] and antiserum to tissue-culture urokinase produced by human kidney.[13]

Standards

Standards of urinary urokinase were from the American National Red Cross, New York, N.Y.[14] Tissue-culture urokinase was from Abbott Laboratories. Tissue-activator standards consisted of preparations from human uteri.[1] Other preparations of urinary urokinase were the high molecular weight form from Choay, and two preparations from Abbott Laboratories consisting, respectively, of high and low molecular weight forms. The latter were obtained by gel filtration in Sephadex G-100 columns of a preparation containing both molecular weight forms.

Assays of Plasminogen Activator Activity

Assays of plasminogen activator activity were performed on fibrin plates prepared with plasminogen-rich bovine fibrinogen,[15] which was obtained according to the method of Brakman [16] or was purchased from Miles Laboratories (Elkhart, Ind.). Plasminogen-independent fibrinolysis was not detected in any of the preparations. Urokinase and tissue-activator standards, prepared freshly with 0.15 M sodium barbital buffer/hydrochloric acid, pH 7–7.5 (SBB), were spotted on the plates in serial dilution; the activity of urokinase was expressed in international units (IU) and of tissue activator in arbitrary units (AU), the lytic area of 1.0 AU corresponding to that of 1.0 IU as shown in Figure 1. Activator from cultures, diluted as necessary with SBB, was assayed quantitatively and examined for immunologic identity with urokinase or tissue activator by quenching assays on fibrin plates containing the respective antisera, or IgG fractions. Inactive form of urokinase was determined by incubating aliquots of culture-produced material with equal volumes of trace amounts of plasmin (0.01–0.02 CTA † U/ml; human plasmin, glycerol-activated, kindly provided by Dr. J. T. Sgouris, Michigan Dept. of Health Laboratories, Lansing, Mich.); [17] trypsin (5–10 BAEE ‡ U/ml; Mann Chemicals, Orangeburg, N.Y.); or buffer alone for 20 min at 37° C, and then assaying for generated urokinase activity on fibrin plates.

† Committee on Thrombolytic Agents.
‡ Bz-Arg-OEt.

Quenching Assays

Antisera to urokinase were incorporated into fibrin plates at the following final dilutions: antiserum to high molecular weight urokinase from Choay, 1:10,000; antiserum to low molecular weight ($5S_1$) urokinase from Dr. W. F.

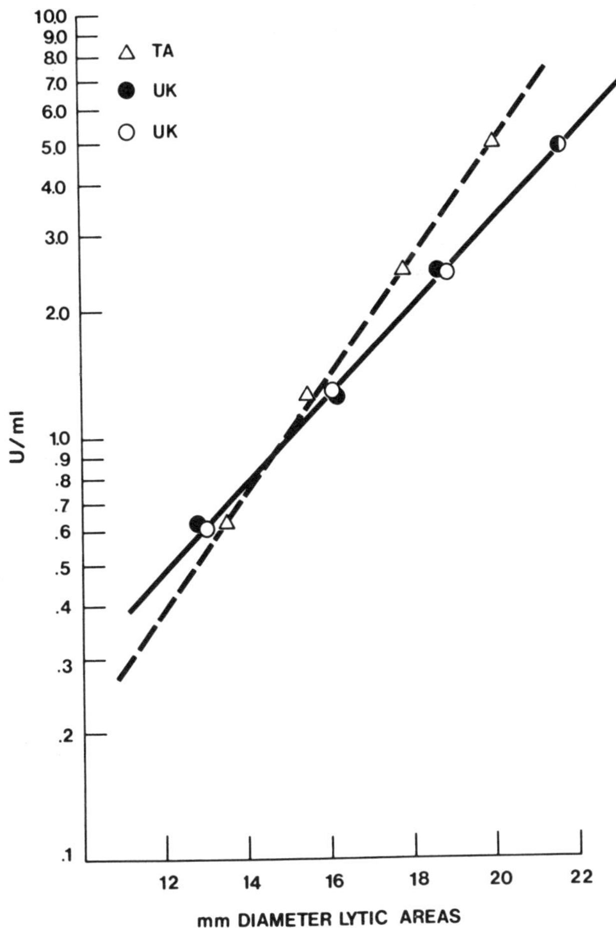

FIGURE 1. Assays of urinary urokinase (—○—), tissue-culture urokinase (—●—), and uterine tissue plasminogen activator (−−△−−) standards on fibrin plates. Diameter of lytic areas in mms is shown in the abscissa and units per ml on the ordinate.

White at 1:20,000; and to tissue-culture urokinase from Abbott Laboratories, 1:5,000. At these concentrations the antisera showed identical degrees of quenching towards the respective antigens as well as towards the various urokinase standards. No effect was observed with control rabbit serum at concentrations of 1:1,000 or less. The IgG fraction from antiserum to tissue activator was at a final dilution of 1.2 μg/ml fibrin plate for assays of gel slices and 0.8 μg/ml fibrin plate for assays of activator material in solution. In assays on the specificity of the antisera used in the experiments, antiserum to tissue activator quenched the activity of the antigen preparation but did not affect the activity of high or low molecular weight urokinase from urine or the activity of culture-produced urokinase. This was in accordance with previous observations.[2,4] In further accordance with these observations, the antisera to urokinase quenched the activity of the various urokinase preparations but not that of tissue activator.

Concentration

Concentration of supernatant medium harvested from cultures was performed in a stirred-cell concentrator (Amicon cell fitted with Diaflo PM 30 membranes) and/or in dialysis tubing (Viking cellulose tubing 12,000 MWCO) in a bed of dry Sephadex, after adding ammonium sulfate (10%, w/vol) to the medium to prevent loss of activator during concentration. Essentially quantitative recovery of bioactivity was obtained from the Amicon cell. Recovery from dialysis tubing ranged from 60–90%.

Chromatography

Column chromatography was performed with Sephadex G-100 or Sephacryl S-200 (Pharmacia Fine Chemicals) using 0.28 M phosphate buffer, pH 6.5, which contained 0.1 M NaCl and 0.08 M ammonium sulfate. Protein standards (aldolase, albumin, ovalbumin, chymotrypsinogen A, and ribonuclease A) and dextran-blue 2,000 to determine void volume were from Pharmacia. Protein determination was performed by the method of Lowry.[18]

Electrophoresis

SDS-polyacrylamide gel electrophoresis (7.5 or 5% gels) were performed according to the method of Weber and Osborn.[19] Running buffer was 0.1 M phosphate, pH 7.2, containing 0.1% SDS. Protein standards, treated with SDS and reducing agents (2-mercaptoethanol, Sigma Chemical Co., St. Louis, Mo.) were bovine albumin, ovalbumin, chymotrypsinogen A, ribonuclease A (from Pharmacia), phosphorylase A, lactic dehydrogenase (from Worthington Biochemicals, Freehold, N.J.), or crosslinked albumin or hemoglobin (Sigma Chemicals). Standards not reduced prior to electrophoresis included albumin monomer (Miles Laboratories), and urinary urokinase standards consisting of high (M_r 55,000) and low (M_r 35,000) molecular weight forms from Abbott Laboratories. Bioactive peaks of urokinase standards and of preparations from tissue culture were located by slicing gels longitudinally and assaying 1-mm segments on fibrin plates. Immunologic identity of activities in the peaks was examined by incubating paired 0.5-mm slices on plates containing antibodies to urokinase or tissue activator. Inactive form of urokinase was located by incubating gel slices with 20 μl plasmin (0.02 CTA U/ml) or trypsin (10 BAEE U/ml) solutions, or buffer alone on fibrin plates.

Accumulation of plasminogen activator in serum-free supernatant medium of various cultures is shown in FIGURE 2. Immunologic identity with urokinase or tissue activator of activities in the medium at harvest time, determined by quenching assays on fibrin plates, is shown in FIGURE 3. Results of quenching by the antisera to high and low molecular weight urokinase from urine or tissue culture were similar and are presented jointly. Cultures from two sources— kidney and HeLa cells—yielded a single immunologic type of activator activity

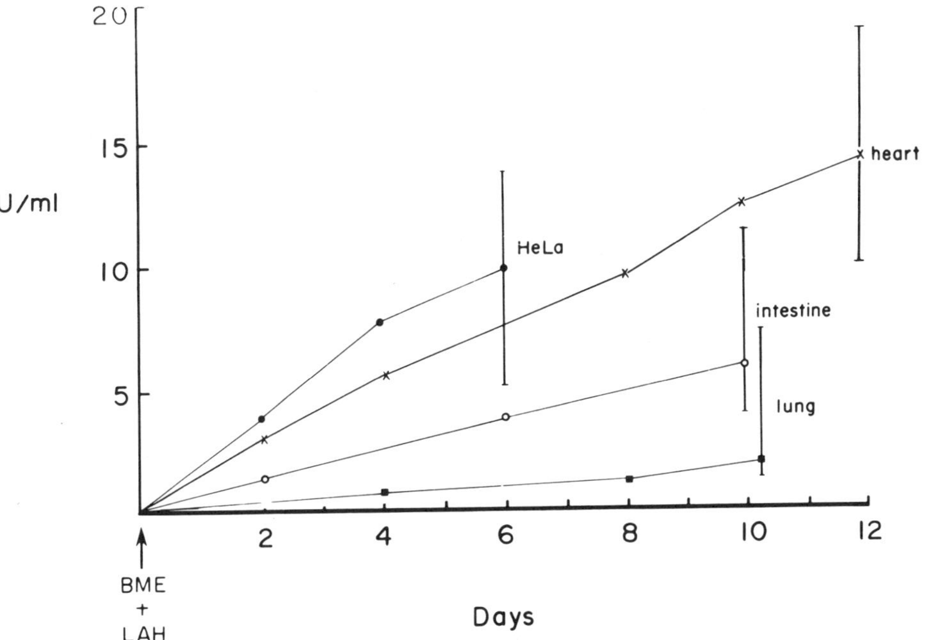

FIGURE 2. Accumulation of plasminogen-activator activity in serum-free supernatant medium of various cultures. At 0′ time, cultures are fed Eagle's basal medium (BME) containing lactoalbumin hydrolysate (LAH); the medium is sampled, assayed on fibrin plates at various intervals, and harvested after 5–15 days. Vertical lines indicate ranges of activator activity in the medium and horizontal lines, average values. Days of observations are shown on the abscissa and accumulation of plasminogen-activator activity in the medium, on the ordinate.

in the supernatant medium (FIGURE 3). As reported previously, activity in cultures of kidney was immunologically identical to urokinase [5, 6] and consisted partly of active and partly of activatable enzyme. In harvests obtained after 10–15 days of culture the two forms were present in an approximate 1:1 ratio (FIGURE 3). In quenching assays on fibrin plates, the biologic activity of both forms was quenched by the anti-urokinase sera to the same extent as urokinase standards. No quenching was observed with antiserum to tissue activator. Activity in culture from HeLa, on the other hand, was quenched completely by this antiserum and was not affected by the anti-urokinase sera. Urokinase-

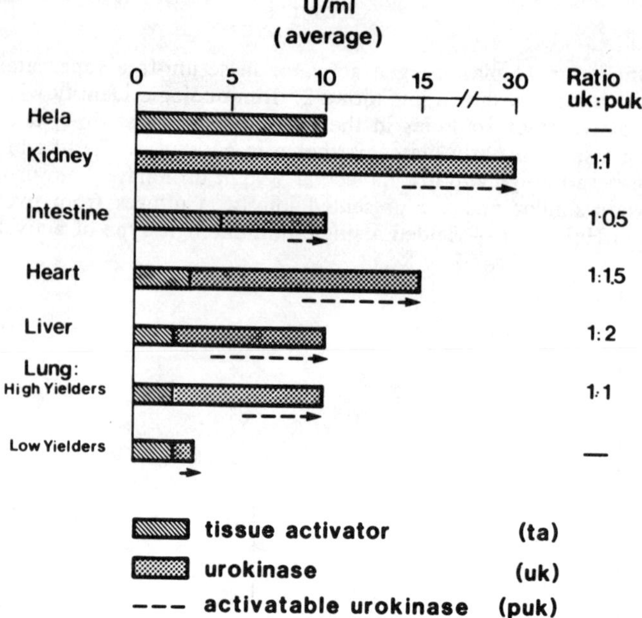

FIGURE 3. Quenching by antiserum to urokinase (UK, dotted areas) or tissue–plasminogen activator (TA, shaded areas) of the biologic activity of plasminogen activators accumulating in the supernatant medium of HeLa (5 day harvests) and other cultures (10–15 day harvests). Urokinase consists of active and activatable enzyme. The latter represents activity generated after incubation of the medium with traces of plasmin or trypsin, and is shown in the graph by the broken lines and arrows (– – →). Ratios of active to activatable enzymes, designated preurokinase (pUK), are shown in the column on the right.

type activity was not detected in HeLa cultures in either active or activatable form.

Cultures from other tissues (i.e., intestine, heart, lung, and liver) yielded both urokinase- and tissue activator-related activities, the former generally predominating (FIGURE 3). Cultures from lung fell into two categories, high and low yielders. The latter consisted of cultures from 3 adult individuals yielding low levels of activator activity in the supernates. Most of this activity was tissue activator-related with only traces of active or activatable urokinase-type activity. The remaining cultures from adult lung and all cultures from fetal lung, designated high yielders, showed relatively high levels of activity (up to 15 U/ml), which appeared to be due primarily to larger accumulations of urokinase-type activator, active and activatable, in the supernatant medium of these cultures (FIGURE 3). Activity in lung and other cultures was quenched completely when assayed on plates containing both antiurokinase and anti-tissue activator sera.

FIGURE 4 shows results of quenching assays of activator harvests from additional sources, normal and neoplastic. Three normal sources—spleen, thyroid, and ureter—are identical to those examined previously [6, 7] with antisera to urokinase alone. Partial quenching of activity from cultures of fetal ureter by antisera to urokinase is confirmed by the present assays, which also demonstrate similar quenching in cultures of adult spleen and thyroid and fetal intestine. Unquenched activity from these various sources is presently shown to be tissue activator-related (FIGURE 4).

In comparative studies of activator from normal and neoplastic sources, cultures derived from the three tumors (carcinoma of the thyroid, kidney, and prostate) yielded activator of the same immunologic type as that formed in the corresponding noncancerous tissue. Thus, cultures from thyroid and prostate tumor yielded both urokinase and tissue activator-related activities in the medium while kidney tumor showed only urokinase-type activity. The heteroploid cell line from kidney, on the other hand, showed little or no urokinase-type activity, as already reported,[6] but yielded tissue activator-related activity. As in cultures from normal sources, urokinase-type activity from tumor tissue consisted both of inactive and active forms, the former frequently predominating.

Study of time-related accumulation of urokinase-type activity in the supernatant medium from four sources—lung, liver, heart, and kidney—demonstrated that this enzyme first appears in the medium in an inactive form, activatable by trypsin or plasmin (FIGURE 5). Active urokinase-type activity

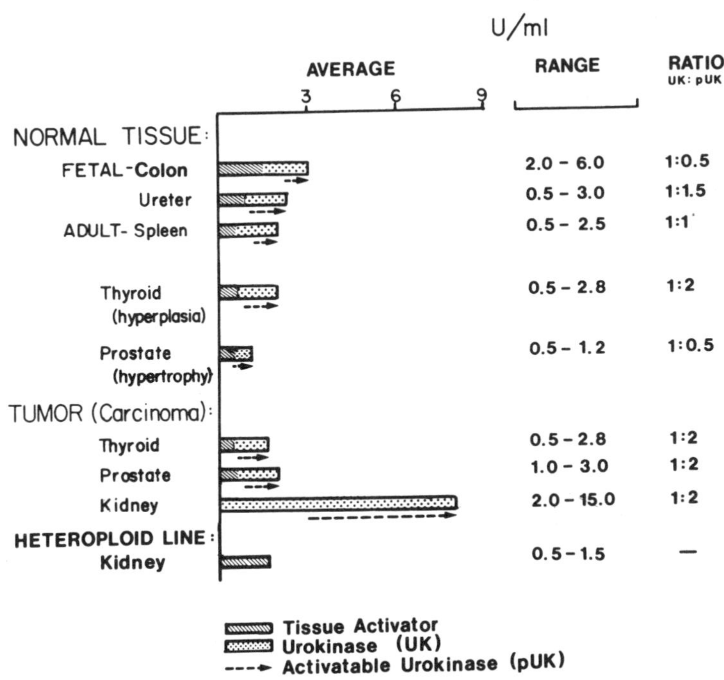

FIGURE 4. Quenching assays in cultures from normal or tumor tissue. Horizontal bars represent average concentrations of urokinase- or tissue activator-related activity in the supernatants of cultures, after 6–10 days. Ranges of total activity in the medium and ratios of active to activatable urokinase (UK:pUK) type activity are given in the columns on the right.

generally was not detected in the medium until one to two days later when traces appeared in most cultures. Concentrations increased thereafter though considerable amounts of unactivated enzyme were still present in the medium after 10–15 days of culture (FIGURE 5). Batches of the latter harvests, which exhibited a high degree (80% or more) of activation upon concentration in the Amicon cell, were used in studies of "spontaneously" activated enzyme. Relatively early, 5–7-day harvests containing little, or not detectable, active enzyme even when concentrated, were selected for study of the inactive enzyme to minimize "spontaneous" activation occurring presumably through plasmin

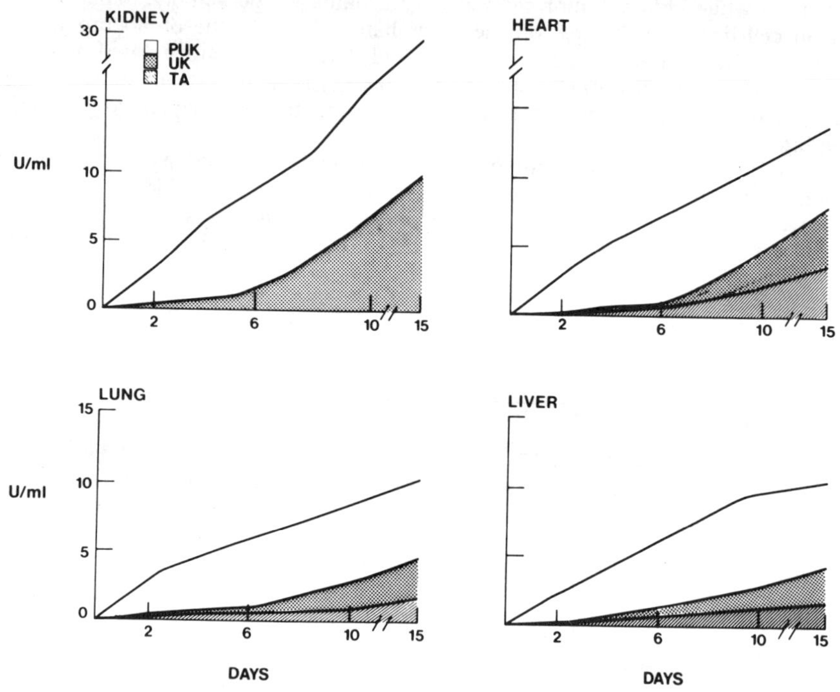

FIGURE 5. Time-related accumulation of active and activatable enzymes in the supernatant medium of various cultures. Active enzymes are urokinase (UK)- or tissue activator (TA)-related. Activatable enzyme, designated preurokinase (pUK), is expressed in IU/ml urokinase generated by incubating samples of the medium with traces of trypsin or plasmin.

generated from plasminogen in the fibrin plate through the action of the active enzyme in the samples.

Location of the active enzymes and immunologic identification of bioactive peaks after SDS-PAGE are shown in FIGURE 6. Activator material from HeLa cells, quenched by antiserum to tissue activator, showed one major peak in the region of 70,000 molecular weight substances and a much smaller peak at approximately 100,000. The urokinase activity in the supernatant media from kidney cultures was located mainly in the region of high (M_r 55,000) molecular weight urokinase from urine. Cultures from adult and fetal kidney showed

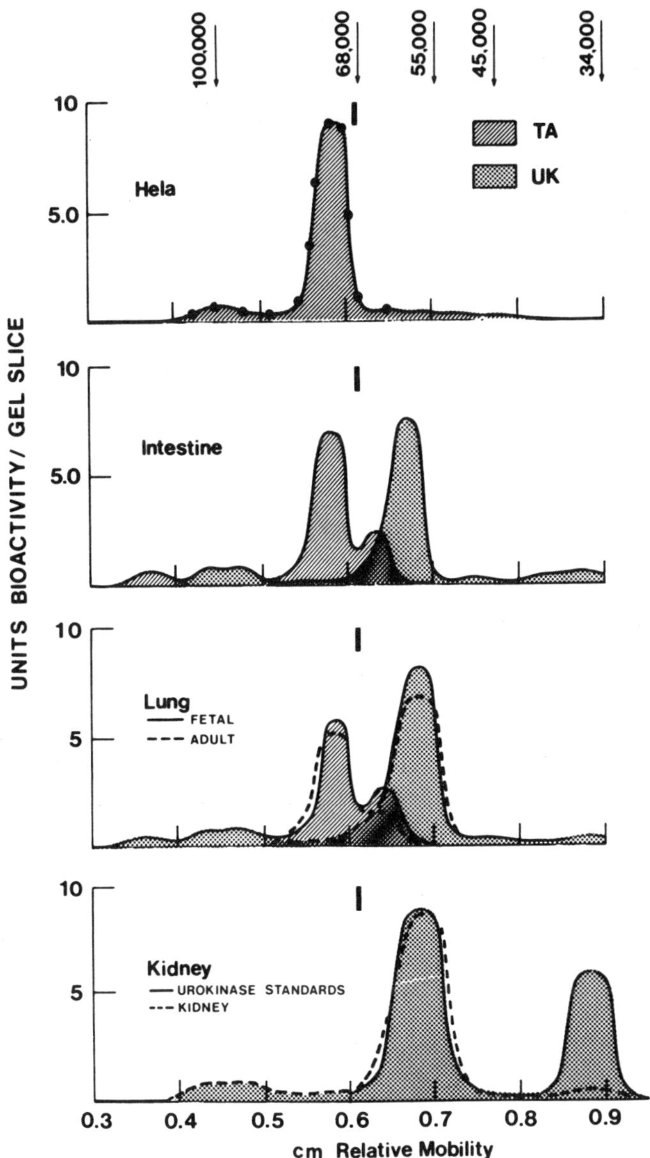

FIGURE 6. Peaks of urokinase- or tissue activator-related activity in concentrated supernates of various cultures, after SDS-polyacrylamide (5% gel) electrophoresis. Activity quenched by antiserum to urokinase is shown by the dotted areas and by antiserum to tissue activator by the shaded. Vertical bars in the region of 68,000 molecular weight substances represent albumin markers in the gels.

similar results. No appreciable activity was observed in either of these cultures, in the region of low (M_r 35,000) molecular weight urokinase, and only minor peaks were detected at molecular weights greater than 55,000 (M_r 90,000–110,000, FIGURE 6).

In contrast to the kidney and HeLa, plasminogen-activator activity in cultures from adult and fetal lung and adult intestine resolved into two major bioactive peaks, a tissue activator-related peak with a mobility similar to that of HeLa ($M_r \sim$ 70,000) and a urokinase-related peak with a mobility similar to that of urokinase from kidney ($M_r \sim$ 55,000). A third peak, tissue activator-related and located immediately behind urokinase ($M_r \sim$ 60,000), was seen less consistently. This peak was observed in approximately 40% of the concentrates from lung or intestine cultures and generally disappeared after storage for several months at $-20°$ C. A minor tissue activator-related peak in the region of 140,000 molecular weight substances also occurred occasionally and was observed mainly in cultures of intestine (FIGURE 6). Cultures from heart (not shown) yielded results similar to those of lung in FIGURE 6: tissue activator-type activity consisted mainly of the 70,000 and urokinase of the 55,000 molecular weight forms. Neither heart nor other cultures showed appreciable activity in the region of low (M_r 35,000) molecular weight urokinase. However, minor urokinase-related peaks, accounting for 10–15% of the total activity applied to the gels, were detected in concentrates from heart, lung, and intestine cultures in the regions of 110,000–90,000 molecular weight substances (FIGURE 6).

Studies of the inactive form of urokinase by gel filtration and SDS-PAGE are shown in FIGURES 7 and 8. On Sephacryl S-200 columns, inactive enzyme from lung eluted in the region adjacent to that of the high (M_r 55,000) molecular weight form of urokinase from urine. Trypsin-activated enzyme from lung coeluted with the latter as did the "spontaneously" activated enzyme from this tissue (FIGURE 7). On SDS-PAGE, the trypsin-activated preparation appeared as a single major peak with mobility undistinguishable from that of the "spontaneously" activated enzyme and the 55,000 molecular weight form of urokinase from urine. The inactive enzyme, activatable in gel slices with either trypsin or plasmin, also appeared as a single major peak adjacent to the peaks of the active preparations. The difference in mobility between active and inactive enzyme was too small to be gauged accurately by bioactivity alone. In comparative studies with enzymes from lung, preparations of harvests from kidney and heart yielded similar results, both forms of the enzyme appearing at or near the 55,000 molecular weight region. In the presently studied 5–7-day harvests, enzyme activatable in gel slices by incubation with trypsin or plasmin, was not detected in appreciable amounts at either higher or lower molecular weight ranges.

DISCUSSION

The production in human tissues of more than one immunologic type of plasminogen activator was first suggested by culture studies[6] that showed that some of the activity accumulating in the supernatant medium of lung and other tissues was quenched, while other activator activity was not affected by antiserum to urokinase. We postulated that the former activity may represent urokinase-type activator and the latter, plasma and/or tissue activator-related

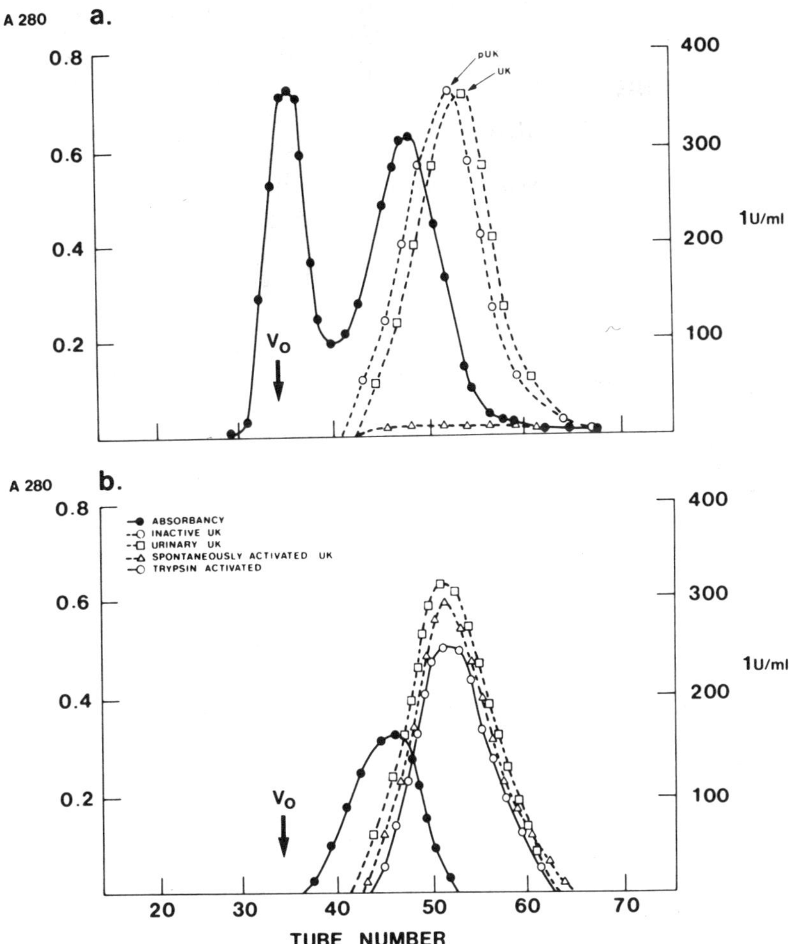

FIGURE 7. a. Elution pattern on Sephacryl S200 column of activatable urokinase-type bioactivity (--O--) and protein (—●—) in harvests from lung cells (Wi38 cell line). Active enzyme (--Δ--) was not detected in appreciable amounts in these harvests. Elution of urinary urokinase (M_r 55,000) bioactivity (--□--) was determined separately in the same column. Inactive enzyme in tubes 45–58 was pooled, concentrated, activated with trypsin (10:1 molar ratio of inactive enzyme to trypsin), and refiltered in the same column. b. Shows elution patterns, examined separately on the same column, of trypsin-activated (--O--) and spontaneously activated (--Δ--) urokinase from lung in relation to the 55,000 molecular weight of urinary urokinase (--□--). Absorption at A280 of protein in the trypsin-activated material is shown by the closed circles (—●—). For both a and b column size: 1.6 × 55 cm; buffer 0.1 M phosphate, pH 6.5 containing 0.08 M ammonium sulfate; flow rate 0.3 ml/min. Volume eluted 1.0 ml/tube.

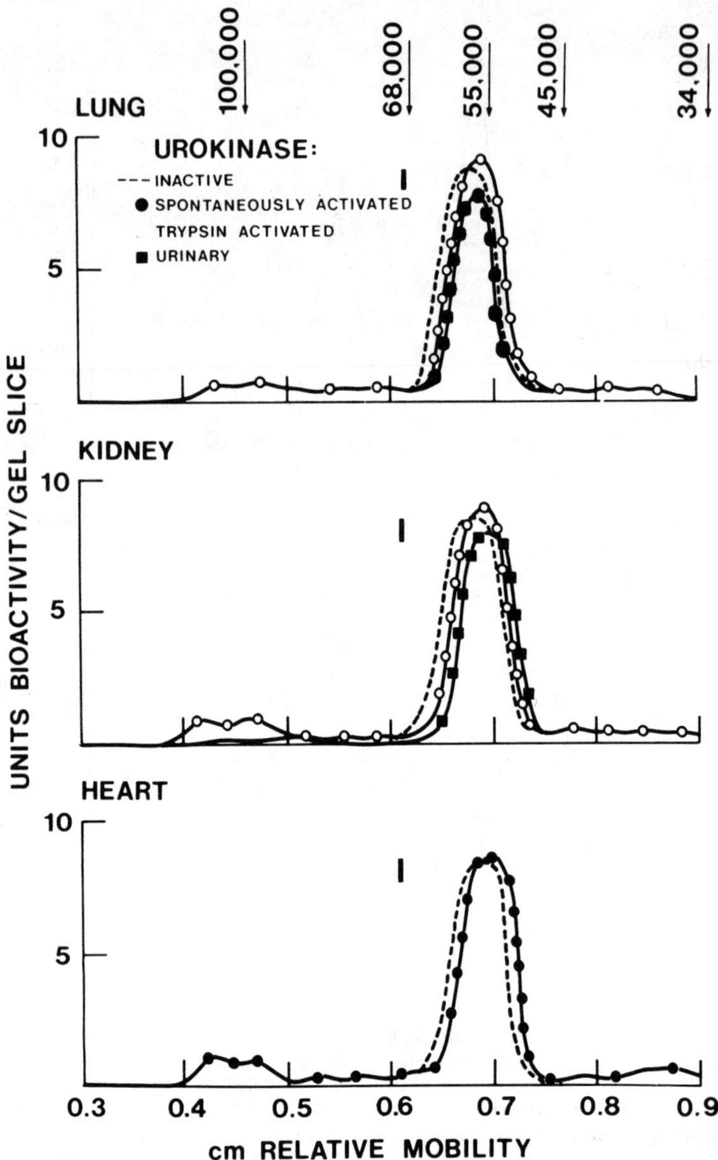

FIGURE 8. Peaks of inactive (......) and activated (–●–●–, –○–○–) urokinase-type bioactivity in concentrated supernates from lung (Wi38), kidney and heart cultures after SDS-polyacrylamide (5% gel) electrophoresis. The various preparations are applied separately to paired gels. Inactive form is assayed by incubating gel slices with traces of plasmin (20 μl of 0.01 CTA U/ml solution). Spontaneously activated (–●–●–) material is similar or identical to that in FIGURE 6. The trypsin-activated preparation from lung (–○–○–) is that used in gel filtration in FIGURE 7. Urinary urokinase is the 55,000 molecular weight form.

activity.[6] Later studies with techniques that combined SDS-electrophoresis with quenching assays suggested multiple molecular weight forms of immunologically distinct plasminogen activators in cultures from various tissues.[10, 20] These activators were recently identified as urokinase- or tissue activator-related.[11] The present study confirms and expands observations on the identity and some of the characteristics of activator material produced by cells of various human tissues.

Antiserum to tissue activator used presently in immunoassays has been shown to quench the activity of the purified antigen from human uteri as well as the activity in homogenates from various other tissues.[2, 4] The antiserum also quenches the activity of vascular activator from perfused cadaver limbs and that in post-venous occlusion plasma which is known for its high vascular-activator content,[3] indicating immunologic relationship between "tissue" and "vascular" activators. No such relationship, however, was found between tissue activator and urokinase in previous[2, 4] or present immunoassays indicating that these activators represent serologically distinct entities.

Tissue and vascular plasminogen activators also differ from urokinase in other criteria. Tissue activator purified from homogenates of human uteri was shown to have a molecular weight of 69,000 by SDS-PAGE and to consist of two polypeptide chains with molecular weight of 38,000 and 31,000, the latter chain apparently containing the active site.[1] A molecular weight of 65–70,000 and a single polypeptide chain were reported for vascular activator from perfused cadaver limbs in studies by SDS-PAGE.[21] Somewhat lesser values (M_r 60,000) were observed both for vascular and tissue activator on gel filtration.[22, 23] In yet other studies also using perfusates from cadaver limbs as the source of vascular activator, the molecular weight of purified preparations was estimated at approximately 56,000.[24] Various molecular weight species have been described for urokinase. The main native species appears to be the 55,000 form, which is comprised of two polypeptide chains with molecular weights of 32,000 and 20,000, the former apparently containing the active site.[25] Forms of lesser molecular weight (32–35,000) have been reported in cultures of fetal kidneys.[9, 20, 26] These forms were observed to occur during certain purification procedures[9] or after prolonged cultures (10 days or more).[26] Varying amounts of activity in the higher molecular weight ranges (approx. 100,000) was reported in harvests obtained after shorter periods of culture (2–7 days).[26] In the present 10 to 15 day harvests from kidney or other tissues (lung, intestine, and heart) the urokinase-type activity appeared to consist mainly of the 55,000 molecular weight form, with only minor peaks at approximately 90,000–110,000 and no significant activity in the range of 30–35,000 molecular weight substances.

Studies on the production of urokinase in cultured tissues have indicated that this enzyme may be produced and released from cells in an inactive form, activatable by various serine proteinases and representing presumably a precursor form of the enzyme.[7-9] This form appears early and may persist, unactivated, in the tissue-culture fluids for prolonged periods of time as shown by Nolan *et al.* in fetal kidney cultures[9] and by the present time-related observations of active and activatable enzyme in kidney and other tissues. Elution patterns of enzymes from lung on gel filtration were similar to that observed in purified preparations from kidney cultures by Nolan *et al.*[9] The apparent minimal differences between active and trypsin- or plasmin-activatable enzyme are presently confirmed by studies with SDS PAGE. These studies demonstrated further that sources of cultured tissues such as lung, kidney, and heart yield essentially identical molecular weight forms of active and inactive enzymes with mobilities in the region of 55,000 molecular weight substances. A lesser molecular weight form ($M_r \sim 35,000$) of inactive enzyme, which in Nolan's studies appeared to derive from the 55,000 form during certain purification procedures (i.e. adsorption to CG-50 resins),[9] was not observed in the present studies. Whether conversion of inactive to active urokinase occurs with the release of a relatively small peptide, or whether, in analogy to another proenzyme,[27] the inactive urokinase elicited hitherto may represent a proteolytically modified, but not activated, proenzyme remains to be determined. The possible production in tissues of an earlier, unmodified precursor form, susceptible perhaps to the action of enzymes or factors other than those examined to date still has to be investigated.

Tissue activator-type activity in supernatants of the present cultures appeared to be mainly of the 70,000 molecular weight form, similar to the molecular weight of purified tissue activator [1] as well as that of the immunologically related vascular activator, according to molecular weight estimates of this activator at 65–70,000 by SDS-PAGE.[21] A second, lesser peak in the region of 60,000 molecular weight substances, occurred less consistently and often disappeared on storage. This peak was observed presently in cultures of lung and intestine but not of HeLa cells, which yielded mainly the 70,000 form. Whether the 60,000 peak represents a molecular weight species of tissue or vascular activator—distinct from and perhaps more labile than the 70,000 form—or a degradation product of the latter form remains to be determined.

Immunologic identity of plasminogen activators produced in and released from tumor tissues, and relationship to the identity of activators formed in the corresponding normal tissues has been examined in a few tumors only. Early observations [6] of diploid and heteroploid cell lines, and of primary cultures and subcultures of normal tissues suggested that "altered" cells may either lose the ability to produce one serologic type of activator while retaining the ability to yield other types, or possibly acquire the ability to produce activator types not generally formed in the tissue of origin. A heteroploid cell line from kidney, which in these early studies was observed to produce activator other than urokinase by immunoassays,[6] is presently shown to yield tissue activator-related activity not usually found in cultures from normal kidneys. In more recent studies by Astedt and collaborators, cells from ovarian carcinomas were shown to yield large amounts of urokinase-related activity,[28] which is not produced in appreciable amounts in cultures from normal ovaries.[28] Urokinase-type activator also was demonstrated in cultures of neoplastic but not of normal or hyperplastic endometrium.[29] Other tumors, however, may reflect essentially the function of the tissue of origin and produce the same immunologic type activator(s) as observed presently in cultures from carcinoma of the kidney, thyroid, and prostate. Somewhat similar observations have been reported in *in vitro* experiments with cell lines transformed by oncogenic virus [30] in which Wi38 cell line from lung continued to yield urokinase-type activator. Continued production of the same immunologic type as that of the tissue of origin also occurred in transformed lung and kidney cultures from hamster.[31] Some of these cultures, however, produced activator of immunologic type other than that of the parental tissue.[31] In the case of human cervical carcinoma, it is of interest that while the present culture of HeLa cells yielded only tissue activator-related activity, another cell line was reported to produce urokinase-type activity.[32] Relationship of these activities to plasminogen activator(s) in parental tissue, however, remains to be determined. Cultures from various human tumors have been shown to yield activator partly [20, 32] or wholly [20, 30] resistant to quenching by antiserum to urokinase. It may be speculated that, whether or not reflecting activator production in the parental tissue, the unquenched activity may be tissue-activator related, as appeared to be the case for all activity resistant to anti-urokinase serum in the present cultures.

REFERENCES

1. RIJKEN, D. C., G. WIJNGAARDS, M. ZAAL-DE JONG & J. WELBERGEN. 1979. Purification and partial characterization of plasminogen activator from human uterine tissue. Biochim. Biophys. Acta **580:** 140–153.
2. RIJKEN, D. C., G. WIJNGAARDS & WELBERGEN. 1979. Biochemical and immunological characterization of plasminogen activator from human tissue. *In* Progress in Chemical Fibrinolysis and Thrombolysis. J. F. Davidson, V. Cepelak, M. Samama & P. C. Desnoyers, Eds. **4:** 349–354. Raven Press.
3. RIJKEN, D. C., G. WIJNGAARDS & J. WELBERGEN. 1980. Relationship between tissue plasminogen activator and the activators in blood and vascular wall. Thromb. Res. **18:** 815–830.
4. RIJKEN, D. C., G. WIJNGAARDS & J. WELBERGEN. 1981. Immunological characterization of plasminogen activator activities in human tissue and body fluids. J. Lab. Clin. Med. **97:** 477–486.
5. BERNIK, M. B. & H. C. KWAAN. 1967. Origin of fibrinolytic activity in cultures of the human kidney. J. Lab. Clin. Med. **70:** 650–661.
6. BERNIK, M. B. & H. C. KWAAN. 1969. Plasminogen activator activity in cultures from human tissues. An immunological and histochemical study. J. Clin. Invest. **48:** 1740–1753.
7. BERNIK, M. B. 1973. Increased plasminogen activator (urokinase) in tissue cultures after fibrin deposition. J. Clin. Invest. **52:** 873–884.
8. BERNIK, M. B. & E. P. OLLER. 1976. Plasminogen activator and proactivator (urokinase precursor) in lung cultures. J. Am. Med. Women's Assoc. **31:** 465–473.
9. NOLAN, C., L. S. HALL, G. H. BARLOW & I. E. TRIBBY. 1977. Plasminogen activators from human embryonic kidney cell cultures. Biochim. Biophys. Acta **496:** 384–400.
10. BERNIK, M. B. 1978. Plasminogen activator differing immunologically from urokinase in cultures from normal and cancer tissues. 17th Congress, Intl. Soc. Hemat. Abstracts (II), p. 631.
11. BERNIK, M. B., D. C. RIJKEN & G. WIJNGAARDS. 1979. Production of two immunologically distinct plasminogen activators by human tissue in culture (Abstract). Thrombos. Haemostas. **42:** 414.
12. WHITE, W. F., G. H. BARLOW & M. M. MOZEN. 1966. The isolation and characterization of plasminogen activators (urokinase) from human urine. Biochem. **5:** 2160–2169.
13. BARLOW, G. H. & L. LAZER. 1972. Characteristics of the plasminogen activator isolated from human embryo kidney cells: comparison with urokinase. Thrombos. Res. **1:** 201–208.
14. JOHNSON, A. J., D. L. KLINE & N. ALKJAERSIG. 1969. Assay methods and standard preparations for plasmin, plasminogen and urokinase in purified systems, 1967–1968. Thromb. Diath. Haemorrh. **21:** 259–262.
15. HAVERKATE, F. & P. BRAKMAN. 1975. Fibrin plate assay. *In* Progress in Chemical Fibrinolysis and Thrombolysis. J. F. Davidson, M. M. Samama & P. C. Desnoyers, Eds. **1:** 151–159. Raven Press. New York, N.Y.

16. BRAKMAN, P. & T. ASTRUP. 1971. The fibrin plate method for assay of fibrinolytic agents. *In* Thrombosis and Bleeding Disorders. N. U. Bang, F. K. Beller, E. Deutsch & E. F. Mammen, Eds. 332–336. Academic Press. New York, N.Y.

17. SGOURIS, J. T., J. K. INMAN, I. B. McCALL, L. A. HYNDMAN & H. D. ANDERSON. 1960. The preparation of human fibrinolysin (plasmin). Vox Sang. **5:** 357–375.

18. LOWRY, O. H., N. J. ROSEBROUGH, A. L. FARR & R. J. RANDALL. 1951. Protein measurement with Folin phenol reagent. J. Biol. Chem. **193:** 265–275.

19. WEBER, K. & M. OSBORN. 1969. Reliability of molecular weight determinations by dodecyl sulfate-polyacrylamide gel electrophoresis. J. Biol. Chem. **244:** 4406–4412.

20. VETTERLEIN, A., P. L. YOUNG, T. E. BELL & R. ROBLIN. 1979. Immunological characterization of multiple molecular forms of human cell plasminogen activator. J. Biol. Chem. **259:** 575–578.

21. BINDER, B., J. SPRAGG & K. F. AUSTEN. 1979. Purification and characterization of human vascular plasminogen activator derived from blood vessel perfusates. J. Biol. Chem. **254:** 1998–2003.

22. KOK, P. 1979. Separation of plasminogen activators from human uterine tissue and a comparison with activators from human urine and porcine tissue. Thrombos. Haemostas. **41:** 718–733.

23. KOK, P. 1979. Separation of plasminogen activators from human plasma and a comparison with activators from human uterine tissue and urine. Thrombos. Haemostas. **41:** 734–744.

24. PEPPER, D. S. & R. ALLEN. 1978. Isolation and characterization of human cadaver vascular endothelial activator. *In* Progress in Chemical Fibrinolysis and Thrombolysis. J. F. Davidson, ed. **3:** 91–98. Raven Press. New York, N.Y.

25. SOBERANO, M. E., E. B. ONG, A. J. JOHNSON, G. SCHOELLMANN & M. LEVY. 1975. Inhibition studies of urokinase with diisopropylphosphoro-fluoridate (DFP) and p-nitrophenyl-p'-guanidinobenzoate (NPGB). Fed. Proc. **34:** 860.

26. ASTEDT, B., G. BARLOW & L. HOLMBERG. 1978. Time-related release of various molecular forms of urokinase in tissue culture. Thromb. Res. **13:** 1031–1037.

27. SODETZ, J. M. & F. J. CASTELLINO. 1975. The mechanism of activation of rabbit plasminogen by urokinase. J. Biol. Chem. **250:** 3041–3049.

28. ASTEDT, B., E. LUNDGREN, G. ROOS & G. ABU SINNA. 1978. Release of various molecular forms of plasminogen activators during culture of human ovarian tumours. Thromb. Res. **13:** 1031–1037.

29. SVANBERG, L. & B. ASTEDT. 1979. Release of plasminogen activator from normal and neoplastic endometrium. Experientia **35:** 818–819.

30. TUCKER, W., W. M. KIRSCH, A. MARTINEZ-HERNANDEZ & L. M. FINK. 1978. Vitro plasminogen activator activity in human brain tumors. Cancer Res. **38:** 297–302.

31. CHRISTMAN, Y. K. 1978. Multiple forms of plasminogen activator. *In* Biological Markers of Neoplasia: Basic and Applied Aspects. R. Ruddon, Ed.: 433–449. Elsevier. New York, N.Y.

32. WU, M. C. & A. A. YUNIS. 1979. Comparative studies on urokinase and plasminogen activator from cultured pancreatic carcinoma. Int. J. Biochem. **10:** 1001–1006.

HUMAN FIBROBLASTS PRODUCE INHIBITOR DIRECTED AGAINST PLASMINOGEN ACTIVATOR WHEN TREATED WITH GLUCOCORTICOIDS *

David J. Crutchley, Lobella B. Conanan, and James R. Maynard

Research Division
Miami Heart Institute
Miami Beach, Florida 33140

INTRODUCTION

Fibrinolysis is a major process by which blood thrombi are degraded. This process can be initiated by the cellular enzyme plasminogen activator, which converts the inactive serum zymogen plasminogen to plasmin. Control of plasminogen activator would therefore have important consequences in the regulation of fibrinolysis. The fibrinolytic activity of cultured cells is sensitive to both metabolic and hormonal control. For example, fibrinolytic activity decreases in cultured rat hepatoma cells,[1] rheumatoid synovial cells,[2] and human embryonic lung cells[3] as well as other cell types when glucocorticoids are included in the culture medium. These suppressive effects may be due to a decreased production of plasminogen activator or alternatively the steroids may stimulate cellular production of a fibrinolytic inhibitor(s). This latter possibility has been suggested as the mode of action of dexamethasone on rat hepatoma cells,[4] although identification of the inhibitor(s) was not attempted. The present studies have been undertaken to assess the relative importance of these two alternatives on the changes in fibrinolytic activity of cultured human foreskin fibroblasts in the presence of two steroids, dexamethasone and hydrocortisone. The results suggest that the fibrinolytic suppressive effects of these compounds are due primarily to enhanced expression of a protease inhibitor. A fibrinolytic inhibitor could be directed against either plasminogen activator or plasmin (or both enzymes). Results consistent with the inhibitor being directed against plasminogen activator and urokinase, but not against plasmin, are presented.

MATERIAL AND METHODS

Cell Culture Techniques

Normal fibroblasts were derived from minced human foreskins as described.[5] Cells were grown to confluence in 35-mm tissue-culture dishes by using medium 199 supplemented with 2 mM L-glutamine, 50 μg/ml streptomycin, 50 units/ml penicillin, and 10% fetal calf serum. Growth medium was removed and replaced with 2 ml fresh serum-free medium with or without glucocorticoids in 0.1% ethanol. After incubation for 18 h, the medium was

* This work was supported in part by Grant HL-25864 from the National Heart, Lung and Blood Institute.

609

removed and centrifuged. Cells were washed with ice-cold saline A containing 20 mM HEPES, pH 7.4, scraped into the same buffer, pelleted by centrifugation, and extracted with 0.1% Triton X-100 in 0.1 M Tris, pH 8.1.

Fibrinolytic Assays

Human plasminogen was purified by affinity chromatography.[6] Bovine fibrinogen was labeled with ^{125}I using chloramine T.[7] [^{125}I]fibrin dishes were prepared as described.[8] Assays for overall fibrinolytic activity contained the following: 50 μl cell extract or conditioned medium, 2 μg plasminogen, and Tris buffer (0.1 M, pH 8.1) in a final volume of 0.5 ml. In assays for antiplasmin activity, plasminogen was substituted by plasmin, which was generated by incubating 1.5 μg/ml of plasminogen with 15 Ploug units/ml of urokinase at 37°C for 1 h. The release of soluble [^{125}I]fibrin-degradation products in these assays was quantitated by liquid scintillation techniques.

Chromogenic Substrate Assay

Urokinase-like activity of cell extracts was assessed by their ability to cleave the synthetic urokinase substrate pyro-Glu-Gly-Arg-p-nitroanilide. Assays run at 37°C contained 20–30 μg cell extract protein, 75 nmol substrate and buffer (50 mM Tris, 38 mM NaCl, pH 8.8) in a total volume of 0.25 ml. Assay sensitivity was increased by coupling the p-nitroaniline product with p-dimethylaminocinnamaldehyde.[9]

Material

Serum and tissue-culture media were products of Gibco, Grand Island, N.Y. Fibrinogen, urokinase, hydrocortisone, dexamethasone, chloramine T, HEPES (N-2-hydroxyethylpiperazine-N'-2-ethanesulfonic acid) and Tris [Tris(hydroxymethyl)aminomethane] were obtained from Sigma Chemical Co., St. Louis, Mo. The synthetic substrate pyro-Glu-Gly-Arg-p-nitroanilide (S2444) was obtained from Ortho Diagnostics, Raritan, N.J.

RESULTS AND DISCUSSION

Suppression of Fibrinolytic Activity by Glucocorticoids

Human foreskin fibroblasts incubated for 18 h with serum-free medium possessed marked fibrinolytic activity, as shown by the ability of cell extracts to solubilize ^{125}I-labeled fibrin. This activity was due to cellular plasminogen activator since fibrinolysis was abolished when plasminogen was omitted from the reaction mixtures. In common with several other cell types, low concentrations of either dexamethasone or hydrocortisone inhibited fibrinolytic activity, dexamethasone being the more potent of the two steroids (FIGURE 1).

Suppression of cellular fibrinolytic activity can be achieved either by failure to synthesize plasminogen activator, by synthesis of a plasminogen activator with reduced catalytic activity, or by increased production of fibrinolytic inhibitors. Therefore, the plasminogen activator in control and steroid-treated cells was tested directly by measuring the ability of cell extracts to liberate *p*-nitroaniline from pyro-Glu-Gly-Arg-*p*-nitroanilide, a synthetic tripeptide substrate for urokinase. Extracts of cells treated with 0.01–1 μM dexamethasone or hydrocortisone cleaved the substrate as readily as did extract of untreated cells (TABLE 1), suggesting that the levels of cellular plasminogen activator are

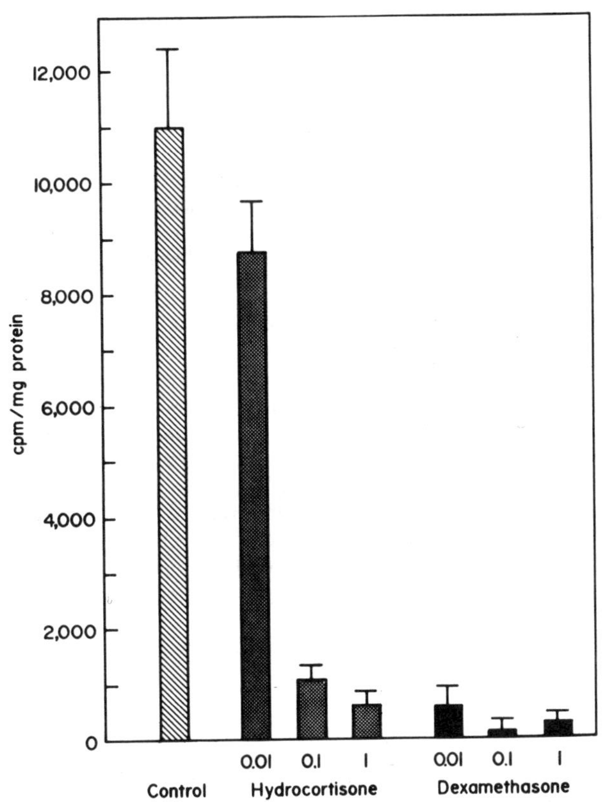

FIGURE 1. Inhibition of cellular fibrinolytic activity by glucocorticoids. Cultures of human skin fibroblasts were incubated for 18 h in medium containing 0.01–1 μM dexamethasone, hydrocortisone, or drug vehicle. After incubation cells were washed, cell extracts were prepared, and fibrinolytic activity was assessed by measuring the ^{125}I-labeled soluble peptides liberated per mg cellular protein in a 3-h fibrin dish assay. Each value is the mean of triplicate incubations. Bars show SEM.

essentially unchanged following glucocorticoid treatment, and therefore, the suppressive effects of these compounds are due to increased fibrinolytic inhibitor production.

In contrast to HeLa cells, which develop high levels of plasminogen activator in both cells and their growth medium,[10] the fibroblasts released little fibrinolytic activity into their serum-free growth medium. However, activity was detected

TABLE 1

HUMAN FIBROBLASTS HAVE UROKINASE-LIKE ACTIVITY WHICH IS
UNALTERED BY EXPOSURE TO STEROIDS

Drug	Dose (μM)	p-Nitroaniline Released (nmol·min^{-1}·mg protein^{-1})
None	–	1.52 ± 0.25
Dexamethasone	1	1.28 ± 0.04
	0.1	2.17 ± 0.05
	0.01	1.87 ± 0.08
Hydrocortisone	1	1.77 ± 0.12
	0.1	1.58 ± 0.10
	0.01	1.66 ± 0.06

NOTE: Cells were incubated for 18 h in serum-free medium containing dexamethasone, hydrocortisone, or vehicle. The p-nitroaniline released by cell extracts from the urokinase substrate pyro-Glu-Gly-Arg-p-nitroanilide was measured.

if the fibrin-dish assays were run for prolonged times (18–24 h), and under these conditions the suppressive effects of glucocorticoids were seen, analogous to those observed with the cell lysates. The very low level of activity of the cell-medium samples allowed them to be directly tested for their fibrinolytic inhibitory activity. Growth medium from cells that were not exposed to steroids had little effect on the plasminogen activator from untreated control cells. However, medium from steroid-treated cells strongly inhibited plasminogen activator, the degree of inhibition being related to the dose of steroid employed (FIGURE 2). Neither steroid directly inhibited the fibrinolytic assay at the concentrations employed. Hence the inhibitory properties of conditioned medium were cell-derived. These results again indicate that the suppressive effects of glucocorticoids on the fibrinolytic activity of human skin fibroblasts are not due primarily to a failure of the cells to synthesize plasminogen activator, but rather are due to the enhanced production of a fibrinolytic inhibitor.

Nature of the Steroid-induced Inhibitor in Conditioned Cell Media

The [^{125}I]fibrin dish assay for fibrinolytic activity is a coupled system involving two enzymic steps: first, the conversion of plasminogen to plasmin and second, the plasmin-catalyzed cleavage of fibrin to soluble degradation products. Either (or both) of these steps could be inhibited by the fibrinolytic inhibitor present in the medium of steroid-treated cells. Separate inhibition assays were therefore used to distinguish between these possibilities.

The presence of plasmin inhibitors in cell media was investigated by mixing samples of media with four concentrations of plasmin over a 20-fold range. The subsequent liberation of ^{125}I-labeled fibrin degradation products from a [^{125}I]fibrin dish was then measured. Conditioned medium from cells treated with 1 μM dexamethasone or hydrocortisone did not possess increased antiplasmin activity relative to medium from untreated cells (FIGURE 3A). This is in marked contrast to the strongly inhibitory properties of steroid-treated cell media when tested against cell plasminogen activator (FIGURE 2), and

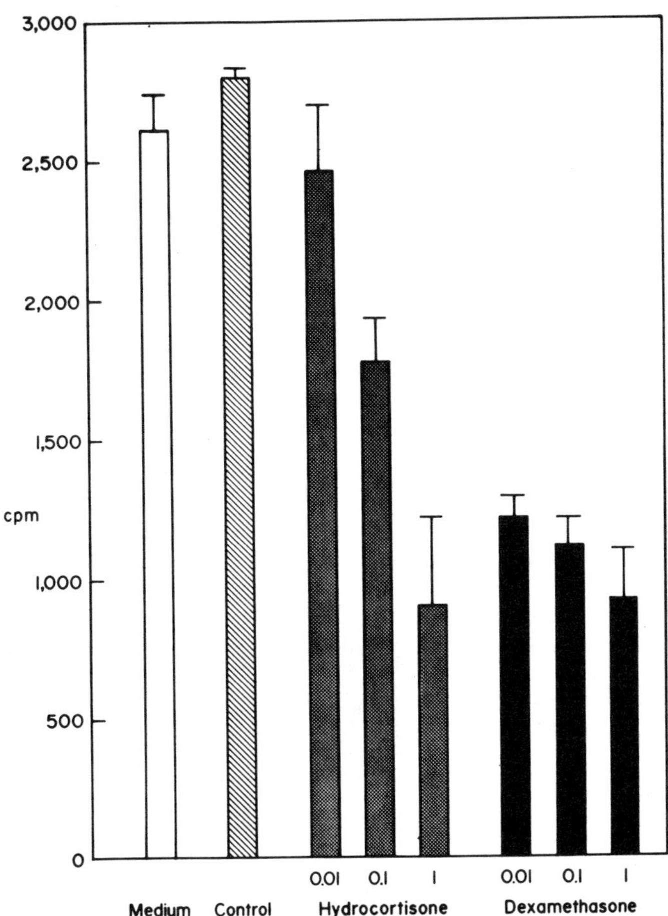

FIGURE 2. Antifibrinolytic activity of conditioned medium from steroid-treated cells. Conditioned medium from cells incubated with 0.01–1 μM dexamethasone, hydrocortisone, or vehicle (Control) was added to a reaction mixture containing 25 μg of control cell extract as a source of plasminogen activator. In all cases the fibrinolytic activity of the conditioned medium in the absence of cell extract was less than 3% of the value for the sample "Medium," which contained cell extracts, and fresh growth medium not exposed to cells. Each value is the mean of triplicate incubations. Bars show SEM.

indicates that the protease inhibitor present in these media is not directed against plasmin. Plasmin inhibitors were also not detected in steroid-treated cell extracts (FIGURE 3B).

These results, taken together, suggest that the glucocorticoids have relatively little effect on intracellular plasminogen activator but rather induce the production of an inhibitor directed against plasminogen activator but not plasmin. Such an inhibitor might be expected to also inhibit urokinase. FIGURE 4 shows that steroid-treated cell media do indeed possess anti-urokinase activity when compared to untreated cell medium.

In conclusion, the present studies have confirmed that the overall fibrinolytic activity of normal cells in culture represents a balance between levels of plasminogen activator and fibrinolytic inhibitor(s). This balance may be altered by changes in growth state of the cells [11] or by the presence of hormones, such as glucocorticoids. The steroid hormones may be particularly important since their effects are seen at low concentrations. Our studies have also provided further evidence on how these compounds exert their antifibrinolytic effects.

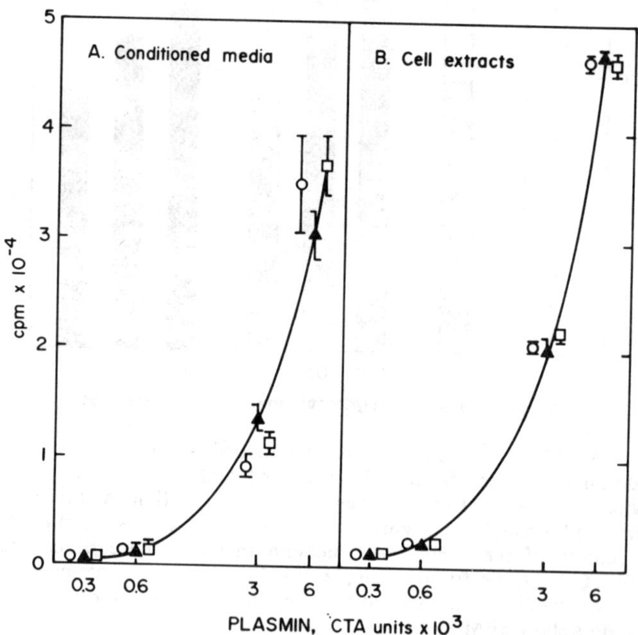

FIGURE 3. Comparison of the antiplasmin activity of cell extracts and growth media from control and steroid-treated cells. Conditioned growth media (Panel A) and cell extracts (Panel B) from fibroblasts exposed to 1 μM hydrocortisone (□) or 1 μM dexamethasone (▲) are indistinguishable from untreated control cells (○) in their effect on urokinase-generated plasmin.

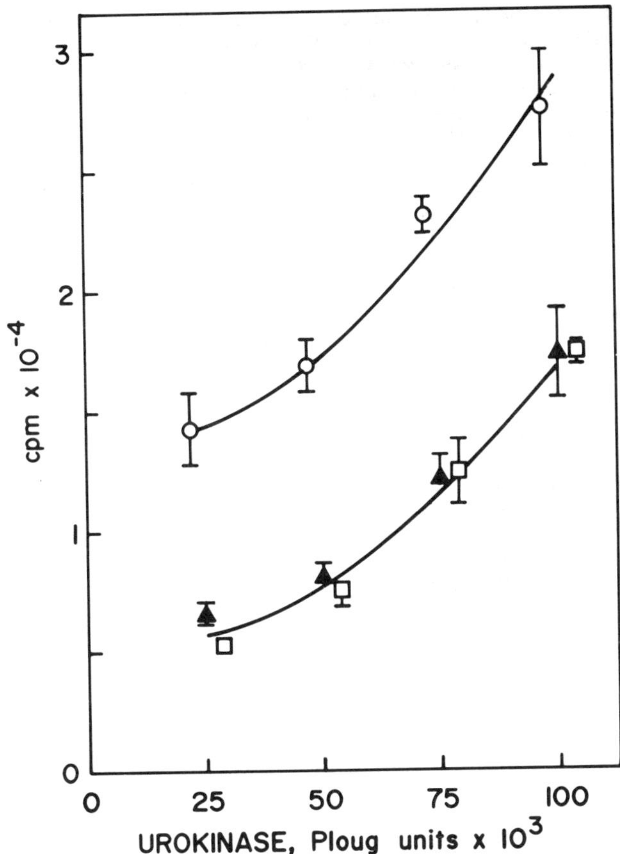

FIGURE 4. Comparison of the anti-urokinase activity of growth media from control and steroid-treated cells. Conditioned media from fibroblasts exposed to 1 μM dexamethasone (▲) or 1 μM hydrocortisone (□) inhibit urokinase activity when compared with untreated cell medium (○).

ACKNOWLEDGMENT

We thank Dr. Jeff Raines for many helpful discussions.

REFERENCES

1. WIGLER, M., J. P. FORD & I. B. WEINSTEIN. 1975. Glucocorticoid inhibition of the fibrinolytic activity of tumor cells. *In* Proteases and Biological Control. E. Reich, D. Rifkin & E. Shaw, Eds.: 849–856. Cold Spring Harbor Laboratory. Cold Spring Harbor, N.Y.
2. WERB, Z., C. L. MAINARDI, C. A. VATER & E. D. HARRIS. 1977. Endogenous activation of latent collagenase by rheumatoid synovial cells. Evidence for a role of plasminogen activator. New Engl. J. Med. **296:** 1017–1023.

3. RIFKIN, D. B. 1978. Plasminogen activator synthesis by cultured human embryonic lung cells: characterization of the suppressive effect of corticosteroids. J. Cell Physiol. **97:** 421–428.
4. SEIFERT, S. C. & T. D. GELEHRTER. 1978. Mechanism of dexamethasone inhibition of plasminogen activator in rat hepatoma cells. Proc. Natl. Acad. Sci. USA **75:** 6130–6133.
5. MAYNARD, J. R., B. E. DREYER, M. B. STEMERMAN & F. A. PITLICK. 1977. Tissue-factor coagulant activity of cultured human endothelial and smooth muscle cells and fibroblasts. Blood **50:** 387–396.
6. DEUTSCH, D. G. & E. T. MERTZ. 1970. Plasminogen: purification from human plasma by affinity chromatography. Science **170:** 1095–1096.
7. HAWKER, R. J. & L. M. HAWKER. 1976. A rapidly produced ^{125}I labeled autologous fibrinogen: *in vitro* properties and preliminary metabolic studies in man. J. Clin. Path. **29:** 495–501.
8. UNKELESS, J. C., A. TOBIA, L. OSSOWSKI, J. P. QUIGLEY, D. B. RIFKIN & E. REICH. 1973. An enzymatic function associated with transformation of fibroblasts by oncogenic viruses. I. Chick embryo fibroblast cultures transformed by avian RNA tumor viruses. J. Exp. Med. **137:** 85–111.
9. KWAAN, H. C., R. B. FRIEDMAN & M. SZCZECINSKI. 1978. Amplification of color yield of chromogenic substrates using *p*-dimethylaminocinnamaldehyde. Thromb. Res. **13:** 5–13.
10. CRUTCHLEY, D. J., L. B. CONANAN & J. R. MAYNARD. 1980. Induction of plasminogen activator and prostaglandin biosynthesis in HeLa cells by 12-*O*-tetradecanoylphorbol-13-acetate. Cancer Res. **40:** 849–852.
11. LEVIN, E. G. & D. J. LOSKUTOFF. 1979. Comparative studies of the fibrinolytic activity of cultured vascular cells. Thromb. Res. **15:** 869–878.

A SENSITIVE, COUPLED ASSAY FOR PLASMINOGEN ACTIVATOR USING A THIOL ESTER SUBSTRATE FOR PLASMIN *

Patrick L. Coleman and George D. J. Green †

Department of Human Genetics
University of Michigan Medical School
Ann Arbor, Michigan 48109

† Biology Department
Brookhaven National Laboratory
Upton, New York 11973

INTRODUCTION

In parallel with the increased interest during the past decade in plasminogen activator involvement in fibrinolysis, tumorigenesis, inflammatory responses, and the expression of hormonal regulation, there has been a rising interest in sensitive and precise methods for the specific assay of plasminogen activator. Several assays for plasminogen activator employ a direct assay method.[1-4] These are remarkably sensitive methods, yet they suffer in comparison to the sensitivity of coupled methods.[5-7] Coupling the assay with plasminogen not only amplifies the sensitivity by the multiplicative effect of plasmin, but insures that only those proteases specific for plasminogen are assayed. The choice of substrate for plasmin is critical. In general, esters are superior to amides in both K_m and k_{cat}, but they suffer a major deficiency in that they are frequently unstable at pH 7–9, the optimum range for plasmin. Green and Shaw [8] synthesized a thiol ester substrate, thiobenzyl benzyloxycarbonyl-L-lysinate (Z-Lys-SBzl), which combines high k_{cat} with alkaline stability relative to the commonly used esters.

In an effort to characterize the plasminogen activator from hepatoma tissue culture (HTC) and its hormonally controlled inhibitor, several of the known direct and coupled methods were found inadequate by reason of either low sensitivity or imprecision. Using Z-Lys-SBzl in a coupled approach we have developed an assay that is superior to the [^{125}I]fibrinolytic assay. It is also extremely sensitive to plasminogen activator ($\sim 2 \times 10^{-17}$ moles of urokinase) and can be used for routine analysis of purification as well as kinetic and binding studies.

MATERIAL AND METHODS

Methods

Plasminogen was prepared from fresh frozen plasma by the method of Deutsch and Mertz.[9] Purified plasminogen was exhaustively dialyzed against

* This work was supported by National Institutes of Health Grant CA 22729 to T. D. Gelehrter (Department of Human Genetics, University of Michigan (P.L.C.)) and the U.S. Department of Energy (G.D.J.G.).

617

1 mM HCl, lyophilized, and stored at $-20°$ C. Concentration was routinely determined by absorbance at 280 nm; $E_{280\,nm}{}^{1\%} = 17.0.$[10] Plasmin, the gift of Dr. David Aronson, was subsequently exhaustively dialyzed against 1 mM HCl and stored at $-20°$ C. Plasmin concentration was determined by active-site titrations using p-nitrophenyl-p-guanidinobenzoate.[11] Urokinase concentration was determined by active-site titrations with methylumbelliferyl p-guanidino-benzoate,[12, 13] using a ratio fluorometer built by Dr. D. Ballou (Dept. of Biological Chemistry).

Fibrinogen was enzymically iodinated[6] using Tris (60 mM)-KCl (300 mM) buffer, pH 7.6. Unbound iodide was separated by chromatography on Dowex 1 (Cl⁻). Specific radioactivity was 9×10^{11} cpm/g. Fibrin plates were prepared and fibrinolysis continuous assays were performed as previously described.[6] Discontinuous fibrinolysis assays were also performed, wherein plasminogen and urokinase were incubated in the absence of the fibrin, then added to the [^{125}I]fibrin well.

Plasminogen activator and inhibitor were prepared from HTC cells as previously described[14] except that serum-free conditioned medium additionally contained bovine serum albumin (1 mg/ml). HeLa-cell plasminogen activator was obtained as serum-free conditioned medium.[6]

Assay

The plasminogen-activator assay is a two-step procedure. In the first step plasminogen is activated to plasmin. The plasmin-catalyzed hydrolysis of Z-Lys-SBzl in the presence of 5,5′-dithiobis (2-nitrobenzoic acid) (DTNB) occurs in the second step. All reactions are typically performed in a 24-well tissue culture dish (each 15 mm diameter). This is not necessary, but convenient when handling many assays simultaneously.

The incubation mixture for the first step typically contains: plasminogen, 1.0 μM; glycine, pH 8.50, 120 mM; bovine serum albumin, 0.5 mg/ml; urokinase, 2.7×10^{-12} M. Total volume is 50 μl. The activity equivalent in plasminogen activator from HTC or HeLa cells may be substituted for urokinase. The reaction is started by the addition of plasminogen to the otherwise complete incubation mixture equilibrated at 37° C. Normally this incubation is allowed to react for 45 min.

The second step is initiated by dilution of the incubation mixture with 950 μl of the plasmin substrate solution: Z-Lys-SBzl, 200 μM; DTNB 220 μM; Triton X-100 0.01%; sodium phosphate (pH 7.50) 200 mM; sodium chloride, 200 mM. Normally the second step is quenched after 60 min by the addition of 100 μl of soybean trypsin inhibitor (1 mg/ml in 1 mM HCl). The absorbance at 412 nm may be read immediately or up to 4 h later. The extinction coefficient of 14,150 cm$^{-1}\cdot$M^{-1} was assumed for the thiophenolate product of the reaction of benzyl mercaptan with DTNB.[15]

Inhibitors were tested by incubation with the first-step incubation mixture prior to the addition of plasminogen. Bimolecular rate constants, $k_{app}/$[I], were determined as previously described.[16] Plasmin standard curves were obtained by substituting plasmin for plasminogen and urokinase in step one.

Other variations from the standard procedure were tested. Z-Lys-SBzl was substituted by D-Val·Leu·Lys p-nitroanilide. 2,2′-dithiodipyridine and 4,4′-dithiodipyridine, dissolved in dimethylformamide, were substituted on an equimolar basis for DTNB. All absorbance measurements were performed on a Gilford spectrophotometer model 2400–2.

Material

Fibrinogen (plasminogen-free), urokinase (B grade) and DTNB were the products of Calbiochem-Behring (La Jolla, CA). 2,2′- and 4,4′-dithiodipyridine were obtained from Aldrich Chemical Co. (Milwaukee). Carrier-free [125I]-(sodium salt) was purchased from Amersham-Searle (Chicago). D-Val·Leu·Lys *p*-nitroanilide was purchased from Kabi Group (Greenwich, CT). Z-Lys-SBzl was synthesized by Peninsula Laboratories (San Carlos, CA) according to the procedure of Green and Shaw.[8] Methylumbelliferyl *p*-guanidinobenzoate and soybean trypsin inhibitor (B grade) were obtained from Sigma Chemical Co. (St. Louis). Phe·Ala·ArgCH$_2$Cl was the gift of Dr. Elliott Shaw. All other chemicals were of reagent grade; 24-well culture plates were purchased from Linbro Co. (Bridgeport, CT).

RESULTS

The sensitivity of the assay depends on the combination of a low "spontaneous" rate of Z-Lys-SBzl hydrolysis with a high enzyme rate. TABLE 1 presents results of a buffer survey in which sodium phosphate yielded both the highest plasmin-catalyzed rate and the lowest "spontaneous" rate. The effect of Triton X-100 (0.001%–2%) on plasmin activity was determined (data not shown). Optimal activity was broadly centered on 0.01% Triton X-100, which was 150% of the rate of the detergent-free control. There was no effect on the "spontaneous" rate. Sodium chloride has an inhibitory effect on urokinase and HeLa and HTC plasminogen activators, but below 250 mM no effect was observed on plasmin activity (data not shown). Thus 200 mM NaCl was added to the plasmin assay solution, which depressed plasminogen activation 78%. FIGURE 1 presents the time- and plasmin concentration-dependence of the reaction. The rates are linear at least two hours if the substrate is not depleted. Under these conditions K_m is 19 μM, k_{cat} is 45 sec^{-1}.

Several modifications of the standard procedure were attempted in search of increased sensitivity (TABLE 2). The rate with 4,4′-dithiodipyridine was comparable to that with DTNB but the control (zero plasmin) absorbance was four-fold higher, thus limiting its utility at low enzyme levels. Doubling the substrates produced a 10% sensitivity gain, but with almost double the blank value.

Optimizations of the first step in the reaction (plasminogen activation) were performed by coupling these experiments to optimal plasmin assay conditions. Sodium glycinate gave the highest urokinase activity (TABLE 1). There was no effect of glycine concentration (20–1600 mM) on urokinase rate nor any effect of Triton X-100 above that attributable to its effect on plasmin (data not shown). FIGURE 2 presents the time- and urokinase concentration-dependence of the reaction. Urokinase activity is not reproducibly linear beyond 45 min, even in the absence of substrate depletion.

A direct comparison was made to a sensitive [125I]fibrin-lysis assay using either a continuous or discontinuous procedure (FIGURE 3). In the discontinuous assays, whether spectrophotometric or radiometric, the rate is directly proportional to the urokinase concentration, thus upward curvature would be expected on semi-log graph paper. In the continuous assays, both proteases are acting simultaneously (two amplifying mechanisms), thus, based on an analysis of the kinetic equations the response presented on semi-log paper should be linear. It is obvious that the spectrophotometric assay is significantly more sensitive than the radiometric assay.

The standard assay was used to evaluate K_m and k_{cat} for the urokinase-catalyzed activation of plasminogen. K_m and k_{cat} values were 1.7 μM and

TABLE 1

EFFECTS OF VARIOUS BUFFERS ON PLASMIN AND
UROKINASE ACTIVITY *

| | Relative Rates of Hydrolysis (% of Rate in Sodium Phosphate) | | |
| | Plasmin | | Urokinase |
Buffer	Enzymic	Non-enzymic	Enzymic
Phosphate (Na)	100	100	100
MOPS †	92	100	118
Barbital †	93	250	—
Tris †	76	420	102
Glycine †	79	220	143
Triethanolamine †	87	290	100
Tricine †	86	290	104
Pyrophosphate †	75	120	69
Phosphate (K) ‡	82	—	100
HEPES *	84	—	126
TES †	92	—	116

* All assays were performed at 37° C. Plasmin activity was determined by continuous recording of A_{412}. Urokinase activity was determined by the standard plasminogen activation assay described herein. In each case the pH profile (6.5–10) for sodium phosphate was obtained for comparison. The pH optima were: plasmin, 7.5; urokinase, 8.5–9.0. There was no variation in the blank rate in the urokinase assay. All buffers are 100 mM. pH was measured before and after incubation, and these values agreed ± 0.05.

† pH 8.50.

‡ pH 7.50.

44 min^{-1}, respectively, in 0.15 M NaCl. These compare favorably with 1.7 μM and 50 min^{-1} reported by Wohl et $al.$[17] for the high molecular weight form of urokinase at pH 7.40, 37° C. The K_m of the HeLa plasminogen activator was 1.8 μM; V_{max} was 0.16 ng plasminogen activated/min/ng HeLa protein.

Inhibition of urokinase activity by Phe·Ala·ArgCH$_2$Cl (FIGURE 4) and the dexamethasone-induced inhibitor from HTC cells (FIGURE 5) was also analyzed. The bimolecular rate constants ($k_{app}/[\text{I}]$) for the inactivation of urokinase by the chloromethyl ketone, whether determined by the coupled plasminogen-activation assay or by the direct urokinase-catalyzed hydrolysis of Z-Lys-SBzl (26 × 10^3 and 24 × 10^3 min^{-1}·M^{-1}, respectively), are in close agreement.

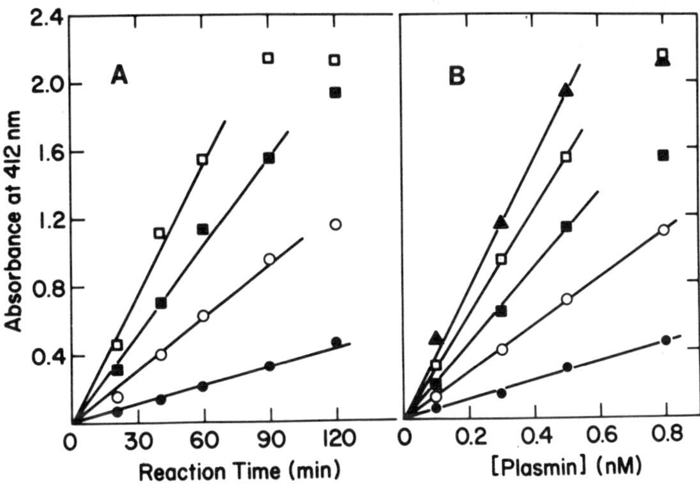

FIGURE 1. The time- and plasmin concentration-dependence of Z-Lys-SBzl hydrolysis. A. Reactions were stopped at the time indicated by addition of soybean trypsin inhibitor. Reaction volume was 1.0 ml. [Z-Lys-SBzl] = 200 μM, [DTNB] = 220 μM. Plasmin concentrations were 0.1 (●), 0.3 (○), 0.5 (■), and 0.8 (□) nM. B. Conditions were as stated in FIGURE 1A. The reactions were stopped at 20 (●), 40 (○), 60 (■), 90 (□), and 120 (▲) min. The lines were determined by linear-regression fit of the data and are drawn to encompass only the linear portion of the data. All data points represent the average of duplicates.

TABLE 2

VARIATIONS ON THE STANDARD PLASMIN-CATALYZED HYDROLYSIS OF
Z-LYS-SBZL COUPLED WITH DTNB *

Substrate/Chromogen	Sensitivity (A/nM)
Z-Lys-SBzl/DTNB	2000
Z-Lys-SBzl/DTNB (2X)†	2260
Z-Lys-SBzl/2,2′-dithiodipyridine ‡	700
Z-Lys-SBzl/4,4′-dithiodipyridine §	2030
D-Val·Leu·Lys p-nitroanilide ¶	600

* Plasmin was varied 0–1 nM in 60 min assays that were terminated by addition of 100 μl soybean trypsin inhibitor as detailed in the Experimental section. DTNB reactions were measured at 412 nm.

† Both reagents were at twice the standard concentrations.

‡ Measured at 270 nm, the wavelength of maximum ΔA.

§ Measured at 324 nm, the wavelength of maximum ΔA.

¶ Measured at 383 nm, the wavelength of maximum ΔA.

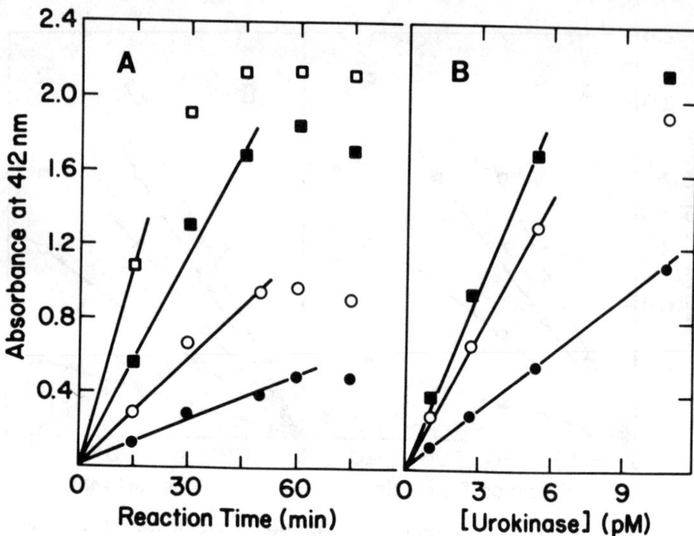

FIGURE 2. The time- and urokinase concentration-dependence of the plasminogen activation reaction coupled to the hydrolysis of Z-Lys-SBzl by plasmin. The conditions for the thiol ester hydrolysis are described in the Experimental section. A. The reaction was terminated at the indicated time by addition of 950 μl of the plasmin reaction solution as described in the text. Urokinase concentrations were 1.08 ($\bullet$), 2.7 ($\bigcirc$), 5.4 ($\blacksquare$), and 10.8 ($\square$) pM. B. Conditions were as described in FIGURE 2A. The activations were quenched at 15 ($\bullet$), 30 ($\bigcirc$), and 45 ($\blacksquare$) min. Data at 60 and 75 min are not presented since the response is not a linear function beyond 45 min (see FIGURE 2A). All times and concentrations relate to the 50 μl activation reaction. The lines represent a linear-regression fit of the data and are drawn to encompass only the linear portion of the data. All data points represent the average of duplicates.

These results differ significantly from those of Kettner and Shaw,[16] 2.9×10^3 min$^{-1} \cdot$M^{-1}, however the pH used here was 1.5 units more basic, which could account for a higher rate. Scatchard analysis of the inhibition of urokinase by the dexamethasone-induced inhibitor from HTC cells yields $K_i \sim 10^{-12}$ M, but the stoichiometry cannot be calculated because the concentration of inhibitor is unknown. A K_i in this range has been previously reported by Green [18] for the association of Kunitz pancreatic inhibitor (aprotinin) with bovine trypsin, but most protease-inhibitor complexes have lower affinities.

DISCUSSION

In general base-catalyzed reactions, such as the "spontaneous" hydrolysis of Z-Lys-SBzl, the choice of buffering agent is often critical if the assay is to be used near its limit of sensitivity. The small list of buffers tested here includes a wide range of "spontaneous" rates and suggests the utility of buffer surveys as a general procedure in assay development.

The standard assay employs 1.0 μM plasminogen which is close to the K_m concentration. An approximately two-fold increase in sensitivity would be realized if a ten-fold higher plasminogen concentration were used, but in most cases the higher sensitivity is not needed, and the use of 10 μM or higher substrate would consume large amounts of plasminogen.

Since there are no pure inhibitors available that are completely selective for plasminogen activators in the presence of plasmin, several other methods were used to depress the activation during the Z-Lys-SBzl step. Primarily, plasminogen activation was inhibited by dilution (20-fold), but the pH shift (1 unit off the optimum) and the addition of chloride yielded substantial additional inhibition (two- and three-fold, respectively). The net activator activity in the second step was less than 1% of its initial value.

The sensitivity with the thiol ester compares favorably with the other substrates tested. As an ester, Z-Lys-SBzl has the advantage of the lowest K_m, and highest k_{cat}. Most of the amide substrates have high K_m and low k_{cat} values. Their chief advantage is their chemical stability. Fluorogenic amide substrates might yield a more sensitive assay based on the greater sensitivity of detection. Were a fluorogenic thiol reagent substituted for DTNB the limit of detection of the hydrolysis of Z-Lys-SBzl might be lowered.

The spectrophotometric assay is considerably more sensitive than the radio-

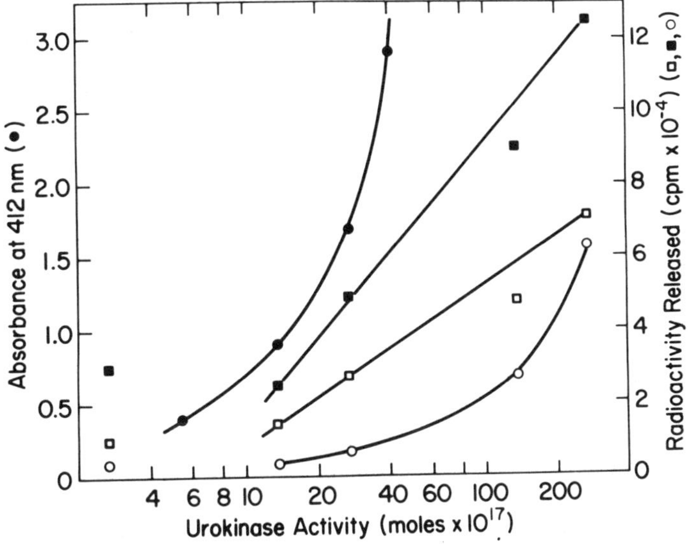

FIGURE 3. A comparison of spectrophotometric and radiometric coupled assays for urokinase. The spectrophotometric assay (●) was performed according to the standard procedures outlined in the text. The volume of continuous radiometric assay is 1.0 ml in 100 mM sodium glycinate, pH 8.50 with 50 nM plasminogen. Total CPM released at 60 (□) and 105 (■) min of incubation are presented. The latter time is the total time required by the discontinuous assays. In the discontinuous radiometric assay (○) plasminogen (1.0 μM) was activated by urokinase in the glycine buffer for 45 min then a 50 μl aliquot was added to the [^{125}I]fibrin-coated well containing 950 μl of 200 mM sodium phosphate and 200 mM NaCl. Total CPM released after 60 min in the presence of fibrin are presented. All reactions were perfomed at 37° C. All radiometric points are averages of triplicates. All spectrophotometric points are averages of duplicates.

metric assay. In the direct comparison (FIGURE 3) there is no difference between 2.7 and 13.5×10^{-17} moles by the radiometric assay, whereas ΔA_{412} is 0.50 between 5.4 and 13.5×10^{-17} moles. Typically in the Z-Lys-SBzl assay the measured difference between 2.7×10^{-17} moles urokinase and the zero urokinase control is >0.100 A_{412}. The assay is also sensitive to other plasminogen activators. 1 ng of protein from HeLa serum-free conditioned medium yields net $\Delta A_{412} = 0.190$. For 1 μg of protein from HTC whole-cell extract the net $\Delta A_{412} = 0.54$. 20 ng of serum-free conditioned medium protein from dexamethasone-induced HTC cells inhibits 90% of the activity present in 7×10^{-16} moles of urokinase.

The wide versatility of the method is demonstrated by the ease of determination of K_m and V_{max} values for plasminogen activation and of inhibition constants for the interaction of the enzyme with natural or synthetic inhibitors. Since the assay is more rapid and sensitive to low levels of enzyme it is more readily adaptable to monitoring enzyme purification than [125I]fibrinolysis.

In summary, the procedure is a sensitive, precise, and rapid method for the analysis and characterization of plasminogen activators. All reagents and materials are inexpensive and commercially available, the colored products are stable, and the measurement is performed on the standard quality spectro-

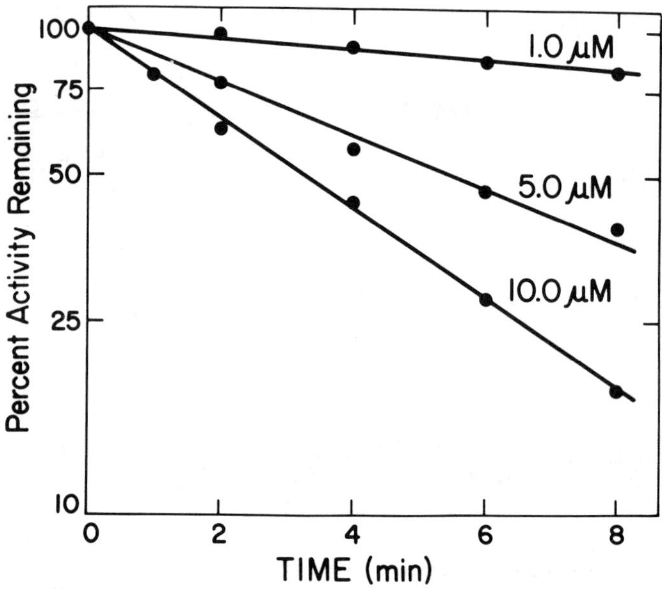

FIGURE 4. The inactivation of urokinase by Phe·Ala·ArgCH₂Cl. Prior to activity determination by the standard assay, urokinase (1.08×10^{-10} M) was incubated with the indicated concentration of the tripeptidyl inhibitor in 80 mM sodium glycinate, pH 8.50 with 1 mg/ml bovine serum albumin, 25° C. At the indicated times, 5 μl of the reaction solution were diluted into 85 μl of the same glycine buffer at 0°. At the completion of the inactivation reaction (8 min) all activation reactions were initiated simultaneously by addition of 10 μl of 10 μM plasminogen and removal to a 37° C incubator. 900 μl rather than 950 μl of plasmin reaction solution was used. $k_{app}/[I] = 260 \times 10^3$ min^{-1}·M^{-1}.

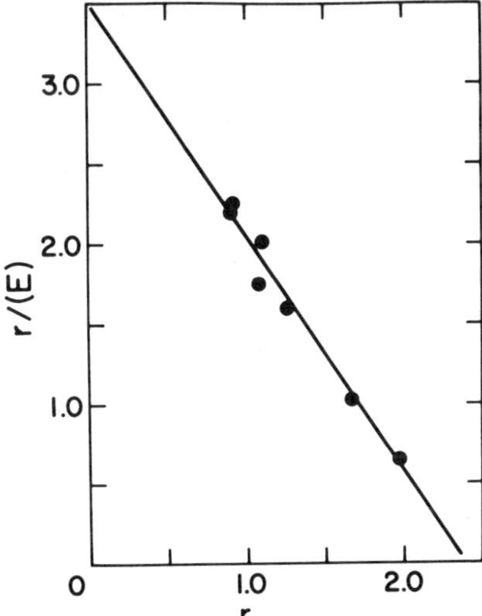

FIGURE 5. Scatchard analysis of the inhibition of urokinase by the plasminogen-activator inhibitor from hepatoma tissue-culture cells. The inhibitor test solution was the serum-free conditioned medium from dexamethasone-induced (10^{-7} M, 16 h) cells. 1–5 μl of test solution were incubated with urokinase (2.7×10^{-16} moles) for 15 min at 25° in 45 μl total volume. The activation reaction was started by the addition of 5μl of 10 μM plasminogen and shifted to 37° C. E is the concentration of active urokinase; r is the concentration of inactive urokinase.

photometer available in almost all laboratories. It is superior to existing methods in its simplicity and ease of manipulation and in the quality of the resultant data—kinetic constants rather than arbitrary units.

ACKNOWLEDGMENTS

We would like to thank Dr. David Aronson (Bureau of Biologics, Public Health Service, Bethesda, MD 20014) for the gift of purified plasmin. We are also grateful to Drs. Elliott Shaw and Charles Kettner (Biology Department, Brookhaven National Laboratory, Upton, NY) for valuable discussions and the gift of Phe·Ala·ArgCH$_2$Cl. We wish to thank Drs. Gelehrter and Shaw for financial support, encouragement, and constructive suggestions.

REFERENCES

1. NIEUWENHUIZEN, W., G. WIJNGAARDS & E. GROENVELD. 1977. Fluorogenic peptide amide substrates for the estimation of plasminogen activators and plasmin. Anal. Biochem. **83:** 143–148.
2. HUSEBY, R. M., S. A. CLAVIN, R. E. SMITH, R. N. HULL & E. L. SMITHWICK, JR. 1977. Studies on tissue culture plasminogen activator. Thrombosis Res. **10:** 679 687.
3. ZIMMERMAN, M., J. P. QUIGLEY, B. ASHE, C. DORN, R. GOLDFARB & W. TROLL.

1978. Direct fluorescent assay of urokinase and plasminogen activators of normal and malignant cells: kinetics and inhibitor profiles. Proc. Natl. Acad. Sci. USA **75:** 750–753.

4. WEHRLY, J. A. 1979. Fluorogenic detection of serine proteases: instrumentation and substrates. Ph.D. Thesis. University of Illinois. Urbana, Ill.

5. UNKELESS, J. C., A. TOBIA, L. OSSOWSKI, J. P. QUIGLEY, D. B. RIFKIN & E. REICH. 1973. An enzymatic function associated with transformation of fibroblasts by oncogenic viruses. J. Exp. Med. **137:** 85–111.

6. COLEMAN, P., C. KETTNER & E. SHAW. 1979. Inactivation of plasminogen activator from HeLa cells by peptides of arginine chloromethyl ketone. Biochim. Biophys. Acta **569:** 41–51.

7. HEUSSEN, C. & E. B. DOWDLE. 1980. Electrophoretic analysis of plasminogen activators in polyacrylamide gels containing sodium dodecyl sulfate and copolymerized substrates. Anal. Biochem. **102:** 196–202.

8. GREEN, G. D. J. & E. SHAW. 1979. Thiobenzyl benzyloxycarbonyl-L-lysinate, substrate for a sensitive colorimetric assay for trypsin-like enzymes. Anal. Biochem. **93:** 223–226.

9. DEUTSCH, D. G. & E. T. MERTZ. 1970. Plasminogen: Purification from human plasma by affinity chromatography. Science **170:** 1095–1096.

10. ROBBINS, K. C. & L. SUMMARIA. 1965. Human plasminogen and plasmin. Meth. Enzymol. **19:** 184–199.

11. CHASE, T., JR. & E. SHAW. 1967. p-Nitrophenyl-p'-guanidinobenzoate·HCl: A new active site titrant for trypsin. Biochem. Biophys. Res. Commun. **29:** 508–514.

12. JAMESON, G. W., D. V. ROBERTS, R. W. ADAMS, W. S. A. KYLE & D. T. ELMORE. 1973. Determination of operational molarity of solutions of bovine α-chymotrypsin, trypsin, thrombin, and Factor X_a by spectrofluorimetric titration. Biochem. J. **131:** 107–117.

13. COLEMAN, P. L., H. G. LATHAM, JR. & E. SHAW. 1976. Some sensitive methods for the assay of trypsin-like enzymes. Meth. Enzymol. **45:** 12–26.

14. SIEFERT, S. C. & T. D. GELEHRTER. 1978. Mechanism of dexamethasone inhibition of plasminogen activator in rat hepatoma cells. Proc. Natl. Acad. Sci. USA **75:** 6130–6133.

15. RIDDLES, P. W., R. L. BLAKELEY & B. ZERNER. 1979. Ellman's reagent: 5,5'—dithiobis (2-nitrobenzoic acid)—a reexamination. Anal. Biochem. **94:** 75–81.

16. KETTNER, C. & E. SHAW. 1979. The susceptibility of urokinase to affinity labeling by peptides of arginine chloromethyl ketone. Biochim. Biophys. Acta **569:** 31–40.

17. WOHL, R. C., L. SUMMARIA & K. C. ROBBINS. 1980. Kinetics of activation of human plasminogen by different activator species at pH 7.4 and 37° C. J. Biol. Chem. **255:** 2005–2013.

18. GREEN, N. M. 1957. Kinetics of the reaction between trypsin and the pancreatic trypsin inhibitor. Biochem. J. **66:** 407–415.

STUDIES ON A HIGHLY POTENT ANTICOAGULANT ANIONIC HIGH MOLECULAR WEIGHT FRACTION ISOLATED FROM PORCINE HEPARIN

Edgar Sache, Jean Choay, and Jawed Fareed *

Institut Choay
75782 Paris Cedex 16, France

** Loyola University Medical Center*
Maywood, Illinois 60153

INTRODUCTION

Since the discovery of heparin,[1,2] many methods for its fractionation have been proposed [3,4] with the hope of obtaining a stronger fraction with potent anticoagulant activity. To date, the results of such fractionation experiments have been mostly obtained by assay methods based on the rate of fibrin formation (i.e., clottting assays). However, the recent introduction of synthetic chromogenic substrates, the *p*-nitroanilides of tri- or tetrapeptides has afforded the possibility of new means for monitoring the fractionation of heparin. Under appropriate conditions, the relative anticoagulant potency of an unknown heparin material can be predicted from the kinetic information obtained from the inhibition of a number of serine proteases of the coagulation cascade. Due to the sensitivity of the chromogenic assays only a small amount of test material is required.

The aim of the present work was to develop newer forms and/or fractions of heparin by methods that are industrially feasible and economically bearable. We have studied the fractionation of USP porcine sodium heparin (PSH) in view of possible differences in the anticoagulant properties of the fractions obtained by various methods. The availability of chromogenic peptide substrates has greatly facilitated these studies.

In this presentation, we report the fractionation of PSH either on gel filtration or ion exchange chromatography columns, which resulted in the isolation of a strongly anionic, high molecular weight, potent anticoagulant fraction in both the *in vitro* and *in vivo* test systems.

MATERIAL AND METHODS

Material

The sodium salts of heparin from porcine intestinal tissues (PSH) were used throughout this work (respectively from Choay, Paris, France, from Diosynth, Oss, Holland, from Cohelfred Laboratories Inc., Chicago, IL, and from Sigma, St. Louis, MO). Samples of heparin calibrated in molecular weight were the kind gift of Dr. G. Van Dedem. The given molecular weights of these samples were 8,200, 12,400, 15,000, 17,300 and 21,000, respectively. Ultrogel (AcA 54) was obtained from Reactifs IBF (Clichy, France), and DEAE-Sephacel from Pharmacia (Uppsala, Sweden). The antithrombin III (AT

0077–8923/81/0370–0627 $01.75/0 © 1981, NYAS

III)-Sepharose gel (purified bovine AT III) was generously provided by Dr. J. C. Lormeau † Thrombin (bovine; 50 NIH—U/mg) was obtained from Hoffmann-LaRoche (Basel, Switzerland, Roche Diagnostica). Russell's viper venom (RVV) was purchased from Wellcome (Beckenham, England). The chromogenic substrates S-2238 (H-D-Phe-Pip-Arg-pNA) and S-2222 (Bz-Ileu-Glu-Gly-Arg-pNA) were purchased from AB-Kabi (Stockholm, Sweden). The fluorogenic substrate (D-Phe-Pro-Arg-5-amidoisophtalic acid dimethyl ester) was from Dade (Miami, Fla.), (Protopath System, with use of a thrombin reagent from bovine origin). Suspensions of cephalin and kaolin were from Stago (Asnières, France), micronized silica (APTT reagent, particulate) from General Diagnostics (Morris Plains, NJ), and ellagic acid from Dade (Dade Actin reagent). Sodium polystyrene sulfonate standards with molecular weights 4,000, 6,500, 16,000, 31,000, and 65,000 were obtained from Pressure Chemical Co. (Pittsburgh, PA).

Heparin Concentration

Heparin concentration in the chromatographic fractions was conveniently estimated by polarimetric measurements using a Perkin-Elmer Model 241 Polarimeter (Uberlingen, W. Germany) with readings at 365 nm (Hg spectral line); $[\alpha]_{365\,nm}^{25°C} = 139° \pm 6$ for the PSH samples referred to above. This technique was used when heparin concentrations exceeded 300 μg/ml. At lower concentrations the carbazole method was employed.

Molecular Weight Estimations

Molecular weight estimations of heparin fractions were carried out by high-pressure liquid chromography (HPLC) of the samples (500 μg/ml) using a Spectraphysics Liquid Chromatograph Model 35000 (Santa Clara, CA) equipped with a model 770 ultraviolet spectrophotometer detector and a set of two stainless steel connected columns (300 $\times$ 4.7 mm) packed with Lichrospher Si 100 Silica gel 10 μ (Merck, Darmstadt, Germany). The mobile phase used was 0.02 M sodium sulfate, at a flow rate of 1 ml/min. The column was calibrated using either heparin standards or sodium polystyrene sulfonate standards. Retention times of these markers were plotted against log molecular weights.

Procedures for Heparin Activity

In Vitro *Methods*

Selected fractions obtained after column fractionation of heparin were assayed for their ability to inhibit thrombin- and FXa-catalyzed amidolysis of chromogenic substrates S-2238 and S-2222, respectively. Outdated transfusion blood collected in citrate-acid–glucose was used as human plasma source. The blood was centrifuged (2000 $\times$ g for 20 min at 4° C) and the plasma removed

† Affiliation of Dr. J. C. Lormeau is: Choay-Chimie, Paris, France.

and stored at −20° C in polystyrene tubes. The buffers used were as indicated in the manufacturer's (AB-Kabi) data sheets, employing human plasma as the source of AT III and of factor X (FX). Activation of FX into FXa was brought about by RVV. A standardized heparin (180 USP U/mg) was used as reference in both the S-2238 and S-2222 assays. In these experiments the amount of heparin was such as to obtain approximately 50% of the amidolytic activity of thrombin or FXa when measured without heparin. In some experiments instead of human plasma, sheep plasma (USP grade) was used for anti-thrombin (S-2238) determinations.

In a typical experiment (anti-thrombin activity using S-2238), 16 μl human plasma are adjusted to 0.6 ml with Tris buffer, pH 8.4 and 0.1 ml thrombin (0.1 NIH unit) is added. After 2-min incubation at 37° C, 0.2 ml of 0.75 mM S-2238 substrate is added and absorbance is read at 405 nm. The same experiment is repeated in the presence of a standardized heparin (0.01 to 0.02 USP units), the decrease in absorbance being related to a known amount of the USP units. Unknown fraction are assayed identically, relating their activity to the heparin standard used. For anti-FXa activity determinations (S-2222), the procedure is very similar, using a 75 μl solution of RVV (5 μg) in 0.1 M NaCl–0.17 M CaCl$_2$, a 2 mM substrate solution, and approximately 0.05–0.1 USP unit of standard heparin.

Thrombin clotting time (TT) and activated partial thromboplastin time (APTT) were measured *in vitro* using equal amounts (2 μg) of PSH and its fractions. Freshly prepared normal human platelet-poor plasma was obtained from healthy normal male and female donors. The thrombelastographic (TEG) studies were carried out using freshly citrated human whole blood (19 parts blood, 1 part sodium citrate, as a 9% solution).

In Vivo *Experiments*

New Zealand white rabbits (average weight, 3 kg) were separated into two groups of 4 animals each. The first group received PSH (control group) and the other group the heparin fraction (see RESULTS). Heparin or its fraction (2.5 mg/kg body weight) was dissolved in 2 ml sterile saline and injected with a 5 ml polypropylene syringe (B-D Plastipak) into the marginal ear vein. Five-ml blood samples were drawn in 3.8% sodium citrate anticoagulant solution (9 parts blood, 1 part sodium citrate). The tests were performed on platelet-poor plasma obtained prior to heparinization and at 1, 3 and 6 hours post-injection time.

Healthy male mongrel dogs weighing 15–20 kg were divided into four groups of 4 animals each. The coagulation profile of each animal was studied and base-line values were obtained in terms of prothrombin time, APTT, TT, and fibrinogen levels. A stock solution (10 mg/ml) of heparin or its fraction was prepared in sterile saline. The heparin was injected through the intracubital vein slowly. Two groups of animals received PSH at 2.5 mg/kg whereas the other groups received the fraction under investigation, also at 2.5 mg/kg. Blood samples were drawn in 3.8% sodium citrate anticoagulant (9 parts blood, 1 part sodium citrate) at 1, 2, 3, 4, and 6 hour intervals, centrifuged at 2000 × g and immediately assayed for coagulation profiles.

In a primate model, monkeys (*Macaca mulatta*; average weight, 5–11 kg) were used. The coagulation profile of each animal was also studied and baseline values obtained as indicated above. PSH and its fraction were injected either intravenously or subcutaneously at 2.5 mg/kg, (10 mg/ml stock solutions) in sterile saline. Blood samples were drawn in 3.8% sodium citrate anticoagulant (9 parts blood, 1 part sodium citrate) prior to injection and at time intervals between 1 and 27 hours, centrifuged immediately at $2000 \times g$ and assayed for coagulation profiles (APTT). For heparin, quantitative measurements after intravenous injection of 0.25, 0.5, and 1 mg/kg of PSH and its fraction, a fluorometric method (Protopath) was used. In some comparative *in vivo* potency studies, APTT assays were carried out using both the particulate (General Diagnostics) and soluble (Dade) activating agents.

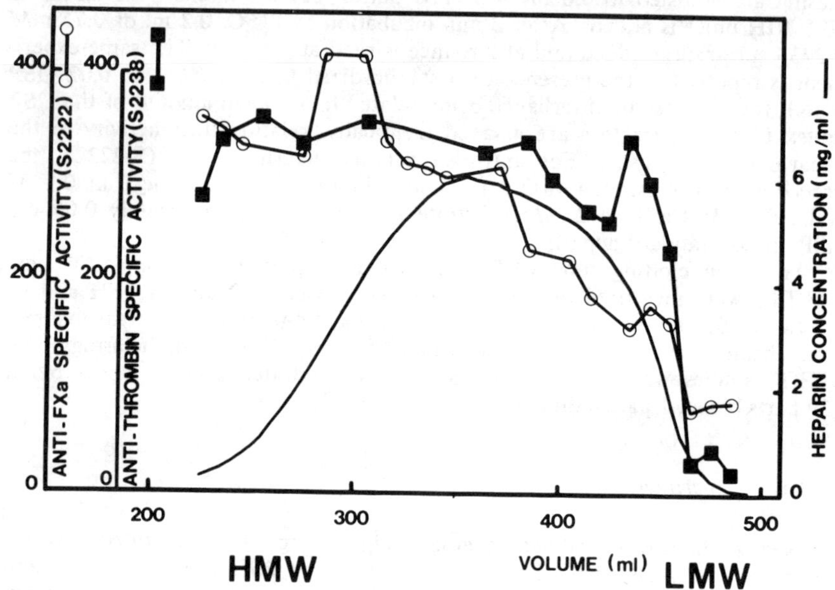

FIGURE 1. Gel filtration on Ultrogel AcA 54 of porcine sodium heparin (PSH). Sample (650 mg) was dissolved in 2 ml of a 0.3 M NaCl solution, pH 6.8, and applied to a column (2.6 × 100 cm), equilibrated and eluted with the same solution; flow rate, 20 ml/h; volume of fractions, 5 ml; temperature 4°C; (———), heparin concentration as determined by polarimetric measurements; (O—O), inhibition of FXa-catalyzed amidolysis of substrate S-2222; (■—■), inhibition of thrombin-catalyzed amidolysis of substrate S-2238. Both inhibition curves are expressed as specific activities (activity per mg weight heparin).

RESULTS

Gel Filtration Fractionation

Gel filtration experiments were carried out on a Ultrogel AcA 54 column as shown in FIGURE 1. Although the anti-thrombin specific activity (using the chromogenic substrate S-2238) is somewhat symmetrically distributed along the whole profile of the elution curve of heparin (FIGURE 1), the anti-FXa specific activity (S-2222) is mainly associated with the fractions eluted in the high molecular weight range (i.e. MW $\simeq$ 20,000), then decreasing more or less sharply on the descending limb of the elution curve of heparin. The activity patterns were very reproducible in a number of experiments where the various samples of heparin in this study were examined. Thus, it appears that heparin when fractionated by gel filtration and assayed with synthetic substrates shows two main regions with respect to its anticoagulant properties: a region of higher molecular weight where anti-thrombin and anti-FXa activities are associated and another region of lower molecular weight, extending from approximately molecular weights 14,000 to 6,000–7,000, with much lower anti-FXa activity and where anti-thrombin activity alone predominates.

Although the overall reproducibility of the anti-thrombin and of the anti-FXa elution curves was generally good in a series of experiments using either sample-to-sample heparin or heparins from different sources, some variations nevertheless could be observed in the detail of both these patterns. In such cases a difficulty was evidently experienced in deciding where to begin pooling the correct fraction(s). For this reason the method was not found completely satisfactory for large-scale fractionation experiments and further preparations were made using ion-exchange methods.

Ion Exchange Chromatography

These experiments were carried out using DEAE-Sephacel (DEAE-cellulose in bead form) columns with sodium chloride gradient elution. Occasionally, other anion exchangers were also used (QAE-Sephadex, TEAE-cellulose). The conditions for a typical experiment are illustrated in FIGURE 2 where human plasma was used as the source of AT III (in the anti-thrombin chromogenic assays) and of FX and AT III (in the anti-FXa chromogenic assays).

Based on the inhibition of serine protease activity patterns, four main chromatographic fractions are usually distinguished: fraction A, eluted with about 0.5–0.6 M NaCl, with negligible anti-thrombin and anti-FXa activities; fraction B, eluted with about 0.6–0.7 M NaCl, with higher anti-thrombin and anti-FXa activities; fraction C, eluted with about 0.7–0.8 M NaCl, with high anti-thrombin and anti-FXa activities; and fraction D, eluted with about 0.8 M NaCl, with very high anti-thrombin and anti-FXa activities.

The four fractions were pooled as indicated in FIGURE 2, dialyzed against six changes of twice-distilled water (until negative reaction to $AgNO_3$, i.e. for 72–96 hours) and lyophilized. These fractions were evaluated in the amidolytic and other coagulation assays to measure heparin activity. The results, as obtained from one representative experiment, are shown in TABLE 1. In all assays the fractions were always compared to the starting material (PSH). The fraction eluted at highest salt molarity, fraction D, was found to possess the strongest activity among the 4 fractions, (or, occasionally, more than 4 fractions) obtained using the ion-exchange method. Interestingly, in the US pharmacopoeial (USP) assays this fraction only possessed 25–30% higher activity than the starting material. However, in the amidolytic and clotting assays, it showed a much higher activity.

In all preparative work, ion exchange was used for the isolation of fraction D and further *in vitro* and *in vivo* studies were conducted using this fraction. It is hereafter referred to as the highly anionic, active fraction (HAF, TABLE 1).

Since sheep plasma is used in the pharmacopoeial standardization, it was

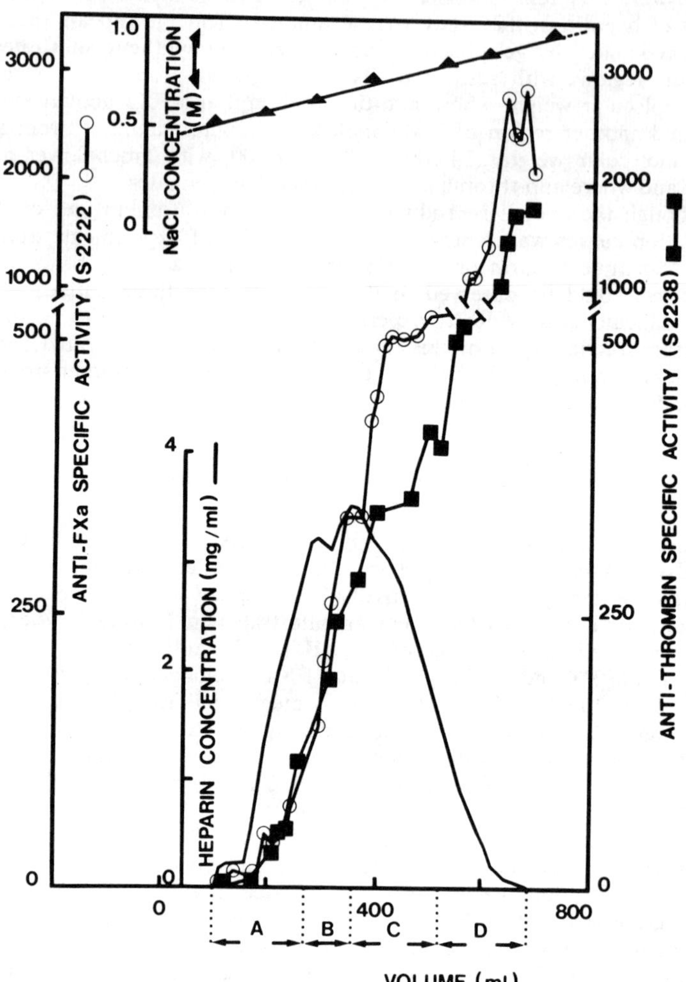

FIGURE 2. Ion-exchange chromatography on DEAE-Sephacel of porcine sodium heparin (PSH). Sample (1g) was dissolved in 10 ml of 0.05 M Tris-HCl buffer–0.4 M NaCl, pH 7.0, and applied to a column (2 × 28 cm) equilibrated with the same buffer; a linear NaCl gradient (0.4 M to 1.4 M) was initiated after the sample was introduced on the column; flow rate, 36 ml/h; volume of fractions, 3 ml; temperature, 4°C; (——), heparin concentration; (○—○), inhibition of FXa-catalyzed amidolysis of substrate S-2222 (using human plasma); (■—■), inhibition of thrombin-catalyzed amidolysis of substrate S-2238 (using human plasma); (▲—▲), NaCl concentration in the gradient.

TABLE 1

SOME PROPERTIES OF HEPARIN FRACTIONATED ON DEAE-SEPHACEL

Properties	Starting Heparin (PSH)	Heparin Fractions			
		A	B	C	D (HAF)
Fraction weight %	100	4	48	17	16
Molecular weight	17,300	7,300	13,200	17,300	20,300
Anti-thrombin activity (S-2238), U/mg					
sheep plasma	227	78	226	274	316
human plasma	304	4	133	396	538
Anti-FXa activity (S-2222) U/mg					
human plasma	283	5	118	395	609
Anti-FXa activity (Yin *et al.*, modified), U/mg	200	—	94	243	317
USP, U/mg	164	37	94	136	211
TT, sec	45 *	17	84	>780	>780
APTT, sec	160 †	61	213	740	>780
TEG (r + k), mm	68 ‡	25	51	84	149

NOTE: The procedure and reagents of the modified Yin *et al.*[6] method were kindly made available to us by Stago Diagnostica, France.

* Saline control : 12 sec.
† Saline control: 48 sec.
‡ Saline control : 23 mm.

felt that the amidolytic anti-thrombin activity monitored in assays supplemented with sheep plasma may provide information comparable to the USP method. A comparative pattern for anti-thrombin activity when sheep and human plasmas where the respective sources of AT III is shown in FIGURE 3. When the assay is supplemented with human plasma, a higher potency is observed, mostly associated with the high molarity elution region. This points to the differences existing in plasmas from different species as a source of AT III in the chromogenic assays and possibly in other anticoagulant tests.

Affinity Chromatography Experiments

These experiments were designed to examine the affinity behavior of heparin fraction D from DEAE-Sephacel (FIGURE 2) on a column of Sepharose-immobilized AT III. The AT III-Sepharose column (1.6×12 cm), with a protein content of about 10 mg/ml of final gel suspension, was equilibrated at 4° C with 0.1 M Tris-HCl buffer–0.2 M NaCl, pH 7.4, as described by Höök et al.[7] A sample of fraction D (2.76 mg in 500 μl of the same solution) was applied to the column, which was successively eluted with 0.2 M NaCl- and 2 M NaCl-containing buffers by a stepwise procedure. The effluent tubes (1 ml) were monitored by polarimetric measurements at 365 nm, by the carbazole reaction, and by assaying their capacity to inhibit thrombin- and FXa-catalyzed amidolysis of the chromogenic substrates S-2238 and S-2222, respectively. No material or activity was found in the breakthrough fraction eluted at 0.2 M NaCl whereas the activity, either assayed with S-2238 or S-2222, was recovered with full yield at 2 M NaCl elution. These results indicate that the highly anionic fraction D (HAF), when subjected to affinity chromatography under the conditions described above, behaves as a high-affinity heparin.

Further Studies on PSH and HAF

Potency equalization studies *in vitro* using the concentrations that were in the linear range of the various assays showed HAF to be at least 2–3 times more potent than the starting material (TABLE 2). Preliminary studies have also shown that HAF requires greater amount of platelet factor 4 (PF-4) for its neutralization, that it is less readily degraded than PSH by heparinase (Flavobacterial heparin lyase, EC 4.2.2.7.), and that it also has less aggregating effect for platelets than PSH (TABLE 2). Compared to PSH, HAF also demonstrated a pronounced effect on the inhibition of factor XIIa (FXIIa). In these experiments fresh normal human pool plasmas were supplemented at a 2.5 μg/ml level either with PSH or HAF and factor levels were determined employing a FXII-deficient plasma. The studies also indicated a possible direct inhibitory (though weak) activity toward FXa.

In Vivo Experiments with HAF

The anticoagulant effects of HAF were studied *in vivo* in rabbits, dogs and monkeys.

Rabbits were divided into a control group receiving PSH and a test group

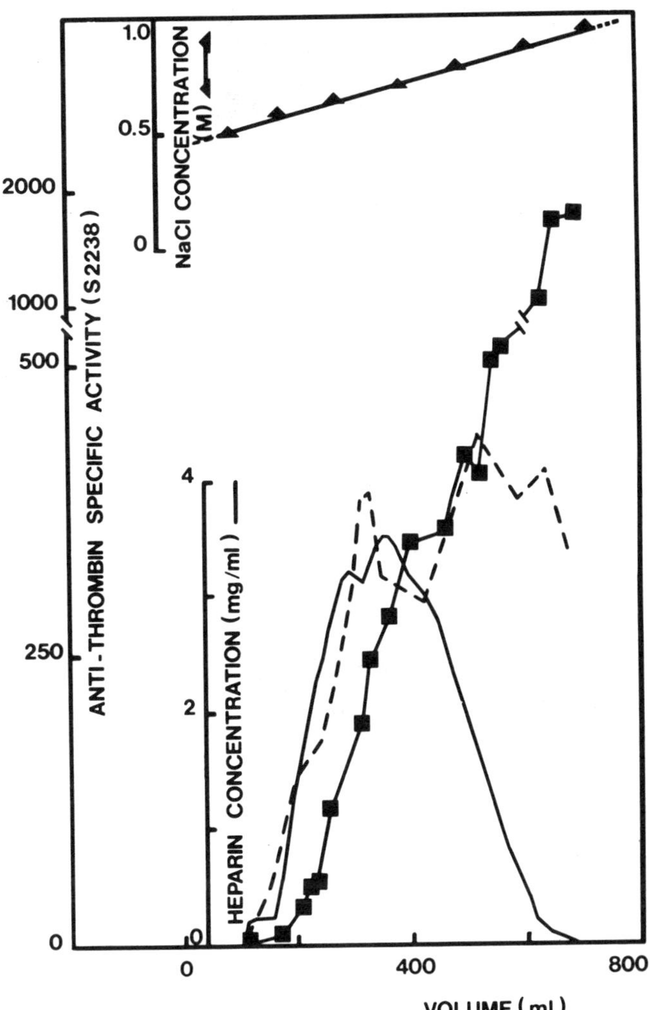

FIGURE 3. Ion-exchange chromatography on DEAE-Sephacel of porcine sodium heparin (PSH). The conditions are those of FIGURE 2. (———), heparin concentration; (■—■), inhibition of thrombin-catalyzed amidolysis of substrate S-2238 (using human plasma); dotted line, inhibition of thrombin-catalyzed amidolysis of substrate S-2238 (using sheep plasma); (▲—▲), NaCl concentration in the gradient.

TABLE 2

A COMPARISON OF PORCINE SODIUM HEPARIN (PSH) WITH ITS HIGHLY ANIONIC
FRACTION (HAF)

Properties	PSH	HAF
USP assays	1.4–1.6 USP U/ml	2–3 USP U/ml
Amidolytic assays *	1.5–2.0 USP U/ml	3–6 USP U/ml
Protamine titration	1.0–2.0 USP U/ml	3–6 USP U/ml
PF-4 neutralization	Readily neutralizable on a mg/mg basis	Resistant to the neutralizing action
Platelet aggregation	Positive in 25% healthy donors	Not seen
Heparinase susceptibility	Readily degraded	Only partially degraded at 2 hours (requires prolonged incubation)
AT III binding	Partially	Totally
Direct FXa inhibition	—	+
FXIIa inhibition	—	±

* Both S-2238 and S-2222 substrates were used in these assays.

receiving HAF. At a 2.5 mg/kg intravenous dose, 1 hour after injection HAF produced a pronounced elevation (3- to 5-fold) of both APTT (FIGURE 4) and calcium clotting time (FIGURE 5). In contrast, only a modest elevation was noted with the starting PSH material. At 3 hours, the PSH anticoagulant action was cleared whereas the animals treated with HAF still showed some anticoagulant activity. These experiments indicate that after intravenous administration of equal weight amounts of PSH and HAF a much more potent anticoagulant effect is exerted by HAF, which also exhibits a slower clearance.

The anticoagulant action and the pharmacokinetics of a 2.5 mg/kg dose of PSH in dogs and its comparison with HAF is shown in FIGURE 6. At one hour, both the PSH and HAF groups showed an APTT level of >100 seconds. At 2 hours the PSH group showed a marked decline in the APTT levels and

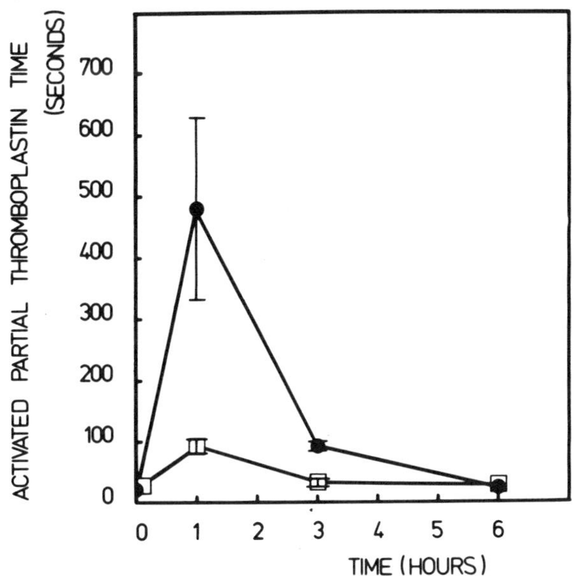

FIGURE 4. Changes (mean ± SEM; $n = 4$) in activated partial thromboplastin time (APTT) following intravenous administration to rabbits of PSH (2.5 mg/kg) (□—□) and HAF (2.5 mg/kg) (●—●). The APTT reagent was cephalin-kaolin (Stago).

progressively reverted to pretreatment level. Samples tested at 6 hours showed almost normal APTT levels. In contrast, the APTT levels remained >100 seconds up to 3 hours in the group receiving HAF, the animals showing a state of anticoagulation (APTT > 2.5 times) for almost 5 hours. A sustained elevated APTT remained for nearly 10 hours. A group tested at 24 hours showed almost no anticoagulant activity.

Phylogenetically, monkey is close to man and *in vitro* heparinization studies showed that monkey blood responds to heparin and its fractions in an identical manner as man. We therefore studied the anticoagulant action and pharmacokinetics of both PSH and HAF in a primate model, *Macaca mulatta*. FIGURE 7 shows that at a 2.5 mg/kg intravenous dose, a very strong initial anticoagulant

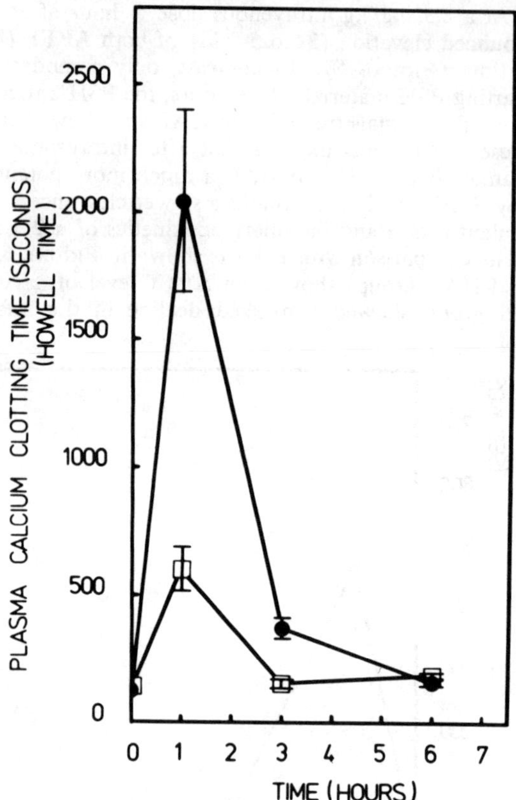

FIGURE 5. Changes (mean ± SEM; $n = 4$) in the calcium clotting time (Howell time) following intravenous administration of PSH (2.5 mg/kg) (□—□) and HAF (2.5 mg/kg) (●—●).

response is produced either by PSH or HAF. However, the anticoagulant action of HAF sustains for a much longer period than that of PSH. FIGURE 8 shows that a 2.5 mg/kg subcutaneous dose of HAF produced a strong, sustained anticoagulant response, whereas PSH only produced a mild anticoagulant response that was cleared within 6 hours.

The determination of heparin levels in monkeys after intravenous administration of PSH and HAF at 0.25, 0.5, and 1 mg/kg is shown in FIGURE 9. The assays were carried out by fluorometric measurements over a 5-hour period. PSH and HAF levels are expressed in terms of USP U/ml. In all of these tests the initial values were higher for animals treated with HAF for which a slower clearance was also observed.

In further experiments, the respective potencies of PSH and HAF were compared *in vivo* in monkeys. The animals were divided into two groups. PSH and HAF were injected intravenously at 1 mg/kg (5 animals) and 0.33 mg/kg (4 animals). The anticoagulant action of both preparations was followed by APTT tests using either a particulate (micronized silica) or a soluble (ellagic acid) reagent (FIGURE 10). These experiments show that nearly equivalent anticoagulant pharmacokinetic patterns are obtained when 1 mg/kg PSH and 0.33 mg/kg HAF are injected. It was also observed that two animals appeared as "low responders" to HAF. There is, however, at present no explanation to this observation.

DISCUSSION

Samples of porcine sodium heparins of USP grade can be fractionated into components differing in their anticoagulant potencies either by gel filtration or ion-exchange chromatography. A simple, powerful, and reproducible technique was found to be fractionation on a column of cellulose ion-exchanger (DEAE-Sephacel), using a linear NaCl gradient elution. The fractionation was monitored employing synthetic chromogenic substrates for the determination of anti-thrombin and anti-FXa activities. The most active anticoagulant fraction, whether assayed *in vitro* with synthetic substrates, by blood clotting determinations, or after *in vivo* administration to rabbits, dogs, and monkeys was always associated with an heparin component eluted at high NaCl (approximately 0.8 *M*) molarity. The yield of this fraction is approximately 15% by weight.

The experiments reported here also show that in the amidolytic as well as in the clotting assays, both the activities of thrombin and FXa are inhibited by this fraction. This material, obtained at high salt molarity with a gradient elution (or by a stepwise procedure, in scaled-up experiments), is highly negatively charged. The material has a high molecular weight, in the range of 20,000. When subjected to affinity chromatography on Sepharose-immobilized AT III columns,[7, 8] the fraction also demonstrates a high-affinity binding behavior. Its anticoagulant potency is 2–3 times that of the starting PSH,

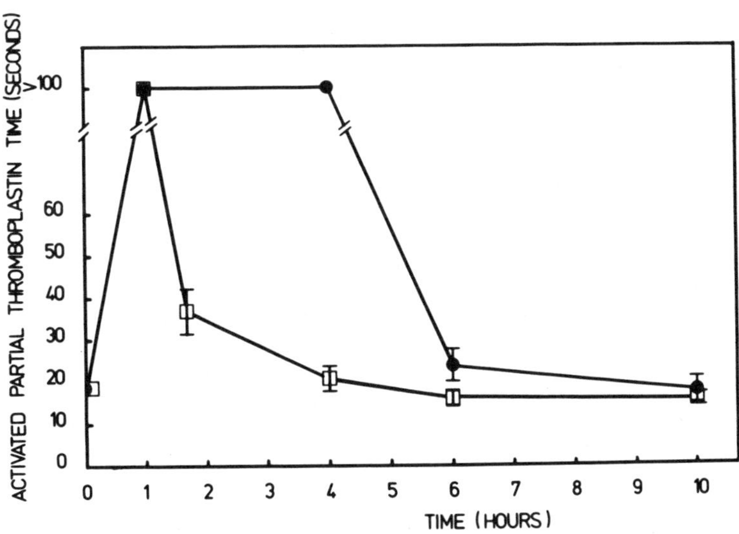

FIGURE 6. Changes in APTT following intravenous administration to dogs of PSH (2.5 mg/kg) (□—□) and HAF (2.5 mg/kg) (●—●). The APTT reagent was ellagic acid (Dade Actin reagent).

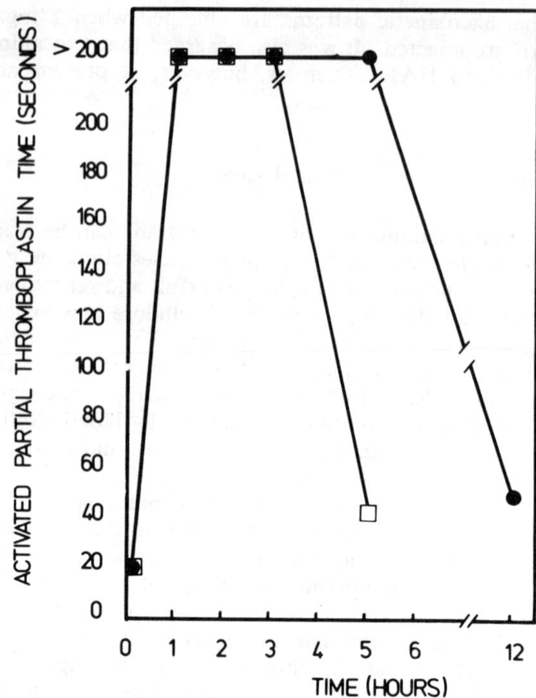

FIGURE 7. Changes in APTT following intravenous administration to monkeys of PSH (2.5 mg/kg) (□—□) and HAF (2.5 mg/kg) (●—●). The APTT reagent was ellagic acid (Dade Actin reagent).

depending upon the type of assays used. *In vivo* studies in three different animal models also showed a stronger anticoagulant response than for PSH. The pharmacokinetics of both heparin and its fraction indicate that the latter not only produces a much stronger anticoagulant action but also sustains for a longer period of time.

Earlier reports have already indicated the efficiency of anion exchange chromatography for obtaining heparin fractions of increased potency.[9-15]

It is also generally assumed that there exists a molecular weight dependency of the anticoagulant activity of heparin, and currently held views seem to indicate that anticoagulant activity increases with increasing molecular weight.[16] Recently, Danishefsky *et al.*[17] isolated very high-activity heparin fractions by chromatography on Biogel P-100 that were of high molecular weight and bound tightly to immobilized AT III. Thus, it seems that a high net negative-charge density, a high molecular weight, and a high affinity for immobilized AT III all represent favorable conditions associated with high anticoagulant potency. It is noteworthy that such conditions are all met within the fraction described here.

While the present work does not bear on other structural features responsible for anticoagulant activity like the distribution of saccharide units along the polysaccharide chain, preliminary experiments by NMR analysis (M. Petitou and B. Casu, personal communication) have clearly shown the occurrence of

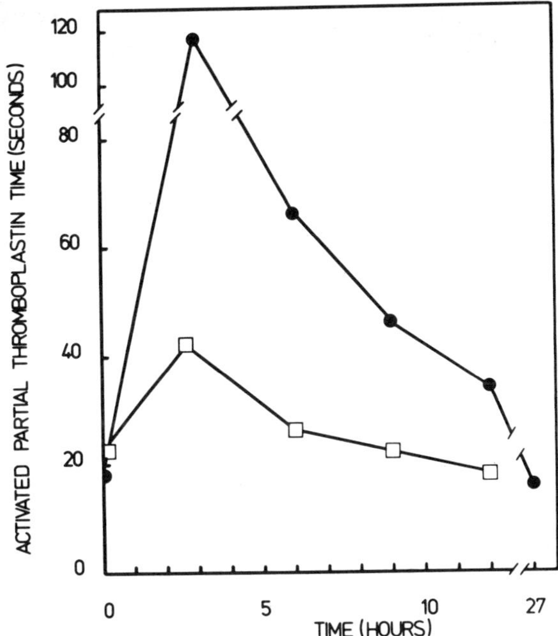

FIGURE 8. Changes in APTT following subcutaneous administration to monkeys of PSH (2.5 mg/kg) (□—□) and HAF (2.5 mg/kg) (●—●). The APTT reagent was ellagic acid (Dade Actin reagent).

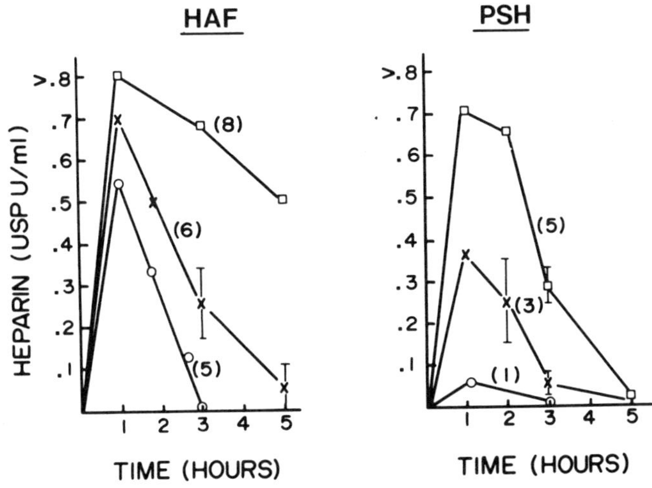

FIGURE 9. Determination of heparin levels in monkeys after intravenous administration of HAF and PSH. Number on each graph is number of animals in each experiment. A fluorometric method was used (Protopath System, Dade) with a thrombin reagent from bovine origin. (□—□), 1 mg/kg; (×—×), 0.5 mg/kg; (○—○), 0.25 mg/kg.

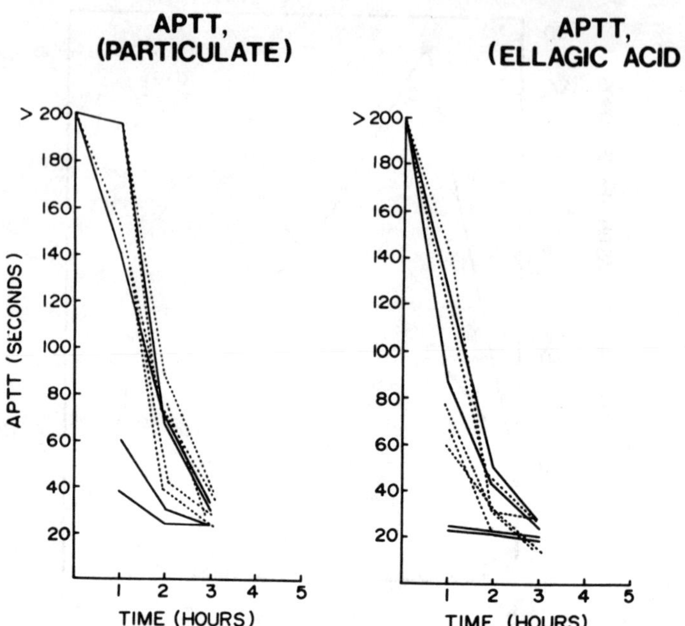

FIGURE 10. The pharmacokinetics of the anticoagulant action of PSH and HAF in monkeys. (– – –), PSH (1 mg/kg); (———), HAF (0.33 mg/kg). The APTT reagent used was either particulate (micronized silica, General Diagnostics) or soluble (ellagic acid, Dade).

N-acetyl groups in HAF. This finding may be relevant to recent studies showing that in porcine intestinal heparins a N-acetylated glucosamine unit is associated with the AT III binding site [18] and/or a tetrahedral sequence structurally critical for anticoagulant activity.[19] The possibility exists that besides having a higher affinity for AT III, HAF may not be, or be less, neutralizable by endogenous protein(s), such as PF-4. It may also be that some presently unknown molecular features favor its sequestration by cells of the reticulo-endothelial system,[20] making it available for a slower release as compared to PSH, with a consequent longer duration of hypocoagulation. Possibly, also, the heparinase complex from liver may not destroy HAF as readily as it destroys PSH.

The present studies suggest that simple chromatographic methods are useful for the fractionation of heparin into more potent fraction(s) and that amidolytic assays using thrombin and FXa-specific substrates can be used to monitor the inhibition of these serine protease activities as well as potency of the fraction(s). While these studies confirm that porcine sodium heparin preparations contain discrete populations of different molecular weight and charge, they also indicate that one of these imparts "heparin" with its anticoagulant properties, as used in clinical practice during anti-thrombotic therapy. The highly anionic, high molecular weight and potent anticoagulant fraction (HAF) described here may thus well represent the main anticoagulant component in porcine heparins.

REFERENCES

1. McLEAN, J. 1916. The thromboplastic action of cephalin. Am. J. Physiol. **41:** 250–257.
2. JAQUES, L. B. 1978. Addendum: the discovery of heparin. Semin. Thromb. Hemostas. **4:** 350–353.
3. BARROWCLIFFE, T. W., E. A. JOHNSON & D. P. THOMAS. 1978. Anti-thrombin III and heparin. Br. Med. Bull. **34:** 143–149.
4. JAQUES, L. B. 1977. Determination of heparin and related sulfated mucopolysaccharides. Methods Biochem. Anal. **24:** 203–311.
5. SVENDSEN, L., B. BLOMBÄCK, A. BLOMBÄCK & P. I. OLSSON. 1972. Synthetic chromogenic substrates for determination of trypsin, thrombin and thrombin-like enzymes. Thromb. Res. **1:** 267–278.
6. YIN, E., S. WESSLER & J. V. BUTLER. 1973. Plasma heparin: a unique, practical submicrogram-sensitive assay. J. Lab. Clin. Med. **81:** 298–310.
7. HÖÖK, M., I. BJÖRK, J. HOPWOOD & U. LINDAHL. 1976. Anticoagulant activity of heparin species by affinity chromatography on immobilized anti-thrombin. FEBS Lett. **66:** 90–93.
8. LAM, L. H., J. E. SILBERT & R. D. ROSENBERG. 1976. The separation of active and inactive forms of heparin. Biochem. Biophys. Res. Commun. **69:** 570–577.
9. GREEN, J. P. 1960. Fractionation of heparin on an anion exchanger. Nature **186:** 472.
10. RINGERTZ, N. R. & P. REICHARD. 1960. Chromatography on Ecteola of sulfate containing mucopolysaccharides. Acta Chem. Scand. **14:** 303–311.
11. TOCCACELI, N. & F. DELLA BERTA. 1961. Fractionnement de l'héparine par une résine cellulosique. Produits Pharmaceutiques. **16:** 212–215.
12. LASKER, S. E. & S. S. STIVALA. 1966. Physicochemical studies of fractionated bovine heparin. I. Some dilute solution properties. Arch. Biochem. Biophys. **115:** 360–372.
13. DI FERRANTI, N. & E. A. POPENOE. 1970. Labeling of acid mucopolysaccharides with tritium:Part II. Purification and fractionation of tritium-labeled heparin. Carbohyd. Res. **13:** 306–310.
14. PIEPKORN, M. W., G. SCHMER & D. LAGUNOFF. 1978. Isolation of high-activity heparin by DEAE-Sephadex and protamine-Sepharose chromatography. Thromb. Res. **13:** 1077–1087.
15. YUE, R. H., T. STARR & M. M. GERTLER. 1979. Preparation of high activity heparin by DEAE-cellulose chromatography. Fed. Proc. **38:** Abstract 4429.
16. BARROWCLIFFE, T. W., E. A. JOHNSON, C. A. EGGLETON & D. P. THOMAS. 1978. Anticoagulant activities of lung and mucous heparins. Thromb. Res. **12:** 27–36.
17. DANISHEFSKY, I., S. RADOFF, M. BENDER & G. VILLANUEVA. 1979. Isolation and characteristics of high-activity heparin. 7th Cong. Thromb. Haem: Abstract 0997.
18. LINDAHL, U., G. BÄCKSTRÖM, M. HÖÖK, L. THUNBERG, L.-A. FRANSSON & A. LINKER. 1979. Structure of the anti-thrombin-binding site in heparin. Proc. Natl. Acad. Sci. USA **76:** 3198–3202.
19. ROSENBERG, R. D., G. ARMAND & L. LAM. 1978. Structure-function relationships of heparin species. Proc. Natl. Acad. Sci. USA **75:** 3065–3069.
20. MAHADOO, J. & L. B. JAQUES. 1979. Cellular control of heparin in blood. Medical Hypotheses **5:** 835–841.

STRUCTURAL STUDIES ON A BIOLOGICALLY ACTIVE HEXASACCHARIDE OBTAINED FROM HEPARIN

Jean Choay, Jean-Claude Lormeau, Maurice Petitou,
Pierre Sinaÿ, and Jawed Fareed *

*Institut Choay
75782 Paris Cedex 16, France, and
Université d'Orleans, France*

** Loyola University Medical Center
Maywood, Illinois 60153*

INTRODUCTION

The isolation from heparin of oligosaccharides active in some specific coagulation assays should allow the study of the minimal critical saccharidic sequences responsible for the various biological effects of this anticoagulant drug. For this purpose, a decasaccharide [1] as well as two octasaccharides [2,3] were recently isolated and characterized. These products have a high anti-factor Xa activity (evaluated by the assay of Yin *et al.*[4] which is related to the ability to bind antithrombin-III (AT-III).

The structural studies carried out on the octasaccharide that we have isolated have led us to propose for this compound the following sequence [2,5]: 4, 5-unsaturated-2-*O*-sulfate uronic acid, *N*-sulfate-D-glucosamine, L-iduronic acid, *N*-acetyl-D-glucosamine, D-glucuronic acid, *N*-sulfate-3-*O*-sulfate D-glucosamine, 2-*O*-sulfate-iduronic acid, *N*-sulfate-D-glucosamine (FIG. 1, A–H). Nuclear magnetic resonance (nmr) studies, originally carried out on the decasaccharide [1] and then on the octasaccharide A-H,[6] revealed the presence in these products of an extra-signal at 57–59 ppm never reported before in heparin. This signal was then related to the presence of an *O*-sulfate group at C-3 of a glucosamine unit.[5-7]

The comparison of the sequences of the two different active octasaccharides led us to postulate that a common hexasaccharidic segment present in both species might be responsible for their biological activity and to propose further the saccharidic sequence of this molecular segment. We also found that further degradation of the octasaccharide A-H by heparinase in specified conditions yielded effectively a hexasaccharide that exhibited potent anti-Xa activity. The primary aim of the present work is to confirm the saccharidic sequence that we proposed for this hexasaccharide.

MATERIALS AND METHODS

Porcine Mucosal Octasaccharide

The octasaccharide A-H (FIG. 1) was obtained from heparin and characterized as already described.[2]

644

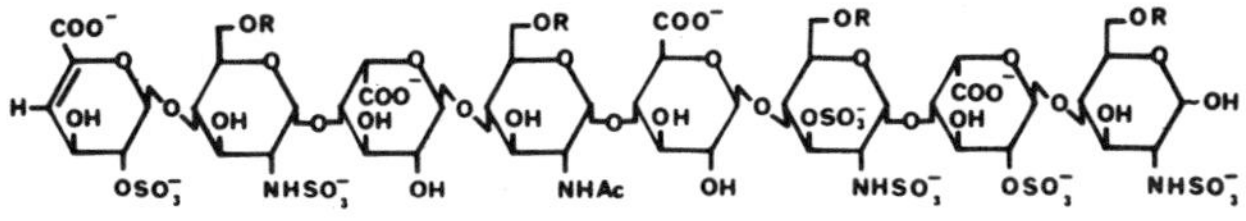

FIGURE 1. Proposed structure for the octasaccharide A-H obtained by enzymatic degradation of heparin by bacterial heparinase.

Enzymatic Degradation of the Octasaccharide

The octasaccharide was incubated in the presence of heparinase as we described for the degradation of heparin,[2] except that a higher amount of enzyme was used (0.5 mg of enzyme per milligram of octasaccharide).

Gel Filtration

The degradation products of the octasaccharide were fractionated on a column of Sephadex G-50 superfine (200 × 2.5 cm) eluted with 0.2 M sodium chloride. The fractionation of the products was monitored by following absorption at 230 nm. The pooled fractions were desalted and lyophilized.

Nitrous Acid Degradation

The degradation was performed according to the method of Shively and Conrad[8] on 0.5 to 1 mg of the material to be analyzed. The degradation products were fractionated on a Sephadex G-50 superfine column (200 × 0.6 cm) eluted with 0.2 M sodium chloride. The fractions were analyzed by previously described methods.[2]

Biological Assays

The entire anticoagulant activity of each fragment was determined by the USP test and the APTT method.[9] The Yin and Wessler method was used to assay the anti-Xa activity.[4] The *in vivo* antithrombotic activity was studied by means of a modified stasis model using rabbit[10] and prothrombin complex concentrate with Russell's viper venom mixture as thrombogenic agents.

RESULTS

Preparation of the Hexasaccharide

We began with the octasaccharide (15 mg) and after enzymatic degradation followed by gel filtration, three major fractions were obtained and were detected by absorption at 230 nm (FIG. 2). The first eluted fraction consisted of unde-

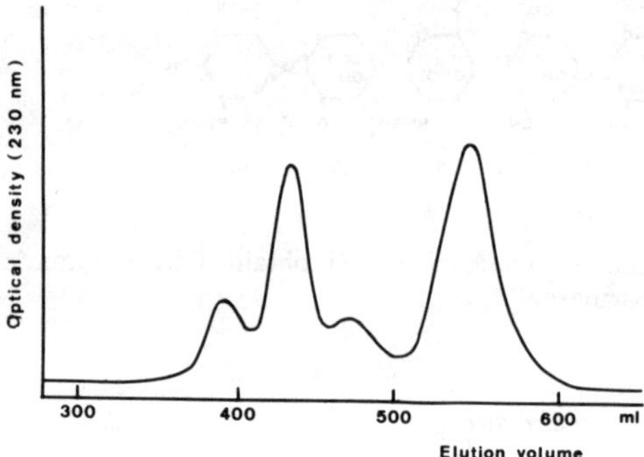

FIGURE 2. Chromatography on Sephadex G-50 of the products obtained by heparinase degradation of the octasaccharide. The hexasaccharide is eluted at 430 ml and the starting material octasaccharide A-H at 390 ml.

graded starting material (4 mg), the second one (7 mg) contained the hexa-saccharide, and the third one contained the disaccharides. A minor fraction was also detectable in the tetrasaccharide region, between the hexa- and the disaccharides.

Structural Analysis

The hexasaccharidic fraction was subjected to nitrous acid treatment under conditions that split all the glycosidic bonds between an *N*-sulfated-glucosamine and the next uronic acid [8] and convert all the sulfated glucosamine units into 2, 5-anhydromannose residues. The hexasaccharide was thus converted into a tetrasaccharide and a disaccharide which were separated by gel filtration (FIG. 3). The fractions eluted from the column were analyzed by optical density at 230 nm as well as for their content in 2, 5-anhydromannose, uronic acids, and glucosamine (for this last component, figures obtained before and after acid hydrolysis were compared, the difference yielding the content in *N*-acetyl-glucosamine). FIGURE 3 clearly shows that all the unsaturated uronic

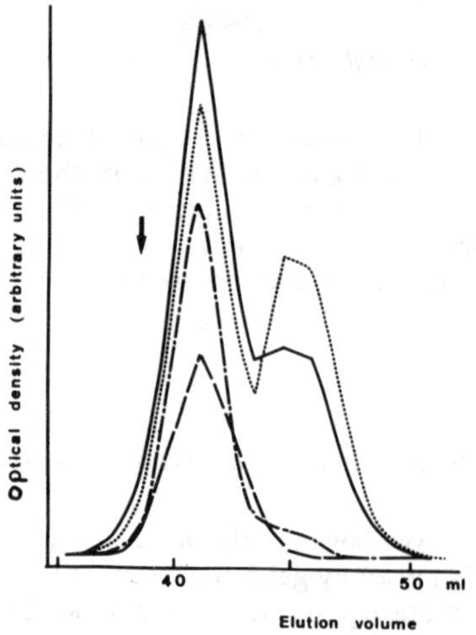

FIGURE 3. Colorimetric analysis of the hexasaccharide C-H fragments obtained by nitrous acid degradation followed by gel filtration. (———) uronic acids; (- - - - -) 2,5 anhydromannose; (— — —) *N*-acetyl-glucosamine; (— · — · —) optical density at 230 nm. The arrow indicates the elution volume for the original hexasaccharide.

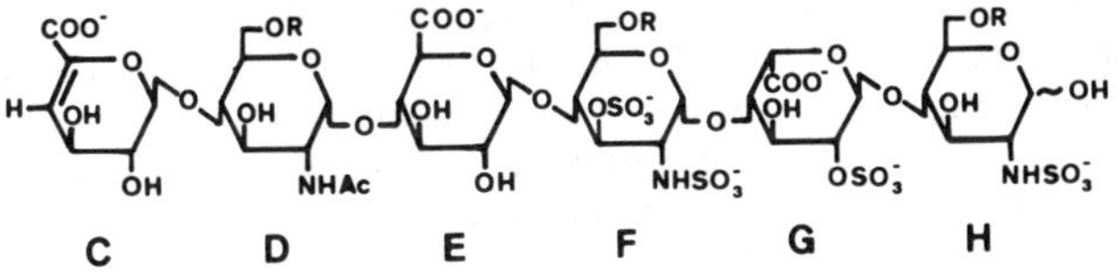

FIGURE 4. Proposed structure for the hexasaccharide C-H obtained by enzymatic degradation of the octasaccharide with bacterial heparinase. The pentasaccharide obtained after incubation with glycuronidase is represented by D-H.

acids that absorb the light at 230 nm are localized in the tetrasaccharide fraction, while the disaccharide segment is practically devoid of such structures. In the same way, as expected, the *N*-acetyl-glucosamine is only present in the tetrasaccharide fraction. The content in uronic acid is twice as high in the tetrasaccharide as in the disaccharide fraction. On the other hand, 2, 5-anhydro-mannose is present in equivalent amount in the two fractions, indicating that disaccharides and tetrasaccharides are obtained in a one to one molar ratio.

These results show that the hexasaccharide is split into two fragments, one of which originates in the reducing end (the disaccharide that does not bear the double bond) and the other in the nonreducing end (the tetrasaccharide).

Further, the hexasaccharide fraction is composed of one very homogeneous species that bears an *N*-sulfate-glucosamine unit at the reducing end, an unsaturated uronic acid at the nonreducing end, and two internal glucosamine units (one of which was *N*-acetylated and next to the unsaturated uronic acid). Consequently, with reference to the known structure of the octasaccharide A-H, it is obvious that the two uronic acid residues that complete the hexa-saccharide are a glucuronic acid and a 2-*O*-sulfated iduronic acid.

These observations along with one obtained on the A-H material, in particular the presence of a 3-*O*-sulfate group at C-3 of the F unit, lead us to propose for the hexasaccharide the following structure: 4, 5-unsaturated uronic acid, *N*-acetyl-D-glucosamine, D-glucuronic acid, *N*-sulfate-3-*O*-sulfate-D-glucosamine, 2-*O*-sulfate-iduronic acid, *N*-sulfate D-glucosamine (FIG. 4, C–H).

Biological Activity

The anti-Xa activity of the octasaccharide A-H and of the hexasaccharide C-H was 2,100 u/mg and 2,400 u/mg, respectively. Both the USP and APTT titers of these two oligosaccharides were lower than 10 u/mg.

In the stasis model in the rabbit, the hexasaccharide C-H was found to produce antithrombotic effects: A dosage of 250 anti-Xa u/kg administered prior to giving a 25 u/kg dosage of the thrombogenic complex was able to prevent clot formation in the jugular veins.

DISCUSSION

Knowing the structure of the octasaccharide A-H used as starting material (FIG. 1), one would expect that after heparinase degradation of this fragment, hexasaccharide A-F would be formed after the splitting of the bond between the sulfated glucosamine unit F and the sulfated iduronic residue G. We provide here strong evidence that the only products obtained result from a cleavage between the sulfated glucosamine unit B and the nonsulfated iduronic acid C. However, the linkage between these two residues was previously found to resist heparinase action; an explanation for this cleavage can be found in the use of a large amount of enzyme. Such an explanation is supported by further experiments showing that the undegraded octasaccharide, when subjected again to heparinase degradation under the same conditions, yields again hexasaccharide and disaccharide, as described above.

Much more unexpected, however, is the resistance to heparinase of the linkage between F and G. This is most probably due to the 3-*O*-sulfated group present on unit F, in the starting octasaccharide, a feature discussed in several recent papers.[5-7] The presence of an *O*-sulfated group at C-3 of an *N*-sulfated glucosamine unit would definitely impair the heparinase action, while such an impairment could be overcome in the case of a nonsulfated iduronic acid.

The hexasaccharide C-H was found to inhibit factor Xa *in vitro* as well as the octasaccharide does. Furthermore, in the stasis thrombosis model this product showed antithrombotic action against various thrombogenic stimuli such as activated coagulant complexes. This observation clearly indicates that the anti-Xa activity measured *in vitro* is related to a specific molecular fragment contained in this hexasaccharide.

Since the C residue modified by heparinase has lost its major chemical characteristics without any effect on the anti-Xa activity, this terminal residue at the nonreducing end is probably useless in this respect. This suggests that the pentasaccharide D-H would still retain a high anti-Xa activity. Preliminary experiments using a glycuronidase prepared according to the method of Warnick and Linker[11] to cleave the unsaturated uronic acid residue, thus yielding the pentasaccharide D-H, seem to confirm this hypothesis. If elimination of unit C proves to have little effect on activity, our results show, in contrast, that a modification of the H residue at the terminal reducing end (borohydride reduction) is accompanied by a decrease in the anti-Xa activity (unpublished results).

Inasmuch as the fine chemical structure of the fragments is critical for their activity, the sulfate groups probably play a crucial role and in this respect it is worth mentioning that the very peculiar sulfated residue F is still present in the hexasaccharide C-H.

In view of the presence of the unit F in the hexasaccharide and in the pentasaccharide, it is to be expected that both of these fragments will show in their nmr spectrum the extra signal at 57–59 ppm that we proposed as a major physicochemical characteristic of this type of oligosaccharide.[5]

References

1. CHOAY, J., J. C. LORMEAU, M. PETITOU, P. SINAY, B. CASU, P. ORESTE & G. GATTI. 1980. Anti-Xa active heparin oligosaccharides. Thromb. Res. **18:** 573–578.
2. CHOAY, J., J. C. LORMEAU & M. PETITOU. 1980. Oligosaccharides de faible poids moleculaire presentant une activité inhibitrice du facteur Xa en milieu plasmatique. Ann. Pharm. Fr. **38:** 475–477.

3. THUNBERG, L., G. BACKSTROM, H. GRUNDBERG, J. RIESENFELD & U. LINDAHL. 1980. The molecular size of the antithrombin-binding sequence in heparin. FEBS Lett. **117:** 203–206.

4. YIN, E. T., S. WESSLER & J. V. BUTLER. 1973. Plasma heparin: A unique practical, submicrogram-sensitive assay. J. Lab. Clin. Med. **81:** 298–310.

5. CASU, B., P. ORESTE, G. TORRI, G. ZOPPETTI, J. CHOAY, J. C. LORMEAU, M. PETITOU & P. SINAY. 1981. The structure of heparin oligosaccharide fragments with high anti-factor Xa activity, containing the minimal antithrombin-binding sequence. Chemical and ^{13}C n.m.r. studies. Biochem. J. In press.

6. CHOAY, J., J. C. LORMEAU, M. PETITOU, J. FAREED & P. SINAY. 1981. Oligosaccharides de faible poids moleculaire presentant une activité inhibitrice du facteur Xa en milieu plasmatique. II. Nouveaux elements de structure et activité antithrombotique. Ann. Pharm. Fr. In press.

7. LINDAHL U., G. BACKSTROM, L. THUNBERG & I. G. LEDER. 1980. Evidence for a 3-0 sulfate D-glucosamine residue in the antithrombin-binding sequence of heparin. Proc. Natl. Acad. Sci. USA **77:** 6551–6555.

8. SHIVELY, J. E. & H. E. CONRAD. 1976. Formation of anhydrosugars in the chemical depolymerization of heparin. Biochemistry **15:** 3932–3942.

9. CAEN, J., M. J. LARRIEU & M. SAMAMA. 1976. *In* L'hemostase. Temps de Cehaline-Kaolin.:169–170. Expansion Scientifique Française. Paris.

10. WESSLER, S., S. M. REIMER & M. C. SHEPS. 1959. Biologic assay of a thrombosis-inducing activity in human serum. J. Appl. Physiol. **14:** 943–946.

11. WARNICK, C. T. & A. LINKER. 1972. Purification of an unusual α-glycuronidase from flavobacteria. Biochemistry **11:** 568–572.

VASCULAR DISTRIBUTION OF INTRATRACHEALLY ADMINISTERED HEPARIN *

J. Mahadoo, L. M. Hiebert, C. J. Wright, and L. B. Jaques †

Department of Surgery, College of Medicine and
† Department of Oral Biology, College of Dentistry
University of Saskatchewan
Saskatoon, Saskatchewan, Canada S7N 0X0

INTRODUCTION

The currently used heparin regimens are not convenient for prolonged anticoagulant therapy because of the short duration of action, fluctuations in the plasma heparin concentration, and the pain associated with repeated injections.[1-4] The search for other modes of administering this drug has led to the development of intrapulmonary heparin as an alternate anticoagulant regimen. A single large dose of heparin can be safely administered in the lungs [5-8] to produce essentially the same anticoagulant effect as single intravenous or subcutaneous injections of small doses repeated over a period of days.[9] We believe that a cellular uptake and eventual slow release of the heparin are responsible for the moderate but protracted hypocoagulation resulting from the administration of a single large dose of the drug in the lungs.[10] We have therefore examined the endothelial tissue after intrapulmonary administration of heparin.

ABSORPTION OF HEPARIN FROM THE LUNGS

The anticoagulant effect observed by several coagulation tests after intrapulmonary administration of sodium heparin to mice, rats, dogs, and humans,[9] the distribution of radioactivity in plasma after tracheal instillation of ^{3}H-labeled heparin [9] and ^{35}S-labeled heparin [11] in rats, and the increased plasma lipoprotein lipase and histaminase activities observed after intratracheal instillation of heparin in mice and rats [12] are all indirect evidence of a pulmonary absorption of heparin. We have now obtained more direct evidence of the absorption of heparin from the lungs. TABLE 1 shows the plasma heparin concentration at various time intervals after intratracheal instillation of sodium heparin (pork intestinal heparin, Diosynth, Inc.) in Wistar rats. The heparin was measured by the procedure described by Penner.[13] The data obtained show that a moderate amount of heparin is present in the plasma for a period of at least 5 days. These plasma heparin concentrations are within the range required for the prophylaxis of thrombosis. Heparin was extracted from dog plasma in a similar experiment and analyzed by agarose gel electrophoresis. It was found to have the same migration rate and number of bands as the pork mucosal heparin that was administered intratracheally to the dogs.[14] A histological examination of the lungs after intratracheal instillation of heparin to

* This work was supported by funds from the Saskatchewan Heart Foundation.

650

mice revealed that the heparin is absorbed via the blood stream and the lymphatic circulation and is also taken up by alveolar macrophages and endothelial tissue of major blood vessels.[15, 16]

Endothelial Uptake of Heparin

The endothelial uptake of heparin has been observed *in vitro* after incubation of rat aorta in heparinized Locke's solution [17] and after incubation of endothelial cells in culture medium with ^{3}H-labeled heparin.[18] This uptake has also been observed *in vivo* after intravenous [19] and intrapulmonary [20] administration of heparin to rats. The detection and measurement of heparin on the endothelium presents one technical problem. The amount of endothelial tissue that can be obtained from the major blood vessels by the Hautchen preparation [21] is quite small. Hence relatively large doses of heparin are usually administered to the animals so that sufficient amount of the drug can be recovered from the endothelium to allow quantitative and electrophoretic

TABLE 1

PLASMA HEPARIN CONCENTRATION AFTER INTRATRACHEAL
INSTILLATION OF HEPARIN (2000 U/KG) IN RATS

Time (hr)	Plasma Heparin (u/ml)
0	0
24	0.26 ± 0.13
48	0.23 ± 0.03
72	0.23 ± 0.09
96	0.07 ± 0.03
120	0.08 ± 0.10

Each value for plasma heparin concentration represents the mean ± 1 standard deviation of data obtained from four rats.

analyses. It should also be pointed out that the minimum intrapulmonary dose at which any heparin is detected in the plasma is about ten times greater than the usual therapeutic intravenous dose.

TABLE 2 shows the amount of heparin recovered from the endothelium of rats to which heparin (19,000 u/kg) was administered intratracheally. The data indicate that at the end of 24 hr the amount of heparin present on the endothelium was still three times higher than the control value. The presence of this amount of heparin in the endothelial tissue may be important in providing an antithrombotic surface to the circulating blood. Besides the antilipemic effect [12] the mere presence of heparin in the endothelium may be an important factor in the control of atherogenesis. This is presently being investigated.

The endothelial uptake of heparin is dose-dependent. FIGURE 1 shows the dose-response relationship between the dose of heparin administered intratracheally to rats and the endothelial heparin concentration. The high correlation (r = 0.99) is a good indication that the uptake of heparin is a genuine

TABLE 2

DOSE OF HEPARIN ADMINISTERED INTO THE LUNGS: 19,000 UNITS/KG

Time After Heparin Administration (hr)	Endothelial Heparin (metachromatic units/cm²)
0	0.003
2	0.119
6	0.119
12	0.042
24	0.009

Each of the values for the endothelial heparin concentration represents heparin recovered from pooled endothelial tissue from four rats.

phenomenon. There is also a good correlation between the plasma and the endothelial heparin concentrations. The endothelial heparin and the heparin administered intratracheally showed similar electrophoretic characteristics.

THE CELLULAR POOL HYPOTHESIS

There are several reports in the literature of a cellular involvement in the distribution of parenterally administered heparin.[15, 19, 20, 22-24] Our own observations on the uptake of heparin by macrophages and endothelial cells after intrapulmonary, subcutaneous, intramuscular, and intraperitoneal administration of the drug[16] confirm these reports. We have recently reviewed the pharmacokinetics of heparin in order to incorporate these features of heparin distribution (FIG. 2). This has led to the formulation of the cellular pool

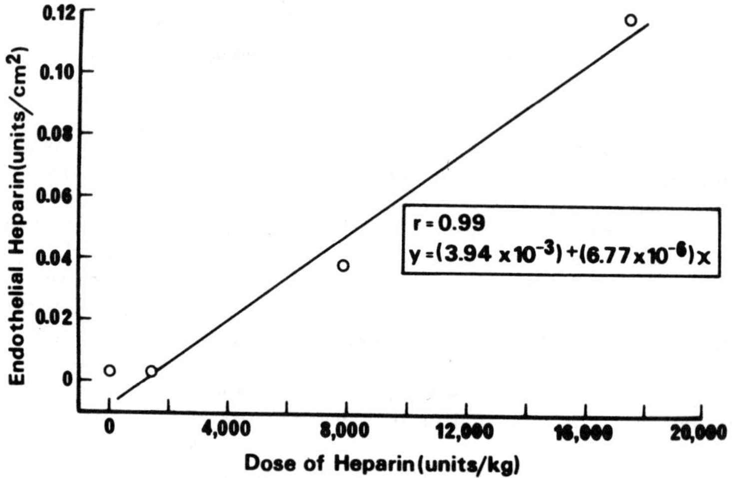

FIGURE 1. Uptake of heparin by aortic endothelium. The units of heparin refer to metachromatic units. Each point represents the heparin concentration from endothelium obtained from four rats.

hypothesis which is essentially based on three assumptions: (a) the uptake of heparin by certain cells; (b) the storage of heparin by these cells and (c) the slow release of this heparin into the circulation. There is sufficient evidence to support the validity of the first assumption.[15–20, 22–28] The second assumption is supported by the data presented here and other reports in the literature.[22, 23, 25, 26] We have yet to obtain direct evidence of a release of the sequestered heparin. An investigation of this aspect of the cellular pool hypothesis is in progress. The size of the population of cells capable of sequestering heparin (macrophages, endothelium, epithelium, etc.) at the site of administration determines the amount of heparin sequestered, stored, and released later. This concept therefore offers a rational explanation for the different types of anticoagulant and other enzymatic responses obtained with the different routes of heparin administration.

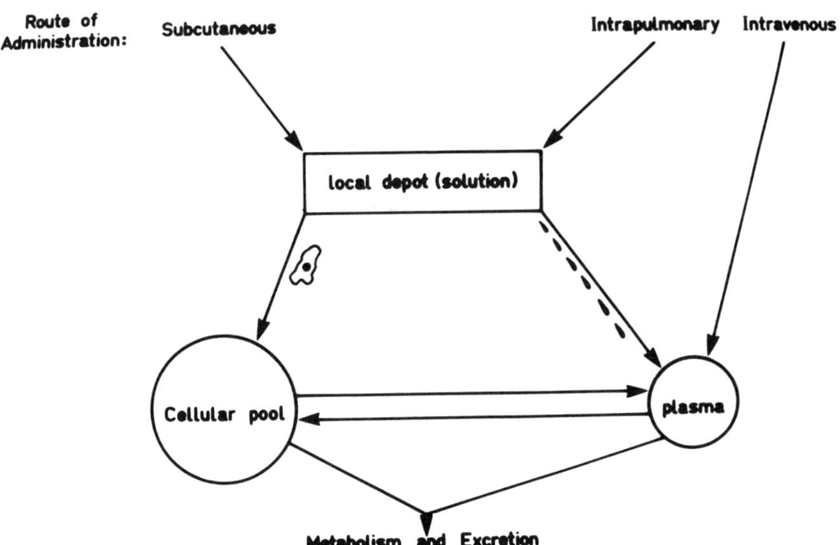

FIGURE 2. Function of the cellular pool in the regulation of plasma heparin. The vascular endothelium forms an integral part of the cellular pool.

CONCLUDING REMARKS

The observations made on intrapulmonary heparin suggest that the macrophages and the endothelial cells are important components of the cellular pool which appears to determine the heparin level in the plasma. The data presented here show that the endothelium can accumulate heparin. The biological significance and the possible clinical applications of this phenomenon are yet to be determined. Investigations of the antithrombotic and antiatherogenic effects of the endothelial bound heparin are in order. A study of the prophylactic use of intrapulmonary heparin for the control of post-surgical thrombosis is in progress.

ACKNOWLEDGMENT

The technical help of Miss Judy Klassen is gratefully acknowledged.

REFERENCES

1. SCHLACHMAN, M. D. & M. CAVUSOGLU. 1959. Practical application of heparin for long-term anticoagulant therapy. N.Y. State J. Med. **59:** 1054–1059.
2. TAKATS, G. D. 1950. The subcutaneous use of heparin. Circulation **II:** 837–844.
3. REFN, I., F. R. SCHOU & L. VESTERGAARD. 1954. Subcutaneous application of heparin. *In* Proceedings of the International Conference on Thrombosis, Basel. Schwabe Publisher.
4. ENGELBERT, H. 1954. Prolonged anticoagulant therapy with subcutaneously administered concentrated aqueous heparin. Surgery **36**(4): 762–770.
5. WRIGHT, C. J. & L. B. JAQUES. 1979. Heparin via the lung. Can. J. Surg. **22**(4): 317–319.
6. WRIGHT, C. J., J. MAHADOO & L. B. JAQUES. 1979. Anticoagulant activity and operative blood loss after intrapulmonary heparin. Br. J. Surg. **66:** 844–847.
7. MAHADOO, J., J. G. HINES & L. B. JAQUES. 1980. Effects of long term treatment of mice with intrapulmonary heparin. Arzneim-Forsch. In press.
8. WRIGHT, C. J. & J. MAHADOO. 1980. Long term toxicity study of intrapulmonary heparin. *In* The Chemistry and Biology of Heparin. R. L. Lundblad, Ed. Elsevier North-Holland Inc. New York. In press.
9. JAQUES, L. B., J. MAHADOO & L. W. KAVANAGH. 1976. Intrapulmonary heparin: A new procedure for anticoagulant therapy. Lancet **ii:** 1157–1161.
10. MAHADOO, J. & L. B. JAQUES. 1979. Cellular control of heparin in blood. Med. Hyp. **5**(8): 835–843.
11. SCHANKER, L. S. & J. A. BURTON. 1976. Absorption of heparin and cyanocobalamine from the rat lung. Proc. Soc. Exp. Biol. Med. **152:** 377–380.
12. MAHADOO, J., C. J. WRIGHT & L. B. JAQUES. 1980. Effect of intrapulmonary heparin on coagulation enzymes, lipoprotein lipase and diamine oxidase. *In* The Chemistry and Biology of Heparin. R. L. Lundblad, Ed. Elsevier North-Holland Inc. New York. In press.
13. PENNER, J. A. 1974. Experience with a thrombin clotting time assay for measuring heparin activity. Am. J. Clin. Pathol. **61:** 645–653.
14. MAHADOO, J. Unpublished data.
15. JAQUES, L. B. & J. MAHADOO. 1978. Pharmacodynamics and clinical effectiveness of heparin. Semin. Thromb. Hemostas. **IV:** 298–325.
16. MAHADOO, J. 1978. Pulmonary absorption of heparin. Ph.D. thesis. University of Saskatchewan, Saskatoon, Saskatchewan, Canada.
17. HIEBERT, L. M. & L. B. JAQUES. 1976. Heparin uptake on endothelium. Artery **2:** 26–37.
18. GLIMELIUS, B., C. BUSCH & M. HÖÖK. 1978. Binding of the heparin on the surface of cultured human endothelial cells. Thromb. Res. **12:** 773–782.
19. HIEBERT, L. M. & L. B. JAQUES. 1976. The observation of heparin on endothelium after injection. Thromb. Res. **8:** 195–204.
20. MAHADOO, J., L. M. HIEBERT & L. B. JAQUES. 1977. Vascular sequestration of heparin. Thromb. Res. **12:** 79–90.
21. PUGATCH, E. M. J. & A. M. SAUNDERS. 1968. A new technique for making Hautchen preparations of unfixed aortic endothelium. J. Ather. Res. **8:** 735–738.
22. ASPLUND, J., U. BOREL & H. HOLMGREN. 1939. Untersuchunger über die Speicherung des Heparins im Tieroganismus sowie über seine Resorptionsmoglichkeitne in Darm und Placenta. A. Mikrosk. Anat. Forsch. **46:** 16–67.

23. MAHADOO, J. 1979. Evidence for a cellular pool for exogenous heparin. *In* Heparin—Structure, Cellular Functions and Clinical Applications. N. M. McDuffie, Ed.: 181–187. Academic Press. New York.
24. MONKHOUSE, F. C., & H. DICKIE. 1954. Physiological factors concerned with the removal of injected heparin from the circulating blood A.m. J. Physiol. **178:** 223–228.
25. MIMS, D. A. 1969. Uptake of heparin by peritoneal macrophages. Aust. J. Exp. Biol. Med. Sci. **47:** 157–158.
26. OH, T. H., S. S. NAIDOO & L. B. JAQUES. 1973. The uptake and disposition of ^{35}S-heparin by macrophages in vitro. J. Reticuloendothel. Soc. **13:** 134–142.
27. KJELLEN, L., A. OLDBERT, K. RUBIN & M. HÖÖK. 1977. Binding of heparin and heparan sulphate to rat liver cells. Biochem. Biophys. Res Commun. **74:** 126–133.
28. KRAEMER, P. M. 1977. Heparin releases heparan sulfate from the cell surface. Biochem. Biophys. Res. Commun. **78:** 1334–1340.

DETERMINANTS OF THE ANTICOAGULANT EFFECT OF HEPARIN *IN VITRO* *

Thorir D. Bjornsson and Katherine M. Wolfram

Division of Clinical Pharmacology
Departments of Pharmacology and Medicine
Duke University Medical Center
Durham, North Carolina 27710

INTRODUCTION

Although heparin has been used for more than 40 years and its clinical efficacy in the treatment and prophylaxis of venous thromboembolism is well established,[1] there are still numerous unanswered questions concerning its optimal use.[2-4] Patients receiving heparin for the treatment of venous thromboembolism require widely varying total daily doses of heparin in order to maintain an anticoagulant effect corresponding to activated partial thromboplastin time (APTT) values of 1½–2½ times control APTT values.[5-7] The total daily dose may vary from about 9,000 to 70,000 units/day.[5-7] This intersubject variation in heparin dose requirements is partly due to differences in its pharmacokinetics,[8, 9] but it is also due to intersubject variability in the anticoagulant response to a given concentration of heparin in plasma or whole blood.[9-11] Presently, neither the relative contribution of pharmacokinetic and pharmacodynamic factors is known with respect to the intersubject variation in the overall therapeutic response to heparin, nor have any determinants of such variabilities been identified. Such information, however, is likely to be clinically useful since heparin requirements in individual patients might be anticipated and heparin therapy thereby made more efficacious and safe.

This study investigates the significance of several possible determinants of the anticoagulant effect of heparin *in vitro*. These include baseline APTT and thrombin time (TT) values, and concentrations in plasma of three serine protease inhibitors. There are two reasons why a baseline coagulation test value may be an important determinant of the anticoagulant response to heparin. Several studies have demonstrated that patients who either have or are at a higher risk of venous thromboembolism have baseline APTT values that are lower than normal control APTT values.[12-14] Other studies have shown that patients with venous thromboembolic disease require higher daily doses of heparin than patients without disease in order to maintain a desired anticoagulant effect as evaluated by APTT.[14] Heparin dose requirements therefore appear to be related to baseline APTT values, but it is presently uncertain if this relationship is due to pharmacokinetic or pharmacodynamic factors, or both.

* Supported in part by National Institutes of Health Grant HL24343. Thorir D. Bjornsson is a recipient of a Pharmaceutical Manufacturers Association Foundation Faculty Development Award in Clinical Pharmacology.

656

MATERIALS AND METHODS

Collection and Preparation of Plasma Samples

Blood samples were obtained by venipuncture from 20 healthy volunteers (10 of each sex; age 30 ± 6 years). The blood was immediately mixed with 3.2% sodium citrate solution to yield 10% citrated blood, which was centrifuged at $1,500 \times g$ for 15 min. The plasma was collected, and series of samples were prepared containing 10% v/v of different heparin standards, or normal saline for the baseline sample, yielding plasma heparin activity between 0.05 and 1.5 units/ml of sample. These plasma samples were kept on ice until assayed for APTT (samples containing 0.05 to 1.0 units/ml) and TT (samples containing 0.1 to 1.5 units/ml). The heparin preparation used was Heparin sodium injection, U.S.P., 1,000 units/ml from beef lung (lot no. 473FU, The Upjohn Company, Kalamazoo, MI). It was diluted with 0.9% sodium chloride solution to produce the heparin standards used.

Determination of APTT and TT

APTT was determined using Automated APTT® (General Diagnostics, Morris Plains, NJ) as the principal reagent. The mixture (0.2 ml) of the plasma sample, with or without added heparin, and Automated APTT® was incubated at 37° C for 5 min, after which 0.1 ml of 0.025 M calcium chloride in water was added to initiate the coagulation process. TT was determined using thrombin purified from bovine plasma (T-6132, Sigma Chemical Company, St. Louis, MO). The lyophilized powder preparation was first dissolved in deionized water to obtain a thrombin concentration of 50 NIH units/ml, and stored in aliquots at $-20°$ C until used. This storage did not result in any reduction in thrombin activity. Immediately prior to use, the frozen thrombin solution was thawed and diluted with 0.025 M calcium chloride in water to yield a thrombin concentration of 25 NIH units/ml and kept on ice. Each plasma sample (0.1 ml), with or without added heparin, was incubated at 37° C for 5 min, after which 0.1 ml of the calcium-enriched thrombin reagent was added to initiate the clotting process. A Fibrometer coagulation timer (Baltimore Biological Laboratories, Cockeysville, MD) was used to determine both APTT and TT. All samples were assayed in duplicates.

Concentrations of the three plasma protease inhibitors, antithrombin III (AT-III), α_1 antitrypsin (α_1AT), and α_2 macroglobulin (α_2MG), and of fibrinogen and α_1 acid glycoprotein (α_1AGP) in plasma were determined by radial immunodiffusion, using M-Partigen® immunodiffusion plates (Calbiochem-Behring Corporation, La Jolla, CA).

Coagulation Times (APTT and TT) Versus Plasma Heparin Activity Curves

An apparent linear relationship was observed on a semilogarithmic plot of both APTT and TT versus heparin activity added to plasma. The individual relationships between the coagulation times (APTT and TT) and plasma heparin activity were therefore determined using linear least-squares regression analysis following transformation of the coagulation time values to their natural logarithmic values. The average coefficient of determination of the linear regression analyses of the relationships between ln APTT and heparin activity was 0.990 ± 0.009. The slopes of these relationships will be referred to as the APTT-heparin and TT-heparin slopes, and they have the unit of ml/unit, i.e., a reciprocal of concentration. FIGURE 1 shows plots of the best-fitted lines of this relationship with respect to APTT for three different subjects, i.e., the ones with the shallowest and the steepest slopes and a subject with an intermediate slope. Because of this semilogarithmic relationship, it follows that the increment in plasma heparin activity or concentration required to double any APTT value, H_d, is simply calculated as:

$$H_d = \frac{0.693}{h}$$

where 0.693 is the natural logarithm of 2 and h represents the APTT-heparin slope. It also follows that the increase in APTT values with increasing plasma heparin activity is simply described by the equation:

$$APTT_{sample} = APTT_{baseline} \times e^{hH}$$

where h and H stand for the APTT-heparin slope and plasma heparin activity, respectively.

RESULTS

Baseline APTT values varied from 28.4 to 59.7 sec, with an average value of 35.9 ± 6.8 sec (mean $\pm$ SD). The average APTT-heparin slope value was 2.167 ± 0.429 ml/unit, with values ranging from 1.488 to 3.427 ml/unit. Baseline TT values varied from 9.2 to 13.7 sec, with an average value of 10.5 ± 1.0 sec. The average TT-heparin slope value was 2.002 ± 0.543 ml/unit, with values ranging from 1.233 to 3.228 ml/unit. There was no statistically significant correlation between baseline APTT and baseline TT values. There was, however, a weak but statistically significant correlation between the APTT-heparin and TT-heparin slope values (r:0.529; $0.02 > p > 0.01$).

The values of the APTT-heparin slopes showed a strong positive correlation with the baseline APTT values (r:0.905; $p < 0.001$). This relationship is shown in FIGURE 2. The relationship between the TT-heparin slope values and baseline TT values was not statistically significant (r:0.417, $0.10 > p > 0.05$).

With respect to plasma concentrations of the protease inhibitors, there was a statistically significant positive correlation between plasma concentrations of $\alpha_2 MG$ and baseline APTT values (r:0.519; $0.02 > p > 0.01$), and also between plasma concentrations of $\alpha_2 MG$ and values of the APTT-heparin slopes (r:0.553; $0.02 > p > 0.01$). Furthermore, there was a statistically significant positive correlation between plasma concentrations of $\alpha_1 AT$ and baseline TT values (r:0.506; $0.05 > p > 0.02$), and also between plasma concentrations of $\alpha_1 AT$ and values of the TT-heparin slopes (r:0.529; $0.02 > p > 0.01$). Neither baseline APTT or TT values nor values of the APTT-heparin or TT-heparin slopes were statistically significantly related to plasma concentrations of AT-III, $\alpha_1 AGP$, or fibrinogen. Concentrations of all proteins were within normal limits.

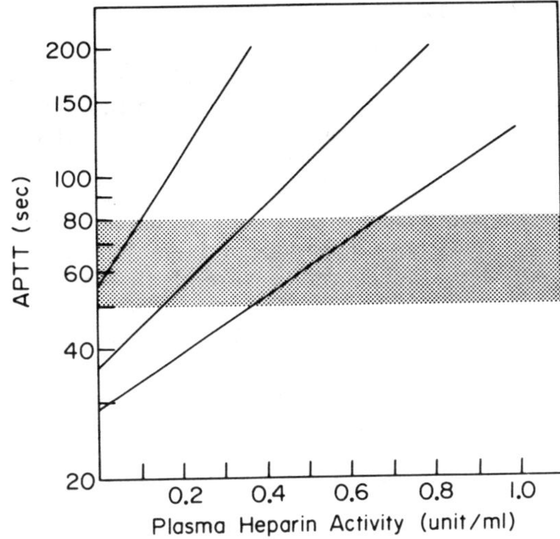

FIGURE 1. Relationship between APTT and heparin activity (in units/ml) added to plasma. Shown are the best-fitted lines of this relationship for three subjects, the ones with the steepest and the shallowest slopes and a subject with an intermediate slope. The stippled area represents a range of commonly observed APTT values during heparin anticoagulation. Note that any given anticoagulant effect is caused by different plasma heparin activities in these three subjects.

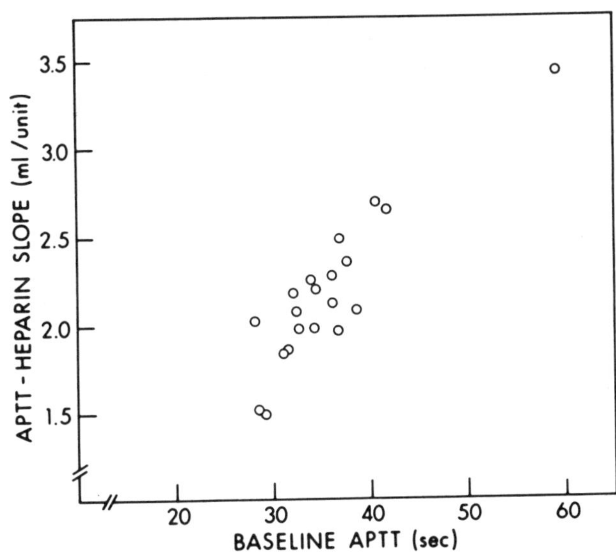

FIGURE 2. Relationship between baseline APTT values and the anticoagulant response to heparin, which is determined as the slope of the relationship between ln APTT versus heparin activity (APTT-heparin slope). Linear regression analysis yields an intercept of 0.111 ml/unit and slope of 0.057 ml/unit $\times$ sec (r:0.905; p $<$ 0.001).

DISCUSSION

This study has demonstrated that the baseline APTT value is a major determinant of the anticoagulant response to heparin *in vitro* as measured by APTT, i.e., low baseline APTT values are associated with shallow APTT-heparin slopes and high baseline APTT values are associated with steep APTT-heparin slopes (FIG. 2). The baseline APTT value alone, which varied from 28.4 to 59.7 sec, accounts for more than 80% of the variability in the APTT-heparin slope values. The study also illustrates a large intersubject variation in the anticoagulant response to heparin *in vitro*, both when the anticoagulant effect was evaluated by APTT and TT. The average value of the APTT-heparin slope was 2.167 ml/unit, indicating that APTT would double for every 0.32 unit/ml increment in plasma heparin activity or concentration (see METHODS). The lowest and highest APTT-heparin slope values were 1.488 and 3.427 ml/unit, indicating that APTT would double for every 0.47 and 0.20 unit/ml increment in plasma heparin activity, respectively. This represents almost 2.5-fold variation in heparin sensitivity based on the APTT-heparin slope values alone. Similar range and variation was also observed with respect to the TT-heparin slope values, but a statistically significant relationship was not observed between baseline TT values and TT-heparin slopes.

The implications of our findings of the relationship between baseline coagulation status and the anticoagulant response to heparin are illustrated in FIGURE 1, where the stippled area represents a range of commonly observed APTT values during heparin anticoagulation, i.e., APTT values of approximately 1½–2½ times control APTT values. It can be seen that any given anticoagulant effect can be caused by a wide range in plasma heparin activity or concentration, depending on the individual anticoagulant response to heparin. For example, an anticoagulant effect of APTT = 70 sec is caused by plasma heparin activity as low as 0.05 unit/ml in the subject with the steepest APTT-heparin slope whereas the subject with the shallowest APTT-heparin slope requires plasma heparin activity as high as 0.6 unit/ml. This represents 12-fold variation in the plasma heparin activity required to elicit a desired anticoagulant effect. Provided that the anticoagulant effect of heparin is the same *in vivo* as it is *in vitro*, this same variation would be expected clinically. Our findings therefore suggest a possible connection between two clinical observations. Several studies have shown that low baseline APTT values are associated with increased risk of venous thromboembolic disease,[12–14] while other studies have shown that patients with verified thromboembolic disease require higher doses of heparin than patients without disease in order to maintain a desired anticoagulant effect as evaluated by APTT.[14] Our results suggest that the lower baseline APTT values in the patient will be associated with smaller anticoagulant response to heparin, i.e., shallower APTT-heparin slopes, requiring higher concentrations of heparin to elicit the same anticoagulant effect, provided that the total clearance of heparin is similar in both groups.

The anticoagulant function of heparin is thought to depend upon its ability to catalyze AT-III.[15, 16] It was therefore of interest to determine if the concentrations in plasma of AT-III, and also of the other serine protease inhibitors, α_2MG and α_1AT were correlated with the baseline coagulation test times and the anticoagulant response to heparin. Neither the anticoagulant response to heparin, i.e., APTT-heparin and TT-heparin slope values, nor their respective baseline values were correlated with plasma concentrations of AT-III, as determined by the immunologic method. However, both baseline APTT values and values of the APTT-heparin slopes were significantly correlated with plasma concentrations of α_2MG, and both baseline TT values and values of the TT-heparin slopes were significantly correlated with plasma concentrations of α_1AT. This suggests that both of these plasma serine protease inhibitors play a role as determinants of baseline coagulation characteristics and the anticoagulant effect of heparin, and it has been suggested that lowered concentrations of α_2MG and α_1AT may be one of several factors that contribute to the development of thrombosis.[17]

In summary, this study has shown that the anticoagulant response to heparin *in vitro* measured by APTT can be predicted with a fair degree of accuracy based on the baseline APTT value alone. During the conduct of this study, a preliminary report [18] confirmed our findings. This study has also demonstrated a wide intersubject variability in the anticoagulant response to heparin.

REFERENCES

1. THOMAS, D. P. 1978. Sem. Hematol. **15:** 1–17.
2. COON, W. W. 1978. Postgrad. Med. **63:** 157–164.
3. DE TAKATS, G. 1976. Am. J. Surg. **132:** 1–3.
4. WESSLER, S. 1976. Ann. Rev. Med. **27:** 313–319.
5. BASU, D., A. GALLUS, J. HIRSH & J. CADE. 1972. N. Engl. J. Med. **287:** 324–327.
6. O'SULLIVAN, E. F., J. HIRSH, R. A. McCARTHY & G. C. DE GRUCHY. 1968. Med. J. Australia **2:** 153–159.
7. SALZMAN, E. W., D. DEYKIN, R. M. SHAPIRO & R. ROSENBERG. 1975. N. Engl. J. Med. **292:** 1046–1050.
8. ESTES, J. W. & P. F. POULIN. 1974. Thrombos. Diathes. Haemorrh. **33:** 329–337.
9. HIRSH, J., W. G. VAN AKEN, A. S. GALLUS, C. T. DOLLERY, J. F. CADE & W. L. YUNG. 1976. Circulation **53:** 691–695.
10. JAQUES, L. G. & A. G. RICKER. 1948. Blood **3:** 1197–1212.
11. ESTES, J. W. 1972. J. Clin. Pathol. **25:** 45–48.
12. GALLUS, A. S., J. HIRSH & M. GENT. 1973. Lancet. **2:** 805–809.
13. POGUE, W. H., M. CRONLUND & F. R. RICKLES. 1978. Clin. Res. **26:** 620A.
14. WHITE, T. M., J. L. BERNENE & A. M. MARINO. 1979. JAMA **241:** 2717–2720.
15. ROSENBERG, R. D. 1977. Sem. Hematol. **14:** 427–440.
16. HOLMER, E., G. SODERSTROM & L.-O. ANDERSSON. 1980. Thrombos. Res. **17:** 113–124.
17. DE BOER, A. C., L. A. M. VAN RIEL & G. J. H. DEN OTTOLANDER. 1979. Thrombos. Res. **15:** 17–25.
18. WHITFIELD, L. R. & G. LEVY. 1980. Clin. Pharmacol. Therap. **27:** 294.

HEPARIN AND OTHER SULFATED POLYANIONS: THEIR INTERACTION WITH THE BLOOD PLATELET *

M. Lois Tiffany and John A. Penner

Simpson Memorial Research Institute
University of Michigan
Ann Arbor, Michigan 48109

INTRODUCTION

Heparin is a heterogeneous mixture of partially sulfated polysaccharide chains. Different subfractions of heparin have been found to interact with platelets to different degrees, which do not parallel the anticoagulant activity of the preparation.[1] There is some suggestion that the low antithrombin III affinity of a subfraction results in more potent platelet interaction. It is, however, extremely difficult to relate function to molecular structure when heterogeneity of molecular species exists. A logical approach is to work with more homogeneous model compounds (sulfated polyanions) in order to understand the molecular features involved in the functions observed and is the basis for the following report.

MATERIALS AND METHODS

The following materials were used: heparin beef lung and intestinal mucosa, Upjohn Company, Kalamazoo, MI and Armour Pharmaceutical Company, Phoenix, AZ; polyvinyl sulfate (molecular weight 100,000), dextran sulfate (molecular weight 500,000 and 40,000), dextran (molecular weight 500,000 and 10,000) and carrageenan (lamda and iota type), Sigma Chemical Company, St. Louis, MO; polyanetholesulfonate, Eastman Kodak Company, Rochester, NY and Roche Diagnostics, Nutley, NJ; cellulose sulfate, Aldrich Chemical Company, Milwaukee, WI; poly methacrylic acid, Polysciences, Warrington, PA; poly-L-glutamic acid, Pilot Chemicals, Inc., Watertown, MA.

Blood was collected in buffered citrate, monojet tubes, final concentrated citrate 0.38% and centrifuged ($160 \times g$, 5 min) to prepare platelet rich plasma. Platelet poor plasma was made by spinning at $1000 \times g$, 10 min. The platelet rich plasma count was adjusted to be 200,000 with plasma or phosphate buffered saline, as desired. To remove plasma as completely as possible, the procedure of albumin density centrifugation followed by Sepharose 2B was followed.[2]

Comparison aggregation studies were using a dual sample aggregometer, Scienco Inc., Morrison, CO. Aggregation with release measured simultaneously was recorded with a lumiaggregometer, Chrono-log Company, Havertown, PA. All polyanions were diluted in phosphate-buffered saline, pH 7.8 and 0.01 ml was added to plasma for pre-incubation studies. This was then added to 0.2 ml of platelet-rich plasma (4×10^5 platelets per μl) and aggregation was recorded at 37° C.

* Supported by The Skillman Foundation, Detroit, Michigan.

RESULTS

Studies discussed in the following portion of the paper are illustrated in FIGURES 1 through 6 which demonstrate the effects of sulfated and nonsulfated polyanions on platelet aggregation under conditions specified.

DISCUSSION

Some insight into the molecular properties required for activation of platelets is derived by our comparative studies of the various polyanions. Dextran sulfate of molecular weight 500,000 was more effective than dextran sulfate of molecular weight 40,000 (FIG. 5C). The degree of sulfation is stated by the manufacturer to be the same. Therefore, chain length is an important factor.

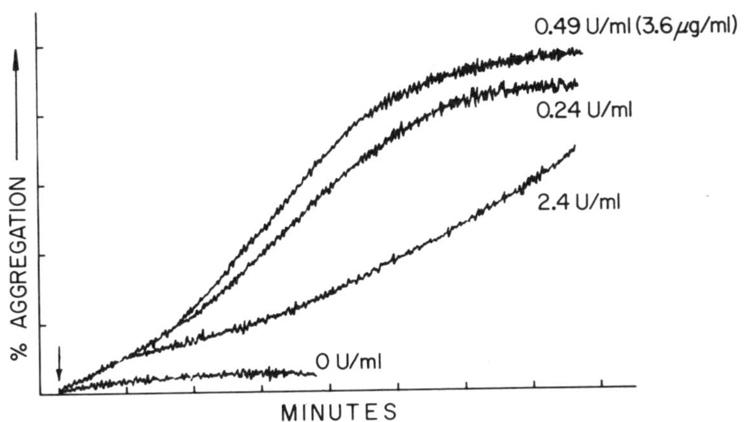

FIGURE 1. Aggregation induced by heparin.

Dextran, sulfated and nonsulfated, of the same molecular weight, 500,000, also were compared. No platelet aggregation was possible with any concentration of dextran when the conditions of observation were 37° C with stirring. If, however, the conditions were room temperature and no stirring, platelets clumped in a high concentration of both forms of dextran (5%). The clumps were easily dispersed by shaking. This is similar to the results reported by Taketomi and Kuramoto.[3] The same percent dextran (5%) completely inhibited platelet aggregation by ADP, epinephrine and collagen, as did similar concentrations of the sulfated polyanions. This inhibition may be a result of coating of the platelet with polymers leading to nonspecific interference with activation of the platelet.

High concentration of polymethacrylic acid (25 μg/ml) was found to induce a slight platelet aggregation response, but another polyanion, poly-L-glutamic acid was without any activity. Thus, a negative charge on the polymer is a necessary, but not a sufficient condition, for activation.

All of the sulfated polyanions studied could induce some platelet aggrega-

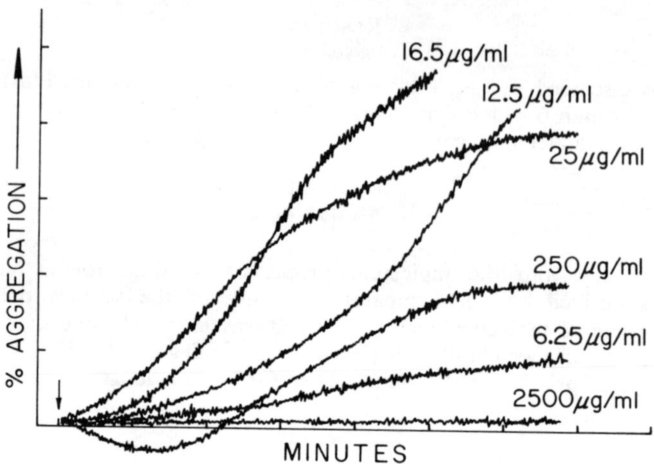

FIGURE 2. Aggregation induced by polyvinyl sulfate.

tion (examples of aggregation studies are given in FIGS. 1, 2, 3 & 4), although only over a limited range of concentrations and in the presence of plasma or serum (example, FIG. 6A). Preincubation of the polyanion either in plasma or in heat-denatured serum enhanced the platelet response (FIG. 6B) suggesting an indirect mechanism of platelet aggregation mediated by a plasma factor. There are a number of reports in the literature which would support a concept that the protease precursor, plasminogen, is the plasma factor responsible. The possible interaction of the sulfated polyanion heparin with an inhibitor to plasminogen activator (thus accelerating plasminogen activation) was postulated by Vairel.[4] Similarly, a "release" of plasminogen activator by sulfated polyanions was suggested by Olesen [5] and Ugar and Mist.[6] On the other hand,

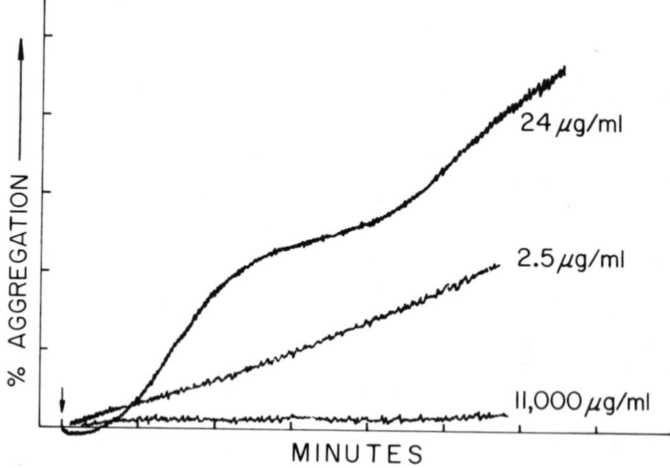

FIGURE 3. Aggregation induced by dextran sulfate.

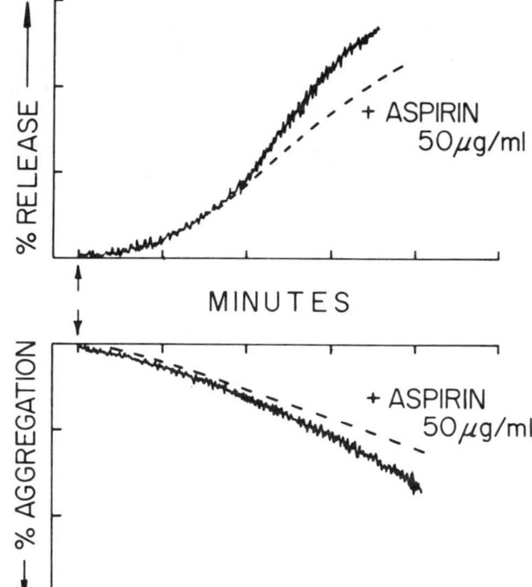

FIGURE 4. Aggregation with concomitant ATP release by relatively high concentration of polyanethol sulfonate (25 μg/ml). Aspirin is not very effective in inhibiting aggregation or release.

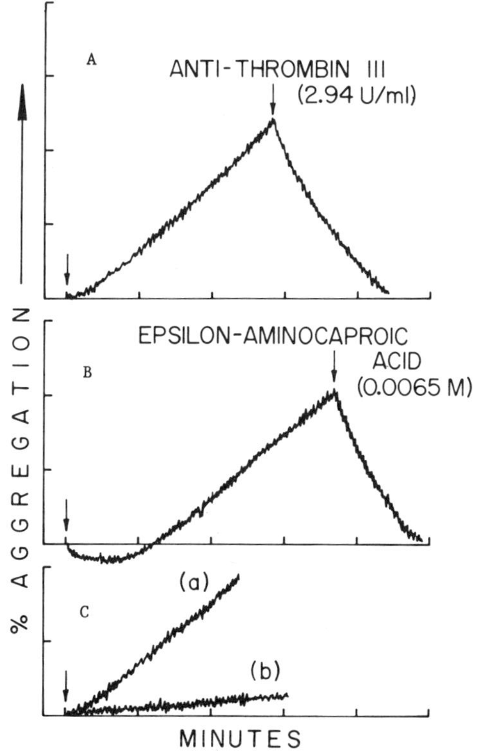

FIGURE 5. (A) Aggregation by 25 μg/ml polyvinyl sulfate is rapidly inhibited and completely reversed by 2.94 U/ml of antithrombin III. (B) Similar inhibition and reversal of aggregation produced by 25 μg/ml of cellulose sulfate is seen with epsilon aminocaproic acid at 0.0065 M. (C) Aggregation is produced at low concentrations with (a) 25 μg/ml of dextran sulfate 500,000 compared to (b) the minimal response by dextran 40,000 under the same conditions of testing.

heparin also was found to accelerate the rate of formation of a complex of antithrombin III with plasmin.[7] This would increase the rate of inhibition of proteolytic and esterolytic activity of this protease. It is possible that low concentrations of heparin increase the formation of plasmin, while excess heparin would interfere with the activity of this enzyme once it is formed. If plasmin is responsible for platelet aggregation produced when polyanions are present, an optimal concentration of polyanion would, therefore, be expected to be most effective in inducing aggregation.

Inhibition of aggregation by the sulfated polyanions occurred at low concentrations of the plasmin inhibitor antithrombin III (2.94 u/ml) (FIG. 5A), as

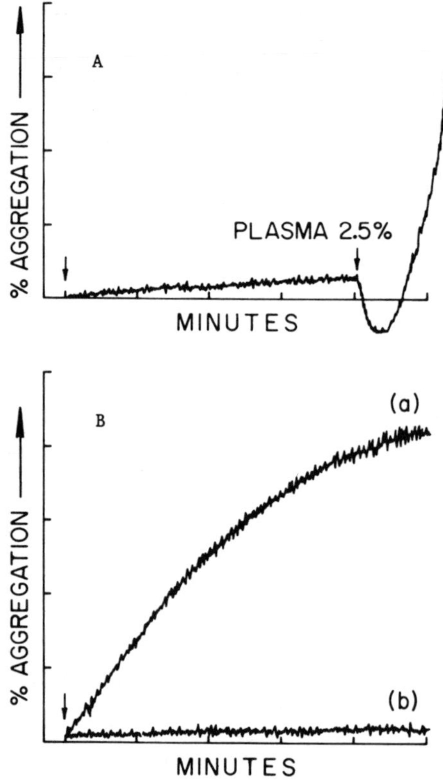

FIGURE 6. (A) Platelets, well washed by albumin density centrifugation followed by gel filtration are not aggregated by λ carrageen (50 μg/ml) until plasma is added, to be 2.5% of final volume. (B) In (a) threshold concentration for aggregation by polyvinyl sulfate exceeds 2.5 μg/ml when the polyanion is first preincubated in plasma or serum for 25 min at room temperature. In control (b) with no preincubation, there is no aggregation response in the first 5 min in contact with the platelets at 37° C.

well as with Cl esterase inhibitor (not shown) and also occurred with low concentration of epsilon aminocaproic acid (0.0065 M) (FIG. 5B), an inhibitor of plasminogen activation.[8, 9] These findings also may be taken as evidence to support the concept that activated plasminogen is capable of inducing platelet aggregation and that the sulfated polyanions exert their action by means of this protease.

In summary, we find sulfated polyanions induce platelet aggregation indirectly by activation of a plasma factor. On a weight basis, the amount of polyanion needed to induce threshold aggregation, is a function of the degree of *polymerization* and the degree of *sulfation* of the polymer. Negative charge on the polymer is a necessary but not sufficient condition for activation. Platelet aggregation is *inhibited* by high concentration (5%) of all poly-saccharides whether they are sulfated or not.

REFERENCES

1. SALZMAN, E. W., R. D. ROSENBERG, M. H. SMITH, J. N. LINDON & L. FAVREAU. 1980. Effect of heparin and heparin fractions on platelet aggregation. J. Clin. Invest. **65:** 64–73.
2. TIMMONS, S. & J. HAWIGER. 1978. Separation of human platelets from plasma proteins including Factor VIII:VWF. Thromb. Res. **12:** 297–306.
3. TAKETOMI, Y. & A. KURAMOTO. 1978. Ultrastructural studies on the surface coat of human platelet aggregated by poly lysine and dextran. Thrombos. Haemostas. (Stuttg.) **40:** 11–23.
4. VAIREL, E. G. 1975. Simple in vitro method for screening fibrinolytic substances. *In* Progress Chemical Fibrinolysis and Thrombolysis, Vol. 2, J. F. Davidson, M. M. Samama & P. C. Desnyers, Eds.: 271–277. Raven Press, New York.
5. OLESEN, E. S. 1961. A fibrinolytic system in human plasma activated by peptone or acid polysaccharides. Scand. J. Clin. Lab. Invest. **13:** 410–415.
6. UNGAR, G. & S. H. MIST. 1949. Observations on the release of serum fibrinolysin by specific antigen, peptone, and certain polysaccharides. J. Exp. Med. **90:** 39–51.
7. HIGHSMITH, R. F. & D. ROSENBERG. 1974. The inhibition of human plasmin by human antithrombin-heparin cofactor. J. Biol. Chem. **249:** 4335–4338.
8. MARKWARDT, F. 1978. Naturally occurring inhibitors of fibrinolysis. *In* Fibrinolytics and Antifibrinolytics. Editor F. Markwardt, Springer-Verlag. Berlin, Heidelberg, New York.
9. ALKAERSIG, N., A. P. FLETCHER & S. SHERRY. 1959. Aminocaproic acid: An inhibitor of human plasminogen. J. Biol. Chem. **234:** 832–837.

BOVINE PLATELET ANTIHEPARIN PROTEIN: PLATELET FACTOR 4 *

Raymond E. Ciaglowski, June W. Snow, and Daniel A. Walz

Department of Physiology
Wayne State University
Detroit, Michigan 48201

INTRODUCTION

Comparative studies involving platelet-rich and platelet-poor plasma indicate that platelets secrete numerous proteins, including: coagulation factors, growth factors, vascular permeability factor, chemotactic factor, and platelet-specific proteins.[1] In humans there are at least four platelet-specific proteins that display antiheparin and/or growth-stimulating activities. These include high affinity platelet factor four (PF-4); low affinity platelet factor four (LA-PF-4); its closely related variant, beta-thromboglobulin (β-TG); and platelet basic protein, a platelet-derived growth factor (PDGF).

As a class these proteins exhibit similar subunit molecular weights (7,000–12,000 daltons), appear localized in the platelet's alpha granules, display release to platelet aggregating agents and show considerable homology in primary structure. Yet they apparently differ considerably in their proportional amounts, physical properties and biologic activities.

Although PF-4 and β-TG have recently been associated with inhibition of collagenase activity [2] and prostacyclin formation,[3] respectively, their specific functional roles remain elusive. Both continue to find importance as markers of platelet activity.[4, 5] Radioimmunoassays for PF-4 and β-TG have been widely employed to monitor various clinical and pathological conditions, indicating both prethrombotic and postthrombotic states.[6]

For a number of years PDGFs have been conditionally implicated in a variety of inflammatory, atherosclerotic and thrombotic processes.[7] One such factor is connective tissue activating peptide-III (CTAP-III), which when isolated from human platelets and added to various connective tissue cell cultures often displays a number of potent mitogenic activities, including stimulation of cellular division, DNA synthesis, and glycosaminoglycan (GAG) synthesis.[8, 9] In 1979 Castor *et al.*, reported that CTAP-III appeared to be similar to LA-PF-4 in mitogenic activities, SDS electrophoretic mobility, amino acid composition and antigenic determinants.[10] They also reported that β-TG did not show similar increases in mitogenic activities. Earlier, Rucinski *et al.*, had reported finding common antigenic determinants between β-TG, LA-PF-4, and CTAP-III, but noted two distinct differences between β-TG and LA-PF-4, namely; a difference in electrophoretic mobilities on cellulose acetate (β-TG migrated in the β-globulin region and LA-PF-4 migrated in the γ-globulin region) and an apparent deletion of four amino acids from the NH_2-terminus of LA-PF-4 for β-TG.[11] Most recently, using preparative isoelectric focusing,

* This work was supported by a Grant-in-Aid from the American Heart Association and its Michigan affiliate.

Niewiarowski *et al.* have reported that LA-PF-4 is probably first secreted by platelets and then converted to β-TG by way of a platelet-derived, heat-labile protease and also that apparently three different materials exist which display immunologic cross-reactivities, *i.e.* LA-PF-4, β-TG, and platelet basic protein.[12]

In an effort to determine whether or not such a diversity of platelet-specific proteins and their activities may exist in other species, studies are under way to identify, isolate and characterize bovine platelet-specific proteins. These studies seek to determine whether or not such proteins can be separated on the basis of different affinities to heparin-sepharose and dextran-sulfate-sepharose resins. They seek to compare differences in pattern of release that might accompany platelet aggregation versus platelet destruction. Finally, they seek to determine whether or not apparent counterparts to the human forms exist, and if so, to what extent their growth factor activities may overlap. Since the earlier works of Deutsch *et al.* introduced bovine PF-4 as a heparin-neutralizing protein, very little remains known regarding its interrelations with other potential bovine platelet-specific proteins.[13–16] Here, with focus on PF-4, preliminary results indicate bovine PF-4 has considerable diversity in primary structure when compared to the well-characterized human PF-4. Initial results suggest that such diversity is not superficial, and may extend throughout this class of bovine platelet-specific proteins.

MATERIALS AND METHODS

Bovine blood was obtained fresh from a slaughter house and anticoagulated with 3.2% sodium citrate. Outdated human platelets were donated by the Southeastern Michigan Chapter of the American Red Cross as concentrates in acid citrate dextrose. Imidazole, Tris-base and heparin were purchased from the Sigma Chemical Co. Gel filtration resins and dextran sulfate were obtained from Pharmacia Fine Chemicals. Porcine mucosa heparin and dextran-sulfate were each coupled to Sepharose 4B by the cyanogen bromide (pH 11–12, 4° C) procedure of Miller-Andersson *et al.*[17] After coupling of the desired ligand the gel was suspended in 1.0 M ethanolamine, followed by washes of distilled water and 1.0 M sodium chloride. Amino acid analysis was by the Spackman, Stein and Moore method[18] employed on a Beckman model 121 M integrating analyzer. Solvents for thin-layer electrophoresis were from Eastman. Gel electrophoresis reagents and sodium dodecyl sulfate (SDS) were obtained from Calbiochem. Acids and inorganic buffer salts were reagent grade from Baker Chemical Co.

FIGURE 1 outlines the experimental procedures described below: Approximately 50 liters of bovine blood was centrifuged at $3000 \times g$ for 15 min. The buffy coats were pooled and recentrifuged at $3000 \times g$ for 15 min. The packed platelets were then suspended in an equal volume of saline wash solution (0.15 M NaCl, 0.05 M Tris-base pH 7.2) and centrifuged at $3000 \times g$ for 5 min. The wash was repeated 2 to 7 times. Approximately 50 milliliters of packed platelets (1 ml/L blood) were stored at $-76°$ C. Treatment of human platelet concentrates has been previously described.[19] All centrifugation was at 4° C. All wash and extraction procedures were carried out at room temperature.

Bovine PF-4 was isolated from platelet concentrates either by freeze-thawing three times or by thrombin (10 U/ml) aggregation and collection of the supernatant following centrifugation at $22,000 \times g$ for 30 min. (Bovine thrombin was generously supplied by Dr. Walter H. Seegers.) Using affinity chromatography (5.0 × 60 cm) on either heparin-Sepharose (HS) or dextran-sulfate-Sepharose (DSS), supernatants were eluted with stepwise increases in buffered sodium chloride concentrations (either 0.05 M Imidazole or Tris-base, pH 7.2). Eluates were ultrafiltered (UM-2 membrane), desalted (Sephadex G-15) with 0.10 M ammonium bicarbonate, and freeze-dried. PF-4 activity was assayed as described by Levine and Wohl.[20] SDS polyacrylamide gel 7.5%

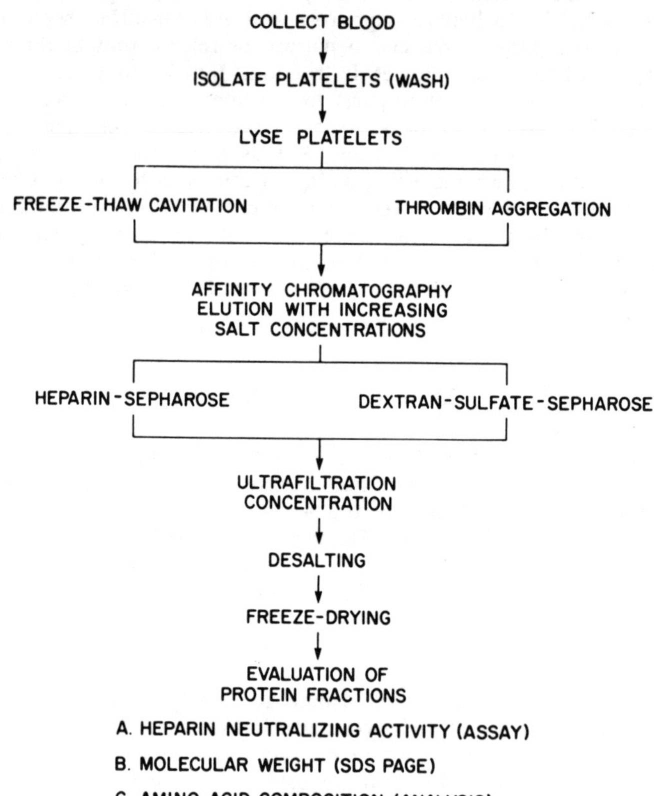

FIGURE 1. Outline of experimental procedures used to prepare bovine platelets.

electrophoresis was carried out according to the method of Weber and Osborn.[21] Samples for amino acid analysis were hydrolyzed *in vacuo* in 6 N HCl at 110° C for 22, 48 or 72 hours. Intact or reduced-alkylated PF-4 were automatically sequenced on a Beckman 890C sequencer. Identification of PTH-derivatives were accomplished as previously cited.[22, 23]

RESULTS

Using heparin-Sepharose affinity chromatography it was previously reported that both human and bovine PF-4s could be obtained from 1-molar sodium chloride eluates. Both gave single bands on SDS gels and both proved to be homogeneous by NH_2-terminal analysis. Reduced human PF-4 on SDS gels had a greater mobility than either the intact or the reduced-alkylated product. Reduced bovine PF-4 and its carboxymethyl derivative both gave a single band having the same molecular weight as the nonreduced product indicating that bovine PF-4 is a single chain polypeptide. Bovine PF-4 has a molecular weight similar to that of prothrombin fragment 2 (12,300), while human PF-4 has an apparent molecular weight of 8,000.[19, 23]

Based on a series of HS chromatograms at varying salt concentrations the elution profile consisted of the following: (1) The 0.15 M and 0.25 M NaCl fractions contained the bulk of the higher molecular weight components; in addition the 0.15 M fraction displayed a low molecular weight component which when gel filtered on Sepharose-4B and Sephacryl-200 corresponded to the alpha/beta chains of hemoglobin; in addition the 0.25 M fraction displayed a β-TG-like protein band. (2) The 0.3 M fraction continued to have high molecular weight components, as well as a predominance of the β-TG-like protein, and sometimes trace amounts of PF-4. (3) The 0.5 M fraction showed trace amounts of higher molecular weight components and substantial PF-4. (4) The 1.0 M fraction contained isolated PF-4. (5) 1.5 M fractions, 2.0 M fractions, or 3.0 M fractions showed no significant amount of protein present. FIGURE 2 compares bovine HS and DSS chromatograms, as well as comparing human DSS chromatography at intermediate salt concentrations.

When similar elution profiles were tried using dextran-sulfate-sepharose a marked difference in distribution of only bovine PF-4 occurred. Whereas the bovine DSS chromatogram gave a clear separation between the β-TG-like protein of the 0.5 M fraction and the PF-4 of 1.5 M fraction, the human DSS chromatogram continued to show an overlap of the β-TG-like protein and PF-4 bands in both the 0.5 M and 1.0 M fractions. Even if intermediate salt concentrations were tried, 0.75 M and 1.25 M, no clear separation was obtainable for human. Attempts to isolate the bovine β-TG-like protein using gel filtration are currently under way.

Amino acid compositions of both 1.0 M HS and 1.5 M DSS fractions showed virtual identity and confirmed bovine PF-4's higher molecular weight (82 amino acids, 9,000 daltons) when compared with human PF-4 (70 amino acids, 7,800 daltons) (TABLE 1). Bovine PF-4 contained more histidine, arginine, aspartate, serine, glutamate, proline and glycine, less alanine, possibly less isoleucine and leucine, and the same amount of lysine, valine, threonine, cysteine and tyrosine. Both PF-4s lack either methionine or tryptophan, and only bovine PF-4 has phenylalanine.

NH_2-terminal sequencing of bovine PF-4 indicated significant diversity from human PF-4 (FIG. 3). Although both had the same NH_2-terminal amino acid, glutamate, only the stable Cys-(Leu)-Cys segment appeared to display any further structural homology, with bovine PF-4 showing an additional 15 amino acids from this point (FIG. 4). It should be further noted that many of the amino acids reported to make up the NH_2-terminus of bovine PF-4 also differed from many of those amino acid residues previously noticed as being different in the amino acid composition studies, indicating further divergence of bovine PF-4 from human.

Studies are also under way to assess each fraction with respect to growth factor activity and corresponding antiheparin activity. These results remain inconclusive.

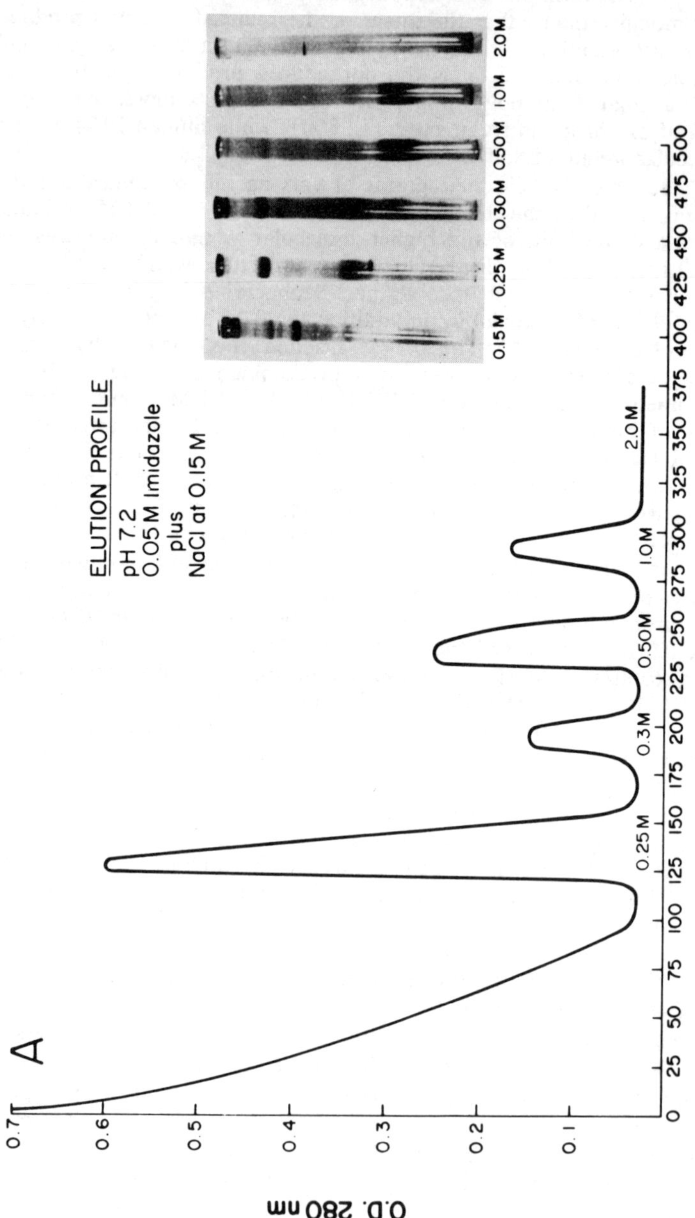

FIGURE 2A. Freeze-thawed bovine platelet lysate chromatogram obtained from step elution of heparin-Sepharose resin. Elution buffers are depicted under the representative protein peaks. Inset is an SDS electrophoresis profile in 7.5% acrylamide (nonreduced).

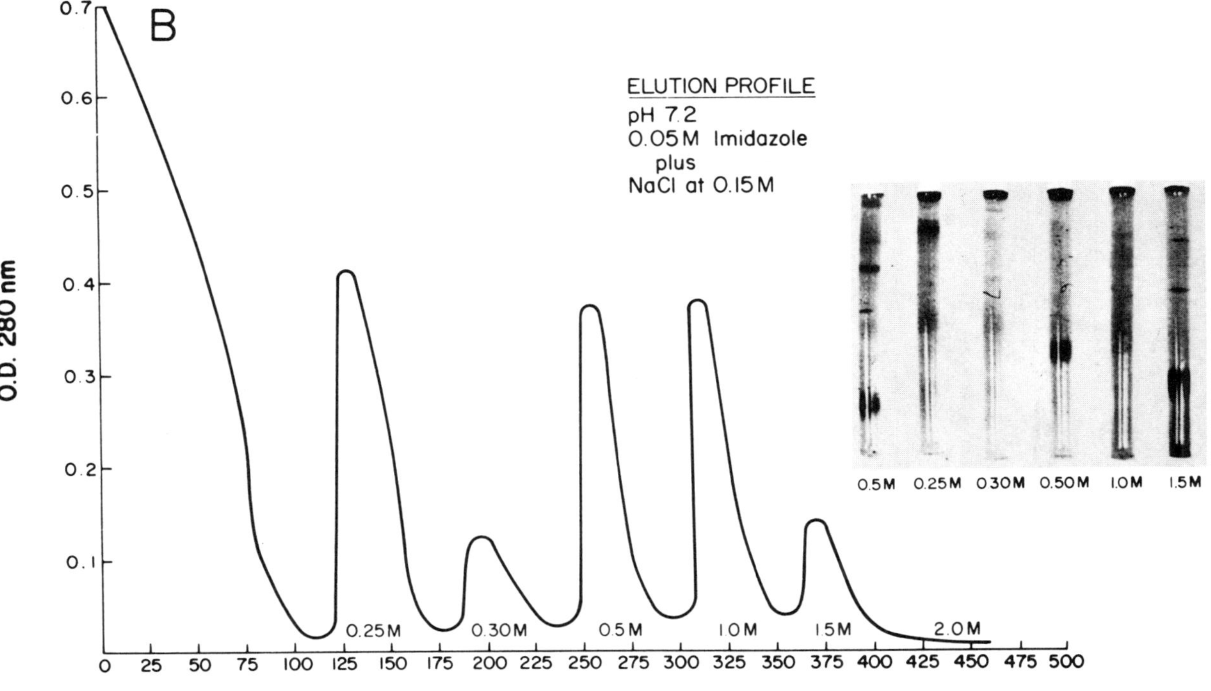

FIGURE 2B. Freeze-thawed bovine platelet lysate chromatogram obtained from step elution of dextran-Sepharose resin. Conditions are similar to those for heparin resin.

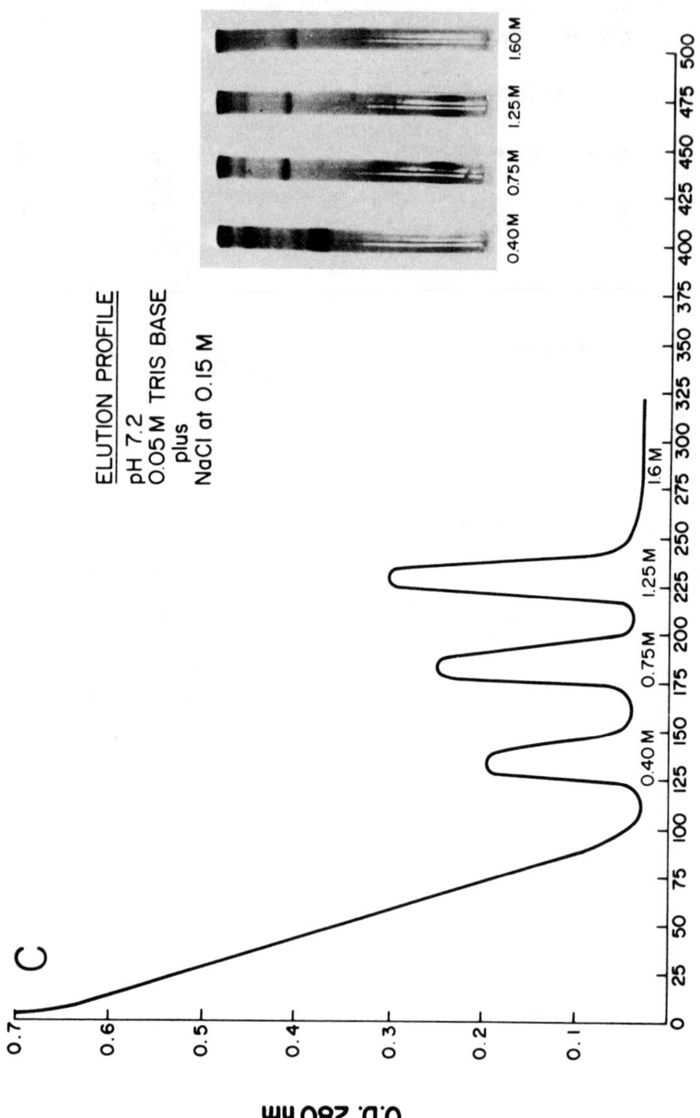

FIGURE 2C. Freeze-thawed human platelet lysate chromatogram obtained from step elution of dextran-Sepharose resin. All chromatography elutions were performed at room temperature with flow rates of 50 ml/hr and collected in 20 ml fractions.

TABLE 1

AMINO ACID COMPOSITIONS OF BOVINE AND HUMAN PLATELET FACTOR FOUR *

	Bovine	Human
Lys	8	8
His	3	2
Arg	4	3
Asx	5	4
Thr	5	5
Ser	8	3
Glx	10	9
Pro	6	4
Gly	5	3
Ala	4	5
Cys	4	4
Val	3	3
Met	0	0
Ile	5	6
Leu	9	10
Tyr	1	1
Phe	2	0
Trp	0	0
Totals	82	70
Calculated Molecular Weight	9046	7772

* Protein samples were hydrolyzed in 6N HCl at 100 C for 22 hours *in vacuo*. No corrections were made for decompositional losses. Each analysis is the average of 6 independent hydrolyses and analyses.

BOVINE PF-4

```
          1     2     3     4     5     6     7     8     9    10    11    12    13    14    15    16
        NH2 - GLU - SER - SER - PHE - PRO - ALA - THR - PHE - VAL - PRO - LEU - PRO - ALA - ASP - SER - GLU

         17    18    19    20    21    22    23    24    25    26    27
        GLY - GLY - GLU - ASP - GLU - ASP -  X  -  X  - CYS (LEU) CYS
```

HUMAN PF-4

```
          1     2     3     4     5     6     7     8     9    10    11    12    13    14    15    16
        NH2 - GLU - ALA - GLU - GLU - ASP - GLY - ASP - LEU - GLN - CYS - LEU - CYS - VAL - LYS - THR - THR

         17    18    19    20    21    22    23    24    25    26    27
        SER - GLN - VAL - ARG - PRO - ARG - HIS - ILE - THR - SER - LEU
```

FIGURE 3. Comparison of the NH₂-terminal sequences for bovine and human PF-4. Each sample was reduced and alkylated and the S-Cm-Cys residues confirmed by quantitation of ³H-CH₃COOH incorporated from the alkylation reaction.

```
PF-4       15'  14'  13'  12'  11'  10'  9'  8'  7'  6'  5'  4'  3'  2'  1'    1    2    3    4    5    6    7    8    9    10   11   12   13   14   15
HUMAN                                                                          GLU - ALA - GLU - GLU - ASP - GLY - ASP - LEU - GLN - CYS - LEU - CYS - VAL - LYS - THR

BOVINE     GLU - SER - SER - PHE - PRO - ALA - THR - PHE - VAL - PRO - LEU - PRO - ALA - ASP - SER - GLU - GLY - GLY - GLU - ASP - GLU - ASP -  X  -  X  - CYS (LEU) CYS -  X  -  X  -  X

RABBIT                                                                   SER - ASX - ASX - PRO - LYS - GLX - SER - GLX - GLY - ASX - LEU - HIS - CYS - VAL - CYS - VAL - LYS - THR

LA-PF-4
HUMAN                                              ASN - LEU - ALA - LYS - GLY - LYS - GLU - GLU - SER - LEU - ASP - SER - ASP - LEU - TYR - ALA - GLU - LEU - ARG - CYS - MET - CYS - ILE - LYS - THR
```

FIGURE 4. Comparison of the NH$_2$-terminal sequences of the PF-4s from human, bovine and rabbit sources, as well as LA-PF-4 from human platelets. Numbering has been referenced to the Cys-Leu-Cys segments of human PF-4.

DISCUSSION

Preliminary results indicate that species differences exist for platelet-specific proteins from human, cow, rabbit, and pig (personal communication).[19, 24] In an effort to determine to what extent platelet factor four and its activity might be broad-based, comparison was drawn between bovine and human PF-4.

It was found that bovine PF-4 could be isolated through one-step affinity chromatography using either heparin-sepharose or dextran-sulfate sepharose, whereas human PF-4 was limited to one-step isolation using only heparin-sepharose. These results indicate that species differences in platelet-specific proteins may require different methods of isolation and separation despite similar tendencies to bind heparin and/or proteoglycan carrier(s).

The need to develop and apply new techniques of separation becomes particularly apparent when viewed with respect to the possibility of distinguishing between overlapping platelet-specific protein activities and possible contaminants. Of particular interest is the need to know whether or not an LA-PF-4 conversion to β-TG may occur in other species. A recent study of avian thrombocytes reported that different aggregating substances (thrombin, serotonin, and collagen) could induce variances in "platelet-specific" protein release, including a β-TG-like protein.[25] It remains unclear, however, to what extent and under what circumstances such changes in the low molecular weight fraction may reflect changes in β-TG-like protein levels. Of further importance is the need to determine to what extent growth-promoting activity may be associated with the β-TG-like proteins in other species and whether or not loss of such activity can be modulated by protease activity. Since low concentrations of platelet-specific protein are often required to stimulate mitogenic activity, the possibility of trace contamination by more potent mitogens continually arises. Comparison of platelet derived growth factors from other species may shed light on the disparity often observed experimentally.

Amino acid compositions of bovine PF-4 account for the increase in SDS subunit molecular weight observed when compared to human PF-4. A substantial increase in polar residues (aspartate, glutamate, serine and threonine) probably accounts for the higher solubility of bovine PF-4 in low ionic strength solutions. The increased affinity of bovine PF-4 for DSS could be associated with an apparent increase of basic residues (lysine, histidine and arginine) towards the carboxyterminus (derived from TABLE 1 and FIG. 3). Although this finding supports the notion that a specific heparin binding site is probably localized in the carboxy-terminal region, it does not resolve the relative importance which lysine residues and primary structure conservation may play in heparin binding.[26] It is hoped that completion of the bovine PF-4 sequence may elucidate the functional importance of amino acid sequence and conformation which may contribute to varying degrees of heparin binding.

Attempts to establish homology both within and between species of platelet-specific proteins remains unresolved.[19, 24, 27] Ginsberg *et al.*, recently reported a high degree of sequence homology between rabbit and human PF-4, but no β-TG-like comparison was similarly made.[24] As indicated in FIGURE 4 a pattern of variable NH_2-terminal extension seems to emerge. The recent finding of protease activity converting LA-PF-4 to β-TG makes the suggestion of different cleavages, post-translational or otherwise, quite plausible. The possibility of identifying some form of species-specific precursor molecule conceivably derived from megakaryocytes needs to be pursued.

ACKNOWLEDGMENT

The authors are indebted to Miss Debra McKinley for her excellent technical assistance.

REFERENCES

1. NIEWIAROWSKI, S. 1977. Proteins secreted by the platelet. Thrombos. Haemostas. (Stuttg.). **38:** 924–938.

2. HITI-HARPER, J., H. WOHL & E. HARPER. 1978. Platelet factor 4: An inhibitor of collagenase. Science **199:** 991–992.

3. HOPE, W., C. N. CHESTERMAN, G. J. DUSTING, I. SMITH, F. J. MORGAN & T. J. MARTIN. 1979. Inhibition by β-thromboglobulin of prostacyclin (PGI$_2$) formation in arterial endothelial cells. Thrombos. Haemostas. (Stuttg.). **42** (1): 8.

4. NIEWIAROWSKI, D., B. RUCINSKI, M. MILLMAN & J. HAWIGER. 1976. Immunoassay of human platelet factor 4 (antiheparin factor) and its significance for evaluation of the platelet function. *In* Platelet Function Testing, Proceedings from Workshop on Platelets entitled The Significance of Platelet Function Tests in the Evaluation of Hemostatic and Thrombotic Tendencies. H. J. Day, H. Holmsen & M. B. Zucker, Eds. DHEW Publication No. (NIH) **78–1087:** 244–266.

5. FAREED, J., H. L. MESSMORE & E. W. BERMES, JR. 1979. Newer methods in the testing of platelet function. *In* Manual of Procedures for the Seminar on Biochemical Hematology. F. W. Sunderman, Ed. **1:** 415–436. Institute for Clinical Science, Inc. Philadelphia, Pa.

6. BROWN, T. R., T. T. S. HO & D. A. WALZ. 1980. Improved radioimmunoassay of platelet factor 4 and β-thromboglobulin in plasma. Clinica Chimica Acta **101:** 225–233.

7. ROSS, R. & A. VOGEL. 1978. The platelet derived growth factor. Cell **14:** 203–210.

8. CASTOR, C. W., M. E. SCOTT, J. C. RITCHIE & S. L. WHITNEY. 1976. Characteristics of a human platelet factor which stimulates DNA and glycosaminoglycan synthesis. Clin. Res. **24:** 575A.

9. CASTOR, C. W., J. C. RITCHIE, M. E. SCOTT & S. L. WHITNEY. 1977. Connective tissue activation. XI. Stimulation of glycosaminoglycan and DNA formation by a platelet factor. Arthritis Rheum. **20:** 859–868.

10. CASTOR, C. W., J. C. RITCHIE, C. H. WILLIAMS, JR., M. E. SCOTT, S. L. WHITNEY, S. L. MYERS, T. B. SLOAN & B. E. ANDERSON. 1979. Connective tissue activation. XIV. Composition and actions of a human platelet autacoid mediator. Arthritis and Rheum. **22**(3): 260–272.

11. RUCINSKI, B., S. NIEWIAROWSKI, P. JAMES, D. A. WALZ & A. Z. BUDZYNSKI. 1979. Antiheparin proteins secreted by human platelets. Purification, characterization, and radioimmunoassay. Blood **53**(1): 47–62.

12. NIEWIAROWSKI, S., D. A. WALZ, P. JAMES, B. RUCINSKI & F. KUEPPERS. 1980. Identification and separation of secreted platelet proteins by isoelectric focusing. Evidence that low-affinity platelet factor 4 is converted to β-thromboglobulin by limited proteolysis. Blood. **55**(3): 453–456.

13. DEUTSCH, E. 1954. Differentiation of certain platelet factors in relation to blood coagulation. Rev, d'hemat. **9:** 483–488.

14. DEUTSCH, E., S. A. JOHNSON & W. H. SEEGERS. 1955. Differentiation of certain platelet factors related to blood coagulation. Circulation Res. **3:** 110–115.

15. DEUTSCH, E., E. WAWERSICH & G. FRANKE. 1957. Ueber das Vorkommen

eines Antiheparin-faktors in Thrombozyten und Geweben, I. Mitteilung. Antiheparinaktivität der Thrombozyten. Thromb. Diath. Haemorrh. **1:** 397–405.

16. DEUTSCH, E. & W. KAIN. 1960. Studies on platelet factor 4. In Henry Ford Hospital International Symposium entitled Blood Platelets. S. A. Johnson, R. W. Monto, J. W. Rebuck & R. C. Horn, Eds. Little Brown Co. Boston. pp. 337–345.

17. MILLER-ANDERSSON, M., H. BORG & L.-O. ANDERSSON. 1974. Purification of antithrombin III by affinity chromatography. Thrombos. Res. **5:** 439–452.

18. SPACKMAN, D. H., W. H. STEIN & S. MOORE. 1958. Automatic recording apparatus for use in the chromatography of amino acids. Anal. Chem. **30:** 1190–1206.

19. WU, V. Y., D. A. Walz & L. E. McCoy. 1977. Purification and characterization of human and bovine platelet factor 4. Preparative Biochemistry **7**(6): 479–493

20. LEVINE, S. P. & H. WOHL. 1976. Human platelet factor 4 (PF-4): Purification and characterization by affinity chromatography. J. Biol. Chem. **251:** 324–328.

21. WEBER, K. & M. OSBORN. 1969. The reliability of molecular weight determination by dodecyl sulfate polyacrylamide gel electrophoresis. J. Biol. Chem. **244:** 4406–4412.

22. WALZ, D. A., D. HEWETT-EMMETT & W. H. SEEGERS. 1977. Amino acid sequence of human prothrombin fragments 1 and 2. Proc. Natl. Acad. Sci. USA **74:** 1969–1972.

23. WALZ, D. A., V. Y. WU, R. DELAMO, H. DENE & L. E. McCoy. 1977. Primary structure of human platelet factor 4. Thrombos. Res. **11** 893–898.

24. GINSBERG, M. H., R. HOSKINS, R. SIGRIST & R. G. PAINTER. 1979. Purification of a heparin-neutralizing protein from rabbit platelets and its homology with human platelet factor 4. J. Biol. Chem. **254**(24): 12365–12371.

25. WACHOWICZ, B. & T. KRAJEWSKI. 1979. The released proteins from avian thrombocytes. Thrombos. Haemostas. (Stuttg). **42:** 1289–1295.

26. HANDIN, R. I. & H. J. COHEN. 1976. Purification and binding properties of human platelet factor four. J. Biol. Chem. **251:** 4273–4282.

27. BEGG, G. S., D. S. PEPPER, C. N. CHESTERMAN & F. J. MORGAN. 1978. Complete covalent structure of human *beta*-thromboglobulin. Biochemistry **17**(9): 1739–1744.

KINETIC STUDIES *IN VIVO* OF ANTITHROMBIN III *

E. Basil Reeve, Bruce Leonard, and Tim Carlson †

Department of Medicine
University of Colorado Health Sciences Center
Denver, Colorado 80262

INTRODUCTION

In this paper we review briefly some of our recent studies of the behavior *in vivo* of antithrombin III (AT) and its interactions with clotting proteases.[1,2] Our studies have been made in dog and man with preparations of dog and human AT labeled with radioactive iodine and the findings have been interpreted with kinetic approaches.[3,4] These have thrown light on the steady state metabolism and distribution of antithrombin III in health and the behavior of complexes of AT with clotting proteases. They have also suggested an important extravascular function for AT. We have also applied steady state kinetics to the interactions of AT with clotting proteases which leads to some surprising and interesting findings.[5]

PREPARATION OF AT LABELED WITH RADIOACTIVE IODINE (*I-AT)

Valid studies of turnover of a plasma protein depend on a preparation that has not suffered alteration of its biological properties during purification or subsequent labeling. Because proteins are often fragile, in general the simpler, gentler, and more rapid the purification and the less destructive the iodination process the better. Until the advent of heparin-agarose affinity chromatography [6,7] the methods of purifying antithrombin III were too long, difficult and potentially damaging to the protein to be satisfactory for turnover studies. The early form of the heparin-agarose method required subsequent ion exchange and gel filtration steps [6] but Damus [7,8] and then we [1,2] found that good preparations of dog, human, rabbit and rat antithrombin III could be obtained by passing citrated plasma through a heparin-agarose column, washing off most of the unwanted protein and eluting with a salt gradient. The resulting AT was in dilute solution but could readily be concentrated on a small heparin-agarose column. With this approach in 24 hours sufficient AT for turnover studies can be prepared from 30 ml citrated plasma. This allows one to study the turnover of a human subject's own autologous AT without risk of infusing him with viruses other than those already present in his plasma.

Iodination of proteins with radioactive iodine (*I) without altering their biological behavior, particularly when the proteins are present in small amount or low concentration, has long presented problems. In general methods suitable for radioimmunoassay, such as the chloramine T method [9] can be ruled out as

* These studies were supported by National Institutes of Health Grants HL 02262, HL 25477, and RR 00051, and by the Colorado Heart Association.

† Now at the Department of Biochemistry, University of New Mexico, Albuquerque, New Mexico 87131.

too damaging to the protein, and the only satisfactory methods are those using lactoperoxidase[10] or iodine monochloride.[11] We find both the latter methods are satisfactory but it is necessary after labeling with the peroxidase method to remove *I-labeled peroxidase and any contaminants from the *I-AT, while the presence of an animal protein (bovine lactoperoxidase) makes the lacto-peroxidase method unsuitable for preparing *I-AT for human studies. Modi-fications of the IC1 method make it usually reliable for labeling small amounts of AT and it then becomes the method of choice for preparing *I-AT. Ideally turnover studies with *I-labeled proteins should use proteins labeled with only one iodine atom per protein molecule. We find that heparin-agarose can separate AT labeled with one iodine atom from that labeled with more than one.[2] Thus after AT radioiodination it is now possible not only to measure the average ratio of iodine atoms to AT molecules in the *I-labeled AT but the ratio of AT molecules with more than one iodine atom to those with one. Preliminary findings suggest that the lactoperoxidase method results in a higher ratio than the iodine monochloride method. Fortunately, the monoiodinated AT can be separated from the polyiodinated on heparin-agarose.

If *I-AT is to provide a satisfactory biological tracer of the physiological behavior of AT it must pass certain *in vitro* and *in vivo* tests. First the prepara-tion should be homogeneous on SDS-PAGE and of essentially the same size and migratory pattern as the unlabeled AT. We find this to be so. Second the *I-AT should have the same heparin cofactor and progressive antithrombin activities as the unlabeled AT. We find that this is so with monoiodinated AT, but some loss of both activities may occur with polyiodinated AT. Third, when *I-AT is added to plasma and the plasma is subject to crossed immunoelec-trophoresis in the presence of heparin,[12] the ratio of *I to the area of antibody bound in the AT peak should approximate the ratio of *I to the area of antibody bound in the AT complex peaks. This we find is true.

The preparation needs also to pass two *in vivo* tests. After i.v. injection, *in vivo* behavior is characterized by 4 patterns: the pattern of loss of *I-AT from the plasma, the pattern of appearance of low MW *I-AT breakdown products in the plasma, the pattern of *I excretion in the urine, and the pattern of whole body radioactivity. In general, irregular patterns with early appear-ance of high levels of radioactive breakdown products in the plasma and their rapid excretion in the urine characterize biologically altered *I-labeled proteins. The patterns following *I-AT injection in man and animals are remarkably consistent and show none of the above hallmarks of altered proteins. A second sensitive test is the effect of "screening" the *I-AT in a "screening" animal on its subsequent behavior in a recipient animal.[13] Screening consists of injecting the *I-AT into an animal in which it remains for 12 to 24 hours after which this animal's plasma serves as the source of screened *I-AT. The "screening" exposes the *I-AT in the screening animal to the cells—including R-E cells— that remove altered protein. We found no significant difference in the *I-AT parameters shown by groups of dogs receiving screened and unscreened *I-AT.[1] Thus our *I-AT by all the above tests appears to be a satisfactory tracer of native AT behavior.

BEHAVIOR OF *I-AT AFTER INTRAVENOUS INJECTION

FIGURE 1 shows typical findings in dog 5a-5 during the 7 days following i.v. injection of *I-AT at time zero. The measured values are shown by the data

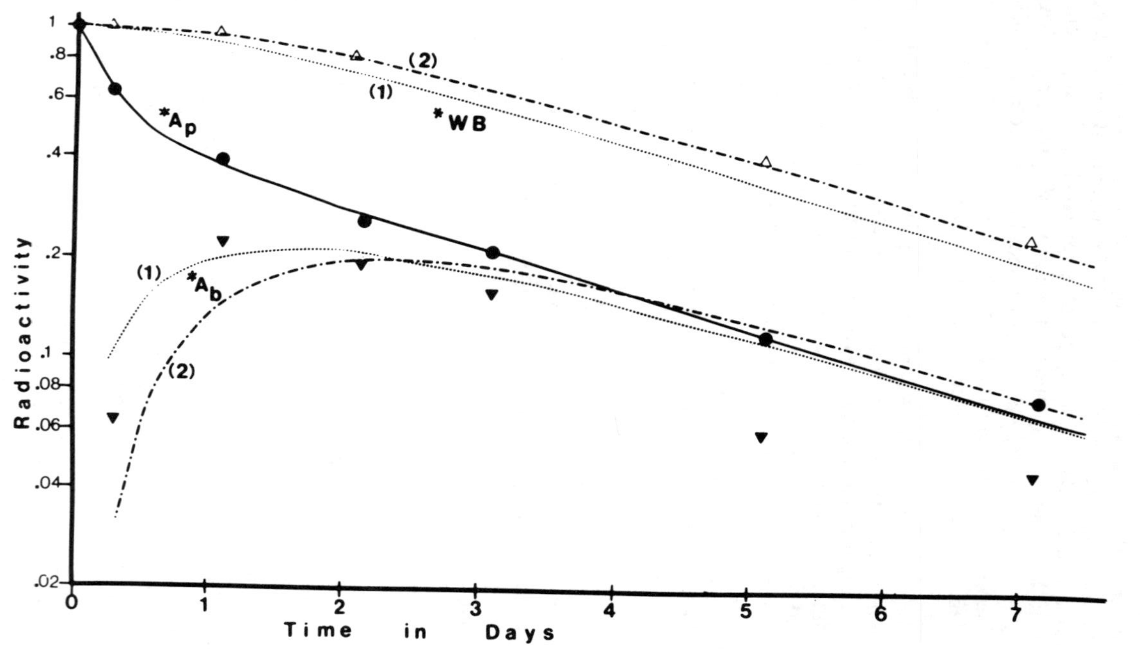

FIGURE 1. Measurements of plasma *I-AT (*filled circles*) connected by a continuous line labeled *A_p. This line is the best fit described by $C_1 e^{-a_1 t} + C_2 e^{-a_2 t} = .494\ e^{-.279t} + 506\ e^{-3.75t}$ obtained by computer fit. Also shown are measurements of *WB indicated by ∇, and of *A_b indicated by $\blacktriangledown$. Predictions of the course of *WB and *A_b obtained with Model 1 are shown by the continuous lines .... and of the course of *WB and *A_b obtained with Model 2 by the continuous lines —·—·. For further discussion see text.

points. Thus the solid circles labeled $*A_p$ are total plasma $*$I-AT, the solid triangles labeled $*A_b$ are total radioactive breakdown products of $*$I-AT and the open triangles labeled $*$WB are whole body radioactivity. We wish to interpret these measurements in terms of the physiological behavior of antithrombin III.

FIGURE 2a shows the standard model of the metabolism and distribution in the animal of a plasma protein such as albumin, which should allow interpretation. In this, specific cells synthesize the protein into the plasma from which it passes through the capillaries to the interstitial fluids and then returns to the plasma by the lymphatics. In a steady state capillary outflow equals lymphatic return. The protein also leaves the plasma to be broken down in catabolic cells, and in a steady state catabolic rate equals synthetic rate. In FIGURE 2a (*upper panel*) A_p denotes total plasma AT, A_e denotes total interstitial AT, j_1A_p denotes transcapillary flux of A_p, j_2A_e denotes lymphatic return of A_e, and j_3A_p denotes catabolic rate of A_p. A_p is measured from the product of plasma AT concentration and plasma volume, but there is no direct measure of A_e or of the fractional rates j_1, j_2 and j_3. If AT is synthesized only in the liver A_s, synthetic rate of AT can be measured with rather elaborate ^{14}C studies.[14, 15]

Denoting $*$I-labeled species by an asterisk ($*$), following i.v. injection (FIG. 2a, *lower panel*) $*$I-AT enters the plasma as $*A_p$, passes to the interstitial fluids at the rate j_1*A_p to form interstitial $*$I-AT, $*A_e$, and returns to the plasma at the rate j_2*A_e. Catabolism at the rate j_3*A_p releases low molecular weight breakdown products, $*A_b$, which are excreted in the urine at the rate k_uA_b. The sum $*A_p + *A_e + *A_b$ termed $*$WB is measured by whole body counting, and since, as shown in FIGURE 1, $*A_p$ and $*A_b$ are measured separately, $*A_e$ is obtained from $*$WB $- *A_p - *A_b$. Thus we have linked the observations of FIGURE 1 to some of the features of the standard models shown in FIGURE 2a.

Assuming that on the average j_1, j_2, j_3 and k_u remain constant the models of FIGURE 2a are defined by linear differential equations. Then, given the equation describing the course of $*A_p$ and a value for k_u the values of A_e, j_1, j_2 and j_3 can be calculated as well as the course of $*$WB and $*A_b$. The equation describing $*A_p$ was obtained by computer fit to the $*A_p$ data points. The two-exponential equation so obtained gave the continuous line in FIGURE 1 which very closely fits the $*A_p$ data points. An average value for k_u was calculated from the $*A_p$, $*A_b$ and $*$WB data points. With these and the equations of the models of FIGURE 2a the course of $*$WB and $*A_b$ was predicted and was shown by the dashed lines labeled (1) in FIGURE 1. It is apparent that these underpredict measured $*$WB but predict adequately $*A_b$. The underpredictions of $*$WB were consistent in many experiments and in a number of experiments early predicted $*A_b$ exceeded measured values. Thus $*$I-AT metabolism is not well described by the usual plasma protein kinetic model, which may be termed Model 1. Model 1 describes quite well the behavior of $*$I-albumin and $*$I-fibrinogen.[4, 17] As compared with the predictions of Model 1 more interstitial (and perhaps intracellular) AT accumulates and less AT is catabolized.

BEHAVIOR OF $*$I-AT COMPLEXES WITH CLOTTING PROTEASES

A possible explanation of these findings was that after i.v. injection of $*$I-AT some of it reacted with clotting proteases (perhaps released by the

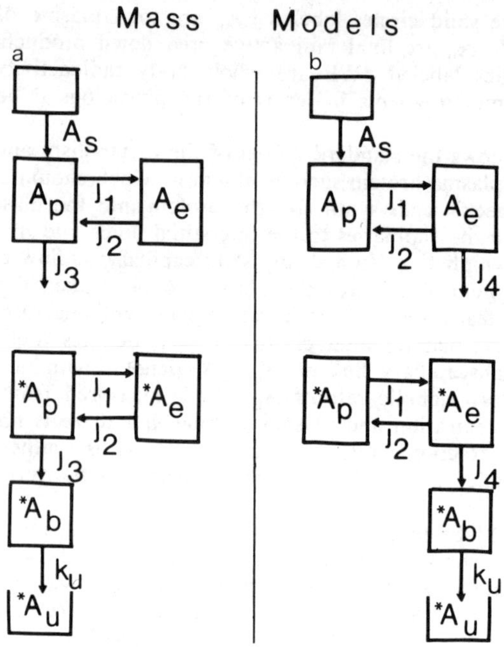

FIGURE 2a (*left side*). Block diagrams of a mass model (*above*) and a tracer model (*below*) of the physiological behavior of albumin and *I-albumin. The j's and k_u are fractional rate constants with dimensions of day^{-1} which when multiplied by the contents of the blocks give rates of mass of protein, *I-protein or *I-protein products transported in the direction of the arrow per day.[4, 17] This model implies breakdown of the plasma protein immediately after it leaves the plasma at the rate $j_3 \cdot A_p$ and is termed Model 1.

FIGURE 2b (*right side*). Block diagrams of mass and tracer models of a plasma protein which though showing similar distribution between plasma and interstitial fluids as Model 1 shows delayed catabolism at the rate $j_4 \cdot A_e$. The delay is pictured as caused by the time required for passage of the plasma protein to interstitial catabolic cells and for catabolism in them. This is termed Model 2. For further description see the text.

venipuncture) and the resulting *I-AT protease complexes entered the interstitial fluids from which they were only slowly removed. We therefore studied the behavior of clotting protease complexes with *I-AT.

AT forms inactive complexes with many clotting proteases including factors XIIa, XIa, Xa, IXa and thrombin.[18, 19] We found that when *I-AT is added to citrated plasma which is then clotted with thromboplastin and calcium a fraction containing AT complexes can be separated by using heparin-agarose and a salt gradient. This fraction contains *I-AT that has lost its heparin cofactor and progressive antithrombin activities and elutes from heparin-agarose well ahead of the uncomplexed *I-AT, which has fully retained these activities. The *I-AT complex fraction has a molecular weight higher than the

AT but a little lower than expected from the sum of the protease and AT molecular weights. FIGURE 3 shows some findings when this fraction is injected i.v. into a dog. The *I-AT complexes are removed very rapidly with a half life of about 30 min. During this rapid removal a very rapid release of radioactive breakdown products is seen, indicating almost immediate catabolism of the complexes. Analysis shows that this behavior cannot explain the interstitial accumulation and delayed catabolism of *I-AT noted above.

POSSIBLE ALTERNATIVE MODEL OF *I-AT METABOLISM

FIGURE 2b shows a block diagram of a second model of plasma protein metabolism, which differs from Model 1 in that catabolism is pictured as occurring at the rate $j_4 A_e$ only after passage of the *I-AT through the interstitial fluids. This is termed Model 2. Assuming that j_1, j_2, j_4 and k_u on the average remain constant, this model is also described by linear differential equations. With these, a value for k_u and the computer-fitted two-exponential equation

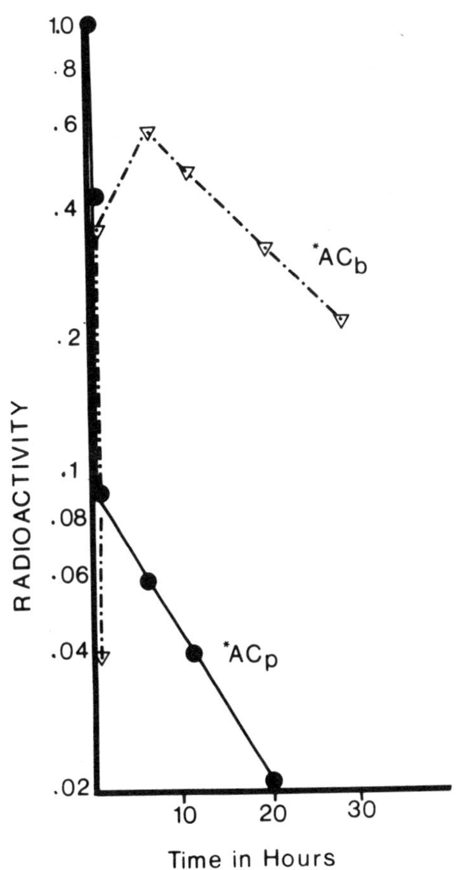

FIGURE 3. Measurements of plasma *I-AT-Protease Complexes, *AC_p, and their low molecular weight breakdown products, *AC_b, following injection at time zero of a preparation of *I-AT-Clotting Protease Complexes. *AC_p leaves the plasma very rapidly and *AC_b appears almost instantaneously. The small tail of *AC_p indicates return of a few percent of the complexes that have briefly passed through the interstitial fluids.

describing $*A_p$, the predictions labeled (2) of the courses of whole body radio-activity, $*WB$, and breakdown product radioactivity $*A_b$, shown in FIGURE 1 were obtained. These fit much better the observed $*WB$ data and reasonably well the less accurate $*A_b$ data. This has been our general finding and Model 2 therefore seems the more appropriate model.

GENERAL FEATURES OF AT METABOLISM

Whether Model 1 or Model 2 applies we can make good measurements of rate of AT breakdown. Further we can obtain fairly good estimates of the ratio of interstitial to plasma AT, A_e/A_p, from the ratio of $*I$-AT in the interstitial compartment, $*A_e$, to that in the plasma, $*A_p$. Some average values obtained in dogs are shown in TABLE 1. When the value of A_e/A_p calculated from Model 2 is compared with that obtained from $*A_e/*A_p$ the latter is only about 10% higher so the values of TABLE 1 are reasonably good estimates of

TABLE 1

FRACTIONAL BREAKDOWN RATE (j_3) AND APPROXIMATE EXTRAVASCULAR/
INTRAVASCULAR AT RATIO ($*A_e/*A_p$) IN DOGS

	Weight (kg)	j_3 (day^{-1})	$*A_e/*A_p$
	All Animals n = 14		
Mean	9.61	.509	1.03
SD	2.76	.056	.13
	Females n = 7		
Mean	8.23	.509	1.04
SD	2.88	.079	.14
	Males n = 7		
Mean	10.99	.509	1.01
SD	1.95	.026	.12

A_e/A_p. TABLE 1 shows that about 50% of the AT in the plasma is catabolized per day while the AT in the interstitial fluids approaches the amount in the plasma.

PHYSIOLOGICAL SIGNIFICANCE OF A_e AND OF THE TWO MODELS OF AT METABOLISM

We try to make this more evident by using the models to make calculations of the effects of a stress. The stress chosen was sudden arrest of synthesis. Calculation of the effects of this in the absence of interstitial stores shows their importance. Calculation of the effects in the presence of Model 1 and Model 2 shows their ability to withstand the stress. The calculations are given in the APPENDIX. The two-exponential plasma $*I$-AT equation defines the js of

Models 1 and 2, which give initial steady state levels of interstitial AT equal to 65% of plasma AT for Model 1 and to 88% of plasma AT for Model 2. With absent interstitial stores, calculation shows that plasma AT falls at a rate of 50% per day and reaches 10% of its initial level after 4.5 days. After 4.5 days Model 1 shows that plasma AT falls to 19.4% and interstitial AT to 18.7% of initial plasma level, while Model 2 shows that plasma AT falls to 24.9% and interstitial AT to 25.4% of initial plasma AT level. Thus, in response to the stress of arrested synthesis AT stores halve the rate of fall of A_p while Model 2 significantly increases the available interstitial and plasma AT as compared with the standard Model 1.

PRELIMINARIES TO THE STUDY OF AT METABOLISM IN DISEASE

We developed methods of making AT turnover studies especially to study the alterations that occur in disease. Low plasma AT levels are common,[20, 21] and understanding the genesis of these requires turnover studies. However, these by themselves give incomplete information since AT reacts with products of other plasma proteins. Thus the metabolism of AT can be much affected by the activation of the clotting proteases of the intrinsic system. To examine some of the effects of this FIGURE 4 presents in a block diagram some relations between the final two clotting proteases and AT. Only steady states are considered, in which transcapillary passage equals lymphatic return of protein so that consideration of interstitial proteins can be omitted. FIGURE 4 shows the noninteracting plasma proteins antithrombin III (A), factor X (X) and prothrombin (P) in their plasma compartments with their plasma levels governed by rates of synthesis, shown with subscript s, and fractional rates of breakdown shown with subscript b. These plasma compartments are enclosed by heavy lines indicating that in health these are the only compartments present, and the metabolism of these three proteins is independent. However, when coagulation is activated factor Xa (Xa) is released from factor X. While free, factor Xa activates prothrombin to thrombin but it is continually being inactivated by complex formation with AT. Thrombin (θ), while free, clots fibrinogen and initiates a number of positive feedback reactions, but thrombin is also continually inactivated by complex formation with AT. Each of these reaction products requires a plasma compartment, outlined with light lines in FIGURE 4. The new compartments contain factor Xa, factor Xa-AT complexes (XaA), thrombin and thrombin-AT complexes (θA). The light lines indicate that the new compartments do not exist in health.

To define the protein flows indicated by the arrows in FIGURE 4 requires some further information. The reactions between factor Xa and AT and thrombin and AT are bimolecular.[18, 22, 23] Thus, using the above symbols, θ for thrombin and A for AT and considering first plasma *in vitro*

$$Xa + A \rightarrow XaA \tag{1}$$

$$\frac{dXaA}{dt} = g \cdot Xa \cdot A \tag{2}$$

$$\theta + A \rightarrow \theta A \tag{3}$$

$$\frac{d\theta A}{dt} = h \cdot \theta \cdot A \tag{4}$$

and the rate of formation of complexes is proportional to the product of Xa or thrombin and AT in the plasma. The bimolecular rate constants g and h, are closely related to those familiar in *in vitro* studies. They have dimensions of $t^{-1} \cdot mol^{-1}$, depend on the temperature and salt environment of the plasma and are increased more than 1000-fold by small concentrations of active heparin.[18, 22, 24] Heparin has similar effects on all intrinsic clotting proteases.[19] With this information the steady state rates in FIGURE 4 can now be inserted. The rate of activation of factor X to factor Xa can be pictured as $k_c X$, where k_c is a constant fractional rate depending on activation processes. The rate of

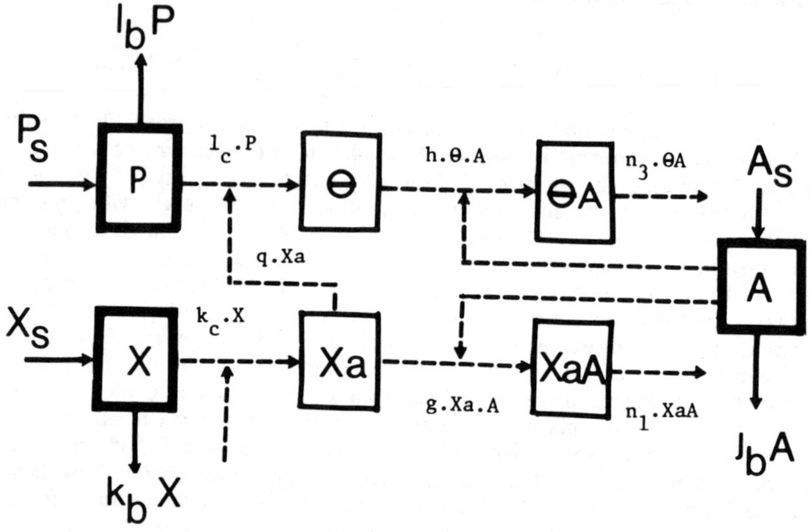

FIGURE 4. Block diagram of steady state relations between factor X (X), factor Xa (Xa), prothrombin (P), thrombin (θ) and antithrombin III (A). In health, only the compartments outlined with heavy lines are present, but activation of coagulation causes the appearance of the other compartments. Activation of factor X at the constant fractional rate, k_c results in a constant level of factor Xa determined by the rate of complex formation with AT. The factor Xa level in turn results in a constant fractional rate, l_c of activation of prothrombin which is equal to $q \cdot Xa$. The complexes of Xa and AT (XaA) and thrombin and AT (θA) are removed from the plasma at the fractional rates n_1 and n_3. The fractional rates k_b, k_c, l_b, l_c, n_1, n_3 and j_b have dimensions of t^{-1}; X, Xa, XaA, P, θ, θA, A have dimensions of mols; g, h and q have dimensions of $mols^{-1} t^{-1}$. For further discussion see text.

inactivation of factor Xa depends on the rate of formation of complexes with AT which is given by $g \cdot Xa \cdot A$. The rate of removal of these complexes from the plasma can be written $n_1 \cdot XaA$ and our experiments with mixtures of complexes suggest it is very fast. In health, as shown in FIGURE 4, AT continually undergoes physiological catabolism but neutralization of Xa will result in additional removal given by $g \cdot Xa \cdot A$. The presence of free Xa results in activation of prothrombin, P, to thrombin, θ, at the rate $l_c \cdot P$. The thrombin reacts with AT to form AT complexes at the rate $h \cdot \theta \cdot A$. The complexes, θA, are removed from the plasma at the rate $n_3 \cdot \theta A$. The utilization of AT for formation of thrombin-AT complexes also results in increased consumption of AT by the rate $h \cdot \theta \cdot A$. We can now use FIGURE 4 to examine some of the parameters controlling plasma antithrombin III concentration given by total plasma AT/plasma volume.

In health total plasma AT, A, is governed by the relation

$$A = A_s / j_b \tag{5}$$

where A_s is daily rate of AT synthesis and j_b is fraction of A catabolized per day.

When activation of factors X and prothrombin occurs FIGURE 4 shows that

$$A = A_s / (j_b + g \cdot Xa + h \cdot \theta). \tag{6}$$

Whether the level of AT falls will depend on how high the levels are of Xa and θ and how much synthetic rate of AT increases. Relation 6 also allows examining the steady state effects of heparin treatment on AT level. Therapeutic doses of heparin enormously increase g and h, $g\uparrow\uparrow$ and $h\uparrow\uparrow$, and it is shown elsewhere [5] that this results in marked reduction of $g \cdot Xa + h \cdot \theta$. Thus if A_s remains constant, AT levels will rise above pretreatment levels.

FIGURE 4 is important because it allows examination of the sort of measurements required for defining the causes of AT alterations in disease. Thus good definition of the features in FIGURE 4 altered in disease could be obtained from measurements of the rate of formation of the complexes XaA and θA, which in a steady state are given by $n_1 \cdot XaA$ and $n_3 \cdot \theta A$, or of levels of plasma X and Xa, II and IIa and the *in vivo* bimolecular rate constants g and h. Other methods of definition will be apparent from the figure.

The steady state kinetics of FIGURE 4 happen also to yield some extraordinarily interesting relations. Remembering that each compartment represents the total amount of the designated protein in the plasma, that the arrows represent the protein flows into and out of the compartment and that in a steady state for each compartment protein inflow = protein outflow so that the sum of the flows represented by the arrows entering and leaving each compartment is zero, from the figure we can write the following relations

$$k_c \cdot X = g \cdot Xa \cdot A = n_1 \cdot XaA \tag{7}$$

This states that the activation rate of factor X, $k_c \cdot X =$ the rate of formation of XaA complexes = the rate of removal of complexes from the plasma $n_1 \cdot XaA$. Rearranging this

$$Xa = \frac{k_c \cdot X}{g \cdot A} = \frac{n_1 \cdot XaA}{g \cdot A} \tag{8}$$

This defines factor Xa level in terms which can be compared with direct measurements.[25] Further it demonstrates that plasma free factor Xa level is inversely proportional to plasma AT level. Thus if plasma AT level falls to one half normal levels and other levels remain constant plasma free factor Xa will double its normal level.

Similar relations apply to thrombin. Thus writing the activation rate of thrombin as $l_c \cdot P$, this equals the rate of formation of complexes, $h \cdot \theta \cdot A$, and also the removal rate of θA complexes from the plasma, $n_3 \cdot \theta A$. This is shown in (9).

$$l_c \cdot P = h \cdot \theta \cdot A = n_3 \cdot \theta A \tag{9}$$

Rearranging (**9**) we obtain (**10**)

$$\theta = \frac{l_c \cdot P}{h \cdot A} = \frac{n_3 \cdot \theta A}{h \cdot A} \tag{10}$$

and this defines θ in measurable terms. However, l_c, activation rate of prothrombin, depends on factor Xa level, i.e., from Fig. 4 $l_c = q \cdot Xa$, where q is a multiplier which relates level of Xa to rate of activation of prothrombin. Thus

$$l_c \cdot P = q \cdot Xa \cdot P \tag{11}$$

However relation 8 also gives $Xa = \dfrac{k_c \cdot X}{g \cdot A}$ and this with relation 11 can then

be substituted in equation 10 to give 12.

$$\theta = \frac{q \cdot Xa \cdot P}{h \cdot A} = \frac{q \cdot k_c \cdot X \cdot P}{g \cdot A \cdot h \cdot A} = \frac{q \cdot k_c \cdot X \cdot P}{g \cdot h \cdot A^2} \tag{12}$$

Relation (**12**) contains much interesting information of great importance in turnover studies. Here we need only note that, other parameters remaining constant, in a steady state level of free thrombin is inversely related to the *square* of AT level! Thus halving the AT level quadruples the free thrombin level in the plasma. This observation may help to explain the great propensity to venous thrombosis shown by patients with hereditary hypoantithrombinemias.

The above is a very simplified exposition of a few features of the steady state kinetics of antithrombin III. We present a much more complete account with much additional information elsewhere.[5]

Discussion

Seegers and collaborators [26] showed that if excess thrombin is incubated with antithrombin the early inactivation of thrombin is later followed by release of some of the inactivated thrombin, presumably from digestion of AT-thrombin complexes by thrombin. More recent studies show that AT-thrombin complexes in test tube experiments may come apart with release of thrombin and altered inactive AT.[27, 28] Clearly any release of active thrombin *in vivo* would be dangerous since it would amplify the consumption of AT by thrombin.

Our studies noted here clearly show the very rapid breakdown of the AT portion of *I-labeled protease-AT complexes. Though in theory the protease portion of the complexes might be treated differently our current studies make this unlikely. Suggestive evidence is also provided by the studies of Vogel *et al.*,[29] which we think that they may have misinterpreted. Their FIGURE 3 shows the time course of whole blood radioactivity after injection of *I-thrombin and *I-AT-thrombin into rabbits, but they did not differentiate between the radioactivity attached to protein and that in the form of small MW breakdown products. As our FIGURE 3 shows, the latter is released very rapidly. Thus the rate of removal of *I-protease AT complexes can only be determined by using the very early parts of their curves. When this is done the rate of removal of the protease part of the complexes from rabbit plasma is even more rapid than the removal of *I-AT complexes from dog plasma. We think that the half lives they quote depend heavily on the rate of excretion of *I-breakdown products and do not mirror the rate of removal of AT protease complexes from the plasma.

The unusual behavior of *I-AT, requiring kinetic Model 2 for its description, is of much interest. This model implies either considerable delay before AT destined for breakdown reaches its breakdown sites or delay in breakdown in the cells catabolizing it, or more generalized breakdown of AT in the interstitial fluids. The last form of breakdown might occur through passage of AT through the cell membranes of the many different cell types distributed through the interstitial fluids. This explanation appeals to us for several reasons. A characteristic and remarkable feature of AT is the enormous increase in its reaction rate with clotting proteases that occurs with heparin.[24] Yet heparin, unless given therapeutically, cannot be demonstrated in the blood [30] and its prime function may be as a binder of vasoactive substances in Mast cells. However, heparan sulfate is widely distributed in cell membranes. Thus AT might well be loosely absorbed to cell membranes and thus rendered very active in neutralizing clotting proteases [31] in the region of cell membranes. Consideration of some properties of the interstitial fluids makes this hypothesis more reasonable. In many tissues the interstitial fluids are only easily permeated by molecules about the size of albumin or smaller,[32] but larger molecules are filtered out. Thus α-2 macroglobulin, factor V and factor VIII should be mainly excluded, but the clotting proteases, most of which are considerably smaller than albumin, should easily enter. In tissue culture thrombin is a dangerous protease which can lead to cell mutations.[33] Thus it becomes important to protect the interstitial cell membranes from attack by thrombin and probably other proteases. The binding of AT by heparan sulfate would greatly speed its rate of complex formation with thrombin and provide an effective mechanism for neutralizing most of the coagulation proteases. Interestingly enough, however, this mechanism would be ineffective in neutralizing factor VIIa, which does not react with AT.[34] If AT is held loosely bound to cell membranes, continuous ingestion of AT with catabolism might be expected, as occurs for instance with low density lipoproteins.[35]

APPENDIX

RATE OF DECLINE OF PLASMA AND INTERSTITIAL ANTITHROMBIN IF SYNTHESIS SUDDENLY CEASES

The general equations are

$$\frac{dA_p}{dt} = S_A + j_2A_e - (j_1 + j_3)A_p$$

$$\frac{dA_e}{dt} = j_1A_p - (j_2 + j_4)A_e$$

The average plasma *I-AT equation is $.537e^{-.294t} + .463e^{-3.814t}$ with t in days.

For Model 1 at time zero $A_p(0) = 100\%$, $A_e(0) = 65\%$

For Model 2 at time zero $A_p(0) = 100\%$, $A_e(0) = 88\%$

By definition S_A, synthetic rate of AT $= 0$

For Model 1 $j_4 = 0$ and

$$A_p = \frac{j_2 A_e(0)(e^{-r_1 t} - e^{-r_2 t})}{r_2 - r_1} + A_p(0)\left\{\frac{j_2 - r_1}{r_2 - r_1}e^{-r_1 t} + \frac{r_2 - j_2}{r_2 - r_1}e^{-r_2 t}\right\}$$

$$A_e = \frac{j_1 A_p(0)(e^{-r_1 t} - e^{-r_2 t})}{r_2 - r_1} + A_e(0)\left\{\frac{r_2 - j_2}{r_2 - r_1}e^{-r_1 t} + \frac{j_2 - r_1}{r_2 - r_1}e^{-r_2 t}\right\}$$

$$j_1 = 1.412, \ j_2 = 2.185, \ j_3 = .513 \ \text{day}^{-1}; \ r_1 = .294, \ r_2 = 3.816$$

For Model 2 $j_3 = 0$ and

$$A_p = \frac{j_2 A_e(0)(e^{-r_1 t} - e^{-r_2 t})}{r_2 - r_1} + A_e(0)\left\{\frac{r_2 - j_1}{r_2 - r_1}e^{-r_1 t} + \frac{j_1 - r_1}{r_2 - r_1}e^{-r_2 t}\right\}$$

$$A_e = \frac{j_1 A_p(0)(e^{-r_1 t} - e^{-r_2 t})}{r_2 - r_1} + A_p(0)\left\{\frac{j_1 - r_1}{r_2 - r_1}e^{-r_1 t} + \frac{r_2 - j_1}{r_2 - r_1}e^{-r_2 t}\right\}$$

$$j_1 = 1.925, \ j_2 = 1.602, \ j_4 = .583 \ \text{day}^{-1}; \ r_1 = .294, \ r_2 = 3.816$$

At $t = 4.5$ days

For Model 1 plasma AT $= 19.4\%$ of $A_p(0)$
       interstitial AT $= 18.7\%$ of $A_p(0)$

For Model 2 plasma AT $= 24.9\%$ of $A_p(0)$
       interstitial AT $= 25.4\%$ of $A_p(0)$

If $A_e(0) = 0$ and there was no interstitial AT
       plasma AT $= 10\%$ of $A_p(0)$ when $t = 4.5$ days

REFERENCES

1. REEVE, E. B., B. LEONARD, S. H. WENTLAND & P. DAMUS. 1980. Studies with ^{131}I-labelled antithrombin in dogs. Thrombos. Res. **20:** 375–389.
2. LEONARD, B., T. CARLSON, A. STEPHENS & E. B. REEVE. 1981. Preparation and turnover of dog ^{131}I-antithrombin III protease complexes. In preparation.
3. JONES, R. H., E. B. REEVE & G. SWANSON. 1981. Fitting and identification of compartmental models with application to plasma protein kinetics. In preparation.
4. REEVE, E. B. & J. E. ROBERTS. 1959. The kinetics of the distribution and breakdown of ^{131}I-albumin in the rabbit—observations on several mathematical descriptions. J. Gen. Physiol. **43:** 415–444.
5. REEVE, E. B. 1980. Steady state relations between factors X, Xa, II, IIa, antithrombin III and alpha-2 macroglobulin in thrombosis. Thrombos. Res. **18:** 19–31.
6. MILLER-ANDERSSON, M., H. BORG. & L.-O. ANDERSSON. 1974. Purification of antithrombin III by affinity chromatography. Thrombos. Res. **5:** 439–452.
7. DAMUS, P. & G. A. WALLACE. 1974. Purification of canine antithrombin III-heparin cofactor using affinity chromatography. Biochem. Biophys. Res. Commun. **61:** 1147–1153.
8. DAMUS, P. & R. D. ROSENBERG. 1976. Antithrombin-heparin cofactor. *In* Methods in Enzymology XLV; Proteolytic Enzymes. B. L. Lorand, Ed.: 653–669. Academic Press. New York.
9. HUNTER, W. M. & F. C. GREENWOOD. 1962. Preparation of iodine[131] labelled human growth hormone of high specific activity. Nature (London) **194:** 495–496.
10. MARCHALONIS, J. J. 1969. An enzymic method for the trace iodination of immunoglobulins and other proteins. Biochem. J. **113:** 299–305.
11. McFarlane, A. S. 1958. Efficient trace-labelling of proteins with iodine. Nature (London) **183:** 53.

12. ANDERSSON, L-O., L. ENGMAN & F. HENNINGSSON. 1977. Crossed immunoelectrophoresis as applied to studies on complex formation. The binding of heparin to antithrombin III and the antithrombin III-Thrombin complex. J. Immunol. Methods **14:** 271–281.

13. MCFARLANE, A. S. 1963. In vivo behavior of I^{131}-fibrinogen. J. Clin. Invest. **42:** 346–361.

14. REEVE, E. B. & J. E. MCKINLEY. 1970. Measurement of albumin synthetic rate with bicarbonate^{-14} C. Am. J. Physiol. **218:** 498–509.

15. KOJ, A. & A. S. MCFARLANE. 1968. Effect of endotoxin on plasma albumin and fibrinogen synthesis rates in rabbits as measured by the ^{14}C-carbonate method. Biochem. J. **108:** 137–146.

16. TAKEDA, Y. 1964. Hormonal effects on distribution and excretion of iodide- ^{131}I in the dog. Am. J. Physiol. **206:** 1237–1243.

17. ATENCIO, A. C., H. R. BAILEY & E. B. REEVE. 1965. Studies on the metabolism and distribution of fibrinogen in young and older rabbits. I. Methods and models. J. Lab. Clin. Med. **66:** 1–19. II. Results J. Lab. Clin. Med. **66:** 20–33.

18. YIN, E. T., S. WESSLER & P. J. STOLL. 1971. Biological properties of the naturally occurring plasma inhibitor to activated factor X. J. Biol. Chem. **246:** 3703–3711.

19. ROSENBERG, R. D. 1977. Chemistry of the hemostatic mechanism and its relationship to the action of heparin. Fed. Proc. **36:** 10–18.

20. ODEGARD, O. R. & U. ABILDGAARD. 1978. Antithrombin III: Critical review of assay methods. Haemostasis **7:** 127–134.

21. KAHLE, L. H., H. G. SCHIPPER, C. S. P. JENKINS & J. W. ten Cate. 1978. Antithrombin III: Evaluation of an automated antithrombin III method. Thrombos. Res. **12:** 1003.

22. BIGGS, R., K. W. E. DENSON, N. AKMAN, R. BORRETT & M. HADDEN. 1970. Antithrombin III, antifactor Xa and heparin. Br. J. Haematol. **19:** 283–305.

23. DOWNING, M. R., J. W. BLOOM & K. G. MANN. 1978. Comparison of the inhibition of thrombin by three plasma protease inhibitors. Biochemistry **17:** 2649–2653.

24. JORDAN, R., D. BEELER & R. ROSENBERG. 1979. Fractionation of low molecular weight heparin species and their interaction with antithrombin. J. Biol. Chem. **254:** 2902–2913.

25. SUOMELA, H., M. BLOMBÄCK & B. BIRGER. 1977. The activation of factor X evaluated by using synthetic substrates. Thrombos. Res. **6:** 267.

26. SEEGERS, W. H., M. YOSHINARI & R. H. LANDABURU. 1960. Antithrombin as substrate for the enzyme thrombin. Thromb. Diath. Haemorrh. (Stuttgart) **4:** 293–298.

27. FISH, W. W., K. ORRE & I. BJORK. 1979. Routes of thrombin action in the production of proteolytically modified secondary forms of antithrombin-thrombin complex. Eur. J. Biochem. **101:** 39–44.

28. JESTY, J. 1979. Dissociation of complexes and their derivatives formed during inhibition of bovine thrombin and activated factor X by antithrombin III. J. Biol. Chem. **254:** 1044–1049.

29. VOGEL, C. N., H. S. KINGDON & R. L. LUNDBLAD. 1979. Correlation of in vivo and in vitro inhibition of thrombin by plasma inhibitors. J. Lab. Clin. Med. **93:** 661–673.

30. JACOBSSON, K. G. & U. LINDAHL. 1979. Attempted determination of endogenous heparin in blood. Thromb. Haemostas. (Stuttgart) **42(1):** 84. Abstr. 0195.

31. THOMAS, D. P., R. E. MERTON, T. W. BARROWCLIFFE, B. MULLOY & E. A. JOHNSON. 1979. Antifactor Xa activity of heparan sulphate. Thrombos. Res. **14:** 507–512.

32. YOFFEY, J. M. & F. C. COURTICE. 1970. Lymphatics, Lymph and the Lymphomyeloid Complex. Academic Press. London.
33. MARTIN, B. M. & J. P. QUIGLEY. 1977. Binding and uptake of thrombin: Possible role in the thrombin-induced mitogenesis of chick embryo fibroblasts. *In* Chemistry and Biology of Thrombin. R. L. Lundblad, J. W. Fenton & K. G. Mann, Eds: 531–544, Ann Arbor Science, Ann Arbor, MI.
34. JESTY, J. 1978. The inhibition of activated bovine coagulation factors X and VII by antithrombin III. Arch. Biochem. Biophys. **185:** 165–173.
35. GOLDSTEIN, J. L. & M. S. BROWN. 1974. Binding of low density lipoproteins by cultured human fibroblasts. J. Biol. Chem. **249:** 5153–5162.

PREPARATION OF
RADIOACTIVE ANTITHROMBIN AND
STUDIES OF ITS REACTION WITH THROMBIN *

Isidore Danishefsky, Lorraine Kuhn, and German B. Villanueva

*Department of Biochemistry
New York Medical College
Valhalla, New York 10595*

INTRODUCTION

Antithrombin, also called heparin-cofactor or antithrombin III, is a circulating glycoprotein that neutralizes the activity of thrombin and a variety of other serine proteases.[1] This effect is produced by the formation of a complex between antithrombin and the respective enzyme, e.g., thrombin. Antithrombin may thus be important in modulating the coagulation process. The principal action of the anticoagulant heparin is to accelerate the interaction between antithrombin and thrombin or other procoagulants.

In order to define various aspects of the mechanism in the action of antithrombin it was desired to label the inhibitor in a manner that would not have any effect on its activity. In a previous publication from this laboratory, it was shown that removal of sialic acid residues from the oligosaccharide chain does not alter the activity of the antithrombin.[2] It was, therefore, reasonable to expect that introduction of a tritium label by modifying the sialic acid would yield an active tagged product. This report gives the details for the preparation of the radioactive antithrombin and describes some of its interactions with thrombin.

EXPERIMENTAL

Materials and Methods

The preparation of human antithrombin, and the assay systems were described previously.[2] Neuraminidase from *Clostridium perfringens* was purchased from Miles Laboratories, Elkhart, IN.

Sodium borotritide (227 mC/millimole), Protosol and Econofluor were purchased from New England Nuclear Corp., Boston, MA.

SDS-polyacrylamide gel electrophoresis was performed with 7.5% gels.[3] The separations were allowed to proceed for approximately 3 hr at 7 mA per tube. The proteins were stained with Coomassie blue. For radioactivity measurements the gels were cut into 1-mm slices and incubated in the counting vials with 3% Protosol in Econfluor for 24 hr at 37° C.

* This work was supported by Grant HL-16955 from the National Institutes of Health.

695

Preparation of Radioactive Antithrombin

A solution of 19.7 mg antithrombin in 20 ml 0.15 M NaCl/0.1 M sodium acetate-acetic acid, pH 7.5, was mixed with 2.2 ml 0.012 M sodium meta-periodate at 4°. After stirring for 15 min, 0.5 ml ethylene glycol was added and the solution was dialyzed overnight against 0.15 M NaCl/0.05 M sodium phosphate, pH 7.5. A small aliquot of the reaction mixture was dialyzed against 0.15 M NaCl/0.01 M Tris, pH 7.5, for subsequent assays and analyses.

The phosphate solution of periodate-oxidized antithrombin was mixed with a solution of 4.2 mg sodium borotritide (227 mC/millimole) in 0.2 ml 0.01 M NaOH. After stirring for 30 min at room temperature, 3.5 mg of $NaBH_4$ were added and the solution was mixed at 4° for 30 min. The reaction mixture was dialyzed against 0.15 M NaCl/0.01 M Tris, pH 7.5, until the dialyzable radioactivity was minimal.

A solution of the modified antithrombin was added to a column containing 8 ml of heparin aminohexyl-Sepharose [4] and the absorbant was washed, sequentially, with water, 0.15 M NaCl, and 0.4 M NaCl, until the eluate showed no radioactivity. Subsequent washing with 1.0 M NaCl yielded a radioactive eluate containing antithrombin activity. The solution was dialyzed against 0.15 M NaCl/0.01 M Tris, pH 7.5, and concentrated to 5 ml by ultrafiltration.

Neuraminidase Digestion

Three ml of tritiated antithrombin were incubated with 53 μg neuraminidase (1.9 u per mg), at pH 5.6 for 18 hr at 30°. The solution was dialyzed against 0.15 M NaCl/0.01 M Tris, pH 7.5, for two days, with several changes of the buffer. This was followed by a second digestion, with 40 μg of the enzyme and the purification was repeated.

RESULTS AND DISCUSSION

Antithrombin was labeled with tritium by mild periodate oxidation followed by reduction with sodium borotritide as outlined in FIGURE 1. The procedure causes a modification of sialic acid residues and introduces the label in carbon-7 of the resultant 5-acetamido-3,5-dideoxy-L-arabino-2-heptulosonic acid derivative.[5] The product obtained after purification by affinity chromatography on heparin-aminohexylsepharose was active in neutralizing thrombin and this activity was accelerated by heparin. The radioactive antithrombin had a specific activity of 2.24×10^6 cpm per mg. It showed a single protein band with the same mobility as unmodified antithrombin, when subjected to sodium dodecyl-sulfate polyacrylamide gel electrophoresis. Analyses of the gels for radioactivity demonstrated that all the label coincided with the antithrombin band (FIG. 2). Treatment with neuraminidase resulted in removal of over 90% of the radioactivity from the protein, indicating that the tritium was located in the modified sialic acid residues (TABLE 1).

The general procedure employed in the synthesis of the radioactive antithrombin results in denaturation of a small, but significant, amount of the protein. The reaction mixture must, therefore, be fractionated to obtain the material with maximum thrombin-inhibitory activity. It should be emphasized that utilization of the tritiated antithrombin without prior purification may lead to erroneous conclusions.

In a previous report from this laboratory,[2] it was shown that preparations of antithrombin contain noncovalently bound glucosylceramide. This glycolipid is not dissociated during the preparation and purification of the tritiated product. However, the glucose associated with the antithrombin is not oxidized by the mild periodate treatment and the label is not introduced into the glycolipid. Thus, extraction of the radioactive antithrombin with chloroform-methanol, which removes the glycolipid, does not extract any tritiated material from the protein.

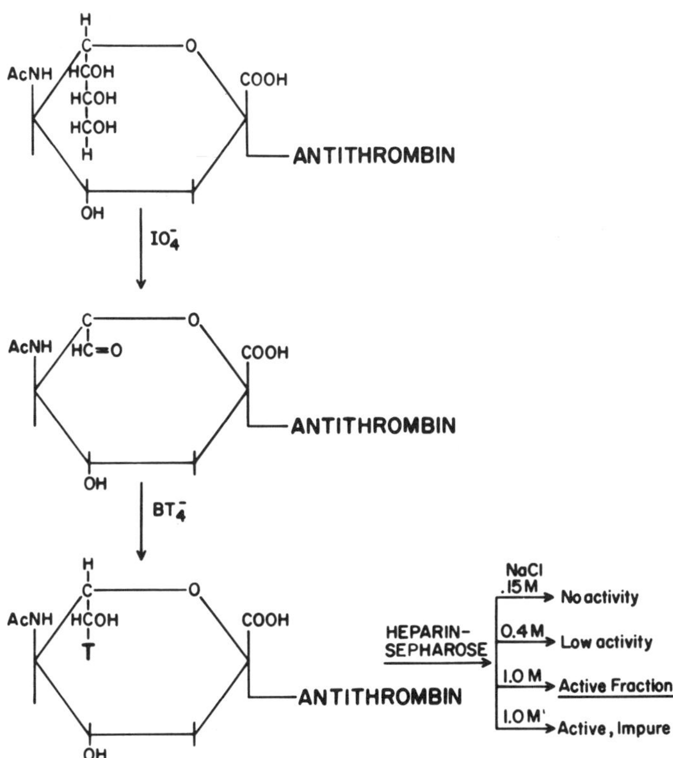

FIGURE 1. Sequence of steps in the preparation of tritiated antithrombin.

Antithrombin combines with thrombin to form a primary complex (C-1) that undergoes degradation to complexes C-2 and C-3 with lower molecular weights.[6] In the present studies, the radioactive antithrombin was incubated with equimolar amounts of thrombin and aliquots obtained after different incubation times were subjected to SDS-polyacrylamide gel electrophoresis. The gels were stained and the proteins quantitated by densitometer analysis. The gels were also sliced in 1 mm samples and analyzed for radioactivity. The results of these experiments are shown in FIGURE 3. It is seen that after a 15-second incubation, protein and radioactivity appear in the primary complex (C-1) and in the unreacted antithrombin. The amount of C-1 was increased after one minute. Subsequently, C-1 decreased and C-2 increased. After 20 min a significant amount of C-3 appeared. Although there were sequential changes

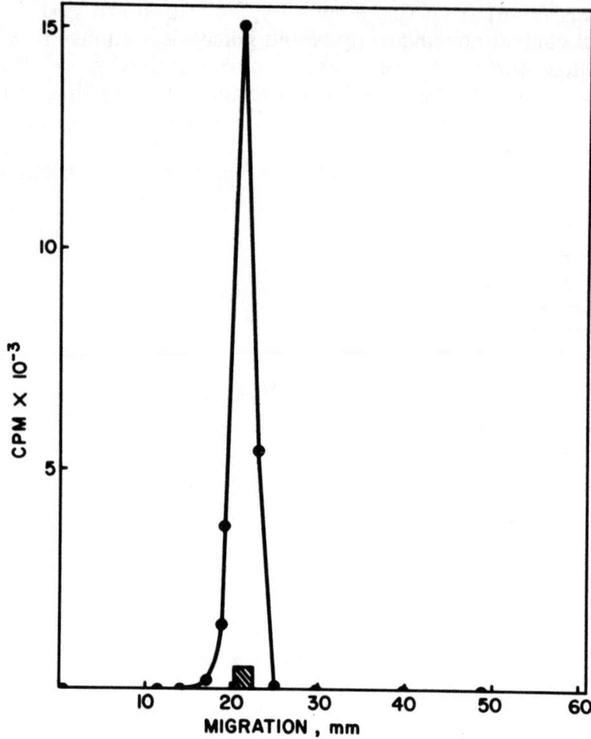

FIGURE 2. Distribution of radioactivity after electrophoresis of tritiated antithrombin. The stippled area shows the position of the stained protein.

in the proteins and in the distribution of radioactivity, the total radioactivity remained constant.

It should be noted that the radioactivity relative to protein differs in each of the measured components. The specific radioactivity is less in C-1 as compared with antithrombin since C-1 is formed from the combination of radioactive antithrombin with nonradioactive thrombin. The conversion of C-1 to C-2 involves the scission of a polypeptide chain from the primary complex. As a result, there is an increase in the specific radioactivity of C-2. Similarly, the relative radioactivity in C-3 is greater than that in C-2. The fact that the total radioactivity does not change significantly indicates that polypeptides that are removed in these transformations do not contain oligosaccharide chains

TABLE 1

EFFECT OF NEURAMINIDASE ON TRITIATED ANTITHROMBIN

Treatment	Total CPM
Tritiated antithrombin	111×10^3
After first digestion	219×10^2
After second digestion	95×10^2

from antithrombin. Considering the difference in molecular weight between C-1 and C-3, the results indicate that the polypeptide that is cleaved from the primary antithrombin-thrombin complex arises from the original thrombin component rather than from the antithrombin. This conclusion is also substantiated by results of other studies in our laboratory.[7]

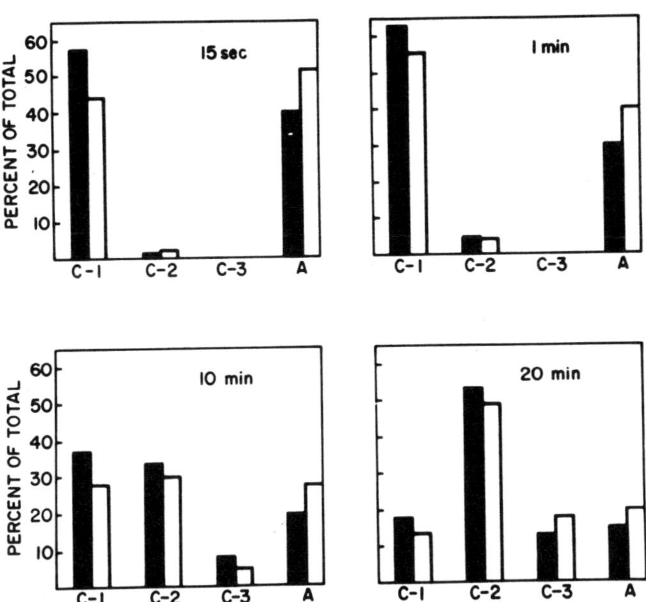

FIGURE 3. Distribution of radioactivity and protein after gel electrophoresis of an incubation mixture consisting of equimolar amounts of thrombin and tritiated antithrombin. For details see text. ■, protein; □, radioactivity.

REFERENCES

1. HARPEL, P. C. & R. D. ROSENBERG. 1976. α_2-Macroglobulin and antithrombin-heparin cofactor, modulators of hemostatic and inflammatory reactions. *In* Progress in Hemostasis and Thrombosis. T. H. Spaet, Ed. Vol. **3:** 145–189. Grune and Stratton. New York.

2. DANISHEFSKY, I., A. ZWEBEN & B. L. SLOMIANY. 1978. Human antithrombin III. Carbohydrate components and associated glycolipid. J. Biol. Chem. **253**(1): 32–37.

3. WEBER, K. & M. OSBORN. 1969. The reliability of molecular weight determinations by dodecyl sulfate-polyacrylamide gel electrophoresis. J. Biol. Chem. **244**(16): 4406–4412.

4. DANISHEFSKY, I. F. TZENG, M. AHRENS & S. KLEIN. 1976. Synthesis of heparin Sepharoses and their binding with thrombin and antithrombin-heparin cofactor. Thromb. Res. **8**(1): 181–140.

5. VAN LENTEN, L. & G. ASHWELL. 1971. Studies on the chemical and enzymatic modification of glycoproteins. J. Biol. Chem. **246**(6): 1889–1894.

6. ROSENBERG, R. D. & P. S. DAMUS. 1973. The purification and mechanism of action of human antithrombin-heparin cofactor. J. Biol. Chem. **248**(18): 6490–6505.

7. DANISHEFSKY, I. & M. BENDER. Manuscript in preparation.

HEPARIN BINDING AND
PROTEASE INHIBITOR ACTIVITY OF
CHEMICALLY MODIFIED ANTITHROMBIN III *

Michael N. Blackburn, Robert L. Smith,
Caroline C. Sibley, and Virginia A. Johnson

*Department of Biochemistry and Molecular Biology
Louisiana State University Medical Center
Shreveport, Louisiana 71130*

Brinkhous *et al.*[1] first demonstrated that the effectiveness of heparin as an anticoagulant requires a plasma component, heparin cofactor, which is now known to be identical to antithrombin III. This disulfide-crosslinked glycoprotein is the major inhibitor of the activated serine proteases of the blood coagulation cascade. The addition of catalytic amounts of heparin greatly accelerates the rate of inactivation of thrombin [2-4] without altering the stoichiometry of the inhibitor-protease complex. Heparin is known to bind to antithrombin III and thrombin, and the enhanced rate of protease inhibition has been attributed to a heparin-induced conformational change in either antithrombin III or thrombin.[3, 5-7] These conformational changes presumably facilitate complex formation.

Studies by Rosenberg and Damus [3] have implicated lysine residues in the binding of heparin to antithrombin III. To further characterize the structural requirements for heparin binding, we initiated a series of experiments to perturb the functional properties of antithrombin III by site-specific chemical modification. Since spectral and fluorescence studies [5, 10] indicate that heparin binding alters the environment of one or more tryptophan residues, we utilized the tryptophan specific reagent dimethyl(2-hydroxy-5-nitrobenzyl) sulfonium bromide [8, 9] to chemically modify antithrombin III. Our initial studies [11] have shown that at low reagent concentrations, one hydroxynitrobenzyl (HNB) moiety is incorporated per molecule of bovine antithrombin III. This derivatized inhibitor does not bind heparin and does not exhibit the heparin-promoted enhancement of thrombin inactivation that is characteristic of native antithrombin III. In the present study, we have extended these observations to the reaction of human antithrombin III with dimethyl(hydroxynitrobenzyl) sulfonium bromide, and the reaction of bovine antithrombin III with *N*-bromosuccinimide. Also, we have demonstrated that HNB modification of antithrombin abolishes the heparin effect on the inactivation of factor Xa as well as thrombin.

MATERIALS AND METHODS

Isolation of Antithrombin III

Antithrombin III was purified from $BaSO_4$ adsorbed bovine or human plasma by chromatography on heparin-Sepharose [11] followed by chromatog-

* This work was supported in part by National Institutes of Health Grant HL24846 and by grants from Research Corporation and The Frost Foundation.

700

raphy on Ultrogel AcA 34 equilibrated with 0.50 M sodium citrate, 0.13 M NaCl, pH 7.4. Preparations of antithrombin III yielded a single band following sodium dodecyl sulfate-gel electrophoresis. Antithrombin III activity was measured by its ability to inhibit the amidolytic activity of purified thrombin or factor Xa [16] using specific chromogenic peptide substrates. Protein concentrations were determined spectrophotometrically at 280 nm using E_{280} of 0.60 ml mg^{-1}cm^{-1} and 0.57 ml mg^{-1}cm^{-1} for bovine and human antithrombin III, respectively.[12]

Modification of Antithrombin III

Dimethyl (2-hydroxy-5-nitrobenzyl) sulfonium bromide (as the solid or dissolved in 1 mM HCl) was mixed with continuous stirring with antithrombin III [11] in 0.20 M phosphate buffer, pH 7.0, containing 0.15 M NaCl. After 15 min at 22° C, the samples were centrifuged to remove insoluble hydroxy-nitrobenzyl alcohol and chromatographed on a column of Sephadex G-25. The extent of derivatization was determined spectrophotometrically [13] in 2 N NaOH at 410 nm with use of a molar extinction coefficient of 1.85×10^4 M^{-1}cm^{-1}.

Oxidation of tryptophan with *N*-bromosuccinimide was performed by the procedure of Spande and Witkop.[14, 15] Aliquots of a 0.01 M solution of *N*-bromosuccinimide were added with stirring to antithrombin III (1.5 mg ml^{-1}) at 25° C in 0.20 M phosphate buffer, pH 7.0, containing 0.15 M NaCl. Absorption spectra of the modified samples were obtained with a Cary 219 spectrophotometer and the change in absorbance at 280 nm, which provides a measure of tryptophan oxidation, was corrected [14] for light scattering by linear extrapolation of the spectral data between 400 and 350 nm. This correction was found to be proportional to the extent of protein modification. The number of tryptophans oxidized was calculated as described by Spande and Witkop.[14]

RESULTS

Modification of Bovine and Human Antithrombin III

Addition of dimethyl(hydroxynitrobenzyl) sulfonium bromide to antithrombin III results in the incorporation of about one HNB group per molecule of antithrombin III. As shown in FIGURE 1, identical amounts of the chromophoric label are incorporated into bovine and human antithrombin III, indicating that both antithrombins contain a reactive tryptophan residue. Heparin was found to protect against tryptophan modification, particularly at low concentrations of reagent (FIG. 2). For example, with 1.1 mM dimethyl (hydroxynitrobenzyl) sulfonium bromide, one-half the number of moles of HNB are incorporated in the presence of heparin (500 units ml^{-1}) compared to that without added heparin. This protective effect can be largely overcome at higher concentrations of reagent (35 mM) where 1.3 moles of HNB are bound in the presence of heparin compared to 1.5 moles without added heparin.

The reactivity of the tryptophan residues of antithrombin III was also examined using *N*-bromosuccinimide. With increasing amounts of *N*-bromosuccinimide substantial oxidation of tryptophan was observed. The overall oxidation of tryptophan is biphasic (FIG. 3), indicating at least two classes of

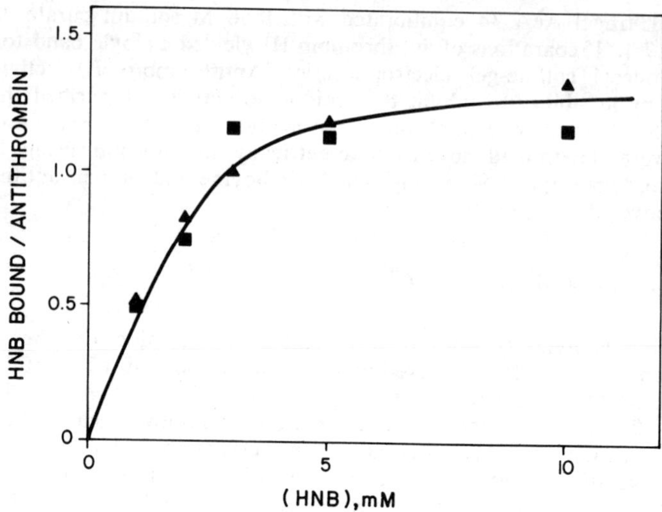

FIGURE 1. Modification of bovine and human antithrombin III with dimethyl(2-hydroxy-5-nitrobenzyl) sulfonium bromide. Antithrombin III was reacted with dimethyl(hydroxynitrobenzyl) sulfonium bromide as described under MATERIALS AND METHODS. A value of 56,600 was assumed for the molecular weight[12] of both antithrombins. The data are presented as moles of HNB bound per mole of bovine (▲) and human (■) antithrombin III as a function of the concentration of modifying reagent.

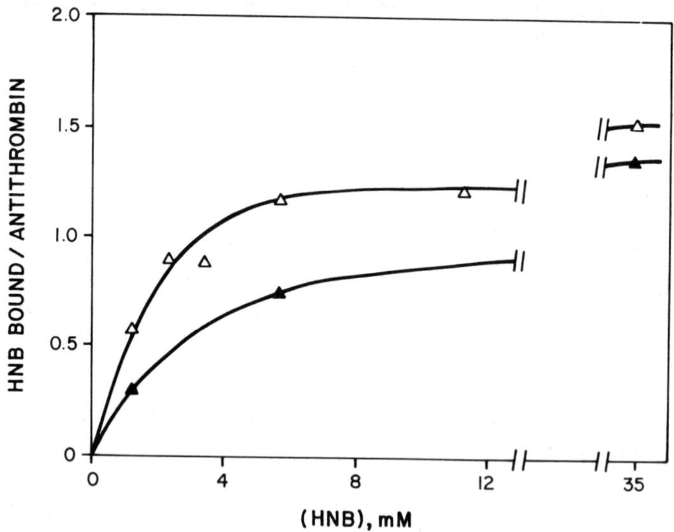

FIGURE 2. HNB-modification of bovine antithrombin III in the presence and absence of heparin. Reaction conditions were as described in MATERIALS AND METHODS. Incorporation of HNB in the absence of heparin (△) and in the presence of 500 units of heparin per ml (▲).

reactive tryptophan residues. The decrease in absorbance at 280 nm indicates that the destruction of tryptophan is approximately linear with the addition of the first 8 moles of *N*-bromosuccinimide per mole of antithrombin III, and corresponds to the loss of about 1.5 tryptophan residues. At higher levels of *N*-bromosuccinimide (15 moles per mole of antithrombin) approximately two residues are modified. When antithrombin III was titrated with *N*-bromosuccinimide in the presence of heparin (500 units ml^{-1}) the extent of tryptophan oxidation was decreased. This indicates that, as in the case of reaction with dimethyl(hydroxynitrobenzyl) sulfonium bromide, heparin provides some protection against modification of tryptophan residues. However, several factors indicate that oxidation with *N*-bromosuccinimide is much less specific than is modification with the active benzyl halide. First, *N*-bromosuccinimide oxidation

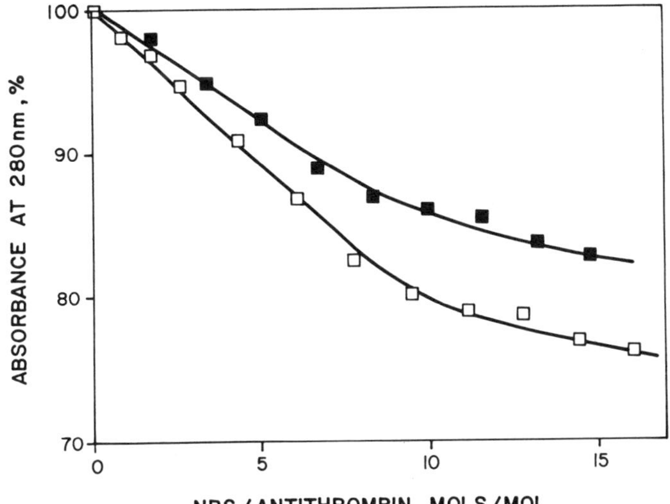

FIGURE 3. *N*-bromosuccinimide oxidation of bovine antithrombin III in the presence and absence of heparin. Antithrombin III was titrated with *N*-bromosuccinimide as described in MATERIALS AND METHODS. The measured decrease in absorbance at 280 nm was corrected for protein dilution and for light scattering. Data are presented as percent of the original absorbance as a function of the mole ratio of *N*-bromosuccinimide (NBS) to antithrombin. Absorbance change in the absence of heparin (□), and in the presence of 500 units of heparin per ml (■).

is accompanied by a significant increase in light scattering, apparently due to aggregation of the oxidized protein. Second, amino acid analysis indicates loss of tyrosine, and to a lesser extent histidine, in addition to the loss of tryptophan. In contrast, HNB-antithrombin does not exhibit an increased tendency towards aggregation, and amino acid analysis following acid and alkaline hydrolysis indicates that tryptophan is the only amino acid altered by this modification procedure.

Functional Properties of Modified Antithrombin III

Native antithrombin III exhibits high affinity for heparin and binds essentially quantitatively (>90%) when chromatographed on heparin-Sepharose affinity columns equilibrated with low ionic strength buffers at neutral pH. In contrast, HNB-antithrombin binds poorly or not at all to these columns. With increasing levels of protein modification, the fraction of inhibitor bound to heparin-Sepharose decreased, and when one or more HNB-groups were incorporated per antithrombin molecule, over 90% of the protein washed through the column. These results indicate that modification of a single tryptophan residue in antithrombin III prevents its binding to heparin. The loss of affinity for heparin-Sepharose is paralleled by a corresponding loss of heparin cofactor activity. However, there is no significant decrease in the progressive antithrombin or anti-factor Xa activity measured in the absence of added heparin. In the presence of heparin, native antithrombin rapidly inactivates thrombin and factor Xa (Figs. 4 and 5, respectively). When assayed with either of these proteases, the rate of inactivation by HNB-antithrombin is not increased by added heparin. Furthermore, the slow loss of thrombin or factor Xa activity due to reaction with native antithrombin III in the absence of heparin is identical to the loss of activity obtained with HNB-antithrombin measured either with or without added heparin. Both thrombin and factor Xa activities are stable in the absence of added antithrombin.

As described above, the addition of heparin to the reaction mixture decreased the apparent reactivity of antithrombin tryptophan residues towards dimethyl(hydroxynitrobenzyl) sulfonium bromide. The functional properties of antithrombin derivatives prepared in the presence of heparin differ signifi-

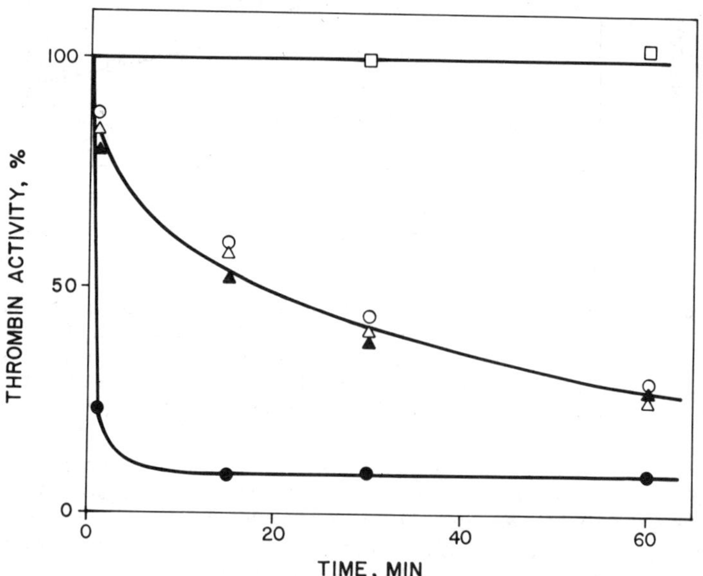

FIGURE 4. Thrombin inactivation by native and HNB-modified bovine antithrombin III. Native and HNB-antithrombin III (modified in the absence of heparin to the extent of 1.2 HNB groups per molecule) were incubated with thrombin. At the indicated times, the residual thrombin activity was measured. Thrombin incubated in the presence and absence of heparin is represented by closed and open symbols, respectively. Native antithrombin III (●,○), HNB-modified antithrombin III (▲,△). Thrombin activity measured in the absence of antithrombin (□).

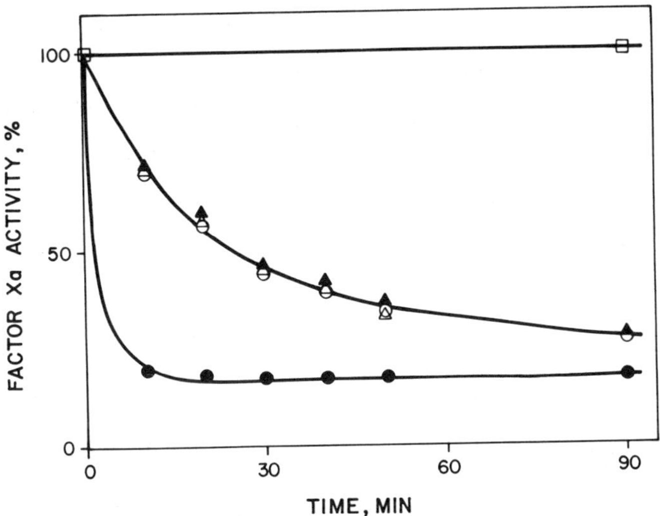

FIGURE 5. Factor Xa inactivation by native and HNB-modified bovine antithrombin III. Native and HNB-antithrombin III (modified with 1.2 HNB groups per molecule) were incubated with factor Xa. At the indicated times the residual factor Xa activity was measured. Factor Xa incubated with antithrombin in the presence and absence of heparin is represented by closed and open symbols, respectively. Native antithrombin III (●,○), HNB-antithrombin III (▲,△). Factor Xa activity in the absence of antithrombin (□).

cantly from those of derivatives prepared in the absence of heparin, even when comparable amounts of HNB are incorporated. Antithrombin modified in the presence of heparin and containing 1.3 to 1.4 moles of HNB per mole of protein exhibit greater than 70% of the heparin cofactor activity of native antithrombin. In contrast, antithrombin modified to the same extent in the absence of heparin retained less than 5% of the heparin cofactor activity of native antithrombin. These results suggest that different tryptophan residues are labeled in the presence and absence of heparin. Peptide mapping experiments with the modified proteins will be required to confirm this conclusion.

DISCUSSION

Although a requirement for heparin in the accelerated inactivation of the blood clotting proteases by antithrombin III has long been recognized,[2] the mechanism of heparin action remains uncertain. Heparin binds to antithrombin[7] as well as to these proteases,[6] but the relative importance of these different interactions has not been defined. The selective modification of one tryptophan residue in antithrombin with dimethyl(hydroxynitrobenzyl) sulfonium bromide blocks heparin binding and the heparin-promoted rate enhancement in the inactivation of both thrombin and factor Xa. These results clearly indicate that binding of heparin to antithrombin is a required step in the mechanism of accelerated protease inhibition, and that the mechanism of enhancement is similar for both proteases.

Antithrombin appears to have two functional domains, the protease binding site and the heparin binding site. Evidence derived from chemical modification studies suggests that these functional domains correspond to separate structural regions within the protein molecule. The protease-binding site contains the reactive center arginine [3] and provides the amino acid residues involved in the stabilization of the inhibitor·protease complex. The heparin binding site contains one or more lysine residues [3] as well as a critical tryptophan.[11] The essential nature of this tryptophan is shown by the total loss of heparin binding capacity and heparin cofactor activity in HNB-modified antithrombin. It is noteworthy that the intrinsic antiprotease activity of antithrombin is not altered by HNB modification. Also, as recently shown by Björk and Nordling,[18] limited N-bromosuccinimide oxidation of tryptophan decreased heparin cofactor activity by 50% without significantly decreasing the progressive antithrombin activity. Our preliminary studies with N-bromosuccinimide agree with their conclusions for the involvement of tryptophan in the heparin binding site. However, secondary reactions arising from N-bromosuccinimide oxidation of antithrombin preclude an unambiguous interpretation of these results. Selective reduction [17] of one of the three disulfide bonds in antithrombin has also been shown to decrease the affinity of antithrombin for heparin, and to prevent the heparin-promoted enhancement in the rate of thrombin inactivation. The reduced inhibitor retains its ability to inactivate thrombin in the absence of heparin, suggesting that this disulfide bond is distant from the protease site. This essential disulfide crosslink may serve to maintain the functional conformation of the heparin binding domain, or it may be required for the expression of the heparin-mediated conformational change in antithrombin III. Although the amino acid sequence of the heparin binding site has not yet been established, the availability of these different chemically modified antithrombin species should allow its identification.

ACKNOWLEDGMENTS

We wish to thank Dr. William Holleman of Abbott Laboratories for the gift of the heparin-Sepharose used in these studies and for helpful advice concerning the purification of antithrombin III.

REFERENCES

1. BRINKHOUS, K. M., H. P. SMITH, E. D. WARNER & W. H. SEEGERS. 1939. The inhibition of blood clotting: An unidentified substance which acts in conjunction with heparin to prevent the conversion of prothrombin into thrombin. Am. J. Physiol. **125:** 683–687.
2. MONKHOUSE, F. C., E. S. FRANCE & W. H. SEEGERS. 1955. Studies on the antithrombin and heparin cofactor activities of a fraction adsorbed from plasma by aluminum hydroxide. Circulation Res. **3:** 397–402.
3. ROSENBERG, R. D. & P. S. DAMUS. 1973. The purification and mechanism of action of human antithrombin-heparin cofactor. J. Biol. Chem. **248:** 6490–6505.
4. BJÖRK, I. & B. NORDENMAN. 1976. Acceleration of the reaction between thrombin and antithrombin III by nonstoichiometric amounts of heparin. Eur. J. Biochem. **68:** 507–511.

5. Villanueva, G. B. & I. Danishefsky. 1977. Evidence for a heparin-induced conformational change on antithrombin III. Biochem. Biophys. Res. Commun. **74:** 803–809.
6. Griffith, M. J. 1979. Kinetic analysis of the heparin-enhanced antithrombin III/thrombin reaction. Reaction rate enhancement by heparin-thrombin association. J. Biol. Chem. **254:** 12044–12049.
7. Jordan, R., D. Beeler & R. Rosenberg. 1979. Fractionation of low molecular weight heparin species and their interaction with antithrombin. J. Biol. Chem. **254:** 2902–2913.
8. Horton, H. R. & W. P. Tucker. 1970. Dimethyl(2-hydroxy-5-nitrobenzyl) sulfonium salts. Water-soluble environmentally sensitive protein reagents. J. Biol. Chem. **245:** 3397–3401.
9. Horton, H. R. & D. E. Koshland, Jr. 1972. Modification of proteins with active benzyl halides. Methods Enzymol. **25:** 468–482.
10. Einarsson, R. & L.-O. Andersson. 1977. Binding of heparin to human antithrombin III as studied by measurements of tryptophan fluorescence. Biochim. Biophys. Acta **490:** 104–111.
11. Blackburn, M. N. & C. C. Sibley. 1980. The heparin binding site of antithrombin III. Evidence for a critical tryptophan residue. J. Biol. Chem. **255:** 824–826.
12. Kurachi, K., G. Schmer, M. A. Hermodson, D. C. Teller & E. W. Davie. 1976. Characterization of human, bovine and horse antithrombin III. Biochemistry **15:** 368–373.
13. London, G. M. & D. E. Koshland, Jr. 1970. The chemistry of a reporter group: 2-hydroxy-5-nitrobenzyl bromide. J. Biol. Chem. **245:** 2247–2254.
14. Spande, T. F. & B. Witkop. 1967. Determination of the tryptophan content of proteins with *N*-bromosuccinimide. Methods Enzymol. **11:** 498–506.
15. Spande, T. F. & B. Witkop. 1967. Tryptophan involvement in the function of enzymes and protein hormones as determined by selective oxidation with *N*-bromosuccinimide. Methods Enzymol. **11:** 506–522.
16. Jackson, C. M., T. F. Johnson & D. J. Hanahan. 1968. Studies on bovine factor X. I. Large-scale purification of the bovine plasma protein possessing factor X activity. Biochemistry **7:** 4492–4505.
17. Longas, M. O., W. S. Ferguson & T. H. Finlay. 1980. A disulfide bond in antithrombin is required for heparin-accelerated thrombin inactivation. J. Biol. Chem. **255:** 3436–3441.
18. Björk, I. & K. Nordling. 1979. Evidence by chemical modification for the involvement of one or more tryptophanyl residues of bovine antithrombin in the binding of high-affinity heparin. Eur. J. Biochem. **102:** 497–502.

THE INTERACTION OF PROTEIN-BOUND
HEPARIN AND ANTITHROMBIN III

J. N. Shanberge and C. N. Sridhar

Thrombosis and Hemostasis Research Laboratory
Department of Clinical Pathology
William Beaumont Hospital
Royal Oak, Michigan 48072

INTRODUCTION

As we have reported before,[1] when a tritium-labeled porcine mucosal heparin is added to defibrinated human plasma and the plasma chromatographed on Sephadex G-200, there is a peak of direct immediate antithrombin activity located between the globulin and albumin peaks as measured by inhibition of the thrombin clotting time of fibrinogen or the hydrolysis of a chromogenic substrate. If whole plasma, which already contains antithrombin III, is used as the substrate, then the thrombin clotting time is inhibited by fractions from the macromolecular area at or near the void volume as well as by the fractions in the albumin-globulin area.

When the anticoagulant activity of the heparinized plasma is neutralized with protamine sulfate and the plasma is then chromatographed, most of the radioactivity shifts to the macromolecular fractions, representing heparin-protamine complexes. When the antithrombin activity is measured by inhibition of a thrombin clotting time of fibrinogen, no inhibitory activity is found in any of the fractions. The progressive inhibition of thrombin by antithrombin III reappears in fractions in the albumin peak where it was located in the original untreated plasma. The macromolecular fractions still retain their antithrombin activity as measured by the immediate inhibition of the thrombin clotting time of whole plasma.

When excess heparin is added to the protamine-neutralized plasma before chromatography, the radioactivity in the first peak increases slightly owing to saturation of the excess protamine originally added. Immediate antithrombin activity reappears in fractions between the globulin and albumin peaks as measured by the thrombin clotting time of fibrinogen or its splitting of a chromogenic substrate. When plasma is used as the substrate for the thrombin clotting time, immediate inhibitory action is found again in both areas.

Since α_2-macroglobulin, like antithrombin III, is a progressive inhibitor of thrombin,[2] it was speculated that this might be the large molecular weight protein which bound fractions of heparin to account for the peak of radioactivity in the macromolecular area and for the activation of antithrombin III by these fractions.

MATERIALS AND METHODS

The tritium-labeled porcine mucosal heparin prepared by the method of Barlow and Cardinal [3] was donated by Abbott Laboratories, North Chicago, IL.

708

Other materials and methods were as described previously.[1, 4] Alpha$_2$-macroglobulin was prepared from defibrinated human plasma by the method of Harpel.[2] Fractions from column chromatography were concentrated with an ultrafiltration apparatus (Amicon Corp., Lexington, MA) using either an XM-100 or UM-10 membrane.

RESULTS

Alpha$_2$-macroglobulin was combined with tritiated heparin (3.9 ml of α_2-macroglobulin plus 0.15 ml heparin — 18.6 U or 3 μCi). The mixture was then chromatographed on Sephadex G-200 yielding two radioactive peaks. The first contained protein but the second, the excess heparin, did not (FIG. 1). The radioactive fractions from the first peak (22–32) were pooled, concentrated by ultrafiltration to 1.2 ml and rechromatographed on Sephadex G-200, yielding a single peak of radioactive protein (FIG. 2). These fractions (24–34) had

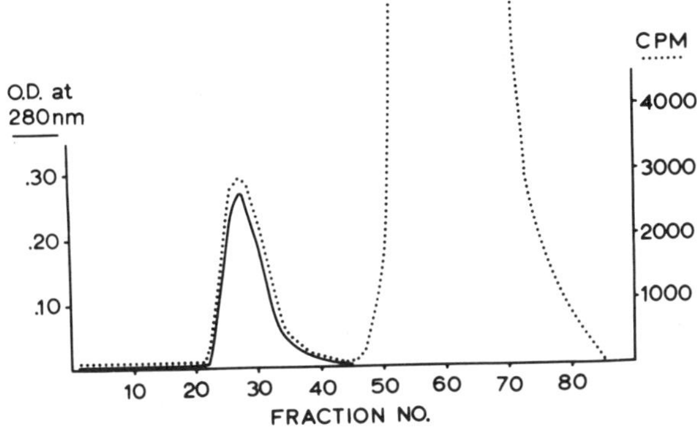

FIGURE 1. Chromatogram of α_2-macroglobulin (3.9 ml) + ^{3}H-heparin (18.6 U).

progressive antithrombin activity when incubated with thrombin and aliquots tested on the clotting time of fibrinogen or the hydrolysis of chromogenic substrates. However, they also had immediate inhibitory activity on the thrombin clotting time of plasma.

Fractions 24–34 were pooled and concentrated to 1.4 ml by ultrafiltration. This was added to 0.5 ml of a pool of fractions from the albumin peak of chromatographed plasma which had only progressive antithrombin activity. This mixture was then chromatographed on a Sephadex G-200 column. Two protein peaks were obtained (FIG. 3). Fractions 22–32 comprising the larger molecular weight fractions were concentrated by ultrafiltration through an XM-100 filter. These fractions were radioactive and had progressive antithrombin activity but did not inhibit the thrombin clotting time of fibrinogen. They did, however, have immediate inhibitory action on the thrombin clotting time of plasma. The lower molecular weight fractions from the second peak were concentrated through a UM-10 filter to approximately 0.5 ml. These were not radioactive but did have immediate inhibitory action on the thrombin clotting time of both fibrinogen and whole plasma.

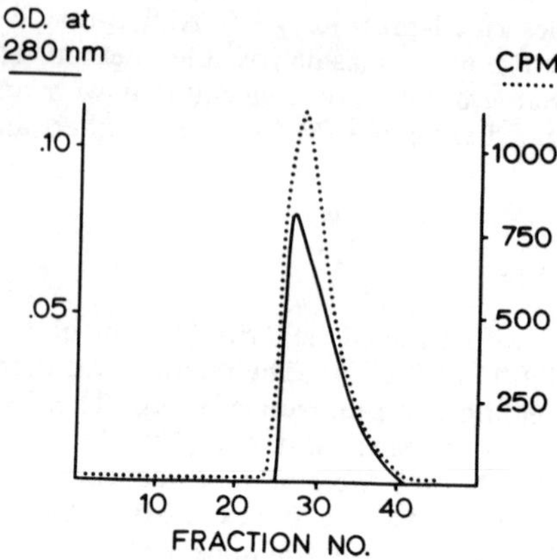

FIGURE 2. Chromatogram of fractions 22–32 from FIGURE 1, pooled and concentrated by ultrafiltration.

DISCUSSION

In 1974, Marciniak [5] reported that in heparinized plasma she found heparin bound only to macromolecular proteins which did not increase the ability of heparin to function as an anticoagulant but did inhibit both thrombin and Xa in the presence of purified antithrombin III. She did not identify the protein to which heparin was attached. However, she found no binding of heparin to antithrombin in plasma or to purified antithrombin. Takeda and Kobayashi [6] also stated that, at least *in vivo*, heparin added to plasma did not complex with antithrombin as much as with other proteins. In a chromatogram of serum and ^{35}S-labeled heparin from a Sephadex G-200 column they found most of the radioactivity in the macromolecular fractions but no determination of anticoagulant activity of any of the fractions was mentioned.

Heparin is a polydisperse substance composed of many different molecular weight polysaccharides having variable anticoagulant properties, particularly in their capacity to modify antithrombin III to become immediate inhibitor of serine proteases. [7]

In recent years investigation has been directed toward those fractions of heparin which have greater or lesser affinity to antithrombin III. [8–13] This is

FIGURE 3. Chromatogram of fractions 23–34 from FIGURE 2 (1.4 ml) + 0.5 ml of a concentrated pool of fractions from the albumin peak of normal human plasma having progressive antithrombin III activity.

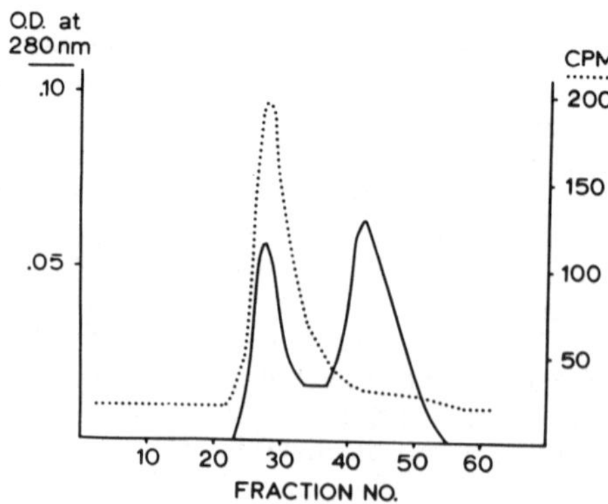

predicated on the theory that a complex must be formed between antithrombin and heparin to activate the inhibitor.[14] Others have proposed that the effect of heparin as an antithrombin may be due to its binding to thrombin or in some way changing it to make it more susceptible to the inhibitory action of antithrombin III.[15] No comparable ideas have been proposed that certain fractions of heparin might have a greater affinity to thrombin than others.

From our own observations it would seem that antithrombin may be activated by heparin fractions in different ways. We can now offer some of the possibilities as diagramed in FIGURE 4. When added to plasma, certain fractions of heparin bind to the α_2-globulin antithrombin III (H-AT III′) possibly bringing about a change in its molecular structure making it a more efficient inhibitor of thrombin (H-AT III$_a$′) as well as other serine proteases. Protamine detaches the heparin from the antithrombin so that it reverts from an immediate to a progressive inhibitor of thrombin (AT III″). This process may be in an equilibrium which can be repeatedly reversed.[1]

At the same time different fraction(s) of heparin may bind to other proteins such as the α_2-macroglobulin (H-X). Unlike antithrombin III, α_2-macroglobulin, another naturally occurring progressive inhibitor of thrombin, is not activated by heparin. Actually its capacity as a progressive inhibitor of thrombin may be decreased in the presence of heparin.[16] However, although bound to the α_2-macroglobulin, the heparin fraction (H-X) is still capable of activating antithrombin III to an immediate inhibitor. Upon the addition of protamine the antithrombin changes back to being a progressive inhibitor of thrombin. Inasmuch as the heparin bound to the α_2-macroglobulin cannot be "neutralized" by protamine, the change in the inhibitory action of the antithrombin must be due to a direct effect of protamine on antithrombin III itself. Although fresh heparin can reactivate "neutralized" antithrombin III (AT III″), the α_2-macroglobulin-heparin fraction (H-X) cannot. This also suggests that a molecular change in the antithrombin may be brought about by protamine.

These findings could be used as another explanation for the heparin "rebound" that has been described in patients in whom the anticoagulant action of heparin had been thought to be adequately counteracted with protamine.[17–19] Although enough protamine may have been administered to overcome the inhibition by heparin-activated antithrombin, the heparin bound to other proteins such as α_2-macroglobulin would remain and be able to activate any fresh antithrombin produced by the patient or given him through infusion of blood or plasma. This would more likely happen if the original heparin dosage had been very high and/or the macroglobulin level were elevated. The newly activated antithrombin, which might enhance bleeding, can be overcome by the administration of additional protamine. Verification of these theories will depend on planned clinical observation.

SUMMARY

When commercially prepared porcine mucosal heparin is added to human plasma, some of the heparin fractions form a complex with antithrombin III activating it to an immediate inhibitor of thrombin as well as of other serine proteases. Certain fractions of heparin may complex with other proteins such as α_2-macroglobulin, another progressive inhibitor of thrombin. Without complexing with antithrombin III, this protein-bound heparin fraction(s) still retains the capacity to activate it to an immediate inhibitor of thrombin. Protamine sulfate inactivates those heparin fractions that bind to antithrombin III but not those bound to α_2-macroglobulin. Activated antithrombin III may undergo a molecular change in the presence of protamine which not only changes it back to a progressive inhibitor but makes it resistant to activation by the protein-bound heparin fraction(s). However, it can still be reactivated by other heparin fractions in fresh whole heparin. The observations presented may help explain heparin "rebound" in patients believed adequately neutralized with protamine.

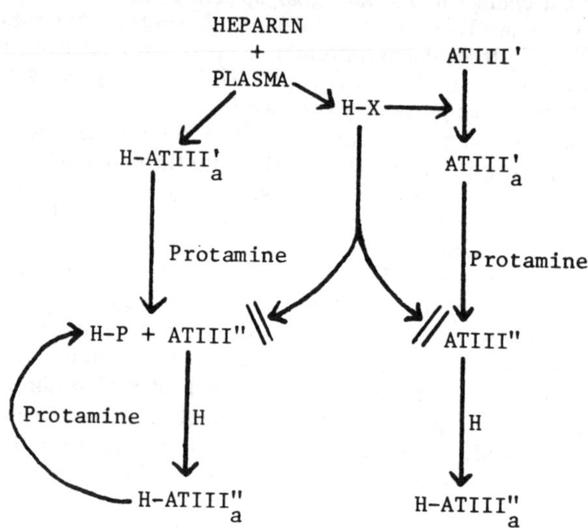

FIGURE 4. Scheme of heparin-antithrombin III interactions. H = heparin fractions; X = protein capable of binding certain heparin fractions (e.g. α_2-macroglobulin); ATIII′ = nonactivated (progressive) antithrombin III; ATIII″ = antithrombin III reconverted to progressive antithrombin by protamine; ATIII$_a$′ or ATIII$_a$″ = activated (immediate acting) antithrombin III.

REFERENCES

1. KITANI, T., S. C. NAGARAJAN, & J. N. SHANBERGE. 1980. Effect of protamine on heparin-antithrombin III complexes. In vitro studies. Thrombos. Res. **17:** 367–374.
2. HARPEL, P. C. 1976. Human α_2-macroglobulin. *In* Methods in Enzymology. L. Lorand, Ed.: 639–652. Academic Press. New York.
3. BARLOW, G. H. & E. V. CARDINAL. 1966. Preparation and characterization of tritiated heparin. Proc. Soc. Exp. Biol. Med. **123:** 831–832.
4. SHANBERGE, J. N., M. GRUHL, T. KITANI, S. AMBEGAONKAR, J. KAMBAYASHI, M. NAKAGAWA & D. LENTER. 1978. Fractionated tritium-labeled heparin studied in vitro and in vivo. Thrombos. Res. **13:** 767–783.
5. MARCINIAK, E. 1974. Binding of heparin in vitro and in vivo to plasma proteins. J. Lab. Clin. Med. **84:** 344–356.

6. TAKEDA, Y. & N. KOBAYASHI. 1977. Studies of heparin affinity to antithrombin III and other proteins in vitro and in vivo. Thrombos. Haemostas. **38:** 685–695.

7. WALTON, P. L., C. R. RICKETTS & D. R. BANGHAM. 1966. Heterogeneity of heparin. Brit. J. Haematol. **12:** 310–325.

8. NORDENMAN, B., A. DANIELSSON & I. BJÖRK. 1978. The binding of low-affinity and high-affinity heparin to antithrombin. Eur. J. Biochem. **90:** 1–6.

9. PEIPKORN, M. W., D. LAGUNOFF & G. SCHMER. 1978. Heparin binding to antithrombin: Variation in binding sites and affinity. Biochem. Biophys. Res. Commun. **85:** 851–856.

10. CHAN, V. & T. K. CHAN. 1979. Heparin-antithrombin III binding. Haemostasis **8:** 373–389.

11. JORDAN, R., D. BEELER & R. ROSENBERG. 1979. Fractionation of low molecular weight heparin species and their interaction with antithrombin. J. Biol. Chem. **254:** 2902–2913.

12. ROSENBERG, R. D., R. E. JORDAN, L. V. FAVREAU & L. H. LAM. 1979. Highly active heparin species with multiple binding sites for antithrombin. Biochem. Biophys. Res. Commun. **86:** 1319–1324.

13. McKAY, E. J. & C. B. LAURELL. 1980. The interaction of heparin with plasma proteins. Demonstration of different binding sites by antithrombin III complexes and antithrombin III. J. Lab. Clin. Med. **95:** 69–80.

14. ROSENBERG, R. D. & P. S. DAMUS. 1973. The purification and mechanism of action of human antithrombin-heparin cofactor. J. Biol. Chem. **248:** 6490–6505.

15. MACHOVICH, R., G. BLASKO & L. A. PALOS. 1975. Action of heparin on thrombin-antithrombin reaction. Biochem. Biophys. Acta **379:** 193–200.

16. FISCHER, A. M., A. BROS, S. RAFOWICZ & F. JOSSO. 1979. Inhibition par l'heparine de l'activite antithrombique de l'α-2-macroglobuline. C. R. Acad. Sc. Paris. **288:** 887–889.

17. HYUN, B. H., R. F. PENCE, J. C. DAVILA, J. BUTCHER & R. P. CUSTER. 1962. Heparin rebound phenomenon in extracorporeal circulation. Surg. Gynecol. Obstet. **115:** 191–198.

18. JAQUES, L. B. 1973. Protamine-antagonist to heparin. C. M. A. J. **108:** 1291–1297.

19. ELLISON, N., C. P. BEATTY, D. R. BLAKE, H. A. WURZEL, & H. MacVAUGH, III. 1974. Heparin rebound. Studies in patients and volunteers. J. Thorac. Cardiovasc. Surg. **67:** 723–729.

NATURAL COAGULATION INHIBITORS: AN ASSESSMENT IN PATIENTS *

Ray Losito, Harry Gattiker, Ginette Bilodeau, and Bernard Longpré

*Department of Medicine
Centre Hospitalier Universitaire
Université de Sherbrooke
Sherbrooke, Québec, Canada*

INTRODUCTION

It is assumed that blood coagulation occurs when an inactive precursor (XII, prothrombin) called the zymogen, is transformed into an active enzymatic form (XII_a and thrombin). In the so-called intrinsic pathway, it is thought that factor XII is activated after there is an injury to the vessel wall endothelium. Factor XII_a then activates factor XI until there is conversion of prothrombin into thrombin. It has also been assumed that various steps in this activation process are regulated by inhibitors, which therefore act as antithrombins.[1] These inhibitors are usually found in the α-globulin fraction of plasma. Besides antithrombin III, there are two other proteins that have been associated with normal physiological antithrombin activity. They are α_2-macroglobulin and α_1-antitrypsin. Low levels of these physiological inhibitors, especially antithrombin III, have been thought to be a possible cause of thromboembolic disease. There is still controversy about the incidence and the role coronary thrombosis plays in various forms of ischemic heart disease. The classic concept supposes that coronary thrombosis precedes the majority of transmural myocardial infarctions. Others postulate that coronary thrombosis is the consequence rather than the cause of acute myocardial infarction. Measurements of blood levels of AT III and the other two inhibitors may help to determine if there is evidence of hypercoagulability in patients with ischemic heart disease. There are still discrepancies between various reports on AT III levels in ischemic heart disease.[2-4] In this report, the measurement of antithrombin III, α_2-macroglobulin and α_1-antitrypsin in a group of patients with an acute episode of ischemic heart disease is presented.

METHODS

Fifty-one patients (TABLE 1) with acute ischemic heart disease were studied over a 2-year period. They were divided into three groups: 26 with unstable angina, 20 patients with acute transmural and 5 with acute subendocardial myocardial infarctions. All patients were initially admitted to an intensive care unit. Samples of blood from each patient were studied on three different occasions: on admission to hospital, before departure from the hospital, and three months after hospitalization. Twenty-two patients received prophylactic

* Supported in part by grants from the Canadian Heart Foundation and the Medical Research Council of Canada.

TABLE 1

SUMMARY OF PATIENTS ACCORDING TO DIAGNOSIS, AGE, SEX, AND TREATMENT *

Diagnosis	Patient Number	Age	Sex	Treatment
Unstable angina				
(26 patients)	1	52	M	Heparin$_1$
	2	60	M	Heparin$_1$
	3	53	M	Heparin$_1$
	5	77	F	Heparin$_1$
	9	37	M	—
	13	53	F	Aspirin$_2$
	16	51	M	—
	17	70	M	Aspirin$_1$
	19	47	M	—
	22	71	M	—
	23	51	M	Heparin$_2$
	24	50	M	—
	25	57	M	—
	26	55	M	Aspirin$_3$
	34	63	M	—
	35	63	F	Heparin$_1$
	36	58	F	—
	38	68	F	Aspirin$_2$
	39	64	M	—
	43	43	M	—
	44	60	M	Heparin$_1$
	46	62	F	Aspirin$_2$
	48	71	M	Heparin$_{1,\,2}$
	49	57	F	Heparin$_{1,\,2}$
	50	49	F	Heparin$_1$, Aspirin$_1$
	51	49	F	—
Transmural myocardial infarction	4	52	M	Heparin$_1$, Aspirin$_1$
(20 patients)	6	45	M	Heparin$_1$, Aspirin$_2$
	8	41	M	Heparin$_1$, Aspirin$_2$
	10	50	M	Heparin$_2$, Aspirin$_2$, Warfarin$_3$
	11	47	M	Heparin$_1$
	12	52	M	Aspirin$_2$
	15	55	M	Heparin$_1$, Aspirin$_2$
	18	73	M	Aspirin$_2$
	21	46	M	—
	27	63	M	Aspirin$_2$
	29	46	M	Aspirin$_2$
	30	56	F	Heparin$_1$
	31	63	M	Aspirin$_2$
	33	57	M	Heparin$_1$
	37	57	M	Heparin$_1$
	40	61	M	Heparin$_2$
	41	46	M	Heparin$_1$, Warfarin$_3$
	42	70	F	Aspirin$_2$
	45	69	M	Aspirin$_2$
	47	60	F	Heparin$_{1,\,2}$, Aspirin$_2$

TABLE 1 (Continued)

Subendocardial myo-cardial infarction				
(5 patients)	7	75	F	Heparin[1]
	14	56	M	Heparin[1], Aspirin[2]
	20	55	F	—
	28	56	F	—
	32	46	M	—

* Subscripts (1,2,3) indicate the times when medication was received: (1) admission; (2) departure; (3) 3 months after.

antithrombotic treatment with subcutaneous heparin during the initial phase of hospitalization. Two patients were on coumadin when investigated at the 3-month interval. Aspirin was given for pain of pericardial origin in some patients. TABLE 1 shows age and sex of the patients and if they received antithrombotic treatment. Antithrombin III, α_2-macroglobulin and α_1-antitrypsin were measured in patients as well as in normal healthy individuals. Measurement of antithrombin III activity was done by clotting, chromogenic, and immunological techniques. The clotting techniques used were those of von Kaulla,[5] Owen and Bollman,[6] and the Thrombo-Screen Antithrombin III Assay™. The chromogenic (amidolytic) method, a combination of clotting and chemical techniques, measured antithrombin III in both plasma and serum (the Quantichrom® AT III diagnostic kit was employed). Antithrombin III was also determined by immunological means by Laurell immunoelectrophoresis [7] and by immunodiffusion employing antibodies to AT III. The levels of α_2-macroglobulin and α_1-antitrypsin were likewise measured by immunodiffusion employing specific antibodies to these proteins. Student's t-test was employed to examine if there was a significant ($p = <0.05$) difference in: (1) inhibitor values between the patients and the controls, (2) inhibitor values within each patient group during the 3-month period, and (3) inhibitor values in patients that received subcutaneous heparin, compared to those who did not receive this treatment.

RESULTS

FIGURE 1 shows the mean values of AT III, α_2-macroglobulin and α_1-antitrypsin in % of the control in patients not receiving coumadin treatment. Values given in the figure are those found on day of admission to hospital (first sample), on day of departure from hospital (second sample) and 3 months later (third sample). The greatest initial decreases in AT III were measured by the von Kaulla method and by immunodiffusion. After separating the patients according to clinical diagnosis, it was found that there was a significant difference between the controls and the patients with unstable angina and transmural myocardial infarction for all three samples employing the von Kaulla method as well as a significant increase of AT III levels within all three groups of patients over the 3-month period. A significant decrease could be seen by immunodiffusion in all samples of the three patient groups when compared to the controls; this technique, however, failed to show any significant changes within the three groups of patients after 3 months. The chromogenic serum

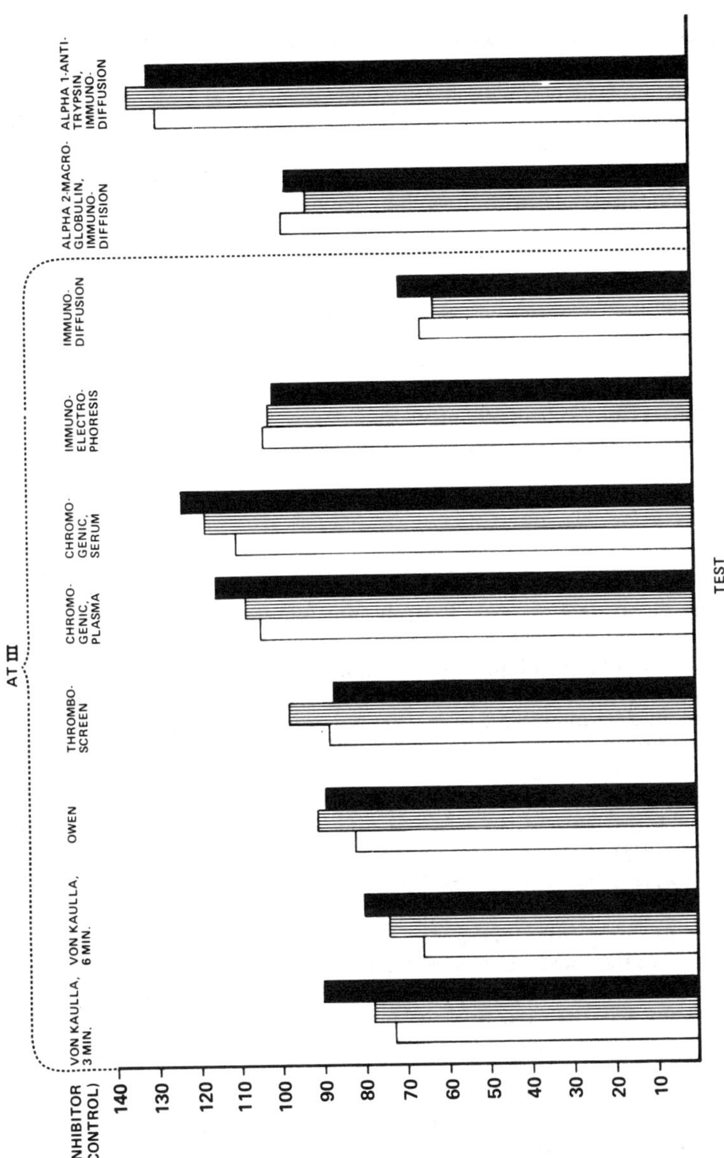

FIGURE 1. Clotting inhibitors in acute ischemic heart disease. Mean values of antithrombin III, α1-antitrypsin and α2-macroglobulin. AT III was determined by immunodiffusion, immunoelectrophoresis and by four functional tests (von Kaulla, Owen, chromogenic, and Thrombo-Screen AT III). Alpha 1-antitrypsin and α2-macroglobulin were determined by immunodiffusion only. Values were determined on admission to hospital (clear bar), on departure from hospital (lined bar) and at 3 months after hospitalization (black bar).

method showed a significant increase in patients with unstable angina and transmural myocardial infarction in samples 2 and 3 after the initial phase when compared to controls. In the transmural and subendocardial infarction groups the values (chromogenic, serum) increased after the acute phase, an observation which was confirmed by the chromogenic plasma method. With the Owen technique, patients with transmural myocardial infarction and subendocardial infarction showed a significant decrease, compared to the controls, at the time of hospitalization only. Thrombo-Screen Assay showed that AT III decreased significantly between the time of hospitalization and at three months in the patients with unstable angina. Immunoelectrophoresis showed a significant increase of AT III in patients with unstable angina as compared to the controls, but failed to change significantly during the course of the study.

On collating the other two inhibitors to controls, only α_1-antitrypsin showed a significant difference. It was increased in all three samples with unstable angina and transmural myocardial infarction and in two samples in the patients with subendocardial myocardial infarction.

Heparin (8000 IU bid subcutaneously) failed to affect the AT III values in patients compared to those not receiving this therapy. On the other hand, coumadin greatly increased the AT III values in the von Kaulla test.

DISCUSSION

Results of the determination of AT III by the different methods show a discrepancy. Antithrombin III was found to be significantly diminished when measured by a functional technique (von Kaulla) in all blood samples of patients with unstable angina and transmural myocardial infarction and by an immunological method (immunodiffusion) in patients with unstable angina, transmural myocardial infarction and subendocardial myocardial infarction. Yet the chromogenic method and another immunological test (immunoelectrophoresis) showed a significant increase in AT III in most of the samples of patients with unstable angina and to a lesser degree, in patients with transmural infarction. Non-significant changes were noted in some blood samples when the other methods were used. It would be intriguing to think that the difference between functional and immunological AT III values may be due to the fact that AT III is almost completely inactivated in the clotting process.[7] Probably more meaningful are the observations obtained after the acute episode of ischemic heart disease: a gradual rise in AT III in patients with transmural myocardial infarction was detected by four techniques (both von Kaulla and both chromogenic), in subendocardial myocardial infarction by three techniques (one von Kaulla and both chromogenic), and in unstable angina by one technique (Thrombo-Screen). Are patients with transmural and subendocardial myocardial infarction more "thrombosis prone" in the acute stage of the disease than patients with unstable angina? These observations may possibly support this assumption.

Studies [8, 9] have shown that intravenous heparin can lower plasma AT III and therefore could be a risk factor for rethrombosis after the cessation of this treatment. We found that minidose heparin given subcutaneously had no significant effect on AT III levels in our patients. This is supported by the work of Aiach and his colleagues [10] who have demonstrated that subcutaneous heparin lowers AT III only when the plasma concentration of heparin in blood reaches a certain level. Oral anticoagulant therapy with coumadin, in contrast, drastically increased AT III when measured by the von Kaulla technique and by immunodiffusion and confirms the observations of other investigators.[5]

The role of the other inhibitors is less certain; it has been implicated that α_1-antitrypsin and α_2-macroglobulin possess some antithrombic activity. Other studies have contradicted this observation.[11] We were surprised to find that all three groups of patients had greatly elevated α_1-antitrypsin levels. The α_2-macroglobulin however did not change. Innerfield *et al.*[3] found α_1-antitrypsin to be abnormal in less than 10% of their patients and α_2-macroglobulin unchanged as in our study. Antithrombin III may be the only physiological clotting inhibitor of importance, but further investigations are needed to clarify the role of these inhibitors and to find the most reliable method for their measurement.

REFERENCES

1. SEEGERS, W. H. & H. P. SMITH. 1943. Antithrombin activity of plasma: Quantitative interrelationshnp. Proc. Soc. Exp. Biol. **52:** 159.
2. YUE, R. H., M. M. GERTLER, T. STARR & R. KOUTROUBY. 1976. Alteration of plasma antithrombin III levels in ischemic heart disease. Thrombos. Haemostas. **35:** 598.
3. INNERFIELD, I., J. D. GOLDFISCHER, H. REICHER-REISS & J. GREENBERG. 1976. Serum antithrombin in coronary-artery disease. Am. J. Clin. Pathol. **65:** 64.
4. LECHNER, K., E. THALER, H. NIESSNER, C. NOWOTNY & H. PARTSCH. 1977. Antithrombin III deficiency and the tendency to thrombosis. Wiener Klin. Wochenschr. **89:** 215.
5. VON KAULLA, E. & K. N. VON KAULLA. 1967. Antithrombin III and diseases. Am. J. Clin. Path. **48:** 69.
6. OWEN, C. A. & J. L. BOLLMAN. 1948. Serum and plasma antithrombin. Proc. Soc. Exp. Biol. **67:** 367.
7. LOSITO, R., R. BEAUDRY, J. C. CARO-VALDERRAMA, L. COUSINEAU & B. LONGPRÉ. 1977. Antithrombin III and factor VIII in patients with neoplasms. Am. J. Clin. Pathol. **68:** 69.
8. MARCINIAK, E. 1975. Adverse effect of heparin in thrombin-antithrombin III interaction. Thrombos. Diathes. Haemorrh. **34:** 748.
9. FISKEN, R. A., O. H. B. GYDE, M. S. KUNDI & D. E. STABLEFORTH. 1977. Venous thrombosis, heparin-induced antithrombin III deficiency and factor VIII (letter). Lancet 2(8050): 1231.
10. AIACH, M., J. BEUVIN, A. MICHAUD & J. N. FIESSINGER. 1978. Modification de l'antithrombine III au cours des traitements par l'héparine. Nouv. Presse Med. **7:** 120.
11. LEARNED, L. A., J. W. BLOOM & M. J. HUNTER. 1976. The antithrombin activity of alpha 1-protease inhibitor: The antitrypsin activity of antithrombin III. Thrombos. Res. **8:** 99.

USE OF FLUOROGENIC SUBSTRATES FOR THE ASSAY OF ANTITHROMBIN III AND HEPARIN

Robert C. Bishop, Patricia M. Hudson, Gary A. Mitchell, and
Sharon P. Pochron

American Dade
Division of American Hospital Supply Corporation
Miami, Florida 33152

Over the past 35 years, the use of heparin in anticoagulant therapy has increased greatly. Clinical usefulness has been proven in a variety of situations, the most common of which are thrombophlebitis, thromboembolism, pulmonary embolism, acute and chronic disseminated intravascular coagulation, extracorporeal circulation, and prophylaxis. Heparin dosage in these situations varies widely, both in the amount given and the route of administration. The range of this variability is exemplified by the last two clinical situations listed above. In extracorporeal circulation, one typically finds heparin levels maintained well in excess of 1 unit per ml by intravenous infusion. When used subcutaneously for prophylaxis, the maximum plasma levels obtained are closer to 0.1 unit per ml.[1]

It has been known for more than 15 years that the capacity of heparin to act as an anticoagulant requires the presence of a naturally occurring inhibitor called antithrombin III (AT-III).[2-4] Heparin exerts its therapeutic effect indirectly by potentiating the activity of this plasma protein. This knowledge has raised many questions about the optimal method of monitoring heparin therapy. It is safe to say there is complete agreement on only one aspect of this problem: the test system used should provide a rational basis for altering dosage as needed to maintain adequate anticoagulation without undue risk of bleeding.[1, 5-7]

Many factors enter into the *in vitro* measurement of heparin anticoagulant activity. The time of sample collection is important, especially if heparin is being given on a bolus injection schedule rather than by continuous infusion where an equilibrium is established. Sample collection and preparation methods are also important in that care should be taken to prevent the release of platelet factor 4, a heparin inhibitor. Lastly, the results obtained are a function of both the test reagent system used and the instrument with which the measurements are made.[1, 5, 8]

According to a recent College of American Pathologists survey, the test most widely used for monitoring heparin therapy is the activated partial thromboplastin time (APTT).[9] The APTT is frequently accepted as a valid assay for heparin, and additionally, has a number of other features to recommend its use in the clinical laboratory.[10] Among the most important of these are its functional, as opposed to immunological, basis, its sensitivity to low levels of AT-III in the presence of heparin, and the fact that it is in routine use.[10-15] On the other side, the APTT has a limited useful range and is sensitive to factor deficiencies, the presence of fibrin degradation products, and other types of anticoagulant therapy.[16, 17] For these latter reasons, it has been suggested that the specific determination of heparin and of AT-III may be the most meaningful way of evaluating heparin therapy.[7] In response to this, our laboratories have developed rapid, specific, functional assays using a fluorogenic substrate.

The principle behind these tests is very straightforward. Rather than measure the rate of fibrin clot formation, which results from thrombin proteolysis of fibrinogen, our assays measure the rate of fluorescent tag release which results from thrombin proteolysis of a synthetic peptide substrate that mimics fibrinogen (FIG. 1).[18-20] The advantage of using this fluorogenic substrate in comparison to other amidolytic methods is its great sensitivity to thrombin.[19, 20]

The test system for our heparin assay is seen in FIGURE 2. Heparin in the patient sample is first reacted with excess AT-III to form the heparin-AT-III complex. This complex is then measured by its ability to inhibit purified thrombin. Any thrombin not neutralized is free to react with substrate, thus producing fluorescence. The two step test procedure can be seen in FIGURE 3. In step 1, 200 μl of 1:40 diluted normal citrated plasma (the source of AT-III) is mixed with 5 μl of heparin-containing test sample, then 50 μl of 1 NIH unit/ml human thrombin is added and the mixture is incubated for 60 sec at 37° C. In step 2, the test mixture is transferred to a cuvette containing 0.3 micromoles of substrate and the reaction is read in a specially designed

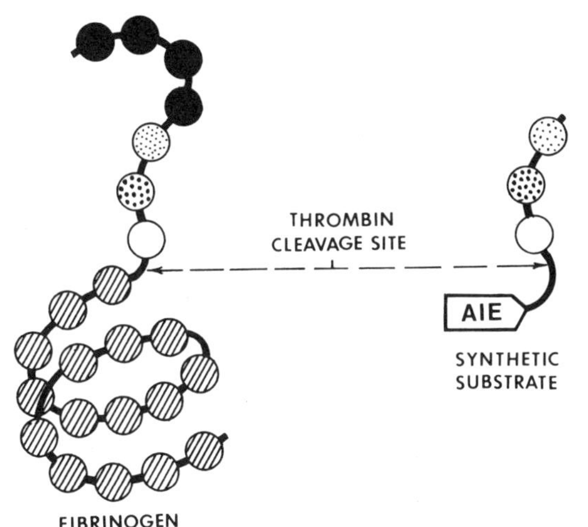

FIGURE 1. Similarity of the synthetic and natural substrates for thrombin.

fluorometer.* Results are expressed in terms of percent thrombin remaining and the heparin concentration of unknown samples is determined by use of a standard curve. FIGURE 4 shows three different curves representing results obtained on three different heparin preparations. On the basis of findings such as these, we previously suggested the need to prepare standard calibration curves with the same heparin used for patient treatment. We have recently confirmed these findings, as can be seen in TABLE 1. Here we see that each of the major heparin manufacturers is internally consistent, but that differences between manufacturers do exist. Overall, the assay precision of this method is excellent. As can be seen in TABLE 2, both within day and day-to-day results show coefficients of variation of less than 5 percent when working at the lower concentra-

---

* Protopath ™ Instrument—available from American Dade, Division of American Hospital Supply Corporation, Miami, Florida, USA.

$$\text{Heparin} \xrightarrow{\text{Excess AT III}} \underset{(\text{COMPLEX})}{\text{AT III} \cdot \text{Heparin}}$$

$$\underset{(\text{COMPLEX})}{\text{AT III} \cdot \text{Heparin}} + \text{Thrombin} \longrightarrow$$

$$\underset{(\text{COMPLEX})}{\text{AT III} \cdot \text{Heparin} \cdot \text{Thrombin}} + \text{Residual Thrombin}$$

$$\text{Residual Thrombin} + \text{D-Phe-Pro-Arg-AIE} \longrightarrow \text{D-Phe-Pro-Arg} + \text{AIE}$$

FIGURE 2. The theory of the fluorogenic substrate assay for heparin.

tions. At values near 0.8 unit/ml, incubation timing errors appear largely responsible for the increased coefficient of variation.

The AT-III assay is based upon analogous principles. As diagramed in FIGURE 5, we react the test sample with excess heparin to form a complex, then measure the complex activity as before. Procedurally, the reaction is carried out in three steps (FIG. 6). First, the test sample is diluted 1:40 in a buffer containing 1 USP unit/ml heparin, then 200 μl of this dilution is mixed with 100 μl of 1 NIH unit/ml human thrombin and finally, after 60 sec of incubation at 37° C, mixed with 2 ml of fluorogenic substrate and the reaction is read in the Protopath™ fluorometer. Results are expressed in terms of percent thrombin inhibited, then converted to percent of normal AT-III by comparison to the inhibition found in a pool of fresh, normal plasma. The precision of this method, as measured by the coefficient of variation for triplicate determinations, averages 3.4%.

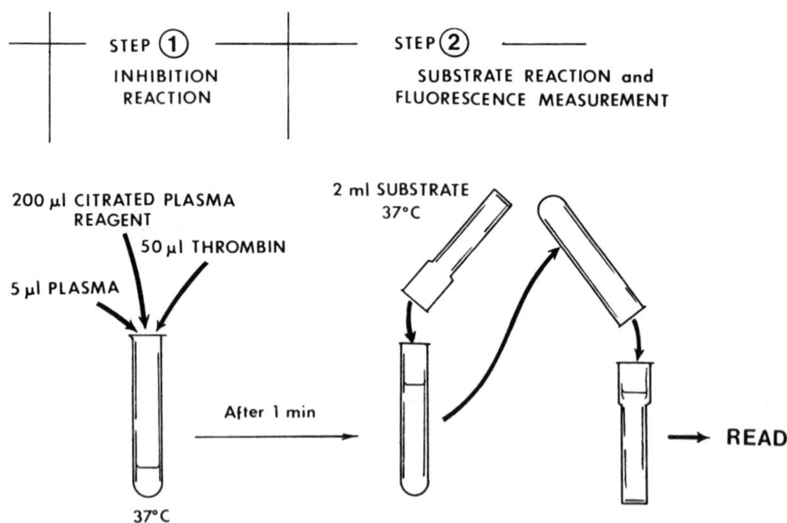

FIGURE 3. Test procedure for the fluorogenic substrate assay of heparin.

Correlation studies have shown a strong relationship between the results obtained by this method and those found with radial immunodiffusion (FIG. 7). Although not further discussed in this paper, the fluorogenic assay for AT-III has obvious utility in areas outside of heparin therapy, especially in the direction of hypercoagulable states.[2, 21-24]

In comparison to the APTT method of measuring heparin, which relies on the patient sample to provide adequate levels of AT-III, the fluorogenic assay for heparin appears to give more accurate results. Evidence for this was found during the assay of 51 normal plasmas to which 0.2 unit/ml of heparin had been added. As seen in FIGURE 8, prior to adding heparin each of these normal plasmas was tested for its "baseline APTT." Subsequent to the heparin addition,

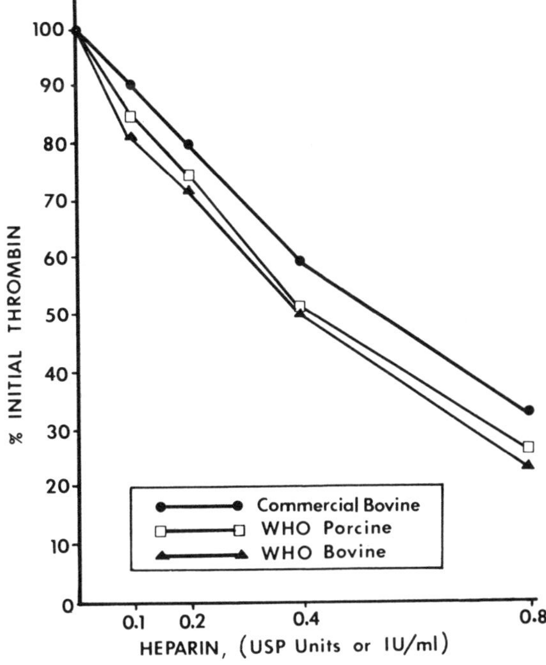

FIGURE 4. Standard curves for the fluorogenic substrate assay of heparin.

each sample was tested by both the fluorogenic and the APTT methods. The results of this study are presented in TABLE 3 and show that when the data are segregated into 2-sec increments of baseline APTT, the value obtained by the APTT method is directly related to the baseline time measured. The reason for this is clear when you consider we are reading values from a calibration curve prepared with pooled plasma. Accurate values would be expected only in that case where the individual patient baseline APTT matched that of the pool. In practice, this is further complicated by the fact that, as seen in FIGURE 9, individual patients may have different dose response curves.

This brings us to reconsider the value of the APTT as an assay for heparin. It is a good general measure of coagulability, but not very specific or accurate

TABLE 1

HEPARIN VARIABILITIES

Abbott Panheparin Lot Numbers	Heparin Standard U.S.P. U/ml	Mean % Thrombin Remaining
06–601–AF	0.1	81 ± 2.6
83–284–AF	0.2	56 ± 1.8
12731–AF	0.4	21 ± 3.0
	0.8	3 ± 0.5
Upjohn Beef Lung Heparin Lot Numbers	Heparin Standard U.S.P. U/ml	Mean % Thrombin Remaining
956–FW	0.1	77 ± 1.7
833–GJ	0.2	49 ± 0.65
443–GY	0.4	18 ± 2.8
	0.8	3 ± 1.3
Lilly Heparin Lot Numbers	Heparin Standard U.S.P. U/ml	Mean % Thrombin Remaining
DEL-80A	0.1	83 ± 1.3
OGX–49A	0.2	63 ± 0.7
3TK–00A	0.4	26 ± 2.7
	0.8	5 ± 0.4

TABLE 2

ASSAY PRECISION FOR STANDARD HEPARIN DETERMINATIONS

Within-day, n = 4		
Heparin, U.S.P. U/ml	Mean % Initial Thrombin	Coefficient of Variation, %
0.1	93.4	1.5
0.2	83.0	3.6
0.4	61.3	4.4
0.8	28.0	10.4
Day-to-day, n = 5		
0.1	91.1	2.9
0.2	79.8	3.3
0.4	59.6	3.1
0.8	30.2	11.8

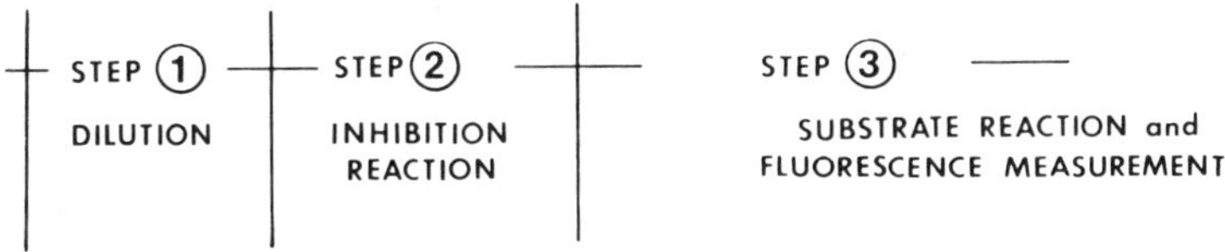

FIGURE 5. The theory of the fluorogenic substrate assay for antithrombin III.

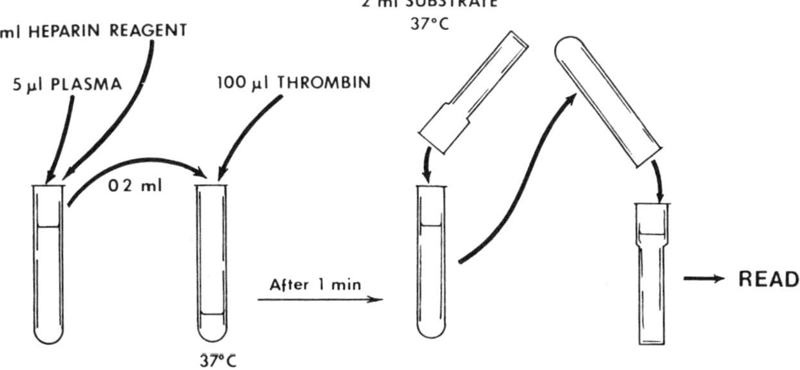

FIGURE 6. Test procedure for the fluorogenic substrate assay of antithrombin III.

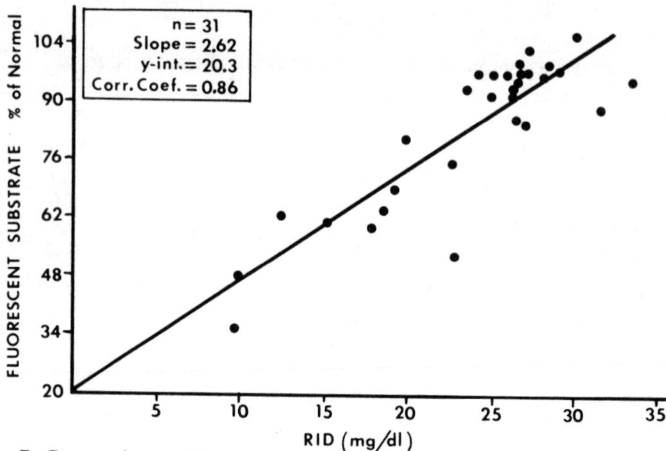

FIGURE 7. Comparison of fluorescent substrate and radial immunodiffusion methods for measuring antithrombin III.

unless you set up a control curve with a sample of the patient plasma obtained before heparinization. We thus expect to find a rather poor correlation between the fluorogenic and APTT methods throughout the range where they can be compared. The data presented in FIGURE 10 shows the results found upon simultaneous testing of 105 patient samples by both methods. As predicted, the correlation coefficient is only 0.6.

It is easy to argue at this point that what you need is not specificity, but a test such as the APTT which is a reliable measure of the patient overall co-agulability. The logic behind this is unassailable and, in fact, the APTT is a reasonable way of assessing the efficacy of medical dose heparin therapy. If it is prolonged as a result of heparin administration, the patient is known to have AT-III and is responding to therapy. The APTT, however, is not a very satis-factory tool for adjusting dosage unless patient baseline values are known.

In summary, it appears that there are several situations in which specific assays of heparin and AT-III are preferable to the more global measures of coagulability. The first of these are those cases in which heparin cannot be measured by the APTT because it is too low, as in minidose prophylaxis, or

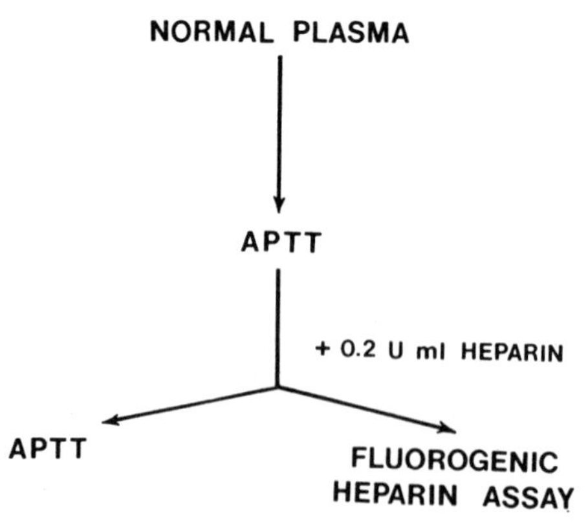

FIGURE 8. Experimental approach to evaluating the relationship between baseline APTT values and heparin assay results by the APTT or fluorogenic assay methods.

TABLE 3

EFFECT OF BASELINE APTT VALUES ON HEPARIN ASSAY VALUES

APTT Range, Seconds	Number of Samples	Heparin, U.S.P. U/ml			
		Fluorescent Substrate		APTT (Auto-Fi® Instrument)	
		Observed Range	Mean	Observed Range	Mean
28.0–29.9	5	0.16–0.28	0.20	0.10–0.26	0.16
30.0–31.9	12	0.15–0.29	0.23	0.09–0.25	0.17
32.0–33.9	16	0.16–0.28	0.22	0.14–0.30	0.21
34.0–35.9	10	0.19–0.29	0.22	0.17–0.29	0.23
36.0–37.9	3	0.21–0.28	0.24	0.31–0.37	0.34
38.0–39.9	3	0.22–0.29	0.25	0.35–0.37	0.36
40.0–41.9	2	0.23–0.25	0.24	0.36–0.40	0.38
28.0–41.9		0.15–0.29	0.23	0.09–0.40	0.26

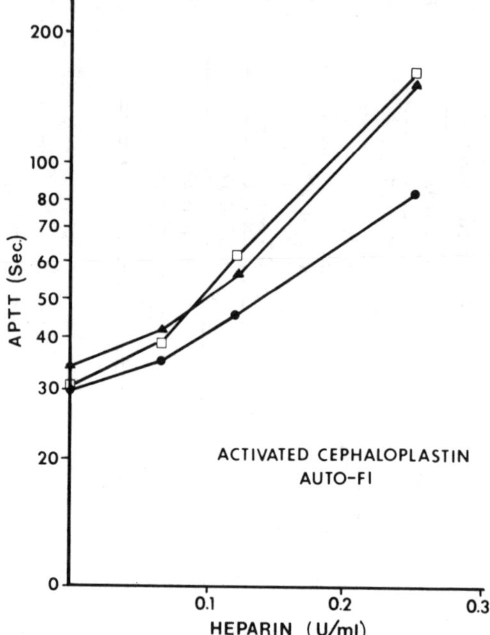

FIGURE 9. Individual *in vitro* response to heparin as measured by the APTT.

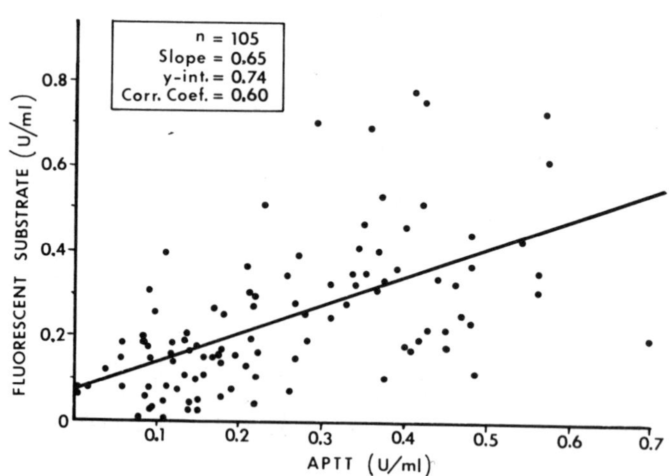

FIGURE 10. Comparison of the fluorescent substrates and APTT methods for measuring heparin.

where the heparin concentration is too high, as in cardiopulmonary bypass. The second situation occurs when a pre-heparinization sample has not been obtained and dosage adjustment is anticipated.

The fluorogenic assays we have developed seem very well suited to meet these testing needs.

REFERENCES

1. PENNER, J. A. & R. G. HISS.   1974.   Heparin therapy in the 70's. Univ. Mich. Med. Ctr. J. **40:** 57–61.
2. ROSENBERG, R. D.   1975.   Actions and interactions of antithrombin and heparin. New Engl. J. Med. **292:** 146–151.
3. BARROWCLIFFE, T. W., E. A. JOHNSON & D. THOMAS.   1978.   Antithrombin III and heparin. Br. Med. Bull. **34:** 143–150.
4. SEEGERS, W. H.   1978.   Antithrombin III. Theory and clinical applications. Am. J. Clin. Pathol. **69:** 367–374.
5. GUREWICH, V.   1976.   Guidelines for the management of anticoagulant therapy. *In* Thrombosis, Platelets, Anticoagulation and Acetylsalicyclic Acid.: 16–36. E. Donoso, J. I. Haft, Eds.: Stratton Intercontinental Book Corp. New York.
6. SOLOWAY, H. B.   1978.   Monitoring heparin therapy: How and why. Diag. Med. **2.**
7. BICK, R. L.   1979.   Monitoring heparin therapy. Diag. Dialog **1.**
8. ISAO, C., T. S. GALLUZZO, R. LO & K. G. PETERSON.   1979.   Whole-blood clotting time, activated partial thromboplastin time, and whole blood re-calcification time as heparin monitoring tests. Am. J. Clin. Pathol. **71:** 17.
9. College of American Pathologists Survey H-C, 1979.
10. LEIEN, A. N. & M. LIE.   1975.   Heparin assay in plasma: A comparison of five clotting methods. Thromb. Res. **7:** 777.
11. SUSSMAN, L. N. & M. BAY.   1974.   Activated partial thromboplastin time (A.P.T.T.) in monitoring heparin therapy. Lab. Med. **5:** 36–40.
12. SCHRIEVER, H. G., S. E. EPSTEIN & M. D. MINTZ.   1973.   Statistical correlation and heparin sensitivity of activated partial thromboplastin time, whole blood coagulation time, and an automated coagulation time. Am. J. Clin. Pathol. **60:** 323–329.
13. BASU, D., A. GALLUS, J. HIRSCH, *et al.*   1972.   A prospective study of the value of monitoring heparin treatment with the activated partial thrombo-plastin time. New Engl. J. Med. **287:** 324–327.
14. STUART, R. K. & A. MICHEL.   1971.   Monitoring heparin therapy with the activated partial thromboplastin time. Can. Med. Assoc. J. **104:** 385–388.
15. SPECTOR, I. & M. CORN.   1967.   Control of heparin therapy with activated partial thromboplastin times. JAMA **201:** 75–77.
16. BERN, M. M.   1975.   Variable response of activated partial thromboplastin time to heparin therapy during hemodialysis. Am. J. Clin. Pathol. **64:** 602–607.
17. LEIAN, A. M. & U. ABILDGAARD.   1976.   On the value of the activated partial thromboplastin time (APTT) in monitoring heparin therapy. Thromb. Hae-mostas. **35:** 592–597.
18. HUSEBY, R. M., G. A. MITCHELL, S. POCHRON, R. J. GARGIULO & P. M. HUDSON.   1978.   Synthetic substrates in blood coagulation and fibrinolysis: current concepts. *In* New Pathways in Laboratory Medicine. S. B. Rosalki, Ed.: 50–61. Hans Huber Publishers. Bern.
19. MITCHELL, G. A., P. M. HUDSON, R. M. HUSEBY, S. P. POCHRON & R. J. GARGIULO.   1978.   Fluorescent substrate assay for antithrombin III. Thromb. Res. **12:** 219–225.
20. MITCHELL, G. A., R. J. GARGIULO, R. M. HUSEBY, D. E. LAWSON, S. P. POCHRON

     & J. A. SEHUANES. 1978. Assay for plasma heparin using a synthetic peptide substrate for thrombin: Introduction of the fluorophore aminoisophthalic acid, dimethyl ester. Thromb. Res. **13:** 47–52.

21. ZUCK, T. F., J. J. BERGIN, J. M. RAYMOND & W. R. DWYRE. 1971. Implications of depressed antithrombin III activity associated with oral contraceptives. Surgery **133:** 609.

22. EGEBERG, O. 1975. Inherited antithrombin deficiency causing thrombophilia. Thromb. Diath. Haemorrh. **13:** 516.

23. LECHNER, K., H. NIESSNER & E. THALER. 1977. Coagulation abnormalities in liver disease. Sem. Thromb. Hemos. **4:** 40.

24. JORGENSEN, K. A. & E. STOFFERSEN. 1979. Antithrombin III and the nephrotic syndrome. Scand. J. Haematol. **22:** 442.

PROPERTIES OF
COMMERCIAL FACTOR IX CONCENTRATES

Michael H. Coan, Michael A. Fournel, and Milton M. Mozen

Cutter Laboratories, Inc.
Berkeley, California 94710

INTRODUCTION

Hemophilia B is a genetic disorder affecting 3000 persons in the United States and more than 30,000 persons worldwide. Some of these patients have had the opportunity to be treated with factor IX concentrates since the 1960s and now most of the patients in the United States use concentrates, often in home infusion programs. The first clinically used concentrate was prepared by Didisheim *et al.*[1] in 1959. Factor IX concentrates are now prepared by manufacturers (both private and state-supported) in almost every major industrialized nation.

In order to conserve maximally the important therapeutic components of plasma, factor IX concentrates are prepared by methods that do not interfere with the recovery of albumin, immune globulins, and factor VIII. This paper will review the biochemical properties of some factor IX concentrates in terms of the proteins contained, the coagulation variables, and the physiologic effects as measured in animal models.

COMMERCIAL FRACTIONATION

The therapeutically useful plasma proteins are separated by methods developed by Cohn *et al.*[2] and Oncley *et al.*,[3] during and directly after World War II, as a result of a need for concentrated plasma expanders. An outline of the process now used is shown in FIGURE 1. It is important to note that pH, temperature, ionic strength and composition, protein concentration, and alcohol concentration must all be rigidly controlled to insure uniformity of product; protein stability, purity, and yield; and performance of the product. This processing method is likely to continue for some time, partly because of regulatory constraints, although newer unit operations are being introduced, such as diafiltration and ultrafiltration.

The concentrate prepared by Didisheim is called PPSB (for the first letters in *P*rothrombin, *P*roconvertin, *S*tuart factor, and *B* factor). In modern nomenclature these are, of course, factors II, VII, X, and IX, respectively. Although this type of concentrate is still made today, it is not suitable for large-scale fractionation. The process requires resin-treated or EDTA-anticoagulated plasma, which cause the destruction of factor VIII, a valuable therapeutic material. Currently used methods for factor IX concentrate production include DEAE-Sephadex® or DEAE-cellulose adsorption from whole plasma (anticoagulated with ACD or citrate), from plasma devoid of cryoprecipitate, or from effluent I. Calcium phosphate adsorption from fraction IV is also used. At Cutter Laboratories, factor IX is prepared as outlined in FIGURE 2.[4]

731

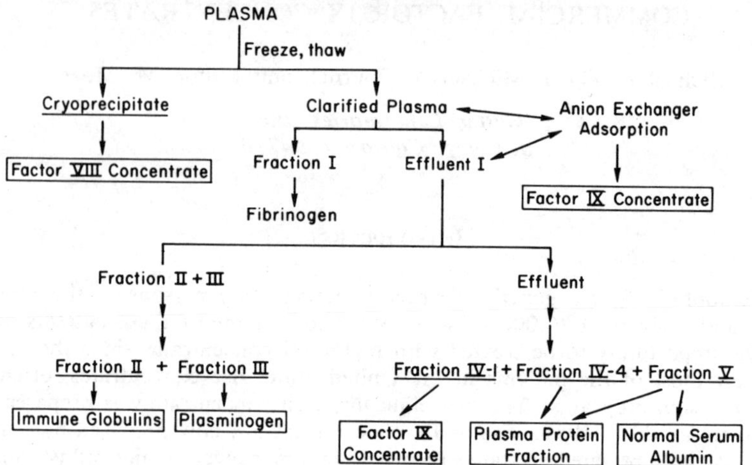

FIGURE 1. A typical plasma fractionation scheme. (Adapted from Cohn *et al.*[2] and Oncley *et al.*[3])

Plasma is obtained solely by plasmapheresis and is anticoagulated with sodium citrate. Effluent I from the Cohn process (alcohol concentration is approximately 8 percent, partially depleted of fibrinogen and factor VIII) is put in contact with DEAE-Sephadex in a batch-type process. Approximately 12 g of ion exchange resin (wet weight) per liter of effluent I are used. The amount of DEAE-Sephadex was chosen to preserve the balance between factor IX yield and albumin yield in subsequent fractionation steps. The "spent" effluent of

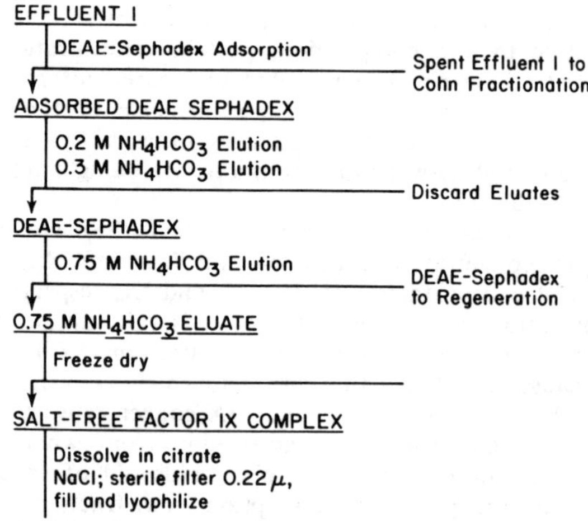

FIGURE 2. Manufacture of Konȳne factor IX complex. (Mozen.[4])

this adsorption is processed further to gamma globulin and albumin. The DEAE-Sephadex is then washed step-wise with increasing concentrations of ammonium bicarbonate: 0.2 *M*, 0.3 *M*, and 0.75 *M*. All of the desired substance is eluted in the last step; and this fraction is lyophilized, resulting in a salt-free protein powder. The protein is dissolved in a sodium-chloride–sodium-citrate solution to achieve a factor IX concentration of 25 units/ml (by a standard one-stage assay, using commercially available activated partial thromboplastin time (aPTT) reagent and naturally occurring factor-IX-deficient plasma). This solution is "sterile-filtered," filled, and lyophilized to yield the Konȳne® product. It is important to note that this process has remained essentially the same since its introduction by Cutter in 1969.

CONTENT OF COMMERCIAL CONCENTRATES

Typically, one vial of a commercial concentrate contains 500 units of factor IX. The concentration of some of the coagulation factors present in two American-manufactured concentrates is shown in TABLE 1. As can be seen, the ratio of the various activities is quite different, depending on the method

TABLE 1

COMPOSITION OF TWO TYPES OF FACTOR IX CONCENTRATES

Product Type	Factor IX (u/ml)	Factor II (u/ml)	Factor VII (u/ml)	Factor X (u/ml)	Thrombin
DEAE-Sephadex (effluent I)	25	20–25	7–11	25	Not detectable
Tricalcium phosphate (fraction IV)	19	9	120	15	Not detectable (heparin present)

of production. This is not at all surprising since the starting materials are so different.

The specific activity of factor IX in Konȳne is close to 1.0 unit per mg protein; thus, factor IX is less than 1 percent pure according to Andersson *et al.*,[5] who reported the specific activity of pure human factor IX to be 142 u/mg. TABLE 1 shows that DEAE-Sephadex type of concentrates contain approximately equal amounts of factors II, IX, and X. The factor VII content is much lower and in some concentrates is nearly absent. The tricalcium phosphate type of concentrate has a totally different ratio of coagulation factors, notably having much more apparent factor VII activity.

Over the years, clinicians have suggested that the Konȳne product has changed. To reiterate: the general process as just described has not changed, although we too, in our laboratories, can measure changes in product. We believe that these may be the result of greater care in blood collection, anti-coagulation, and freezing and shipping of plasma in order to preserve more effectively factor VIII. The major changes noted *in vitro* are in the factor VII concentration and the nonactivated partial thromboplastin time (NAPTT). Factor VII is assayed in a standard manner using naturally deficient plasma. The NAPTT is measured according to the method of Kingdon *et al.*[5] These changes are illustrated in TABLE 2. The factor VII content has fallen more than two-fold, and the NAPTT is now longer. The decrease in factor VII may be related to the greater relative concentration of citrate as a result of revised bleeding regulations enacted in March 1976. Factor VII is more loosely bound to DEAE-Sephadex than are the other prothrombin complex factors. The longer NAPTT may reflect more rapid freezing of plasma after collection and greater temperature control during frozen storage. Where Konȳne has been used to promote coagulation in patients with hemophilia A who also have naturally occurring inhibitors, we have been informed that recent lots may be less effective. It should be noted that such use of Konȳne is not indicated. So far, no consistent correlative patterns have emerged relating effectiveness and *in vitro* measurements.

THROMBOGENICITY OF FACTOR IX PRODUCTS

Many papers have been published proposing methods for evaluating "thrombogenic potential" of factor IX concentrates. The goal has been to correlate *in vivo* (clinical or animal model) studies with certain *in vitro* tests.

Kingdon and coworkers [6] initially proposed that the NAPTT test could be used to predict thrombogenicity because there was an apparent correlation with the Wessler [7] stasis model. This was later shown to be not always true.[10] Hedner and coworkers [8] have proposed an infusion model (using dogs) wherein factor IX concentrates were differentiated on the basis of *in vivo* effects. Fibrinogen, fibrin and fibrinogen degradation products, antithrombin III, platelets, and factors V, VIII, and IX were monitored. Also, activated partial thromboplastin time, prothrombin time (PT), and ethanol gelation tests were performed. Typically, the effects noted after administration of some concentrates were those that might be attributed to diffuse intravascular coagulation (DIC); however, the authors concluded that these *in vitro* measurements were not predictive of clinical effect. Sas *et al.*[9] have proposed that the TG_{t50} test might correlate with thrombogenicity. Later Pepper *et al.*[10] showed that the TG_{t50} and the NAPTT did not necessarily correlate.

Various investigators have proposed at one time or another that any of the activated coagulation factors are the cause of thrombogenicity.[11-14] These include factors VIIa, IXa, Xa, and XIa. There are no consistent results. The actual thrombogenic agent may be none, one, several, or all of the above.

At Cutter Laboratories, we have compared several factor IX products with respect to coagulation variables and these findings are summarized in TABLE 3. We had hoped to gain some insight into the causes of thrombogenicity. Initially,

TABLE 2

APPARENT CHANGES IN KONȲNE FACTOR IX CONCENTRATE

Year of Production	Factor IX (u/ml)	Factor VII (u/ml)	NAPTT (sec at 1:100)*
1970	25	25	120
1980	25	10	250

* Blank time >300 seconds.

TABLE 3

COMPARISONS OF COAGULATION ACTIVITIES OF SEVERAL FACTOR IX CONCENTRATES
(BOTH UNACTIVATED AND ACTIVATED)

Product	Factor IX (u/ml)	Factor X (u/ml)	Factor II (u/ml)	Factor VII (u/ml)	Factor Xa (u/ml)	Thrombin (u/ml)	NAPTT (sec at 1:100)
Konȳne® (Cutter)	24	27	23	7	<0.1	0	245
Konȳne (Cutter)	25	26	18	11	Not detected	0	164
Preconativ (Kabi)	19	16	15	8	Not detected	0	207
Christmassin (Green Cross)	22	26	23	0.5	Not detected	0	316
Proplex® * (Hyland)	19	15	9	120	<0.1	0	Not determined
DEFIX (SNBTS)	23	25	21	0.4	<0.1	0	Not determined
FEIBA † (Immune)	25	6	13	48	<0.1	1.6	80
Autoplex® * (Hyland) †	134	12	6	270	1.8	5.7	37
Laboratory-prepared "activated" factor IX concentrate	80	25	34	160	1.0	0.2	39

* These products contain heparin.
† Activated for use in patients with factor VIII inhibitor.

we thought that certain assays or ratios of activities would be useful, but in practice the comparisons shown shed little light on the problem of thrombogenicity and only underscore the differences among the products. We see that all concentrates have little or no thrombin and factor Xa. Both the factor VII levels and the nonactivated partial thromboplastin times vary widely. The factor VII levels are very low, by design, in Christmassin and DEFIX. Studies that could prove to be more useful are those that would involve animal models.

PHYSIOLOGICAL TESTING OF FACTOR IX CONCENTRATES

Initial investigations in our laboratories centered upon both a modified Wessler venous stasis assay [7] (ipsilateral vessel ligation and inspection enhances control of experimental artifact) and observation in an acute toxicity test in mice.[15] The latter was eventually abandoned because of relative nonspecificity; however, it remains a unique feature of these concentrates that high doses in mice induce intravascular thrombosis and significant necrosis, particularly of the liver, due to vascular occlusion.

Recent studies have concentrated upon the development of an infusion model in rabbits, which are essentially adaptations of the studies reported by Cash *et al.*[16] and Hedner *et al.*[8] Factor IX concentrates are intravenously infused into anesthetized, cannulated rabbits in a standard dosage of 100 units factor IX per kilogram body weight at a rate of approximately 25 units factor IX per minute. A 6-hour postinfusion observation period ensues, with blood samples taken hourly for monitoring variables of interest. Presently, these include platelets,[17] plasma fibrinogen,[18] and the clotting tests, activated partial thromboplastin time (aPTT) and prothrombin time (PT). Additional variables being considered include antithrombin-III (AT-III), α_2-macroglobulin (α_2M), factor X and fibrinogen/fibrin degradation product (FDP) levels. Infusion of thrombin, 200 units per kilogram body weight over 6 hours, results in near-complete depletion of platelets (>80 percent), total defibrinogenation, and near-incoagulability in either clotting test. Significant declines at AT-III and factor X are likewise found. Injection of thrombin (Stat) at a similar dose is uniformly lethal, most probably because of intravascular thrombus formation and embolization. Infusion of 2.5 percent serum albumin (human) in factor IX concentrate buffer (0.5 *M* citrate, 0.09 *M* NaCl) was without significant effect upon any variable monitored, save for a decline in platelets over time. These results are summarized in FIGURE 3.

Infusion of factor IX concentrate preparations in this model results in reproducible and specific effects upon the monitored variables ranging between the extremes described in the controls. Results of four preparations from three manufacturers are presented in FIGURE 4 to provide some indication of their range. Significantly, there is general correlation within the model between assay variables such that a sample that substantially reduces platelet counts and fibrinogen levels also affects the clotting tests. A striking and presently not understood observation was the time-related prolongation of the PT with some factor IX preparations, while more variable clot times were observed with the PTT.

We have studied a number of factor IX concentrates with this animal model and find some to have virtually no activity (that is, asymptomatic results equivalent to the albumin control), while others exert thrombin-like effects with the characteristics of disseminated intravascular coagulation (DIC) and lethality. To date, correlative investigations attempting to isolate specific *in vitro* variables (such as the coagulation factor assays presented in TABLE 3) that show a relationship to "thrombogenicity" as determined in the rabbit model have not been successful: no single *in vitro* variable appears to indicate a potential for induction of DIC in this animal model. Nonetheless, several leads have been found, some of which are described below.

"Activated" factor IX preparations, such as FEIBA (Immuno) or Autoplex® (Hyland), do not present any significantly greater activity in this model than "unactivated" factor IX concentrates, despite a very substantial increase in Wessler venous stasis activity (when compared on a unit factor II per kilogram body weight basis, the "activated" material possesses at least ten times the activity of "unactivated" concentrates) and markedly shorter NAPTT values (TABLE 3). This relationship agrees with that of Kingdon *et al.*[6] showing the correlation of the NAPTT and Wessler activity. Thus, not only is there a lack of correlation between the animal model systems, but also activation *per se* does not appear to induce thrombogenicity in the rabbit infusion model. These

Effects of Thrombin Infusion

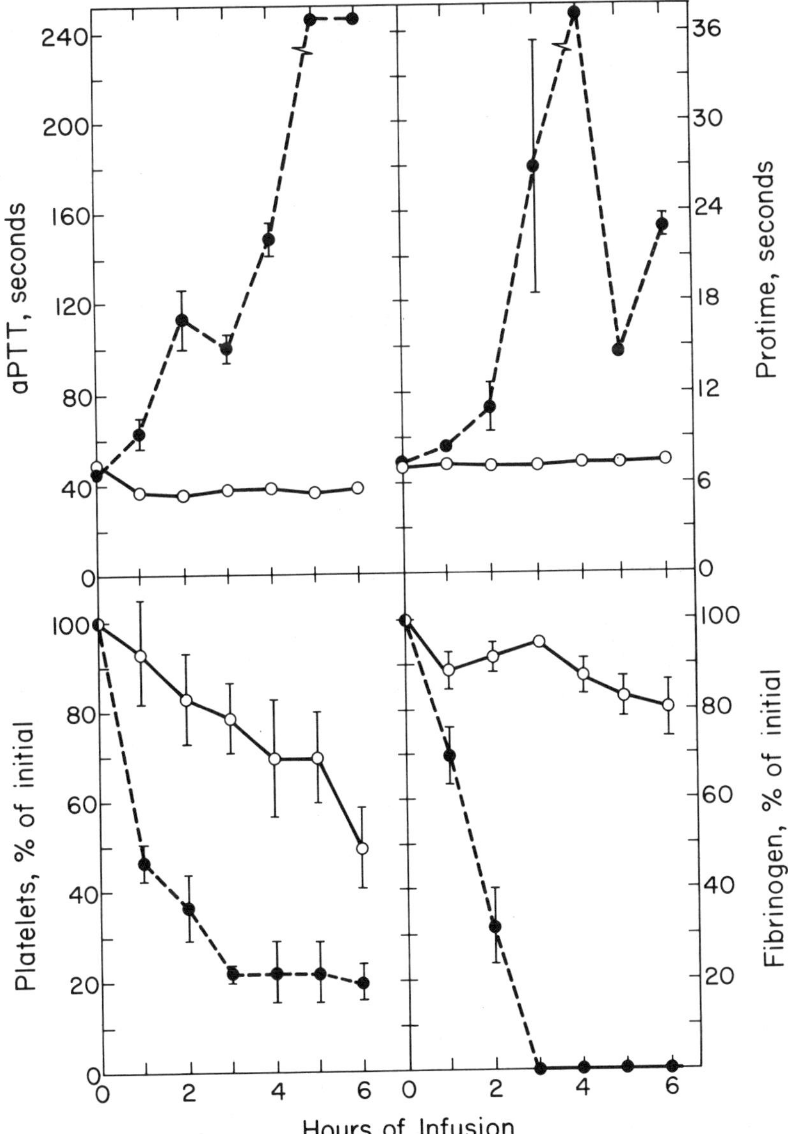

FIGURE 3. Effects of thrombin infusion. Effects of thrombin (●—●, 200 u/kg/per hr) or 2.5 percent human serum albumin in saline-citrate buffer (○—○, 4 ml/kg; 1 ml/min) upon indicated variables in the rabbit infusion model. (n = 4 for all; standard error of the mean is indicated.)

Effects of Factor IX Concentrate Infusion

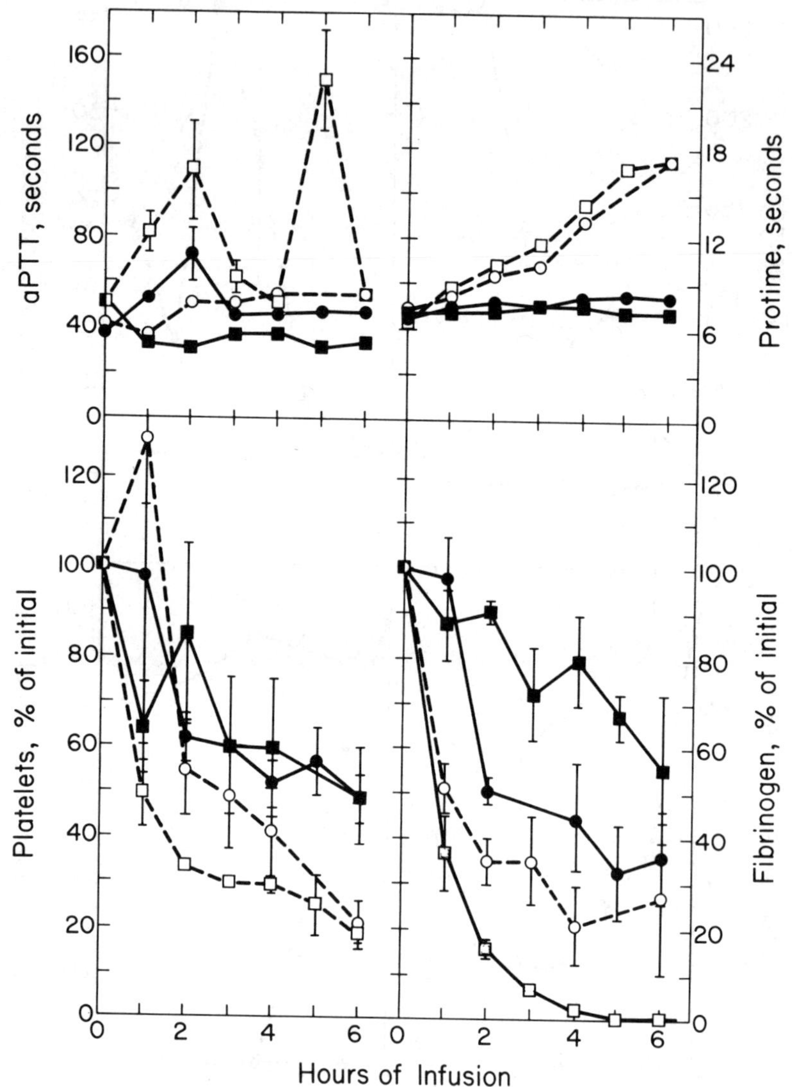

FIGURE 4. Effects of factor IX concentrate infusion. Effects of infusion of four representative factor IX concentrates (100 units factor IX/kg; 1 ml/min; 25 units/min; □—□, Konȳne; ■—■, Konȳne; ●—●, Preconativ [Kabi]; ○—○, Proplex [Hyland]. (n = 4 for all; standard error of the mean is indicated).

data also suggest that "activated" factor IX concentrates will not cause DIC generically (at least in rabbits).

Laboratory-prepared factor IX concentrates in contact with various ion-exchange materials appear to possess differential activity; for example, SP-Sephadex appears to induce increased activity in this model and also in the Wessler venous stasis model without altering *in vitro* characteristics save for a reduction in thrombin concentration. QAE-Sephadex contact has a similar effect, while reducing factor VII concentration. These results and others suggest that some as yet unidentified component of the factor IX preparations may well be involved in the occurrence of thrombogenic reactions independent of the state or concentration of the major vitamin-K-dependent factors.

Efforts to refine the model by enhancing the monitoring profile have included assay of inhibitor and procoagulant activities. Functional AT-III levels, determined by an adaptation of the method of Ødegard *et al.*,[19] have shown some changes after factor IX concentrate infusion, but further study is necessary to validate and quantitate these findings; estimation of α_2 macroglobulin activity is also under investigation. Monitoring of factor X levels to date has revealed a slight shift in activity slopes with factor IX concentrate infusions, suggesting activation *in vivo;* both an amidolytic assay [20] and a radiometric assay [21] using ^{3}H-Factor X are being studied. Fibrinogen degradation products, which Hedner, *et al.*[8] found to be significantly increased after factor IX concentrate injection in dogs, are likewise being investigated to provide yet another indication of the extent and nature of thrombogenic activity.

This animal model, which appears to mimic the development of DIC after infusion of some factor IX concentrates, may enable the identification and elimination of thrombogenicity from these concentrates and provide some criteria for the *in vitro* screening of concentrates for thrombogenicity.

OTHER PROTEINS IN FACTOR IX CONCENTRATES

Factor IX concentrates contain a host of other plasma proteins. As noted earlier, the factor IX in Konȳne is only about 1 percent pure. We have evidence [22, 23] that the factor IX antigen concentration is higher than the coagulant activity. Presumably, all the coagulant activity does not survive the isolation process. Low levels of factor VIII:C(Ag) have been measured by Onder and Hoyer [24] and Reisner.[25]

In our laboratories, we have shown that Konȳne contains immunologically detectable low and variable levels of antithrombin-III and α_2-macroglobulin. We have not been able to measure active AT-III and suspect that it is present in complex with enzymes.

Konȳne does contain traces of amidolytic and esterolytic activities. The levels of activity found are low and variable and are not due to free thrombin. The results of a survey of several lots of Konȳne are shown in TABLE 4. In these experiments the chromogenic peptide substrates (Kabi) were used according to the manufacturer's directions. Konȳne (25 μl) was assayed in a 1.0-ml cuvette. (S-2238 is designed to be specific for thrombin, S-2251 for plasmin, and S-2302 for kallikrein).

Inspection of these results shows no pattern. The spectrum of activity does not correspond to the known activities of any single enzyme (plasmin, factor Xa, thrombin, factor XIIaβ). The activity seen in Konȳne likely results from a mixture of small amounts of several active amidases.

An enzyme responsible for some of this activity has been purified from Konȳne by a combination of benzamidine-Sepharose® and heparin-Sepharose affinity chromatography.[26] FIGURE 5 shows the elution pattern of Konȳne applied to benzamidine-Sepharose (details are described in the legend). The lysine gradient was found to effect a good separation of factors IX and X. An enzyme, hereafter called the S-2238 hydrolase, eluted at high concentrations of NaCl. The active fractions were pooled and dialyzed prior to final purification by heparin-Sepharose affinity chromatography. The elution pattern is shown in FIGURE 6 and chromatography details are described in the legend. The resulting protein preparation is practically homogeneous, as shown by polyacrylamide gel electrophoresis in the presence of sodium dodecylsulfate (FIG. 7). The molecular weight is approximately 70,000 daltons, and after the preparation was reduced in 5 percent (v/v) β-mercaptoethanol, we could detect two peptide species of molecular weight 45,000 and 25,000 daltons. This enzyme does not react with antisera to factor X, factor IX, or prothrombin, nor does it react with antisera to the first and third complement components. Some further properties of this enzyme are summarized in TABLE 5. The hydrolase seems to be a new entity. It was conceivable that S-2238 hydrolase might be activated human protein C; thus, the amidolytic activities of activated

TABLE 4

SOME AMIDOLYTIC ACTIVITIES PRESENT IN KONYNE *

Lot Number	S-2238	S-2251	S-2302
1	0.10	0.04	0.02
2	0.03	0.03	0.01
3	0.15	0.07	0.04
4	0.16	0.06	0.05
5	0.13	0.03	0.03

* The change in absorbance at 405 nm in 10 minutes is given.

bovine protein C [27, 28] were compared with the activities of this hydrolase. The data shown in TABLE 6 confirm that the enzymes are not at all similar. A further comparison of the properties of the two enzymes is shown in TABLE 7. These properties confirm that the hydrolase is indeed a new enzyme; however, the *in vivo* function remains to be determined.

CONCLUSION

Factor IX concentrates have been available for 20 years, during which time thousands of patients have been treated successfully. In that same span of time, the biochemistry of the individual coagulation factors has been thoroughly examined, but in practice little of that knowledge has been applied to the preparation of concentrates and to the treatment of patients. It is only in recent years that this is being done.

At Cutter Laboratories, we have been producing Konȳne, a factor IX concentrate, since 1969. Konȳne is most similar to other DEAE-Sephadex-adsorbed concentrates, and it contains equivalent levels of the coagulation

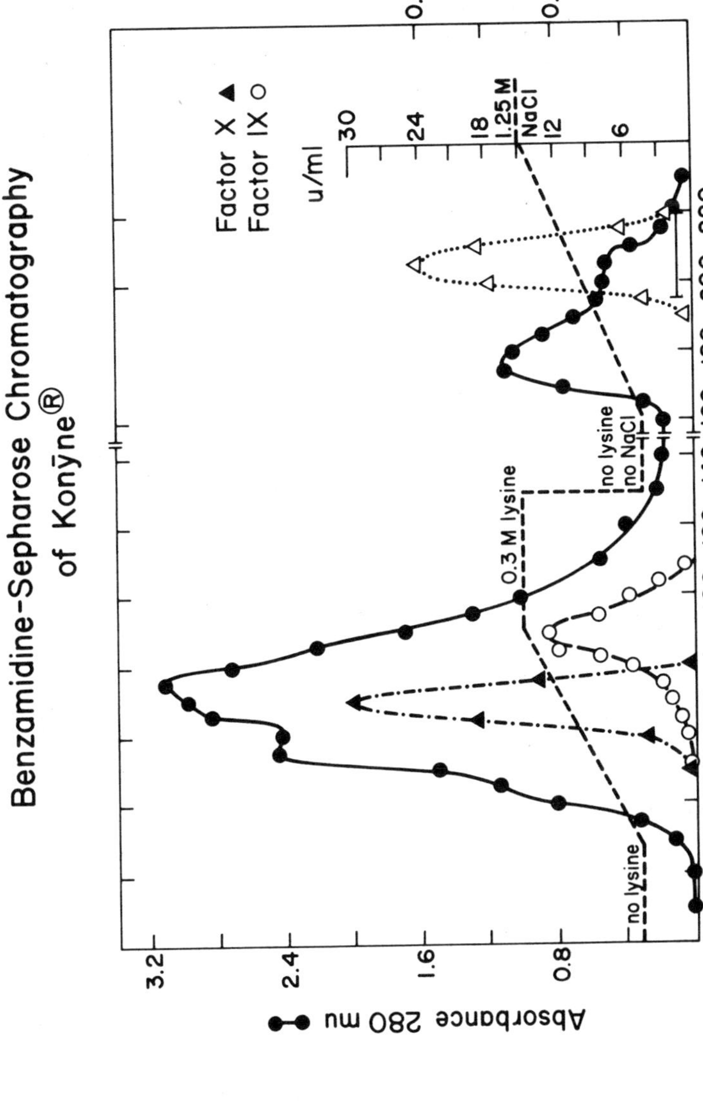

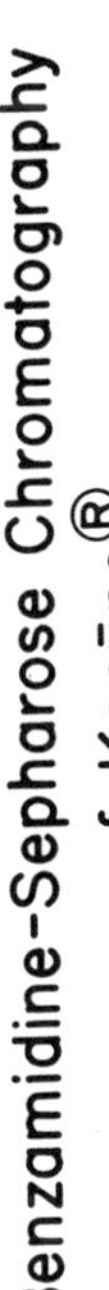

FIGURE 5. Benzamidine-Sepharose chromatography of Konȳne®. The column (2.5 × 25 cm) was equilibrated with 0.025M sodium acetate (pH 5.6). Sample was applied and the column was washed with 200 ml equilibration buffer. These fractions were discarded. Then a linear gradient (800 ml) to 0.3M lysine in the acetate buffer was initiated, collecting 8.0 ml fractions. The column was then washed with 300 ml 0.3M lysine, 0.025M sodium acetate, pH 5.6, followed by 100 ml of 0.025M sodium acetate. Then a 600-ml linear gradient (to 1.25M NaCl) was initiated, collecting 8.0 ml fractions.

factors. It differs in several detectable ways from factor IX concentrates prepared from Cohn fraction IV. Both *in vivo* (animal) and *in vitro* comparisons have been made of variables that may be associated with thrombogenicity of factor IX concentrates. The *in vivo* model we have developed does differentiate between factor IX concentrates and among batches of factor IX concentrates, but no one single *in vitro* variable has been implicated. It is evident that further studies of these complex systems are needed, and progress along those lines is being made at Cutter.

Further, we have shown that factor IX concentrates (specifically Konȳne) contain a variety of other plasma proteins. Konȳne also contains a mixture of

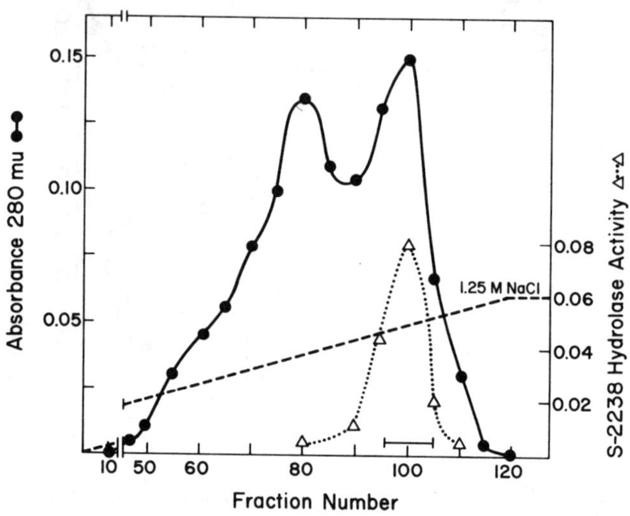

FIGURE 6. Heparin-Sepharose chromatography of S-2238 hydrolase. The column (2.5 × 25 cm) was equilibrated with 0.025*M* sodium acetate (pH 5.6), 0.01*M* NaCl. Sample was applied and the column was washed with 100 ml equilibration buffer, collecting 8.0 ml fractions. Then a linear gradient to 1.25*M* NaCl in the acetate buffer was initiated. The total volume of the gradient was 800 ml.

unidentified esterolytic and amidolytic activities in trace amounts. There is as yet no evidence that any of these proteins has direct effect on the potential thrombogenicity or putative factor VIII inhibitor bypassing activity of the product. A new hydrolase has been purified (S-2238 hydrolase), but its *in vivo* functions remain to be determined.

In our laboratories we are continuing to investigate the properties of factor IX concentrates, and major emphasis has been placed on further development of *in vivo* and *in vitro* assays of potential thrombogenicity and on the detailed characterization of the other proteins contained in these products.

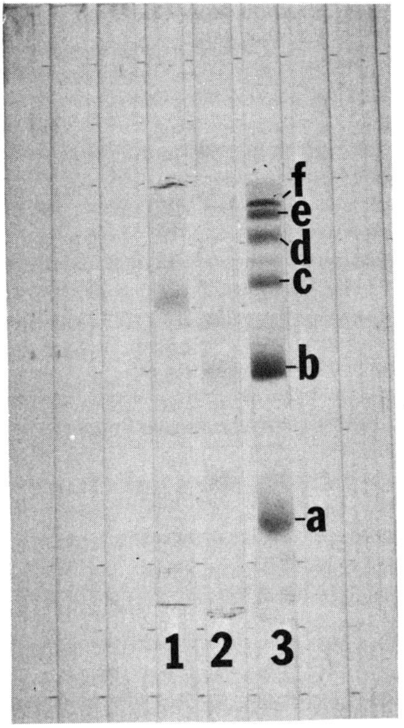

FIGURE 7. SDS-polyacrylamide electrophoresis of S-2238 hydrolase in 8.5 percent polyacrylamide. Gel 1 shows the S-2238-hydrolase. Gel 2 shows the enzyme after reduction with β-mercaptoethanol. Gel 3 shows modified ISG, with major bands at approximately 23,000 (a), 55,000 (b), 78,000 (c), 110,000 (d), 133,000 (e), and 156,000 (f) daltons.

TABLE 5

OTHER PROPERTIES OF HYDROLASE

1. Not readily inhibited by active-site specific trypsin inhibitors such as N-α-tosyl-L-lysylchloromethyl ketone (TLCK) or *p*-amidinophenacyl bromide (APB).

2. Inhibited by Trasylol®.

3. Has no effect on fibrinogen (by SDS-PAGE and clotting test).

4. Has no effect on plasminogen (by SDS-PAGE and activity).

5. Has no effect on factors II, VII, IX, X, XI, and XII.

6. Has no effect on prekallikrein.

7. Inhibits platelet aggregation (at 10 μg enzyme per ml).

8. Does not react with antisera to prothrombin, or factors IX and X.

9. Has pH maximum at 7.4, but is unstable at a more alkaline pH.

10. K_m is approximately 0.1 mM for S-2238.

TABLE 6

RELATIVE ACTIVITY OF HYDROLASE AND PROTEIN C
TOWARDS SEVERAL CHROMOGENIC SUBSTRATES

Substrate	S-2238 Hydrolase	Protein C
S-2238	1.00	1.18
S-2160	0.10	1.00
S-2302	0.11	0.68
S-2251	0.75	0.00
S-2222	0.14	0.10

TABLE 7

COMPARISON OF S-2238 HYDROLASE AND BOVINE PROTEIN C

	Human S-2238 Hydrolase	Bovine Protein C
2 chain	45K, 25K	41K, 21K
DFP:	Poor inhibitor	Readily inhibits
AT-III	Inhibits	Has no effect
AT-III + heparin:	Provides better inhibition	Has no effect
Soybean trypsin inhibitor:	Provides no inhibition	Provides no inhibition
$CaCl_2$	Enhances activity	Enhances activity
EDTA:	Kills activity	Removes Ca^{2+} effect
	Activates bovine factor V	Destroys bovine factor V and not human factor V
	Activates and degrades human factors V and VIII	

ACKNOWLEDGMENTS

We thank N. Pancham, S. Wada, D. Lee, E. Erde, S. Bernhard, M. Lebedev, J. Beaver, J. Newgren, A. Bubnic, and C. Zuffi for assistance in performing the experiments reported. Dr. D. D. Schroeder, Dr. W. J. Brockway, Dr. S. P. Bajaj, and Mr. R. Guzman contributed many valuable ideas during the course of these studies

REFERENCES

1. DIDISHEIM, P., J. LOEB, C. BLATRIX & J. P. SOULIER. 1959. Preparation of a human plasma fraction rich in prothrombin, proconvertin, Stuart factor, and PTC and a study of its activity and toxicity in rabbits and man. J. Lab. Clin. Med. **53**: 322–330.
2. COHN, E. J., L. E. STRONG, W. L. HUGHES, D. L. MULFORD, J. N. ASHWORTH, M. MELIN & H. L. TAYLOR. 1946. Preparation and properties of serum and plasma proteins. IV. A system for the separation into fractions of the

protein and lipoprotein components of biological tissues and fluids. J. Am. Chem. Soc. **68:** 459–475.

3. ONCLEY, J. L., M. MELIN, D. A. RICHERT, J. W. CAMERON & P. M. GROSS, JR. 1949. The separation of the antibodies isoagglutinins, prothrombin, plasminogen, and β_1-lipoprotein into subfractions of human plasma. J. Am. Chem. Soc. **71:** 541–550.

4. MOZEN, M. M. 1976. The development and use of the coagulation concentrates Factor IX (Konȳne®) and Factor VIII (Koāte ™). Presented at the Twenty-Fourth Annual Wayne State University Symposium on Blood, Detroit, Michigan, January 22 and 23, 1976.

5. ANDERSSON, L. A., H. BORG & M. MILLER-ANDERSSON. 1975. Purification and characterization of human factor IX. Thromb. Res. **7:** 451–459.

6. KINGDON, H. S., R. L. LUNDBLAD, J. J. VELTKAMP & D. L. ARONSON. 1975. Potentially thrombogenic material in factor IX concentrates. Thromb. Diath. Haemorrh. **33:** 617–631.

7. WESSLER, S., S. M. REIMER & M. C. SHERS. 1959. Biologic assay of thrombosis-inducing activity in human serum. J. Appl. Physiol. **14:** 943–946.

8. HEDNER, U., I. M. NILSSON & S-E. BERGENTZ. 1976. Various prothrombin complex concentrates and their effect on coagulation and fibrinolysis *in vivo.* Thromb. Haemostas. **35:** 386–395.

9. SAS, G., R. E. OWENS, J. K. SMITH, S. MIDDLETON & J. D. CASH. 1975. *In vitro* spontaneous thrombin generation in human factor IX concentrates. Br. J. Haematol. **31:** 25–35.

10. PEPPER, D. S., D. BANHEGYI, A. HOWIE & J. D. CASH. 1977. *In vitro* thrombogenicity tests of factor IX concentrates. Br. J. Haematol. **36:** 573–583.

11. HULTIN, M. B. 1979. Activated clotting factors in factor IX concentrates. Blood **54:** 1028–1038.

12. SELIGSOHN, U., C. K. KASPER, B. ØSTERUD & S. I. RAPAPORT. 1979. Activated factor VII: Presence in factor IX concentrates and persistence in the circulation after infusion. Blood **53:** 828–837.

13. KANG, E. P. & D. C. TRIANTAPHYLLOPOULOS. 1974. Intrinsic activation of prothrombin potentiated by celite and reduced by kaolin. Thromb. Diath. Haemorrh. **32:** 600–606.

14. ELÖDI, S. & K. VARADI. 1978. Activation of clotting factors in prothrombin complex concentrates as demonstrated by clotting assays for Factors IXa and Xa. Thromb. Res. **12:** 797–807.

15. GUZMAN, R. J., R. G. RAMUS & J. HIDALGO. 1976. A mouse model for studying thrombogenicity of prothrombin complex concentrates (PCC). Fed. Proc. **35:** 805.

16. CASH, J. D., R. G. DALTON, S. MIDDLETON & J. K. SMITH. 1975. Studies on the thrombogenicity of Scottish factor IX concentrates in dogs. Thromb. Diath. Haemorrh. **33:** 632–639.

17. BULL, B. S., M. A. SCHNEIDERMAN & G. BRECHER. 1965. Platelet counts with the Coulter counter. Am. J. Clin. Pathol. **44:** 678–688.

18. MILLAR, H. R., J. G. SIMPSON & A. L. STALKER. 1971. An evaluation of the heat precipitation method for plasma fibrinogen estimation. J. Clin. Pathol. **24:** 827–830.

19. ØDEGARD, O. R., M. LIE & U. ABILDGAARD. 1975. Heparin cofactor activity measured with an amidolytic method. Thromb. Res. **6:** 287–294.

20. SUOMELA, H., M. BLOMBÄCK & B. BLOMBÄCK. 1977. The activation of factor X evaluated by using synthetic substrates. Thromb. Res. **1:** 267–281.

21. SILVERBERG, S. A., Y. NEMERSON & M. ZUR. 1977. Kinetics of the activation of bovine coagulation factor X by components of the extrinsic pathway. J. Biol. Chem. **252:** 8481–8488.

22. PECHET, L. Personal communication.

23. THOMPSON, A. Personal communication.

24. ONDER, O. & L. W. HOYER. 1979. Factor VIII coagulant antigen in factor IX complex concentrates. Thromb. Res. **15:** 569–572.
25. REISNER, H. Personal communication.
26. COAN, M. H., D. D. SCHROEDER & M. M. MOZEN. 1979. Isolation of a new enzyme from human plasma fractions and its effects on coagulation. Presented at the VII International Congress on Thrombosis and Haemostasis, London.
27. KISIEL, W., L. H. ERICSSON & E. W. DAVIE. 1976. Proteolytic activation of protein C from bovine plasma. Biochemistry **15:** 4893–4900.
28. KISIEL, W., W. M. CANFIELD, L. H. ERICSSON & E. W. DAVIE. 1977. Anticoagulant properties of bovine plasma Protein C following activation by thrombin. Biochemistry **16:** 5824–5830.

PROTHROMBIN COMPLEX CONCENTRATES: CLINICAL USE *

Doris Menache

American Red Cross Blood Services Laboratories
Bethesda, Maryland 20014

Factor IX concentrates, factor IX complex concentrates, prothrombin complex concentrates and PPSB (prothrombin, proconvertin, Stuart factor and antihemophilic B factor) are the names currently used to designate the plasma derivative that contains the vitamin K-dependent clotting factors. The preparation and clinical use of PPSB (Centre National de Transfusion Sanguine, Paris, France), the first concentrate used extensively for the treatment of hemophilia B, were initiated more than 20 years ago in France.[1]

All purification methods for the preparation of prothrombin complex concentrates take advantage of the specific adsorbability of the vitamin K-dependent clotting factors. Prothrombin complex concentrates for clinical use were first produced from blood collected on ion exchange resin. The plasma was adsorbed either with tricalcium phosphate [1] or barium sulfate.[2] The occurrence of side effects after the injection of barium sulfate eluates [3] prompted its abandonment and replacement by DEAE-cellulose.[4] At the same time, the original technique [1] was modified by the introduction of EDTA as anticoagulant [5] in order to allow large-scale fractionation that could not be achieved using plasma collected through an ion exchange resin column. Small-scale fractionation using aluminum hydroxide as adsorbent was also effective.[6] Another approach was developed in Oxford [7] that used, as source material for the first time, G-2, a byproduct of ether fractionation.

The need to recover red cells and platelets for clinical use, together with the increased knowledge of the characteristics of the vitamin K-dependent clotting factors, and the advent of new technology, have contributed to the development of improved methods for the production of prothrombin complex concentrates. The most common production method utilized today is purification by DEAE adsorption (for review see Bidwell *et al.*[8]). The source material is either whole plasma or the supernatant plasma after removal of the antihemophilic factor by cryoprecipitation or the removal of Cohn fraction I.[9] Another approach is adsorption of Cohn fraction IV-1 by tricalcium phosphate. Concentration of the various eluates is achieved by either lyophilization, ultrafiltration, or PEG-4000.

All DEAE preparations have relatively low levels of factor VII and about equal levels of factors II and X, as compared with factor IX. In contrast, the level of factor VII seems higher than that of factor IX in tricalcium phosphate preparations.[1, 10]

While *in vivo* infusion of other coagulants (factors II, VII and X) predictably yields almost quantitative recoveries in plasma samples taken within a short time of infusion, factor IX shows a striking deviation from this rule. In essentially all such studies in a great number of laboratories, the *in vivo*

* Contribution No. 491 from the American Red Cross.

747

recovery of infused factor IX is between 25 and 50 percent. It does not seem to make any difference whether the factor IX is infused as plasma or a concentrate. Some have proposed that the poor recovery of factor IX is a feature of the disease and not of the nature of the material infused,[11] while others have interpreted this to mean that factor IX is distributed in a larger extravascular volume than are the other vitamin K-dependent factors.[12]

Clinical use of prothrombin complex concentrates for replacement therapy in patients with vitamin K-dependent clotting factors deficiencies was based on the knowledge that these products contained concentrated factors II, VII, IX and X. The indications for their use included both congenital and acquired deficiencies.

Of all the conditions for which these concentrates have been used, hemophilia B (Christmas disease) is the one for which the most clinical data exist, clearly demonstrating efficacy in the treatment of hemorrhagic episodes and prevention of hemorrhage after surgery. Hemophilia B remains the major clinical indication for the use of factor IX concentrates. Although congenital diseases of the other vitamin K-dependent clotting factors are rarer and fewer data are available, the efficacy of prothrombin complex concentrates for replacement therapy in patients deficient in either prothrombin, factor VII, or factor X is generally accepted (for review see Menache and Guillin [13]).

In acquired deficiencies prothrombin complex concentrates have been used in a variety of pathologic conditions. While the clinical efficacy for reversal of coumarin's drug effect is documented,[14] the risk of transmission of hepatitis in patients with low exposure to blood products has been shown to be very high.[15-18] Thus the benefit/risk ratio for a given patient has to be considered in each instance. Many patients with chronic and acute liver disease have been treated with prothrombin complex concentrates and there is substantial evidence of side effects, including disseminated intravascular coagulation (DIC). There is no evidence for a beneficial effect in patients with chronic liver disease and it would not seem appropriate, therefore, to use the concentrates in such patients. Patients with acute hepatic failure undergo a dramatic and catastrophic DIC, and prothrombin complex concentrates are clearly contraindicated.

The increasing availability of prothrombin complex concentrates has considerably extended their use and has focused attention on the onset of complications, the most common of which, as outlined previously, remains the transmission of hepatitis. Recent studies have shown that factor IX concentrates may transmit not only hepatitis type B, but also hepatitis type non-A non-B.[19]

Another adverse effect has been the occurrence of thromboembolic complications and DIC. During the early studies of factor IX concentrates, the concept of thrombogenicity as a potential hazard was clearly recognized. The occurrence of acute DIC and subsequent death in a patient with liver disease substantiated this danger.[20] Although in most subsequent reports on the clinical use of such preparations this problem did not appear to arise, other reports clearly documented the relationship between these concentrates and thrombohemorrhagic complications. The occurrence of DIC and/or thromboembolic complications has been reported in pathologic conditions with acquired deficiencies of the vitamin K-dependent factors, particularly liver disease.[13, 21-27] In patients with hemophilia B these complications have occurred after the use of factor IX concentrates for the prevention of postoperative hemorrhage. Analysis of the data indicates various manifestations such as DIC, superficial vein thrombosis, deep vein thrombosis, pulmonary embolism, and myocardial infarction.[28-33] Activated prothrombin complex concentrates have been reported to induce transient blindness in a patient with hemophilia A with inhibitors[34] and DIC in another.[35] In addition, we are aware of two patients with hemophilia A (16 and 17 years old) with inhibitors in whom myocardial infarction developed (which was fatal in one) after the use of large doses of standard prothrombin complex concentrates (referred to by Luscher *et al.*[36]).

Further evidence for thrombotic and/or DIC complications resulting from infusion of factor IX concentrates comes from animal experiments. An animal model using the venous stasis technique of Wessler *et al.*[37] has been outlined for testing the thrombogenicity of factor IX concentrates,[38] and thrombosis was prevented by the addition of heparin, but not by the addition of soybean trypsin inhibitor or by diisopropyl fluorophosphate, suggesting that the responsible factor was IXa. In addition, a correlation was found between the nonactivated partial thromboplastin time (NAPTT) and the *in vivo* assays in products not containing heparin.[39] However, more recent data[40] indicate that the *in vitro* test that correlates more closely with the *in vivo* test is the thrombin generation test, TGt_{50}. A nonstasis rabbit model has also been used to evaluate thrombogenicity of these concentrates. Infusion of concentrates into healthy rabbits resulted in a decrease in platelet count and in concentrations of fibrinogen, factor V, and factor VIII (suggesting the occurrence of DIC), with subsequent death in 34 percent of the animals infused.[41] It is of interest that in these experiments, the route of administration of the product affected the incidence of death (82 percent when the animal was injected in the jugular vein through a catheter versus 17 percent when injected into the marginal vein of the ear), suggesting that the use of a catheter may have resulted in an "activation" of the clotting factors. Infusion of a variety of factor IX concentrates in a nonstasis rabbit model showed that those concentrates active in *in vitro* thrombogenicity tests induced DIC.[42]

Experiments in dogs have shown that commercially available concentrates can activate the coagulation process *in vivo* with doses equivalent to those used in the treatment of patients. Coagulation changes did not occur immediately after infusion, but were most marked in the samples obtained at least 30 minutes[43] or 4 hours[44] after infusion, indicating a gradual generation of thrombin *in vivo*. Heparin in the concentrates had no effect,[43, 44] whereas the addition of both antithrombin-III and Trasylol® (Bayer, Leverkusen, Germany) prevented almost all changes in dogs.[45] The clinical significance of these canine observations remains to be established.

The nature of the species present in factor IX concentrates and responsible for inducing thrombotic complications has not yet been established with certainty. Prothrombin complex concentrates that markedly shorten the NAPTT were shown to correlate with a tendency towards thrombosis *in vivo*.[39, 46] Further studies have implicated factors Xa, IXa, VIIa and factors of the contact phase,[38, 47-51] while other studies implicate factor XIIa activation of prekallikrein as the initial reaction responsible for thrombogenicity.[52] However, experiments performed in mice indicate that some adverse effect of factor IX concentrates may result from high levels of zymogens rather than the small amounts of active enzymes.[53]

Although the question remains unanswered, several attempts have been made to devise methods both for the detection of potential thrombogenicity in factor IX concentrates and for the improvement of the safety of these products.

Initially most investigators relied on tests for the detection of thrombin activity, using either fibrinogen or whole plasma as substrate. Although good clinical results favored the efficacy of these tests, the occurrence of thrombotic complications showed the need for more sensitive methods, which were developed later. These include the effect of a concentrate on the NAPTT of normal plasma [39] and on the recalcification time of celite-exhausted plasma.[54] Another approach has been to evaluate the *in vitro* generation of thrombin (TGt_{50}) after recalcification of factor IX concentrates.[54] Studies have revealed that the latter two tests are sensitive to different activities since it has been possible to separate them by gel filtration,[55] and no correlation was found during routine quality-control testing.[56] The method of choice to detect potential thrombogenicity of a given product will require the identification of the responsible factor(s). However, it has recently been suggested that of the presently available *"in vitro"* tests for potential thrombogenicity of factor IX concentrates, a combination of NAPTT, TGt_{50} and factor VIII inhibitor bypassing activity tests would be sufficient to demonstrate the presence of any activation in factor IX concentrates, and that in some cases the Xa generation test may be more relevant than the TGt_{50}.[57]

The presence in prothrombin complex concentrates of a factor VIII inhibitor bypassing activity needs to be emphasized. The observation in 1969 by Breen and Tullis [58] of the hemostatic effect (accompanied by a shortening of the silicone clotting time) of a factor IX concentrate in a patient with factor VIII deficiency is the first evidence that prothrombin complex concentrates contain a substance which is able to bypass antihemophilic factor in the coagulation process. This was substantiated in 1972 by Fekete *et al.*[59] and in 1974 by Kurczynski and Penner,[60] who described the use of an "activated prothrombin complex" (Auto Factor IX, Hyland, Costa Mesa, CA) to control bleeding in several patients with hemophilia A with inhibitors. Abildgaard *et al.*[61] provided further evidence in 1976 by reporting the effectiveness of a standard preparation, Konȳne® (Cutter, Berkeley, CA), in the treatment of patients with inhibitors.

Since that time many patients with factor VIII inhibitors have been treated with several preparations of prothrombin complex concentrates, including two activated products, Autoplex® (Hyland, Costa Mesa, CA), initially referred to as Auto IX, and FEIBA® (Immuno, Vienna, Austria), initially referred to as Fraction R. A few patients have also been treated in Australia with an activated Prothrombinex® (Commonwealth Laboratories, Melbourne, Australia).

The results of a survey conducted by the International Committee on Thrombosis and Haemostasis indicated that standard and activated prothrombin complex concentrates were effective in one-third of the bleeding episodes treated.[62]

The results of a recent multicenter therapeutic trial unequivocally established, for the first time, the beneficial effect of standard prothrombin complex concentrates in the treatment of hemorrhage in hemophilia A patients with inhibitors.[63] This trial consisted of a controlled, randomized, blind study of the effectiveness of Konȳne and Proplex® (Hyland, Costa Mesa, CA) in the treatment of 157 episodes of hemarthrosis in 51 hemophiliacs with antibodies to factor VIII. The results indicated that approximately 50 percent of the episodes treated with a single dose (factor IX 75 u/kg) of prothrombin complex concentrates, compared with 20 percent of episodes treated with placebo, were effectively treated. This difference is significant at $p < 0.01$. Each prothrombin complex concentrate was more effective than placebo ($p < 0.05$) and no significant difference was seen between the two concentrates.

No controlled clinical trial with activated factor IX concentrates has been reported. An uncontrolled trial of Autoplex showed that by subjective evaluation, a good or excellent clinical response was achieved in 85 percent of episodes (90/105).[64]

Several extremely important questions remain to be answered. What is the effective component(s) responsible for this ability to establish hemostasis with an inhibitor to factor VIII? Factor VIIa has been invoked and found to remain in the circulation for some hours after the infusion of the activated concentrate, Auto IX.[51] However, in the multicenter clinical trial, both Proplex and Konȳne had the same effect, despite the fact that the activity of factor VII in those concentrates differs 10-fold. Some reports have indicated that the activated concentrate, FEIBA, enhances platelet coagulant activity,[65] while others indicate that platelets enhance the factor VIII bypassing activity of Auto IX.[66] A relationship has been suggested [65, 66] between these observations and the fact that fresh platelet transfusions in hemophilia A patients with inhibitors result in an alleviation of the coagulation defect.[67]

It should be emphasized that there is no laboratory test that correlates well with the *in vivo* effect of the infusion of factor IX concentrates into patients with inhibitors. Some laboratories have reported significant, if not dramatic, shortening of activated partial thromboplastin time (APTT) and the prothrombin time, while others do not see these changes. The relationship between thrombogenicity and factor VIII inhibitor bypassing activity, if any, is not established.

The use of factor IX concentrates in the treatment of hemophilia A patients with inhibitors has induced anamnestic responses in many instances. Among 136 patients for whom inhibitor titers have been followed,[61, 68–80] 54 patients had anamnestic responses,[68, 70–72, 76–80] which represents an incidence of 40 percent. These responses occurred after the infusion of PPSB, Konȳne, Proplex, FEIBA, and Autoproplex. Significant factor VIII coagulant antigen (VIII C:Ag) has been identified in prothrombin complex concentrates [81] and accounts for the anamnestic responses observed in the hemophilia A patients.

Prothrombin complex concentrates have now been used clinically for over 20 years, but the basic method for their preparation has not changed. In addition to our previous knowledge that these products contain concentrated coagulation factors II, VII, IX and X, we have to consider that they may also contain these factors in an activated form as well as additional proteins, such as the F VIII-related antigens, F VIII R:Ag and F VIII C:Ag. A new biological activity—the factor VIII bypassing activity—has been identified, and we can assume, on the basis of their characteristics, that proteins C,[82] S,[83] and M [84] are also present in these concentrates. To our previous knowledge that the clinical indication for prothrombin complex concentrates was replacement therapy in vitamin K-dependent clotting factor deficiencies, we have to recognize the danger of using these products in some acquired deficiencies, such as liver disease (particularly acute liver failure). In addition, we now know that these products are efficacious in some hemophilia A patients with inhibitors.

REFERENCES

1. DIDISHEIM, P., J. LOEB, C. BLATRIX & J.-P. SOULIER. 1959. Preparation of a human plasma fraction rich in prothrombin, proconvertin, Stuart factor, and PTC and a study of its activity and toxicity in rabbits and man. J. Lab. Clin. Med. **53:** 322–330.

2. SURGENOR, D. M., M. MELIN, B. B. STEELE, L. WHEATON & R. B. PENNELL. 1959. Preparation of barium sulfate eluate of plasma for physiological studies in humans. Vox Sang. **4:** 71–72.

3. TULLIS, J. L., P. JURIGIAN & M. MELIN. 1964. Clinical studies with human prothrombin complexes. Vox Sang. **9:** 228.

4. MELIN, M., J. W. JANSKY, G. LEONARDOS, A. DI FRANCESCO, R. B. PENNELL & J. L. TULLIS. 1964. The preparation of a prothrombin-containing fraction from human plasma by chromatography. Vox Sang. **9:** 227.

5. SOULIER, J.-P., C. BLATRIX & M. STEINBUCH. 1964. Fractions "coagulantes" contenant les facteurs de coagulation adsorbables par le phosphate tricalcique. Presse Med. **21:** 1223–1228.

6. HOAG, M. S., P. M. AGGELER & A. H. FOWELL. 1960. Disappearance rate of concentrated proconvertin extracts in congenital and acquired hypoproconvertinemia. J. Clin. Invest. **39:** 554–563.

7. BIGGS, R., E. BIDWELL, D. A. HANDLEY, R. G. MACFARLANE, J. TRUETA, A. ELLIOT-SMITH, G. W. R. DIKE & B. J. ASH. 1961. The preparation and assay of a Christmas-factor (factor IX) concentrate and its use in the treatment of two patients. Br. J. Haematol. **VII:** 349–364.

8. BIDWELL, E., G. W. R. DIKE & T. J. SNAPE. 1976. Therapeutic materials. *In* Human Blood Coagulation, Haemostasis and Thrombosis, 2nd ed. R. Biggs, Ed.: 249–309. Blackwell Scientific Publications, Oxford.

9. MIDDLETON, S., L. BENNETT & J. SMITH. 1973. A therapeutic concentrate of coagulation factors II, IX and X from citrated factor VIII depleted plasma. Vox Sang. **24:** 441–456.

10. DIKE, G. W. R., E. BIDWELL, C. R. RIZZA. 1972. The preparation and clinical use of a new concentrate containing factor IX, prothrombin and factor X and of a separate concentrate containing factor VII. Br. J. Haematol. **22:** 469–490.

11. BIGGS, R. 1966. Christmas disease. *In* Treatment of Haemophilia and Other Coagulation Disorders. R. Biggs & R. G. Macfarlane, Eds.: 222–239. F. A. Davis Company. Philadelphia, PA.

12. ZAUBER, N. P. & J. LEVIN. 1977. Factor IX levels in patients with hemophilia B (Christmas disease) following transfusion with concentrates of factor IX or fresh frozen plasma (FFP). Medicine **56:** 213–224.

13. MENACHE, D. & M. C. GUILLIN. 1975. The use of factor IX concentrates for patients with conditions other than factor IX deficiency. Br. J. Haematol. **31**(Suppl.): 247–257.

14. TABERNER, D. A., J. M. THOMSON & L. POLLER. 1976. Comparison of prothrombin complex concentrate and vitamin K_1 in oral anticoagulant reversal. Br. Med. J. **2:** 83–85.

15. HELLERSTEIN, L. J. & D. DEYKIN. 1971. Hepatitis after Konȳne administration. N. Engl. J. Med. **284:** 1039–1040.

16. FARIA, R. & N. J. FIUMARA. 1972. Hepatitis B associated with Konȳne. N. Engl. J. Med. **287:** 358–359.

17. SANDLER, S. G., C. E. RATH & A. RUDER. 1973. Prothrombin complex concentrates in acquired hypoprothrombinemia. Ann. Int. Med. **79:** 485–491.

18. GRAMMENS, G. L. & R. T. BRECKENRIDGE. 1974. Complications with Christmas factor (factor IX) concentrates. Ann. Int. Med. **80:** 666–667.

19. WYKE, R. J., A. THORNTON, B. PORTMANN, A. J. ZUCKERMAN, K. N. TSIQUAYE, Y. WHITE, P. K. DAS & R. WILLIAMS. 1979. Transmission of non-A non-B

hepatitis to chimpanzees by factor-IX concentrates after fatal complications in patients with chronic liver disease. Lancet **1**: 520–524.

20. MENACHE, D., R. FAUVERT & J.-P. SOULIER. 1959. Utilisation en hepatologie d'une fraction contenant la prothrombine, le complexe proconvertine-facteur Stuart et le facteur anti-hemophilique B (P.P.B.). Path. Biol. **7**: 2515–2523.

21. TULLIS, J. L. & F. A. BREEN. 1970. Christmas factor concentrates. The clinical use of several preparations. *In* Proceedings of the 5th Congress of the World Federation of Hemophilia, Montreal, 1968; Bibl. Haemat. **34**: 40–51. Karger. Basel.

22. GUILLIN, M. C., D. MENACHE, J. BARGE, B. RUEFF & R. FAUVERT. 1971. Les troubles de l'hemostase au cours des hepatites virales graves : Etude clinique, anatomique et biologique. Ann. Med. Int. **122**: 605–612.

23. CEDERBAUM, A. I. & H. R. ROBERTS. 1973. Complications of the use of prothrombin complex concentrates in liver disease. Clin. Res. **21**: 92A.

24. GAZZARD, B. G., M. L. LEWIS, G. ASH, C. R. RIZZA, E. BIDWELL & R. WILLIAMS. 1974. Coagulation factor concentrate in the treatment of the haemorrhagic diathesis of fulminant hepatic failure. Gut **15**: 993–998.

25. CEDERBAUM, A. I., P. M. BLATT & H. R. ROBERTS. 1976. Intravascular coagulation with use of human prothrombin complex concentrates. Ann. Int. Med. **84**: 683–687.

26. DAVEY, R. J., G. G. SHASHATY & C. E. RATH. 1976. Acute coagulopathy following infusion of prothrombin complex concentrates. Am. J. Med. **60**: 719–723.

27. MARASSI, A., V. MANZULLO, V. DI CARLO & P. M. MANNUCCI. 1978. Thromboembolism following prothrombin complex concentrates and major surgery in severe liver disease. Thromb. Haemostas. **39**: 787–788.

28. LOELIGER, E. A., A. HENSEN, M. J. MATTERN, J. J. VELTKAMP, P. F. BRUNNING & H. C. HEMKER. 1967. Treatment of haemophilia B with purified factor IX (PPSB). Folia Med. Neerl. **10**: 112–125.

29. KASPER, C. K. 1973. Postoperative thromboses in hemophilia B. N. Engl. J. Med. **289**: 160.

30. STEINBERG, M. H. & B. J. DREILING. 1973. Vascular lesions in hemophilia B. N. Engl. J. Med. **289**: 592.

31. EDSON, J. R. 1974. Prothrombin-complex concentrates and thromboses. N. Engl. J. Med. **290**: 403.

32. MARCHESI, S. L. & R. BURNEY. 1974. Prothrombin-complex concentrates and thromboses. N. Engl. J. Med. **290**: 403–404.

33. CAMPBELL, E. W., S. NEFF & A. J. BOWDLER. 1978. Therapy with factor IX concentrate resulting in DIC and thromboembolic phenomena. Transfusion **18**: 94–97.

34. RASCHE, H., H. BINDEWALD, W. KÖHLE, R. SCHECK, R. HEINRICH & K. SEIBERT. 1977. Emergency treatment of haemophilia A with factor VIII inhibitors using activated prothrombin complex concentrates. Dtsch. Med. Wochenschr. **102**: 319–323.

35. STEINBJERG, S. & J. JORGENSEN. 1977. Disseminated intravascular coagulation and infusion of factor-VIII-inhibitor bypassing activity. Lancet **1**: 360.

36. LUSCHER, J. M., S. S. SHAPIRO, J. E. PALASCAK, A. V. RAO, P. H. LEVINE, P. M. BLATT & THE HEMOPHILIA STUDY GROUP. 1980. Prothrombin complex concentrates in hemophiliacs with inhibitors. A multicenter therapeutic trial. N. Engl. J. Med. **303**: 421–425.

37. WESSLER, S., S. M. REIMER & M. C. SHEPS. 1959. Biologic assay of a thrombosis-inducing activity in human serum. J. Appl. Physiol. **14**: 943–946.

38. ARONSON, D. L. 1974. Inhibition of thrombotic effect of factor IX. N. Engl. J. Med. **290**: 861.

39. KINGDON, H. S., R. L. LUNDBLAD, J. J. VELTKAMP & D. L. ARONSON. 1975.

    Potentially thrombogenic materials in factor IX concentrates. Thromb. Diath. Haemorrh. **33:** 617–631.

40. CASH, J. D., R. OWENS, R. G. DALTON & R. J. PRESCOTT. 1978. Thrombogenicity of factor IX concentrates: *in vitro* and *in vivo* (rabbit) studies. Vox Sang. **35:** 105–110.

41. TRIANTAPHYLLOPOULOS, D. C. 1972. Intravascular coagulation following injection of prothrombin complex. Am. J. Clin. Path. **57:** 603–610.

42. PROWSE, C. V. & A. R. WILLIAMS. 1979. A non-stasis rabbit model for the detection of factor IX concentrate thrombogenicity. Thromb. Haemostas. **42:** 327.

43. CASH, J. D., R. G. DALTON, S. MIDDLEDON & J. K. SMITH. 1975. Studies on the thrombogenicity of Scottish factor IX concentrates in dogs. Thromb. Diath. Haemorrh. **33:** 632–639.

44. HEDNER, U., I. M. NILSSON & S.-E. BERGENTZ. 1976. Various prothrombin complex concentrates as demonstrated by cloting assays for factors IXa and Xa. Thromb. Res. **12:** 797–807.

45. HEDNER, U., I. M. NILSSON & S.-E. BERGENTZ. 1979. Studies on the thrombogenic activities in two prothrombin complex concentrates. Thromb. Haemostas. **42:** 1022–1032.

46. BLATT, P. M., R. L. LUNDBLAD, H. S. KINGDON, G. MCCLEAN & H. R. ROBERTS. 1974. Thrombogenic materials in prothrombin complex concentrates. Ann. Int. Med. **81:** 766–770.

47. KANG, E. P. & D. C. TRIANTAPHYLLOPOULOS. 1974. Intrinsic activation of prothrombin potentiated by celite and reduced by kaolin. Thromb. Diath. Haemorrh. **32:** 600–607.

48. WHITE, G. C., H. R. ROBERTS, H. S. KINGDON & R. L. LUNDBLAD. 1977. Prothrombin complex concentrates: Potentially thrombogenic materials and clues to the mechanism of thrombosis in vivo. Blood **49:** 159–170.

49. ELÖDI, S. & K. VARADI. 1978. Activation of clotting factors in prothrombin complex concentrates as demonstrated by clotting assays for factors IXa and Xa. Thromb. Res. **12:** 797–807.

50. HULTIN, M. B. 1979. Activated clotting factors in factor IX concentrates. Blood **54:** 1028–1038.

51. SELIGSOHN, U., C. K. KASPER, B. ØSTERUD & S. I. RAPAPORT. 1979. Activated factor VII: Presence in factor IX concentrates and persistence in the circulation after infusion. Blood **53:** 828–837.

52. CHANDRA, S. & M. WICKERHAUSER. 1979. Contact factors are responsible for the thrombogenicity of prothrombin complex. Thromb. Res. **14:** 189–198.

53. MAGNER, A. & D. ARONSON. 1979. Toxicity of factor IX concentrates in mice. Proceedings of International Symposium on Test Methods for the Quality Control of Plasma Proteins, 1979. Edited by the International Association of Biological Standardization. Developments in Biological Standardization **44:** 185–188. Karger, Basel.

54. SAS, G., R. E. OWENS, J. K. SMITH, S. MIDDLETON & J. D. CASH. 1975. *In vitro* spontaneous thrombin generation in human factor-IX concentrates. Br. J. Haematol. **31:** 25–35.

55. PEPPER, D. S., D. BANHEGYI, A. HOWIE & J. D. CASH. 1977. *In vitro* thrombogenicity tests of factor IX concentrates. Br. J. Haematol. **36:** 573–583.

56. PROWSE, C. V., D. S. PEPPER, J. D. CASH & M. PATTERSON. 1977. Thrombogenicity screening of factor IX concentrates. Thromb. Haemostas. **38:** 728–729.

57. PROWSE, C. V., A. CHIRNSIDE & R. A. ELTON. 1979. In vitro thrombogenicity tests of factor IX concentrates. 1. A survey of available assays. Thromb. Haemostas. **42:** 1355–1367.

58. BREEN, F. A. & J. L. TULLIS. 1969. Prothrombin concentrates in treatment of Christmas disease and allied disorders. J. Am. Med. Assoc. **208:** 1848–1852.

59. FEKETE, L. F., S. L. HOLST, F. PEETOOM & L. L. DE VEBER. 1972. "Auto" factor IX concentrate: A new therapeutic approach to treatment of hemophilia A patients with inhibitors (abstract 295). XIV Congress International Society of Haematology, Sao Paulo, Brazil.

60. KURCZYNSKI, E. M. & J. A. PENNER. 1974. Activated prothrombin concentrate for patients with factor VIII inhibitors. N. Engl. J. Med. **291:** 164–167.

61. ABILDGAARD, C. F., M. BRITTON & J. HARRISON. 1976. Prothrombin complex concentrates (Konȳne) in the treatment of hemophilic patients with factor VIII inhibitors. J. Pediat. **88:** 200–206.

62. BLATT, P. M., D. MENACHE & H. ROBERTS. 1980. A survey of the effectiveness of prothrombin complex concentrates in controlling hemorrhage in patients with hemophilia and anti-factor VIII antibodies. Thromb. Haemostas. **44:** 39–42.

63. LUSCHER, J. M., S. S. SHAPIRO, J. E. PALASCAK, A. V. RAO, P. H. LEVINE & P. M. BLATT. 1980. Prothrombin complex concentrates in treatment of hemophiliacs with Factor VIII inhibitors—A multicenter therapeutic trial. Clin. Res. **28**(2): 548A.

64. Proceedings of Workshop, "Activated Factor IX". National Institutes of Health, Bureau of Biologics, Bethesda, MD, April 27, 1979.

65. VERMYLEN, J., J. SCHETZ, N. SERMERARO, F. MERTENS & M. VERSTRAETE. 1978. Evidence that "activated" prothrombin concentrates enhance platelet coagulant activity. Br. J. Haematol. **38:** 235–242.

66. CASTALDI, P. A. & I. L. SMITH. 1980. The effect of platelets on the *in vitro* response to prothrombin complex concentrates in F.VIII inhibitor plasma. Pathology **12:** 111–118.

67. BLOOM, A. L. & R. D. HUTTON. 1975. Fresh-platelet transfusions in haemophilic patients with factor-VIII antibody. Lancet **2:** 369–370.

68. ALLAIN, J. P. & G. R. KRIEGER. 1975. Prothrombin-complex concentrate in treatment of classical haemophilia with factor-VIII antibody. Lancet **2:** 1203.

69. KELLY, P. & J. A. PENNER. 1976. Antihemophilic factor inhibitors. Management with prothrombin complex concentrates. J. Am. Med. Assoc. **236** (18): 2061–2064.

70. MANNUCCI, P. M., R. BADER & Z. M. RUGGERI. 1976. Concentrates of clotting-factor IX. Lancet **1:** 41.

71. BLATT, P. M., G. C. WHITE, II, C. W. MCMILLAN & H. R. ROBERTS. 1977. Treatment of anti-factor VIII antibodies. Thromb. Haemostas. **38:** 514–523.

72. PRESTON, F. E., R. C. W. DINSDALE, D. J. SUTCLIFE, G. BARDHAN, P. J. WYLD & J. F. HAMLYN. 1977. Factor VIII inhibitor by-passing activity (FEIBA) in the management of patients with factor VIII inhibitors. Thromb. Res. **11:** 643–651.

73. PRICE, D. A., S. D'SOUZA & H. EKERT. 1977. The use of non-activated prothrombin concentrate in the management of haemophilia A with factor VIII antibodies. Aust. N.Z. J. Med. **7:** 286–290.

74. STENBJERG, S. & J. JORGENSEN. 1977. Resistance to activated F IX concentrate (FEIBA). Scand. J. Haematol. **18:** 421–426.

75. BUCHANAN, G. R. & S. V. KEVY. 1978. Use of prothrombin complex concentrates in hemophiliacs with inhibitors: Clinical and laboratory studies. Pediatrics **62:** 767–774.

76. LECHNER, K., C. NOWOTNY, B. KRINNING, M. ZEGNER & E. DEUTSCH. 1978. Effect of treatment with activated prothrombin complex concentrate (FEIBA) on factor VIII-antibody level. Thromb. Haemostas. **40:** 478–485.

77. PARRY, D. H. & A. L. BLOOM. 1978. Failure of factor VIII inhibitor by-passing activity (FEIBA) to secure haemostasis in haemophilic patients with antibodies. J. Clin. Path. **31:** 1102–1105.

78. STENBJERG, S. & J. JORGENSEN. 1978. Activated factor IX concentrate (FEIBA) used in the treatment of haemophilic patients with antibody to F VIII. Acta Med. Scand. **203:** 471–476.

79. HESSELING, P. B. 1979. Inactivated Proplex for the haemophiliac with inhibitors. A case report. S.Afr. Med. J. **56:** 108–110.
80. KASPER, C. K. & THE HEMOPHILIA STUDY GROUP. 1979. Effect of prothrombin complex concentrates on factor VIII inhibitor levels. Blood **54:** 1358–1367.
81. ONDER, O. & L. W. HOYER. 1979. Factor VIII coagulant antigen in factor IX complex concentrates. Thromb. Res. **15:** 569–572.
82. KISIEL, W. 1978. Isolation and partial characterisation of human plasma protein C. Circulation **58:** 822.
83. DI SCIPIO, R. G., M. A. HERMODSON, S. G. YATES & E. W. DAVIE. 1977. A comparison of human prothrombin, factor IX (Christmas factor), factor X (Stuart factor), and protein S. Biochemistry **16:** 698–706.
84. SEEGERS, W. H., A. GHOSH & W. VAN-YU. 1979. Function of previously unrecognized plasma protein M in thrombin generation. *In* Vitamin K Metabolism and Vitamin K-Dependent Proteins. J. W. Suttie, Ed.: 96–101. University Park Press. Baltimore, MD.

PHARMACOLOGIC CONTROL OF BLOOD COAGULATION BY SYNTHETIC, LOW MOLECULAR WEIGHT INHIBITORS OF CLOTTING ENZYMES

F. Markwardt

Institute of Pharmacology and Toxicology
Medical Academy Erfurt
Erfurt, German Democratic Republic

The reaction principle of the clotting system consists of a successive activation of proenzymes to specific proteolytic enzymes. The sequence of enzyme reactions involves biologic amplification and feedback mechanisms. The inhibition of clotting enzymes represents an effective interference in this chain of reactions. At present, pharmacologic control of blood coagulation in this way is possible only with the aid of the mammalian acidic polysaccharide, heparin. This anticoagulant has certain disadvantages. Apart from needing parenteral administration, heparin exerts its inhibitory effect on the clotting enzymes indirectly via potentiation of the inhibitory function of antithrombin-III. Therefore, its inhibitory activity depends on the blood level of this plasma protein. Furthermore, heparin interacts with other blood constituents such as platelets, fibrinolytic components, and lipoproteinases.

The answer to the pharmacologic problem was seen as the development of selective inhibitors that block the clotting enzymes directly. We attempted initially to solve this problem by isolation and pharmacologic characterization of naturally occurring inhibitors from blood-sucking animals such as leeches, which produced the specific thrombin inhibitor, hirudin, a highly effective anticoagulant.[1] Because of difficulties in production, the use of these high molecular weight polypeptides was limited. A decisive advance was the development of synthetic, low molecular weight inhibitors of clotting enzymes, because such substances could find potential use as orally active, rapidly and directly acting anticoagulants.[2, 3] The inhibitors are also of importance in the biochemical analysis of the function and structure of clotting enzymes. They are especially employed as probes of the topographic differences between their active sites. The inhibitors are also used in affinity chromatography for enzyme isolation.

DESIGN OF INHIBITORS

The design of such inhibitors is based on the knowledge of the catalytic function of the clotting enzymes and particularly on the findings of the past several years on the structure of their active sites, which are the receptors for inhibitory drugs. Thus, the use of the inhibitors became possible, and studies on structure-activity relationships have allowed a goal-oriented synthesis of a new type of anticoagulant.

Thrombin and other enzymes of the clotting system, such as the activated clotting factors X, VII, IX and XII, belong to the group of trypsin-like serine-histidine proteinases. The specificity of the enzymes is achieved by the charac-

757

teristic structure of their substrate binding sites, in which these proteinases are built according to the same principle.

Imitating the amino acid arginine of natural and synthetic substrates, signifying the primary specificity, inhibitors can be produced that enter into a covalent or noncovalent bond with the active site of the enzymes (TABLE 1). Potent competitive inhibitors were found among the aliphatic and aromatic amines, guanidines, and amidines.[4] By estimating the inhibitors under the aspect of a possible anticoagulant effect, it could be shown that among the reversible competitive inhibitors of thrombin, the N_α-substituted arginine amides[5] and benzamidine derivatives[6,7] are most suitable for the chemical control of thrombin activity in the blood. The inhibitors are assumed to be fixed at the active site of the enzyme on the grounds of their structural relationships to the substrate. Quantitative structure-activity relationships of series of benzamidines[8] have shown that benzamidines with a carbonyl function occupy the specificity pocket and interact with the catalytic center via a tetrahedral arrangement. Hydrophobic residues are required for additional bond formation at one side of the specificity pocket. Benzamidines that possess a second basic group (bis-benzamidines) are assumed to interact with a secondary cationic binding site in this region.[6] Inhibitors that extend to both sides of the specificity pocket are the ω-amidinophenyl-α-aminoalkylcarboxylic acid amides and the N_α-substituted arginine amides. Structure-activity relationships showed that compounds of both series with a hydrophobic N_α-residue and a secondary cyclic amide component on the carboxyl group are particularly effective.[9]

Another type of inhibitor is the active-site-directed irreversible inhibitor. The reaction sequence involves the initial formation of a reversible enzyme-inhibitor complex which is converted into an irreversible one. The inhibitors are equipped with reactive groups that bind specifically to one of the amino acids at the active site of the enzymes, most commonly to either histidine or serine. It was shown that competitive inhibitors after combining with chemically reactive groups may be converted into inhibitors that form a stable covalent bond with the enzyme. Starting from the competitive inhibitor benzamidine, compounds with a reactive fluorosulfonyl moiety at the aromatic ring (4-amidino benzenesulfonyl fluorides) were obtained whose inhibitory effects on thrombin surpassed those of the organophosphates, which are commonly used as irreversible inhibitors of serine proteinases.[10] The velocity of inactivation by these compounds is so low that they are not able to prevent the effect of clotting enzymes in blood. Inhibitors are required to interfere with the immediately starting reaction of the clotting enzymes with the permanently present substrate. Therefore, the only inhibitors that are effective are those whose reaction rate equals or surpasses that of the enzyme-substrate reaction. The peptidyl-arginyl-chloromethanes[11] and the peptidyl argininals,[12] which have proved to be highly effective thrombin inhibitors, comply with these requirements.

The question arises which of the clotting enzymes should be inhibited in order to interfere most effectively with coagulation. Since the blockade of thrombin represents an effective interference, the studies on synthetic inhibitors were focused on their antithrombin effects. Thrombin initiates not only the formation of insoluble fibrin, but also further reactions that are of decisive importance in hemostasis and thrombosis. It activates the clotting factors required for prothrombin conversion and factor XIII, which stabilizes the fibrin clot formed. Moreover, it causes drastic changes in the permeability of platelet membrane followed by aggregation of platelets and the release of their biologically active components.

Besides thrombin, the other serine proteinases of the clotting system are considered points of attack of the synthetic inhibitors. In this context, factor Xa is of special interest. It plays a central role in coagulation since it is activated in either the intrinsic or extrinsic pathway. Only a few investigations have been made of the inhibition of factor Xa by synthetic compounds.[6, 13]

In order to judge the inhibitory effect, the fact that further arginine-specific serine proteinases exist in the blood, such as plasmin, serum kallikrein, and C_1-esterase, must be taken into account. In principle, they can also be inhibited.[14] However, investigations on the influence of synthetic inhibitors on these enzymes have shown that some of them possess a preference for one enzyme over another.[15-17] The different extent of inhibition is caused by topographic variation in the secondary binding sites of the various enzymes. On the basis of these facts, successful searches for selective inhibitors were made. Moreover, maps of the binding sites of the enzymes may be obtained from structure-activity relationship studies for series of chemically related inhibitors.

PHARMACOLOGY OF SYNTHETIC INHIBITORS

In order to evaluate the potential usefulness of synthetic inhibitors as anticoagulants, a special program of *in vitro* and *in vivo* investigations was established (TABLE 2). The first criterion for usefulness was the inhibitory activity measured in isolated enzyme-substrate systems and expressed as dissociation constants of the enzyme-inhibitor complex. In the case of representative inhibitors, these constants are in the range of 10^{-8} to 10^{-6} M and thus compare with the values for the naturally occurring inhibitors. The inhibitors of the mentioned groups interfere with the hydrolytic activity of thrombin in isolated enzyme-substrate systems as well as with its clotting function in blood. Their anticoagulant effect *in vitro* reaches or surpasses that of heparin and hirudin. To estimate the anticoagulant effect *in vivo*, different clotting variables were measured after intravenous and oral administration in experimental animals. The effect of the inhibitors *in vivo* depends decisively on their level in the blood since blood not only transports these drugs, but is also the site of their action, too. To assess the anticoagulant and antithrombotic effects of these inhibitors, *in vivo* investigations of the pharmacokinetics as well as pharmacotoxicologic examinations are necessary.

The antithrombotic effect of synthetic thrombin inhibitors was studied in experimental thrombosis in which the pathologic mechanism corresponds to that of arterial deposition thrombi and venous clotting thrombi in man. In experimental animals, lethal effects caused by thrombin infusion and the incidence of thrombosis induced by activation of the clotting system and by stasis of the jugular vein were prevented (TABLE 3).

The inhibitors were also effective in endotoxin- and thrombin-induced disseminated intravascular coagulation (DIC) (FIG. 1). The effect of synthetic inhibitors on DIC is of special interest. Studies on the pathogenesis of DIC have shown that activation of the clotting system and of other biochemical systems such as fibrinolysis, kininogenesis, and complement system has been triggered. In viewing these facts we must keep in mind that the benzamidine

TABLE 1

REPRESENTATIVE INHIBITORS OF THROMBIN

Compound (Type)	Moieties of Inhibitor Molecules Occupying the Binding Sites of the Enzyme *			
	C′	A	B	C″
Nα-dansyl-L-arginine 4-methylpiperidide (substituted arginine)				
Nα-tosyl-(4-amidinophenyl)- alanine piperidide (benzamidine derivative)				

H-D-Phe-Pro-Arg-H
(peptidyl argininal)

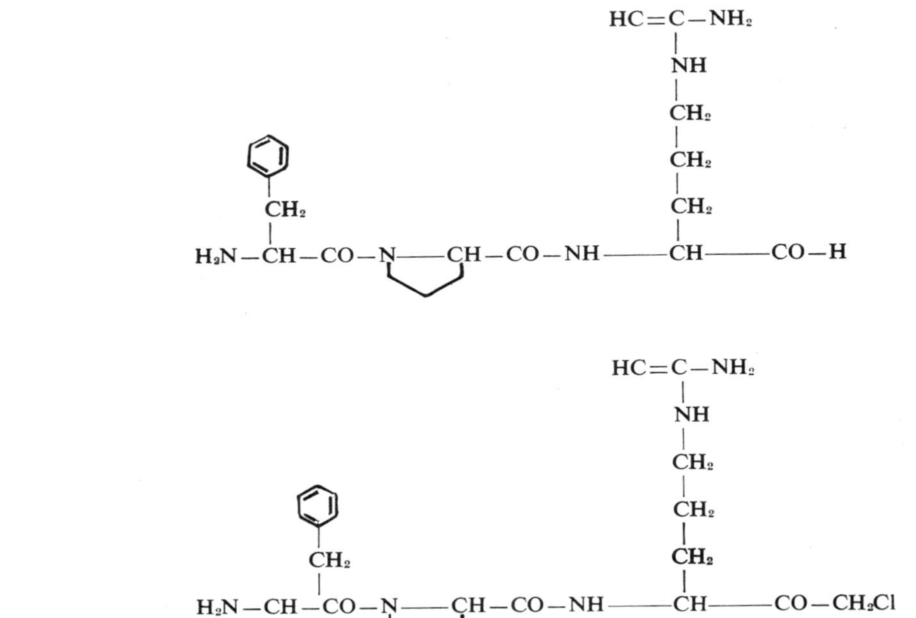

H-D-Phe-Pro-Arg-CH₂Cl
(peptidyl arginyl
chloromethane)

* A = specificity pocket; ionic and hydrophobic interactions. B = catalytic center; hydrogen bonds, tetrahedral arrangement. C', C" secondary binding sites; hydrogen bonds and van der Waals interactions.

TABLE 2

PHARMACOLOGIC SCREEN FOR THE DEVELOPMENT OF SYNTHETIC
INHIBITORS OF CLOTTING ENZYMES

	Subject	Procedure	Information
In vitro	Isolated enzymes	Biochemical methods: inhibition of enzyme activity	Type of inhibition, affinity, specificity, structure-activity relationship
	Blood or plasma	Coagulation tests: inhibition of enzyme function in blood in vitro and in vivo	Anticoagulant effect, dose-effect relationship
In vivo	Experimental animal	Pharmacotoxicologic standard methods, experimental thrombosis and disseminated intravascular coagulation	Tolerance, toxicity, pharmacodynamics, pharmacokinetics, antithrombotic effect

derivatives inhibit not only thrombin, but also other serine proteinases of the blood involved in DIC. This effect might contribute to the potency of the synthetic inhibitors in DIC.

Although in biochemical investigations a great number of highly potent thrombin inhibitors were found, only a few of them are currently under pre-clinical testing. Extensive studies were performed on the benzamidine derivative, 4-amidinophenylpyruvic acid, and this inhibitor has reached the state of clinical evaluation.[18] Furthermore, several N_α-substituted arginine amides and new benzamidine derivatives known as selective competitive thrombin inhibitors were tested for toxicity and anticoagulant effects *in vivo*.[5, 19]

TABLE 3

EFFECT OF N_α-TOSYL-(3-AMIDINOPHENYL)-ALANINE PIPERIDIDE ON
THROMBUS FORMATION IN RATS *

Infusion Rate ($mg \times kg^{-1} \times min^{-1}$)	Plasma Level ($\mu g/ml$)	Animals with Thrombi †
0.3	6.6	9
0.4	10.2	6
0.5	14.4	2

* Induced by systemic injection of heterologous serum followed by stasis of the juglar vein.

† Groups of ten each.

FINAL REMARKS

The objective of the development of synthetic inhibitors of clotting enzymes is to obtain alternatives to heparin and the oral anticoagulants, the coumarins. Pharmacologic studies have shown that blood coagulation *in vitro* and *in vivo* as well as intravascular thrombus formation is prevented by synthetic thrombin inhibitors. The differences from the known anticoagulants are apparent since the inhibitors are synthetic, low molecular weight compounds with a direct action and they can be administered orally. The development of such inhibitors leads to fundamental questions. In attempting clinical trials of the efficacy of synthetic thrombin inhibitors as antithrombotics we recognize that, so far, no anticoagulant with a similar mode of action has been introduced into clinical medicine. Therefore, it is difficult to determine dosages that will prevent thrombosis. Since the inhibitors are required to maintain constant levels in the blood after oral administration, their pharmacokinetics, particularly with

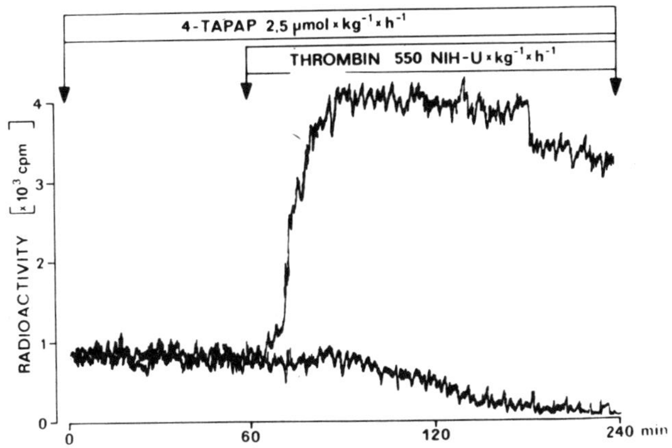

FIGURE 1. Prevention of thrombin-induced microthrombosis in rats by Nα-tosyl-(4-amidinophenyl)-alanine piperidide (4-TAPAP). Counts taken over the lung after injection of [^{125}I]fibrinogen indicate an increase in fibrin deposition.

regard to gastrointestinal absorption, must be improved. Finally, clinical trials have to be carried out to determine special indications for the use of synthetic inhibitors. Congenital and acquired antithrombin III deficiency might be such an indication.

It is concluded that certain synthetic inhibitors of clotting enzymes could play a major role in the treatment of thrombosis.

REFERENCES

1. MARKWARDT, F. 1970. Hirudin as an inhibitor of thrombin. *In* Methods in Enzymology. S. P. Colowick & N. O. Kaplan, Eds. Vol. **19:** 924–932. Academic Press. New York, N.Y.
2. LORAND, L. & J. L. G. NILSSON. 1972. Molecular approach for designing inhibitors to enzymes involved in blood clotting. *In* Drug Design. J. Ariens, Ed. Vol. **3:** 415–447. Academic Press. New York, NY.

3. MARKWARDT, F. 1974. Synthetic, low molecular thrombin inhibitors. A new concept of anticoagulants? Haemostasis **3:** 185–202.
4. MARKWARDT, F. & H. LANDMANN. 1971. Blutgerinnungshemmende Proteine, Peptide und Aminosäurederivate. *In* Handbuch der Experimentellen Pharmakologie. F. Markwardt, Ed. Vol. **27:** 76–142 (Anticoagulantien). Springer. Berlin.
5. HIJIKATA, A., S. OKAMOTO, E. MORI, K. KINJO, R. KIKUMOTO, S. TONOMURA, Y. TAMO & H. HARA. 1976. In vitro and in vivo studies of a new series of synthetic thrombin-inhibitors (OM-inhibitors). Thromb. Res. **8**(Suppl. II): 83–89.
6. GERATZ, J. D. & R. R. TIDWELL. 1978. Current concepts on action of synthetic thrombin inhibitors. Haemostasis **7:** 170–176.
7. MARKWARDT, F., H. LANDMANN & P. WALSMANN. 1968. Comparative studies on the inhibition of trypsin, plasmin and thrombin by derivatives of benzylamine and benzamidine. Eur. J. Biochem. **6:** 502–506.
8. STÜRZEBECHER, J., F. MARKWARDT, G. WAGNER & P. WALSMANN. 1976. Synthetische Hemmstoffe der Serinproteinasen. 13. Quantitative Struktur-Wirkungsbeziehungen bei der Hemmung von Trypsin, Plasmin und Thrombin durch 4-Amidinophenylverbindungen mit Ketonstruktur. Acta Biol. Med. Ger. **35:** 1665–1676.
9. MARKWARDT, F., G. WAGNER, J. STÜRZEBECHER & P. WALSMANN. 1979. Nα-Arylsulfonyl-ω-(4-amidinophenyl)-α-aminoalkylcarboxylic acid amides—novel selective inhibitors of thrombin. Thromb. Res. **17:** 425–431.
10. WALSMANN, P., M. RICHTER & F. MARKWARDT. 1972. Inaktivierung von Trypsin und Thrombin durch 4-Amidinobenzolsulfofluorid und 4-(2-Aminoäthyl)-benzolsulfofluorid. Acta Biol. Med. Ger. **28:** 577–585.
11. KETTNER, C. & E. SHAW. 1979. D-Phe-Pro-ArgCH$_2$Cl—a selective affinity label for thrombin. Thromb. Res. **14:** 969–973.
12. BAJUSZ, S., E. BARABÁS, P. TOLNAY, E. SZÉLL & D. BAGDY. 1978. Inhibition of thrombin and trypsin by tripeptide aldehyde. Int. J. Pept. Protein Res. **12:** 217–221.
13. STÜRZEBECHER. J., F. MARKWARDT & P. WALSMANN. 1976. Synthetic inhibitors of serine proteinases. XIV. Inhibition of factor Xa by derivatives of benzamidine. Thromb. Res. **9:** 637–646.
14. MARKWARDT, F. 1977. Pharmacological control of hyperproteolytic states in blood by enzyme inhibitors. Acta Biol. Med. Ger. **36:** 1855–1861.
15. HAUPTMANN, J. & F. MARKWARDT. 1977. Inhibition of the haemolytic complement activity by derivatives of benzamidine. Biochem. Pharmacol. **26:** 325–329.
16. MARKWARDT, F., Ed. 1978. Handbuch der Experimentellen Pharmakologie. Vol. **46:** Fibrinolytics and Antifibrinolytics. Springer. Berlin.
17. MARKWARDT, F., J. DRAWERT & P. WALSMANN. 1974. Synthetic low molecular weight inhibitors of serum kallikrein. Biochem. Pharmacol. **23:** 2247–2256.
18. MARKWARDT, F. & H.-P. KLÖCKING. 1972. The antithrombotic effect of synthetic thrombin inhibitors. Thromb. Res. **1:** 243–252.
19. HAUPTMANN, J., B. KAISER, F. MARKWARDT & G. NOWAK. 1980. Anticoagulant and antithrombotic action of novel specific inhibitors of thrombin. Thromb. Haemostas. **43:** 118–123.

INHIBITION OF SERINE PROTEASES BY LOW MOLECULAR WEIGHT PEPTIDES AND THEIR DERIVATIVES

Jawed Fareed, Harry L. Messmore, Gisela Kindel,
and John U. Balis

Departments of Pathology, Pharmacology and Medicine
Loyola University Medical Center
Maywood, Illinois 60153; and
Department of Pathology
University of South Florida
Tampa, Florida 33612

INTRODUCTION

During the past decade considerable progress has been made in understanding the molecular mechanisms by which the coagulation, fibrinolytic, and kallikrein pathways are regulated, and in defining their relationship to the generation of serine protease enzymes and low molecular weight peptides with bioregulatory functions. TABLE 1 shows the role of various serine proteases in the regulation of blood coagulation, fibrinolytic, kallikrein, and complement-mediated pathways. The coagulation cascade is now known to be a complex network of serine protease zymogens and their activators and inhibitors. In this network the clotting, fibrinolytic, kallikrein, and complement enzymes interact to regulate such crucial functions as hemodynamics, hemostasis, and immune responses.[1-5] FIGURE 1 illustrates the interaction of the coagulation and fibrinolytic enzymes with the kallikrein and complement systems. Most of the active enzymes involved in this cascade mimic trypsin in their ability to cleave certain amide bonds and are classified as serine proteases. Certain basic amino acid esters and amides are therefore used as substrates to determine their activities.[6-10] The application of synthetic peptide substrates to coagulation testing is discussed extensively elsewhere in this volume. While working on the determination of plasma prekallikrein and kallikrein, employing the synthetic peptide substrates chromozym PK (Bz-Pro-Phe-Arg-pNA) and S-2302 (H-D-Pro-Phe-Arg-pNA), we found that these substrates strongly antagonized the bradykinin-induced contraction of isolated guinea pig ileum and rat uterus.[11] We therefore modified the amino and carboxy terminals of these peptides in order to study the structure-activity relationship. A detailed account of the synthesis of low molecular weight peptide analogs of bradykinin was reported earlier.[12] While developing various chromogenic peptide derivatives, the Scandinavian groups have synthesized many structural variant forms of peptide substrates for numerous serine proteases. Some of these peptides and their derivatives are listed in TABLE 2. We screened the antiserine protease actions of these peptides on clotting and amidolytic assays and found that some of these peptides are relatively specific inhibitors of thrombin, factor Xa, and glandular kallikrein.[13-15] These studies prompted us to evaluate the naturally occurring low molecular weight peptides with arginine and lysine at the carboxyl terminal and their derivatives for any modulating effects on serine protease

765

TABLE 1

SERINE PROTEASES AND THEIR ROLE IN PHARMACOLOGY, PATHOLOGY, AND
PHYSIOLOGY OF HEMOSTASIS AND RELATED SYSTEMS

System	Enzyme	Inhibitors	Physiology	Pathology	Pharmacology
Blood coagulation	Thrombin, trypsin coagulation factors: VIIa, IXa, Xa, XIa, XIIa, XIIIa	AT-III, Anti-factors α_1-AT	Hemostasis	Thrombosis, hyper-coagulation	Anticoagulants, antithrombotics
Fibrinolysis	Plasmin, plasmin-ogen activators	α_2-macroglobulin, antiplasmins, other inhibitors	Regulation of fibrinolysis	DIC, primary and secondary fibrinolysis	Antifibrinolytics (EACA, etc), hemostyptics
Kallikrein-kinin	Kallikrein	Antikallikreins	Regulation of hemodynamics	Shock, inflammation	Antishock drugs, antiphlogistics
Complement pathways (C_1'-esterase)	Mediation of immune reactions	Anticomplements	Mediation of immune complex disease	Anticomplement action	Immunosuppressive agents

enzymes and related systems. Numerous other derivatives of these peptides were also synthesized by conventional methods and were evaluated in standard systems.

It has been reported that a low molecular weight peptide isolated from plasmin-digested products of bovine fibrinogen markedly elevated the partial thromboplastin time.[16, 17] Takagi and coworkers reported on the anticoagulant activity of low molecular weight peptides obtained from human fibrinogen degradation by plasmin.[18] Uszyski described the anticoagulant action of a peptide isolated from human placental homogenates.[19] Bajusz and coworkers have also reported on the inhibitory effect of certain peptide aldehydes on thrombin and trypsin.[20] Many investigators have synthesized the arginine analog of natural and synthetic substrates of thrombin to develop potential anticoagulant drugs. Aliphatic and aromatic amines, quinidines, and amidines have been found to be strong inhibitors of the thrombin-fibrinogen reactions

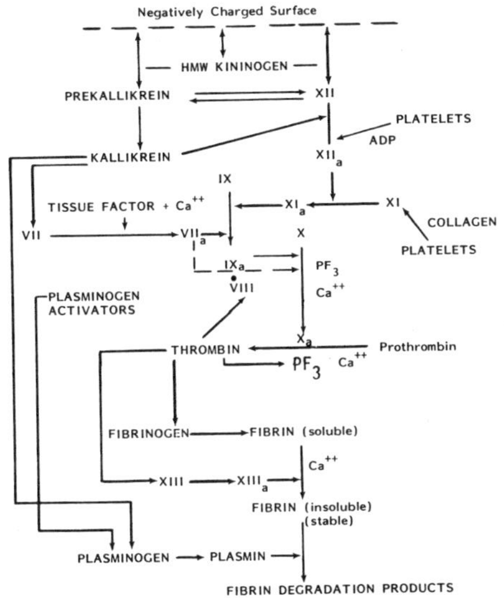

FIGURE 1. Present status of coagulation cascade. Interaction between kallikrein and plasminogen is also illustrated.

and certain serine proteases.[21–25] *N*-α-dansylarginine amide developed by Okamoto and coworkers is a competitive inhibitor of thrombin.[26] New derivatives of benzamidine (*N*-α-arylsulfonyl-ω-amidinophenyl-α-aminoalkyl-carboxylic acid amides) have been found to be highly potent inhibitors of thrombin.[27] In a recent report Tidwell and coworkers identified 1, 2-di(5-amidino-2-benzyfuranyl) ethane (DABE) as a preferential inhibitor of bovine factor Xa and α, α′-bis (4-amidino-2-iodophenoxy) *p*-xylene as a selective inhibitor of human thrombin.[28]

Materials and Methods

Peptide Substrates and Inhibitors

Specific synthetic chromogenic substrates for various serine protease enzymes were obtained from Kabi, Inc. (Greenwich, CT), Abbott Laboratories

TABLE 2

CHEMICAL STRUCTURE OF VARIOUS SYNTHETIC PEPTIDE SUBSTRATES

S-2166	H-Phe-Arg-pNA
S-2446	H-D-Phe-Phe-Arg-NHiPR
S-2447	H-D-Phe-Phe-Arg-NH-C_6H_{11}
S-2448	H-D-Phe-Phe-Arg-NH_2
S-2455	H-D-Phe-Phe-Arg-NH-heptyl
S-2456	H-D-Pro-Phe-Arg-OiPR
S-2457	H-D-Pro-Phe-Arg-NH-lauryl
S-2462	H-Arg-O-heptyl
S-2325	H-D-Val-Phe-Arg-pNA
S-2320	H-D-Pip-Phe-Arg-pNA
S-2354	H-D-Val-Leu-Arg-Ser-pNA
S-2261	H-L-Pro-Phe-Arg-pNA
S-2249	Bz-L-Pro-Phe-Arg-pNA
S-2171	Bz-Phe-Phe-Arg-pNA
S-2404	pyro-Glu-Phe-Arg-pNA
S-2168	H-Phe-Phe-Arg-pNA
S-2385	H-D-Phe-Phe-Arg-pNA
S-2432	H-D-Phe-Tyr-Arg-pNA
S-2316	H-D-Pro-Phe-Lys-pNA
S-2390	H-D-Val-Phe-Lys-pNA
S-2429	Bz-Glu-Phe-Arg-pNA
S-2434	H-D-Gln-Tyr-Arg-pNA
S-2436	H-Pro-Phe-Arg-OH
S-2437	H-Pro-Phe-Arg-OH·2HCl
S-2438	H-Ser-Pro-Phe-Arg-OH·2HCl
S-2439	H-Phe-Ser-Pro-Phe-Arg-OH
S-2440	H-D-Pro-Phe-Arg-O-heptyl
S-2441	H-D-Pro-Phe-Arg-NH-heptyl
S-2442	H-D-Pro-Phe-D-Arg-OH·2HCl
S-2443	H-D-Pro-Phe-Arg-NH_2·2HCl
Chromozym-TH	Tos or CBz-Gly-Pro-Arg-pNA
S-2160	Bz-Phe-Val-Arg-pNA
S-2238	H-D-Phe-Pip-Arg-pNA
Abbott "?"	H-Gly-Pro-Arg-pNA
S-2222	Bz-Ile-Glu(γ-OR)-Gly-Arg-pNA
S-2237	Bz-Ile-Glu(γ-O-Piperidyl)-Gly-Arg-pNA
S-2251	H-D-Val-Leu-Lys-pNA
Chromozym-P	Tos-Gly-Pro-Lys-pNA
S-2322	H-D-Val-Gly-Arg-pNA
S-2302	H-D-Pro-Phe-Arg-pNA
Chromozym-PK	Bz-Pro-Phe-Arg-pNA
S-2266	H-D-Val-Leu-Arg-pNA
Chromozym-UK	Bz-Val-Gly-Arg-pNA
S-2444	Pyro-Glu-Gly-Arg-pNA
Chromozym-Try (2)	H-D-Val-Gly-Arg-pNA
	Cbo-Val-Gly-Arg-pNA

NOTE: Peptides with a suffix S were obtained from Kabi Peptide Group, Molndal, Sweden, whereas substrates of the chromozym series were obtained from Pentapharm, Basel, Switzerland.

(North Chicago, IL), and Pentapharm (Basel, Switzerland) and were a generous gift from Drs. Lars Melstam and Goran Claeson of Peptide Research Group Kabi AB (Molndal, Sweden). All of the chromogenic substrates were obtained in powdered form and a stock solution of 2.5×10^{-3} M was prepared in sterile distilled water, except for S-2160 where only a 10^{-3} M concentration was used. All solutions were kept at $4°$ C for periods of up to 3 months. All of the derivatives of synthetic peptides listed in TABLE 2 were obtained from Kabi AB and Pentapharm AG and were dissolved to make a 1×10^{-3} M solution. Fluorogenic peptide substrates were obtained from Peninsula Laboratories (San Carlos, CA). Most of these were kept frozen at $-70°$ C for periods of up to 1 year and thawed at room temperature prior to use.

Kinin-related peptides such as kassanin, ranatensin, xenopsin and litorin, and bombesin and their analogs, basic peptides such as tuftsin, IgE peptide III, liver cell growth factor, contraceptive tetrapeptide, proctolin, leupeptin, antipain, and chymostatin were purchased from Peninsula Laboratories. Polybasic amino acids such as polylysine and polyarginine were purchased from Sigma Chemical Co. (St. Louis, MO). Analogs of D-Phe-Pro-Arg-OH, D-Phe-Pro-Arg-NH$_2$, D-Phe-Phe-Arg-NH$_2$, D-Phe-Phe-Arg-OH, and Val-Leu-Lys-COOH were synthesized by Peninsula Laboratories. The tripeptide aldehydes H-D-Phe-Pro-Arg-H and Boc-D-Phe-Pro-Arg-H were a gift from Dr. S. Bajsuz of the Research Institute for Pharmaceutical Chemistry (Budapest, Hungary). Serine protease enzymes and molecular variants of human thrombins were a gift from Dr. John Fenton, II (New York State Department of Health, Albany, NY). Commercially available lyophilized human thrombin (Fibrindex) was purchased from Ortho Diagnostics, (Raritan, NJ). Bovine factor Xa preparations were purchased from Sigma Chemical Co. and from Diagnostic Reagent (Oxon Thame, England). Human plasmin was purchased from Kabi, Inc., and was a gift from Dr. K. Robbins of Michael Reese Hospital (Chicago, IL). Glandular kallikrein preparations were obtained from Dr. G. Haberland of Bayer Leverkusen (West Germany) and were also purchased from Sigma Chemical Co. Factor XIIa and plasma kallikrein were gifts from Dr. J. J. Pisano of the National Institutes of Health (Bethesda, MD). Trypsin was obtained from the Sigma Chemical Co. and urokinase (Abbokinase) from Abbott Laboratories.

Blood Plasma

Venous blood from 10 healthy male and female subjects (five in each group) was collected by the standard double-syringe venipuncture method in 3.8 percent sodium citrate (9 volumes of blood with 1 volume of anticoagulant) and centrifuged at $2500 \times g$ for 15 minutes and the plasma was removed. In all studies, freshly prepared plasma was used.

Reagents for Clotting Assays

Thromboplastin-C for the prothrombin time and Actin brand of activator cephaloplastin reagent for activated partial thromboplastin time were obtained from American Dade (Miami, FL). Thromboquik® bovine thrombin reagent for thrombin time was obtained from General Diagnostics (Morris Plains, NJ). A commercially available kit for prekallikrein quantitation was obtained from Diagnostica Stago (Ansiers, France).

Amidolytic Assays for Serine Protease Enzymes and Their Inhibitors

A stock solution of each serine protease enzyme was prepared in terms of assigned units/ml (for example, NIH u/ml for thrombin, Denson units for Xa, CTA units for plasmin, and TAME units for trypsin) and stored at 4° C for periods of up to 8 hours. 0.1 ml of the active enzyme was incubated with 0.7 ml of specific buffer and mixed and equilibrated at 37° C for 1 minute, and the inhibitor peptide was added at different concentrations (10^{-4}–10^{-6} M) and mixed well, and ΔA_{405}/min was measured in a recording spectrophotometer. The degree of inhibition was calculated by comparing the ΔA_{405}/min of the control enzyme with the one obtained in the presence of inhibitor.

Dextran-activated plasma amidolytic activity assay to evaluate the pre-kallikrein and factor XIIa was performed by a modified method described previously.[29]

In data analysis, where K_i values were required, kinetic variables were obtained by plotting the reciprocals of the initial reaction velocity at two different concentrations against different inhibitor concentrations.[30]

Coagulant Assays

Normal human pooled plasma was supplemented with various amounts (1–100 μg/ml) of test peptides, mixed and incubated at 37° C for 30 minutes, and tested in the prothrombin time (PT), activated partial thromboplastin time (APTT), and thrombin time (TT) assays using standard procedures.[31]

To measure the fibrinogen clotting time, 40, 80, and 100 mg/dl buffered fibrinogen solutions, supplemented with test peptides, were assayed by thrombin time test using 5, 10 and 20 NIH u/ml human thrombin.

Anti-Xa activity was measured using anticoagulant free bovine plasma reagent and a modified Xa assay.[32]

The effect of various peptides on euglobulin clot lysis time was measured by adding various amounts of peptides to the euglobulin fraction prepared by standard methods.[33, 34] Plasminogen activator assays were performed employing a simple method described by Conrad.[35]

RESULTS

Initially we screened the effect of various synthetic peptides on the routine coagulant assays such as those of activated partial thromboplastin time (APTT), prothrombin time (PT), and thrombin time (TT). TABLE 3 shows that peptides with H-D-Phe-Pro-Arg- sequence produced some prolongation of these variables, suggesting that these peptides inhibit some of the steps in the extrinsic and intrinsic pathways. TABLE 4 shows the effect of various tripeptides on coagulant assays. Of all the seven tripeptides studied, only D-Phe-Pro-Arg-OH produced prolongation of the APTT, TT, and recalcification time, suggesting that the amino acid sequence D-Phe-Pro-Arg- is necessary for their anticoagulant effects. Only weaker anticoagulant effects were observed with D-Phe-Phe-Arg-OH. TABLE 5 surveys the inhibitory activities of various D-Phe-Pro-Arg-derivatives. All of these peptide derivatives were found to possess varying inhibitory actions on the amidolytic and coagulant properties of thrombin, although they showed other effects as well. D-Phe-Pro-Arg-OH and D-Phe-Pro-

TABLE 3

EFFECTS OF VARIOUS PEPTIDES ON COAGULANT ASSAYS

Peptide	PT	APTT	TT
H-D-Phe-Phe-Arg-NHiPR	↑	↑	↑
H-D-Phe-Phe-Arg-NHC$_6$H$_{11}$	↑	↑	↑
H-D-Phe-Phe-Arg-NH$_2$	−	−	−
H-D-Phe-Pro-Arg-NH-heptyl	↑	↑	↑
H-D-Phe-Pro-Arg-COOH	↑	↑	↑
H-D-Pro-Arg-NH-lauryl	−	−	−
H-Arg-O-heptyl	−	−	−
H-Pro-Phe-Arg-OH·2HCl	−	−	−
H-Ser-Pro-Phe-Arg-OH·2HCl	−	−	−
H-Phe-Ser-Pro-Phe-Arg-OH·	−	−	↑
H-D-Pro-Phe-Arg-O-heptyl·	↑	↑	↑
H-D-Pro-Phe-Arg-NH-heptyl·	↑	↑	↑
H-D-Pro-Phe-D-Arg-OH·2HCl	−	−	−
H-D-Pro-Phe-Arg-NH$_2$·2HCl	−	−	−

NOTE: ↑=prolongation; −=no effect; PT=prothrombin time; APTT=activated partial thromboplastin time; TT=thrombin time.
All peptides were tested at 10 μg/ml final concentration in normal human plasma.

TABLE 4

SCREENING OF THE ANTICOAGULANT ACTION OF VARIOUS PEPTIDES

Peptide	PTT	TT (5 NIH units)	Recall Time
D-Pro-Phe-Arg-COOH	36.7	11.9	280
D-Phe-Pro-Arg-COOH	57.9	29.8	>500
D-Phe-Phe-Arg-COOH	37.3	11.8	390
D-Pro-Pro-Arg-COOH	38.7	12.8	290
D-Pro-Phe-Lys-COOH	37.5	11.7	280
D-Pro-D-Phe-Lys-COOH	35.1	12.9	310
D-His-Phe-COOH	35.3	13.0	360
Control	34.6	12.8	280

NOTE: PTT=partial thromboplastin time. All peptides were added to freshly drawn normal human plasma at a 50 μg/ml. Routine methods were used to evaluate the effect of these peptides.

TABLE 5

STRUCTURE-ACTIVITY RELATIONSHIP OF THE PEPTIDE INHIBITORS

Structure		Activity
D-Phe-Pro-Arg-COOH	($> \mu M$)	Mild inhibitor of serine proteases
D-Phe-Pro-Arg-NH$_2$	($> \mu M$)	Mild inhibitor of serine proteases
D-Phe-Pro-arginal	($< \mu M$)	Potent inhibitor of serine proteases
D-Phe-Pro-Arg-S-CH$_2$-C$_6$H$_5$	($< \mu M$)	Potent antiplatelet agent
D-Phe-Pro-Arg-NH-heptyl	($> \mu M$)	Potent inhibitor of kallikreins
D-Phe-Pro-Arg-O-heptyl	($> \mu M$)	Potent inhibitor of kallikreins
D-Phe-Pro-Arg-lactam	($< \mu M$)	Potent inhibitor of serine proteases

Arg-NH$_2$ at submicromolar levels showed only weak inhibitory actions toward thrombin and trypsin, but D-Phe-Pro-arginal showed a very potent activity towards thrombin ($K_i = <10^{-7} M$). H-D-Phe-Pro-Arg-S-CH$_2$-C$_6$H$_5$ produced a strong inhibition of platelet aggregation by arachidonic acid and thrombin. D-Phe-Pro-Arg-NH-heptyl and D-Phe-Pro-Arg-O-heptyl derivatives produced varying degrees of inhibition of glandular and plasma kallikreins, whereas D-Phe-Pro-Arg-lactam produced a strong inhibition of serine proteases such as thrombin and trypsin. However, the potency of this inhibitor was much weaker than that observed for D-Phe-Pro-arginal.

In our studies we found that H-D-Pro-Phe-Arg-NH-heptyl was also an active inhibitor of some serine proteases and possessed some other pharmacologic properties. TABLE 6 summarizes some of these properties of this peptide. Since we reported on the inhibitory properties of this peptide on smooth muscle contractile activity [11] in various isolated tissue preparations, properties which were thought to be due to inhibition of serine protease enzymes, studies were undertaken on isolated serine protease system. At a submicromolar level this peptide was found to inhibit glandular kallikrein, trypsin, and XIIa. TABLE 7

TABLE 6

SOME PROPERTIES OF H-D-PRO-PHE-ARG-NH-HEPTYL

Pharmacologic
Inhibits the smooth muscle contractile action of bradykinin and angiotensins on the isolated guinea pig ileum and rat uterus preparation.
Inhibits the oxytocic actions of oxytocin, vasopressin, pituitrin, and their derivatives.
Inhibits the spontaneous contractions of the isolated rat uterus.

Biochemical
Inhibits glandular kallikrein ($K_i = < 10^{-6}$).
Inhibits trypsin.
Inhibits XIIa.

shows a composite of the serine protease inhibitory spectrum of various synthetic peptide derivatives. All of these substrates were tested at the μM level. Although varying inhibitory actions were produced by some of the peptides listed in TABLE 7, certain peptides showed specific inhibitory actions toward one enzyme. For example, S-2455 (H-D-Phe-Arg-NH-heptyl) and related peptides produced strong inhibition of bovine Xa activity, whereas S-2441 (H-D-Pro-Phe-Arg-NH-heptyl) was found to be a strong inhibitor of glandular kallikrein. Other peptides were found to produce varying degrees of inhibition of plasmin, plasma kallikrein, Hageman fragment, and thrombin. FIGURE 2 shows the effect of various H-D-Phe-Phe-Arg- derivatives on the amidolytic action of bovine Xa using a peptide substrate (H-D-Val-Gly-Arg-pNA). All of the peptides studied produced varying degrees of inhibition of factor Xa, although S-2455 (H-D-Phe-Phe-Arg-NH-heptyl) produced the strongest inhibition of this enzyme. At a higher substrate concentration, a lesser inhibition of the amidolytic action of Xa was observed. These data are suggestive of some competitive mechanisms involved in producing this inhibition.

TABLE 7

SERINE PROTEASE INHIBITORY SPECTRUM OF VARIOUS SYNTHETIC PEPTIDES
AS STUDIED ON AMIDOLYTIC ASSAYS USING PURIFIED ENZYMES

Substrate	X_a	Trypsin	Plasmin	Glandular Kallikrein	Plasma Kallikrein	Hageman Fragment	Thrombin
S-2447	42	30	19	—	—	—	15
S-2443	—	36	13	30	—	—	66
S-2435	—	21	20	—	—	—	—
S-2442	—	49	5	—	—	—	35
S-2171	—	10	—	—	—	—	—
S-2446	54	21	23	—	—	—	—
S-2440	—	3	8	—	32%	—	14
S-2441	—	31	7	71%	—	—	14
S-2456	—	36	—	—	—	60	—
S-2438	—	19	11	—	—	—	—
S-2448	42	5	11	—	—	—	—
S-2439	—	26	30	—	—	—	—
S-2455	57	—	—	—	—	—	—
S-2457	—	9	40	—	—	—	—
CBZ-GLY-Pro-Arg-MNA	—	10	36	—	—	—	—
TFA-D-Val-Leu-Lys	—	10	36	—	—	—	—
TFA-D-Pho-Arg-Try	—	40	19	—	—	30	—
S-2430	2	—	—	—	—	—	90

NOTE: All synthetic peptides were screened at a 10^{-6} *M* concentration.

TABLE 8 summarizes the antithrombotic and anticoagulant actions of H-D-Phe-Pro-arginal and Boc-D-Phe-Pro-arginal. Both of these peptides produced a strong anticoagulant action when studied by routine assays. Supplementation of whole blood (human) with 5 µg/ml peptides produced marked prolongation of the clotting time; APTT, PT, and TT were also prolonged. Factors XI and XII were also suppressed. Furthermore, dextran-activated amidolytic activity was inhibited by this peptide. Both of these peptides produced a marked inhibition of thrombin-induced aggregation of platelets, they had only weaker inhibi-

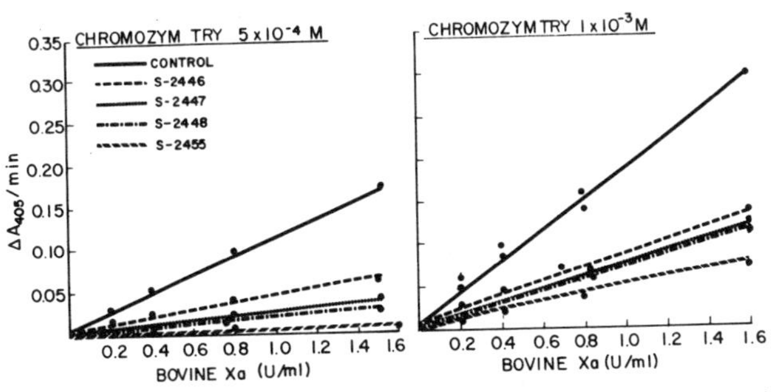

FIGURE 2. Inhibition of the amidolysis of H-D-Val-Gly-Arg-pNA (chromozym TRY) by synthetic peptide analogs of H-D-Phe-Phe-Arg-NH₂. (pH 8.4, 0.05 *M* Tris HCl buffer, 37° C.).

TABLE 8

A SUMMARY OF ANTITHROMBOTIC-ANTICOAGULANT ACTIONS OF H-D-PHE-PRO-ARG-H
AND BOC-H-D-PHE-PRO-ARG-H

Assays	H-D-Phe-Pro-Arg-H	Boc-D-Phe-Pro-Arg-H
Whole blood clotting time (< 5 μg/ml)	Prolonged	Prolonged
APTT (< 5 μg/ml)	Prolonged	Prolonged
PT (< 5 μg/ml)	Prolonged	Prolonged
TT (<5 μg/ml)	Prolonged	Prolonged
Factor XI (< 5 μg/ml)	Suppressed	Suppressed
Factor XII (< 5 μg/ml)	Suppressed	Suppressed
Dextran-activated amidolytic activity	Suppressed	Suppressed
Euglobulin lysis time (5 μg/ml)	Suppressed	Suppressed
Platelet aggregation		
Thrombin (< 5 μg/ml)	Inhibited	Inhibited
Arachidonic acid (< 5 μg/ml)	No action	No action
ADP (< 10 μg/ml)	Weak inhibition	Weak inhibition
Ristocetin ($<$ μg/ml)	No action	No action

tory actions on ADP and ristocetin-induced aggregation of human platelets.
TABLE 9 shows the inhibitory characteristics of these two peptide arginals for
various serine protease enzymes. All results presented in this Table were
obtained by amidolytic assays. Both of these peptides possessed broad-spectrum
inhibitory activity. Boc-D-Phe-Pro-Arginal appears to be a stronger inhibitor of
serine proteases, which suggests that the presence of Boc grouping may influence
the inhibitory properties of a peptide. Thrombin, Xa and trypsin were strongly
inhibited, whereas varying degrees of inhibition of other serine proteases was
observed. The inhibitory concentration at which 50 percent of the enzymatic
activity was reduced was designated as $(I)_{50}$ and was calculated using a plot
method for both of these peptides.

TABLE 9

INHIBITION OF VARIOUS SERINE PROTEASE BY H-H-PHE-PRO-ARG-H
AND BOC-D-PHE-PRO-ARG-H

Enzyme	H-D-Phe-Pro-Arg-H $(I)_{50}$*	Boc-D-Phe-Pro-Arg-H $(I)_{50}$
Thrombin (Human α)	$5.0 \times 10^{-7}\,M$	$4.0 \times 10^{-7}\,M$
Bovine Xa	$2.0 \times 10^{-6}\,M$	$3.2 \times 10^{-7}\,M$
Plasmin	$2.0 \times 10^{-6}\,M$	$1.0 \times 10^{-6}\,M$
† Kallikrein (plasma)	2.0×10^{-5}	1.6×10^{-5}
† Kallikrein (glandular)	1.0×10^{-5}	8.0×10^{-7}
† Urokinase	1.0×10^{-6}	7.5×10^{-7}
† SK-Plasminogen complex	2×10^{-6}	$1.3 \times 10^{-6}\,M$
† Trypsin	1×10^{-7}	6.1×10^{-8}
† XIIa	1.5×10^{-6}	1.0×10^{-6}

* The concentration of peptides at which 50 percent of the enzymatic activity was
inhibited is designated as $(I)_{50}$ and was calculated by a plot method.

† All enzymes were found to be inhibited at varying levels of $(I)_{50}$ and the K_i is to
be calculated.

NOTE: The data presented in this table are obtained using amidolytic assays.

TABLE 10 shows the inhibitory action of another arginal peptide, leupeptin, on fibrinogen clotting by thrombin and the activated partial thromboplastin time of normal human citrated plasma. This peptide produced a prolongation of thrombin time when added in varying amounts to buffered fibrinogen substrate, suggesting that the coagulant activity of thrombin is inhibited. This effect was concentration-dependent and was observed at two different concentrations of thrombin. Supplementation of NHP with this peptide also produced a prolongation of APTT, although this effect was not as pronounced as the one observed with thrombin times. TABLE 11 shows the data on the inhibition of trypsin by leupeptin and antipain. Both of these peptides produced strong inhibition of trypsin, but antipain produced a much stronger effect.

TABLE 12 shows the inhibitory spectrum of various lysine- and arginine-containing peptides and leupeptin on the amidolytic action of thrombin and plasmin. Contraceptive peptide (Thr-Pro-Arg-Lys-COOH) was found to inhibit plasmin, but have no effect on thrombin. Leupeptin inhibited the actions of both thrombin and plasmin. All of the other peptides showed no significant

TABLE 10

EFFECT OF LEUPEPTIN ON THROMBIN'S COAGULANT ACTION ON FIBRINOGEN AND
APTT OF NORMAL HUMAN PLASMA

Concentration (μg/ml)	Thrombin Times (FIB)		APTT (NHP)
	(5 NIH units)	(10 NIH units)	
100	>100	>100	75.8
50	>100	92.2	46.6
25	105.2	62.5	40.4
12.5	71.9	42.4	36.8
6.25	53.9	32.6	34.1
3.25	46.2	26.4	31.3
0	17.4	26.5	30.8

NOTE: Thrombin times were determined on buffered fibrinogen (80 mg/dl IMCO) supplemented with varying amounts of leupeptin, whereas APTT was determined on fresh citrated normal human plasma supplemented with leupeptin.

inhibitory activity. TABLE 13 shows the effect of Val-Leu-Lys-analogs on the plasmin-supplemented englobulin lysis time. Euglobulin fraction obtained from normal human plasma was clotted with thrombin and supplemented with these peptides at 10 μg/ml, and 100 μl of a 10-caseinolytic unit plasmin was added to this mixture and the lysis time was noted. H-D-Val-Leu-Lys-NH-heptyl produced a marked prolongation of the euglobulin lysis clot, whereas D-Val-Leu-Lys-TFMCA produced only mild prolongation. D-Val-Leu-Lys-COOH and D-Val-Leu-Lys-pNa did not produce any significant effect. These results indicate that D-Val-Leu-Lys-derivatives may be able to inhibit the action of plasmin.

TABLE 14 shows the effect of various peptides on the dextran-activated amidolytic activity of normal human plasma. This experiment was designed to study the possible inhibitory effect of the peptides on factor XII fragments and dextran-XIIa-mediated plasma kallikrein activity. In this test system H-D-Pro-Phe-Arg-NH-heptyl and H-D-Pro-Phe-Arg-O-heptyl produced a strong inhibition of dextran-activated amidolytic activity at a final concentration of 10^{-4} M. The free and acid forms of H-D-Phe-Pro-Arg- and H-D-Pro-Phe-Arg- did not produce any significant inhibition.

TABLE 11

INHIBITION OF TRYPSIN BY ANTIPAIN AND LEUPEPTIN (Ac-Leu-Leu-l-Arginal)

Concentration (μg/ml)	Antipain	Leupeptin
62.5	92	89
31.25	87	79
15.5	78	68
7.8	66	58
3.9	56	38
2.0	45	19
1.0	21	11
0.5	11	6

NOTE: Various amounts of antipain and leupeptin were mixed with a known amount of trypsin and incubated for 1 min; then 100 μl S-2222, 2.5 $\times$ 10^{-3} M, was added and the ΔA_{405}/min was monitored using a recording spectrophotometer.

TABLE 12

INHIBITION OF THROMBIN AND PLASMIN BY VARIOUS BASIC PEPTIDES

Peptide	Thrombin	Plasmin
Thr-Lys-Pro-Arg COOH (tuftsin)	−	−
Phe-Ser-Trp-Gly-Ala-Glu-Gly-Arg COOH (EAE)	−	−
Asp-Ser-Asp-Pro-Arg COOH (IgE peptide)	−	−
Thr-Pro-Arg-Lys-COOH (contraceptive peptide)	−	+
Gly-His-Lys-COOH (liver cell growth factor)	−	−
Acet-Leu-Arginal (leupeptin)	+	+

NOTE: All peptides were tested at 10 μg/ml final concentration; purified human thrombin and plasmin preparations were used to study the inhibitory action of these peptides. H-D-Phe-Pip-Arg-pNA was used to assay thrombin and D-Val-Leu-Lys-pNA was employed to assay plasmin.

TABLE 13

EFFECT OF VAL-LEU-LYS- ANALOGS ON THE PLASMIN-SUPPLEMENTED EUGLOBULIN LYSIS TIME

Peptide	Euglobulin Lysis Time (min)
D-Val-Leu-Lys-NH-heptyl	>300
D-Val-Leu-Lys-COOH	90
D-Val-Leu-Lys-TFMCA	180
D-Val-Leu-Lys-pNA	>90
Control	90

NOTE: Euglobulin fraction from freshly prepared normal human plasma was prepared by acidification, clotted with bovine thrombin, and supplemented with test peptides (10 μg/ml); 100 μl of a 10-caseinolytic-unit plasmin was added to the mixture and lysis time was recorded.

DISCUSSION

Our studies on low molecular peptides and their derivatives suggest that these agents through molecular manipulation may lead to the design of broad- and narrow-spectrum serine protease inhibitors. Many recent reports have appeared on the anticoagulant and antithrombotic actions of peptide derivatives.[36-38] In initial screening experiments we found that peptides containing the D-Phe-Pro-Arg-sequence show inhibitory actions towards thrombin, whereas peptides containing H-D-Pro-Phe-Arg-sequence exerted inhibitory action towards kallikreins. Both of these peptides bear resemblance to the sites of the natural substrates where these two enzymes act and this principle is utilized in the development of synthetic peptide substrates.[7] The presence of a dextro form of an amino acid at the amino terminal and a long-chain hydrophobic grouping at the carboxyl end tends to increase the inhibitory potency of these peptides.

It had been reported that D-Phe-Pro-arginal and D-Phe-Pro-Arg-CH_2Cl

TABLE 14

INHIBITION OF DEXTRAN-ACTIVATED AMIDOLYTIC ACTIVITY
OF NORMAL HUMAN PLASMA BY VARIOUS PEPTIDES

Peptides	$\Delta A_{405}/min$	Inhibition (%)
H-D-Pro-Phe-Arg-NH-heptyl	0.0120	92
H-D-Pro-Phe-Arg-O-heptyl	0.010	93
H-D-Pro-Phe-Arg-COOH	0.130	8
H-D-Pro-Phe-Arg-NH₂	0.130	8
H-D-Phe-Pro-Arg-COOH	0.125	11
H-D-Pro-Phe-Arg-NH₂	0.130	8
Control saline solution	0.140	0

NOTE: 0.1 ml of a $10^{-3} M$ solution of a given substrate is mixed with 0.9 ml of freshly prepared normal human plasma. Plasma is activated in cold with dextran and the resultant amidolytic activity is determined using chromozym PK.

inhibit the action of thrombin and trypsin.[20, 36-38] However, these peptides are broad-spectrum serine protease inhibitors and probably exert their action via an irreversible mechanism. Although many reports on their biologic actions are available, their mechanism of action is not well understood.

Our studies also reveal that H-D-Phe-Pro-Arg- can be molecularly manipulated at the amino terminal to produce varying inhibitory actions. The thiobenzyl ester form of D-Phe-Pro-Arg- is found to be a potent inhibitor of thrombin and also suppresses the action of arachidonic acid and thrombin on platelets. The regulating role of serine proteases is believed to mediate through the kallikreins, fibrinolytic coagulant enzymes, and the complement proteases, although no information on their influence on platelet function is available. Our results suggest that these proteases may also be involved in the regulation of platelet function. Only the aldehyde, lactam, or amino group protected forms of various peptides were found to be biologically active. The free carboxylic and amino-group-containing peptides only produced minimal effects. This suggests that the presence of the hydrophobic group enhances the affinity of a peptide to a serine protease, resulting in a modification of the active site, and thereby rendering it nonactive. In the structure-activity studies we found that the lysine and arginine residues at the carboxyl terminus are important in producing the biologic activity. In the amidolytic assay using Xa-specific synthetic peptide substrates, studies with Xa inhibitor peptides suggest that the mechanism of their inhibitory action may be competitive. When the chromogenic substrate concentration is increased, the inhibition produced by some of these peptides is weaker. On a molar basis the substrates that produced maximal effects contain a longer hydrophobic hydrocarbon chain at the carboxyl end.

A great deal of interest has been shown in the study of D-Phe-Pro-arginal and D-Phe-Pro-Arg-CH$_2$Cl. Most of the studies done with these agents employed trypsin and thrombins.[20, 36, 38] Our studies show that these are nonselective broad-spectrum inhibitors of serine proteases. In the *in vitro* assays the aldehyde and chloromethyl ketones produced prolongation of APTT, PT, and TT when added to NHP at μg levels. At 5-μM levels these agents produced strong inhibition of thrombin, plasmin, factor Xa, kallikreins, trypsin, and related enzymes. This suggests that the *in vivo* actions of these agents may not be specifically antithrombotic, but that these aldehydes also inhibit other physiological pathways regulated by serine proteases and that one should be cautious in classifying these agents as antithrombotics.

Although preliminary, our studies suggest that these peptide aldehydes are nonspecific inhibitors of trypsin-like enzymes, although their peptide sequences can be modified to develop relatively specific inhibitory actions. In contrast to the tripeptide aldehyde with potent antiserine protease activity, leupeptin and antipain were found to be relatively weaker inhibitors of serine proteases. However, both of these aldehydes produced strong inhibition of trypsin and thrombin. Furthermore they produced a prolongation of APTT and inhibited the clotting action of thrombin on fibrinogen.

Most of the coagulation enzymes belong to lysine- or arginine-directed esteroproteases, that is, serine proteases that are characterized by their ability to cleave synthetic ester or amide substrates involving either of the two cationic amino acids. Despite this common feature, various clotting enzymes are quite different in their biologic functions. The high degree of specificity is presumably determined by the difference in the secondary binding sites outside the specificity pocket adjacent to the active site. Geratz and coworkers have provided some data that support this hypothesis.[39] Oligopeptide analogs with a bulky side chain may influence both the primary and secondary binding sites, thereby altering the entire catalytic area of a given serine protease and provide us with the unique opportunity to design specific inhibitors of serine proteases.

Our studies on the derivatives of H-D-Phe-Arg-OH and H-D-Phe-Phe-Arg-OH are suggestive that these tripeptides can be molecularly manipulated to obtain inhibitors with selective inhibitory action towards thrombin. The N-α-dansyl-arginine amides reported by Okamoto are also selective competitive inhibitors of thrombin.[26] They are comparable in their potency and structure to N-α-arylsulfonyl-ω-(4-amidinophenyl)-α-aminoalkylcarboxylic acid amides reported by Markwardt.[27] Both of these classes of inhibitors allow structural variations and provide models for the study of the structure-activity relationship. These derivatives are believed to inhibit thrombin competitively and therefore are presumed to occupy the same site as the natural substrates. The oligopeptide inhibitors studied by us are much more specific in this regard and may help in topographical studies of the binding sites on serine protease enzymes.

Numerous basic oligopeptides play an important role in the physiological regulation of various body processes and are formed upon a physiological trigger. Although these peptides contain arginine and lysine at the carboxyl terminus, they do not exhibit any significant inhibitory activities. Furthermore, molecular manipulation of naturally occurring basic peptides such as tuftsin, IgE peptide, liver cell growth factor, and related peptides may result in the development of modulators of serine protease enzymes. Our studies on D-Val-Leu-Lys- derivatives suggest that selective inhibitors of the action of plasmin can also be developed and the information can be used to synthesize a specific substrate for plasmin.[40] Once again the free peptide did not seem to possess any inhibitory activity, although the introduction of an aromatic side chain or a hydrocarbon chain resulted in the development of an inhibitor. These tripeptide analogs do carry some information on the affinity to serine proteases, but the introduction of a bulky group or other molecular manipulation alters their effect on the enzyme. Besides binding to the active site, which may primarily be determined by the tripeptide sequence, the presence of a D amino acid and side chain may modify the active site of a given serine protease enzyme, thus rendering it nonactive.

Dextran activation of normal human plasma normally results in the activation of factor XII and subsequent activation of prekallikrein. The amidolytic activities generated by this process represent collective actions of a number of active enzymes. We found that H-D-Pro-Phe-Arg-NH-heptyl and H-D-Pro-Phe-Arg-O-heptyl produce strong inhibition of these enzymes in systems where these enzymes are present or generated. This system certainly mimics contact activation, which is manifested by a number of pathologic conditions. If a peptide inhibitor selectively inhibited the contact factors, it may be very useful in controlling contact-mediated pathophysiologic responses.

Another interesting finding during our study was the inhibitory action of some of these peptide derivatives on platelet function. The fact that some of these serine protease inhibitors also inhibit platelet function suggests that serine proteases may play some role in the regulation of platelet function. However, there may be certain additional factors in view of the fact that the serine protease inhibitory action of some of these peptides did not always correspond with their antiplatelet effect. For instance, the peptide arginals reported by Bajsuz[20] do not show any significant antiplatelet action, although they possess strong antiserine protease actions. On the other hand, the thiobenzyl esters of D-Phe-Pro-Arg- exhibit both the thrombin inhibitory and antiplatelet actions. It is therefore conceivable that some of the peptides may have multiple actions.

We have developed an extensive test battery for the study of the inhibition of serine proteases by amidolytic assays and clot-based methods. TABLE 15 surveys the methods that have been used to study the antiserine protease spectrum of a peptide. The development of newer methods for the analysis of coagulation function has greatly facilitated our knowledge in this area and has provided us with simpler methods to study the inhibitory characteristic of a given peptide. In this regard, the synthetic peptide substrates are very useful. Not only are they useful to assay a given serine protease, but they also provide information on the composition of the sites of a serine protease, which can be used to develop an inhibitor.

The role of various serine proteases in the regulation of complement, coagulation, kallikrein, and fibrinolytic pathways is depicted in FIGURE 3. Factor XII plays a central role in the modulation of all of these systems. In

TABLE 15

STUDY OF THE INHIBITION OF SERINE PROTEASES BY
LOW MOLECULAR WEIGHT PEPTIDES

Serine Protease	Method of Study
Thrombins	
α	Plasma and fibrinogen clotting, amidolytic and esterolytic assays
β	Amidolytic and esterolytic assays
γ	Amidolytic and esterolytic assays
Glandular kallikrein	Release of kinins (bioassays), amidolytic and esterolytic assays
Plasma kallikrein	Release of kinins (bioassays), amidolytic and esterolytic assays
Bovine Xa	Procoagulant assays and amidolytic assays
Human Xa	Procoagulant assays and amidolytic assays
Plasmin	Fibrinolytic bioassays, amidolytic and esterolytic assays
Urokinase	Activation of plasminogen (bioassays) and amidolytic assays
Trypsin	Amidolytic and esterolytic assays
Tissue Activator of Plasminogen	Amidolytic assays
XII_f	Amidolytic assays
XII_a	Coagulant assay (NAPTT)

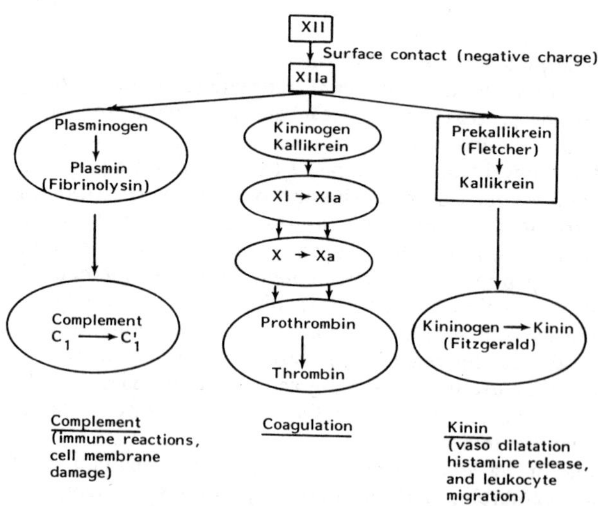

FIGURE 3. Factor XII modulation of serine proteases.

many pathologic conditions activation of various serine protease systems results in such conditions as disseminated intravascular coagulation, shock, hypercoagulable state, and complement-mediated reactions. It is conceivable that a single peptide inhibitor may be able to inhibit all factor-XII-mediated pathologic responses, thus providing a useful mean to control many disease processes. Preliminary evidence in our laboratories with endotoxemic and bacteremic shock has provided some data to support this hypothesis. However, further work on the antiserine protease properties of these peptides is warranted. Our studies suggest that molecular manipulation of low molecular weight synthetic peptide analogs of biologically active proteins, active sites of serine proteases, and endogenous oligopeptides may result in the design of useful selective inhibitors of serine protease enzymes and their activators.

SUMMARY

Numerous derivatives and various molecular forms of H-D-Pro-Phe-Arg-NH$_2$, H-D-Pro-Phe-Arg-OH, H-D-Phe-Pro-Arg-NH$_2$, H-D-Phe-Pro-Arg-OH, H-Phe-Phe-Arg-NH$_2$, H-D-Phe-Phe-Arg-OH, L-Pro-Phe-Arg-NH$_2$, L-Pro-Phe-Arg-OH, kinin-related peptides such as kassinin, ranatensin, xenopsin and litorin, Bombesin and their analogs, certain basic peptides such as tuftsin (Thr-Lys-Pro-Arg), IgE peptide III (Asp-Ser-Asp-Pro-Arg), liver cell growth factor (Gly-His-Lys), contraceptive tetrapeptide (Thr-Pro-Arg-Lys), protolin (Arg-Tyr-Leu-Pro-Thr), leupeptin (Ac-Leu-Leu-arginal), antipain and chymostatin, synthetic analogs of angiotensin, bradykinin, and certain polybasic amino acids (MW < 2000) were screened for their inhibitory effects in clotting assays such as those of prothrombin time (PT), partial thromboplastin time (PTT), activated partial thromboplastin time (APTT) using various activators, thrombin time (TT) using bovine and human thrombins with fibrinogen and citrated human, pooled plasma as substrates, thrombin-induced aggregation of human platelets, Xa coagulant assays, amidolytic/esterolytic assays for thrombin, Xa, plasmin, glandular and plasma kallikrein, urokinase, tissue activator of plasminogen and trypsin. H-D-Phe-Pro-Arg-OH and H-D-Pro-Phe-Arg-NH-heptyl inhibited the amidolytic action of glandular kallikrein ($K_i = 10^{-6}$ M), plasma kallikrein ($K_i = 10^{-5}$ M) and they blocked the release of kinins from HMW kininogen. H-D-Phe-Phe-Arg-NH$_2$ and its derivatives produced varying degrees of inhibition of the coagulant and amidolytic actions of bovine and human Xa. Amidolytic activity of activated plasma and activated factor XII were also blocked by H-D-Pro-Phe-Arg-NH-alkyl and H-D-Phe-Phe-Arg-NH-alkyl derivatives. All of the peptides with inhibitory action towards serine proteases showed varying degrees of inhibition of trypsin. Peptides containing lysine at the carboxyl terminus showed varying degrees of the inhibition of the amidolytic action of plasmin, SK-plasminogen complex, and tissue activator of plasminogen.

ACKNOWLEDGMENTS

We wish to thank Drs. Goran Claeson and Lars Melstam of Kabi AB Peptide Group, Molndal, Sweden and Dr. R. Hart of Kabi, Inc., Greenwich, CT, for donating chromogenic peptide substrates and for making helpful suggestions. We further thank Dr. Lars Svendsen of Pentapharm AG, Basel,

Switzerland, for his valuable input and critique during this project. We are thankful to M. Brauer and Cher Gurtler for their skillful help in the preparation of this manuscript, and we gratefully acknowledge the encouragement and support to pursue our studies from Professor Martin G. Lewis, chairman of the Department of Pathology of the Stritch School of Medicine of Loyola University.

REFERENCES

1. JACKSON, C. M. 1970. Blood coagulation. Ann. Rev. Biochem. **49:** 765–811.
2. MESSMORE, H. L. 1981. Advances in clinical hemostasis and thrombosis. *In* Perspectives in Hemostasis. (J. Fareed *et al.*, Eds.: 1–21. Pergamon Press. New York, NY.
3. BAUGH, R. F. & C. HOUGIE. 1979. The chemistry of blood coagulation. Clin. Hem. **8**(11): 3–30.
4. DAVIE, E. W., K. FUJIKAWA, K. KURACHI & D. V. KISSEL. 1979. The role of serine protease in blood coagulation cascade. Advan. Enzymol. **49:** 277–318.
5. DAVIE, E. W., K. FUJIKAWA, M. E. LEGAZ & H. KATO. 1975. E. Reich *et al.*, Eds.: 79–84. Role of protease in blood coagulation. *In* Proteases and Biological Control. Cold Spring Harbor Symposium. Cold Spring Harbor, NY.
6. FAREED, J., H. L. MESSMORE & E. W. BERMES. 1980. New perspectives in coagulation testing. Clin. Chem. **26**(10): 1380–1391.
7. HUSEBY, R. M. & R. E. SMITH. 1980. Synthetic oligopeptides substrates: Their diagnostic application in blood coagulation, fibrinolysis, and other pathologic states. Semin. Throm. Hemostas. **VI**(3): 173–314.
8. KAKKAR, V. V. & M. F. SCULLY, Eds. 1979. Chromogenic Peptide Substrates. Churchill Livingstone. Edinburgh.
9. I. WITT Ed. 1977. New Methods for the Analysis of Coagulation Using Chromogenic Substrates. Walter de Gruyter. Berlin.
10. LASKOWSKI, M., JR. & I. KATO. 1980. Protein inhibitors of proteases. Ann. Rev. Biochem. **49:** 593–626.
11. FAREED, J., G. KINDEL, H. L. MESSMORE & J. U. BALIS. 1979. *In* Current Concepts in Kinin Research. G. L. Haberland & U. Hamberg, Eds.: 237–247. Pergamon Press. Oxford.
12. CLAESON, G., J. FAREED, G. KINDEL, A. ARIELLY, R. SIMONSSON & C. LARSSON. 1979. Inhibition of the contractile action of bradykinin on isolated smooth muscle preparation by derivatives of low molecular weight peptides. *In* Kinin II: Systemic Proteases and Cellular Function. H. Morita *et al.*, Eds.: 691–713. Plenum Press. New York, NY.
13. MESSMORE, H. L., J. FAREED, J. GALLAGHER & P. ORFEI. 1979. Inhition of the amidolytic and procoagulant action of bovine factor Xa by H-D-Pro-Phe-Arg-OH (S-2430) and their derivatives. Throm. Haemostas. **42**(1): 206.
14. FAREED, J., H. L. MESSMORE, D. L. JANOTA, P. ORFEI, J. GALLAGHER & J. U. BALIS. 1979. Studies on the inhibition of glandular and plasma kallikreins by derivatives of low molecular weight peptide analogues of bradykinin. Thromb. Haemostas. **42:** 399.
15. FAREED, J., H. L. MESSMORE, J. GALLAGHER, P. ORFEI, Z. A. PARVEZ & J. W. FENTON. 1979. Inhibition of thrombin by H-D-Pro-Phe-Arg-OH (S-2430), H-D-Pro-Phe-Arg-NH$_2$ (S-2448) and their derivatives. Thromb. Haemostas. **42**(1): 399.
16. TAKAGI, A., M. ISHIGURO & M. FUNATASU. 1972. Anticoagulant peptides obtained from fibrinogen degradation products by plasmin I isolation of the peptide. Proc. Jpn. Acad. **48:** 528.

17. TAKAGI, A., S. YOSHITAKA, M. ISHIGURO & M. FUNATASU. 1972. Anticoagulant peptide obtained from fibrinogen degradation products by plasmin II sequence determination of the peptide. Proc. Jpn. Acad. **48:** 534.

18. TAKAGI, K., S. SUZUKI & T. KAWAI. 1979. Anticoagulant peptides obtained from human fibrinogen degradation products by plasmin. Thromb. Res. **16:** 737–746.

19. USZYNSKI, M. 1979. Anticoagulant activity of peptides from the human placenta. Thromb. Res. **16:** 689–694.

20. BAJUSZ, S., E. BARABAS, P. TOLNAY, E. SZELL & D. BAGDY. 1978. Inhibition of thrombin and trypsin by tripeptide aldehyde. Int. J. Peptide Protein Res. **12:** 217–221.

21. MARKWARDT, F. 1974. Synthetic low molecular weight thrombin inhibitors. A new concept of anticoagulants. Haemostasis 3: 185–202.

22. STURZEBECHER, J., F. MARKWARDT, G. WAGNER & D. WALSMANN. 1976. Synthetische Hemmstoffe der Serinproteinasen. 13. Quantitative Struktur-Wirkungs-Beziehungen bei der Hemmung von Trypsin, Plasmin und Thrombin durch 4-Amidinophenylverbindungen mit Ketonstruktur. Acta Biol. Med. Germ. **35:** 637–646.

23. GERATZ, J. D. & R. R. TIDWELL. 1977. The development of competitive reversible thrombin inhibitors. *In* Chemistry and Biology of Thrombin. R. L. Lundblad, J. W. Fenton, II & Mann, K. G., Eds.: 179–196. Ann Arbor Science Publishers. Ann Arbor, MI.

24. WALSMANN, P., H. HORN, F. MARKWARDT, P. RICHTER, J. STURZEBECHER, H. VIEWEG & G. WAGNER. 1976. Synthetische Inhibitoren der Serinproteinasen. 11. Uber die Hemmung von Trypsin, Plasmin und Thrombin durch neue Bisamidinoverbindunger. Acta Biol. Med. Germ. **35:** K1–K8.

25. STURZEBECHER, J., F. MARKWARDT & P. WALSMANN. 1976. Synthetic inhibitors of serine proteinases. XIV. Inhibition of Factor Xa by derivatives of benzamidine. Thromb. Res. **9:** 637–646.

26. OKAMOTO, S., A. HIJIKATA, K. IKEZAWA, K. KINJO, R. KIKUMOTO, S. TONOMURA & Y. TUMOA. 1976. A new series of synthetic thrombin inhibitors (OM-inhibitors) having extremely potent and selective action. Thromb. Res. **8:** (Suppl. II) 77–82.

27. MARKWARDT, F., G. WAGNER, J. STURZEBECHER & P. WALSMAN. 1980. N-α-arylsulfonyl-ω-(4-amidinophenyl)-α-aminoalkylcarboxylic acid amides. Novel selective inhibitions of thrombin. Thromb. Res. **17:** 425–431.

28. R. R. TIDWELL, W. P. WEBSTER, S. R. SHAVER & J. D. GERATZ. 1980. Strategies for anticoagulation with synthetic protease inhibitors Xa inhibitors versus thrombin inhibitors. Thromb. Res. **19:** 339–349.

29. SORIA, J., C. SORIA, M. R. BOISSEAU, P. HOURDILLE & G. SANCHES. 1979. Measurement of prekallikrein. Clinical application to patients suffering from burns, and the relationship between platelet nucleotide and prekallikrein level in chromogenic substrates. *In* Chromogenic Peptide Substrates. V. V. Kakkar, & M. F. Scully, Eds.: 93–101. Churchill Livingstone. Edinburgh.

30. DIXON, M. 1953. The determination of enzyme inhibitor constants. Biochem. J.: 170–171.

31. OWEN, C. A., E. J. W. BOWIE, P. DIDISHEIM & H. THOMPSON, Eds. 1969. The Diagnosis of Bleeding Disorders. Little, Brown, Boston, MA.

32. YIN, E. T., S. WESSLER & J. BUTLER. 1973. Plasma heparin: A unique practical submicrogram sensitive assay. J. Lab. Clin. Med. **81:** 298.

33. BUCKELL, M. 1958. The effect of citrate on euglobulin methods of estimating thrombolytic activity. J. Clin. Pathol. **11:** 403–405.

34. CHAKRABARTI, R., H. BIELAWIEC, J. F. EVANS & G. R. FLARNLEY. 1968. Methodological study and a recommended technique for determining the euglobulin lysis time. J. Clin. Pathol. **21:** 698–701.

35. CONRAD, J. 1976. Plasma plasminogen activator clot lysis assay technique.

In Progress in Chemical Fibrinolysis and Thrombolysis, vol. 2. J. F. Davidson, M. M. Samama & P. C. Deshoyers, Eds.: 15–23. Raven Press. New York, NY.

36. HAMPTON, J. & F. MARKWARDT. 1980. Studies on the anticoagulant and antithrombotic action of an irreversible thrombin inhibitor. Thromb. Res. **20:** 347.

37. KETTNER, C. & E. SHAW. 1979. D-Phe-Pro-Arg-CH₂Cl—a selective affinity label for thrombin. Thromb. Res. **14:** 969.

38. KETTNER, C. & E. SHAW. 1977. The selective inactivation of thrombin by peptides of arginine chloromethyl ketone. *In* Chemistry and Biology of Thrombin. R. L. Lundblad, J. W. Fenton, II & K. G. Mann, Eds.: 129–143. Ann Arbor Publishers. Ann Arbor, MI.

39. GERATZ, J. D., F. M. STEVENS, K. L. PALAKOSKI, R. F. PARRISH & R. R. TIDWELL. 1979. Amidino substitute aromatic hetrarocycle as probes of the specificity pocket of trypsin like proteases. Arch. Biochem. Biophys. **197:** 551.

40. CLAESON, G., L. AURELL, G. KARLSSON, S. GUSTAVSSON, P. FRIBERGER, S. ARIELLY & R. SIMONSSON. 1979. Design of chromogenic peptide substrates. *In* Chromogenic Peptide Substrates. V. V. Kakkar & M. F. Scully, Eds.: 20–31. Churchill Livingstone. Edinburgh.

SYNTHETIC SUBSTRATE ASSAYS OF THE COAGULATION ENZYMES AND THEIR INHIBITORS. COMPARISON WITH CLOTTING AND IMMUNOLOGIC METHODS FOR CLINICAL AND EXPERIMENTAL USAGE

Harry L. Messmore, Jr., Jawed Fareed, Judith Kniffin,
Grace Squillaci, and Jeanine Walenga

Departments of Pathology and Medicine
Loyola University Medical Center
Maywood, Illinois 60153

INTRODUCTION

The application of newly developed synthetic peptide substrate, enzymologic, and immunologic methods to the analysis of the coagulation proteins offers many alternatives to traditional clotting methods. In some instances these methods may soon replace the traditional methods because of greater sensitivity, specificity, accuracy, and simplicity. In special clinical circumstances, more than one method may be clinically useful, such as in comparing the functional and immunologic levels in suspected hereditary deficiencies of an enzyme or inhibitor. The basic principles of the methods will be briefly discussed and their clinical applications reviewed.

SYNTHETIC PEPTIDE SUBSTRATES

The introduction of synthetic substrates for the testing of coagulation enzymes and their inhibitors began in the 1950s and 1960s with the introduction of the esters of basic amino acids, arginine and lysine. The arginine esters were useful to assay thrombin,[1] factor Xa,[2] XIa,[3] XIIa,[4] and the prekallikrein-kallikrein system.[5] Lysine esters were useful to assay plasmin.[6]

The lack of specificity of these substrates resulted in their being replaced by the oligopeptide substrates (3–4 amino acids in sequence) such as *N*-benzoyl-L-nitrophenyl-alanyl-L-valyl-L-arginin-paranitroaniline hydrochloride. This substrate was introduced by Svendsen and his coinvestigators in 1972.[7] It is sensitive to thrombin, plasmin, and trypsin. The substrate was synthesized on the basis of the known structure of the alpha chain of fibrinopeptide A and the cleavage sites and binding sites of thrombin. Another important feature of this compound is the chromophore paranitroaniline, which is linked to the C-terminal end of the molecule in an *amide* linkage. Splitting of this group from the tripeptide results in rapid development of a yellow color in the 405-nm range of the visible spectrum. This reaction may be stopped at a given time with acetic acid (end-point method) or recorded as a reaction rate on a recording spectrophotometer.[8] The method is readily automatable for the measurement of coagulation enzymes and their inhibitors [9–11] or even for chromogenic partial thromboplastin time.[12] The basic reaction with release of the chromophore is shown in FIGURE 1.

The amino terminal (N-terminal) end of the molecule can be manipulated

785

$$\text{B-AA-AA-AA-pNA} \xrightarrow{\text{enzyme}} \text{B-AA-AA-AA-COOH} + \text{pNA (yellow)}$$

FIGURE 1. Basic biochemical reaction of the chromogenic substrates. The released pNA is read in a spectrophotometer at 405 nm. B = blocking group (BZ, CBZ, tos, etc.); AA = amino acid; pNA = chromophore-paranitroaniline; enzyme = thrombin, Xa, plasmin, kallikrein, tissue activator, urokinase, etc.

to add specificity, solubility, and stability. This has been done in a variety of ways, such as by the use of D-amino acids, p-toluenesulfonyl (tos), N-α-benzyloxycarbonyl (CBz), and t-butyloxycarbonyl (Boc) groups. A list of commercially available chromogenic substrates and their clinical applicability is found in TABLE 1.

Fluorogenic substrates were introduced in 1975 by Mitchell, Huseby, and Hudson.[13] They synthesized the thrombin-sensitive fluorescent substrate CBz-Gly-Pro-Arg-4-methoxy-beta naphthylamide (β-NA) for the assay of antithrombin-III. Other fluorophores found to be useful are the amino-isophthalic acid diester (AIE) and 4-methyl coumaryl amide (MCA). For a list of

TABLE 1

SYNTHETIC CHROMOGENIC PEPTIDE SUBSTRATES AND THEIR APPLICATIONS

Substrate *	Chemical Structure	Applications
Chromozym-TH	Tos or CBz-Gly-Pro-Arg-pNA	Prothrombin, antithrombin-III, antithrombins, monitoring of oral anticoagulants, heparin platelet factor 3 and platelet factor 4
S-2160	Bz-Phe-Val-Arg-pNA	
S-2238	H-D-Phe-Pip-Arg-pNA	
S-2366	Pyro-Glu-Pro-Arg-pNA	
Abbott "?"	CH3-Gly-Pro-Arg-pNA	
S-2222	Bz-Ile-Glu(γ-OR)-Gly-Arg-pNA	X, Xa, anti-Xa and platelet factor 4
S-2337	Bz-Ile-Glu-(γ-O-piperidyl)-Gly-Arg-pNA	
S-2251	H-D-Val-Leu-Lys-pNA	Plasmin, plasminogen, antiplasmin, and plasminogen activators
Chromozym-P	Tos-Gly-Pro-Lys-pNA	
S-2322	H-D-Val-Gly-Arg-pNA	Tissue activator of plasminogen
S-2288	H-D-Ile-Pro-Arg-pNA	
S-2303	H-D-Pro-Phe-Arg-pNA	Plasma kallikrein, antikallikrein and kallikrein activators
Chromozym-PK	Bz-Pro-Phe-Arg-pNA	
S-2266	H-D-Val-Leu-Arg-pNA	Glandular kallikrein, antikallikrein and kallikrein activators
Chromozym-UK	Bz-Val-Gly-Arg-pNA	Urokinase
S-2444	Pyro-Glu-Gly-Arg-pNA	
Chromozym-Try	H-D-Val-Gly-Arg-pNA	Trypsin and antitrypsin
	Cbo-Val-Gly-Arg-pNA	
S-2422	Bz-Ile-Glu-Gly-Arg-pNA	Endotoxin, *Limulus* procoagulant enzyme
S-2433	Acet-Ile-Gly-Gly-Arg-pNA	

* The substrates of the chromozym series are manufactured by Pentapharm (Basel, Switzerland) and the substrates of the "S" series are manufactured by Kabi AB (Stockholm, Sweden) and supplied in the United States by Kabi Group, Inc., Greenwich, CT.

commercially available fluorogenic substrates, see TABLE 2. The basic reaction is shown in FIGURE 2.

Biochemical investigations for the selection of various oligopeptide sequences, detector groups, and blocking groups have been developed over the past 8 years by a variety of investigators.[14-18] The results of these studies are summarized by Huseby and Smith in an extensive review.[19]

CLINICAL APPLICATIONS OF SYNTHETIC SUBSTRATE ASSAYS

We have been utilizing the synthetic chromogenic substrate assays in our laboratories since 1974, when we started to use S-2160 to assay for plasminogen. It was much simpler than the caseinolytic method and the fibrin plate method and so much faster than the immunologic method and we were very eager to assess its accuracy. It compared well with other methods. We have since then replaced S-2160 with more sensitive, more soluble, and more specific substrates, but we still find it more convenient to assay plasminogen by a chromogenic substrate method than by any other. Clinical application of each of these substrates is listed in TABLE 3.

ANTITHROMBIN-III ASSAYS

Antithrombin-III (AT-III) assays utilizing factor Xa or thrombin-sensitive substrates have been available as chromogenic[8-10] or fluorogenic[13] methods and we find them to be useful in our laboratory on a daily basis. Disorders associated with antithrombin-III deficiency on an acquired basis are listed in TABLE 4. TABLE 5 is a comparison of AT-III levels in various pathologic states seen in our hospital. Inherited AT-III deficiency[20, 21] and hereditary defects in the AT-III molecule[22] may cause thromboembolic disease.

These assays are automatable[8-10] and can be readily employed in assessing thrombotic disease prior to institution of therapy. The basic reaction of the AT-III assay is shown below in A or B, depending upon whether exogenous thrombin or factor Xa is used:

A. Thrombin (human) or (bovine)

$$\text{Thrombin (excess)} + \text{test plasma * (AT-III)} \longrightarrow \text{thrombin residual}$$
$$+ \text{thrombin AT-III complex}$$
$$\text{Thrombin (residual)} + \text{R} \cdot \text{pNA} \longrightarrow \text{R} \cdot \text{COOH} + \text{pNA}$$
$$\text{R} \cdot \text{pNA} = \text{S-2238, chromozym Th, S-2266, Quantichrome}^® \text{ (Abbott)}$$

B. Factor Xa

$$\text{Factor Xa (excess)} + \text{test plasma † (AT-III)} \longrightarrow \text{Xa residual}$$
$$+ \text{Xa} \cdot \text{AT-III complex}$$
$$\text{Xa residual} + \text{R} \cdot \text{pNA} \longrightarrow \text{R} \cdot \text{OH} + \text{pNA}$$

* The test plasma is in heparinized buffer. An identical amount of thrombin is added to a 100 percent control, which is a pool of 10 or more samples of fresh normal plasma or a standard AT-III supplied in the kit. The method of calculation is shown above (reaction rate method) in FIGURE 3.

† Test plasma is in heparinized buffer. Factor Xa is added to standard AT-III provided or to fresh normal human pooled plasma (NHP) to determine the percentage of normal.

Calculations (Fig. 3):

$$\Delta A405/\text{min with saline solution} = A$$
$$\Delta A405/\text{min with normal pooled plasma (NHP)} = B$$
$$\Delta 405/\text{min with test sample} = C$$

$$\% \text{ AT-III} = \frac{A - C}{A - B} \times 100$$

PLASMINOGEN AND ANTIPLASMIN ASSAYS

Plasminogen assays are useful in detecting the fibrinolytic state or the depression of plasminogen in association with liver disease, asparaginase therapy,[23] or DIC syndrome, for example. We may also wish to assay plasmino-

$$B\text{-AA-AA-AA-AIE} \xrightarrow{\text{enzyme}} B\text{-AA-AA-AA-COOH} + \text{AIE (fluor)}$$

FIGURE 2. Basic biochemical reaction of the fluorogenic substrate assays. AIE = fluorophore-amino-iso-phthalic acid ester.

TABLE 2

SYNTHETIC FLUOROGENIC SUBSTRATES AND THEIR APPLICATIONS

Enzyme	Chemical Structure	Applications
Thrombin	Boc-Val-Pro-Arg-MCA * CBz-Gly-Pro-Arg-βNA H-D-Phe-Pro-Arg-AIE *	Prothrombin, antithrombin-III, monitoring of oral anti-coagulants, heparin, platelet factor 3 and 4
Factor Xa	Boc-Ile-Glu-Gly-Arg-MCA †	X, Xa, anti-Xa, platelet factor 4, heparin and endotoxin
Urokinase	Glut-Gly-Arg-MCA †	Urokinase, urokinase activators and inhibitors
Plasmin	H-D-Val-Leu-Lys-AIE * Boc-Gly-Leu-Lys-MCA † Boc-Val-Leu-Lys-MCA †	Plasminogen, antiplasmin, plasmin, and plasminogen activators
Urinary kallikrein	Pro-Phe-Arg-MCA †	Kallikrein and antikallikrein
Pancreatic kallikrein	Pro-Phe-Arg-MCA †	Glandular kallikrein and prekallikrein
Plasma kallikrein	Z-Phe-Arg-MCA †	Plasma kallikrein and prekallikrein
Limulus clotting enzyme	Boc-Leu-Gly-Arg-MCA †	Endotoxin, bacterial activators
IXa, XIIa	Boc-Phe-Ser-Arg-MCA † Boc-Leu-Thr-Arg-MCA †	Contact factors

*Substrate available in the Dade Protopath Kits.
† Substrate available from Peptide Institute, Protein Research Foundation, Osaka, Japan.

TABLE 3

CURRENT STATUS OF SYNTHETIC SUBSTRATE ASSAYS FOR CLINICAL USE

Coagulation Test or Assay	Status
Antithrombin III	Equivalent to clotting methods; readily available; clinically relevant.
Plasminogen	Equivalent to caseinolytic, fibrin plate and immunologic methods; readily available and clinically relevant.
α_2 Antiplasmin	Equivalent to immunologic methods; available and clinically relevant.
Heparin assay	Equivalent to clotting methods; available; clinical relevance not solidly established.
Prothrombin assay	Equivalent to clotting methods if proper activator is used and prothrombin molecule is normal (hereditary dysprothrombinemia may give false results).
Factor X assay	Equivalent to clotting and immunologic methods.
Factor VII assay	Results comparable to clotting method; not influenced by "cold activation" phenomenon observed with clotting assay.
Factor VIII assay	Equivalent to clotting method; clinical trials in progress; not readily available; requires IXa as a reagent, S-2222 as substrate for factor X.
Factor XI assay	Equivalent to clotting method, but standard assay kit not readily available.
Factor XII assay	In process of development and clinical correlations; based on conversion of XII $\longrightarrow$ XIIa and XIIa converting pre-kallikrein to kallikrein and utilizing a kallikrein-sensitive substrate.
Prekallikrein	Readily available in kit form; easier than clotting methods; deficient plasma not needed for the chromogenic assay, which is a great advantage.
Platelet factor 3	Easily performed utilizing Russell's viper venom to activate factor X; rate of activation is measured by release of pNA from a factor Xa substrate, S-2337; no kit readily available.
Platelet factor 4	Best assayed by RIA method; the chromogenic and clotting methods are good if the concentration in the blood is sufficiently high.

TABLE 4

PHYSIOLOGIC AND DISEASE STATES ASSOCIATED WITH LOW LEVELS OF
ANTITHROMBIN III (AT-III)

Low levels of AT-III: Physiologic states
    1. Pregnancy
    2. Neonatal period

Low levels of AT-III: Hereditary
    1. Decreased levels
    2. Abnormal molecule dysfunction

Low levels of AT-III: Acquired
    Drug-related
        Heparin therapy (intravenous, prolonged)
        Oral contraceptives
        L-asparaginase therapy
    Surgery-related
        Major surgery (especially hip surgery)
    Trauma
        Crushing injuries, burns
    Malignancy (disseminated types)
        Hypercoagulable state; disseminated intravascular coagulation (DIC); thromboembolic disease
    Infection
        Disseminated infection with DIC or thromboembolism
    Liver disease
        Impaired production and/or DIC
    Nephrotic syndrome
        Loss in urine resulting in a hypercoagulable state

TABLE 5

ANTITHROMBIN-III LEVELS AS OBSERVED IN
VARIOUS PATHOLOGIC STATES AT LOYOLA MEDICAL CENTER *

Pathologic State	AT-III Level (% of Normal Value)
Disseminated intravascular coagulation (9)	76.4 ± 4.6
Liver cirrhosis (25)	27.8 ± 3.9
Congenital antithrombin-III deficiency (2)	31.8 ± 4.6
Neonates (5)	48.4 ± 19.2
Gram-negative septicemia (3)	36.8 ± 11.6
Oral contraceptives (5)	64.4 ± 24.1

* Number of patients given in parentheses.

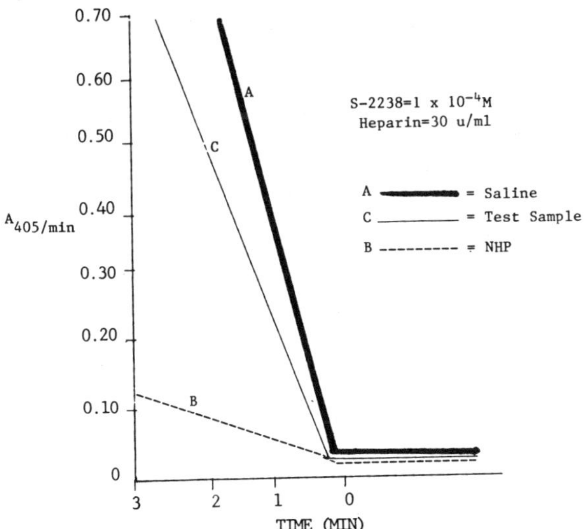

FIGURE 3. Sample curves obtained on kinetic analyzer in the analysis of anti-thrombin-III by chromogenic substrate methods.

gen in the blood of patients who have a thrombotic disorder of unknown cause. Low levels of *functional* plasminogen as determined by these assays along with normal levels determined by an immunologic method are strongly suggestive of a qualitatively abnormal plasminogen molecule.

α_2-antiplasmin can be assayed readily by chromogenic substrate methods utilizing the same substrates (see *D* below) as those used for plasminogen assay (see *C* below). This assay is clinically useful in detecting hereditary α_2-anti-plasmin deficiency, an hereditary bleeding disorder similar to hemophilia.[24] The principle of the plasminogen assay is as follows:

C.   Plasminogen (plasma) + streptokinase⟶ SK·plasminogen complex

$$R \cdot pNA \xrightarrow[\text{R·pNA = S-2251, chromozym P ‡}]{\text{SK·plasminogen complex}} R \cdot COOH + pNA$$

D. α_2-antiplasmin (plasma) + plasmin (excess added) ⟶
      α_2-antiplasmin·plasmin complex + plasmin (residual)

$$R \cdot pNA \xrightarrow{\text{plasmin}} R \cdot COOH + pNA$$
$$R \cdot pNA - \text{S-2251, chromozym P §}$$

‡ S-2251 and chromozym P are hydrolyzed equally well by either plasmin or the SK·plasminogen complex. The inhibitor α_2-antiplasmin (see above) does not inhibit the SK·plasmin complex.

§Incubation is short in this assay to avoid interaction of the residual plasmin with α_2-macroglobulin.

Clotting Factor Assays

Other uses of the chromogenic substrates are to determine individual enzymes (zymogens) and coenzymes of the coagulation cascade. Individual factor assays currently available are for factors XII,[25] XI,[26] prekallikrein,[27] VII,[28] VIII,[29] X,[30] and II.[31] The substrates used in these assays are listed in Table 3. The principles are essentially the same as those shown in Figures 1 and 2.

It has recently been shown that certain pitfalls may exist in the assays of coagulation factors by synthetic substrate methods. One of these is that an abnormal molecule such as prothrombin may be converted to an abnormal thrombin that has normal amidolytic activity on a synthetic substrate such as S-2238, but has reduced ability to convert fibrinogen to fibrin. The assay for prothrombin with this substrate and a variety of activators is satisfactory[32] when there is a pure hereditary deficiency or a deficiency due to liver disease. Warfarin therapy and vitamin K deficiency will give rise to erroneous results due to PIVKA if the direct activators staphylocoagulase, *Echis carinatus*, or Taipan snake venom are used.

It is fair to say that these methods may eventually be accepted for clinical use in the proper setting, but their limitations have yet to be determined, and it is premature to recommend their routine use.

Heparin Assays

The chromogenic and fluorogenic methods lend themselves well to the assay of heparin since the functional activity of heparin is directly related to its effect on antithrombin-III in the usual clinically encountered heparin concentrations.

The principle of the assays is shown in *A* (thrombin method) or *B* (Xa method).

A.
Heparin || + AT-III (excess) $\longrightarrow$ heparin·AT-III
Heparin AT-III + thrombin (excess) $\longrightarrow$ heparin·AT-III·thrombin + thrombin excess
Thrombin excess + R·pNA $\longrightarrow$ R·COOH + pNA

B.
Heparin # + AT-III (excess) $\longrightarrow$ heparin·AT-III complex
Heparin·AT-III + factor Xa $\longrightarrow$ AT-III·heparin-Xa + excess Xa
Excess Xa + R·pNA $\longrightarrow$ R·COOH + pNA

Heparin assays using factor Xa and an Xa-sensitive chromogenic or fluorogenic substrate are available commercially.[33] Kits utilizing thrombin-sensitive substrates in chromogenic[34] or fluorogenic systems[35] are also commercially

---

|| Heparin in plasma is rapidly neutralized by platelet factor 4 (PF-4), and care in drawing the blood and separating the platelets by centrifugation is essential for accuracy. Frozen and thawed samples have lower heparin values due to release of PF-4.

\# Heparin curves are made from *the same heparin* supplemented to fresh pooled plasma (carefully drawn nonpooled plasma) in serial dilutions to contain heparin in 0.0, 0.2, 0.4 and 0.6 units/ml final concentration.

available for heparin assay. The fluorogenic method appears to be quite sensitive and precise in lower heparin concentrations. Linearity is a problem with wide-ranging concentrations of heparin, and the appropriate dilutions are made in the standard curves to assure linearity at that concentration.

The question is becoming critical of whether all heparin preparations in the future will be assayed by the same system and labeled in USP, British, or International units in terms of anticoagulant, antithrombin, or anti-factor Xa. Some low molecular weight fractions have minimal antithrombin activity. Since such heparins have "antithrombotic" activity but little "anticoagulant" activity, the question of how they are to be labeled for potency remains to be determined.

The clinical utility of "heparin levels" remains to be determined. A recent study[36] showed a good correlation between thrombin times and heparin levels and less correlation between either of these and the activated partial thromboplastin time. The influence of factor VIII levels and the type of activator used on the activated partial thromboplastin time probably accounts for the lack of correlation of this test with heparin levels and the thrombin time. One has to decide what information is desired before selecting a method for monitoring heparin therapy since each method measures something different. We prefer the activated partial thromboplastin time or the activated whole blood clotting time (ACT)[37, 38] as reflecting the overall anticoagulated state of the blood better than heparin levels or thrombin time. Eventually a global type of chromogenic substrate method, as discussed later, might be utilized for monitoring heparin therapy.

GLOBAL ASSAYS

The measurement of the prothrombin time and activated partial thromboplastin time by means of chromogenic substrates is currently undergoing clinical evaluation. Several clinical studies have been reported for the prothrombin time equivalent, some utilizing a thrombin-sensitive chromogenic substrate[39, 40] and others utilizing an Xa-sensitive substrate.[41] They appear to be most adaptable to long-term anticoagulant therapy and correlate well with current clotting assays, provided that a "suitable" activator is used and the substrate is relatively specific for factor Xa or thrombin. Another factor to be considered in the development of these assays is the inhibition of factor Xa by the free acid form of some thrombin-sensitive substrates.[42]

These assays have been found to be quite sensitive and precise and are automatable. Their use in the setting of long-term oral anticoagulant therapy remains to be fully explored, but they appear to be promising. The use of snake venom (*Echis carinatus*) or staphylocoagulase for prothrombin activation has its drawbacks because they detect the PIVKA material as well as functionally active prothrombin; but when parallel testing is done with natural activators (Xa-mediated), the ratio of the natural to unnaturally activated assay provides knowledge of vitamin K deficiency or warfarin effect. An assay employing activation of the intrinsic system (activated PTT) and a thrombin-sensitive substrate is reported by Aiyappa in this volume.

These global assays lack the specificity of coagulation assays at the point where the final enzyme activity acts on the substrate. They therefore have limited usefulness in screening for bleeding disorders and disease states involving dysprothrombinemia [32] or hypofibrinogenemia. Inhibitors of fibrin polymerization are also impossible to detect with these newer synthetic substrate assays. This would include certain proteinopathies and systemic lupus with inhibitors of this specific type.

PLATELET-RELATED ACTIVITIES

The synthetic substrates have been utilized to measure the functional activity of platelet factor 3 (PF 3) and platelet factor 4 (PF 4).

Since PF 3 is an accelerator of the extrinsic pathway and since its contribution to factor X activity and its ability to activate prothrombin are easily measured, a test was devised combining Stypven (Russell's viper venom) as an activator of factor X and a thrombin-sensitive substrate, S-2238.[43] This was found to be 10 times more sensitive than the clotting assay using the same activator. PF 3 activity is absent in some acquired platelet disorders and in certain rare hereditary platelet defects, usually in conjunction with some other problem of the platelet.[44] PF 4 assays can be performed with chromogenic substrates since PF 4 is an inhibitor of heparin, and heparin can be assayed as discussed earlier. Clotting assays and chromogenic substrate assays are less specific and not nearly as sensitive as currently available radioimmunoassays for PF 4.[45]

PLASMINOGEN ACTIVATOR ASSAYS

Specific substrates for urokinase, S-2444, and chromozym UK have little clinical utility at this time since urokinase therapy is monitored by observing for a lytic state by thrombin times, prothrombin time, or partial thromboplastin times.

It may be useful to detect *inhibitors of urokinase* and other tissue activators, but such an assay is not yet clinically available. The structure of the substrate S-2444 is shown in TABLE 1.

Substrates for other tissue activators of plasminogen, S-2288 and S-2322,[46–48] are also listed in TABLE 1. They are useful in coagulation research and may be useful in the future in clinical study of hereditary and acquired vascular defects related to endothelial function and to pathologic disorders such as malignancy related to abnormal tissues.

CONCLUSION

Synthetic chromogenic and fluorogenic peptide substrates are proving to be extremely useful tools in the investigative and clinical aspects of the analysis of coagulation-related proteins, such as enzymes, inhibitors, activators and accelerators.

Many studies are in progress to further clarify the role of these peptide substrates in clinical coagulation analysis, and as they are more clearly understood, these substrates will be utilized selectively to improve the quality of medical care.

REFERENCES

1. TROLL, W., S. SHERRY & J. WACHMAN. 1954. The action of thrombin on synthetic substrates. J. Biol. Chem. **208:** 85–93.
2. ESNOUF, M. P. & W. J. WILLIAMS. 1962. The isolation and purification of a bovine plasma protein which is a substrate for the coagulation fraction of Russell's viper venom. Biochem. J. **84:** 62–71.
3. KINGDON, H. S., E. W. DAVIE & O. RATNOFF. 1964. The reaction between activated plasma thromboplastin antecedent and diisopropyl-phosphorfluoridate. Biochemistry 3: 166–173.
4. NIEWIAROWSKI, S., J. STACHURSKA & Z. WEGRZYNOWNCZ. 1962. Arginine esterase activity of the contact (Hageman) factor. Thromb. Diath. Haemorrh. **7:** 514–522.
5. COLMAN, R. W., L. E. MATTLER & S. SHERRY. 1969. Studies on the prekallikrein (kallikreinogen)–kallikrein enzyme system of human plasma. J. Clin. Invest. **48:** 11–32.
6. SHERRY, S. & W. TROLL. 1954. The action of plasmin on synthetic substrates. J. Biol. Chem. **208:** 95–105.
7. SVENDSEN, L., B. BLÖMBACK, M. BLÖMBACK & P. OLSSON. 1972. Synthetic chromogenic substrates for the determination of trypsin, thrombin, and thrombin-like enzymes. Thromb. Res. **1:** 267–278.
8. ODEGARD, O., M. LIE & U. ABILDGAARD. 1975. Heparin cofactor activity measured with an amidolytic method. Thromb. Res. **6:** 287–294.
9. CONARD, J., P. BARBIER & M. SAMAMA. 1979. Automated amidolytic method for AT-III determination. Thrombos. Haemostas. (Stuttgart) **42:** 1350–1352.
10. ØDEGARD, O., B. ROSENLUND & E. ERVICK. 1978. Automated antithrombin III assay utilizing a centrifugal analyzer. Haemostasis **1:** 202–209.
11. YAMADA, K. & T. MEGURO. 1979. Novel method of APTT using an Autoanalyzer (abstract 0530). VII International Congress on Thrombosis and Haemostasis. Thromb. Haemost. **42:** 225.
12. FAREED, J., H. MESSMORE & E. BERMES. 1980. New perspectives in coagulation testing. Clin. Chem. **26:** 1380–1391.
13. MITCHELL, G., P. HUDSON, R. HUSEBY, S. POCHRON & R. J. GARGIULO. 1978. Fluorescent substrate assay for antithrombin III. Thromb. Res. **12:** 219–225.
14. BANG, N. U. & L. E. MATTLER. 1978. Sensitivity and specificity of serine protease chromogenic substrates. Haemostasis **7:** 98–104.
15. MATTLER, L. E. & N. U. BANG. 1977. Serine protease specificity for peptide chromogenic substrates. Thrombos. Haemostas. **38:** 776–792.
16. CLAESON, G., L. AURELL, G. KARLSSON & P. FRIBERGER. 1977. Substrate structure and activity relationship. *In* New Methods for the Analysis of Coagulation Using Chromogenic Substrates. Witt.: 37. Walter de Gruyter. Berlin.
17. ABILDGAARD, U., M. LIE & O. ODEGARD. 1976. A simple amidolytic method for the determination of functionally active antithrombin III. Scand J. Clin. Lab. Invest. **36:** 109–112.
18. AURELL, L., P. FRIBERGER, G. KARLSSON & G. CLAESON. 1977. A new sensitive and highly specific chromogenic substrate for factor Xa. Thromb. Res. **11:** 595–609.
19. HUSEBY, R. M. & R. E. SMITH. 1980. Synthetic oligopeptide substrates: Their diagnostic application in blood coagulation, fibrinolysis and other pathologic states. Semin. Thromb. Hemostas.: 173–314.
20. EGEBERG, O. 1965. Inherited antithrombin deficiency causing thrombophilia. Thromb. Diath. Haemorrh. **13:** 516–530.
21. MARCINIAK, E. & FARLEY, L. 1973. Familial thrombosis due to antithrombin III deficiency. J. Clin. Invest.: 52–54a.

22. SAS, G., S. PEPPER & J. CASH. 1975. Further investigation on antithrombin III in the plasmas of patients with the abnormality of "antithrombin III Budapest." Thromb. Diath. Haemorrh. **33:** 564–572.
23. PRIEST, J., N. RAMSAY, R. LATCHAU, L. LOCKMAN, D. HASEGAWA, T. COATES, P. COCCIA, R. EDSON, M. NESBIT & W. KRIVIT. 1980. Thrombotic and hemorrhagic strokes complicating early therapy for childhood acute lymphoblastic leukemia. Cancer **46:** 1548–1554.
24. KOIE, K., T. KANIYA, K. OGOTA, J. TAKAMATSU & M. KOHAKURA. 1978. Miyasato's disease. Lancet **11:** 1334–1335.
25. VINAZZER, H. 1979. Assay of total factor XII and of activated factor XII in plasma with a chromogenic substrate. Thromb. Res. **14:** 155–166.
26. IWANAGA, S., H. KATO, I. MURAYAMA, N. ADACHI, Y. OHNO, K. TAKADA, T. KIMURA & D. SAKAKIBARA. 1979. Fluorogenic peptide substrates for proteases in blood coagulation, kallikrein-kinin and fibrinolysis systems. Substrate for plasmin and factor XIa (abstract 0105). VII International Congress on Thrombosis and Haemostasis.) Thromb.-Haemostas.: 42–49.
27. EGBERG, N. & K. BERGSTROM. 1978. Studies on assays for plasma prekallikrein and for monitoring of Coumarol therapy. Haemostasis **7:** 85–91.
28. AVVISATI, G., J. TEN CATE, E. VAN WIJK, L. KAHLÉ & G. MARIANI. 1980. Evaluation of a new chromogenic assay for factor VII and its application in patients on oral anticoagulant treatments. Br. J. Haematol. **45:** 343–352.
29. SEGHATCHIAN, M. 1979. The usefulness of chromogenic substrates in the diagnosis of hemophilia and control of blood products. *In* Chromogenic Peptide Substrates. M. Scully & V. Kakkar, Eds.: 102–118. Churchill Livingstone. London.
30. A. FAMODIE, G. INGRAM & S. DARBY. 1979. Anticoagulant control with chromogenic measurements of factor X and VII (abstract 0688). (VII International Congress on Thrombosis and Haemostasis. Thromb. Haemostas. **42:** 292.
31. KIRCHOF, R., C. VERMEER & H. HEMKER. 1978. The determination of prothrombin using synthetic chromogenic substrates: Choice of a suitable activator. Thromb. Res. **13:** 219–232.
32. GEROLAMI, A., P. GIOVANNI, F. TOFFANIN & L. SAGGIN. 1980. Chromogenic substrate (S-2238) prothrombin assay in prothrombin deficiencies and abnormalities. Am. J. Clin. Path. **74:** 83–87.
33. TEIEN, A., M. LIE, & U. ABILDGAARD. 1976. Assay of heparin in plasma using a chromogenic substrate for activated factor X. Thromb. Res. **8:** 413–416.
34. LARSEN, M., U. ABILDGAARD, A. TEIEN & K. GJESDAL. 1975. Assay of plasma heparin using thrombin and the chromogenic substrate H-D-phe-phe-pip-arg-pNA (S-2238) Thromb. Res. **13:** 285–288.
35. MITCHELL, G., R. GARGIULO, R. HUSEBY, D. LAWSON, S. POCHRON & J. SCHUANES. 1978. Assay for plasma heparin using a synthetic peptide substrate for thrombin: Introduction of the fluorophore aminoisophthalic acid, dimethyl ester. Thromb. Res. **13:** 47–52.
36. BOUNEMEAUX, H., G. MARBET, L. BERNHARD, R. EICHLISBERGER & F. DUCKERT. 1980. Comparison of thrombin time, activated partial thromboplastin time and plasma heparin concentration and analysis of the behavior of antithrombin III. Am. J. Clin. Path. **74:** 68–73.
37. MATTOX, K., G. GUINN, P. RUBIO & A. BEALL. 1975. Use of the activated clotting time in intraoperative heparin reversal for cardiopulmonary by-pass. Ann. Thorac. Surg. **19:** 634–637.
38. BABKA, R., C. COLBY, A. EL-ETR & R. PIFARRE. 1977. Monitoring of intraoperative heparinization and blood loss following cardiopulmonary by-pass surgery. J. Thorac. Cardiovasc. Surg. **73:** 780–782.
39. BERGSTRÖM, K. & M. BLÖMBACK. 1974. Determination of plasma prothrom-

bin with a reaction rate analyzer using a synthetic substrate. Thromb. Res. **4:** 719–729.

40. BAUGHMAN, D. & A. LYTWYN. 1979. A novel chromogenic assay equivalent to the one stage prothrombin time (P.T.) (Abstract 0687). (VII International Congress on Thrombosis & Haemostasis.) Thromb. Haemostas. **42:** 291.

41. VAN WIJK, E., L. KAHLÉ & J. TEN CATE. 1980. Mechanized amidolytic technique for determination of factor X and factor-X antigen and its application patients being treated with oral anticoagulants. Clin. Chem. **26:** 885–890.

42. MESSMORE, H., J. FAREED, J. WALENGA, A. ANDERSEN & L. SVENDSEN. Amidolytic equivalent assays for prothrombin time (PT) and partial thromboplastin (PTT). Selection of a suitable substrate (abstract 42). (Sixth International Congress on Thrombosis of the Mediterranean League Against Thrombotic Disease.) Monte Carlo, October 23–25.

43. SANDBERG, H. & L. ANDERSON. 1979. A highly sensitive assay of platelet factor 3 using a chromogenic substrate. Thromb. Res. **14:** 113–124.

44. MINKOFF, I., K. WU, J. WALASEK, B. LIGHTFOOT & C. AMITH-KEARN. 1980. Bleeding disorder due to an isolated platelet factor 3 deficiency. Arch. Int. Med. **140:** 366–367.

45. WOHL, H., M. KUJAWA & L. PRAGER. 1978. Assay of platelet factor 4 (PF4) using synthetic thrombin substrates. Thromb. Res. **13:** 289–295.

46. SVENDSEN, L. 1977. Estimation of urokinase activity by means of a highly susceptible synthetic chromogenic substrate. *In* New Methods for Analysis of Coagulation using Chromogenic Substrates. I. Witt, Ed. 251–262. Gruyter. Berlin.

47. MORITA, T., H. KATO, S. IWANAGE, K. TAKADA, T. KIMURA & S. SAKAKIBARA. 1977. New fluorogenic substrates for a thrombin, factor Xa, kallikrein, and urokinase. J. Biochem. **82:** 1495–1498.

48. CLAESON, G., L. AURELL, G. KARLSSON, S. GUSTAVSSON, P. FRIBERGER, S. ARIELLY & R. SIMONSSON. 1979. Design of chromogenic peptide substrates. *In* Chromogenic Peptide Substrates. M. F. Scully & V. V. Kakkar, Eds.: 20–31. Churchill Livingstone. London.

SMALL SYNTHETIC PEPTIDES WITH AFFINITY FOR PROTEASES IN COAGULATION AND FIBRINOLYSIS: AN OVERVIEW

Göran Claeson and Leif Aurell

Kabi AB
Research & Development Division
Stockholm, Sweden; and
Peptide Research
Mölndal, Sweden

INTRODUCTION

Simple esters and amides of amino acids have been used for more than 20 years as synthetic substrates for serine proteases in the field of coagulation and fibrinolysis.[1,2] Their use has, however, been limited, mainly because of their low specificity. These amino acid derivatives reflect the primary site of the natural substrates. One would expect that an amino acid sequence rather than a single amino acid could also imitate secondary sites of the natural substrate. This would increase the affinity and improve the selectivity with regard to a particular enzyme and give substrates with more sensitivity and specificity.

The first synthetic peptide with a pronounced affinity for thrombin was prepared in 1968[3,4] and developed as a chromogenic substrate in 1972.[5-7] It has since been followed by the development of a large number of short peptides with affinity for several proteases in coagulation and fibrinolysis. This paper will give an overview of the development of such peptides and will describe how they have been used to form different chromogenic and fluorogenic substrates and also reversible as well as irreversible inhibitors.

PEPTIDES WITH AFFINITY FOR THROMBIN

The synthesis of the first synthetic peptide imitating the natural substrate of thrombin was based on the sequence studies done by Blombäck in the 1950s, which revealed the high degree of homology of the carboxyl terminal of fibrinopeptide A throughout evolution. Blombäck postulated that this homology persists in order to provide specific interaction sites for thrombin.[8]

Synthetic studies in collaboration with the Kabi group showed that the subsites Arg (P_1) and Phe (P_9) in fibrinopeptide A were important for the substrate-enzyme interaction.[3,4] Shortening the distance between them led to weaker interactions. However, the short peptide, H-Phe-Val-Arg-OMe, with Phe in P_3, also had a pronounced inhibiting effect on thrombin. The suggested interpretation was that the space distance between Phe and Arg in the tripeptide is similar to the P_1 to P_9 distance in fibrinopeptide A, provided that this part of the molecule has a helical structure. An ordered structure of fibrinopeptide A was later demonstrated by Huseby[9] and Marlar,[10] and Sheraga's extensive studies of peptide sequences around the cleavage sites in fibrinogen[11] have

798

confirmed the importance of Phe (P_9) for the thrombin-fibrinogen interaction. Subsequently, the tripeptide mimicking important parts of the natural substrate was transformed into a chromogenic substrate, Bz-Phe-Val-Arg-pNA.[5, 7]

An interesting observation by Claeson *et al.* was that although the replacement of Bz-L-Phe by Bz-D-Phe or H-L-Phe in position P_3 in this substrate resulted in drastically diminished hydrolysis, replacement by H-D-Phe in this position led to practically no decrease in susceptibility to thrombin (TABLE 1). The same phenomenon has been observed with other tripeptide substrates not only for thrombin, but also for several other serine proteases,[12-14] and has played an important role in the designing of new substrates. Christensen has studied the change of kinetic parameters of the aforementioned substrates with variation of the P_3 position and has indicated a possible explanation.[15] By means of nuclear magnetic resonance spectroscopy (nmr), Scheraga has studied the conformation of the same substrates.[16]

Besides the Arg-16-Gly-17 bond, the Arg-19-Val-20 bond in the Aα chain (FIG. 1) is also susceptible to hydrolysis by thrombin.[17] Dorman found that the tripeptide H-Gly-Pro-Arg-OH, containing the sequence preceding the Arg-19-Val-20 bond, was an inhibitor of thrombin,[18] and Svendsen used the same sequence to synthesize a good chromogenic thrombin substrate, Tos-Gly-

TABLE 1

RELATIVE SENSITIVITY OF A THROMBIN SUBSTRATE WITH A FREE OR
PROTECTED N-TERMINAL AMINO ACID OF DIFFERENT CONFIGURATIONS

Substrate	Relative Reaction Rate of Thrombin
Bz-Phe-Val-Arg-pNA	100
H-Phe-Val-Arg-pNA	5
Bz-D-Phe-Val-Arg-pNA	5
H-D-Phe-Val-Arg-pNA	95

Pro-Arg-pNA.[19] Also, other proteins besides fibrinogen have specific bonds that are cleaved by thrombin[8, 20-22]; for example, in both factor XIII and prothrombin, Pro occurs in the P_2 position (FIG. 2). Thus, the Pro-Arg sequence seems to constitute important binding sites for thrombin. Very good kinetic data have also been shown for the substrate H-D-Phe-Pip-Arg-pNA,[12, 23] where Pip is pipecolic acid, a six-membered homolog to Pro. Recently Gray modified the aforementioned Tos-protected substrate and obtained Me-Gly-Pro-Arg-pNA.[24]

The chromophore, *p*-nitroaniline, is the leaving group in all the aforementioned substrates. Since fluorescence usually can be measured with higher sensitivity than uv light absorbance, there has been great interest in changing chromogenic substrates to fluorogenic substrates. The first fluorophores studied in this connection were 2-naphthylamine (βNA) and 4-methoxy-2-naphthylamine (MβNA). They have been widely used, mainly in combination with single amino acids. Mitchell *et al.*[25] have used the thrombin substrate Cbo-Gly-Pro-Arg-MβNA. The carcinogenicity of β-naphthylamine, however, will probably prevent development of this type of marker.

Zimmerman introduced 7-amino-4-methylcoumarin (MCA) as a sensitive

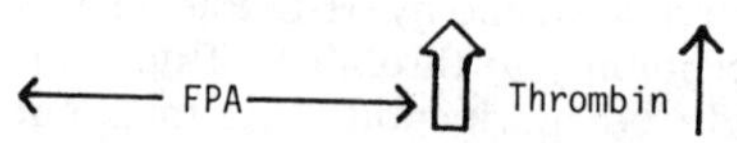

FIGURE 1. The primary structure of the N-terminal part of the Aα chain of fibrinogen and the cleavage sites of thrombin.

leaving group for chymotrypsin substrates [26] and Morita applied it to peptide substrates for proteases in coagulation and fibrinolysis.[27] The substrate, Boc-Val-Pro-Arg-MCA, mimicking the thrombin cleavage site of factor XIII, turned out to be a sensitive substrate for thrombin. Huseby recently introduced a new fluorophore, 5-amino-isophthalic acid dimethyl ester (AIE), which with the already known thrombin-susceptible peptide, Phe-Pro-Arg, gave a good thrombin substrate, H-D-Phe-Pro-Arg-AIE.[28] (For formulas see FIGURE 3.) Suggested substrates for thrombin, together with available kinetic data, are listed in TABLE 2.

In 1974, Bajusz synthesized reversible peptide inhibitors for thrombin. He utilized the thrombin-sensitive sequences, Phe-Val-Arg, Gly-Pro-Arg, Ile-Pro-Arg, and Val-Pro-Arg, and changed the carboxyl group of arginine (Arg-OH) to an aldehyde (Arg-H), using the leupeptins as models. The inhibitors obtained in this way are transition state analogs and show very good inhibiting capacity. The most potent one was H-D-Phe-Pro-Arg-H.[29, 30]

Kettner and Shaw have synthesized a large number of irreversible peptide inhibitors for serine proteases containing a C-terminal lysine or arginine chloromethyl ketone. Just like Bajusz, they obtained good inhibitors using the amino acid sequences at the sites cleaved by thrombin in its physiologic substrates.[31, 32] The very best, a highly effective irreversible thrombin inhibitor, H-D-Phe-Pro-Arg-CH$_2$Cl (K$_i$ 10^{-10}), also had the same sequence as the best aldehyde inhibitor. The structures of the thrombin inhibitors mentioned are listed in TABLE 3.

PEPTIDES WITH AFFINITY FOR FACTOR Xa

Factor Xa activates bovine prothrombin by splitting two bonds (FIG. 4), preceded by identical tetrapeptide sequences.[22] The same sequences are found in human prothrombin, except that the Glu residue is replaced by an Asp in the C-terminal part of the A chain.[33] This indicates the great importance of this sequence for the enzyme-substrate interaction and was further established by the synthesis of the chromogenic substrates, Tos-Ile-Glu-Gly-Arg-pNA[22]

FIGURE 2. Amino acid sequences preceding bonds cleaved by thrombin.

BONDS CLEAVED BY THROMBIN

P9	P3	P2	P1	Substrate
Phe...	Gly-	Val-	Arg↓Gly	Fibrinogen (Aα)
	Gly-	Pro-	Arg-Val	-"- (Aα)
	Val-	Pro-	Arg-Gly	F XIII
	Ile-	Pro-	Arg-Ser	Prothrombin

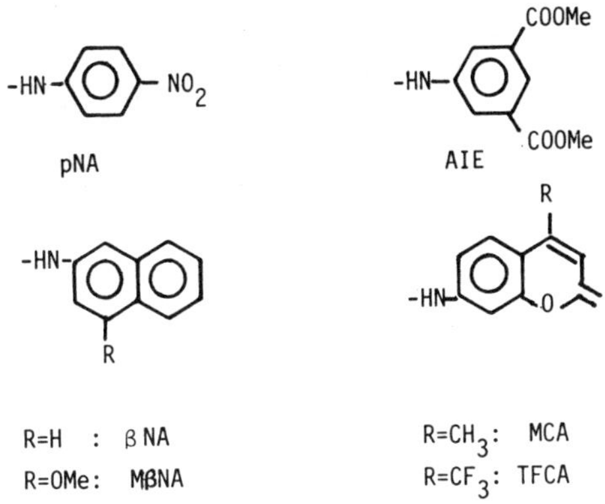

FIGURE 3. Formulas of chromophoric and fluorophoric leaving groups commonly used in synthetic substrates.

and Bz-Ile-Glu-Gly-Arg-pNA.[34] This particular amino acid sequence makes the substrates sensitive to and quite specific for human as well as bovine factor Xa and the corresponding tripeptide derivative is only very slowly hydrolyzed.[34] When ester or amide derivatives were made of the γ-carboxyl group of the glutamyl residue, the substrate could be made even more sensitive.[35] Morita changed the p-nitroanilide in the factor Xa substrate to a 4-methyl-coumaryl-7-amide,[27] thus obtaining the fluorogenic substrate, Boc-Ile-Glu-Gly-Arg-MCA.

It is interesting that the *Limulus* clotting enzyme has similar substrate requirements, as has factor Xa.[36] Boc-Ser-Gly-Arg-MCA and Boc-Ser(O-Bzl)-Gly-Arg-MCA, which were originally designed as substrates for that enzyme, also showed very good substrate properties for factor Xa.[27] An irreversible chloromethyl ketone inhibitor has also been prepared for factor Xa: H-Ile-Glu-Gly-Arg-CH$_2$Cl.[37]

PEPTIDES WITH AFFINITY FOR KALLIKREIN

Plasma kallikrein and glandular kallikrein release bradykinin and lysyl-bradykinin (kallidin), respectively, from the kininogen molecule (FIG. 5). The

TABLE 2

KINETIC CONSTANTS FOR VARIOUS THROMBIN SUBSTRATES *

Thrombin Substrate	K_m (mol/L)	V_{max} (mol/min·NIH)
Bz-Phe-Val-Arg-pNA	$11\cdot10^{-5}$	$4\cdot10^{-8}$
H-D-Phe-Pip-Arg-pNA	$0.7\cdot10^{-5}$	$20\cdot10^{-8}$
H-D-Phe-Pro-Arg-AIE	$5\cdot10^{-5}$	
Tos-Gly-Pro-Arg-pNA	$1\cdot10^{-5}$	
Me-Gly-Pro-Arg-pNA		
Cbo-Gly-Pro-Arg-MβNA	$8\cdot10^{-5}$	
Boc-Val-Pro-Arg-MCA	$2\cdot10^{-5}$	$3\cdot10^{-8}$

* The figures in this and in the following tables are taken from the references (see text) and are not always exactly comparable because the experimental conditions are not identical.

TABLE 3

CHRONOLOGIC ORDER OF REPORTING OF DIFFERENT TYPES OF PEPTIDE
INHIBITORS OF THROMBIN

Peptide Inhibitor	Investigator	Year
H-Phe-Val-Arg-OMe	Blombäck	1968
H-Gly-Pro-Arg-OH	Dorman	1972
H-D-Phe-Val-Arg-H	Bajusz	1974
H-Gly-Pro-Arg-H	Bajusz	1974
H-D-Phe-Pro-Arg-H	Bajusz	1974
H-Val-Pro-Arg-CH₂Cl	Kettner	1977
H-D-Phe-Pro-Arg-CH₂Cl	Kettner	1979

first chromogenic substrate for plasma kallikrein, Bz-Pro-Phe-Arg-pNA, based on the sequence preceding one of the scissile bonds, was synthesized by Amundsen.[38] As for many other tripeptide substrates, the N-terminal H-D-form, H-D-Pro-Phe-Arg-pNA, was shown by Claeson [39] to be advantageous.

The last-mentioned substrate was cleaved by glandular kallikrein to a much lesser degree than it was by plasma kallikrein. In our experience, imitation of the amino acid residues preceding the bonds cleaved by glandular kallikrein gave no satisfactory substrate for this enzyme. Especially chromogenic substrates with the amino acid sequence Ser-Leu-Met were split very poorly by glandular kallikrein.[39] This is also confirmed by Fiedler, who studied a series of peptides and among them a corresponding tripeptide ester.[40] Iwanaga, however, has reported that a small kininogen fragment containing kallidin extended at its N-terminal end with the aforementioned sequence is cleaved by pancreatic kallikrein at the methionyl bond.[41] Stewart [42] recently synthesized one octadeca- and one octapeptide (TABLE 4) based on the primary structure of bovine kininogen and containing the sequences on both sides of the N-terminal part of kallidin. These peptides were also cleaved at the Met-Lys bond by rat urinary kallikrein. It is evident that interactions between glandular kallikrein and some part of the substrate within the kallidin sequence are important for the unique cleavage of the Met-Lys bond.

Because our attempts to imitate the natural substrate gave poor results in the case of glandular kallikrein, we instead tried to establish structure-activity correlations by systematic variation of the amino acid residues of the peptides (TABLE 5). In this way, the chromogenic substrate H-D-Val-Leu-Arg-pNA for glandular kallikrein was obtained.[39, 43] Fiedler, however, has shown [44] that the

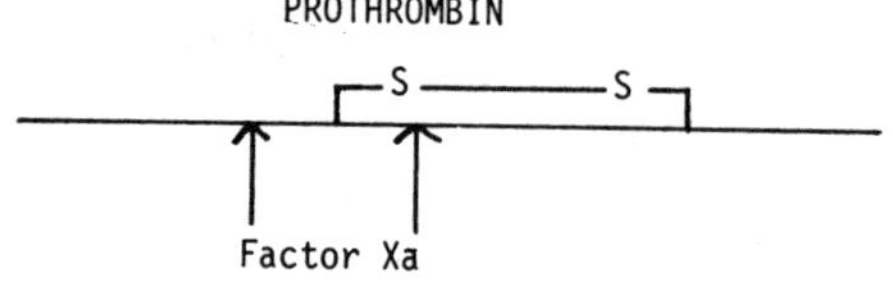

FIGURE 4. Schematic representation of the enzymatic cleavage of the bovine prothrombin molecule by factor Xa.

FIGURE 5. Amino acid sequences around the bonds cleaved in kininogen by plasma and glandular kallikreins.

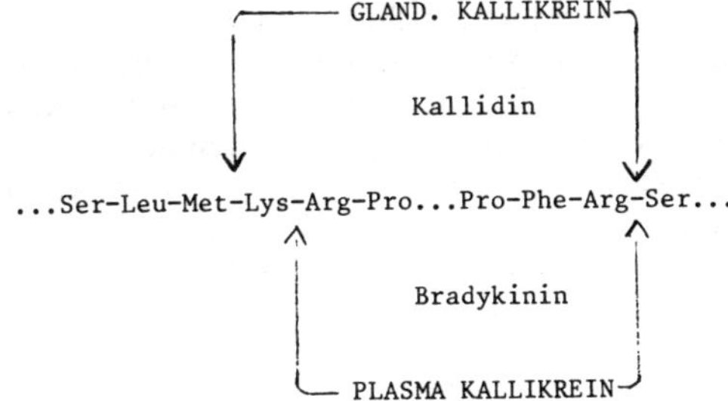

TABLE 4

KINETIC CONSTANTS FOR VARIOUS KALLIKREIN SUBSTRATES

Substrate	K_m	k_{cat}	K_{cat}/K_m
Human urinary kallikrein			
H-Pro-Phe-Arg-[³H]-anilide	$8 \cdot 10^{-7}$	290	$3700 \cdot 10^5$
H-Pro-Phe-Arg-MCA	$2 \cdot 10^{-4}$	23	$1 \cdot 10^5$
Porcine pancreatic kallikrein			
Ac-Phe-Arg-OMe	$3 \cdot 10^{-5}$		$310 \cdot 10^5$
Ac-Pro-Phe-Arg-OMe			$350 \cdot 10^5$
H-D-Val-Leu-Arg-OMe	$2 \cdot 10^{-5}$		
↓			
Ac-Ser-Leu-Met-Lys--Arg-Pro-Pro-Gly-NH₂	$1 \cdot 10^{-4}$		

TABLE 5

INFLUENCE OF STRUCTURAL VARIATIONS UPON THE SUBSTRATE SENSITIVITY TOWARDS GLANDULAR KALLIKREIN

Substrate $P_3\ P_2\ P_1$	Relative Reaction Rate of Glandular Kallikrein
Bz-Phe-Val-Arg-pNA	100
Bz-Val-Val-Arg-pNA	320
Bz-Leu-Val-Arg-pNA	150
Bz-Ile-Val-Arg-pNA	115
Bz-Phe-*Leu-Arg*-pNA	880
Bz-Val-Leu-Arg-pNA	2,600
Bz-Leu-Leu-Arg-pNA	1,400
Bz-Ile-Leu-Arg-pNA	2,300
Bz-Phe-Ile-Arg-pNA	15
Bz-Val-Ile-Arg-pNA	180
Bz-Leu-Ile-Arg-pNA	85
Bz-Ile-Ile-Arg-pNA	90

dipeptide ester, Ac-Phe-Arg-OEt, is a very sensitive substrate for glandular kallikrein (TABLE 4), 40 times more sensitive than H-D-Val-Leu-Arg-pNA. The drawback in using this substrate in a kallikrein assay, however, is the need for a coupled enzymatic determination of ethyl alcohol. Fluorogenic substrates for kallikreins have been prepared by Iwanaga,[45] who found that Cbo-Phe-Arg-MCA functions well for plasma kallikrein and H-Pro-Phe-Arg-MCA for pancreatic and urinary kallikreins.

An extremely sensitive assay for urinary kallikrein has been developed by Chung,[46] using H-Pro-Phe-Arg-[³H]-benzylamide or H-Pro-Phe-Arg-[³H]-anilide as substrates (TABLE 4). An important finding arising from these studies is also that both substrates inhibit human urinary kallikrein when used at concentrations greater than 10 μM.

Another important finding was made by Fareed.[47] He observed that the substrate H-D-Pro-Phe-Arg-pNA, imitating the C-terminal end of bradykinin, had an antagonistic effect on the bradykinin-induced contraction of isolated smooth muscles. Claeson et al.[48] changed the C-terminal end group and obtained a higher effect with H-D-Pro-Phe-Arg-NH-heptyl.

Irreversible inhibitors to human plasma kallikrein have been synthesized by Kettner.[49] H-Ala-Phe-Arg-CH$_2$Cl has a somewhat better K$_i$ than H-Pro-Phe-Arg-CH$_2$Cl, but the latter is more specific.

Peptides With Affinity for Plasmin

In its physiologic function, plasmin splits a great number of Arg and Lys bonds of fibrin. Of these amino acids, the enzyme seems to prefer Lys. Substrates with only this amino acid have been synthesized. The chromogenic thrombin substrate Bz-Phe-Val-Arg-pNA was used by Amundsen[50] as a plasmin substrate for the determination of plasmin inhibitors in plasma. The first amino acid sequence especially suitable for plasmin was obtained through structure-activity correlations by the Kabi group.[13, 51] This sequence was used with the pNA chromophore, H-D-Val-Leu-Lys-pNA. Later the same sequence was used with fluorophoric leaving groups: D-Val-Leu-Lys-AIE,[52] Boc-Val-Leu-Lys-MCA,[45] and H-D-Val-Leu-Lys-TFCA.[53] It is worth mentioning that the amino acid sequence -Leu-Lys- is a common C-terminal sequence of early plasmic fragments of fibrinogen. Also, other sequences give good substrates for plasmin, such as Tos-Gly-Pro-Lys-pNA,[54] H-D-Ala-Leu-Lys-TFCA,[51] Boc-Glu-Lys-Lys-MCA,[45] H-pyro-Glu-Phe-Lys-pNA,[55] and succinoyl-Ala-Phe-Lys-MCA,[56] which are all similar to amino acid sequences preceding bonds split in natural plasmin substrates. Kinetic data for some of the synthetic substrates are given in TABLE 6. Shaw has also prepared irreversible inhibitors to plasmin, such as H-Ala-Phe-Lys-CH$_2$Cl.[57]

Peptides With Affinity for Plasminogen Activators

The plasminogen-streptokinase (Plg·SK) complex and plasmin were found by Friberger[55] to have similar substrate requirements, as judged from studies with synthetic tripeptide p-nitroanilides. The good plasmin substrate H-D-Val-Leu-Lys-pNA is an even better substrate for Plg·SK.[55] Also, Boc-Val-Leu-Lys-pNA is hydrolyzed by both enzymes.[45] However, Iwanaga[45] has reported that

TABLE 6

KINETIC CONSTANTS FOR VARIOUS PLASMIN SUBSTRATES

Plasmin substrate	K_m (mol/L)	V_{max} (mol·min^{-1}·CU^{-1})
H-D-Val-Leu-Lys-pNA	$2 \cdot 10^{-4}$	$5 \cdot 10^{-7}$
H-D-Val-Leu-Lys-TFCA	$6 \cdot 10^{-4}$	$1 \cdot 10^{-7}$
Boc-Val-Leu-Lys-MCA	$3 \cdot 10^{-4}$	$6 \cdot 10^{-7}$
H-Val-Leu-Lys-AIE	$3 \cdot 10^{-4}$	
Boc-Glu-Lys-Lys-MCA	$5 \cdot 10^{-4}$	$6 \cdot 10^{-7}$
Tos-Gly-Pro-Lys-pNA	$3 \cdot 10^{-4}$	

the plasmin substrate, Boc-Glu-Lys-Lys-MCA, imitating the C-terminal sequence of the N-terminal fragment released in the plasmin-mediated transformation of Glu-plasminogen to Lys-plasminogen,[58] is not hydrolyzed by the Plg·SK complex.

By means of limited proteolysis, plasminogen is activated by various activators. The structure around the activation bond is shown in FIGURE 6. Magnusson[59] and the Kabi group[55] have prepared Bz-Pro-Gly-Arg-pNA. It was found to be a substrate for urokinase and also for tissue activator (Wallén), but not a good one for either enzyme. The Kabi group has also synthesized longer peptides having the sequence found in the natural substrate. However, none was satisfactory as a substrate for urokinase or tissue activator. Magnusson has studied several peptide fragments containing the bond to be cleaved. He obtained a good substrate for urokinase when the disulfide bridge around the activation cleavage site was intact,[60] indicating that the tertiary structure is important for the enzyme-substrate interaction.

By structure-activity correlations, reasonably good chromogenic substrates for urokinase have been obtained (H-Glu-Gly-Arg-pNA,[39] Bz-Val-Gly-Arg-pNA,[61] pyro-Glu-Gly-Arg-pNA[55]) as have fluorogenic substrates (H-Val-Gly-Arg-βNA,[62, 63] glutaryl-Gly-Arg-MCA,[45] and Cbo-Gly-Gly-Arg-TFCA[53]). Substrates for plasminogen tissue activators that are sufficiently good for plasma assays are not yet available, but H-D-Val-Gly-Arg-pNA,[55] Boc-Val-Gly-Arg-βNA,[62] and Cbo-Gly-Gly-Arg-MCA[64] function well in purified systems.

Kettner and Shaw[65, 66] made a careful study of the susceptibility of urokinase and plasminogen activator to peptides of arginine chloromethyl ketone. They found that the "natural" sequence Pro-Gly-Arg is far from optimal for a chloromethyl ketone inhibitor. This is also in agreement with the results obtained by Magnusson[59] and Friberger,[55] who found that Pro-Gly-Arg does not form good substrates for urokinase and plasminogen activators. The best inhibitor for urokinase is H-Glu-Gly-Arg-CH$_2$Cl[65] and the best for the plasminogen activator from HeLa cells is dansyl-Glu-Gly-Arg-CH$_2$Cl.[66] Kettner

Plasminogen activators

↓

-Lys-Lys-Cys-Pro-Gly-Arg-Val-Val-

←——Heavy chain   Light chain——→

FIGURE 6. Amino acid sequence around the bond cleaved in plasminogen by plasminogen activators.

et al. point out that plasminogen activator seems to be more susceptible to those peptide inhibitors where P_4 is an amino acid or acyl group rather than a free amino group at P_3. These results are consistent with results obtained by Nieuwenhuizen [62, 63] with plasminogen activator substrates having the sequence Val-Gly-Arg. Kettner and Shaw as well as Friberger have demonstrated that urokinase and plasminogen activators have different susceptibility patterns towards a series of inhibitors and substrates, thus showing that these enzymes are not identical.

PEPTIDES WITH AFFINITY FOR FACTORS IXA AND XIA

A chromogenic tetrapeptide substrate imitating the sequence preceding the cleavage site of factor X cleaved by factor IXa—Bz-Gln-Val-Val-Arg-pNA—has been synthesized by the Kabi group. Suomela [67] and others, however, found the substrate very insensitive towards factor IXa.

Bovine factor IX is converted to factor IXa by factor XIa in a two-step

TABLE 7

AMINO ACID SEQUENCES PRECEDING BONDS CLEAVED IN FACTOR X
AND FACTOR IX BY THEIR ACTIVATING ENZYMES *

Enzyme	Natural Substrate	Sequence Preceding Scissile Bond
Factor IXa	Factor X (bovine)	-Glu-Val-Val-Arg- ↓
Factor XIa	Factor IX (bovine)	-Lys-Leu-Thr-Arg-
Factor XIa	Factor IX (bovine)	-Glu-Phe-Ser-Arg-

* Factor IXa and Factor XIa, respectively.

reaction. The amino acid sequences preceding the bonds split (TABLE 7) are known.[68] Iwanaga has synthesized fluorogenic tripeptide substrates on the basis of these sequences.[45] These substrates are hydrolyzed by factor XIa, but the reaction rate seems too slow to be of great practical value.

DISCUSSION

Interest in small synthetic peptides that are recognized by proteolytic enzymes in a manner similar to that of natural substrates has grown rapidly during the last decade. In coagulation and fibrinolysis the interest originated from attempts to synthesize thrombin inhibitors [3, 4, 18] and from the finding that for thrombin very important enzyme-substrate interaction could be localized to the tertiary structure of the natural substrate immediately preceding the bond split by thrombin.[8] This was shown to be true also for other serine proteases, and often a direct imitation of the primary amino acid sequence preceding the susceptible bond gave satisfactory properties to the synthetic substrate.[14, 45]

The sensitivity of these short synthetic peptide substrates is often quite good, even compared to that of the natural ones. The thrombin substrate Bz-Phe-Val-Arg-pNA has, for example, a specificity constant (k_{cat}/K_m) comparable to that of fibrinogen, and this constant for H-D-Phe-Pip-Arg-pNA is even two powers of ten higher.[23]

In order to obtain good kinetic constants, the amino acid sequence is of course the most important feature in the structure of these substrates. TABLE 5 gives a good illustration of how the small structural changes obtained when varying the P_2 position between Val, Leu, and Ile give rise to very great changes in the susceptibility of the substrates to the enzyme.

The importance of the configurations of the amino acids and the N-terminal groups of the peptides is clearly shown in TABLE 1. Variation of the C-terminal leaving group can also drastically change the kinetic constants of the substrates. It is well known that esters give in general better leaving groups than amides. But also, changing the C-terminal amido group can change both K_m and k_{cat}. The plasmin-sensitive sequence H-D-Val-Leu-Lys has, for example, a specificity constant that is 15 times higher with the chromophore pNA than with the fluorophore TFCA (cf. TABLE 6). That means that replacing the chromophore with a fluorophore in a given amino acid sequence will not always give a more sensitive substrate. The gain in going to fluorescence spectroscopy may be completely lost because of the interior kinetic constants obtained when changing from a chromogenic to a fluorogenic substrate. An extreme example of the importance of the C-terminal end group is shown in TABLE 4, where it is seen that the amino acid sequence, H-Pro-Phe-Arg, for urinary kallikrein gives substrates with k_{cat}/K_m differing by four powers of ten, depending upon the C-terminal leaving group.

Not only the sensitivity, but also a certain amount of specificity can be built into these short amino acid sequences. But, of course, when one goes from the large natural substrate to the small synthetic peptide, one loses many interaction sites as well as the tertiary structure corresponding to the natural substrate. Thus, partially degraded, isolated enzymes can lose part of their biological activity, and this might not be fully reflected in their activity towards a smaller synthetic substrate.[69]

The development of chromogenic peptide substrates for most of the enzymes in coagulation and fibrinolysis has been advanced mainly by the work of the Kabi and Pentapharm groups. Great attention has also lately been devoted to fluorogenic substrates. All the amino acid sequences produced as p-nitroanilides and several original ones have been furnished with fluorogenic leaving groups. In this area, Iwanaga and associates have been leading, but much interesting work has also been done in the United States, such as that of Smith and the groups at Dade and Merck.

The application of these chromogenic and fluorogenic substrates toward the determination of enzymes, proenzymes, and antienzymes in the coagulation, fibrinolysis, and kallikrein-kinin systems is steadily increasing, especially as research tools, but also in the clinical laboratory.[70, 71] In the coming years, we will probably see peptide substrates as diagnostic tools for proteolytic enzymes within other areas.

The development of specific inhibitors for the proteolytic enzymes seems very promising. The transition state analog inhibitors synthesized by Bajusz and the irreversible chloromethyl ketone inhibitors studied by Kettner and Shaw have pointed to the potential development of such peptides in the therapeutic field.

SUMMARY

In order to synthesize peptide derivatives with affinity for rather specific proteases, such as those in the coagulation cascade, valuable information can be obtained from the primary sequence of their natural substrates. Thus, the development of peptide substrates for thrombin has to a great extent been based on the primary sequences preceding the thrombin-sensitive bonds in fibrinogen. Likewise, the determination of the primary structure of prothrombin—and the definition of the bonds split by factor Xa—made it possible to synthesize tetrapeptide substrates sensitive to, and quite specific for, factor Xa. Another example of this procedure is that of the C-terminal tripeptide of bradykinin, which contains enough structural information to make it function well as an affinity handle in chromogenic substrates for plasma kallikrein.

Less success was achieved in the attempt to develop substrates for urokinase, factor IXa, and glandular kallikrein along the same line. Instead, structure—activity correlations were obtained by systematic variation of the amino acid residues of the peptides. Thus, the requirements of different enzymes for the substrate positions P_1, P_2, and P_3 were evaluated. In this way substrates for enzymes such as urokinase, plasmin, and glandular kallikrein could be obtained.

The amino acid sequences with affinity for different enzymes obtained in the aforementioned ways have been utilized not only to make chromogenic substrates (*p*-nitroanilides), but also to synthesize various kinds of fluorogenic substrates (for example, derivatives of β-naphthylamines, aminoisophthalic acid, and aminomethylcoumarin). Several very good reversible and irreversible inhibitors have also been synthesized from the aforementioned peptides. This has been accomplished by changing the C-terminal carboxyl group to an aldehyde and a chloromethyl ketone, respectively.

REFERENCES

1. SHERRY, S. & W. TROLL. 1954. J. Biol. Chem. **208:** 95–105.
2. TROLL, W., S. SHERRY & J. WACKMAN. 1954. J. Biol. Chem. **208:** 85–95.
3. BLOMBÄCK, B., M. BLOMBÄCK, P. OLSSON, L. SVENDSEN, B. AF EKENSTAM & G. CLAESON. 1967. Swedish Patent Application. U.S. 3,826,739.
4. BLOMBÄCK, B., M. BLOMBÄCK, P. OLSSON, L. SVENDSEN & G. ÅBERG. 1969. Scand. J. Clin. Lab. Invest. **24**(Suppl. 107): 59–64.
5. BLOMBÄCK, B., M. BLOMBÄCK, G. CLAESON & L. SVENDSEN. 1972. Swedish Patent Application. U.S. 3,884,896.
6. CLAESON, G., G. KARLSSON & L. SVENDSEN. 1972. Swedish Patent Application. U.S. 3,886,136.
7. SVENDSEN, L., B. BLOMBÄCK, M. BLOMBÄCK & P. OLSSON. 1972. Thromb. Res. **1:** 267–278.
8. BLOMBÄCK, B., B. HESSEL, D. HOGG & G. CLAESON. 1977. *In* Chemistry and Biology of Thrombin. R. L. Lundblad, J. W. Fenton, II & K. G. Mann, Eds.: 275–290. Ann Arbor Science Publishers. Ann Arbor, MI.
9. HUSEBY, R. M. 1973. Physiol. Chem. Phys. **5:** 1–12.
10. MARLAR, R. A., D. A. WALZ, J. W. FENTON & W. H. SEEGERS. 1977. Abstract 99. American Chemical Society, Div. Biol. Chem. 174th National Meeting.
11. SCHERAGA, H. A. 1977. *In* Chemistry and Biology of Thrombin. R. L. Lundblad, J. W. Fenton, II & K. G. Mann, Eds.: 145–158. Ann Arbor Science Publishers. Ann Arbor, MI.

12. CLAESON, G., L. AURELL & G. KARLSSON. 1975. Swedish Patent Application. U.S. 4,137,225.
13. CLAESON, G., L. AURELL, G. KARLSSON, S. GUSTAVSSON & A. OLAUSSON. 1975. Swedish Patent Application. U.S. 4,137,225.
14. CLAESON, G., L. AURELL, G. KARLSSON, S. GUSTAVSSON, P. FRIBERGER, S. ARIELLY & R. SIMONSSON. 1977. *In* Chromogenic Peptide Substrates. Chemistry and Clinical Usage. M. Scully & V. V. Kākkar, Eds.: 20–31. Churchill Livingstone. London. 1979.
15. CHRISTENSEN, U. & H.-E. IPSEN. 1979. Biochem. Biophys. Acta **569:** 177–183.
16. RAE, I. D. & H. A. SCHERAGA. 1978. Private communication.
17. BLOMBÄCK, B., M. BLOMBÄCK, B. HESSEL & S. IWANAGA. 1967. Nature **215:** 1445–1448.
18. DORMAN, L. C., R. C. CHOW & F. N. MARSHALL. 1972. *In* Chemistry and Biology of Peptides. J. Meinhofer, Ed.: 455–459. Ann Arbor Science Publishers. Ann Arbor, MI.
19. SVENDSEN, L. & K. STOCKER. 1977. *In* New Methods for Analysis of Coagulation Using Chromogenic Substrates. I. Witt, Ed.: 23–35. Walter de Gruyter. Berlin.
20. NAKAMURA, S., S. IWANAGA & T. SUZUKI. 1975. J. Biochem. **78:** 1247–1266.
21. WALZ, D. A., W. H. SEEGERS, J. REUTERBY & L. E. MCCOY. 1974. Thromb. Res. **4:** 713–717.
22. MAGNUSSON, S., T. E. PETERSEN, L. SOTTRUP-JENSEN & H. CLAEYS. 1975. *In* Proteases and Biological Control. E. Reich, D. B. Rifkin & E. Shaw, Eds.: 123–149. Cold Spring Harbor Press. Cold Spring Harbor, NY.
23. CLAESON, G., L. AURELL, G. KARLSSON & P. FRIBERGER. 1977. *In* New Methods for Analysis of Coagulation Using Chromogenic Substrates.[19] pp. 37–54.
24. GRAY, A. J., K. A. UHLMEYER & E. J. FEDOR. 1979. Thromb. Haemostas. (Stuttgart) **42:** 225.
25. MITCHELL, G. A., P. M. HUDSON, R. F. HUSEBY, S. P. POCHRON & R. J. GARGIULO. 1978. Thromb. Res. **12:** 219–225.
26. ZIMMERMAN, M., E. C. YUREWICZ & G. PATEL. 1976. Anal. Biochem. **70:** 258–262.
27. MORITA, T., H. KATO, S. IWANAGA, K. TAKADA, T. KIMURA & S. SAKAKIBARA. 1977. J. Biochem. (Tokyo) **82:** 1495–1498.
28. MITCHELL, G. A., R. J. GARGIULO, R. M. HUSEBY, D. E. LAWSON, S. P. POCHRON & J. A. SEHUANES. 1978. Thromb. Res. **13:** 47–52.
29. BAJUSZ, S., É. BARABÁS, E. SZÉLL, AND D. BAGDY. 1974. Hungarian Patent No. 169870.
30. BAJUSZ, S., É. BARABÁS, P. TOLNAY, E. SZÉLL & D. BAGDY. 1978. Int. J. Pept. Protein Res. **12:** 217–221.
31. KETTNER, C. & E. SHAW. 1977. *In* Chemistry and Biology of Thrombin. R. L. Lundblad, J. W. Fenton, II & K. G. Mann. Eds.: 129–143. Ann Arbor Science Publishers. Ann Arbor, MI.
32. KETTNER, C. & E. SHAW. 1979. Thromb. Res. **14:** 969–973.
33. WALZ, D. A. & W. H. SEEGERS. 1974. Biochem. Biophys. Res. Commun. **60:** 717–722.
34. AURELL, L., G. CLAESON, G. KARLSSON & P. FRIBERGER. 1976. *In* Peptides 1976. Proceedings of the 14th European Peptide Symposium, Weipon, Belgium. A. Loffet, Ed.: 191–195. Edition de l'Université de Bruxelles. Brussels.
35. AURELL, L., R. SIMONSSON, S. ARIELLY, G. KARLSSON, P. FRIBERGER & G. CLAESON. 1978. Haemostasis **7:** 92–94.
36. IWANAGA, S., T. MORITA, T. HARADA, S. NAKAMURA, M. NIWA, K. TAKADA, T. KIMURA & S. SAKAKIBARA. 1978. Haemostasis **7:** 183–188.
37. KETTNER, C., S. SPRINGHORN, E. SHAW, W. MÜLLER & H. FRITZ. 1978. Hoppe Seyler's Z. Physiol. Chem. **359:** 1183–1191.

38. AMUNDSEN, E., L. SVENDSEN, M. M. VENNEROD & K. LAAKE. 1976. *In* Chemistry and Biology of the Kallikrein-Kinin System in Health and Disease. J. J. Pisano and K. F. Austen, Eds.: 215–220. Fogarty International Center Proceedings No. 27. U.S. Government Printing Office. Washington, D.C.

39. CLAESON, G., L. AURELL, P. FRIBERGER, S. GUSTAVSSON & G. KARLSSON. 1978. Haemostasis **7:** 62–68.

40. FIEDLER, F. & G. LEYSATH. 1979. *In* Kinins: II: Biochemistry, Pathophysiology, and Clinical Aspects. S. Fujii, H. Moriya & Suzuki, Eds.: 261–271. Plenum Press. New York, NY.

41. IWANAGA, S., Y. N. NAH, H. KATO & T. SUZUKI. 1977. *In* Kininogenases-Kallikrein, Vol. 4. G. L. Haberland, J. W. Rohen & T. Suzuki, Eds.: 79–90. FK. Schattauer Verlag. Stuttgart.

42. STEWART, J. M. & D. H. MORRIS. 1978. *In* Kinins: II: Biochemistry, Pathophysiology, and Clinical Aspects.[40] pp. 213–218.

43. AMUNDSEN, E., J. PÜTTER, P. FRIBERGER M. KNÖS, M. LARSBRAATEN & G. CLAESON. 1978. *In* Kinins: II: Biochemistry, Pathophysiology, and Clinical Aspects.[40] pp. 83–95.

44. FIEDLER, F., R. GEIGER, C. HIRSCHAUER & G. LEYSATH. 1978. Hoppe-Seyler's Z. Physiol. Chem. **259:** 1667–1673.

45. IWANAGA, S., T. MORITA, H. KATO, T. HARADA, N. ADACHI, T. SUGO, I. MARUYAMA, K. TAKADA, T. KIMURA & S. SAKAKIBARA. 1978. *In* Kinins: II: Biochemistry, Pathophysiology, and Clinical Aspects.[40] pp. 147–163.

46. CHUNG, A., J. W. RYAN, G. PENA & N. B. OZA. 1978. *In* Kinins: II: Biochemistry, Pathophysiology, and Clinical Aspects.[40] pp. 115–125.

47. FAREED, J., G. KINDEL, H. L. MESSMORE & J. U. BALIS. 1979. *In* Current Concepts in Kinin Research. G. L. Haberland & U. Hamberg, Eds.: 237–247. Pergamon Press, Oxford.

48. CLAESON, G., J. FAREED, C. LARSSON, G. KINDEL, S. ARIELLY, R. SIMONSSON, H. L. MESSMORE & J. U. BALIS. 1979. *In* Kinins: II: Systemic Proteases and Cellular Function. S. Fujii, H. Moriya & T. Suzuki, Eds.: 691–713. Plenum Press, New York, NY.

49. KETTNER, C. & E. SHAW. 1978. Biochemistry **17:** 4778–4784.

50. AMUNDSEN, E., L. SVENDSEN & A. VEFLING. 1973. Abstract 22. IVth International Congress on Thrombosis and Haemostasis, Vienna, Austria.

51. FRIBERGER, P., M. KNÖS, S. GUSTAVSSON, L. AURELL & G. CLAESON. 1977. *In* Chromgenic Peptide Substrates. Chemistry and Clinical Usage.[14] pp. 121–127.

52. POCHRON, S. P., G. A. MITCHELL, I. ALBAREDA, R. M. HUSEBY & R. J. GARGIULO. 1978. Thromb. Res. **13:** 733–739.

53. SMITH, R. E., E. R. BISSELL, A. R. MITCHELL & K. W. PEARSON. 1980. Thromb. Res. **17:** 393–402.

54. GALLIMORE, M. J., E. AMUNDSEN, A. O. AASEN, M. LARSBRAATEN, K. LYNGAAS & L. SVENDSEN. 1979. Thromb. Res. **14:** 51–60.

55. FRIBERGER, P., G. CLAESON, M. KNÖS, L. AURELL, S. ARIELLY & R. SIMONSSON. 1979. *In* Progress in Chemical Fibrinolysis and Thrombolysis, Vol. 4, J. F. Davidson, Ed.: 149–153. Churchill Livingstone. Edinburgh.

56. PIERZCHALA, P. A., C. P. DORN & M. ZIMMERMAN. 1979. Biochem. J. **183:** 555–559.

57. SHAW, E. 1975. *In* Proteases and Biological Control. E. Reich, D. B. Rifkin & E. Shaw, Eds.: 445–465. Cold Spring Harbor Press. Cold Spring Harbor, NY.

58. WIMAN, B. 1973. Eur. J. Biochem. **39:** 1–9.

59. MAGNUSSON, S., L. SOTTRUP-JENSEN, T. E. PETERSEN, G. DUDEK-WOJCIECHOWSKA & H. CLAEYS. 1976. *In* Proteolysis and Physiological Regulation. D. W. Ribbon & K. Brew, Eds.: 203–238. Academic Press. New York, NY.

60. SOTTRUP-JENSEN, L., H. CLAEYS, M. ZAJDEL, T. E. PETERSEN & S. MAGNUSSON. 1978. *In* Progress in Chemical Fibrinolysis and Thrombolysis, Vol. 3, J. F.

Davidson, R. M. Rowan, M. M. Samama & P. C. Desnoyers, Eds.: 191–209.
Raven Press. New York, NY.
61. SVENDSEN, L. 1977. *In* New Methods for Analysis of Coagulation Using Chromogenic Substrates.[19] pp. 251–262.
62. NIEUWENHUIZEN, W., G. WIJNGAARDS & E. GROENEVELD. 1978. Haemostasis **7:** 146–149.
63. NIEUWENHUIZEN, W., G. WIJNGAARDS & E. GROENEVELD. 1977. Thromb. Res. **11:** 87–89.
64. ZIMMERMAN, M., J. QUIGLEY, B. ASHE, C. DORN, R. GOLDFARB & W. TROLL. 1978. Proc. Natl. Acad. Sci. USA **75:** 750–753.
65. KETTNER, C. & E. SHAW. 1979. Biochem. Biophys. Acta **569:** 31–40.
66. COLEMAN, P., C. KETTNER & E. SHAW. 1979. Biochem. Biophys. Acta **569:** 41–51.
67. SUOMELA, H., M. BLOMBÄCK & B. BLOMBÄCK. 1977. Thromb. Res. **10:** 267–281.
68. TITANI, K., D. L. ENFIELD, K. KATAYAMA, L. H. ERICSSON, K. FUJIKAWA, K. A. WALSH & H. NEURATH. 1977. Thromb. Haemostas. (Stuttgart) **38:** 116.
69. GAFFNEY, P. J., LORD K. & BRASHER, M. 1977. Thromb. Res. **10:** 549–556.
70. STORMORKEN, H. 1976. Thrombos. Haemostas. (Stuttgart) **36:** 299–301.
71. DUCKERT, F. 1979. Med. Lab. (Stuttgart) **32:** 25–32.

CHROMOGENIC SUBSTRATE SPECTROPHOTOMETRIC ASSAYS FOR THE MEASUREMENT OF CLOTTING FUNCTION

P. Ashok Aiyappa

Cardiovascular Research and Development
Diagnostics Division
Abbott Laboratories
North Chicago, Illinois 60064

INTRODUCTION

Specific tripeptide substrates with detectable leaving groups have been used extensively for the measurement of proteolytic activities of serine proteases.[1–3] Several assay systems employing the chromogenic substrates, D-Phe-Pip-Arg-pNA (S-2238) for thrombin and CBz-Ile-Glu-Gly-Arg-pNA (S-2222) for factor Xa, have been described for the determination of prothrombin and factor X levels in plasma.[4–6] These assay systems, although representing an improvement in sensitivity over that of the clotting time assay (prothrombin time), are not substitutes for the clotting time assays because of their inability to measure all the factor activities involved in the intrinsic clotting mechanism.

The present report describes the development of spectrophotometric assays for the measurement of all the coagulation factor activities in plasma, employing a relatively thrombin-specific chromogenic substrate, sarcosine-Pro-Arg-pNA. These tissue-factor-activated and surface-activated spectrophotometric assays offer improvements over the prothrombin time (PT) and activated partial thromboplastin time (APTT) assays, which are based on the present theories of extrinsic and intrinsic coagulation mechanisms, respectively.

MATERIALS AND METHODS

All the deficient plasma samples were purchased from George King Biomedical, Inc. (Overland Park, KS). Rabbit-brain powder was purchased from Pel-Freez Biologicals, Inc. (Rogers, AK). Ellagic acid, soybean trypsin inhibitor (SBTI), and hirudin were purchased from Sigma Chemical Co. (St. Louis, MO). S-2238 was purchased from Ortho Diagnostics (Raritan, NJ) and serum reagent from Dade Diagnostics (Miami, FL), and Simplastin and Platelin plus activator reagents were purchased from General Diagnostics (Morris Plains, NJ).

Tissue Thromboplastin

Rabbit-brain thromboplastin was prepared by a saline extraction technique, as described by Biggs.[7]

Phospholipids

Phospholipids from rabbit-brain powder were extracted with chloroform, as described by Bell and Alton.[8] The phospholipid suspension in saline solution was stored at −80° C.

812

Tissue Factor Activator Reagent

Tissue factor activator reagent consisted of rabbit-brain thromboplastin and Ca^{++} in Tris-HCl buffer at pH 7.4.

Surface Activator Reagent

Surface activator reagent consisted of ellagic acid, brain phospholipids, and Ca^{++} in Tris-HCl-saline buffer pH 7.4.

Chromogenic Substrate Reagent

Chromogenic substrate reagent consisted of sarcosine-Pro-Arg-pNA and soybean trypsin inhibitor (SBTI) in Tris-HCl-saline buffer at pH 7.4.

Blood Collection

Blood samples were collected using a standard two-syringe technique, employing a 19-gauge butterfly needle with 12-inch tubing and plastic syringes. One to 3 ml of the blood were collected into the first syringe and discarded. The blood sample for the test was then collected into the second syringe. Nine volumes of blood was transferred to a plastic tube containing 1 volume of 3.8 percent sodium citrate (pH 9.1) as an anticoagulant. The blood samples were stored in ice after gentle mixing.

Plasma Preparation

Blood samples were centrifuged within 1 hr of venipuncture, at $2000 \times g$ for 15 min at 2–8° C. The plasma was separated using a plastic pipette and kept at 2–8° C in polypropylene tubes or stored at −80° C.

Assay Procedures

The assays were performed either manually or by an automated spectrophotometer. 5 μl of the plasma sample (50 μl of a 1:10 dilution for manual assay method) was mixed with 500 μl of the tissue factor activator (extrinsic system) or surface activator reagent (intrinsic system) and incubated for 5 min at 37° C. Subsequently, 200 μl of the chromogenic substrate reagent was added to the reaction mixture. The change in absorbance for 5 min at 405 nm was measured by means of a kinetic spectrophotometer. In the manual method the reaction was stopped by the addition of 500 μl of 50 percent acetic acid. The amount of color produced was read at 405 nm.

RESULTS

Specificity of Thrombin Activity on Chromogenic Substrates

Five μl of the plasma sample was incubated with 500 μl of surface activator reagent for 5 min at 37° C. 10 μl of 1×10^{-7} M hirudin was added to the reaction mixture and incubated for 1 min. Subsequently, 500 μl of 2×10^{-4} M S-2238 or 2×10^{-3} M Sarc-Pro-Arg-pNA was added. The initial rates of amidase activity were measured at 405 nm using a kinetic spectrophotometer (FIG. 1). Hirudin inhibited 96 percent of the amidase activity with both the substrates. Similarly the assay was performed using prothrombin (factor II)-deficient plasma and without the addition of hirudin.

Only about 5 percent of the normal plasma activity could be generated by the factor II-deficient plasma (TABLE 1). This residual activity was inhibited by 1×10^{-8} M soybean trypsin inhibitor, added along with the substrates (TABLE 1).

Sensitivity and Specificity of the Tissue-Factor-activated Assay System

Normal, pooled plasma collected from 20 donors was serially diluted with Tris-saline buffer (pH 7.4) containing 10 mg/ml bovine serum albumin (BSA) to give 12.5, 25, 50, 75 and 100 percent of the total factor activities. Similarly, the normal plasma was diluted with specific factor-deficient plasmas of the extrinsic system (factors VII, V, X and prothrombin). Assays were performed using the tissue factor activator reagent. FIGURES 2 and 3 show the relative sensitivity of the assay system for multifactor levels and individual factor levels. Under these assay conditions plasma samples deficient in factor XII, prekallikrein, and factors XI, IX and VIII showed normal levels of activity and plasma samples deficient in factors VII, X, and V and prothrombin showed gross abnormal levels of thrombin generation (TABLE 2).

Sensitivity and Specificity of the Surface-activated Assay System

Normal, pooled plasma was serially diluted with specific factor-deficient plasma samples of the intrinsic system (factors XII, XI, IX, PK, VIII, X, V and II) to give various factor levels (12.5, 25, 50, 75, and 100 percent of the

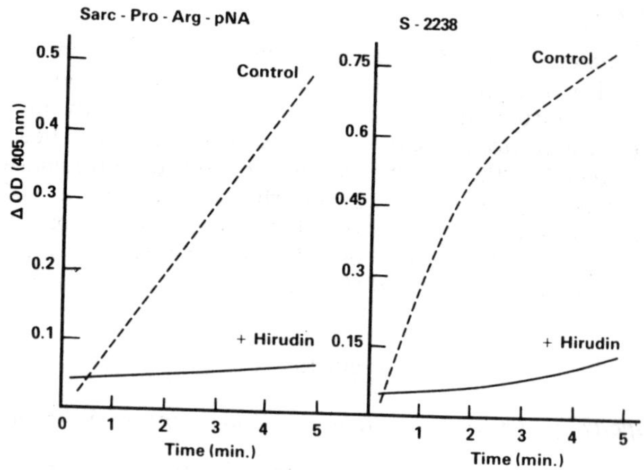

FIGURE 1. Inhibition of amidase activity by 2×10^{-8} M hirudin.

TABLE 1

SPECIFICITY OF CHROMOGENIC SUBSTRATES

Plasma Sample	(Optical density/min)*			
	S-2238	S-2238 + SBTI	SPA-pNA	SPA-pNA + SBTI
Normal	0.17	0.165	0.06	0.055
Factor-II-deficient	0.0025 (1.4%)	0.00	0.0035 (5.8%)	0.00

NOTE: Factor-II-deficient plasma was incubated with the surface activator reagent for 5 min at 37° C before the addition of the substrate or substrate plus soybean trypsin inhibitor (SBTI) reagents. The initial rates of reactions were measured at 405 nm.

* At 405 nanometers.

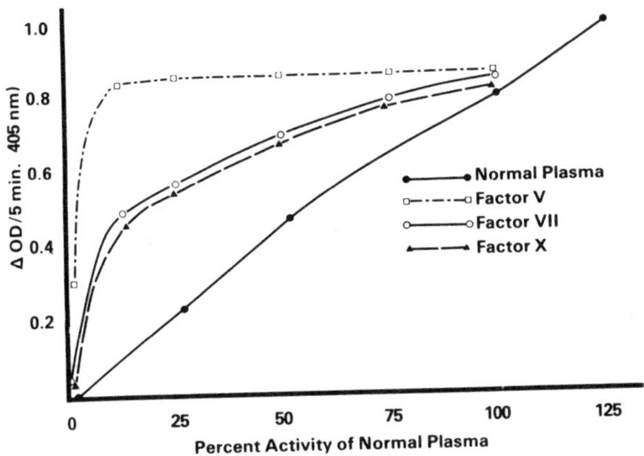

FIGURE 2. Sensitivity of the spectrophotometric assay for the tissue-factor-activated clotting system. Normal, pooled plasma was serially diluted with Tris-HCl buffer (pH 7.4) containing 10 mg/ml BSA. The plasma was also diluted with specific factor-deficient plasmas to generate different levels of factor deficiencies.

FIGURE 3. Improved sensitivity of the spectrophotometric assay for the tissue-factor-activated clotting system for factors VII, X, V, and II levels. The assay was performed using the tissue factor activator reagent, which was diluted 1:1 with Tris-HCl buffer containing 10 mg/ml BSA. Assay details are as for FIGURE 1.

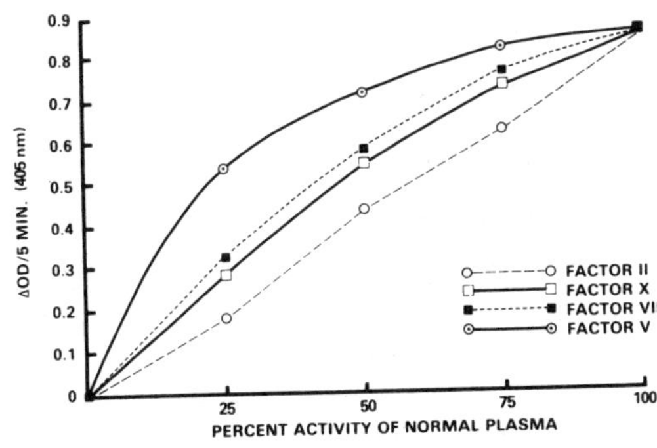

normal levels). Assays were performed using the surface activator reagent. FIGURES 4, 5, and 6 show the sensitivity of the assay system to the individual factor levels of the intrinsic system. All the deficient plasma samples showed abnormal levels of thrombin generation (TABLE 2).

Sensitivity of the Surface-activated Assay System to Factor VII Levels

Factor-VII-deficient plasma showed total abnormal level of thrombin generation when used in this surface-activated assay system (TABLE 2). Serial dilution of the normal plasma with factor-VII-deficient plasma (FIG. 7) generated a curve similar to that of other factors of the intrinsic system. To further establish this observation, assays were performed by means of aluminum-hydroxide-adsorbed plasma (source of factors V, VIII, XI, and XII) and serum reagent (source of factors VII, IX, X, XI, and XII) in a 1:1 combination with the factor-VII-deficient plasma. Adsorbed plasma failed to correct the factor VII deficiency, whereas the serum reagent corrected the factor VII deficiency and showed an increased thrombin generation activity (TABLE 3). The factor-VII-deficient plasma used in these experiments showed normal APTT and abnormal PT values by clotting time assays, thus establishing the authenticity of factor-VII-deficiency.

Effect of Heparin

FIGURE 8 shows the sensitivity of both tissue-factor-activated and surface-activated assay systems for heparin in plasma. The surface-activated assay system appeared to be very sensitive to heparin concentrations in the therapeutic range (0.1 to 0.4 units/ml) and showed proportionate lowering of thrombin generation. The tissue-factor-activated assay system is affected only at higher levels of heparin (above 0.4 u/ml) in plasma.

TABLE 2

SPECIFICITY OF SPECTROPHOTOMETRIC ASSAYS FOR VARIOUS CLOTHING FACTORS

Plasma Sample	Surface-activated Assay (OD/5 min at 405 nm)	Tissue-Factor-activated Assay (OD/5 min at 405 nm)
Normal	0.95	0.85
Factor XII⁻	0.14	0.65
Factor XI⁻	0.10	0.70
PK⁻	0.15	0.74
Factor IX⁻	0.029	0.58
Factor VIII⁻	0.05	0.55
Factor VII⁻	0.013	0.009
Factor X⁻	0.006	0.016
Factor V⁻	0.014	0.004
Factor II⁻	0.021	0.02
Normal range	0.4 to 1.0	0.4 to 0.9

NOTE: Assays were performed on the factor-deficient plasmas (Factor⁻) and on normal plasma as described in the text.

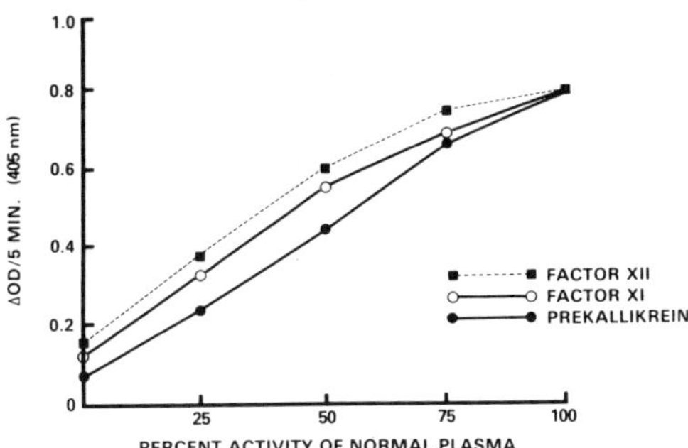

FIGURE 4. Sensitivity of the spectrophotometric assay for the surface-activated clotting system for factors XII and XI and prekallikrein (PK) deficiencies. Normal, pooled plasma was serially diluted with plasma deficient in factors XII and XI and prekallikrein to give various levels of factor deficiencies.

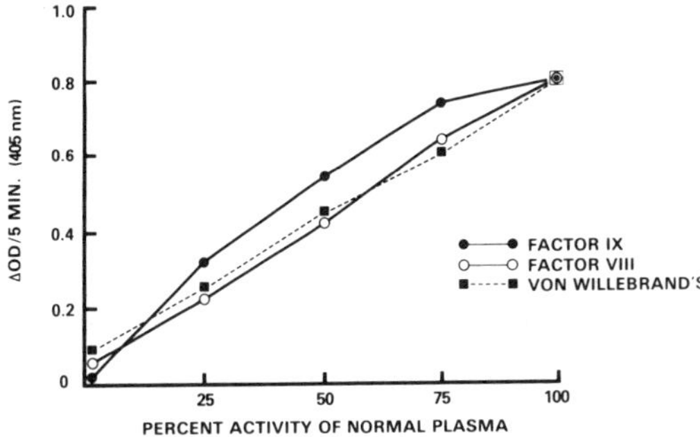

FIGURE 5. Sensitivity of the spectrophotometric assay for the surface-activated clotting system for factors VIII and IX and von Willebrand's deficiencies. Assay details are as for FIGURE 4.

FIGURE 6. Sensitivity of the spectrophotometric assay for the surface-activated clotting system for Factors X and V and prothrombin deficiencies. Assay details are as for FIGURE 4.

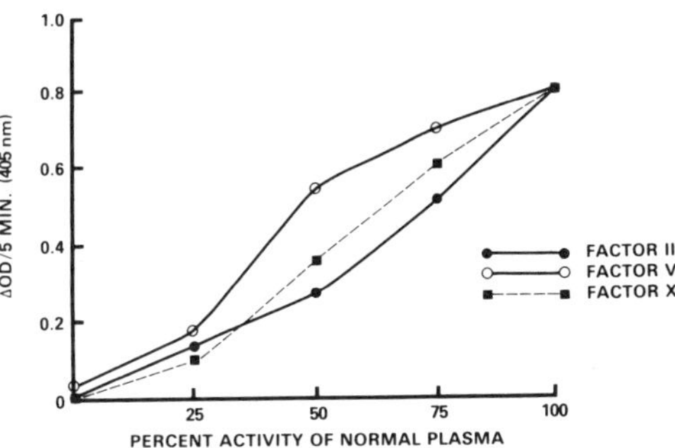

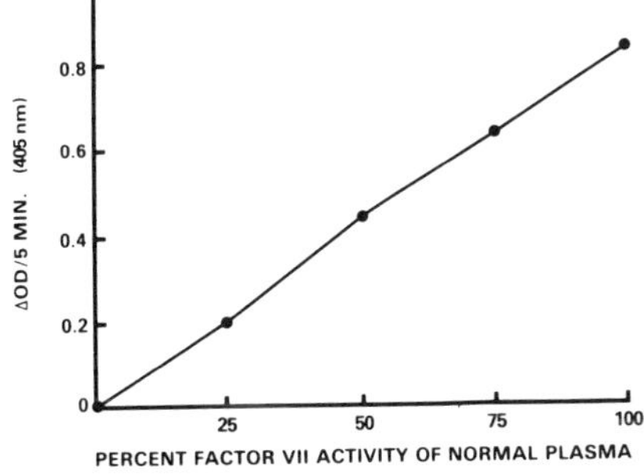

FIGURE 7. Sensitivity of the spectrophotometric assay for the surface-activated clotting system for factor VII deficiency. Assay details are as for FIGURE 4.

TABLE 3

SENSITIVITY OF THE SURFACE-ACTIVATED ASSAY SYSTEM TO FACTOR VII DEFICIENCY

Sample	OD/5 min
Factor-VII-deficient plasma	0.01
Adsorbed plasma *	0.01
Serum reagent †	0.02
Factor-VII-deficient plasma + adsorbed plasma (1:1)	0.012
Factor-VII-deficient plasma + serum reagent (1:1)	0.482

NOTE: Assays were performed using factor-VII-deficient plasma, serum reagent, and adsorbed plasma as described in the text.

* Source of factors V, VIII, XI and XII.

† Source of factors VII, IX, X, XI, and XII.

DISCUSSION

The two-stage assay system using a synthetic tripeptide substrate to measure the activity levels of all the known coagulation factors in plasma is based on the following principle: In the first stage of the tissue-factor-activated system, factor VII is thought to be activated by the tissue factor, which leads to the subsequent activation of factor X and prothrombin using factor V as the cofactor.[9]

In the surface-activated system, as it is understood at the present time, factor XII is activated in a surface phenomenon involving prekallikrein and high molecular weight kininogen.[9] Subsequently, factors XI, IX, and X and prothrombin are activated using factors VIII and V as cofactors. In the second stage, the amount of thrombin generated is quantitated by the addition of a chromogenic substrate relatively specific for thrombin and measurement of the chromogen released at 405 nm. The kinetics of these assay systems are such that the amount of thrombin generated is proportional to the concentration of coagulation factors present in the plasma (FIGS. 2, 3, 4, 5, and 6).

Hirudin inhibition of the amidase activity on chromogenic substrate Sarc-

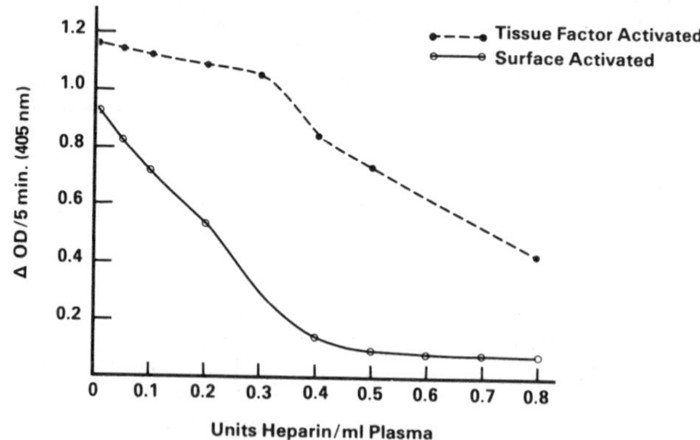

FIGURE 8. Effect of heparin on the spectrophotometric assays for tissue-factor-and surface-activated clotting systems. Heparinized plasma samples were prepared by the direct addition of various heparin levels to pooled, normal plasma.

Pro-Arg-pNA as well as S-2238 suggests that proteases other than thrombin have minimal activity on these substrates under the assay conditions (FIG. 1). The residual activity of other proteases on the chromogenic substrate, as evidenced by the use of factor-II-deficient plasma (TABLE 1), is inhibited by the use of soybean trypsin inhibitor along with the substrate reagent. Thus, the amidase activity measured is essentially due to the activity of thrombin on the chromogenic substrate. Since the plasma is diluted 100-fold, the low concentration of fibrinogen in the reaction mixture prevents any substantial clot formation that might interfere in the spectrophotometric measurements of the chromogen released.

The tissue-factor-activated assay system has the same specificity as that of the prothrombin time clotting assay and can monitor the levels of factors VII, X, and V and prothrombin activities in plasma (TABLE 2). However, the spectrophotometric assay offers a higher degree of sensitivity to these factor levels (FIGS. 2 and 3) as compared with that of the prothrombin time clotting assays. The clotting time assays are usually sensitive only below 25 percent of the normal factor levels (FIGS. 9 and 10).

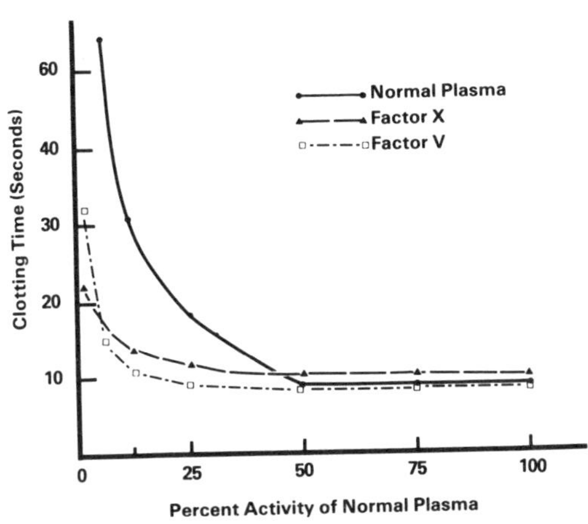

FIGURE 9. Prothrombin time (PT) assay. The clotting assays were performed using Simplastin reagent according to the manufacturer's instructions on serial dilution of normal plasma with Tris-saline buffer and specific factor-deficient plasmas.

The surface-activated spectrophotometric assay system also provides a higher degree of sensitivity as compared with that of the APTT clotting time assay method (FIGS. 4, 5, and 6). This assay system can be used to monitor the factor levels involved in the intrinsic clotting cascade, namely, factors XII, PK, XI, IX and VIII, in addition to factors V and X and prothrombin, which are common to both extrinsic and intrinsic pathways (TABLE 2).

Factor-VII-deficient plasma showed abnormal thrombin generation in the surface-activated assay system (TABLE 2, FIG. 7). The ability of the serum reagent, but not the aluminum-hydroxide-adsorbed plasma, to correct the factor VII deficiency in this assay system (TABLE 3) also substantiates the observation that factor VII is essential for thrombin generation under the assay conditions. Several investigators have reported the involvement of factor VII in the intrinsic coagulation cascade in recent years,[10, 11] thus questioning the validity of two separate mechanisms for *in vivo* blood coagulation. Segligsohn *et al.*[12] in 1979 suggested a pathway where factor IXa functions as a principal activator of factor VII. Such a mechanism might be in force under the assay conditions described herein. The involvement of factor VII in thrombin generation under these assay conditions may not have any bearing on the *in vivo* coagulation mechanism. Nevertheless, it offers an *in vitro* method for studying and better understanding of the interrelationship among the various possible coagulation mechanisms.

The amidolytic efficiency of thrombin (K_{cat}/K_m) on Sarc-Pro-Arg-pNA at the optimal substrate concentration is lower (1×10^5 $M^{-1} \cdot sec^{-1}$) than that on the most specific substrate, D-Phe-Pip-Arg-pNA (2.5×10^6 $M^{-1} \cdot sec^{-1}$). Thus, the reaction linearity of amidolysis by thrombin on Sarc-Pro-Arg-pNA under the assay conditions is much longer than on D-Phe-Pip-Arg-pNA (FIG. 1). The prolonged linearity of the reaction allows increased incubation times in the performance of the assays, which provides the advantage of simultaneous multiple sample analysis in automated systems and a lower percentage of errors in manually timed methods.

From a practical standpoint, the development of these spectrophotometric assays is aimed at improving upon the existing prothrombin time (PT) and activated partial thromboplastin time (APTT) tests. Efforts to develop assays equivalent to PT and APTT tests using chromogenic substrates S-2160,[13] Chromozym TH,[14] and S-2238 [15] have been reported. The assay systems de-

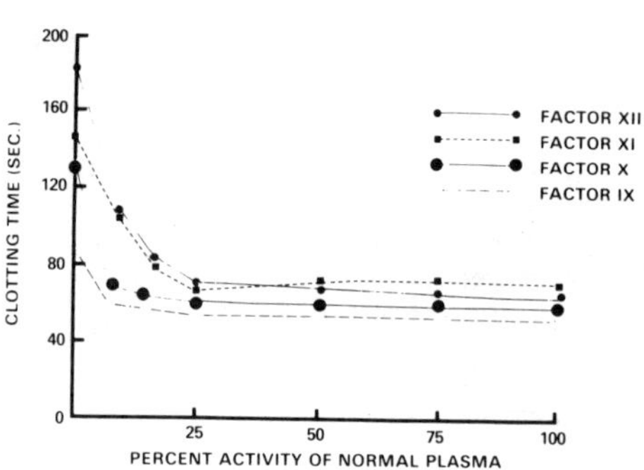

FIGURE 10. Activated partial thromboplastin time (APTT) assay. The clotting assays were performed using Platelin plus activator reagent according to the manufacturer's instructions on serial dilution of normal plasma with specific factor-deficient plasmas.

scribed herein, however, offer a higher degree of sensitivity for factor levels as compared with that of the clotting time assays. This should prove to be helpful in monitoring mild factor abnormalities, for which the clotting time assays are presently insensitive. The tissue-factor-activated spectrophotometric assay system can be used as a sensitive and rapid method for monitoring the effects of coumarin therapy as well. The spectrophotometric assay for the surface-activated clotting system can be used for global screening of all factor deficiencies because of its ability to measure the factor VII levels in addition to the other clotting factors measured by the conventional clotting time assays. Furthermore, this assay system provides a sensitive method for monitoring heparin therapy.

SUMMARY

Spectrophotometric assays for the measurement of coagulation factor activities in plasma have been developed using a relatively specific chromogenic substrate for thrombin. The tissue-factor-activated assay system involves the activation of factors VII and X and prothrombin. The surface-activated assay system involves the activation of factors XII, PK, XI, IX, VII, X and prothrombin using factors V and VIII as cofactors. The thrombin generated subsequent to activation in these two assay systems is measured via its activity on the chromogenic substrate Sarc-Pro-Arg-pNA. These spectrophotometric assays provide a higher degree of sensitivity as compared with the clotting time assays. The tissue-factor-activated system provides a sensitive method for monitoring coumadin therapy. The surface-activated assay system can detect deficiencies of all the factors measured by the conventional APTT assay system, as well as factor VII. Furthermore, this assay provides a sensitive method for monitoring heparin therapy.

ACKNOWLEDGMENTS

I wish to thank Diane Edlefson, Donna Carmody, and Ming-Chu Chen for their excellent technical assistance and Dr. Alfred Gray for his suggestions during the course of this study.

REFERENCES

1. SVENDSEN, L. *et al.* 1972. Synthetic chromogenic substrates for determination of trypsin, thrombin and thrombin-like enzymes. Thromb. Res. **1:** 267.
2. MATTLER, L. G. & N. U. BING. 1977. Serine protease specificity for chromogenic substrates. Thromb. Haemostas. **38:** 776.
3. POCHRON S. *et al.* 1978. A fluorescent substrate assay for plasminogen. Thromb. Res. **13:** 733–739.
4. BERGSTROM, K. & N. EGBERG. 1978. Determination of vitamin K-sensitive coagulation factors in plasma: Studies on three methods using synthetic chromogenic substrates. Thromb. Res. **12:** 531–547.
5. KIRCHHOF, G., E. VERMEER & H. HEMKER. 1978. The determination of prothrombin using synthetic chromogenic substrates: Choice of a suitable activator. Thromb. Res. **13**(2): 219–232.
6. KIRCHHOF, B., A. MULLER, C. VERMEER & H. HEMKER. 1979. Control of anticoagulant therapy with a chromogenic substrate. Haemostasis **8:** 1–7.
7. BIGGS, R. 1976. Human Blood Coagulation, Haemostasis and Thrombosis. R. Biggs, Ed. Blackwell. Oxford.
8. BELL, W. N. & H. ALTON. 1954. A brain extract as a substitute for platelet suspensions in the thromboplastin generation test. Nature, **174:** 880–881.
9. DAVIE, E. W. & K. FUGIKAWA. 1975. Basic mechanisms in blood coagulation. Ann. Rev. Biochem. **44:** 799–829.
10. ØSTERUD B. & S. RAPAPORT. 1977. Activation of factor IX by the reaction product of tissue factor and factor VII: Additional pathway for initiating blood coagulation. Proc. Natl. Acad. Sci. USA **74**(12): 5260–5264.
11. LAAKE, K. & B. ØSTERUD. 1974. Activation of purified plasma factor VII by human plasmin, plasma kallikrein and activated components of the human intrinsic blood coagulation system. Thromb. Res. **5:** 759–772.
12. SELIGSOHN U., B. ØSTERUD, S. BROWN, J. GRIFFIN & S. RAPAPORT. 1979. Activation of human factor VII in plasma and in purified systems. J. Clin. Invest. **64:** 1056–1065.
13. ROKA, L., R. KOCH & H. BLEYL. 1977. Studies on the determination of prothrombin with S-2160. *In* New Methods for the Analysis of Coagulation Using Chromogenic Substrates. I. Witt, Ed. Walter de Gruyter. New York, NY.
14. WITT, I. 1977. Determination of plasma Prothrombin with Chromozym TH. *In* New Methods for the Analysis of Coagulation Using Chromogenic Substrates. I. Witt, Ed. Walter de Gruyter. New York, NY.
15. YAMADA, K. & T. MEGURO. 1979. A new APTT assay employing a chromogenic substrate and a centrifugal analyzer. Thromb. Res. **15:** 351–358.

EFFECT OF SERA ON
THROMBIN ACTIVATION RATE CONSTANTS:
A ONE-STAGE ASSAY OF THE EXTRINSIC SYSTEM

D. J. Baughman and Ann Lytwyn

Ortho Diagnostic Systems, Inc.
Raritan, New Jersey 08869

INTRODUCTION

There is a need to improve the methods of standardizing tissue thromboplastins used in the one-stage prothrombin assay (PT) for monitoring oral anticoagulant therapy.[1] Improved standardization of thromboplastins would lead to better standardization of therapeutic limits for monitoring oral anticoagulant therapy. The development of chromogenic substrates [2] introduced the possibility of significantly improving the standardization of thromboplastins and the monitoring of oral anticoagulant therapy. Although several chromogenic assays for monitoring oral anticoagulants have been described, most of these assays do not use thromboplastins. In addition, they do not correlate well with clotting assays over the range from normal to therapeutic levels of oral anticoagulants.[3-8]

A one-stage chromogenic assay has been described that uses tissue thromboplastin and the thrombin-sensitive substrate, S-2238.[9] After reagents are combined, there is a lag phase during which no substrate hydrolysis occurs. After the lag phase, the log (absorbance at 405 nm/min) is linear with time. The linearity extends up to the maximal thrombin concentration for all types of extrinsic system clotting factor deficiencies. The linear slope, b, of this time dependency was called the thrombin activation rate constant (TARC). The linearity implies that thrombin production is proportional to thrombin concentration. The least complicated explanation of the linearity is that the final rate-limiting step is a thrombin enzymic activation producing more thrombin, that is, positive feedback of thrombin activation. After appropriate log transformations, linear relationships exist for all types of plasma deficiencies between b and PT and between b and plasma factor concentrations. Thus, b can be converted to PT and *vice versa*.

Because of these properties the one-stage chromogenic assay is sensitive to clotting factors in the extrinsic system and its results correlate well with those obtained by the PT assay from the normal to the therapeutic level of oral anticoagulants.

Under the conditions described,[9] the lag phase can vary from 2 to more than 10 minutes for some types of plasmas. The variability in the lag phase makes it difficult to perform the assay on currently available automatic instruments. It would be desirable to reduce the variation in the lag phase without altering the other important properties of the assay system. This report describes the methods and properties of certain types of sera or clotted plasma supernatants that achieve this desired result. Some of the implications of these results on the kinetics of thrombin production are also discussed.

822

MATERIALS AND METHODS

Reagents

Russell viper's venom (RVV) and hirudin (leeches, Gr III) were obtained from Sigma Chemical Co. (St. Louis, MO); Polybrene® (1,5-dimethyl-1,5-diazaudecamethylene polymethobromide) from Aldrich Chemical Co. (Milwaukee, WI); antithrombin-III (AT-III) standard and activated partial thromboplastin, activated Thrombofax® from Ortho Diagnostics, Inc. (Raritan, NJ); and heparin (Vitrum) from Kabi (Stockholm, Sweden). Other reagents have been described elsewhere.[8] All chemicals were reagent grade.

RVV solutions were prepared at 0.12 mg/ml in 0.1 M NaCl; aliquots were frozen and stored at $-20°$ C. After thawing at $37°$ C, fresh solutions of RVV were prepared daily by combining 1 volume of $CaCl_2$ (0.4 M) and 2 volumes of thawed RVV. Hirudin (minimal activity = 10 units) was reconstituted with 1.0 ml distilled water. Heparin/AT-III was prepared by combining 2.4 ml of reconstituted AT-III and 0.10 ml of heparin diluted to 25 units/ml in 0.154 M NaCl.

Sera

Sera A

Normal human blood was collected in (red-top) J-VAC® Tubes from Jelco Labs (Raritan, NJ) and allowed to clot at room temperature for at least 2 hours. The supernatant was collected after centrifugation at 5000 × g for 15 minutes.

Sera B

Nine volumes of citrated human plasma were combined with 0.33 volumes $CaCl_2$ (0.28 M) and 0.67 volumes of tissue thromboplastin. The mixture was allowed to clot at $5°$ C for 2 hours and the supernatant was collected after centrifugation at 5000 × g for 15 minutes at $5°$ C.

Sera C

Nine volumes of citrated human plasma were combined with 0.33 volumes of activated partial thromboplastin and with 0.67 volumes $CaCl_2$ (0.15 M). The mixture was clotted and collected in a manner identical to that of sera B.

Sera D

Nine volumes of citrated human plasma were combined with 1 volume of $CaCl_2$ (0.10 M) and the mixture was clotted and collected in a manner identical to that of sera B.

Sera E

Nine volumes of citrated human plasma were combined with 1 volume thrombin (10 units/ml), and the mixture was clotted and collected in a manner identical to that of sera B.

All sera were either stored frozen at $-55°$ C or lyophilized and stored at $5°$ C.

Procedures

Barium Citrate Adsorption

Barium citrate adsorption [10] was performed by slowly adding 1 volume $BaCl_2$ (1.0 M) to 10 volumes sera with gentle stirring. After 15 minutes at $5°$ C, the mixture was centrifuged at $3000 \times g$ for 30 minutes at $5°$ C. The supernatant was collected and either stored frozen at $-55°$ C or lyophilized and stored at $5°$ C.

Chromogenic Extrinsic System Assay

Chromogenic extrinsic system assay consists of combining diluted citrated plasma with S-2238 and tissue thromboplastin. The absorbance at 405 nm (A_{405}) is monitored. The linear slope of log (A_{405}/min) versus time is either computed automatically or obtained from appropriate chart recordings. The linear slope, b, is called TARC. The details of the chromogenic assay and of the one-stage prothrombin time methods are described elsewhere.[9] When sera were used, the assay was performed by adding 0.05 ml of diluted sera (usually 40 percent v/v with saline solution) to a mixture of 1.60 ml S-2238/buffer and 0.40 ml of tissue thromboplastin at $37°$ C. Immediately, 0.05 ml of plasma was added, mixed, and inserted into the spectrophotometer. The linear slope, b, from log (A_{405}/min) versus time is called the thrombin activation rate constant (TARC).

The lag phase, the time from adding the last reagent until the log (A_{405}/min) becomes linear, was determined from strip-chart recordings by either of two methods: (1) direct measurements from the strip chart or (2) determination of the time to $A_{405} = 0.1$, which was an absorbance just above the background. T_{max} is the maximal thrombin concentration.

Chromogenic Total Factor X and Factor Xa Assays

Chromogenic total factor X and Xa assays [11] used S-2222 as substrate. For the total factor X assay, 1.0 ml of Tris-saline buffer (0.05 M Tris, pH $= 7.0$, $I = 0.25$, 0.1 mg/ml Polybrene) was combined with 0.1 ml sample (sera). Then, 0.20 ml of the diluted sera and 0.20 ml of RVV in $CaCl_2$ were combined at $37°$ C for exactly 60 seconds. Finally, 0.50 ml of heated ($37°$ C) S-2222/buffer (1.5 volumes Tris-saline buffer [0.05 M Tris, pH $= 8.6$, $I = 0.25$] and 1.0 vol 4 mM S-2222) were added. The absorbance at A_{405} was monitored with a Gilford spectrophotometer model 250 (Gilford Instrument Laboratories,

Inc., Columbia, MD) with automatic strip-chart recorder (model 6050, Gilford). The initial A_{405}/min was determined from the recording. Assays for factor Xa were identical, except that RVV was replaced with buffer.

S-2238 Sera Hydrolytic Activity

S-2238 sera hydrolytic activity was measured by combining 0.05 ml of serum, 1.75 ml Tris-saline buffer (0.05 M Tris, pH = 8.5, I = 0.15), and 0.25 ml 2 mM S-2238. All reagents except sera were maintained at 37° C. Rates of A_{405}/min were monitored as in the factor X assay. When appropriate, 0.40 ml tissue thromboplastin replaced 0.40 ml Tris-saline buffer in the assay.

Factors V, VII, X, and II

Factors V, VII, X, and II were assayed using the one-stage prothrombin clotting assay in which 1 volume of unknown sample (or saline dilutions of pooled normal plasma as standards) were combined with 1 volume of a specific factor-deficient plasma. Assays were performed with 0.1 ml of the factor-deficient plasma diluted sample and 0.2 ml tissue thromboplastin. The factor-deficient plasmas were assumed to have zero factor concentration. The unknown factor concentration was determined from standard curves of log (factor concentration) versus clotting time.

RESULTS

Clotting Factor Effects on Lag Phase

The lag phase was measured for different dilutions of each clotting factor in the extrinsic system. The results are summarized in FIGURE 1. Normal plasma is included as a reference. Factors VII and X have significant effects on the lag phase, whereas factor V does not. Factor II has an intermediate effect. With low levels of factor II, the resulting low rates of thrombin production make measurement of the lag phase more difficult. Because of the low levels of thrombin and because of the smaller effects of factor II on the lag phase, the factor II effect is probably not of the same origin as the effects due to factors X and VII. Thus, these results suggest that some product of the factor VII and X interactions probably decrease the lag phase.

Thrombin and Sera

The lag phase was measured in the presence of thrombin and sera from clotted whole blood (sera A) for different dilutions of normal plasma. The results are shown in FIGURE 2. Both thrombin and sera significantly shorten the lag phase. Sera are more effective than thrombin since they produce a shorter lag phase over a wider range of plasma dilutions. The rates of A_{405} production for 25 percent normal plasma in the presence and absence of serum are shown in FIGURE 3. As can be seen, the lag phase is almost totally elimi-

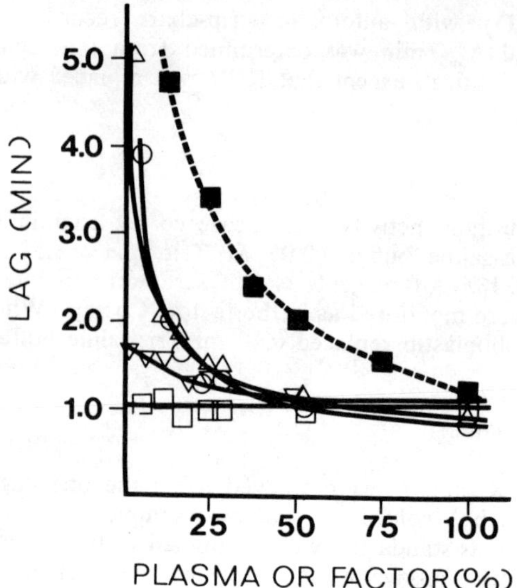

FIGURE 1. Results of lag phase measurement for different dilutions of each clotting factor.

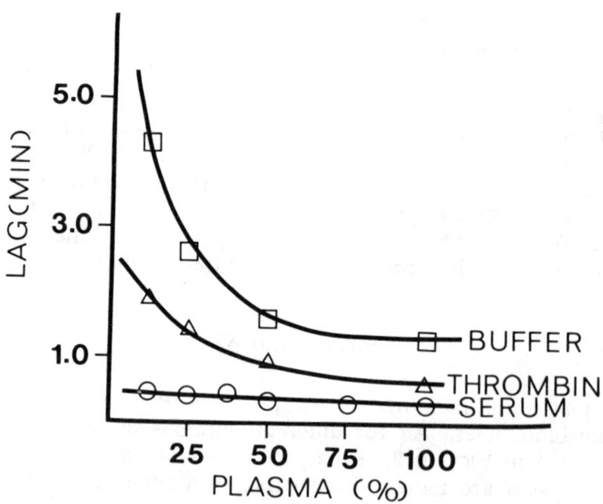

FIGURE 2. Results of lag phase measurement in presence of thrombin and sera from clotted whole blood.

nated with little or no effects on the TARC (the rate of A_{405}/min) or T_{max}. Similar results on b and T_{max} were obtained for other plasma dilutions. Also, similar results were obtained for plasmas deficient in each of the extrinsic system clotting factors when diluted with normal plasma. Thus, sera from whole blood and to a lesser extent, thrombin, can shorten the lag phase without markedly altering the rate of thrombin production.

Different Sera Types

The effects of other types of sera on the lag phase were examined. These sera were compared for their effects on the lag phase, linearity of b (log A_{405}/min versus time), and T_{max}. Sera B and sera C behaved just like sera A, but sera D and E did not. Sera D and E demonstrated increased T_{max} and

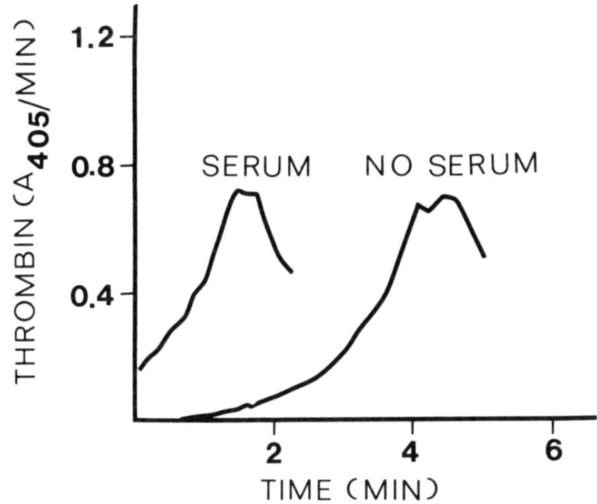

FIGURE 3. Rates of A_{405} production for 25 percent normal plasma in the presence and absence of serum.

produced nonlinear responses for log (A_{405}/min) versus time. Also, when the concentrations of sera A, B and C were increased, there was little change in the observed b. When the concentrations of sera D and E were increased, the observed b's were increased. Thus, sera types A, B and C appeared to be satisfactory; sera D and E did not. Sera B were used for most of the other studies described. These results strongly suggest that the activity that reduces the lag phase is a product of the clotting process.

Quantitative Comparison of Sera and Buffer

Several important properties of sera were determined by comparing sera with buffer in the assay system. During one year, eleven experiments were performed at different times using different sera preparations. Normal plasma samples at 100 percent and 25 percent were used in all experiments. Three sera B and four sera A samples were used. Sera concentrations ranged from 10 percent to 100 percent of undiluted sera. Buffer control experiments were always performed.

From these experiments the effects of the linearity of log (A_{405}/min) versus time were determined. The average residual variance of the regressions were 5.53×10^{-3} and 6.05×10^{-3} for buffer and sera, respectively. Their respective degrees of freedom were 736 and 1289. These average residuals are equivalent to a correlation coefficient of $r = 0.997$. Only 20 percent of these r values were less than 0.990 and half occurred during one experiment. Thus, it is concluded that sera do not affect the extent of the linearity of log (A_{405}/min) versus time and the kinetic properties of TARC have been preserved.

From the same data, the quantitative reproducibility of T_{max} was also examined. In the eleven experiments, the average variances between replicates of T_{max} for buffer or sera were 0.356 and 0.365, with 21 and 93 degrees of freedom, respectively. The differences between the average T_{max} of buffer and sera at 25 percent and 100 percent were 0.04 and 0.64, respectively. The average values for T_{max} were 2.4 (25 percent) and 10.4 (100 percent). The presence of sera gave a significantly greater T_{max} at 100 percent, but not at 25 percent plasma. Also, the average differences varied between experiments depending on the source of the sera or plasma. Thus, sera has not altered the relationship between T_{max} and plasma concentration, but does produce ~6 percent greater T_{max}.

Some of the quantitative effects of sera on b were determined by comparing normal plasma dilution curves in buffer and sera. A direct comparison was made on nine occasions using nine different normal plasmas, six different sera A and three different sera B. One example of these curves is shown in FIGURE 4. The results of both log b versus log (plasma) and log b versus log PT are summarized in TABLE 1. None of the differences between sera and

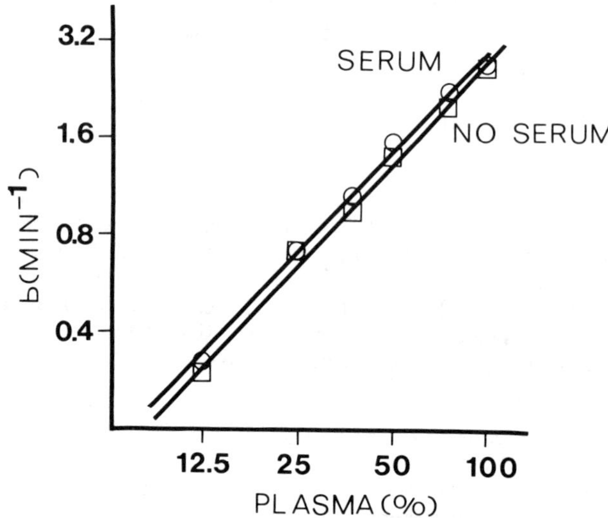

FIGURE 4. Results of comparison of normal plasma dilution curves in buffer and sera.

TABLE 1

REPRODUCIBILITY OF NORMAL PLASMA DILUTION CURVES

	Sera	Buffer
Log (b) versus log (plasma)		
Number of curves	9	12
Average slope	2.85	3.35
Average residual variance	2.65×10^{-4} *	3.68×10^{-4}
Degrees of freedom	30	40
Log (b) versus log (PT)		
Number of curves	7	10
Average slope	1.80	3.12
Average residual variance	3.21×10^{-3} *	3.75×10^{-3}
Degrees of freedom	19	22

* Not significantly different from buffer curves within 95 percent confidence limits.

buffer is statistically significant. From the agreement between the average residual variances, it is concluded that the linearity and precision of both curves are not affected by sera. Not shown is the observation that in the presence of sera the value of b can be increased by 20 percent more than the corresponding buffer value. This increase in b has not affected the precision or linearity of the dilution curve.

Characterization of the Sera

In order to characterize the activity in sera that reduces the lag phase, the concentration of different clotting factors was examined. Thromboplastin was added to each sera and an increased rate of hydrolytic (S-2238) activity was used to detect the presence of prothrombin. Although sera D and E demonstrated significantly increased hydrolysis rates upon thromboplastin addition, sera A, sera B, and sera C did not for at least 5 minutes. Thus, it was concluded that sera D and sera E contain significant amounts of prothrombin and that sera A, B, and C did not.

Some sera, unlike plasmas, possess S-2238 hydrolyzing activity. For example, samples of sera A, sera B, and sera C averaged 0.2 A_{405}/min hydrolysis, whereas samples of sera D and sera E averaged 0.04 A_{405}/min hydrolysis. The effects of hirudin and heparin/AT-III on this residual hydrolytic activity were examined. The results for each thrombin inhibitor are summarized in TABLE 2. Thrombin (0.1 u/ml) solutions were used as controls. As can be seen, these thrombin inhibitors had little effect on the rates of hydrolysis. Thus, it is concluded that free thrombin is not present in these sera.

The sera were also tested for factor Xa and total factor X activity before and after adsorption with barium citrate. The results are shown in TABLE 3. These results indicate that sera contains significant amounts of factor X which can be removed by adsorption. After adsorption, a small amount of total factor X remains. Most of the remainder is assumed to be factor Xa. Thus, the residual S-2238 activity and, presumably, the reduction of the lag phase is probably not arising from factor X or factor Xa.

TABLE 2

EFFECTS OF HIRUDIN AND HEPARIN/AT-III ON SERA
S-2238 HYDROLYTIC ACTIVITY

	(A_{405}/min)	
	Thrombin (0.1 u/ml)	Sera (1%)
No hirudin	0.112	0.189
Hirudin (0.48 u/ml)	0.042	0.198
No heparin/AT-III	0.102	0.235
Heparin/AT-III	0.012	0.232

The clotting activity of factors VII, V and X were assayed in the sera before and after barium citrate adsorption. The results are given in TABLE 4. With respect to factor X behavior, these results confirm the results of the chromogenic assays for factor X and factor Xa. However, there does appear to be a large amount of factor VII in sera. This amount is probably due to the presence of factor VIIa, which remains after adsorption. Some factor V is lost during adsorption, and the remainder would seem to be too small to account for the effects seen in these sera. Thus, if the sera effect is due to one of the known extrinsic system factors, it would appear to be a result of factor VIIa.

Factor-Deficient Dilution Curves

The effects of barium-citrate-adsorbed sera on the b versus log (factor concentration) dilution curves were examined. Factor-deficient plasmas were diluted with normal plasma. The results are summarized in FIGURE 5. Normal plasma dilutions were included as an estimate of factor II activity. Even when sera is used to control the lag phase, the assay is still sensitive to all factors in the extrinsic system. Factor II is probably the most sensitive and factor V is the least sensitive factor. The linearity of the factor V and factor VII curves is reduced at low factor concentrations, probably because of the presence of the residual factor V and factor VII in the sera. By use of barium-citrate-adsorbed sera, the linearity of factor X was preserved. All factor concentrations of

TABLE 3

AMOUNT OF TOTAL FACTOR X AND FACTOR Xa BEFORE AND
AFTER BARIUM CITRATE ADSORPTION

	Factor X (average ± SD *)	Factor Xa (average ± SD *)
Preadsorption data †	68% ± 7%	7% ± 2%
Postadsorption data ‡	5.9 % ± 0.1%	4% ± 1%

* SD = standard deviation.
† From 5 experiments.
‡ From 2 experiments.

TABLE 4

CLOTTING FACTOR ACTIVITY (% OF NORMAL VALUES) IN SERA
BEFORE AND AFTER BARIUM CITRATE ADSORPTION

	Unadsorbed	Adsorbed
Factor V	31%	17%
Factor VII	415%	173%
Factor X	117%	4%

15–20 percent or less were easily detected by this assay system. Similar results were obtained when the log b versus log PT were examined: Linearity at high-factor concentrations was preserved, but at low-factor concentrations, b values tended to be constant except for normal plasma. Thus, it was concluded that sera can be used in the chromogenic assay to detect potential hemorrhagic abnormalities in the extrinsic system.

Dicumarolized Plasmas

The correlation between the chromogenic assay using sera and one-stage prothrombin time (PT) was obtained using 62 different dicumarolized samples. These data are summarized in FIGURE 6. The regression of log b versus log (PT) yielded a slope $= -1.97$ and r $= -0.84$. Since the PT is more sensitive to factor VII and the chromogenic assay more sensitive to factor II, the largest discrepancies would be expected to occur during the earliest days of therapy. To examine this possibility, a series of regressions were performed. First those patients with only one day's therapy, then two days', and so on, were successively deleted from the regression analysis. The results are summarized in TABLE 5. As can be seen, both the slope and the r value increases as patients

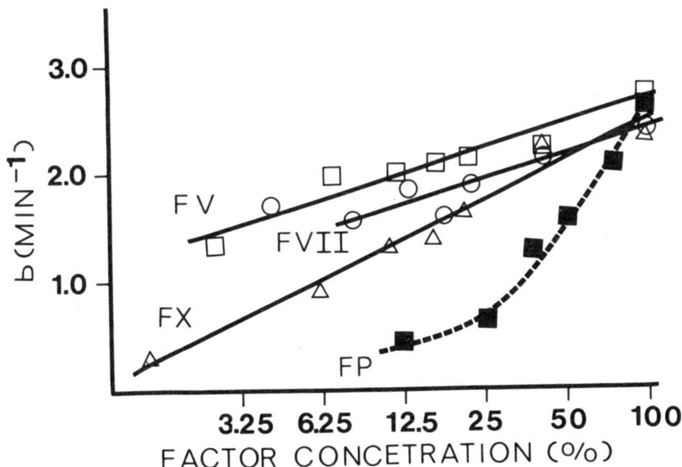

FIGURE 5. Effects of barium-citrate-adsorbed sera on the b versus log (factor concentration) dilution curves.

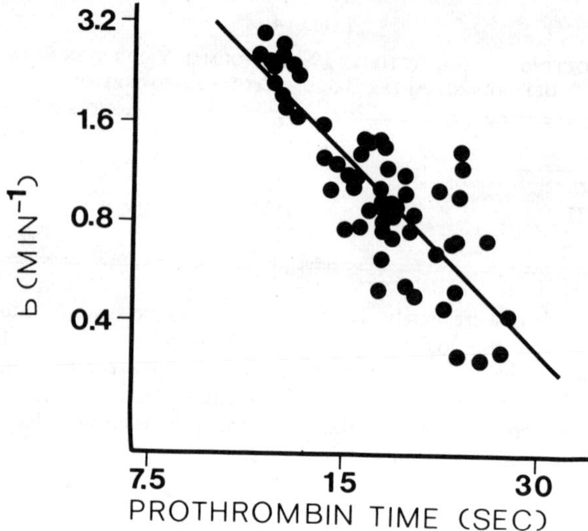

FIGURE 6. Correlation between chromogenic assay using sera and one-stage prothrombin time (PT) test in 62 dicumarolized samples.

TABLE 5

CORRELATION BETWEEN SERA-CHROMOGENIC AND CLOTTING
ASSAYS ON DICUMAROLIZED PATIENTS

Days * on Therapy	N †	r ‡	Slope §
	62	−0.844357	−1.97
1 day	61	−0.849758	−2.07
2 days	58	−0.858462	−2.07
3 days	51	−0.893245	−2.22
4 days	49	−0.893768	−2.22
5 days	48	−0.890764	−2.23
6 days	43	−0.896628	−2.22
7 days	41	−0.934744	−2.37
9 days	39	−0.940469	−2.39
10 days	38	−0.943797	−2.41
11 days	37	−0.943875	−2.41

* Patients receiving therapy for this time have been removed from the regression.
† Number of samples in regression.
‡ Linear regression coefficient.
§ Slope of log b versus log PT.

with only 1 to 2 days of therapy are removed. There is another change in slope and r value between days 6 and 7, which may be coincidental. Thus, it is concluded that the chromogenic assay can be used to monitor patients on anticoagulant therapy. In addition the correlation is particularly high after the first one to two days of therapy. In order to compare these results with another chromogenic assay, the same samples were assayed for total factor X. Similar results were obtained, except that both the regression slopes and the r values were lower. Thus, the slope of log (nkat/ml) versus log (PT) was -1.69 and the r value was -0.786 for 62 patients. Consequently it was concluded that factor X assays do not correlate as well with the PT assay as the one-stage assay described here.

DISCUSSION

The one-stage chromogenic assay previously described was difficult to automate because the lag phase, or time when thrombin appeared, was so variable.[9] The current data showed that the lag phase was dependent on the products of factor X and VII reactions (FIG. 1). Both thrombin and whole blood sera could significantly shorten the lag phase, but sera were better (FIG. 2). Under most conditions sera appear to shorten the lag phase without significantly altering the properties of the assay. Successful sera appear to contain significant amounts of factor VIIa, some factor V, less factor X, no prothrombin, and no free thrombin (TABLES 2 to 4). Residual S-2238 activity does not appear to arise from free thrombin.

When chromogenic assays with and without sera were compared quantitatively, they appeared to be identical in most respects. The log (A_{405}/min) versus time was linear, giving a slope called TARC or b. Both assays were sensitive to all hemorrhagic levels of the extrinsic system clotting factors. Both gave linear relationships for log b versus log (plasma concentration), indicating that normal plasma could be used as a standard for the assays. Both assays gave linear log b versus log PT responses for all types of plasmas, indicating that one variable could be used to measure the other. Both gave linear plots of b versus log (factor concentration), indicating they could be used for quantitative factor assays. Most importantly, both assays gave the same regression slope for log b versus log PT when monitoring oral anticoagulants.[9] The correlation is particularly good after one to two days' therapy and is significantly better than that of the assay for factor X. Under most conditions both assays yielded the same T_{max}. These data strongly suggest that sera do not alter the inherent nature of the thrombin activation reactions.

The addition of sera in the assay system results in two important differences from assays not containing sera. For some sera the resulting values for b can be significantly larger by 20 percent. Also, the sensitivity to very low levels of factors VII and V are reduced. Both of these differences are due, presumably, to the presence of factors V and VII in the sera. Neither of these differences affects the similarities between the assays described earlier. Also, because of the hydrolytic activity of sera, the order of adding reagents must be more carefully controlled when sera are used.

From a practical point of view, adding sera to the assay simplifies the assay procedure. In the presence of sera, b can be determined by recording absorbancies at two times after final reagent addition, for example, at 1.0 and 1.25

minutes. Under these conditions the assays with sera can be used for screening for factor-deficient patients and monitoring oral anticoagulant plasmas. Under conditions requiring maximal quantitative results, an assay without sera can be used. Such situations would include standardization of thromboplastin and assaying for low levels of clotting factors. Under all conditions, normal plasmas can be used as a standard. These two chromogenic assays in combination with assays for T_{max} and assays for factor X could allow development of diagnostic and quantitative assay methods for all extrinsic system clotting factors without requiring the need for deficient plasmas, except, possibly, for confirmation.

From a kinetic viewpoint, some of these results do not appear to agree with the cascade theory of prothrombin activation.[12] From the cascade theory, both factor V and prothrombin would be expected to affect the lag phase as well as factors VII and X. Also, it would seem that factor Xa or active factor V and not factor VIIa (or unknown factor), would be the appropriate product with which to shorten the lag phase. The activation of thrombin behaves more as if it were a highly coiled spring or an explosive primed for release, for example, thrombin position feedback. Once the releasing mechanism occurs, thrombin activation proceeds at a constant exponential rate. The releasing mechanism seems to be a product of the factor VII and factor X interactions, but not of factor V or prothrombin. Some types of sera can provide this release. The releasing factor could be something not yet known or factor M, just recently described.[13] If the releasing factor is a known extrinsic system factor, it is most likely factor VIIa. Presumably, it is not free thrombin.

SUMMARY

A one-stage chromogenic assay sensitive to all factors of the extrinsic system has been developed. Diluted plasma is combined with tissue thromboplastin in the presence of S-2238, a thrombin-sensitive substrate. After a lag phase, log (A_{405}/min) is linear with time up to the maximal thrombin concentration. The linear slope, b, is called the thrombin activation rate constant (TARC). Log b, or b, is linearly related to log transformations of plasma dilutions, of factor concentrations, of dicumarolized plasmas, and of one-stage prothrombin times.

Since the lag phase can vary from 2 to more than 10 minutes, it is difficult to perform the assay on current automated equipment. Results show that factors VII and X affect the lag phase, while factors V and II do not. Small amounts of sera or thrombin, to a lesser extent, can shorten the lag phase to near zero without altering the relationships between TARC and plasma dilutions and between TARC and prothrombin times for dicumarolized plasmas and for dilutions of factor-deficient plasmas. The only effects of some sera are to increase b by ~20 percent. Successful sera can be made from clotted whole blood or supernatants of sera from citrated plasma clotted with tissue or partial thromboplastins. These sera appear to have minimal amounts of factor X, undetectable prothrombin, and undetectable free thrombin. The sera contain excesses of factor VII and/or factor VIIa and nearly 20 percent of factor V. If the sera activity arises from the extrinsic system, it is probably due to factor VIIa.

ACKNOWLEDGMENTS

We would like to acknowledge our appreciation of the assistance given by Fae Parker in producing the tables and graphs and the technical assistance given by Kathy Gilbert Dumas.

REFERENCES

1. ICTH/ICSH EXPERT PANEL (INGRAM, G.I.C., Chairman. 1979. Prothrombin time standardization: Report of the expert panel on oral anticoagulation control. Thromb. Haemostasis **42:** 1073–1114.
2. SVENDSEN, L., B. BLOMBÄCK, M. BLOMBÄCK & P. OLSSON. 1972. I. Synthetic chromogenic substrates for determination of trypsin, thrombin and thrombin-like Enzymes. Thromb. Res. **1:** 267–278.
3. BERGSTRÖM, K. & M. BLOMBÄCK. 1974. Determination of plasma prothrombin with a reaction rate analyzer using a synthetic substrate. Thromb. Res. **4:** 719–729.
4. AXELSSON, G., K. KORSAN-BENGTSEN & J. WALDENSTRÖM. 1976. Prothrombin determination by means of a chromogenic peptide substrate. Thromb. Haemostas. **36:** 517–524.
5. KORSAN-BENGTSEN, K., I. AXELSSON & J. WALDENSTRÖM. 1977. Determination of plasma prothrombin and the chromogenic peptide substrate H-D-Phe-Pip-Arg-pNA (S-2238). *In* New Methods for the Analysis of Coagulation Using Chromogenic Substrates: 155–169. I. Witt, Ed. W. deGruyter. New York, NY.
6. KIRCHHOF, B. R. J., C. VERMEER & H. C. HEMKER. 1978. The determination of prothrombin using synthetic chromogenic substrates. Choice of a suitable activator. Thromb. Res. **13:** 219–232.
7. BERGSTRÖM, K. & N. EGBERG. 1978. Determination of vitamin K-sensitive coagulation factors in plasma: Studies on three methods using chromogenic substrates. Thromb. Res. **12:** 531–547.
8. FRANCIS, J. L. 1979. A new chromogenic assay for the specific determination of prothrombin. J. Clin. Pathol. **32:** 651–654.
9. BAUGHMAN, D. J. & A. LYTWYN. 1980. Thrombin activation rate constant: One-stage chromogenic assay for the extrinsic system. Submitted for publication.
10. LEWIS, M. L. & WALL, A. G. 1953. Proc. Soc. Exp. Biol. Med. **84:** 636.
11. AURELL, L., P. FRIBERGER, G. KARLSSON & G. CLAESON. 1977. A new sensitive and highly specific chromogenic peptide substrate for factor Xa. Thromb. Res. **11:** 595–609.
12. NEMERSON, Y. & F. A. PITLICK. 1972. The tissue factor pathway of blood coagulation. Prog. Haemostas. Thromb. **1:** 1–37.
13. SEEGERS, W. H. & A. GHOSH. 1980. Activation of prothrombin and factor X: Function of previously unrecognized plasma protein. Thromb. Res. **17:** 71–81.

α-HALOGENMETHYL CARBONYL COMPOUNDS
AS VERY POTENT INHIBITORS OF
FACTOR XIIIa *IN VITRO*

Gerd Reinhardt

Bayer AG, Institut für Biochemie
Pharma-Forschungszentrum
5600 Wuppertal 1, Federal Republic of Germany

Fibrin stabilization inhibitors can be subdivided grossly into two categories: one group blocks the crosslinking enzyme (F XIIIa) and the other one blocks the substrate (fibrin monomers).

F XIIIa is known to be a sulfhydryl enzyme.[1] Therefore, "sulfhydryl reagents" such as organomercurials, disulfides, and iodoacetic acid belong into the first category. They are able to form a covalent bond with the active site of the enzyme and thus inhibit its activity. These substances do not specifically react with F XIIIa and so high concentrations are necessary to obtain a considerable inhibition.

To elucidate the action of the second group of substances, a schematic representation of the chemical events that occur during the crosslinking process is given in FIGURE 1. Initially, the active SH-group of the enzyme reacts with a glutamine residue of one fibrin molecule to form a thio ester ("S-acyl enzyme"); ammonia is released in this step. The second step involves the aminolysis of the thio ester by a lysine residue of a second fibrin molecule releasing the free enzyme. This results in the covalent linkage of the two fibrin molecules. Since every fibrin molecule has several of such crosslinking sites, an indefinite network of covalently connected fibrin molecules is formed (fibrin polymer). Most of the compounds belonging to the second category of inhibitors have a primary amino group that is able to compete for the lysine residues during the aminolysis of the thio ester intermediate.

These "competitive substrates" terminate the polycondensation reaction chain by rendering the crosslinking sites in the fibrin monomers unsusceptible to further reaction. Consequently, the formation of polymeric fibrin is prevented. As shown in FIGURE 2, the most efficient substrate competitors are structurally related to the lysine residue, which is the natural substrate. The aromatic nucleus and the $-SO_2-$group are of additional importance. Obviously this combination provides a primary interaction between these molecules and the enzyme molecules, the exact nature of which is not known. A compilation of the molecular features of this class of substances has been given by Lorand and Nilsson.[2] These compounds can be regarded as quite specific. Nonetheless, high concentrations must be available to produce a measurable inhibition, since they have to compete with the substrate, which itself is present in high concentration compared with that of the enzyme.

To produce more effective inhibitors of the fibrin stabilization, the notion was had of combining the selectivity of the substrate-like amines with the chemical reactivity of the sulfhydryl reagents. As the result of these considerations, the general structure given in FIGURE 3 was designed. The group R′–X– (with an aromatic nucleus in the position R′ and $-X- = -SO_2-$) represents

836

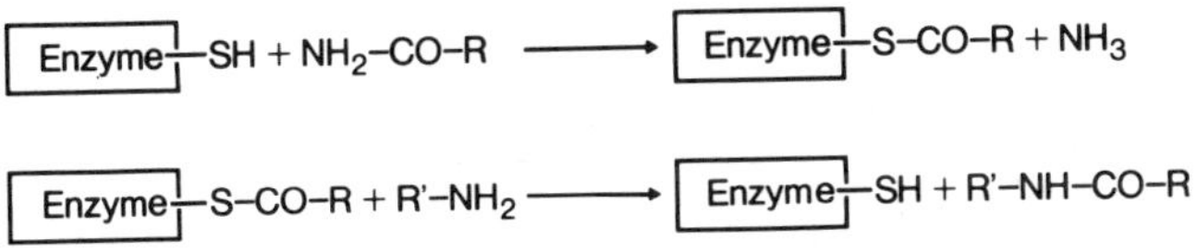

$$\boxed{Enzyme}\!-\!SH + NH_2\!-\!CO\!-\!R \longrightarrow \boxed{Enzyme}\!-\!S\!-\!CO\!-\!R + NH_3$$

$$\boxed{Enzyme}\!-\!S\!-\!CO\!-\!R + R'\!-\!NH_2 \longrightarrow \boxed{Enzyme}\!-\!SH + R'\!-\!NH\!-\!CO\!-\!R$$

FIGURE 1. Schematic representation of the fibrin crosslinking reaction. (After Lorand and Nilsson.[2])

the point of primary interaction, thus providing a specific attraction of the inhibitor by the enzyme. Once this interaction has taken place, the group $-CO-CH_2-Z$ $(Z = Cl, Br)$ can approach the sulfhydryl group very easily, allowing the formation of a covalent bond. This halogenmethyl carbonyl group has already been used very successfully in the development of specific protease inhibitors.[3] Both parts of the molecule are connected by the spacer group $-(CH_2)_n-Y-$ $-Y-=-O-, -NH-, -CH_2-)$, which keeps the functional groups at an optimal distance by variation of n. Theoretically its chain length should correspond to the length of a lysine residue.

FIGURE 4 provides an example of a synthesis route for one of the most promising compounds, 1-chloro-7-tosylamido heptan-2-one.[2] 6-Aminohexanoic acid and tosyl chloride are condensed by the Schotten-Baumann reaction. The carboxylic acid is converted into the acid chloride by means of $SOCl_2$, which, in turn, is reacted with ethereal diazo methane solution to yield the diazo methyl ketone. This is treated with gaseous HCl to produce the target product.

To quantify the degree of fibrin stabilization, purified bovine fibrin monomers, dissolved in 2 percent aqueous acetic acid, and a crude plasma fraction from bovine blood as a source of F XIII are used. F XIII is activated for 10 minutes by means of thrombin in imidazole buffer containing $CaCl_2$; at this point the test substances, which have been dissolved in dimethyl formamide at such a concentration as to keep the amount of dimethyl formamide in the assay system below 1 percent, are added. After another 10 minutes, these mixtures are poured into the fibrin monomer solution. At the same time, imidazole solution is added, the quantity of which has been exactly adjusted to bring the final pH of the assay mixture to 7.2. After an incubation period of 30 minutes, the reaction is stopped by means of monochloroacetic acid solution, which also dissolves the nonstabilized fibrin. The insoluble (that is, stabilized) fibrin is centrifuged down and dissolved in 30 percent NaOH solution. The protein content of this solution is estimated by a biuret method.[4] A similar assay method has already been described by Lorand et al.[5]

The degree of fibrin stabilization is expressed as the proportion of insoluble

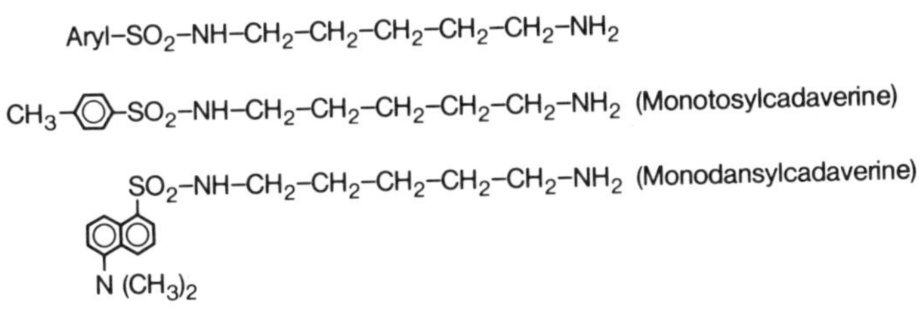

$$Aryl-SO_2-NH-CH_2-CH_2-CH_2-CH_2-CH_2-NH_2$$

$$CH_3-\bigcirc-SO_2-NH-CH_2-CH_2-CH_2-CH_2-CH_2-NH_2 \quad (Monotosylcadaverine)$$

$$SO_2-NH-CH_2-CH_2-CH_2-CH_2-CH_2-NH_2 \quad (Monodansylcadaverine)$$

N (CH_3)_2

FIGURE 2. Examples of fibrin stabilization inhibitors acting as substrate competitors.

$$R' - X - \overset{\overset{\displaystyle R}{|}}{N} - (CH_2)_n - Y - CO-CH_2 - Z$$

R'= Aryl −	X= −SO$_2$−, −CO−	R= −H, n−Alkyl, Benzyl	n= 2 − 6 and 9	Y= −CH$_2$−, −NH−, −O−		Z= −Cl, −Br

FIGURE 3. Outline for general structural features of proposed F XIIIa inhibitors.

fibrin per total fibrin. A plot of these ratios against different concentrations of an inhibitor produces curves such as those shown in FIGURE 5. The descending part of these curves is of particular interest since it allows one to estimate the efficiency of an inhibitor. The inhibitory threshold concentration of a substance, as indicated by the arrows in FIGURE 5, is taken as a measure of its activity.

Such inhibitory threshold concentrations of chloromethyl carbonyl compounds having the tosyl group in the position R'–X– (FIG. 3) are given in TABLE 1. All substances of this series are inhibitors of the fibrin stabilization. A pronounced dependency of the inhibitory activity on the structural features can be observed. The chain length of the spacer group is of striking importance. The highest inhibitory activity is achieved with compounds having a distance of about five atoms between the tosyl group and the chloromethyl carbonyl function. The nature of the heteroatom (–Y–) is also most important. An oxygen atom in this position endows the compounds with relatively low activity only; the nitrogen atom is more favorable, and the most active substances contain a mere hydrocarbon spacing. For comparison, this Table also includes the inhibitory threshold concentrations of reference substances that are the most effective inhibitors of the fibrin stabilization known up to now. Several of our newly synthesized substances with optimal molecular properties prevent the fibrin stabilization in concentrations that are about 100-fold lower.

TABLE 2 shows the corresponding bromo derivatives. A comparable dependency of the activity on the chain length and on the nature of the heteroatom (–Y–) is observed. Since the bromo atom, however, is known to be a better leaving group than the chloro atom in nucleophilic substitution reactions, the bromo compounds are generally active at even lower concentrations than

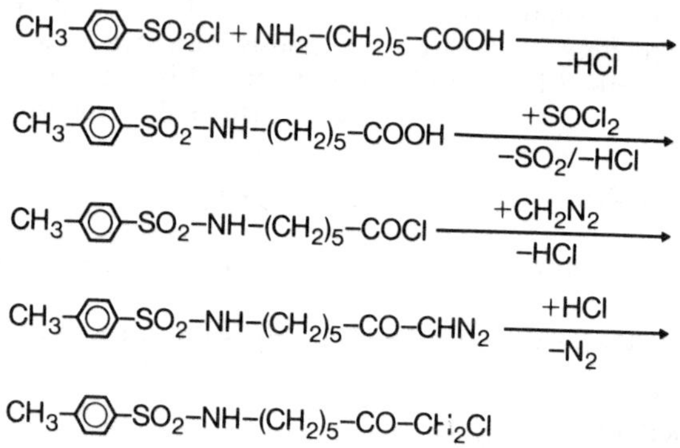

$$CH_3-\langle \bigcirc \rangle-SO_2Cl + NH_2-(CH_2)_5-COOH \xrightarrow[-HCl]{}$$

$$CH_3-\langle \bigcirc \rangle-SO_2-NH-(CH_2)_5-COOH \xrightarrow[-SO_2/-HCl]{+SOCl_2}$$

$$CH_3-\langle \bigcirc \rangle-SO_2-NH-(CH_2)_5-COCl \xrightarrow[-HCl]{+CH_2N_2}$$

$$CH_3-\langle \bigcirc \rangle-SO_2-NH-(CH_2)_5-CO-CHN_2 \xrightarrow[-N_2]{+HCl}$$

$$CH_3-\langle \bigcirc \rangle-SO_2-NH-(CH_2)_5-CO-CH_2Cl$$

FIGURE 4. Synthesis route for 1-chloro-7-tosylamido heptan-2-one.[2]

the chloro compounds. But, remarkably, the lowest level of inhibitory threshold concentrations (approximately 0.05 µg/ml) that has been attained by the chloro derivatives cannot be further lowered by the analogous bromo derivatives. This unexpected observation still needs an explanation.

TABLE 3 shows the activity of a number of further substances with the general structure outlined in FIGURE 3. The optimal chain length, the methylene group in the position –Y–, and the chloromethyl carbonyl function have been kept constant, whereas the other features of the molecule have been varied. With increasing size of the alkyl group R, the inhibitory activity is reduced progressively. Possibly the bulky residues prevent the mutual attraction between the two molecules by steric hindrance. A replacement of $-SO_2-$ by $-CO-$ also impairs the activity, which has already been shown in the case of the competitive amines.[2] Obviously the aromatic nucleus can be subjected to variation without considerably changing the activity of these compounds.

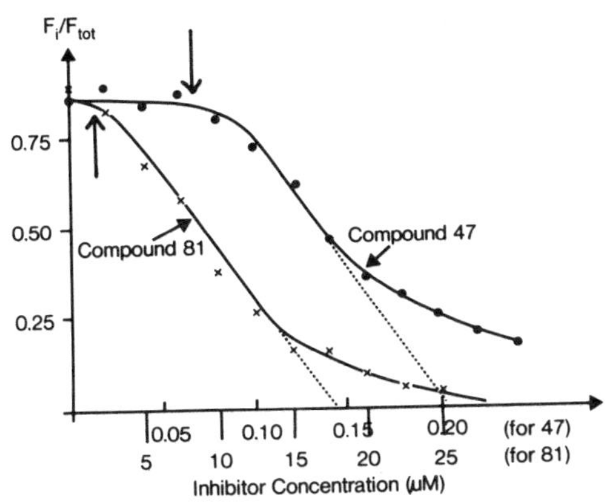

FIGURE 5. Decrease of the relative amount of insoluble fibrin (ratio of insoluble fibrin per total fibrin, F_i/F_{tot}) with increasing concentrations of fibrin stabilization inhibitors. Compound 47: CH_3—⬡—SO_2—NH—$(CH_2)_5$—CO—CH_2Cl. Compound 81: CH_3—⬡—SO_2—NH—$(CH_2)_5$—NH—CO—CH_2Cl.

In conclusion, we have been able to confirm our hypothesis that compounds with the general formula shown in FIGURE 3 are very potent inhibitors of fibrin stabilization *in vitro*. The most active substances of this category prevent the formation of stabilized fibrin in much lower concentrations than the best inhibitors known today. 1-chloro-7-tosylamido heptan-2-one [2] is particularly promising in this respect. The high inhibitory activity and, in addition, the strong dependency of this activity on the molecular features of these substances are strong indications that compounds of this type can be used as affinity labels of F XIIIa. One might consider introducing a chromophoric, a fluorescent, or a radioactive marker into these molecules, preferably into the aromatic nucleus R′. It is hoped that substances like these can become valuable tools for further investigations of the structure and the mode of action of F XIIIa.

TABLE 1

INHIBITORY THRESHOLD CONCENTRATION OF SUBSTANCES
WITH THE GENERAL STRUCTURE:

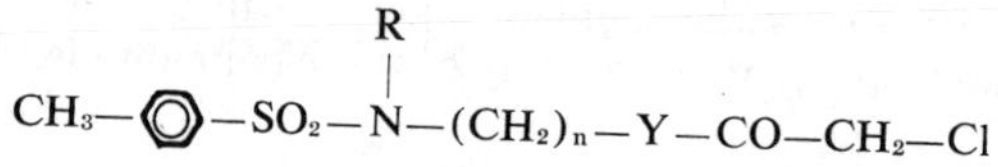

$$CH_3 - \bigodot - SO_2 - \overset{\overset{\textstyle R}{\textstyle |}}{N} - (CH_2)_n - Y - CO - CH_2 - Cl$$

R	n	Y	Threshold Concentration (μg/ml)
–H	2	–O–	250
–H	3	–O–	60
–H	4	–O–	40
–H	5	–O–	30
–H	2	–NH–	250
–H	3	–NH–	60
–H	4	–NH–	15
–H	5	–NH–	3
–H	6	–NH–	5
–CH$_3$	2	–CH$_2$–	3
–CH$_3$	3	–CH$_2$–	1
–H	4	–CH$_2$–	0.05
–H	5	–CH$_2$–	0.1
–H	6	–CH$_2$–	0.1
–H	9	–CH$_2$–	50

For Comparison:

Structure	Threshold Concentration (μg/ml)
$J - CH_2 - COOH$	6
$O_2N - \bigodot - S - S - \bigodot - NO_2$, HOOC ... COOH	15
$(CH_3)_2N - \bigodot$ $\bigodot - SO_2 - NH - (CH_2)_5 - NH_2$	50

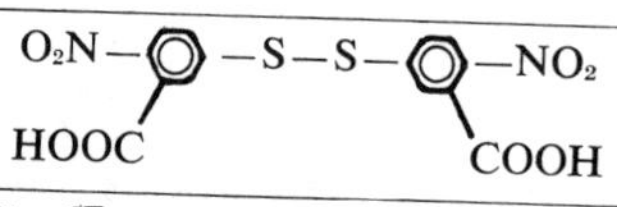

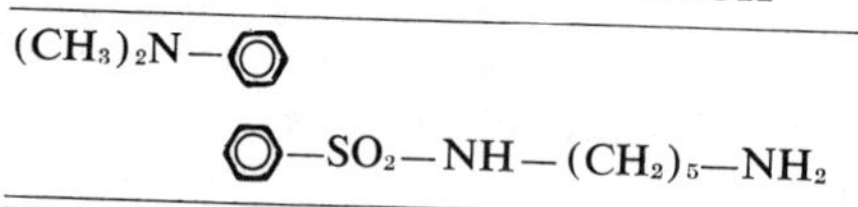

TABLE 2

INHIBITORY THRESHOLD CONCENTRATION OF SUBSTANCES
WITH THE GENERAL STRUCTURE:

$$CH_3-\text{⬡}-SO_2-\underset{\overset{|}{R}}{N}-(CH_2)_n-Y-CO-CH_2-Br$$

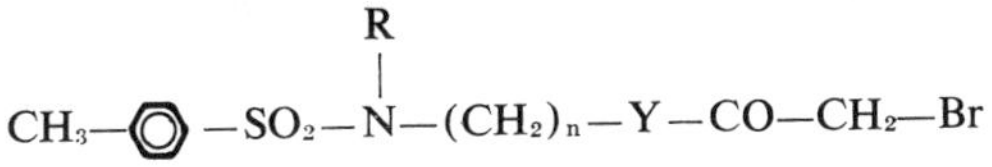

R	n	Y	Threshold Concentration (μg/ml)
–H	2	–O–	10
–H	3	–O–	3
–H	4	–O–	0.8
–H	5	–O–	0.5
–H	2	–NH–	5
–H	3	–NH–	1.5
–H	4	–NH–	0.05
–H	5	–NH–	0.05
–H	6	–NH–	0.05
–H	4	–CH$_2$–	0.05

TABLE 3

INHIBITORY THRESHOLD CONCENTRATIONS OF SUBSTANCES
WITH THE GENERAL STRUCTURE:

$$R'-X-\underset{\overset{|}{R}}{N}-(CH_2)_5-CO-CH_2-Cl$$

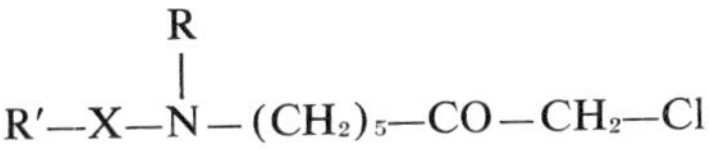

R'	X	R	Threshold Concentration (μg/ml)
CH$_3$–⬡–	–SO$_2$–	–H	0.05
CH$_3$–⬡–	–SO$_2$–	–CH$_3$	0.1
CH$_3$–⬡–	–SO$_2$–	–CH$_2$–CH$_3$	0.4
CH$_3$–⬡–	–SO$_2$–	–(CH$_2$)$_2$–CH$_3$	1.0
CH$_3$–⬡–	–SO$_2$–	–(CH$_2$)$_3$–CH$_3$	1.0
CH$_3$–⬡–	–SO$_2$–	–(CH$_2$)$_4$–CH$_3$	3.0
CH$_3$–⬡–	–SO$_2$–	–CH$_2$–⬡	8.0
CH$_3$–⬡–	–CO–	–H	0.8
Cl–⬡–	–SO$_2$–	–H	0.2
NO$_2$–⬡–	–SO$_2$–	–H	0.2
⬡⬡	–SO$_2$–	–H	0.2

REFERENCES

1. HOLBROOK, J. J., R. D. COOKE & I. B. KINGSTON. 1973. The amino acid sequence around the reactive cysteine residue in human plasma factor XIII. Biochem. J. **135:** 901–903.
2. LORAND, L. & J. L. G. NILSSON. 1972. Molecular approach for designing inhibitors to enzymes involved in blood clotting. Med. Chem. **11:** 415–447.
3. SHAW, E. 1967. Site-specific reagents for chymotrypsin and trypsin. Methods Enzymol. **XI:** 677–686.
4. ITZHAKI, R. F. & D. M. GILL. 1964. A micro-biuret method for estimating proteins. Anal. Biochem. **9:** 401–410.
5. LORAND, L., C.-H.J. CHOU & I. SIMPSON. 1972. Thiolester substrates for transamidating enzymes: Studies on fibrinoligase. Proc. Natl. Acad. Sci. USA **69:** 2645–2648.

DISSEMINATED INTRAVASCULAR COAGULATION: A CLINICAL/LABORATORY STUDY OF 48 PATIENTS

Rodger L. Bick

San Joaquin Hematology Oncology Medical Group
Bakersfield, California 93301

Wayne State University
Detroit, Michigan 48201

UCLA Center for the Health Sciences
Los Angeles, California 90024

Disseminated intravascular coagulation (DIC), which is also referred to as consumptive coagulopathy or the defibrination syndrome, is a frequently seen clinical entity and may present as a spectrum of disease ranging from a moderately severe bleeding disorder to a catastrophic fulminant and often fatal form associated with thrombosis and/or hemorrhage. In spite of recent awareness of this syndrome, the pathophysiology and clinical and laboratory diagnosis as well as the general concepts of management are often confusing and sometimes controversial. In addition, relatively few series of patients with acute or chronic DIC have been discussed in the literature and so it is more difficult to derive guidelines with respect to clinical findings, reliable laboratory diagnostic aids, effective management, or survival rates. This paper presents a group of patients with acute and chronic DIC and critically evaluates their clinical presentations, pertinent laboratory findings, efficacy of therapy, and overall survival.

MATERIALS AND METHODS

All patients were diagnosed as having disseminated intravascular coagulation, either chronic or acute, using generally accepted clinical features and noting the appropriate type of bleeding and/or thrombosis in the appropriate clinical setting.[1] In all instances, the clinical diagnosis was made by the same observer. The following tests and determinations were carried out in all patients before initiation of therapy and at the time of clinical diagnosis: prothrombin time, activated partial thromboplastin time, reptilase R time, thrombin time, fibrin(ogen) degradation products, platelet count, protamine sulfate test for soluble fibrin monomer, fibrinogen determination and biological AT-III levels. In all instances, the techniques used were routine and have been previously published.[2] In addition, these same hemostasis laboratory methods were used to monitor patients during and after therapy. Further, all patients were subjected to an SMA 18/60 biochemical screening survey, complete blood count, and other clinical, laboratory, and radiographic studies, as was deemed necessary by the particular clinical situation. In acute DIC the aforementioned laboratory tests were repeated at 4-hour intervals and in chronic DIC these tests were repeated at 24-hour intervals. Management was sequential[3, 4] and consisted of treatment of the underlying disease process, followed by antiprocoagu-

843

lant therapy, if indicated, and followed by component replacement, if indicated; no patients received antifibrinolytic therapy. The summary of findings in all patients with acute DIC is given in TABLE 1. This includes all of the pretreatment laboratory data, the "trigger" thought to be responsible for initiating disseminated intravascular coagulation, the specific antiprocoagulant therapy delivered, and 4-hour post-therapy repeat hemostasis variables. The findings in all patients with chronic DIC are given in TABLE 2 with the same parameters as those listed in TABLE 1.

RESULTS

In this series of 48 patients, DIC was acute in 38 and chronic in 10 patients. With respect to laboratory findings, it was noted at the time of diagnosis that the prothrombin time (PT) was prolonged in 76 percent of patients, the partial thromboplastin time (PTT) was prolonged in only 63 percent, the reptilase R time was prolonged in 58 percent, the thrombin time was abnormal in 81 percent, fibrin(ogen) degradation products (FDPs) were elevated in 100 percent, thrombocytopenia was present in 97 percent, soluble fibrin monomer was present in 92 percent, hypofibrinogenemia was present in 79 percent, and a biological antithrombin-III level was abnormal in 97 percent of patients. Thus, the probability of a pretreatment abnormality in acute DIC is as follows: FDP > AT-III = platelet count > soluble fibrin monomer > thrombin time > protime > fibrinogen level > PTT > reptilase R time. The probability of noting a pretreatment and posttreatment abnormality in acute DIC using these generally accepted laboratory diagnostic aids is depicted in TABLE 3. The most reliable tests would be those that are most likely to be abnormal before therapy and would be most likely to be normal after therapy, indicating the efficacy of therapy in causing cessation of the intravascular clotting process.[5] From these variables it would appear that in acute DIC the most reliable of these tests are the determinations of fibrin(ogen) degradation products, antithrombin-III level, and the platelet count followed by the detection of soluble fibrin monomer and a prolonged thrombin time. However, the FDP level is not likely to correct itself as quickly after therapy as is the antithrombin-III level, and the platelet count is even less likely to be corrected after therapy. The probability of noting a pretreatment and posttreatment abnormality in acute DIC is shown in TABLE 3. When we examine the probability of a pretreatment abnormality compared with the probability of posttreatment correction, we see that the most reliable tests appear to be the antithrombin-III level and reptilase R time. There is a high probability of noting a pretreatment FDP elevation and the presence of soluble fibrin monomer; however, these only show a moderate probability of correction after specific therapy, that is, 50 percent in the case of FDPs and 50 percent and 20 percent, respectively, will remain abnormal after successful therapy. Thus, in chronic DIC the probability of pretreatment abnormalities was as follows: 80 percent of patients had an abnormal prothrombin time, 30 percent had an abnormal partial thromboplastin time, 70 percent had a prolonged reptilase R time, 30 percent had an abnormal thrombin time, 100 percent had elevated FDPs, 50 percent had thrombocytopenia, 80 percent demonstrated the presence of soluble fibrin monomer, 30 percent had hypofibrinogenemia, and 70 percent had decreased biological AT-III levels. Thus, the probability of pretreatment abnormalities to aid in the diagnosis of

TABLE 1

SUMMARY OF FINDINGS IN PATIENTS WITH ACUTE DISSEMINATED INTRAVASCULAR COAGULATION

Patient No.	Pretreatment Findings									Diagnosis
	PT	PTT	RT	TT	FDPs	PL	PSO$_4$	Ø	AT-III	
1	18.2	70.7	52	28	>40	70	+	75	137	Malignancy
2	22.0	64.4	41	18	>40	32	+	43	31	Malignancy/sepsis
3	16.3	38.0	12	21	>80	105	+	108	76	Malignancy/sepsis
4	14.8	51.5	16	16	>40	28	+	156	68	Malignancy/sepsis
5	15.2	62.7	26	14	<40>10	56	+	42	80	Malignancy/sepsis
6	19.0	74.7	38	34	>40	72	+	115	55	Malignancy/sepsis
7	14.4	54.5	29	28	>40	30	0	215	33	Malignancy/sepsis
8	12.8	48.0	19	28	>40	16	+	105	77	Malignancy/sepsis
9	17.6	38.4	21	18	>40	78	+	128	68	Shock/arrest
10	16.4	27.1	18	16	>40	92	+	144	75	Shock/arrest
11	21.0	61.6	26	19	>80	120	+	97	17	Shock/arrest
12	18.4	74.8	36	22	>80	17	+	82	64	Shock/hemolysis
13	16.4	55.2	30	38	>80	63	+	44	73	Shock/hemolysis
14	14.0	61.0	12	66	>40	41	+	68	50	Shock/hemolysis
15	12.6	38.9	34	37	>80	97	+	110	58	Trans Rx.
16	13.6	49.0	48	18	<40>10	114	+	137	47	Shock/sepsis
17	14.8	63.4	23	22	>40	72	0	144	50	Shock
18	16.2	58.9	22	24	>40	70	0	74	36	Shock
19	18.4	74.0	28	12	>80	29	+	168	60	Shock
20	11.8	52.5	32	18	>40	58	+	117	56	Shock
21	17.4	66.4	23	16	>40	38	+	79	21	Shock
22	16.4	73.9	44	24	>40	104	+	122	80	PV disease
23	11.2	59.0	18	33	>40	131	+	146	72	PV disease
24	14.8	63.7	24	18	>80	63	+	90	65	PV disease
25	12.6	89.0	33	63	>40	20	+	78	75	Kasabach-Merritt disease
26	14.2	32.4	14	10	>40	140	+	215	77	
27	16.4	59.1	16	23	>40	18	+	168	12	CVD

TABLE 1—(Continued)

28	15.2	48.1	28	22	>80	74	+	118	65	CVD
29	14.4	28.8	18	11	<40>10	102	+	265	60	Hip fracture
30	14.8	55.9	36	43	>40	97	+	68	73	Polycythemia vera
31	14.6	54.0	49	21	>40	18	+	28	19	Missed AB
32	13.6	45.4	16	19	>40	23	+	82	44	Shock
33	12.4	33.0	19.4	11.7	>40	65	+	450	57	Malignancy/sepsis
34	13.4	50.0	14.7	10.2	>40	150	+	126	30	Malignancy/sepsis
35	14.7	58.6	20.0	12.0	>80	23	+	500	60	Shock/sepsis
36	39.0	92	29	24	>40	51	+	56	50	Malignancy/sepsis
37	47.6	49.0	23	19	>40	40	+	112	67	Shock/sepsis
38	13.0	46.2	30	28	>40	38	+	38	60	Shock/sepsis
$\bar{x}$	16.8	55.8	26.8	23.8	↑	64.6	+	129	57.8	

Patient No.	Treatment	Posttreatment Findings								
		PT	PTT	RT	TT	FDPs	PL	PSO$_4$	Ø	AT-III
1	Mini-heparin	14.6	40.1	21	9	<10	128	0	241	167
2	Mini-heparin	14.0	38.7	19	8	<10	134	0	190	86
3	Mini-heparin	12.5	38.2	14	16	<10	225	0	244	105
4	Mini-heparin	14.5	41.7	15	20	<10	168	0	350	98
5	Mini-heparin	11.9	48.0	22	14	<10	155	0	168	114
6	Mini-heparin	14.0	54.4	19	14	<10	124	0	240	76
7	Mini-heparin	13.8	32.7	16	12	<10	150	0	368	58
8	Mini-heparin	12.8	33.0	14	9	<10	105	0	241	191
9	Heparin	14.9	54.8	21	28	<10	250	0	256	93
10	Mini-heparin	14.0	30.1	19	14	<10	355	0	176	107
11	Mini-heparin	11.9	51.2	28	20	>40	350	+	154	93
12	Mini-heparin	14.0	33.0	21	14	<10	98	0	105	131
13	Mini-heparin	14.4	64.2	18	21	<40>10	263	0	210	124
14	Mini-heparin	14.2	41.7	16	13	<10	168	0	156	98
15	Mini-heparin	13.0	38.6	15	15	<10	403	0	216	100

16	Heparin	11.8	68.2	19	39	<10	215	0	168	104
17	Mini-heparin	14.4	30.9	19	7	<10	290	+	205	90
18	Heparin	13.2	59.9	17	34	<40>10	156	0	312	10?
19	Mini-heparin	15.0	50.2	14	13	<40>10	190	0	183	123
20	Mini-heparin	11.8	41.1	20	11	<10	138	0	208	127
21	Mini-heparin	15.4	33.7	19	14	<10	207	0	160	73
22	Mini-heparin	16.0	34.0	23	12	<10	256	0	214	148
23	Mini-heparin	11.4	43.1	16	15	<40>10	360	0	315	115
24	Mini-heparin	12.0	29.8	20	9	<40>10	244	0	222	128
25	Mini-heparin	12.3	43.7	19	8	<10	120	0	169	93
26	ASA/dipyridamole	14.4	32.0	16	11	<40>10	468	+	215	100
27	Mini-heparin	15.0	40.9	13	15	<10	240	0	97	100
28	Mini-heparin	15.4	45.0	18	13	<10	323	0	254	95
29	ASA/dipyridamole	12.0	29.0	20	11	<10	430	0	305	98
30	D & C	14.0	32.4	19	14	<10	375	0	300	100
31	Mini-heparin	14.0	58.6	36	22	>40	19	+	58	54
32	Mini-heparin	14.6	50.2	18	22	>40	63	+	104	89
33	Mini-heparin	12.6	36.0	16.0	12.0	<40>10	105	+	440	72
34	Mini-heparin	12.4	49.0	14.2	12.0	<10	240	0	246	75
35	Mini-heparin	16.0	58.0	22	14	>40	17	+	436	23
36	Mini-heparin	12.0	32.6	22	17	<10	60	0	140	98
37	AT-III	14.6	36.0	19	25	<10	106	0	200	107
38	AT-III	12.4	36.6	19	16	<10	74	0	141	98
	$\bar{x}$	13.6	42.4	18.8	15.6	↑	204	+	221	101.4

NOTE: PT = prothrombin time; PTT = partial thromboplastin time; RT = reptilase time; TT = thrombin time; FDPs = fibrin-(ogen) degradation products; PL = platelet; PSO_4 = (SFM) soluble fibrin monomer; ϕ = fibrinogen; PV = peripheral vascular; CVD = cardiovascular disease.

TABLE 2

SUMMARY OF FINDINGS IN PATIENTS WITH CHRONIC DIC

Patient No.	Pretreatment Findings									
	PT	PTT	RT	TT	FDP	PL	PSO₄	Ø	AT-III	Diagnosis
1	16.2	32.4	18	11	>40	98	+	475	90	Malignancy
2	15.8	48.6	24	14	>40	445	+	240	105	Malignancy
3	11.2	31.7	23	33	>40	302	+	650	80	Malignancy
4	12.3	68.8	36	28	>10	77	+	105	65	Malignancy
5	14.1	28.4	30	14	>40	58	+	328	80	Malignancy
6	14.6	52.5	29	8	>40	380	0	127	145	Malignancy
7	15.2	65.3	18	12	>80	205	+	92	66	Malignancy
8	13.3	25.0	60	33	<40>10	158	+	460	80	Malignancy
9	16.6	46.7	16	9.7	>40	104	0	482	62	PV Disease
10	14.6	40.0	24	15.0	>40	64	+	254	59	PV Disease
x̄	14.4	43.9	27.8	17.7	↑	190	+	321	83.9	

Patient No.	Treatment	Posttreatment Findings								
		PT	PTT	RT	TT	FDP	PL	PSO₄	Ø	AT-III
1	ASA/Dipyridamole	13	30.0	18	9	<40>10	228	0	420	130
2	ASA/Dipyridamole	12.4	29.0	17	11	<40>10	400	0	300	176
3	ASA/Dipyridamole	12.0	28.8	15	8	<10	400	0	290	97
4	ASA/Dipyridamole	12.0	29.9	15	12	<40>10	188	+	248	99
5	ASA/Dipyridamole	11.9	28.4	21	14	<40>10	128	0	405	160
6	ASA/Dipyridamole	13.8	34.4	22	14	<40>10	360	0	268	163
7	ASA/Dipyridamole	12.8	58.3	18	13	<10	350	0	240	104
8	ASA/Dipyridamole	13.8	25.2	17	14	<10	205	0	340	160
9	ASA/Dipyridamole	12.4	44.2	17	12	<10	122	0	460	82
10	ASA/Dipyridamole	12.0	36.4	22.0	12.0	<10	155	+	360	101
x̄		12.6	34.5	18.2	11.9	5↑	254	0	333	116.8

TABLE 3

PROBABILITY OF PRETREATMENT AND POSTTREATMENT
ABNORMALITIES IN ACUTE DIC

Patient No.		Pretreatment Rx	Posttreatment Rx
1	FDP	100%	24%
2	AT-III	97%	16%
3	PL	97%	34%
4	SFM	92%	18%
5	TT	81%	32%
6	Fibrino	79%	16%
7	PT	76%	58%
8	PTT	63%	24%
9	RT	58%	8%

NOTE: FDP > AT-III = PL > SFM > TT > Ø > PT > PTT > RT.

chronic DIC is as follows: FDP > soluble fibrin monomer = prothrombin time > AT-III level = reptilase R time > platelet count > fibrinogen level = thrombin time; however, only 50 percent of patients with elevated FDPs will have corrected levels after therapy and 20 percent of patients demonstrating soluble fibrin monomer before therapy will still have these species present after therapy, leaving the antithrombin-III level as the test most likely to be abnormal and yet to become corrected after successful therapy to halt the intravascular clotting process. The probability of noting pre- and posttreatment abnormalities in chronic DIC is seen in TABLE 4. Clinical findings in this population of patients with disseminated intravascular coagulation are presented in TABLE 5. It can be seen that all patients with DIC, either chronic or acute, presented with hemorrhage. In addition, 53 percent of patients with acute DIC presented with some clinical evidence of thrombosis, usually manifest as increasing creatinine and blood urea nitrogen (BUN) levels compatible with renal microvascular thrombosis [6]; 80 percent of patients with chronic DIC likewise presented with clinical evidence of thrombosis. It will further be noted that the mortality rate

TABLE 4

PROBABILITY OF PRETREATMENT AND POSTTREATMENT
ABNORMALITIES IN CHRONIC DIC

Patient No.		Pretreatment Rx	Posttreatment Rx
1	FDP	100%	50%
2	SFM	80%	20%
3	PT	80%	30%
4	AT-III	70%	10%
5	RT	70%	0%
6	PL	50%	30%
7	Fibrino	30%	0%
8	PTT	30%	10%
9	TT	30%	0%

NOTE: FDP > AT-III = PL > SFM > TT > Ø > PT > PTT > RT.

in acute DIC was 26 percent and in chronic DIC 0 percent, giving a total overall *survival rate* of 79 percent. The vast majority of patients with acute DIC were treated with "mini-dose" heparin therapy [7] and all patients with chronic DIC were treated with antiplatelet agents delivered in the form of 600 mg aspirin orally twice a day with 30 cc of liquid antacid plus 50 mg dipyridamole orally four times a day. The survival data would suggest that mini-heparin therapy is the anticoagulant modality of choice in acute DIC and that antiplatelet therapy [8] is the modality of choice for antiprocoagulant therapy in chronic DIC.

SUMMARY

In summary, this series of 48 patients with acute and chronic DIC demonstrates the reliability of laboratory tests in both aiding a diagnosis of DIC and in offering reasonable predictability of efficacy of therapy, as noted by the correction of abnormalities after delivery of antiprocoagulant therapy for this syndrome. It appears that the diagnostic tests most likely to aid in diagnosis and to reliably inform the clinician when the intravascular clotting process has been stopped are those that determine the antithrombin-III level, the presence of soluble fibrin monomer, and the finding of elevated fibrin(ogen) degradation products, thrombocytopenia and a prolonged thrombin time in the face of the appropriate type of bleeding in the appropriate clinical setting. In addition, it would appear that mini-dose heparin therapy is highly effective in controlling the intravascular clotting process in acute DIC, whereas antiplatelet therapy utilizing two agents is effective in chronic DIC. In addition, in this population, patients with acute disease demonstrated a 74 percent survival rate and those with chronic disease had a 100 percent survival rate from this disseminated intravascular clotting process.

TABLE 5

SURVIVAL RATE IN PATIENTS WITH DIC HAVING
HEMORRHAGE OR THROMBOSIS

| Patients with: | Survival after: | | Mortality |
	Hemorrhage	Thrombosis	
Acute DIC (38)	100%	53%	26%
Chronic DIC (10)	100%	80%	0%
Total population (48)	100%	58%	21%

REFERENCES

1. BICK, R. L. & T. ADAMS. 1974. Disseminated intravascular coagulation: etiology, pathophysiology, diagnosis and management. Med. Counterpoint 6(8).
2. BICK, R. L. 1980. Laboratory procedures in hemostasis. *In* Current Concepts of Hemostasis and Thrombosis. R. L. Bick, Ed. American Society of Clinical Pathology, Manual #5548.
3. BICK, R. L. 1978. Disseminated intravascular coagulation and related syndromes: Etiology, pathophysiology, diagnosis and management. Am. J. Hematol. 5: 265.
4. BICK, R. L. 1980. Disseminated intravascular coagulation and related syndromes: Etiology, pathophysiology, diagnosis and management. *In* Current Concepts of Hemostasis and Thrombosis. Rodger L. Bick and Gene Murano, Eds. CRC Press, West Palm Beach, FL.
5. BICK, R. L., M. D. BICK, & L. F. FEKETE. 1980. Antithrombin III patterns in disseminated intravascular coagulation. Am. J. Clin. Pathol. 73: 577.
6. BICK, R. L. 1981. Disseminated intravascular coagulation (DIC) and related syndromes. *In* Perspectives in Hemostasis. Jawed Fareed, Ed. Pergamon Press, New York, NY.
7. BICK, R. L. 1979. Monitoring heparin therapy. Diag. Dialog 1(4).
8. BICK, R. L. 1976. Treatment of bleeding and thrombosis in the patient with cancer. *In* Management of the Patient with Cancer, 2nd ed. Thomas F. Nealon, Ed.: 48. W. B. Saunders. Philadelphia, PA.

HEREDITARY HEMORRHAGIC TELANGIECTASIA AND DISSEMINATED INTRAVASCULAR COAGULATION: A NEW CLINICAL SYNDROME

Rodger L. Bick

San Joaquin Hematology Oncology Medical Group
Bakersfield, California 93301

Wayne State University
Detroit, Michigan 48201

UCLA Center for the Health Sciences
Los Angeles, California 90024

Hereditary hemorrhagic telangiectasia (HHT) is a relatively common disorder and is the most common hereditary vascular disorder that is associated with a bleeding or thrombotic diathesis. The disorder is inherited as an autosomal dominant with 70 percent of individuals having a positive family history; in addition, the homozygous state is thought to be lethal.[1] Additionally, there is evidence that the gene responsible for HHT is somehow linked to blood group O. The hallmark characteristic of this disease is epistaxis, which may be profuse and usually begins in early childhood. However, the classic telangiectatic lesions of HHT may not appear until later in life, commonly the second or third decade. The classic diagnostic triad of HHT is: (1) a hereditary basis, (2) telangiectasia, and (3) bleeding from telangiectatic lesions.[2] Chronic blood loss, commonly from the gastrointestinal tract, is often severe enough to be manifest as a significant iron-deficiency anemia of unknown etiology and the diagnosis is not made until endoscopy is performed. Telangiectatic lesions of HHT may be of three types: pinpoint, nodular, and spider-like. These lesions are nonpulsatile, distinguishing them from those seen in chronic liver disease.[3] The number of telangiectasia as well as the episodes of clinical bleeding usually increase with advancing age; however, epistaxis often decreases with age. Bleeding of HHT may be occult and it may represent common causes of gastrointestinal hemorrhage, genitourinary hemorrhage, hemoptysis, or heavy menstrual flow. In some individuals, only mucosal membrane bleeding is noted and no telangiectasia of the skin are present, making the diagnosis most difficult. Approximately 20 percent of patients develop arteriovenous fistulae of the lungs.[4] In addition, there is an inordinantly high incidence of Laennec's type of cirrhosis occurring in these persons. Hematomas of the liver and spleen may also be associated with HHT.[5] The basic pathology of this disorder is poorly understood; however, most studies have shown that elastic fibers are depleted in vascular walls.[6] There are few characteristic laboratory findings in HHT. The tourniquet test and template bleeding time may be normal or abnormal, depending upon the integrity of the vessel wall in the particular area where the test is performed; there are no other characteristic laboratory abnormalities. The diagnosis is suggested by a history of recurrent epistaxis, occult gastrointestinal bleeding, and the noting of the appropriate type of telangiectasia most commonly found in the skin, sublingual or subungual areas or oral mucosa.

851

0077–8923/81/0370–0851 $01.75/0 © 1981, NYAS

Disseminated intravascular coagulation is an intermediary mechanism of disease which is commonly known throughout all medical disciplines. The etiology, pathophysiology, diagnosis, and management of this syndrome have recently been reviewed.[6, 7] DIC is almost always associated with an initial triggering disease state and is rarely, if ever, a disease or event unto itself. There are many recognized triggers for disseminated intravascular coagulation, one group of which encompasses vascular disorders.[8] We are familiar with the association of giant cavernous hemangiomas and disseminated intravascular coagulation, the so-called Kasabach-Merritt syndrome.[9] The triggering event for the development of DIC in patients with giant cavernous hemangiomas remains poorly understood, but one could readily imagine that altered blood flow in the abnormal endothelial-lined cavernous hemangiomatous lesions could readily set off the clotting sequence and/or platelet release reaction, which would provide a trigger for disseminated intravascular coagulation in these patients. Forty-seven patients with classical hereditary hemorrhagic telangiectasia have been studied over the past two years. An inordinantly high incidence of associated defects in hemostasis has been noted, but most pronounced is the finding of DIC in many of these patients. This report summarizes the clinical and laboratory aspects in these 47 patients and emphasizes the necessity for recognizing this new syndrome of HHT and DIC.

Materials and Methods

All forty-seven patients were referred to San Joaquin Hematology Oncology Medical Group for a hematology/hemostasis consultation after they were found to have a disorder of hemostasis or severe chronic iron-deficiency anemia of unknown origin. In rare instances a patient was referred with a known diagnosis of HHT, but in the vast majority of cases the cause of the bleeding or thrombotic diathesis was unknown. All patients referred were evaluated with a thorough history and physical examination, with particular search for the characteristic telangiectasia of HHT especially to be noted in the skin, sublingual areas, subungual areas, and oral mucosa. All patients were subjected to an SMA 18/60 biochemical screening survey, prothrombin time test, activated partial thromboplastin time, platelet count, platelet adhesion and platelet aggregation studies to rule out a platelet function defect versus a vascular defect. The patients also had a routine complete blood count. In addition, a template bleeding time was determined in all individuals. If adhesion or aggregation prothrombin time or PTT abnormalities were found, additional investigation was instituted as dictated by the particular clinical picture. If the prothrombin time or partial thromboplastin time were prolonged, the patient was subjected to a DIC work-up consisting of a thrombin time, reptilase R time, protamine sulfate test for soluble fibrin monomers, fibrin(ogen) degradation product titer, antithrombin-III level, and fibrinogen level. Methods for all of these testing systems have been published previously.[10]

Results

TABLE 1 summarizes findings in all 47 patients who have HHT and a dissociated defect of hemostasis. Especially noteworthy is the high incidence of disseminated intravascular coagulation seen in 51 percent (24 patients). Also noteworthy is the association of HHT and factor XI deficiency and HHT and von Willebrand's syndrome type II. TABLE 2 summarizes findings in all patients

TABLE 1

HEREDITARY HEMORRHAGIC TELANGIECTASIA AND ASSOCIATED
HEMOSTASIS DEFECTS (TOTAL POPULATION)

No. of Patients with Hereditary Hemorrhagic Telangiectasia	Associated Defect
21	None
24	DIC
1	MvW type II
1	Hemophilia C

NOTE: MvW = Mild von Willebrand's disease.

TABLE 2

HEREDITARY HEMORRHAGIC TELANGIECTASIA AND DISSEMINATED
INTRAVASCULAR COAGULATION

Patient No.	Type of DIC	Manifestations
1	Acute	Hemorrhage/DVT
2	Acute	Hemorrhage/DVT
3	Acute	Hemorrhage/DVT
4	Acute	Hemorrhage/MVT
5	Acute	Hemorrhage/MVT
6	Acute	Hemorrhage/MVT
7	Acute	Hemorrhage/MVT
8	Acute	Hemorrhage/MVT
9	Acute	Hemorrhage/MVT
10	Acute	Hemorrhage/MVT
11	Acute	Hemorrhage/MVT
12	Acute	Hemorrhage/MVT
13	Acute	Hemorrhage/MVT
14	Acute	Hemorrhage/MVT
15	Acute	Hemorrhage/MVT
16	Acute	Hemorrhage/MVT
17	Acute	Hemorrhage/MVT
18	Acute	Hemorrhage/MVT
19	Acute	Hemorrhage/MVT
20	Acute	Hemorrhage/DVT/PE
21	Chronic	Hemorrhage/DVT/PE
22	Chronic	Hemorrhage/DVT/PE
23	Chronic	Hemorrhage/MVT
24	Chronic	Hemorrhage/MVT

NOTE: DVT = deep venous thrombosis; MVT = microvascular thrombosis; PE = pulmonary embolus.

with HHT and DIC. Of particular interest are the numerous episodes of acute DIC manifest as fulminant hemorrhage in 19 individuals. In all instances of acute DIC, the patients responded to mini-dose heparin therapy or antiplatelet therapy. Five patients had only chronic DIC in association with their HHT and these individuals were treated with antiplatelet agents. Six of the patients with HHT and DIC presented with diffuse, recurrent venous thromboses and three individuals suffered pulmonary emboli.

SUMMARY

In summary, 47 patients with documented HHT and a bleeding problem were referred to San Joaquin Hematology Oncology Medical Group over a 2-year period. Fifty-one percent of patients were noted to have an associated DIC syndrome and of these 24 patients, 19 had acute DIC episodes, six had chronic DIC, six presented with diffuse, recurrent deep venous thrombosis and of these six, three suffered pulmonary emboli. Other defects were also noted and were thought to be coincidental defects. This syndrome should be readily considered and searched for when seeing patients with HHT, especially if significant hemorrhage or thrombosis is present. It should further be appreciated that many patients with HHT and bleeding are candidates for the development of acute or chronic DIC and thus a "mini" Kasabach-Merritt syndrome. When patients with HHT present with undue bleeding, this syndrome should be appreciated, searched for from the clinical and laboratory standpoint and, when found, treated in the appropriate manner with supportive therapy, mini-heparin or antiplatelet therapy as the clinical situation dictates.

REFERENCES

1. HARRISON, D. F. N. 1964. Familial haemorrhagic telangiectasis. Quart. J. Med. **33:** 25.
2. OLSER, W. 1901. On a family form of recurrent epistaxis associated with telangiectasia of the skin and mucous membranes. Bull. Johns Hopkins Hosp. **12:** 33.
3. OSLER, W. 1907. On multiple hereditary telangiectasia with recurrent hemorrhages. Quart. J. Med. (October): 53.
4. HODGSUM, C. H. & R. L. KAYE. 1963. Pulmonary arteriovenous fistulae and hereditary hemorrhagic telangiectasis. Dis. Chest **43:** 449.
5. FITZ-HUGH, T. 1931. Splenomegaly and hepatic enlargement in hereditary hemorrhagic telangiectasis. Am. J. Med. Sci. **181:** 261.
6. BICK, R. L. 1979. Vascular disorders associated with thrombohemorrhagic phenomena. Semin. Thromb. Hemostas. **5:** 167.
7. QUICK, A. J. 1966. Telangiectasia. *In* Hemorrhagic Diseases and Thrombosis. Lea and Febiger. Philadelphia, PA.
8. BICK, R. L. 1978. Disseminated intravascular coagulation and related syndromes: Etiology, pathophysiology, diagnosis and management. Am. J. Hematol. **5:** 265.
9. INCEMAN, S. & Y. TANGUN. 1969. Chronic defibrination syndrome due to a giant hemangioma associated with microangiopathic hemolytic anemia. Am. J. Med. **46:** 997.
10. BICK, R. L. 1980. Coagulation laboratory procedures. *In* Current Concepts of Hemostasis and Thrombosis. Rodger L. Bick, Ed. Am. Soc. Clin. Path. Manual #5548.

Index of Contributors

855